Evidence-Based Sexual and Reproductive Health Care

Policies, Clinical Procedures, and Related Research

Theodora D. Kwansa, PhD, MEd, MTD, Diploma in Higher Education HE Nursing (CT), RN, RM
Programme Tutor MSc Health Studies
MSc Sexual & Reproductive Health Studies
Lecturer
Abertay University
Dundee, Scotland, United Kingdom

Jill Stewart-Moore, PhD, MSc, RN, RM, Diploma in Nursing (Lond), PGCEA, MTD
Lecturer
Contraception and Sexual and Reproductive Health Nurse
Brook Coleraine and Belfast Health and Social Care Trust
Belfast, Northern Ireland, United Kingdom

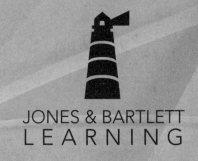
JONES & BARTLETT
LEARNING

World Headquarters
Jones & Bartlett Learning
5 Wall Street
Burlington, MA 01803
978-443-5000
info@jblearning.com
www.jblearning.com

Jones & Bartlett Learning books and products are available through most bookstores and online booksellers. To contact Jones & Bartlett Learning directly, call 800-832-0034, fax 978-443-8000, or visit our website, www.jblearning.com.

Substantial discounts on bulk quantities of Jones & Bartlett Learning publications are available to corporations, professional associations, and other qualified organizations. For details and specific discount information, contact the special sales department at Jones & Bartlett Learning via the above contact information or send an email to specialsales@jblearning.com.

Production Credits

VP, Product Management: David D. Cella
Product Manager: Teresa Reilly
Product Assistant: Christina Freitas
Associate Production Editor: Alex Schab
Marketing Communications Manager: Katie Hennessy
Production Services Manager: Colleen Lamy
Product Fulfillment Manager: Wendy Kilborn
Composition: S4Carlisle Publishing Services
Cover Design: Michael O'Donnell
Media Development Editor: Troy Liston

Director of Rights & Media: Joanna Gallant
Rights & Media Specialist: Wes DeShano
Cover Image (Left to Right, Top to Bottom): © Galina Barskaya/Shutterstock, © ESB Professional/Shutterstock, © NorthGeorgiaMedia/Shutterstock, © Thinkstock/Stockbyte/Getty, © Diana Lundin/Dreamstime.com, © Rubberball Productions, © Digital Vision/Photodisc/Getty, © Adkasai/iStock/Getty Images Plus, © AbleStock, © michaeljung/Shutterstock
Printing and Binding: Edwards Brothers Malloy
Cover Printing: Edwards Brothers Malloy

Library of Congress Cataloging-in-Publication Data
Names: Kwansa, Theodora, author. | Stewart-Moore, Jill, author.
Title: Evidence-based sexual and reproductive health care / Theodora Kwansa and Jill Stewart-Moore.
Description: Burlington, Massachusetts : Jones & Bartlett Learning, [2019] | Includes bibliographical references.
Identifiers: LCCN 2017044947 | ISBN 9781284114942
Subjects: | MESH: Reproductive Health | Evidence-Based Practice | Reproductive Health Services
Classification: LCC RG110 | NLM WQ 200.1 | DDC 618.1--dc23
LC record available at https://lccn.loc.gov/2017044947

6048

Printed in the United States of America
22 21 20 19 18   10 9 8 7 6 5 4 3 2 1

Contents

Part Synopses

The contents of *Evidence-Based Sexual and Reproductive Health Care* are grouped into five parts by topic.

Part I

Part I chapters explore the concept of evidence-based practice (EBP) and related challenges. Thus, the rationale and principles of EBP are addressed in an attempt to capture practitioners' interest, motivation, and commitment in implementing EBP competently. The processes involved in systematic review, including meta-analysis and metasynthesis, are examined to enhance practitioners' understanding of this concept. Clear conception of the development, implementation, and evaluation processes strengthen practitioners' sense of ownership and interactions among multidisciplinary team members to ensure that EBP application becomes more meaningful and more conscientious.

Part II

The links among the chapters in Part II are intended to encourage further exploration and increase professional knowledge about specific sexually transmitted infections (STIs), reproductive tract infections (RTIs), and human immunodeficiency virus/acquired immunodeficiency syndrome (HIV/AIDS). The chapters examine the clinical manifestations, current recommended therapeutic interventions, treatment efficacy, and patient outcomes and also explore efficient communication of patient information.

The scientific aspects of reproductive physiology underpin explanation of pathological damage and disease caused to sexual and reproductive structures due to specific infections. Supportive research evidence relating to the ovarian/endometrial cycles and contraception are also explored as evidence for substantiating patient information about STIs/RTIs, HIV/AIDS, conception, subfertility, and the different methods of contraception. Other findings may also be relevant for health promotion and education purposes in providing more efficient instruction to patients and their sexual partners on the correct techniques of male and female condom application.

Emerging trends in contraception and contraceptive services are examined. These enable practitioners to emphasize the need for compliance with, and the benefits of, correct use of the different contraceptive methods. Moreover, practitioners are better informed and able to reinforce the importance of uptake of STI/HIV screening and available contraceptive services. This part of the text is intended to enhance practitioners' cognizance of the significant influence of organizational, national, and international policy guidelines and recommendations. Thus, the U.S. Centers for Disease Control and Prevention's current regulations, recommendations, and guidelines on key aspects of sexual and reproductive health (SRH) care are explored, and factors that influence implementation in different states are also examined.

For reflective considerations, specific conditions, clinical scenarios, and algorithms are presented as appropriate to encourage ongoing reflection with regard to practice relating to the care and treatment interventions that patients receive.

Part III

Part III chapters examine the support services in SRH care. Thus, services available to young people and special client groups are examined. Sexual health issues relating to lesbian, gay, transgender, bisexual, and questioning dispositions are explored in terms of lifestyle behaviors and related sexual health implications; male sexual health services are explored as well.

The roles of clinical and health psychologists and the significance of counseling in sexual health care are considered together with psychotherapeutic support. Additionally, the role of sexual health advising and partner services provision as diversifying yet significant supportive services is also examined in relation to partner notification, partner management, and contact tracing. Health promotion and health education are considered important components of sexual history taking and patient education within sexual healthcare provision with the goal of providing adequate insight about the significance of effective interactions, collaboration, and referral systems.

Part IV

Part IV chapters explore the significance of research and clinical audit. Research is an imperative professional requirement although many practitioners find the entire process rather daunting. Nonetheless, the need for ongoing research in this field must be recognized and diligently embraced. Practitioners' competence and confidence in research utilization and development is crucial for gaining understanding of the impact of the different sexual health problems. The impact of sexual ill health on individuals, families, communities, and societies emphasizes the importance of research and clinical audit for continual evaluation and improvement on the effectiveness of care and treatment and improved patient outcomes.

SRH care is fraught with ethical issues and dilemmas and the imperative regulation of professional practice in this field is recognized. Therefore, in addition to exploring ethical concepts and principles, relevant professional codes defining the standards of conduct, performance and ethics are also explored. Professional regulation in this field of practice is complex and attributed to the different professional disciplines in the multidisciplinary teams. Therefore, the importance of building a competent nursing workforce is also considered.

Part V

Part V chapters represent ongoing efforts in resource-constrained developing countries. The initiatives in two sub-Saharan African countries, Lesotho and Ghana, are presented to demonstrate exemplars at different ends of the spectrum of multiple resource limitations. The insight gained enables practitioners in developed countries to better understand the impact of cultural principles and practices, economic and religious influences, and educational/literacy attainment presented by migrant or ethnic minority patients who access SRH care.

Preface

The impetus for developing this text evolved from the recognition of apparent lack of a comprehensive text that addresses evidence-based practice (EBP) within the clinical field of sexual and reproductive health (SRH) care and service provision. Nevertheless, the concept is recognized, advocated, and implemented, albeit rather disconnectedly in some aspects of this field of practice. The centers of excellence in SRH care and services diligently provide sound research and evidence-based recommendations to guide practice. Yet in some areas of practice, apparent uncertainty persists in the comprehension and competent implementation of EBP.

Arguably, a clear conception of the rationale, principles, and evolution of EBP is imperative at all levels to ensure correct and conscientious implementation of this approach to clinical practice. EBP should be overtly incorporated into all aspects of SRH care and should be recognized as involving all levels of professional practitioners in the multidisciplinary team.

While acknowledging the importance of detailed reference texts by leading experts on evidence-based healthcare professional practice, there is, undoubtedly, a need for an all-encompassing yet relatively simple text for SRH practitioners. This text is written with the aim of providing the kind of comprehensive text that explores EBP in a way that can be realistically interpreted and translated for practical application. Therefore, the key elements examined include the processes of identification and categorization of different types and levels of research studies and other approved clinical expertise, patient experiences, preferences, standards of performance, and patient outcomes. The importance of familiarity with the relevant policies and approaches employed for evaluation and how these are effected through the strength and quality of leadership are examined. Additionally, the importance of establishing a recognizable and functional evidence-based in-house philosophy and ethos is also considered with leadership facilitation, effective organizational management, support for practitioners, and continuing professional education. The emphasis on continual improvement of quality clinical care, safeguarding of performance standards, better outcomes of healthcare service delivery, and implementation of change demands commitment and sound accountability.

Standards of quality clinical care and performance are substantiated by best available evidence, which derive from efficient systematic reviews. These are crucial not only for benchmarking required standards of quality care provision and establishing levels of professional practice, but also for communicating examples of excellence in clinical practice. Identification of best available evidence serves as substantive basis for implementation of change to accomplish desired clinical care improvement. Thus, practitioners should be familiar with the aims of the sexual health strategies and the key principles of clinical governance (clinical effectiveness, education and training, research and development clinical audit, openness, risk management, and information management, which thread through the different aspects of evidence-based SRH). The relevance to stakeholders should also be considered, including the commissioning authority at the national level, primary and secondary sectors, education sectors, multidisciplinary teams, and individual practitioners, as well as patients/clients, their representatives, relevant agencies, and voluntary organizations.

This text is intended to provide an effective resource for practitioners of varied backgrounds in SRH care in the United Kingdom and United States, as well as most other countries that seek to implement or re-examine their in-house conception and implementation of evidence-based approach to care. The suggested reflective considerations lend themselves to small group interactions and discussions of specific issues (research evidence and clinical audit findings by colleagues in the multidisciplinary teams or an individual practitioner).

Introduction

Sexual and reproductive health (SRH) has consistently been a mutual public health concern shared by all countries and hence the consensus resolution to address these at a global level. *Evidence-Based Sexual and Reproductive Health Care* is intended to enhance the awareness of practitioners and researchers in this field about global initiatives that influence national and international policy decisions, recommendations, and guidelines on SRH care, monitoring, and surveillance. The importance of identifying and dealing with the multiple interconnected social, cultural, economic, and religious influences is acknowledged. Collaboration occurs among governmental and healthcare organizations, nongovernmental agencies, and voluntary organizations in their joint commitment toward better sexual health for all people in all countries. Various national and international campaigns and ongoing initiatives are continually launched together with endeavors in recognition of human rights, empowerment, respect, and responsibility among individuals, communities, population groups, and societies. Thus, the wider context of SRH care is explored.

It is crucial that practitioners and researchers in this field strive together to bring about improvements through ongoing research activities and clinical audit endeavors. The emphasis on evidence-based practice (EBP) is demonstrated by examination of related policies, professional practice regulations, recommendations, and guidelines. The intention is to encourage SRH practitioners to embrace EBP with more commitment to provide high-quality care with continual improvement in patient outcomes.

The chapters on sexually transmitted infections, human immunodeficiency virus (HIV), and contraception have been developed from the perspective of clinical care provision and incorporate screening and follow-up care, substantiated by sound research evidence. Other related aspects of the care provision are addressed in relevant chapters including applied sexual and reproductive science, clinical and health psychology, counseling, sexual health advising, and partner services provision. Young people and special client groups, health promotion clinical governance, research, clinical audit, and ethics in sexual health care are also discussed.

This text provides a versatile resource for an extended target audience of SRH practitioners of varied professional disciplines in developed countries (United Kingdom, United States, and others) and many developing countries. International and national recommendations; policies, professional regulations, and procedure guidelines, together with code of conduct, ethics, and standards of practice, reflect stipulations of the World Health Organization, Centers for Disease Control and Prevention, and the British Association for Sexually Transmitted Infections and HIV as well as National Institute for Health and Care Excellence and the Scottish Intercollegiate Guidelines Network, based on best available evidence. The content lends itself to interpretation and translation to the reality of care and service provision, and is therefore applicable within the different contexts of SRH care and acquired immunodeficiency syndrome (HIV/AIDS) services. The intention is to constantly enhance mindfulness among SRH multidisciplinary teams regarding the broad framework of EBP in this field of clinical practice.

Crucially, this text aims to encourage quality evidence-based SRH and HIV/AIDS care and services to safeguard the welfare and interest of the patients. Examples of excellence in sexual health clinical practice are presented and hypothetical scenarios with problems and questions are suggested as a way of challenging practitioners who read this text to reflect critically on their professional decisions and actions.

Acknowledgments

Sincere appreciation goes to Dr. Wilhelmina Kwansa and Mr. James Stewart-Moore for their encouragement and support throughout the development of this project.

Contributors and Reviewers

Tina Campbell, MSc, BD (Hons), PGCE
National Safeguarding Coordinator for the Roman
    Catholic Church in Scotland
Scottish Catholic Safeguarding Service
Former Head of Counselling Services,
Sandyford NHS Greater Glasgow & Clyde
Scotland, United Kingdom

Hannah L. Dale, MSc, BPS, BSc (Hons)
Health Psychologist
NHS Fife
Scotland, United Kingdom

Mandy J. Forbes, DClinPsychol, MA (Hons), MSc,
    AFBPsS
Clinical Psychologist
Psychology Department
NHS Fife
Scotland, United Kingdom

Lorraine Forster, MPC, BSc (Hons), RN, RM
Head of Nursing, Sexual & Reproductive Health
Sandyford
NHS Greater Glasgow & Clyde
Scotland, United Kingdom

Linda A. Graf, DNP, CNM, WHNP-C, APN, RN
Clinical Assistant Professor, Nursing
School of Nursing
DePaul University
Chicago, Illinois

Elizabeth D. Kennedy, MBChB, MRCGP, FRACGP,
    MSc, MIPM, FFSRH
General Practitioner
University of Melbourne
Shepparton Medical Centre
Victoria, Australia

Theodora D. Kwansa, PhD, MEd, MTD, Diploma in
    Higher Education HE Nursing (CT), RN, RM
Programme Tutor MSc Health Studies, MSc Sexual &
    Reproductive Health Studies
Lecturer
Abertay University
Dundee, Scotland, United Kingdom

Regina M. Mpemi, MSc, BS, SRNM
Lecturer (HoD-Nursing)
National University of Lesotho
Lesotho

Philip Okai Odonkor, PhD, MBChB, BSc (Hons)
Professor and Associate Dean
School of Medicine
University of Namibia
South Africa

Sally-Ann Ohene, MBChB, MPH, FGCPS
Fellow of the Ghana College of Physicians and Surgeons
Public Health Physician
Accra, Ghana

Maseabata V. Ramathebane, MPharm (Hons), MPharm
    (Pharmacy Practice)
Member of Lesotho Medical Dental and Pharmacy
    Council
Lecturer of Pharmacy Practice, National University of
    Lesotho
Consultant Pharmacist, Baylor College of Medicine,
    HIV/AIDS
Lesotho

Fred Stephen Sarfo, PhD, MBChB, FWACP, BSc
Senior Lecturer, Department of Medicine
School of Medical Sciences
Senior Physician Specialist
Department of Medicine
Komfo Anokye Teaching Hospital
Kumasi, Ghana

Kevin R. Smith, PhD, BSc (Hons)
Senior Lecturer
School of Contemporary Sciences
Abertay University
Dundee, Scotland, United Kingdom

Jill Stewart-Moore, PhD, MSc, RN, RM, Diploma in
    Nursing (Lond), PGCEA, MTD
Lecturer
Contraception and Sexual and Reproductive Health
    Nurse
Brook Coleraine and Belfast Health and
    Social Care Trust
Belfast, Northern Ireland, United Kingdom

Reviewers

Vicki Aaberg, PhD, RNC
Assistant Professor of Nursing
Seattle Pacific University
Seattle, Washington

Michelle Collins, PhD, CNM, FACNM
Professor and Director, Nurse-Midwifery
    Program
School of Nursing
Vanderbilt University
Nashville, Tennessee

Janna Figg Edrington, MSN, RNC, ARNP
Assistant Professor
Luther College
Decorah, Iowa

Melicia Escobar, MSN, CNM, WHNP-BC
Clinical Faculty Director
Instructor
Georgetown University
Washington, DC

Eva Fried, DNP, WHNP-BC
Assistant Professor
Otterbein University
Columbus, Ohio

Gay L. Goss, PhD, APRN-BC
Professor
California State University, Dominguez Hills
Carson, California

Catherine Jennings, DNP, MSN, APN
Associate Professor
Felician University
Lodi, New Jersey

Stefanie LaManna, PhD, MPH, ARNP, FNP-C
Associate Professor
Clinical Coordinator of the APRN Program
Nova Southeastern University
Fort Lauderdale, Florida

Susan Scott Ricci, ARNP, MSN, MEd, CNE
Concurrent Nursing Program Coordinator
University of Central Florida
Orlando, Florida

Debbie Ringdahl, DNP, RN, CNM
Clinical Associate Professor
School of Nursing
University of Minnesota
Minneapolis, Minnesota

Maria Ruud, DNP, APRN, WHNP-BC
Clinical Assistant Professor
School of Nursing
University of Minnesota
Minneapolis, Minnesota

Diane Ryan, AGPCNP-BC, FNP-BC
Associate Professor
Daemen College
Amherst, New York

Melissa A. Saftner, PhD, CNM
Clinical Associate Professor
School of Nursing
University of Minnesota
Minneapolis, Minnesota

Dr. MaryAnn Troiano, DNP, APN-C
Professor
Monmouth University
West Long Branch, New Jersey

I

Exploration of the Concept of Evidence-Based Practice and Related Challenges

Clinical Governance in the United Kingdom and the U.S. National Strategy for Quality Improvement: Interrelationships with the Principles of Evidence-Based Practice

THEODORA D. KWANSA

THEODORA D. KWANSA

CHAPTER OBJECTIVES

The main objectives of this chapter are to:
- Examine and clarify the concept of evidence-based practice (EBP)
- Explore what clinical governance entails
- Identify each of the core components of clinical governance
- Examine the ways in which those core elements interrelate with the principles of EBP

Introduction

Clinical governance—a U.K.-based health services accountability system—is rather complex. It is underpinned by evidence-based practice (EBP) that are incorporated to achieve standardization of high-quality care and service provision. Moreover, health systems in the United States strive to incorporate EBP into practice. To meet expected professional standards, practitioners must understand the link between EBP and clinical governance. Thus, practitioners should examine the rationales for the core elements of clinical governance together with the principles of evidence-based practice. Therefore, the rationales for clinical effectiveness, education and training, research and development, clinical audit, openness, risk management, and information management are presented in this chapter.

Similar principles conveyed in the U.S. National Strategy for Quality Improvement are also presented. Practitioners are encouraged to consider these concepts and principles in tandem as they try to fulfill organizational requirements for care and service provision. It is necessary, as well, to carefully examine the complexity of accountability and shared responsibility among multidisciplinary teams of sexual and reproductive care and service providers.

Concept of Clinical Governance Explained

As stated, clinical governance ensures the quality of sexual health care. Essentially, clinical governance represents joint responsibility and accountability for clinical success. Thus, professional self-regulation and practitioner judgments should not be replaced by clinical governance because these are critical components of health care and promote high-quality clinical care.

In its 2013 description of clinical governance, the U.K. Department of Health (DH) used the original definition of the concept, placing emphasis on the organization's accountability for realization of excellence in healthcare. Three essential elements are included in the DH's definition of clinical governance:

1. High standards of care
2. Continuous and effective improvement in care and services
3. Optimal patient outcomes

Joint responsibility and collaboration of activities within the organizational systems are crucial to realize the desired standards of care and service delivery. Thus, the concept of "integrated governance" is currently advocated by the healthcare organization as a more apt conception of governance in its entirety. Various documents have been published to clarify key elements of good integrated clinical governance, including the updated versions of the Healthcare Quality Improvement Partnership's *Good Governance* Handbooks (Bullivant, Burgess, Corbett-Nolan, & Godfrey, 2012; Corbett-Nolan et al., 2015). Integrated governance represents a system within healthcare organizations that embraces integrated schemes of "management of inputs, structures and process," which ensure clinical excellence by striving to achieve effective outcomes of care and service delivery (Bullivant et al., 2012; Corbett-Nolan et al., 2015; Department of Health [DH], 2013a; Som, 2004).

Accountability, Leadership, and Concerted Decision-Making

While accountability does not feature as one of the seven core elements of clinical governance, it does, nonetheless, thread through the core elements. The clinical governance framework sets out indicators for continuous improvement of health care through evidence-based practice to achieve better outcomes for patients and other service users. This fundamental aim assures the general public by maintaining confidence and trust in the healthcare professions and the services provided. Professional codes consistently remind practitioners of not only their ethical and moral responsibilities and duties but also their legal obligations. The operational structure of a healthcare organization lends itself to an obvious hierarchical system with varying levels of accountability. In the United Kingdom, accountability cascades from the Department of Health to the healthcare units, even down to the patients, care providers, and their representative groups, relevant service users, and the stakeholders. Allen (2000) describes downwards accountability, upwards accountability, and horizontal accountability, with upwards accountability taking precedence. The actual mechanisms that influence accountability depend on the nature of answerability, the associated resource implications, and other factors. In relation to clinical governance, Allen (2000) noted that clinical governance would broaden practitioners' accountability beyond their existing schemes of legal and professional accountability. However, there exists an inherent ambition among the healthcare professional disciplines to establish distinctive delineations of their specialism. This can create obstacles for a unified or shared accountability among multidisciplinary teams.

Savage and Moore (2004) pointed out the National Health Service's (NHS) encouragement for collaboration among healthcare professionals in the realization of more flexible role boundaries. These authors contend that accountability becomes obscured where role boundaries are blurred. There is clearly a need for more thorough exploration of the changing roles, professional autonomy, and accountabilities of nurses and other practitioners within the framework of clinical governance. The domains of accountability are explained later.

Mechanisms That Shape and Regulate Professional Accountability

The mechanisms relate to answerability in terms of who is accountable and to whom. The tiers of accountability within the healthcare system differ in different countries. Readers are advised to explore the relevant system in the country in which they live and work to understand local policies regulating practice. A brief overview is provided here relating to the U.K. system.

Systems for Standardizing Accountability

Particular formal schemes have been instituted that hold the providing organizations to account through a system of regulators. The key regulatory body in the United Kingdom—the Care Quality Commission (CQC)—regulates health service providers, while the NHS Foundation Trusts operate in a rather independent capacity. Therefore, while the current clinical commissioning groups (CCGs) commission their services via contracts, the regulation of the Foundation Trusts is undertaken by a different regulatory body. Professional regulators are independent, and their principal responsibility is to protect the safety of the general public and regulate the quality of care that practitioners provide to patients. The professional regulators are responsible to Parliament, which registers and regulates the training practices of each of the different healthcare professionals. These professional bodies perform various key roles and responsibilities, including the certification of new practitioners. They have the responsibility of ensuring that practitioners maintain standards and remain fit to practice (National Health Service [NHS], 2009).

At the local level, NHS commissioning boards are accountable to involve and report to the public any plans for specific health services. Furthermore, they are expected to report proposals for changes in the provision of services and to report decisions that may affect the ways in which the services operate. The current CCGs are also under legal obligation to report publicly on the ways in which they involved the public in their various activities and decisions. Similarly, they have an obligation to report on how their consultations with the public impacted their decisions (DH, 2013a; NHS, 2009).

Individual practitioners are expected to report proposals for any changes in the provision of the services as well as reporting decisions that may affect the ways in which the services operate and how consultations with the public impact on the major decisions that are made. The complex nature of accountability within the wider context of the health service organization is quite recognizable, and the perspective of the individual practitioner should be made clear. Allen (2000) maintains that the legal obligation for the individual professional to provide a high standard of care will always exist in healthcare provision. Statutory bodies of the different professional disciplines provide additional mechanisms and support for regulating and monitoring professional conduct, performance, and accountability (e.g., the General Medical Council [GMC], the Nursing and Midwifery Council [NMC], and the general social care council). These bodies regulate issues that may adversely affect the standard of patient care and outcomes, such as professional negligence. Moreover, they hold other disciplinary powers in dealing with matters relating to misconduct, malpractice, and other misdemeanors in professional practice (Allen, 2000; General Medical Council [GMC], 2013; Nursing and Midwifery Council [NMC], 2015; Savage & Moore, 2004).

Tension arises where clinical governance advocates collective responsibility for quality care provision and professional accountability. Additionally, clinical governance advocates the notion that groups of professionals should be accountable to one another regarding each other's performance (Allen, 2000). Clearly, there is a need for thorough exploration of the changing roles, professional autonomy, and accountabilities of the practitioners.

Ambiguity in the Interpretation of Accountability

Krautscheid (2014) noted that the multiple levels of responsibility within the healthcare system have resulted in variations in the domains and dimensions of accountability. The multiplicity of the professional disciplines also creates varied perceptions of accountability. Distinctions in academic and professional qualifications create apparent elitism and differences in perception associated with the traditional inflexible demarcations among the professional disciplines. In many areas, these are perpetuated by the disconnected and exclusive post-registration (post-graduate) continuing professional development activities. As a result, a somewhat hierarchical view exists among healthcare professionals that certain levels of responsibility and accountability are more significant and therefore command more respect than others (Savage & Moore, 2004).

There is clearly a need for clarification of the domains of accountability, and a brief overview is presented here.

Domains of Accountability

The domains of accountability are explained as follows:

- **Process accountability**, which emphasizes that appropriate systems should be used in the delivery of care for the right patients at the right time and in the right way in fulfilment of the governance principles. The applied system should be carefully recorded. That means that care delivery procedures must be based on appropriate, nationally stipulated guidelines and policies, and approved local standards must be adhered to in structured and coordinated care provision. In this way, process accountability allows for professional self-assessment of performance against the set standard.
- **Program accountability** is the mechanism of quality improvement relating to specific activities, including development of annual reports, and the coordination and dissemination of findings from clinical audits conducted within particular areas of care and service provision (Allen, 2000).
- **Structural accountability** occurs in financial resourcing and collaborative implementation of the clinical governance agenda and principles (Royal College of Nursing [RCN], 2008; Savage & Moore, 2004). The employers/service providers and commissioners have a responsibility to invest in their employees who form the multidisciplinary teams of practitioners. This ensures that the practitioners gain adequate familiarity with the stipulated employment standards, policies, procedures, and guidelines. The individual professionals have the obligation to acquire the essential knowledge and development of their roles and responsibilities. Appropriate provision should therefore be made for the necessary education and training support with opportunities for continuing professional development (RCN, 2008). Provision of such resources serves as a means to clarify any uncertainties about professional and legal accountability, and practitioners should be aware of their obligations in different contexts (Savage & Moore, 2004).

Savage and Moore (2004) examined the ways in which accountability is interpreted among healthcare practitioners and noted that in certain specialties, such as family planning and contraception services, where the practitioners frequently have to make immediate decisions to take urgent actions, they may find themselves confronted with conflicts of interest. Practitioners face the challenge of not overstepping professional boundaries in situations of compliance with the moral, ethical, and legal obligations imposed by the employer–employee relationship and their accountability to the professional bodies/regulators. It is therefore important to carefully examine the accountability statements in the internal policy guidelines as well as the expectations and recommendations of their professional bodies/regulators.

The challenges of having multiple leads in an interdisciplinary team should be carefully explored in the context of shared accountability and shared responsibility. That shared accountability would require establishing ongoing interdisciplinary communication in the team's working relationships. This would help facilitate decision-making while minimizing the risk of clinical errors caused by inaccurate unilateral decisions. The role and responsibilities of a team lead or manager should be made clear to all members of the multidisciplinary team. There is no doubt that lack of clarity about multidisciplinary team leadership and accountability, answerability for roles, and responsibilities can hinder achieving these principles.

Collaboration, Collective Responsibility, and Accountability

It is important for practitioners to understand the principles of professional collaboration, shared responsibility, and accountability. The concept of collaborative decision-making within a multidisciplinary team is complicated and many practitioners find it confusing. Failures in this regard are attributed to a lack of opportunity for colleagues to engage in joint clinical decision-making. Ongoing interdisciplinary communication in the team's working relationships is required and should be thoroughly explored (Savage & Moore, 2004).

Shared accountability should involve sound communication and joint decision-making strategies. Specifications of practice protocols; care interventions; and departmental, unit, or ward policies should involve input from team members of the various professional disciplines to achieve collective decision-making (O'Grady & Jadad, 2010). In addition to organizing meetings to obtain staff viewpoints, some staff members may be contacted individually for their input. Lack of familiarity with identified patients' special needs, diagnostic appraisal, and the complexity of holistic interventions could result in limited contributions to team decision-making (Allen, 2000; RCN, 2008; Savage & Moore, 2004). Consequently, individuals may have reservations about the expectation to participate in decision-making activities.

Accountability and Decision-Making: Potential Implications of Independent Decision-Making

Decision-making in the multidisciplinary team context involves members of staff of varied professional backgrounds functioning at different levels, inevitably constituting varied levels of input. Staff members with higher or more advanced expertise tend to hold positions of leadership and/or authority. They are therefore likely to be perceived as having the required professional knowledge to initiate and lead key decisions about patient care or deemed to have the professional authorization and accountability to make decisions. Moreover, they are recognized as having the status and professional readiness to accept the consequences for the decisions and actions taken (Savage & Moore, 2004).

Leadership and Accountability

Leadership occurs at all levels of the health service structure and therefore the principles of shared accountability and joint decision-making should be addressed at each level. This is particularly complex at the clinical practice level in a multidisciplinary team. The notion that team leads should be the only ones to make decisions or take particular actions for which they can claim accountability and answerability is debatable. Team leads may show bias in decision-making or make an error in suggesting action to be taken (O'Grady & Jadad, 2010).

Concerted Decision-Making

The notion of joint decision-making should be thoroughly explored, and the benefits, risks, and alternatives carefully

examined. Additionally, collaborative decision-making in partnership with healthcare professionals, the patients, their care providers, representative groups, and relevant stakeholders (RCN, 2008) is crucial.

Reflective Considerations

- How much collaboration in decision-making is practical and realistic within the multidisciplinary team context of care provision?
- What clinical interventional issues in terms of care and procedural interventions, policies, and protocols should be considered for shared decision-making by the team of professional practitioners?
- What issues should be appropriately considered for collaborative decision-making in partnership arrangement with stakeholders?

To achieve efficient participation, productive meetings, and accurate clinical decisions for efficacious outcomes and improvement of patient care and safety, consider the following questions carefully:

- What criteria should be in place for determining which members of staff will attend specific shared decision-making meetings?
- Which stakeholders should be invited to attend meetings of specific collaborative decision-making in partnership arrangement?
- What key factors should influence the timings for each of these meetings?
- What factors should be taken into account to guide the choice of venue for each of these meetings?

Main Benefits of Concerted Decision-Making

The main benefits to a concerted decision-making process are the following:

- Collective ideas enhance mutual respect and consideration of each individual's contributions, thus fostering a sense of personal responsibility within the team.
- The processes encourage interdisciplinary cooperation, empowerment, and increased staff motivation to participate in decision-making activities and in implementation of actions.
- Integration of multidisciplinary perspectives in the interventional and policy decisions ensures achievement of more effective outcomes.
- Collective policy decision-making encourages motivation and commitment to implement strategies to achieve the desired standard of quality care provision.

- Shared and concerted decision-making fulfills team ownership of the outcomes from the decision-making activities and it fosters the confidence to acknowledge related responsibility and answerability.
- Collaborative decision-making yields more impartial and constructive evidence-based interventional actions, and better patient outcomes.

The multidisciplinary team should acknowledge their responsibility to accomplish the principles of quality care provision in terms of patient safety and compliance with set standards toward effectiveness. Admittedly, a significant responsibility of the service providers, the regulators, and the service commissioners is the provision of efficient and sustainable services and support. The aim is to ensure delivery of the desired standard and quality of patient care (RCN, 2008). However, practitioners must be aware of employer requirements as well as responsibility to their statutory professional body. Savage and Moore (2004) identified the need for a consensus statement by the main professional regulatory bodies to provide clarification of the type, level, and boundary of accountability of the different disciplines. The emphasis on team-based working suggests multidisciplinary decision-making, which threads through the components of both EBP and clinical governance. The equivalent governance initiative in the United States, the National Quality Strategy (NQS), is examined in the following section and a boxed detail of the United Kingdom's parallel approach is also presented.

U.S. Department of Health and Human Services (HHS): National Strategy for Quality Improvement in Health Care

Like the United Kingdom's Department of Health, the United States' HHS upholds equivalent principles conveyed in its NQS. This evolved from the Patient Protection and Affordable Care Act (PPACA) or, concisely, ACA (2010), that pledges the intent to increase, expand, and support accessibility for high-quality affordable health care for all Americans (Agency for Healthcare Research and Quality [AHRQ], 2011). The NQS slogan "Working for Quality: Achieving Better Health and Health Care for all Americans" (U.S. Department of Health and Human Services [HHS], 2014) conveys this goal. The HHS endorses collaborative efforts that draw together federal and state government agencies, healthcare payers, purchasers, providers, consumers, and other affiliates in a framework for healthcare quality improvement.

Key Organizations

Key organizations participating in this framework comprise the California Department of Health Care Services, together with various HHS agencies, including the Centers for Medicare and Medicaid Services (CMS). These organizations have adopted, interpreted, and translated the aims and priorities of the NQS as the basis for developing their particular healthcare quality improvement policies. They represent the key leading providers of health care and services for a larger population of Americans; therefore, the healthcare quality improvement strategies that they advocate are widely influential.

The NQS upholds the value of partnership in care provision that is underpinned by best available evidence. Consequently, joint participation comprises the different states; licensing, healthcare professional specialty, and accrediting organizations; consumers and their advocates; and private sector purchasers. Collaboration in various healthcare initiatives among the stakeholders is also advocated to address specific issues including prevention of healthcare-associated infections and accountability in care provision and to implement community preventative activities.

Currently, several U.S. systems exist for measuring healthcare quality improvement and for interpreting and evaluating performance, which creates confusion for providers, payers, patients, and consumers alike. The need for consistency resulted in the establishment of the Measurement Policy Council, which examined the numerous existing measures to establish a streamlined system. Their foci for improved systems of measurement include control of hypertension; prevention of hospital-acquired conditions and coordination of patient care; patient experience; smoking cessation; perinatal care; human immunodeficiency virus (HIV)/acquired immune deficiency syndrome (AIDS); obesity; and depression.

NQS Aims and Priorities

The original NQS published in 2011 (AHRQ, 2011) and updated in 2014 outlined three key aims and six priorities in its guiding principles. U.S. practitioners should understand how the key elements and related principles have been interpreted and applied by their employing healthcare organizations, as slight variations may exist among purchaser/provider, and state and local organizational policies and regulations.

The three aims are as follows:

1. **Better care:** patient-centered, reliable, and accessible care and services, as well as improved patient safety
2. **Healthy people/healthy communities:** evidence-based, sanctioned interventions targeting behavioral, social, and environmental health factors
3. **Affordable care:** lower-cost, good quality health care

The six priorities are as follows:

1. Reducing harm with safer care delivery
2. Partnering with individuals and families in care provision

3. Using effective communication and coordination of care

4. Using the most effective prevention and treatment practices for the leading causes of death, particularly cardiovascular disease

5. Working with communities to foster best healthy living practices

6. Ensuring affordable, good quality health care by innovating new models of healthcare delivery

The Ethics and Standards of Patient Care Principles

Evidence-based practice principles, clinical governance, and the NQS cannot be addressed discretely in healthcare practice, as they share professional codes of conduct, standards of performance, and ethical principles for high-quality patient care. Common among them is the inherent ethos to take account of the concerns, views, and values of the individual patient, care providers, and the general public. An important practitioner obligation is to ensure that inadvertent negligence as well as inappropriate and inefficient care and service provision are avoided. Simply going through the motions of responding to the requirement to implement EBP is bound to fall short and fail to achieve expected outcomes. Each part of the healthcare organization—for example, the sexual health care and service providers—should aim to devise more carefully thought out, sustainable strategies to implement EBP.

Implementation of EBP in the NQS

In examining the "Efforts to identify and disseminate effective interventions in the United States," Biglan and Ogden (2008) single out the Blueprints for Healthy Youth Development project as the most efficient and productive scheme for circulating EBPs. Specific selection criteria are applied by the reviewing agencies/researchers. Moreover, in 2001 the HHS advocated the Substance Abuse and Mental Health Services Administration's (SAMHSA) approach to identifying evidence-based interventions as the selection benchmark. SAMSHA stipulates that the intervention deemed most effective should be the consensus among experts based on their understanding of theory, research, and practice. The views of key community prevention leaders and identified cultural leaders are also acknowledged.

Careful consideration is given to the dissemination process to ensure effective implementation. The selected sites for implementation should have essential resources, commitment, staff training, provision of technical assistance, and effective ongoing monitoring of compliance and consistency of implementation (Biglan & Ogden, 2008). In addition to these guiding principles, the individual characteristics for each setting should be carefully considered, and a combination of different strategies may have to be used to implement EBP (Shojania & Grimshaw, 2005).

Titler's (2006) definition and critical examination of EBP in the United States are largely comparable to that of the United Kingdom. Scientific evidence from empirical research based on randomized controlled trials together with descriptive and qualitative studies are emphasized, as well as case reports, scientific principles, and expert opinion.

The following are the key objectives of the AHRQ's model of the stages of knowledge transfer:

- Development and refinement of knowledge
- Dispersal and distribution
- Organizational adoption and implementation

The Patient Safety Research Coordinating Committee is particularly important in accomplishing these goals. As Titler and Everett (2001) explain, the Translation Research Model postulates that adoption of innovations is influenced by four key factors: (1) the type and strength of evidence in terms of identified clinical topic, (2) the method of communication or dissemination, (3) the particular users of the evidence, and (4) organizational system or context of care delivery—for example, the social system.

Comparable Elements in the Clinical Governance

Comparable elements in the clinical governance are that key parties for joint participation in the provision of care and services include commissioning organizations, local authorities, professional organizations, practitioners, and the voluntary sector (DH, 2013a). The shared objective is to improve the sexual health not only of individuals but society at large by targeting sexual health inequalities and better outcomes. At the same time, the aim is to establish an open culture based on honesty and transparency. It also aims at empowering individuals to make informed and responsible decisions and choices in their sexual relationships while recognizing the impact of poor sexual health on local communities (DH, 2013a).

Clinical governance in the U.K. framework emphasizes the responsibility of the NHS commissioning boards and other commissioning organizations to continually improve and maintain high standards of care and services. That means providing a nurturing climate of excellence in clinical practice with identification and prioritization of the education and development needs of practitioners to ensure an appropriately skilled workforce. The importance of establishing systems to support EBP in terms of clinical effectiveness and research governance is emphasized (DH, 2013b; Scally & Donaldson, 1998).

In addition, clinical governance portrays a milieu for clearly observable high standards of quality care delivery. It is characterized by an obligation to maintain standards as well as active and ongoing improvement (Bullivant et al., 2012; Corbett-Nolan et al., 2015; DH, 2013b; Galbraith & Department of Health, 1998).

Seven Core Elements of Clinical Governance

The seven core elements of clinical governance are the following:

1. Clinical effectiveness
2. Education and training
3. Research and development
4. Clinical audit
5. Openness
6. Risk management
7. Information management

See new and updated CQC's 2016 "Good Governance" (http://www.cqc .org.uk/guidance-providers/regulations-enforcement/regulation-17-good -governance#guidance-links). See also http://www.gov.uk/government /publications/records-management-code-of-practice-for-health-and-social-care.

Similar key elements are outlined in the DH (2013b) sexual health clinical governance document, grouped into three broad areas: (1) patient safety, including incident and risk management; (2) clinical effectiveness, which includes EBP, National Institute for Health and Care Excellence (NICE) guidance, clinical guidelines, clinical audits, education, and training; and (3) patient/public experience, which includes patient/public needs, consent, patient/public information, and complaints management.

These elements ensure that integrated clinical governance becomes an achievable and transparent operation. Each key element is examined in the following sections and their interrelationship with EBP is explored.

Clinical Governance and EBP Implementation

An evidence-based culture ensures that care provision is underpinned by substantiated evidence. Although skepticism persists among some experts regarding what counts as evidence in EBP, a broader view is generally tolerated in current practice. Thus, expert opinion, endorsement of practice by an authorized professional body, or organization and committee reports also constitute substantive evidence. Evidence from clinical experience and practitioner performance should be consistent with other factors. The circumstances, requirements, and personal preferences of patients or identified groups of care and service users may also constitute acceptable forms of evidence if indisputably substantiated (Harris et al., 2001).

Findings from systematic reviews provide insight into the best available evidence and serve as the basis for EBP. Therefore, in addition to professional knowledge and competence, evidence-based practitioners must acquire expertise in the critique of research and appraisal of systematic review reports, which enables them to efficiently explore the best available evidence for treatment interventions, the most effective mode of administering particular treatments, timeliness for interventions, and the most suitable environments.

Therefore, effective dissemination of such information both formally and informally by various means, including written and verbal processes, is crucial in clinical practice. It also requires making relevant data available in comprehensible language to all concerned. Practitioners should develop an understanding of systematic reviews and meta-analyses. Reasonable statistical knowledge and skills for interpreting and synthesizing data from research and clinical audits is also important. Training for such activities may be coordinated at the organizational level, unit, or in-house level to prepare practitioners for undertaking EBP with confidence and efficiency.

Broughton and Rathbone (2001) maintain that the likelihood of guidelines being followed depends on the way they are formulated, the processes of application involved, and the effectiveness of supervision. These elements of EBP are examined together with the core elements of clinical governance to establish the rationale, significance, and the interrelationship in the principles. In the next section, specific components of the 2013 changes in England's NHS are examined.

Implications for Specific Organizational Changes

Although the following outline represents the U.K. context, practitioners and readers in other countries are encouraged to understand the regulatory structure and commissioning of their healthcare and service provision. In particular, readers are encouraged to investigate how equivalent principles of clinical governance are translated and linked to EBP nationally and internationally.

- The main changes emphasize who has responsibility for making the most crucial decisions about the services and who has responsibility for commissioning providers and allocating funding. The regulating and monitoring responsibilities are also specified.

- Since April 2013, the primary care trusts (PCTs) have been replaced by newly formed commissioning bodies, and CCGs have assumed most of the functions of the PCTs. Additionally, the CCGs have responsibility for the services provided by general practitioners (GPs), nursing, and other health professionals. They also have authority to contract service providers who are considered to be cost-effective and efficient contributors to meet the predetermined NHS organizational standards. This means that providers must fulfill the expected requirements of high-quality care and services. They are expected to respond to the guidelines and recommendations issued by NICE and CQC.

- The commissioning organizations must also demonstrate that they involve stakeholders, including patients, care providers, and members of the general public, in decisions about the commissioned services.

- The NHS commissioning boards undertake responsibilities that include ensuring improvement of the quality of care and outcomes, contracting of primary care and specialist services, and allocation of resources. Providers within the NHS are expected to register with the CQC as well as with Monitor—the health sector regulatory body in the United Kingdom—to be eligible to function in the capacity of providers of healthcare services.

- Monitor has the responsibility of regulating the providers of health and adult social care services. Professional regulation continues to be undertaken by the relevant professional bodies including the GMC, NMC, General Dental Council, and the Health and Care Professions Council. The Department of Health, however, retains its official leadership responsibility for both the health and social care systems.

- The role of the local authorities has now expanded and in addition to contracting providers, their current role incorporates public health responsibilities together with the related budgeting.

- Health and Wellbeing Boards have the responsibility to facilitate integration of commissioned health and social care services. These boards are intended to strengthen the working relationships between health and social care while also boosting representation of input into key decisions from its own and other perspectives.

- Public Health England (PHE) currently undertakes leadership for the public health team and part delivery of evidence-based public health services across the country. Additionally, PHE is expected to have mechanisms in place to help people make informed choices toward achievement of better health and lifestyle.

- Another organization referred to as "Healthwatch" undertakes a representative role to support public views about the provision of health and social care services. Healthwatch has the responsibility to represent public opinion in specific decisions and report the service users' experiences. It is expected that Healthwatch England would work alongside the CQC in this role.

In essence, while many functions reflect existing principles, the actual contracting, regulating, and monitoring have undergone significant changes since 2013. These responsibilities are no longer undertaken by PCTs, but by the commissioning boards and the CQC, which regulates health and social care services provided by the NHS Commissioning Boards, the Clinical Commissioning Groups, local authorities, and private and voluntary organizations.

To supplement the (2013a) Framework for Sexual Health Improvement in England, the DH developed Sexual Health–Clinical Governance (2013b). Examining the section on "Improving outcomes through effective commissioning" is particularly useful for more insight about the regulation of care and service provision. What each of the key elements of clinical governance entails is examined here.

Clinical Effectiveness

Clinical effectiveness was launched under the ideals of the quality improvement campaign as a means to measure and report on the efficacy and proficiency of the system of management. In essence, clinical effectiveness affords a means to measure not only the efficacy of treatment interventions but also the related economic value, and ensures that clinical practice undergoes continuous improvement and that patient and care provider welfare is safeguarded. Clinical effectiveness is generally considered as representing the extent to which clinical interventions fulfill their intended purpose. However, a more pertinent conception was later proposed that emphasizes the use of expert/specialist knowledge, emerging research evidence, sanctioned or approved clinical expertise, and patient choices for the realization of best practice (DH, 2013b). The challenge for practitioners is how to determine clinically effective care and service provision. The essential components as defined by experts are summarized here.

Essential Components and Requirements of Clinical Effectiveness

The key principles are described in these terms (DH, 2013b):

- Doing the right thing
- For the right person
- In the right way
- At the right time
- At the right place (within the right environment and facilities of care provision) with the aim of achieving the best possible outcomes
- At the right cost.

The essential requirements are the following (DH, 2013b):

- Developing a culture of evidence-based practice within the organization
- Ensuring appropriate professional competence and relevant skills
- Providing treatment/services when the patient needs them
- Ensuring appropriate environments and accessible locations of treatment/services
- Maximizing health gain for the patients/clients in terms of clinical effectiveness

- Effective communication system with effective diffusion of information among the professional practitioners and the patients/clients
- Ensuring effective implementation of standards, clinical guidelines, protocols, and recommendations
- Achieving effective outcomes
- Ensuring efficient use of resources for the achievement of cost effectiveness
- Responding appropriately to the obligatory requirement of regular clinical audits

Outcome measures should reflect both positive and negative effects of specific clinical interventions on the recipient. Nevertheless, directly attributing a patient's state of health to a specific intervention could prove to be complex or even impossible. The issue of cost effectiveness is determined through the predictions of health economics whereby effective use of resources, financial disbursement, and expenditure are examined in detail. This principle of clinical effectiveness advocates efficient use of resources in the provision of high standards of care with positive interventional outcome(s) (DH, 2013b).

Assessing and providing trustworthy information about a particular aspect of health care through service evaluation enables the patients and care providers to make confident decisions and choices in their uptake of that service. Feedback from healthcare service users informs practitioners and organizational managers through the care recipient viewpoints.

Clinical effectiveness also requires practitioners to use critical thinking to ascertain if the desired standards and level of performance are being achieved and where appropriate changes to care provision are necessary. From the organizational level to the multidisciplinary team and individual practitioners, all are accountable and are overseen by the National Service Framework (NSF) and NICE, the key authorized bodies providing appropriately substantiated recommendations (Bullivant et al., 2012; Corbett-Nolan et al., 2015; Starey, 2001). However, in order to achieve successful outcomes from any clinical effectiveness audit, meticulous assessment and discussion among the multidisciplinary team of professional practitioners becomes necessary (**Box 1-1**).

Evaluation of Clinical Effectiveness

In the evaluation of clinical effectiveness, all key aspects of the project should be critically examined. The complexity of the challenge is created by the different groups of service users, including the patients, care providers, and their related representative groups. Nevertheless, economical use of resources and cost effectiveness should be demonstrated in meeting the expected goals of care and service provision.

Clearly, clinical effectiveness audit projects provide a means of assessing the degree to which set standards have been achieved. At the same time, the process allows for

---

BOX 1-1 Clinical Effectiveness Audits: Main Issues Taken into Consideration

The following list offers questions that can guide clinical effectiveness audits.

- What issue, aspect of care, or topic has been identified for the clinical effectiveness audit project?
- What was the incentive or trigger for considering this project?
- Is the topic or problem significant enough to be prioritized at national level for a clinical effectiveness project?
- Has there been clear evidence of best practice published in the recommendations and/or guidelines of the field to indicate a need for this audit project?
- What proportion of patients and/or practitioners are affected by the problem?
- Is there any indication that patients and/or staff are at high risk due to the problem?
- Who else has previously expressed concerns about the problem and proposed a clinical effectiveness project?
- In what way is it envisioned that clinically effective care can be realistically improved further?
- To what extent does this incentive for clinical effectiveness audit project receive the support and commitment of the multidisciplinary team?
- How realistically can the required change be effected if the problem is confirmed to exist and deemed to be significant enough to warrant a clinical effectiveness audit project?
- What potential ethical considerations are likely to emerge that would need to be addressed?
- How confident is the team about its efficiency and competence to undertake a clinical effectiveness audit project and make changes for improvement?
- What resources are in place for providing different levels of education and training support for the multidisciplinary team?

---

judging the degree of improvement achieved in relation to specific performance indicators. Thus, clinical effectiveness projects foster team cohesion and enhance decision-making among the organizational board of managers, the various stakeholders, and the clinical care providers. Moreover, the principles provide effective means of disseminating recommendations (DH, 2013b).

Similar to the United Kingdom's clinical governance, the U.S. NQS stipulates 10 key principles to guide achievement of the three aims mentioned previously.

NQS Core Principles

"Working for Quality: Achieving Better Health and Health Care for All Americans" (http://www.ahrq.gov/working forquality/nqs/principles.htm) stipulates that healthcare delivery should conform to a set of standard principles used by all stakeholders. This approach attempts to achieve better healthcare delivery and affordable health care for all Americans. The 10 principles, in brief, are the following:

1. Person-centeredness and family involvement
2. Specific health considerations
3. Elimination of disparities in care
4. Alignment of the efforts of public and private sectors
5. Quality improvement
6. Consistent national standards
7. Bigger focus on primary care
8. Enhancement of coordination
9. Integration of care delivery
10. Providing clear information.

Box 1-2 shows policies and infrastructure that support NQS priorities.

The United States recognizes that potential variations occur in the conversion or translation of guidelines, policies, and principles into practical application. Moreover, there are differences in regulations at state and local health organizational levels. For these reasons, U.S. practitioners are strongly encouraged to familiarize themselves with the stipulations and policy/procedural guidelines of their employer and ensure appropriate compliance. There are several key elements for successful quality improvement (Hughes, 2008):

- Fostering and sustaining a culture of change and safety
- Developing and clarifying an understanding of the identified problem or limitation
- Involving key stakeholders
- Testing relevant change strategies
- Continuous monitoring of performance and reporting of findings to sustain the change.

Generic Questions for Clinical Effectiveness Project Appraisal

The following questions could serve as the basis for appraising a completed clinical effectiveness audit project and for considering further projects. The questions are by no means prescriptive or exhaustive; therefore, they can be adapted to develop a more comprehensive and purposeful evaluative tool for the particular clinical effectiveness audit project.

BOX 1-2 Policies and Infrastructure for Supporting the NQS Priorities

1. Payment arrangements offering greater value for high-quality health care, with innovations, evidence-based practices, and professional efficiency. These should be monitored, appropriately measured, and evaluated.

2. Public reporting schemes allow for comparisons of the costs, patient care and treatment outcomes, and patient satisfaction.

3. Quality improvement/technical assistance enhances public and private support of the providers to deliver high-quality health care. This policy requires that the provider organizations, clinical specialty groups, and quality improvement organizations should work together with physicians, hospitals, nursing homes, home health agencies, and other parties. Moreover, this facilitates dissemination of research evidence and sharing of best practice and others' experiences. The role of the HHS is to contract quality improvement organizations to bring about quality improvement through state and local level collaborative endeavors.

4. Certification, accreditation, and regulation via professional certification by state, federal, and federally authorized accrediting organizations. In their regulatory capacity, the state and federal agencies supervise and monitor provider organizations and facilities to safeguard patient safety through sustained quality improvement measures.

5. Consumer incentives and benefit designs. This policy emphasizes the requirement for clinicians and relevant healthcare practitioners to be well informed about available evidence supporting better health practices and adherence to recommended medications. In relation to this, the HHS advocates value-based insurance models.

6. Measurement of care processes and outcomes. This policy involves the collaboration of public and private stakeholders in devising accurate measures for the quality of health care and services through monitoring quality improvement endeavors and data collection on care delivery, patient experience, and patient outcomes. The HHS advocates the coordination of quality measurement endeavors that address the six priorities of the NQS.

7. Health information technology. This policy relates to extensive use of electronic health records with

a view to reducing the amount of paperwork and related costs such as prescription drug savings. Electronic documentation provides a useful and efficient clinical decision support system toward improving care delivery.

8. Evaluation and feedback. This policy ensures that clinicians and providers are appropriately informed about ways to identify gaps in healthcare provision and elimination of risks. These can be supported by the patient safety organizations, which inform the healthcare organizations on a voluntary basis regarding innovations to improve healthcare provision.

9. Training, professional certification, and workforce and capacity development. This policy emphasizes the importance of making best use of the professional training and acquired skills. Lifelong learning is strongly emphasized. Dedicated funding is made available toward expansion of the National Health Service Corps (NHSC), an addition to the previous investment made through the American Recovery Reinvestment Act of 2009. From September 2010, special consideration was also given to increase primary healthcare professionals and sites within communities across the United States considered to be lacking in those services. Furthermore, the NHSC supports physicians, nurse practitioners, physician assistants, and other healthcare professionals with financial aid through loans and scholarships. These enable the professionals to pursue lifelong learning and ongoing enhancement of their professional knowledge and competencies. The Health Resources and Services Administration's National Center for Health Workforce Analysis identifies areas of shortages and best use of resources.

In their capacity as authorized professional regulatory bodies, the American Boards of Medicine and nursing and other health professional bodies also endorse endeavors toward quality improvement in patient care. Practitioners must fulfill their obligation to update their professional knowledge and skills for efficient performance in their fields of practice.

10. Promoting innovation and rapid-cycle learning. This policy recognizes the impact of innovations, collaborative endeavors, and functional communication regarding the uses of emerging new diagnostic techniques for disease detection with new models of care and treatment. It emphasizes the significant role of the Center for Medicare and Medicaid Innovation. Working together with many public and private sectors, these support wider implementation of groundbreaking practices and novel models of care to bring about changes in healthcare settings for quality improvement. The significance of implementing patient safety curricula throughout lifelong learning and rapid-cycle learning in health professional education and training programs is endorsed by the World Health Organization (WHO). A highly recommended reading for practitioners is the WHO. (2011). Patient safety curriculum guide: Multiprofessional edition. The absence of preventable harm caused as a direct consequence of the process of health care is considered an issue of global importance (WHO, 2011).

Reflective Considerations: Questions for Appraisal of the Clinical Effectiveness Project

- *What problem, clinical issue, or aspect of care was the impetus for the current clinical effectiveness project?*

- *How prioritized within that healthcare organization was the particular issue to achieve outcome improvement?*

- *How significant is the endeavor toward development of best practice in the specific aspect of clinical care?*

- *How prioritized is the project toward achievement of set targets, effective use of resources, and provision of the funding allocation?*

- *What clinical practice guidelines and recommendations were drawn upon to substantiate the decision for the project and from what authorized body?*

- *What systems of decision-making were employed in terms of group decision-making, open or closed?*

- *What processes were involved and how were the meetings convened?*

- *What evidence substantiates the clinical issue for the project?*

- *If related to services, what system was applied to organizing the services and how were these implemented and delivered?*

- *What limitations have emerged within the system and how have these impacted care and service provision, professional practice and patient outcomes?*

- *What health economic technique(s) were employed to assess disbursement of the funding, the cost of specific care and/or services, and equipment/resource use?*

(continues)

Reflective Considerations: Questions for Appraisal of the Clinical Effectiveness Project *(continued)*

- *Overall, what significant improvements have been achieved and in which aspects of care and services?*

- *What system is or should be put in place within the health service organization, units, and the actual contexts of care provision to effectively collect and interpret clinical information that can be used to plan, implement, improve, and monitor the quality of patient care?*

- *What specific limitations in terms of performance as measured by the practitioners' effectiveness and efficiency were identified through the project and in what area/aspects of care and service provision?*

- *What is the anticipated plan of action to be taken to resolve those limitations and achieve improvement*

and better interventional outcomes for the specific patient/client group?

- *Who should be involved for expert guidance and support in setting realistic and achievable goals and for the actual implementation of the plan? (Consider the decision-making system.)*

- *What measures should be taken to monitor and review the implementation?*

- *What is the target for submission of the full report?*

- *To whom should the relevant details in the report be disseminated and in what format (e.g., full details, summarized details, in written format, verbal format, or both)?*

- *Overall, who should be involved in the relevant decisions and actions at different stages?*

Practitioners are encouraged to explore various examples of audit projects that have been implemented in aspects of sexual health care and services. Systematic review reports of relevant clinical effectiveness projects also provide very useful sources to learn from.

Rationale for Education and Training in Clinical Governance

The requirement for continuing professional education and training applies to all qualified healthcare practitioners. Employing healthcare organizations have a responsibility to make it possible for clinical practitioners to fulfill their continuing education requirements.

Requirement for Continuing Professional Development (CPD) Programs

Continuing professional development programs focus on emerging professional knowledge, new developments in technology, and new procedures and skills for upholding professional conduct, ethics, and behavior. Therefore, there should be adequate capacity for training support and supervision of newly qualified practitioners.

New theories and concepts are continually verified and substantiated through ongoing research, thus enhancing the existing knowledge in clinical practice. As Starey (2001) argued, the professional knowledge and practical skills acquired during undergraduate education become outmoded in time. They are superseded by emerging new knowledge, innovative concepts, and more contemporary ways of practice. New procedures emerge in clinical practice through research and advances in medical technology, while changes in society create complex challenges in care and service provision. Consequently, these influence professional regulations, guidelines, policies, and recommendations

relating to care and service provision at international, national, and local levels. They also influence expectations in professional practice in terms of conduct, decision-making, and actions.

In view of all these, U.K. practitioner performance has to be closely regulated to maintain the desired improvements in the quality of patient care (DH, 2013b). Practitioners must be mindful of ongoing societal changes and their obligation to continually update their knowledge, their overall professional competency, and their day-to-day practical skills.

The endorses the importance of an appropriately educated and well-informed health workforce to provide the best health care and services to populations worldwide to achieve best health for all. The continuing professional development, education, and training requirements are necessary to encourage and assist clinical practitioners to fulfill their obligation to stay up-to-date with new professional knowledge, technology, and procedures.

Certain CPD courses are generic and cater to education and training needs for mixed groups of professional practitioners and these may be delivered at national and local levels. The NMC's post-registration education and practice (PREP) stipulated CPD education and training requirements for qualified nursing professionals. This was replaced by the revalidation of registration in 2016. Various other CPD programs are designed for specific disciplines of allied health professionals (AHPs) including physiotherapists, pharmacists, social workers, and occupational therapists. Another emerging concept is the educational conference program, "Nursing in Practice," launched in April 2016. This is designed to support nurses in the primary care sector who need to further develop and update their professional knowledge and practical skills. The Nursing in Practice programs should help practitioners fulfill expectations in their professional development portfolio stipulated by the NMC.

In view of certain differences in the professional disciplines, the funding for education and training endeavors remains a complex matter within the organization and particularly in the wider context of sexual and reproductive health (SRH) care. Nevertheless, the objective of the mandatory education and training requirement is to ensure that all practitioners continually update and enhance the scope and depth of their knowledge and competencies. This is recognized and endorsed by all the professional bodies, and practitioners must respond accordingly to this requirement. In some disciplines specialist practitioners must fulfill this requirement to retain their professional accreditation.

The concept of CPD in the United Kingdom shares common elements with the professional regulation in the United States regarding training, professional certification, credentialing, workforce, and capacity development. The requirement for practitioners to engage in lifelong learning activities is strongly advocated by the U.S. medical and nursing professional bodies.

Related documents published by the GMC include *Good Medical Practice* (2013) and *Promoting Excellence: Guidance for Medical Education and Training* (2016). The Royal College of General Practitioners (RCGP) and the Committee of General Practice Education Directors (CGPED) have also published their new guidance on standards for GP specialty training (RCGP/CGPED, 2014). Similarly, the NMC has launched the revalidation requirement guidance document that replaces the requirement for post-registration education ending March 2016. Practitioners are encouraged to find out more details regarding the education and training and the revalidation requirements stipulated by their professional bodies for continuing professional development.

Continuing professional education is recognized as essential to development and enhancement of proficiency in professional practice (Dickenson, 2010; Ni et al., 2014; Skees, 2010), hence the current emphasis on the requirement to demonstrate appropriate response to ongoing professional education and training (Institute of Medicine 2010; American Nurses Association 2010). Medical and nursing practitioners have a professional and legal obligation to update their knowledge and seek to enhance their professional competencies (American Nurses Association, 2010; Institute of Medicine, 2010). Despite this requirement, Schweitzer and Krassa (2010) found that practitioners may fail to attend and participate in CPD programs due to duration of the course or training sessions, together with child care responsibilities and other domestic commitments.

Research and Development in the United Kingdom

Clinical governance research and development encompasses the continuous search for new knowledge, innovative approaches, and advances in therapeutic interventions to achieve improvement in health. The establishment of centers of excellence ensures coordination of high-standard scientific medical research studies conducted by experts who provide guidance about the economic implications of such accomplishments. They provide information and recommendations to guide practice toward achievement of better patient outcomes. The research and development (R&D) centers of excellence inform the organizational management, practitioners, and service users about the quality of specific aspects of care and service delivery.

Other research activities performed or guided by centers of excellence include exploration of the efficacy of pharmaceutics, outcomes of specific therapeutic procedures involving use of new specialist equipment, and the resource implications. Evaluative research allows for studying the impact of national and local policies and recommendations on professional practice. Moreover, exploration of the service users' perspectives on the care and services that they receive enables the centers to determine improvements for better patient outcomes and better health. These centers possess the level of knowledge and expertise to facilitate and support education and training activities at local and national levels. They may also provide invaluable expertise to support clinical studies conducted by teams of healthcare practitioners to ensure efficient use of evidence-based findings from research.

Gerrish and Lathlean (2015) reiterate the interpretation of research as an endeavor to produce new knowledge that is generalizable by exploring clearly defined problems/topics through the application of meticulous processes. Thus, research within the context of care and service provision allows for detailed investigations to gain deeper understanding of existing interventions while seeking alternative ways to achieve further improvements. The challenge for the NHS organizations, units of care providers, ancillary departments, and multidisciplinary teams is to acknowledge their responsibilities in this component of clinical governance. Appropriate funding and protected time are crucial for realization of essential research activities. While the NHS organizations embrace the ethos of research governance and the related tenets, managers and practitioners must also embrace their responsibilities to acquire knowledge and competencies.

From January 2015, the health research authority (HRA) replaced the research governance framework for health and social care and took over its roles and policies. The governance stipulated the regulations and protocols that must be complied with for research projects within the NHS organization. It aimed at protecting research participants from potential risks directly associated with the conduct of investigative studies. In this way, it ensured that the principles of health and safety would be conscientiously implemented.

Another aim was to ensure that the ethical review procedures were functional and effective. The governance framework emphasized transparency for ethical approval, recording, and monitoring of all activities employed in conducting research investigations. That includes respect for confidentiality, anonymity and privacy of each study participant and the general public. It also stipulated that participant information and reports supplied to relevant stakeholders should be clear, unambiguous, and comprehensible in terms of language and use of terminology. Overall, the conduct of the study must be scrupulous and reflect excellence in healthcare professional practice. In assuming the responsibilities of the previous Research Governance Framework (RGF), the HRA collaborates with the Research Ethics Committees (RECs) to execute their new process of assessing governance and legal compliance and in implementing a more simplified approval process to prevent duplication of applications as well as stipulating the policy guidelines and regulation for ethical reviews. Readers are encouraged to examine the requirements stipulated by their equivalent health research authority to make comparisons of key elements in their research governance.

Rationale for Regular Clinical Audits

As Kapp (2006) pointed out, the HHS stipulated the regulations to be applied to all patient safety research and are employed by most U.S. healthcare institutions. The core element of common rule emphasizes protection of human participants.

Clinical audit is defined in the DH (2013b) sexual health clinical governance document as a means of assessing if health or social care is being provided according to the required standards. The DH's specification of standards for integrated sexual health services recommends the use of clinical audits for indicators of quality outcomes (DH, 2013b). The complex link between clinical audit and clinical governance is conveyed in the statement that clinical audit forms an integral part of the core of clinical governance (Burgess & Moorhead, 2011). Clinical audit offers a system whereby the quality of care provision can be systematically assessed on a regular basis. In the United Kingdom, commissioners may specify the minimum number of clinical audits that providers should carry out annually. It is also recommended that the focus of the audit(s) for each year should be determined at the beginning of that particular year. Therefore, most providers develop an annual timetable or schedule of clinical audit projects. The audits should include assessment of the practitioners' competences, performance attributes and professional updates (DH, 2013b). Clinicians and other healthcare practitioners are expected to participate in clinical audit projects (National Quality Board [NQB], 2013).

Core Element of Openness

Openness relates to processes of quality assurance that require substandard and unacceptable practice to be exposed and subjected to public inquiry (DH, 1998; Starey, 2001). The importance of openness is emphasized in the publication, "Openness and Honesty When Things Go Wrong: The Professional Duty of Candour." Openness provides assurance to the general public that the health service organization is committed to meeting the healthcare needs of the population. Therefore, its collaboration with the departments of public health, the local authorities, and local communities is crucial.

Core Element of Risk Management

Risk management may relate to patients, practitioners and service providers, and the health service organization. Specific statutory regulations ensure that neither the patients nor the practitioners or members of the general public are exposed to potential risks. The system of reporting faults, specific incidents, and slip-ups in procedures that can adversely affect patients has certain crucial advantages. It becomes possible for other teams of practitioners in different units, healthcare sectors, and specialties to learn of the potential risks that may be inherent in their own practices. The 2014 publication, *Quality and Safety Governance Development: Sharing Our Learning* makes recommendations that commissioners, health service providers, and policy makers may consider for underpinning their local action plans (Health Service Executive, 2014).

Related Policies and Protocols

In both the United Kingdom and the United States, different protocols and policies for guarding against clinical and other related risks are controlled by specific regulations and it is important that practitioners conscientiously comply with the recommended protocols and guidelines. In Scotland, risk management forms a crucial element in the provision of safe and effective care. In the United Kingdom, appropriate guidelines and recommendations are outlined in the Clinical Governance and Risk Management Standards: National Overview. The Healthcare Improvement Scotland replaced the National Health Service Quality Improvement Scotland (NHS QIS) in 2011. One of its objectives is to assure healthcare safety through risk-based scrutiny of care and service provision.

Successful management of clinical risks is vital because of the potential impact on individuals' lives. This can be achieved through correct identification and careful assessment of the possible health impacts, effective system of reporting, careful planning, and meticulous implementation of appropriate measures to minimize or eliminate the risks. Hickey's (2005) distinction between clinical risk management and patient safety is noteworthy. This author argues that clinical risk management reflects competence and is individual- or clinician-oriented, reflecting a voluntary code of moral, ethical, and personal values, beliefs, and principles. Patient safety, on the other hand, reflects performance and therefore is typically team- and systems-oriented. It is underpinned by regulatory framework and therefore exemplifies a patient-centered orientation. Establishment of the National Reporting and Learning System (NRLS) in 2012 in place of the National Patient Safety Agency 2003 was intended to enhance improvement of the safety and quality of care.

Similarly, in the United States, the NQS Patient safety portfolio emphasizes making care safer by reducing the harm that can be caused in patient care delivery and the costs associated with hospitalizations due to healthcare associated infections. Standardization of the NQS policies and procedures among the different healthcare organizations and hospitals helps to prevent, mitigate, and decrease medical/clinical errors, risks to patient safety, hazards, and the potential harmful effects on patients. The AHRQ provides evidence-based tools that can be implemented to improve patient safety. To evaluate the various components of the patient safety portfolio, quantitative and qualitative measures are used. Outcome data, reporting systems, survey data, and interviews with stakeholders provide the evidence-based information to substantiate development of the policy and procedure guidelines and required changes.

Related publications that examine patient safety and risk management in the U.S. healthcare systems highlight national policies, standards, and protocols for healthcare organizations and hospitals both for inpatient and ambulatory settings. To ensure appropriate compliance with recommended practices and guidelines for patient safety, quality care provision, and risk management as well as avoid potential litigations, healthcare practitioners should seek their employing organizations' guidance. Recommended publications examining patient safety and risk management policies and procedures for healthcare organizations include the following:

- Irving, A.V. (2014). Policies and procedures for health care organizations: A risk management perspective. *Patient Safety & Quality Health Care*. Retrieved from https://www.psqh.com/analysis/policies-and-procedures-for-healthcare-organizations-a-risk-management-perspective/
- Association of periOperative Registered Nurses (AORN). (2013). Perioperative standards and recommended practices for inpatient and ambulatory settings; 311 pp. Denver, CO: AORN Journal
- Destache D.M. (2013). Hospital policies: Will they be a burden or a benefit to you in litigation? *Midwest Legal Advisor*. Retieved from http://ldmmedlaw.com/hospital-policies-will-they-be-a-burden-or-a-benefit-to-you-in-litigation/.
- Hughes R.G. (Ed.). (2008). *Patient safety and quality: An evidence-based handbook for nurses*. Rockville, MD: Agency for Healthcare Research and Quality.

A brief outline of common clinical risks and the main considerations for assessment and analysis of risks can be found in **Box 1-3**.

Risks to Patients

Every practitioner has a responsibility to participate in risk identification and analysis. In order to effectively manage

---

BOX 1-3 Common Clinical Risks

Common clinical risks include the following:

- Faulty and unsafe equipment
- Contaminants (i.e., agents and chemicals); contaminated surfaces and items
- Handling and storage of hazardous agents and materials
- Errors in medication prescription and administration
- Rushed procedures

Factors that influence risk identification include the following:

- Complexity of the specific area of care provision and the structure and profile of the multidisciplinary team
- Feedback from brainstorming activities that enable all grades of staff to highlight potential risks
- Findings from detailed and accurate staging of patient journeys and the potential risks identified at each stage
- Prioritization of the significance and verification of each identified risk
- Detailed documentation to be submitted for discussion with the risk management and clinical governance staff

---

risks to patients, regulations such as the Data Protection Act 1998, the Control of Substances Hazardous to Health (COSHH), and the safe management of healthcare waste were put into effect as protective measures (RCN, 2007). Practitioners have an obligation to comply with these regulations. The ethical codes stipulated by the medical, nursing, and allied health professional organizations serve as important means of regulating practice (GMC, 2013; NMC, 2015). Critical event audits and the patients' complaint system provide additional means of reviewing and questioning the degree of practitioners' compliance.

Risks to Practitioners

Management of risk to practitioners includes practitioner immunization against infectious diseases, safe work environments, and keeping practitioners up-to-date on safe practice. As previously mentioned, various measures and guidance are in place, including the control of substances hazardous to health and the safe management of healthcare waste (RCN, 2007).

Risks to the Organization

Organizational risks are complex, and the impact of risks on the overall performance could have implications for patient safety. Variations in staffing levels due to staff turnover and shortages may result in the risk of employing staff rather hurriedly. Without proper detailed assessment of qualifications, extent of practical experience, and level of competence and skills, the risk of poor supervision, errors, and various incidents becomes unpredictable. Employment of highly and appropriately qualified staff is vital in the healthcare system and the practices involving locum clinicians and agency nurses should consistently involve strict scrutiny. The financial position of the organization could create constraints in the employment of staff, as well as the choice and supply of high-quality equipment and other essential resources.

Core Element of Information Management

Information management also forms a significant component of clinical governance. Apart from the standard data compiled about the general population, communities, and specific groups in terms of demographic and socioeconomic profiles, other more personal information is also retained. The sensitivity of specific records relates to the ethical and legal implications that surround them. Patient records contain personal and clinical details that may be required for decision-making on clinical interventions, related guidelines, and policies and recommendations. Accurate collection of those details is crucial to enable the healthcare organization to determine the trend of health problems within the population for which it provides services.

It is important that the collection, handling, storage, and use of all clinical information are addressed with great caution and thoroughness. While regulations such as the Data Protection Act 1998 and the Caldicott principles are in place to protect the confidentiality of patient information, they also allow for controlled use of specific information for research purposes. Similar elements as outlined above also appear as key elements in the United Kingdom's 2013 sexual health clinical governance.

The ensuing sections provide overviews of the national frameworks for improvement in SRH care. The U.S. public health approach to sexual health care is followed by the United Kingdom's SRH framework that is widely recognized as a model/commendable exemplar.

National Framework of Public Health Approach to Sexual Health Care in the United States

The RAND Corporation study (Auerbach et al., 2012) commented on the fragmentation of SRH care delivery and the disconnection from primary care and public health. Nonetheless, the point is made that the public health approach portrays a shift of focus to a broadly integrated health promotion approach to sexual health care (Satcher Hook, & Coleman, 2015). Comprehensive implementation

of the sexual health framework should be apparent across multiple levels of the health impact pyramid. Therefore, counseling and education, clinical interventions, long-lasting protective interventions, changing the context to make individuals' default decision healthy, and socioeconomic factors are crucial issues.

For the requisite health impact assessment (HIA), the key elements that need to be considered comprise screening to determine the likelihood of successful sexual health strategy; scoping, to identify potential risks and benefits; assessment of the baseline sexual health of the population; and prediction of the potential health effects. Recommendations of practical solutions with feasible implementation strategies require careful consideration. Reporting ensures appropriate dissemination of the findings to decision-makers, the relevant communities, and stakeholders. Finally, monitoring and evaluation of the changes in sexual health and associated risk factors together with evaluation of the efficacy of the processes and entire HIA are also required. Thus, disease control and prevention features as fundamental in the public health–focused SRH strategy.

The U.S. Centers for Disease Control and Prevention (CDC) prioritized working with prevention partners and providers to identify specific opportunities for sexual health framework to enhance their work (Douglas, 2011). The framework highlights complex factors at the individual relationship, community, and societal levels that influence health outcomes and shape individuals' ability to be sexually healthy across the lifespan. Douglas (2011) examined the rationale and options for the implementation of a national framework within the context of public health. Consultations on this initiative received great support as being appropriate, optimistic, constructive, and empowering. The key recommendations urge the following actions:

- Developing a CDC definition of sexual health and publishing a white paper
- Outlining the key objectives and stipulating the national SRH indicators
- Exploring the right milieu and tone of communication for achieving maximal acceptance
- Convening a national partnership of advocates, including faith-based organizations

Rationale for Establishing a National Sexual Health Framework

U.S.-based sexual health care and services were fragmented due to differences in state legislatures, diverse regulations and policies, and variations in care system structures. The SRH care system has predominantly been operating a disease-focused scheme. It is envisioned that a more contextualized national sexual health framework may encourage more open, normalized discussion on sexuality and sexual behavior, upheld by public health policy, contraception service, and SRH education in schools and at home. A sexual health framework in the public health context has the potential to reach youth and specific population groups and, essentially, the general public at appropriate levels on appropriate terms. Therefore, risk factors associated with adolescent pregnancy should be more extensively explored and carefully addressed. An exemplar of good practice prevention program is the U.S. Navy's sexual health and responsibility program (SHARP) implemented in 2000 based on the existing HIV prevention program.

U.S. Navy Sexual Health and Responsibility Program (SHARP): An Exemplar of Good Practice

The SHARP program is endorsed by the U.S. Department of the Navy; it is mandatory and supported. The program advocates planned pregnancy, sexually transmitted infection (STI) and HIV prevention, and elimination of syphilis. These goals are further enhanced by appropriate clinical care and counseling support, together with partner services, and access to contraception services and condoms. Thus, a strategic and comprehensive approach to sexual health promotion should provide a means of HIV prevention among special groups, including men who have sex with men. It emphasizes extensive education of the American public about HIV prevention and reduction of stigma/discrimination (Douglas, 2011). It is envisaged that the existing U.S. national HIV/AID strategy could provide a basis for advancing a public health approach to sexual health that includes HIV prevention. The framework could support, streamline, and enhance existing disease control and prevention using its four pillars of primary focus: (1) healthy and safe community environments, (2) preventive clinical and community endeavors, (3) empowerment of individuals, and (4) abolishing health disparities (Swartzendruber & Zenilman, 2010).

Issues for Consideration in Relation to STI Prevention in the SRH Strategy

Each state must address system-level barriers to timely treatment of partners of persons infected with an STI. This includes implementation of expedited partner therapy for the treatment of chlamydia. Variables, including gender/sex of the infected person's sex partner(s), are essential to understanding the epidemiology of STIs as well as guiding preventive efforts.

Innovative communication schemes are critical in addressing issues of disparities, facilitating uptake of services such as HPV vaccination, and normalizing perceptions of sexual health and STI prevention. In particular, these help reduce health disparities. It is necessary to coordinate STI prevention efforts with the healthcare delivery system to leverage new developments provided by health reform legislation. Social, economic, and behavioral factors that affect the spread of STIs include racial and ethnic disparities, poverty and marginalization, access to health care, substance abuse, sexuality, and secrecy in sexual networks.

The national prevention strategy (NPS) prioritizes SRH and upholds the following principles:

- Appropriate knowledge practices and care are crucial in enabling individuals to fulfill their capability and community stability.
- Safe and responsible sexual practices are associated with reduction in sexual violence, spread of HIV, viral hepatitis, and STIs.
- Planned and healthy pregnancy is vital to the well-being of the mother and child.
- Implementation of effective sexual health strategy could prove significant for addressing the burden of teen pregnancy and related consequences on educational attainment, employment, and financial stability.

The recommendations emphasize the following goals:

- Provision of effective sexual health education for youth
- Empowerment to make informed healthy choices and decisions on the uptake of SRH services
- Enhancing early detection of HIV, viral hepatitis, and STIs for appropriate linkage to care interventions
- Increasing use and uptake of preconception and prenatal care.

Sexual assault prevention is maintained and appropriate response intervention provided together with drug/alcohol abuse prevention (Douglas, 2011). The CDC's definition of sexual health states: "Sexual health requires a positive and respectful approach to sexuality and sexual relationships, as well as the possibility of having pleasurable and safe sexual experiences, free of coercion, discrimination and violence CDC, 2016)."

Framework for the United Kingdom's Sexual Health Improvement 2013

The DH describes sexual health as offering advice and providing services for supporting contraception, relationships, STIs, HIV infection, and abortion. It embraces the complexity of SRH care and services within diverse settings, including general practice settings, community services, acute hospitals, pharmaceutical service, and the voluntary, charitable, and independent sectors. To further improve the sexual health among communities and the wider society, a detailed re-examination and reassessment was carried out to establish evidence-based efficient service provision through appropriate change.

The 2013 framework for sexual health care comprised at its core partnerships and joint participation among the commissioning organizations to accomplish high-quality sexual health services and better patient/client outcomes. This undertaking, described as Joint Strategic Needs Assessments (JSNAs) was supported by Joint Health and Wellbeing Strategies (JHWSs) to fulfill the identified needs.

The evidence-based information obtained was intended to guide the local commissioning of care and services by the relevant local authorities, the NHS commissioning boards (NHS CBs), and the CCGs. The local authorities were expected to commission open-access sexual health, STI, and contraception services to fulfill the requirements of their local communities (DH, 2013a).

The Department of Health acknowledged the improvements that have been achieved over the past few years. Nevertheless, other issues have been identified as needing further attention, such as sexual health-related stigma, discrimination, and prejudices, and implementation of evidence-based preventive measures and treatment initiatives to reduce the rate of STIs. Effective patient/client access to the full range of contraception services and family planning together with guidance and support regarding unwanted and unplanned pregnancies are also identified. HIV prevention with increased access to early diagnosis and early treatment are also considered as requiring further attention, as is integration of cost-effective, evidence-based, high-quality care (DH, 2013a).

Attention to Focal Needs

Taking account of the main sexual health needs of the general population, the measures to improve sexual health outcomes were recognized in the DH (2013a) framework as follows:

- Pertinent, trustworthy, and correct information provided at the most appropriate time for making informed decisions about sexual relationships, sexual health, and sex
- Protective processes to foster empowerment, self-respect, and self-confidence to make informed choices for better health
- Quick or urgent access that is personal and private, integrated care and support by relevant professionals, at opportune times in a variety of settings
- Evidence-based approved and effective diagnosis and treatment of STIs and HIV infections together with partner notification and partner management
- Collaboration and continuity of care across gynecology, antenatal, and HIV care and services within the primary, secondary, and community care sectors in different settings

Issues of Particular Concern

Certain issues of concern included the high incidence of unplanned pregnancies, the persistently high rate of chlamydia among young adults, the high prevalence of HIV infections and late diagnosis of newly infected patients due to delays in seeking consultations, the increasing rate of syphilis, and emerging strains of resistant gonorrheal infections. The high incidence of abortion and the persistence of sexual assaults among vulnerable groups of women at high risk also need to be prioritized for special attention (DH, 2013a).

Areas for Priority Action

In relation to these concerns certain key areas were identified for priority action with specified objectives. These included measures to reduce sexually transmitted infections through provision of evidence-based information, sexual health promotion/education, and support for people of all age groups; implementation of preventive programs, including testing and treatment interventions aimed at reducing HIV infections; and further improvement of contraception services to reduce the rate of unwanted pregnancy among all women of fertile age. Reduction of the abortion rate with counseling support and prevention of teenage pregnancy were also priority areas (DH, 2013a).

Commissioning and the Proposed Changes

The broad context of commissioning (or contracting) involves contribution from the local authority commissioning, CCGs, and NHS commissioning boards. The DH (2013a) framework sets out guiding principles that should be applied in the contracting process by each of the three commissioning bodies.

Role of Local Authorities in Clinical Governance

In their role as major commissioning bodies, the local authorities have to ascertain that the contracting providers have effective clinical governance systems in place. The providers have an obligation to comply with the standards set by authorized organizations for guiding clinical care and service provision. Monitoring procedures are in place, set by the local authorities to ensure that the providers correctly implement all elements specified in the clinical governance principles. This may be a nonmandatory public health services contract set by the Department of Health in collaboration with relevant stakeholders including public health professionals. In addition, the DH has issued a standard service specification for integrated sexual health services that outlines quality indicators and performance measures to be used to ascertain that the principles of clinical governance are properly implemented (DH, 2013a). As part of the tendering process, the local authority commissioners assess the adequacy of the structures and capacity for meeting the requirements of clinical governance. In their role as chief adviser on health for the local authority the Director of Public Health is consulted for advice on the public health perspective of the clinical governance mechanisms. Specialized medical and pharmaceutical contributions are also considered in the contracting and tendering processes. This allows for carefully examining the clinical governance requirements for safe and effective use of medicines in relation to the patient group directions (PGDs).

Quality surveillance groups examine shortcomings in the quality of SRH care in relation to clinical governance. It is proposed that an informal facilitative process can also be undertaken by the local health and wellbeing board. The establishment of provider events is allowed to encourage open and transparent opportunities for development of new models of care and service delivery. These may help to substantiate new approaches to SRH care and service delivery (DH, 2013a).

Role of Providers in Clinical Governance

Recognition is given to shared responsibility for ongoing improvement in healthcare delivery and for dealing with inadequate or deficient quality standards. Nonetheless, the view of experts is that the ultimate responsibility should be carried by the leadership of the provider organization. A designated lead for clinical governance is recommended for genitourinary medicine (GUM) and reproductive healthcare services. Providers are required to register with the Care Quality Commission, which functions as the statutory regulator to confirm that they are formally regulated SRH care and services providers.

The Department of Health (2013a) stipulates six key guiding principles that the commissioners are expected to apply toward achievement of best practice:

1. Prioritizing prevention of poor sexual health through health-promotion techniques: This draws on insights from behavioral science in adopting change in lifestyle behaviors toward better sexual health.

2. Establishing a strong and effective leadership team should comprise members from each of the three commissioning authorities: Their partnerships with relevant parties from the voluntary and community sectors should help strengthen their commitment to improve sexual health throughout the local area.

3. Focusing on outcomes based on accurate data, determining outcome measures, and carrying out needs assessment: The findings can be used with other best available evidence to plan and implement actions to reduce inequalities in sexual health and well-being.

4. Continuously monitoring the improvement to help in assessing and maintaining cost effectiveness of the interventions and the related services.

5. Carefully examining the wider determinants of sexual health.

6. Considering the associations between sexual health and various factors identified as determinants of health—alcohol, misuse of drugs, violence against women, and mental health.

To ensure their effective implementation, the local authority commissioners are required to register with the CQC, who inspects and monitors the services to see that they are complying with the required standards of care and service provision through the principles of clinical governance (DH, 2013a).

Commissioning of High-Quality Providers of Correct Interventions and Services

These should take place in a variety of settings at flexible times that are acceptable to patients and delivered by appropriately trained, qualified, and well-informed practitioners. Moreover, the interventions should reflect best practice. Therefore, feedback from the service users should be considered important. Provision of high-quality training through approved courses is crucial to prepare and support practitioners for competent performance of their roles. Examples are programs, courses, and modules provided by the Faculty of Sexual and Reproductive Health and the British Association of Sexual Health & HIV. Effective referral systems and commissioned services offered at easily accessible sites are emphasized.

Meeting the needs of population groups at higher risk is another stipulated principle. The vulnerable groups include those with special needs and at risk of poor sexual health as well as people with learning disabilities; young people; the lesbian, gay, bisexual, and transsexual (LGBT) community; and specific ethnic minority groups. This overview of the 2013 Sexual Health Framework attempts to establish links to the core elements of clinical governance previously examined in this chapter.

Patient Group Directives (PGDs): Role Extension of Pharmacists

Two important elements in sexual health care are examined here. To begin with the importance of confidentiality, PGDs are explored as outlined in DH *Sexual Health: Clinical Governance* (DH, 2013b), followed by the implementation of PGDs.

Respect for Patient Confidentiality

Respect for confidentiality is an important component of professional practice in healthcare. Relevant documents include the National Health Service's Confidentiality: NHS *Code of Practice* (NHS, 2003), *Confidentiality: NHS Code of Practice Supplementary Guidance: Public Interest Disclosure* (NHS, 2010) and the Health Insurance Portability and Accountability Act of 1996 (HIPAA). The latter provides supportive interpretation of the key principles specified in the code of practice to guide practitioners when faced with decisions of disclosure of patient confidentiality. Practitioners employed in the National Health Service are expected to comply with the Caldicott principles of confidentiality (Brook et al., 2013; Faculty of Sexual and Reproductive Healthcare of the Royal College of Obstetricians and Gynaecologists [FSRH], 2015). The professional regulatory bodies also issue guidelines on confidentiality; the Nursing and Midwifery Council, for example, provides *The Code: Standards of Conduct Performance and Ethics for Nurses and Midwives* (NMC, 2015). These regulatory bodies stipulate standards for safeguarding patient/client confidentiality and dealing with confidential information justifiably, with discretion, honesty, and respect as specified in the Caldicott principles.

In certain situations, however, public interest requires that particular infections should be notified, which may involve disclosure of confidentiality. The rationale for this is to protect the public from the risk of acquiring the infections by putting in place measures to control the rate of spread and acquisition. The United Kingdom's Faculty of Sexual and Reproductive Health (FSRH, 2015) cautions about violation of confidentiality, mishandling of patients' records, potential professional consequences, and the possibility of litigation. Therefore, practitioners must be made aware of this and the related disciplinary action in their contracts of employment. Details of patients' sexual history should not be divulged to third parties, and the preferred mode of correspondence should be respected and used as the individual requests. Furthermore, a practitioner should not inadvertently breach doctor–patient confidentiality by asking an individual's medical general practitioner to divulge specific personal details. The use of identifiable items including personal details and photographs must be consented by the individual. Various ethical dilemmas arise in relation to the duty of confidence and it is possible that protecting the confidentiality of one patient or the sexual contacts could have damaging consequences for other individuals. The FSRH (2015) outlines standard statements on confidentiality training, the rights of patients to confidentiality, disclosure without consent, duty of confidentiality to young people, sharing, and disposal of confidential information. These are contained in the *Service Standards on Confidentiality* (FSRH, 2015).

Beckley and Szilagyi (2013) also provide useful insight into the ethical issues relating to detailed health history taking. Practitioners may find it useful to critically analyze these to consider how best these can be interpreted and translated into practical application. It is also useful to reflect on some of the moral and ethical dilemmas and conflicts that may arise in the partner notification process and the potential legal implications.

Patient Group Directives: Requirements and Processes

Patient Group Directives are explained in the Health Service Circular (HSC) as "a written instruction for the supply or administration of medicines to groups of patients who may not be individually identified before presentation for treatment" (Medicines & Healthcare products Regulatory Agency, 2017). This means that a named registered practitioner who is functioning under the regulations of a professional body may supply and/or administer a specific medicine to individuals of identified patient groups. Thus, a formal prescription for a particular patient may not be required. However, the specified set of criteria must be fulfilled in the PGDs guidelines. In SRH care, PGDs are specifically used for the supply and administration of certain types of contraception and for treatment of chlamydia. While PGDs offer quick and easy access to treatment, patient safety is strongly emphasized and must supersede all other aspects of this practice.

Regulations and Guidelines on PGDs

The regulation stipulates that PGDs require the signature of registered authorized practitioners—in particular a physician or pharmacist—and they must be endorsed by the appropriate authorizing body stated in the PGD guidelines. Independent and voluntary sector providers may also supply and administer medicines. However, they must be registered with the Care Quality Commission and endorsed by the relevant commissioning body such as the local authorities. It is important that all practitioners involved in PGDs have received the required additional training for this role and be appropriately qualified. Of equal importance, providers must comply with careful reviews and renewal of expired PGDs. Practitioners are encouraged to read the comprehensive guidance issued by NICE in its good practice guidance regarding PGDs and to examine the recommendations for reporting incidents of errors relating to patient safety (DH, 2013b).

Confidentiality: An Essential Element in Sexual and Reproductive Health Care

Apart from situations relating to a criminal offense, the legal regulation emphasizes that information that can identify a patient should not be shared between authorities without the individual's consent. In relation to STI testing, the degree of safeguarding an individual's confidentiality is even stricter. A new code of practice developed by the DH and the Health and Social Care Information Center replaces existing regulations and guidelines. The Caldicott (2013) publication— Information: To Share or Not to Share"—is highly recommended reading (http://www.gov.uk/government/publications/the-information-governance-review). Practitioners would find it particularly useful to critically examine the data protection act and the guidance on the law and regulations relating to safeguarding the rights, consent, privacy, and confidentiality of individual patients (DH, 2013b).

The Department of Health's (2013b) *Sexual Health: Clinical Governance* emphasizes patient safety, clinical effectiveness, and patient/public experiences of sexual health. The main action points relating to each element are stated. The aim is to achieve improved sexual health service provision by maintaining efficient and high-quality services and favorable outcomes (DH, 2013b).

The FSRH document *Service Standards on Confidentiality* (2015) provides excellent guidelines on confidentiality standards.

Rationale for Standardization of the Directives for SRH Treatment

It is important that practitioners are aware of the rigor by which policy regulations, recommendations, and guidelines are developed. Relevant authorities ensure that the best available evidence from various sources is meticulously examined. Within this field the involvement of SRH professional experts and the stakeholders is also secured. Thus, contributions and reviews are made by GUM physicians and other specialists, sexual health nursing practitioners, sexual health advisers, the association of pharmacists, and relevant patient group representatives.

The key rationale for standardizing the principles, guidelines, and procedures for treatment is to ensure that the treatments provided for specific STIs are based on best available evidence. Moreover, standardization allows for accomplishing control and prevention of spread and recurrence of specific infections among members of the community. Consistency in the application of the recommended evidence-based guidelines ensures efficient management to avoid long-term adverse health, social, and economic consequences. The interactions between sexual health physicians, other practitioners, and the patients help to initiate preliminary measures toward change in sexual behaviors while encouraging uptake of available sexual health services, including screening.

The WHO urges that all countries establish their national standards, protocols, and recommended guidelines for the treatment of STIs. This ensures consistency in care and service provision with all patients receiving the appropriate recommended treatment and support. Moreover, standardization requires that practitioners undergo purposefully designed education and training to acquire appropriate knowledge and skills for efficiency in practice. These are crucial for correct implementation of the different procedures and treatment interventions in all aspects of STI care. Standardized national protocols should reflect carefully assessed epidemiological status and antimicrobial drug sensitivity results among the population of each country. Thus, the expertise and guidance of bacteriologists, biochemists, and pharmacists should be sought. The following section briefly examines the role of pharmacy in the provision of STI and reproductive tract infection (RTI) treatment, care, and support.

Significance of Pharmacy Services in SRH Care and Service Provision

Pharmacy services contribute a crucial role toward the overall SRH care and services. Service provision within the community settings ensures that accessibility to comprehensive pharmaceutical support can be extended beyond the inpatient sector of secondary care and outpatient clinics. In this way, pharmacy services in STI/RTI care clearly demonstrate the concept of integrated primary and secondary care and service provision for the general public. Apart from the practicality and ease of access to obtain prescribed medication, the extended role of pharmacists contributes toward enhancement of care and service provision for SRH patients/clients.

As the pharmacy profession continues to evolve, becoming more clinically focused with specialization in areas such as sexual health, pharmacists are able to provide invaluable specialist support. The Royal Pharmaceutical Society of Great Britain publishes relevant evidence-based guidelines, and readers who are members of the society are encouraged to explore the most current Sexual Health Toolkit publication.

Clinical pharmacists with qualifications up to consultant level may be employed within the HIV care and services sector. Apart from providing specialist advice to the SRH physicians and patients on important aspects of drug therapy, they also monitor safety in drug treatment for the patients. In the United Kingdom, clinical pharmacists may function in the independent or supplementary capacity to prescribers with additional direct responsibility for caseloads and patient management (Royal Pharmaceutical Society [RPS], 2014).

Extended Role of Pharmacists: Significance in Sexual Health Care and PGDs

The extended role of pharmacists incorporates implementation of PGDs. The PGDs policy allows for the supply and administration of prescription-only medicines (POMs) under certain circumstances, and it ensures enhancement of patient care. As mentioned, PGDs may be authorized by the healthcare provider registered with the Care Quality Commission. In practice, the directives may be determined and authorized by NHS bodies such as the current CCG-qualified physicians, dentists, hospitals, and clinics in compliance with legislation relating to the Medicines Act 1968. Pharmacists are in a position to provide support and advice within primary and secondary care in the preparation of PGDs. Additionally, pharmacists may be involved in the development of formularies and the related policies for the management of medicines in community contraception services and local GUM services (RPS, 2014).

Furthermore, community pharmacists may provide a range of comprehensive supportive roles in sexual health services depending on the disbursement of local and national funding. An additional role involves providing advice on, dispensing, and supplying medications and other sexual health products directly to the public. This role may necessitate private consultations in response to increased public demand and the willingness of individuals, specific social groups, and community members to consult pharmacists on sensitive issues relating to STIs/RTIs. The continuously increasing variety of medicines and over-the-counter products invariably necessitates the provision of specialist advice to sexual health clinicians and practitioners with direct private patient consultations.

Qualified pharmacists who have acquired additional specific qualifications through prescribed specialist training programs in identified clinical areas such as STIs/RTIs and GUM have remits to perform particular roles. These may include managing common uncomplicated sexually transmitted infections by carrying out specific screening and diagnostic tests, such as chlamydia and gonorrhea screening within both NHS and private sectors. Provision of STI treatment in the extended role of the pharmacist may involve dispensing and/or administering treatment for infections such as chlamydia, genital warts, and genital candidiasis. Supply and instructions on correct handling and application of the different types and products of condoms and HBV vaccination are additional potential roles. Other extended remits may involve referral of patients for specialist care and treatment and, to some extent, participating in the process of partner notification and preliminary health promotion (RPS, 2014).

The issue of professional, ethical, and legal importance is that these roles should be recognized as guided and regulated by statutory acts, and the PGDs should be defined by the relevant healthcare providing organization. Compliance with the regulations is obligatory and should reflect the accountability of pharmacists within the wider context of SRH care, particularly STI/RTI care and service provision.

Compliance in Relation to PGDs and POM

Regular reviews of PGDs are stipulated to occur at least every two years. The type and classification of the particular prescription-only medication to which the PGDs relate should be clearly stated and complied with. Moreover, the clinical conditions and indications for which the particular POM can be used to treat and the criteria for eligibility for the treatment or exclusion from it should be fulfilled as specified in the PGDs. There should be clear stipulation of the circumstances for which advice should be sought from a specialist physician or the relevant medical officer. The form of the POM, the prescribed strength and dosage, as well as the mode and frequency of administration must be strictly complied with. Of equal importance, the minimum and maximum duration and relevant precautions relating to the particular POM is vital for protecting the safety of patients. Circumstances for which follow-up action would be required and the related referral systems to be employed for further medical intervention should each be clearly stated in the PGDs and complied with accordingly. Accurate record keeping should be regarded as a professional obligation. The requirement for detailed information should be complied with including the sale, supply, and administration of specific medication under the PGDs regulations.

Details of patient/client assessment should incorporate the information that the individual provides by completing the prescribed pro-forma indicating the name, date of birth, and contact details. Additionally, record should clearly indicate the name of the medication, the dosage, and quantity supplied to the particular patient. The advice and supplementary information provided to the individual including specific leaflets given to him/her should all be recorded accurately together with the date and signatures of the patient and the pharmacist (RPS, 2014).

Participation in HIV and AIDS care and service provision involves working with the multidisciplinary team. The specialist clinical pharmacist may be consulted for advice regarding specific drug treatments and drug interactions. The consultant pharmacist may have a role in post-test counseling while he/she may also be involved in HIV clinical services in the secondary care context and management of medicines in the primary care setting. The pharmacist's involvement in community HIV/AIDS care and services may entail provision of advice and support to the patients (RPS, 2014).

It is envisaged that the role and contribution of pharmacists in STI care will continue to extend beyond the current policy restrictions to allow for involvement of pharmacists in a wider range of screening tests. HPV vaccination by pharmacists may increase, and the provision of post-exposure HIV prophylaxis may also be considered in the remit of the community pharmacist (RPS, 2014).

Increasing Public Demands for On-Site Testing and Treatment

The concept of integrated STI/RTI care and service provision within the primary and secondary care sectors aimed at providing comprehensive and accessible care confirms the need for wide-ranging professional expertise. STI/RTI together as a unified structure undergoes constant evolution with fluctuating epidemiologic patterns of the infections and related consequences. The evolving characteristics of the different infections should be carefully considered in the provision of treatment, guidance, and support in order to achieve effective outcomes. The range of treatment also varies widely and continues to expand, getting increasingly complex in response to laboratory discovery of resistant microorganisms. Correspondingly, the pharmaceutical industries have had to respond to the emergence of new and more virulent species and strains of microorganisms, viruses, and bacteria. To keep up, the industries are manufacturing more specific/complex drugs with appropriate strength and sensitivity to deal effectively with the emerging strains of organisms. With the discovery of concomitant organisms, the choice of treatments, combinations of antimicrobials, and the mode of administration and the schedules of the regimens have to be constantly reviewed and updated. The emergence of more sophisticated scientific techniques has enabled specialist laboratories to perform more complex tests with more reliable results. At the same time, relatively simple yet sensitive tests have emerged with appropriate tool-kits that can be employed in performing specific tests on self-collected specimens. Undoubtedly, these ongoing changes are associated with increasing public demand for on-site testing and treatment.

These situations clearly demonstrate a scenario of multidisciplinary collaboration in STI/RTI care and service provision and therefore the need for standards and consistency of patient care and support. Clearly, the role of pharmacists spans across the wider context of STI/RTI care and service provision and the importance of confidentiality is clearly evident. Pharmacists at specific levels of professional practice who have undertaken extended role preparation relating to specific aspects of sexual health care would be in the best position to participate in STI/RTI care in more diverse ways. The role extension may allow the qualified pharmacist to participate in community based on-site testing and treatment in accordance to the organizational policy and regulations.

All-Embracing SRH Services Across Public Health and Primary Care: Endorsement by the WHO

The WHO's definition of SRH embraces the reproductive health of men and women throughout the lifespan, as well as preconception, contraception, and pregnancy. Also included are women's health and routine gynecological care, specialist gynecological assessments such as infertility, men's genitourinary conditions, and sexual health promotion. The all-inclusive SRH spans across pre- and post-reproductive years and is associated with socio-cultural factors, gender roles, and human rights and protection (WHO, 2011). Aligned with public health and primary care, integrated SRH services should provide the full extent of SRH obligations and accountabilities, including prevention services. Brief outlines of the core competencies of SRH are presented here (**Box 1-4**).

Domains of the Requisite SRH Core Competencies

Thirteen competencies are categorized into four domains as synopsized here (WHO, 2011):

- Domain 1 focuses on the practitioner's knowledge of ethics and principles, which influences all other competencies. Essentially this domain is required for fulfilling the human rights of each patient.
- Domain 2 represents the leadership and managerial roles and attributes. This domain is intended for program leaders and managers but may also be applicable at other levels. This domain requires managerial responsibility for establishing an atmosphere of high motivation with support for continuing education, facilities, and appropriate resources to provide high-quality SRH care and services.

BOX 1-4 Key Elements of SRH

- Enhancing antenatal, perinatal, postpartum and neonatal care
- Providing high-quality family planning services and infertility services
- Abolishing unsafe abortions
- Preventing sexually transmitted infections including HIV, reproductive tract infections (RTIs), cervical cancer, and other SRH conditions
- Promoting sexual health
- Increasing capacity for supporting and sustaining research and program development (as construed from WHO [2011] SRH core competencies in primary care)

Modified from WHO. (2011). *Sexual and reproductive health care competencies in primary care.* Geneva: Author.

- Domain 3 comprises four general SRH competencies for healthcare providers and includes working with the community, health education, counseling, and efficient assessment of the client.
- Domain 4 comprises seven specific clinical competencies for different types of SRH care provision. This domain outlines a minimum package of care and service provision that is accessible to every individual patient.

Ideally, education and training programs focused on providing efficient high-quality SRH care and services should be consistent at national level. Arguably, certain variations may emerge in implementation at the state level. Nonetheless, key elements in the SRH education and training curricula programs could lend themselves to interdisciplinary teaching and learning. Clinical practice placement opportunities and acquisition of a shared set of competencies in the development of practical experience within the integrated primary healthcare context have received positive recognition (Newhouse & Spring, 2010). The shared competencies that should thread through all the SRH and other programs encompass human attitudes, knowledge, ethics, human rights, leadership, management, teamwork, community work, education, counseling, clinical settings, and service provision. These could be considered key elements in the concept of "interprofessional competencies in integrative primary health care," examined by Kligler et al. (2015). A careful collaborative effort among the relevant educators, academic institutions, and professional disciplines is required to address variation among the different disciplines (Kliger et al., 2015; Newhouse & Spring, 2010). Berg, Woods, Kostas-Polston, and Johnson-Mallard (2014) examine the concerns about the adequacy of the curricular content of the SRH preparatory education and training programs for women's health nurse practitioners (WHNPs). They strongly suggest that educators involved in NP primary care specialty programs should carefully examine the adequacy of the SRH content for developing the essential competencies as proposed by the Royal College of Nursing and the WHO. Feedback from graduates could also be obtained to establish their views about the adequacy of their preparatory program for meeting the SRH needs of the men and women encountered in their practice. They also suggest determining if SRH care provision within primary care adequately meets the needs of men and women patients/clients. Collaborating with certification and accreditation programs would ensure creating benchmarks for measuring SRH competencies in the primary care specialties. Offering residency programs should help to enhance the knowledge that primary care NPs acquire (Berg et al., 2014). Wisby and Capell (2005) also examined how sexual health competencies can be implemented and identified challenges relating to the academic and practice contexts as they recognized the increasing interest in interdisciplinary learning.

Conclusion

Challenges relating to the preparation of practitioners for efficient performance and high-quality care in SRH should be continually addressed. Moreover, the potential benefits of interdisciplinary learning and shared common core competencies should be more extensively examined. The perspectives explored in this chapter with exemplars may help practitioners to explore the ongoing developments within national and local levels of health care and service provision. An overview of the ongoing initiatives in the United States to establish a sexual health strategy should be complemented by further exploration of national and state-level endeavors. Practitioners may find it useful to compare developments within the systems of SRH care and service provision in the United States, United Kingdom, and other countries to learn from examples of best practice.

• • • REFERENCES

Agency for Healthcare Research and Quality (AHRQ). (2011). *2011 report to congress: National strategy for quality improvement in health care*. Rockville, MD: Author. Retrieved from http://www.ahrq.gov/workingforquality/reports/2011-annual-report.html

Allen, P. (2000). Accountability for clinical governance: developing collective responsibility for quality in primary care. *The BMJ, 321*(7261), 608–611.

American Nurses Association (2010). *Scope and standards of practice* (2nd ed.). Silver Spring, MD: Author.

Auerbach, D. I., Pearson, M. L., Taylor, D., Battistelli, M., Sussell, J., Hunter, L. E., . . . Schneider, E. C. (2012). *Nurse practitioners and sexual and reproductive health services: An analysis of supply and demand*. Santa Monica, CA: Rand Corporation. Retrieved from https://www.rand.org/pubs/technical_reports/TR1224.html

Berg, J. A., Woods, N. F., Kostas-Polston, E., & Johnson-Mallard, V. (2014). Breaking down silos: The future of sexual and reproductive health care—An opinion from the Women's Health Expert Panel of the American Academy of Nursing. *Journal of the American Association of Nurse Practitioners, 26*(1), 3–4.

Bickley, L. S., Szilagyi, P. G., Bates, B. (2013). *Bates' guide to physical examination and history-taking* (11th ed.) Philadelphia PA: Wolters Kluwer Health/Liillincott Williams & Wilkins

Biglan, A., & Ogden, T. (2008). The evolution of evidence based practices. *European Journal of Behavioral Analysis, 9*(1), 81–95.

Brook, G., Bacon, L., Evans, C., McLean, H., Roberts, C., Tipple, C., . . . Sullivan, A. K. (2013). UK national guide to consultations requiring sexual history taking. Clinical Effectiveness Group British Association of Sexual Health and HIV. *International Journal of STD and AIDS, 25*(6), 391–404.

Broughton, R., & Rathbone, B. (2001). *What makes a good clinical guideline?* Retrieved from http://www.evidence-based-medicine.co.uk

Bullivant, J., Burgess, R., Corbett-Nolan, A., & Godfrey, K. (2012). *Good governance handbook*. London, United Kingdom: Healthcare Quality Improvement Partnerships Ltd.

Burgess, R., & Moorhead, J. (2011). *New principles of best practice in clinical audit* (2nd rev. ed.). London, United Kingdom: Radcliff.

Centers for Disease Control and Prevention (CDC). (2016). *Sexual Health*. Retrieved from https://www.cdc.gov/sexualhealth/default.html

Centers for Medicare and Medicaid Services (CMS). *CMS quality strategy 2016*. Retrieved from https://www.cms.gov/Medicare/Quality-Initiatives-Patient-Assessment-Instruments/QualityInitiativesGenInfo/Downloads/CMS-Quality-Strategy.pdf

Corbett-Nolan, A., Bullivant, J., Godfrey, K., Marrett, H., Sutton, D., & Baltruks, D. (2015). *Good governance handbook*. London, United Kingdom: Healthcare Quality Improvement Partnerships Ltd.

Department of Health (DH). (1998). *A first class service: Quality in the New NHS*. London, United Kingdom: Author.

Department of Health (DH). (2013a). *A framework for sexual health improvement in England*. London, United Kingdom: Author.

Department of Health (DH). (2013b). *Sexual health: Clinical governance*. London, United Kingdom: Author.

Dickenson, P. S. (2010). Continuing nurses' education: enhancing professional development. *Journal of Continuing Education in Nursing, 41*(2), 100–101.

Douglas, J. M., Jr. (2011, August). *Advancing a public health approach to improve sexual health in the United States: A framework for national efforts*. Presented at the Implications of a Sexual Health Approach for HIV Prevention: National HIV Prevention Conference, Atlanta, GA.

Faculty of Sexual and Reproductive Healthcare of the Royal College of Obstetricians and Gynaecologists (FSRH). (2015). *Service standards on confidentiality*. Retrieved from https://www.fsrh.org/documents/clinical-standards-service-standards-confidentiality/clinical-standards-service-standards-confidentiality.pdf

Galbraith, S., & Department of Health. (1998). *A first class service: Quality in the new NHS*. London, United Kingdom: The Stationery Office.

General Medical Council (GMC). (2013). *Good medical practice*. Retrieved from http:www.gmc-uk.org/static/documents/content/GMP_.pdf

General Medical Council (GMC). (2013). *Good Medical Practice: Working with doctors Working with patients*. Manchester, United Kingdom: Author.

General Medical Council (GMC). (2016). *Promoting excellence: standards for medical education and training.* Retrieved from http://www.gmc-uk.org/education/standards.asp

Gerrish, K., & Lathlean, J. (Eds.). (2015). *The research process in nursing* (7th ed.). Oxford, United Kingdom: Wiley-Blackwell.

Harris, R.P., Helfand, M., Woolf, S.H., Lohr, K.N., Mulrow, C.D., Teutsch, S.M., . . . Third US Preventive Services Task Force. (2001). Current methods of the US Preventive Services Task Force: A review of the process. *American Journal of Preventive Medicine, 20*(Suppl. 3), 21–35.

Health Service Executive. (2014). *Quality and safety governance development: Sharing our learning.* Retrieved from http://www.hse.ie/eng/about/who/qualityandpatientsafety/Clinical_Governance/sharing/sharingourlearning.html

Hickey, J. (2005). Risk management, patient safety and a medical protection organization. In J. Hickey, K. Hayes, & M. Thomas (Eds.), *Clinical risk management in primary care.* Oxford, United Kingdom: Radcliffe.

Hughes, R. G. (2008). Tools and strategies for quality improvement and Patient safety. In R. G. Hughes (Ed.), *Patient safety and quality: An evidence-based handbook for nurses.* Rockville, MD: Agency for Healthcare Research and Quality.

Institute of Medicine. (2010). *Redesigning continuing education in the health professions.* Retrieved from http://www.nap.edu/openbook.php?record_id=12704.

Kligler, B., Brooks, A. J., Maizes, V., Goldblatt, E., Klatt, M., Koithan, M. S., . . . Lebensohn, P. (2015). Interprofessional competencies in integrative primary healthcare. *Global Advances in Health and Medicine, 4*(5), 33–39.

Krautscheid, L. (2014). Defining professional nursing accountability: A literature review. *Journal of Professional Nursing, 30*(1), 43–47.

Medicines & Healthcare products Regulatory Agency. (2017). *Patient group directions: who can use them.* Retrieved from http://www.gov.uk/government/publications/patient-group-directions-pgds/patient-group-directions-who-can-use-them

National Health Service (NHS). (2003). *Confidentiality: NHS Code of Practice.* Retrieved from http://www.gov.uk/government/publications/confidentiality-nhs-code-of-practice

National Health Service (NHS). (2010). *Confidentiality: Supplementary Guidance: Public Interest Disclosure.* Retrieved from http://www.gov.uk/government/publications/confidentiality-nhs-code-of-practice-supplementary-guidance-public-interest-disclosures

National Health Service (NHS). (2009). *Statement of accountability.* London, United Kingdom: Department of Health.

National Health Service (NHS). (2013). *Caldicott review: information governance in the health and care system.* Retrieved from https://www.gov.uk/government/publications/the-information-governance-review

National Quality Board (NQB). (2013). *Quality in the new health system—Maintaining and improving quality from April 2013.* NQB January 2013.

Newhouse, R. P., & Spring, B. (2010). Interdisciplinary evidence-based practice: Moving from silos to synergy. *Nursing Outlook* 2010, *58*(6), 309–317.

Ni, C., Hua, Y., Shao, P., Wallen, G. R., Xu, S., & Li, L. (2014). Continuing education among Chinese nurses: A general hospital-based study. *Nurse Education Today, 34*(4), 592–597.

Nursing and Midwifery Council. (2015). *The code for nurses and midwives.* Retrieved from http:www.nmc.org.uk/standards/code/

Nursing and Midwifery Council (NMC). (2015). *The NMC Code: Professional standards of practice and behaviour for nurses and midwives.* London, United Kingdom: Author.

O'Grady, L., & Jadad, A. (2010). Shifting from shared collaborative decision making: A change in thinking and doing. *Journal of Participatory Medicine, 2,* e13.

Royal College of General Practitioners and Committee of GP Education Directors. (2014). *Guidance for Deaneries/LETBs on Standards for GP Specialty Training.* Retrieved from http://www.rcgp.org.uk/-/media/Files/GP-training-and-exams/Information-for-deaneries-trainers-supervisors/Guidance-for-deaneries-on-standards-for-GP-training-Jan-2014.ashx?la=en

Royal College of Nursing (2007) (RCN). *Understanding benchmarking.* London, United Kingdom: Author.

Royal College of Nursing (RCN). (2008). *Principles to inform decision making: Quality, accountability, equality, partnership.* London, United Kingdom: Author.

Royal Pharmaceutical Society (RPS). (2014). *Professional standards for public health practice for pharmacy.* Retrieved from https://www.rpharms.com/Portals/0/RPS%20document%20library/Open%20access/Professional%20standards/Professional%20standards%20for%20public%20health/professional-standards-for-public-health.pdf

Satcher, D., Hook, E. W. III, & Coleman, E. (2015). Sexual health in America: Improving patient care and public health. *JAMA, 314*(8), 765–766.

Savage, J., & Moore, L. (2004). *Interpreting Accountability: An ethnographic study of practice nurses' accountability and multidisciplinary team decision-making in the context of clinical governance.* London, United Kingdom: Royal College of Nursing.

Scally, G., & Donaldson, L. J. (1998). Clinical governance and the drive for quality improvement in the new NHS in England. *BMJ, 317*(7150), 61–65.

Schweitzer, D. J., & Krassa, T. J. (2010). Deterrents to nurses' participation in continuing professional development: An integrative literature review. *Journal of Continuing Education in Nursing, 41*(10), 441–447.

Shojania, K. G., & Grimshaw, J. M. (2005). Evidence-based quality improvement: The state of the science. *Health Affairs, 24*(1), 138–150.

Skees, J. (2010). Continuing education a bridge to excellence in critical care nursing. *Critical Care Nursing Quarterly, 33*(2), 104–116.

Som, C.V. (2004). Clinical Governance: A fresh look at its definition. *Clinical Governance: An International Journal, 9*(2), 87–90.

Starey, N. (2001). *What is clinical governance? (Evidence-based medicine).* Kings Hill, United Kingdom: Hayward Group.

Swartzendruber, A., & Zenilman, J. M. (2010). A national strategy to improve sexual health. *JAMA, 304*(9), 1005–1006.

Titler, M. G. (2006). *Developing an evidence-based practice* (6th ed.). St Louis, MO: Mosby.

Titler, M. G., & Everett, L. Q. (2001). Translating research into practice: Considerations for critical care investigators. *Critical Care Nursing Clinics of North America, 13*(4), 587–604.

U.S. Department of Health and Human Services (HHS). (2014). National Quality Strategy – Better care, affordable care, healthy people/healthy communities: Working for quality, achieving better health and health care for all Americans. Retrieved from http://www.ahrq.gov/workingforquality/priorities-in-action/index.html

Wisby, D., & Capell, J. (2005). Implementing change in sexual health care. *Nursing Management, 12*(8), 14–16.

World Health Organization (WHO). (2011). *Sexual and reproductive health core competencies in primary care.* Geneva, Switzerland: Author.

World Health Organization. (2011). *Patient Safety Curriculum Guide: Multi-professional edition.* WHO Patient Safety. Geneva, Switzerland. Author.

• • • SUGGESTED FURTHER READING

Baker, G. R. (2011). *The roles of leaders in high performing healthcare systems.* Retrieved from http://www.kingsfund.org.uk/publications/articles/leadership_papers/the_roles_of_leaders.html.

Currie, L., Morrell, C., & Scrivener, R. (2003). *Clinical governance: An RCN resource guide.* London, United Kingdom: Royal College of Nursing.

Department of Health (DH). (2005). *Research governance framework for health and social care* (2nd ed.). London, United Kingdom: Author.

Department of Health (DH). (2010). *Research governance framework: Resource pack for social care* (2nd ed.). London, United Kingdom: Author.

Department of Health (DH). (2011). *Research governance arrangements for research ethics committees: A harmonised edition.* London, United Kingdom: Author.

Department of Health (DH). (2013). *Information: To Share or not to Share – Government Response to the Caldicott Review.* Retrieved from http://www.igt.hscic.gov.uk/KnowledgeBaseNew/Government%20Response%20to%20Report%20of%20the%20Caldicott2%20Review.pdf

Entwistle, F. (2013). Framework for improving sexual health outcomes. *Nursing Times, 109*(22), 22.

Ford, J. V., Barnes, R., Rompalo, A., & Hook, E. W. III. (2013). Sexual health training and education in the U.S. *Public Health Report, 128*(1), 98–101.

Gallagher, L. (2006). Continuing education in nursing: A concept analysis. *Nurse Education Today, 27*(5), 466–475.

Gaw, A., & O'Neill, F. H. (2014). Ethics in research: Practice and respect. *Nursing Times, 110*(20), 12–13.

Healthcare Quality Improvement Partnership (HQIP). (2011). *Criteria and indicators of best practice in clinical audit.* London: Healthcare Quality Improvement Partnership. pp. 4–13. Retrieved from http://www.healthcareimprovementscotland.org.

Healthcare Quality Improvement Partnership (HQIP) (2016). Best Practice in Clinical Audit. Retrieved from https://www.rcr.ac.uk/sites/default/files/hqip_guide_for_best_practice_in_clinical_audit.pdf

Healthcare Improvement Scotland (2011). *Healthcare quality standard: Assuring person centred, safe and effective care: Clinical governance and risk management.* Retrieved from http://www.healthcareimprovementscotland.org/previous_resources/standards/healthcare_quality_standard.aspx.

Irving, A. (2014). Policies and procedures for healthcare organizations: A risk management perspective. *Patient Safety and Quality Healthcare.* Retrieved from https://www.psqh.com/analysis/policies-and-procedures-for-healthcare-organizations-a-risk-management-perspective/

General Medical Council (GMC). (2012). *Continuing professional development: Guidance for all doctors.* Manchester, United Kingdom: Author.

General Medical Council (GMC). (2016). *Promoting excellence: Guidance for medical education and training.* London, United Kingdom: Author.

Health and Social Care Information Centre. (2013). *A guide to confidentiality in health and social care: Treating confidential information with respect.* Retrieved from http://content.digital.nhs.uk/media/12822/Guide-to-confidentiality-in-health-and-social-care/pdf/HSCIC-guide-to-confidentiality.pdf

Healthcare Quality Improvement Partnership (HQIP). (2012). *Criteria and indicators of best practice in clinical audit.* Retrieved from https://www.hqip.org.uk/resources/best-practice-in-clinical-audit-hqip-guide/

Kapp, M. B. (2006) Ethical and legal issues in research involving human subjects: Do you want a piece of me? *Journal of Clinical Pathology, 59*(4): 335–339.

Jacobs, K. (2008). Accountability and clinical governance in nursing: a critical overview of the topic. In S. Tilley & R. Watson (Eds.), *Accountability in nursing and midwifery* (2nd ed.). Oxford, United Kingdom: Blackwell Science.

Monitor: Independent Regulator of NHS Foundation Trusts. (2011). *Compliance framework 2011/12.* Retrieved from http://www.gov.uk/government/organisations/monitor

National Institute for Clinical Excellence. (2002). *Principles for best practice in clinical audit.* Oxon, United Kingdom: Radcliffe Medical Press.

Nieva, V., Murphy, R., Ridley, N., Donaldson, N., Combes, J., Mitchell, P., . . . Carpenter, D. (2005). From science to service: a framework for the transfer of patient safety research into practice. In K. Henriksen, J. B. Battles, D. I. Lewin, & E. Marks (Eds.), *Advances in patient safety: From research to implementation* (pp. 441–453). Rockville, MD: Agency for Healthcare Research and Quality.

Nursing and Midwifery Council (NMC). (2017). Revalidation. Retrieved from http://revalidation.nmc.org.uk

Rogers, E. M. (2003). *Diffusion of innovations* (5th ed.). New York, NY: The Free Press.

Royal College of Nursing (RCN). (2009a). *Research ethics: RCN guidance for nurses.* London, United Kingdom: Author.

Royal College of Nursing (RCN). (2009b). *Sexual health competencies: An integrated career and competence framework for sexual and reproductive health nursing across the UK.* London, United Kingdom: Author.

Royal College of Nursing (2011). (RCN). *Informed consent in health and social care research: RCN guidance for nurses* (2nd ed.). London, United Kingdom: Author.

Santelli, J. S., & Schalet, A. T. (2009). *A new vision for adolescent sexual and reproductive health.* Retrieved from https://ecommons.cornell.edu/handle/1813/19323

Titler, M. G., Kleiber, C., Steelman, V. J., Rakel, B. A., Budreau, G., Everett, L. Q., . . . Goode, C. J. (2001). The Iowa model of evidence-based practice to promote quality care. *Critical Care Nursing Clinics of North America, 13*(4), 497–509.

Titler, M. G. (2008). The Evidence for evidence-based implementation. In R. G. Hughes (Ed.), *Patient Safety and Quality: An evidence-based handbook for nurses. AHRQ Publication* No. 08-0043; Section II: Chapter 7: pp.1–49. Rockville, MD: U.S. Government Printing Office.

The Royal College of General Practitioners. (2013). *The Royal College of General Practitioners' guide to the revalidation of general practitioners* (Version 8.0). London: RCGP Author. Retrieved from.

World Health Organization (WHO). (2006). *Quality of care: A process for making strategic choices in health systems.* Geneva, Switzerland: Author.

World Health Organization (WHO). (2007). *Introducing WHO's sexual and reproductive health guidelines and tools into national programs. Principles and processes of adaptation and implementation WHO 2007.* Geneva, Switzerland: Author.

World Health Organization (WHO). (2009). *Sexual and reproductive health strategic plan 2010–2015 and proposed programme budget for 2010–2011.* Geneva, Switzerland: Author.

CHAPTER

2

Overview of the Key Concepts and Guiding Principles of EBP as Applied in Sexual and Reproductive Health Care

THEODORA D. KWANSA

Introduction

The processes outlined in this chapter may be useful for selecting appropriate studies from the abundance of published research in clinical practice. As necessary, the application of specific processes applied in the implementation of evidence-based practice (EBP) is demonstrated with examples. Readers should note that the components of the examples are not by any means exhaustive and should be read with a critical mind.

For nearly 2 decades, the influence of evidence-based practice in healthcare has created widespread familiarity with the concept. Nevertheless, the extent of knowledge, understanding, and insight of the principles of EBP varies among professional practitioners. Misconceptions, inadequate

interpretations, and ambiguous insight about the essential components, the rationale, and related principles hamper the standard and quality of practice. This chapter sets out to analyze and translate EBP into simple, more pragmatic terms to enable practitioners to make more competent application.

Brief Overview of the Original Conception

The term *evidence-based practice* and its variations emerged from the original conception of evidence-based medicine (EBM). In this chapter, the term *EBP* is predominantly used. Sackett, Rosenberg, Gray, Haynes, and Richardson's (1996) explanation of evidence-based medicine is still worth considering. They suggested that the concept involves "the conscientious, explicit, and judicious use of current best evidence in making decisions about the care of individual patients." (p.71) Further elaboration on this definition provides indications of what constitutes significant evidence.

The authors pointed out the necessity to integrate the professional expertise of the practitioner with the best findings from current research in the field. However, while intuitive knowledge acquired from several years of experience in a specific clinical specialty may arguably constitute evidence, this is questionable. Years of experience alone as evidence may lack the desired substantiation of seminal findings from extensive research. Other interpretations of EBP emphasize putting an end to impulsive and unreasoned decision-making based on unfounded intuition or on the mainstream, unquestioned practices. The principle of using sound, proven, and supported evidence ensures that care provision remains consistently competent, safe, and beneficial, while also being cost effective.

Patient values are related to the individual's anxieties and desires, personal expectations, and preferences (Sackett et al., 1996; Sackett, Straus, Richardson, Rosenberg, & Haynes, 2000). The principles of EBP emphasize the importance of recognizing these and integrating patient concerns into care and treatment decisions and actions to achieve better patient outcomes and satisfaction.

Significant Elements

Despite slight differences in the interpretation of EBP, key elements are inherent (DiCenso, Cullum, Ciliska, & Guyatt, 2005; Levine, 2004; McKibbon & Marks, 1998; Polit & Beck, 2011; Sackett et al., 1996; Sackett et al., 2000).

- Ongoing scientific research is essential and should form a significant standard component of EBP. This means that the claim to evidence-based practice should be upheld to be valid through research guided by clear and precise criteria.
- The specific health problem identified should be methodically examined in separate fragments by asking explicit relatable clinical questions.
- Extensive literature search and critical reading are crucial to gain adequate insight and understanding of the problem and the current treatment and care interventions.

- Detailed systematic reviews and evaluation of relevant published studies is required to establish the best results achieved with specific treatment regimens, therapeutic techniques, and procedures in care provision. The appraisal should be guided by a valid set of criteria to identify the strongest empirical evidence. It is important to use approved guidelines for correctly translating and implementing the evidence from appropriate literature.
- The identified evidence should be specifically relevant for making accurate decisions about the choice of treatment to resolve the problems and needs of the patient.
- EBP requires conscientious critical examination of the findings from research to guide decisions about the care of an identified client group with a specific clinical problem.
- Practitioners should responsibly employ the best available evidence in making practical and carefully reasoned clinical decisions in their care provision.
- Implementation of treatment regimens, care procedures, and interventions should be supported by convincing evidence and aimed at producing the most favorable outcomes.
- Professional expertise should be supported by attributes that demonstrate high standards of performance in practice toward professional excellence.

Figure 2-1 represents an illustrative summary of the key elements of EBP.

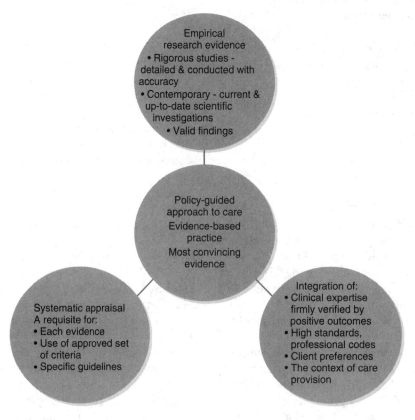

Figure 2-1 Snapshot of EBP Key Elements

Ethical Arguments About EBP

It is ethically justified that healthcare service users should receive the most effective high-quality care and treatment available as confirmed by extensive research. For example, when cheaper condoms are considered the only options to offer groups of sexually active adolescents and commercial sex workers for the simple reason of rationing the cost implications, it would be considered to be ethically unjustified. Nevertheless, it could also be argued that the availability of more sophisticated and more expensive products for those who can afford them increases the range of options to allow more freedom of choice with the additional advantages of scientific technological advancements and appropriately qualified staff. It is argued that clinicians and other healthcare professional practitioners who disregard the principles of EBP/EBM risk making the wrong therapeutic decisions and giving incorrect advice to patients. Similar risks may occur when individuals' moral/ethical values, beliefs, choices, and personal involvement in decisions about their own care and treatment are disregarded (Ciliska, DiCenso, Melnyk, & Stetler, 2005; Guyatt, Cook, & Haynes, 2004; Rees, 2010; Rycroft-Malone & Bucknall, 2011). Apart from accurate interpretation and efficient application of research findings, practitioners are expected to substantiate the explanations that they provide to patients. This ensures that information about the condition, treatments, and procedures will be factual, trustworthy, and unambiguous. That assurance gives individuals the confidence to make informed decisions about the care, treatment, and support that they need.

Ascertaining Compelling Evidence

The concern for many practitioners is how to determine what exactly constitutes convincing and valid evidence. EBP/EBM is perceived as embracing a reasoned and unbiased means of establishing excellence and safe standards in clinical practice. It therefore demands professional competency, appropriate motivation, adequate professional knowledge, insight, and understanding to apply it efficiently. Moreover, EBP and EBM emphasize diligence, accountability, and conscientiousness in professional practice (Barker, 2010). Correspondingly, EBH represents the broader context of evidence-based healthcare. Jordan, Lockwood, Aromataris, and Munn (2016) define EBH as "clinical decision-making that considers the feasibility, appropriateness, meaningfulness and effectiveness of healthcare practices. The feasibility, appropriateness, meaningfulness and effectiveness of healthcare practices may be informed by the best available evidence, the context in which the care is delivered, the individual patient, and the professional judgment and expertise of the health professional." These authors explain Feasibility in terms of the practicability and viability of an intervention in a particular context; Appropriateness in terms of how fitting the particular

intervention is for the given context; Meaningfulness in terms of the extent to which the intervention produces a favorable experience for an individual or patient group; and Effectiveness in terms of achievement of the expected outcomes. These core elements represent the FAME scale that underpins different healthcare research endeavors as well as providing a structure and framework that guides and directs different types of reviews.

The Rationale for Prioritizing Research Evidence

The role of research in EBP is to identify the best available interventions that have been proven through systematic reviews of randomized controlled trials (RCTs) to achieve best possible outcomes. Apart from the clinical condition, account should also be taken of the social circumstances, values, reactions, and preferences of the patients. While these are not exactly stated in any of the categories, at higher levels they do, nonetheless, constitute important evidence. In various modified rating systems, qualitative studies are classified as levels V and VI (Guyatt & Rennie, 2002; Harris et al., 2001; Melnyk & Fineout-Overholt 2005, 2014). This means that relevance and applicability must be central in translating research evidence into care and treatment interventions.

However, Melnyk and Fineout-Overholt (2005, 2014) argue that science and art can and should merge in EBP. The suggestion is that this process helps to accomplish highly successful patient outcomes. Combining the evidence from scientific research together with the evidence from clinical expertise of professional practitioners is crucial to achieve high-quality care, satisfaction, and better outcomes.

Quantitative studies involving concrete and objective measurements of identified factors—the positivist paradigm—tend to be upheld as more scientific with trustworthy evidence. The investigation involves RCTs, whereby the effectiveness and outcomes of a particular treatment or intervention is scientifically tested and precisely measured with comparisons among sample groups from the patient population. Such studies are placed at the top end of the rating of research studies. However, as Saks and Allsop (2007) point out, the quantitative research design of RCT may not be applicable to certain problems/phenomena in the fields of health care and social sciences. Rubin and Rubin's (2005) argument that quantitative research design is neither practical nor applicable for exploring people's lived experiences and the meanings they attach to these supports that observation.

The lower end evidence includes qualitative descriptive studies, opinions about clinical expertise, case reports, and committee reports. Detailed appraisal of this evidence allows one to determine what is best to guide decisions about a specific clinical intervention of particular interest.

Classifications and Levels of Evidence

Various classifications and levels of what constitutes compelling and persuasive evidence have been devised and ranked. While some classifications focus on the type of research,

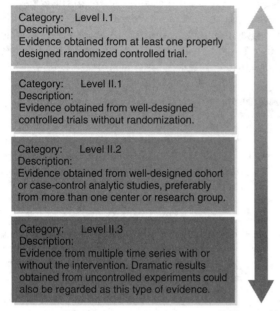

Figure 2-2 Hierarchies of Research Evidence

others emphasize the quality of the study or its relevance or compatibility to the patient situation. The following are examples of rating systems showing the hierarchy or grading of research evidence.

Figure 2-2, derived from Harris et al. (2001), represents a hierarchical rating of evidence. The levels of evidence show the higher grades of scientific studies at the top. The less scientific descriptive studies based on professional expertise are placed at the bottom. However, detailed examination of each evidence material on its own merit is important.

Exemplar of Practical Application of the Rating System

The following example presents quality grading and rating of a survey study that explored how prevalent is simultaneous use of dual methods for preventing unintended/unwanted pregnancy and protection against STIs/HIV infection among female sex workers (Yam et al., 2013). Readers are encouraged to read the research paper then examine the example of rating on the study with a critical mind. It must be noted that the despite the use of specific tools for assessing research studies, the extent of detail may depend on the practitioners' professional and research knowledge and expertise, and the amount of information provided in the research report.

Study Assessed

- Yam, E.A., Mnisi, Z., Mabuza, X., Kennedy, C., Kerrigan, D., Tsui, A., Baral, S. (2013). Use of dual protection among female sex workers in Swaziland. *International Perspectives on Sexual and Reproductive Health, 39*(2), 69–78.

The exemplar of quality assessment applied to Yam et al.'s (2013) study draws on the Research Connections Quantitative Research Assessment Tool, which can be accessed at:

The Research Connections Research Assessment Tools http://www.researchconnections.org/content/childcare /understand/research-quality.html#resources

The rating scores of {1}, {0}, {−1}, and {NA} and the overall grading of Good, Fair, and Poor have been applied.

Study domain: Mixed domain survey; therefore, this could be graded as level 3.

Quality rating:

Study population identified. However, it represents a rather limited, selective subgroup of the population of interest: female sex workers in Swaziland. {0}

Non-random sampling. "Snowballing" pattern of recruitment of study participants. {0}

Eligibility criteria outlined though somewhat lacking in precision to allow for accurate and consistent inclusion and exclusion. The key factors included age, occupation as sex worker over the previous 12 months, and education/literacy status.

Sample size. The sample consists of 329 participants. Although the sample characteristics specify the proportion of participants by age, education/literacy, marital status, number of children, financial income, and HIV status, comparison to other similar studies is unclear. {−1}

Intervention used. The intervention involved use of double methods for dual-protection against STIs and unwanted pregnancy described as dual-method use.

The dual methods were condoms plus other non-barrier modern contraceptive methods—oral contraceptive pill, injectable or intrauterine contraceptive device (IUD) implant, or sterilization.

The data collection by use of survey questionnaire interviews involved multiple interviewers and apparent biases that emerged were reported as limitations of the study. Therefore, design-specific risk of bias assessment was also explained.

Measurements. Dependent and independent variables are explained in reasonable detail, and these match adequately to the variables in the tables. {1}

Patterns of condom use were categorized in relation to new clients, regular clients, and non-commercial partners, or as always used with each type of sexual partner.

Outcome categories were quantified as: 0 = inconsistent condom use; 1 = consistent use of condoms only; 2 = use of non-barrier methods alone or with inconsistent condom use; 3 = use of dual-methods (i.e. consistent condom use and reported current use of non-barrier methods).

Statistical analysis. Adequate rigor seemed to have been applied, the statistical techniques employed for data analysis were rationalized, and the caveats were reasonably well conveyed. {1}

Discussion and conclusion. A reasonable attempt is made to demonstrate direct links to the results. However, certain weaknesses are evident. Internal validity seems rather questionable and the researchers' claims based on the findings are not compelling enough. The findings from the study do not convincingly establish a significantly strong and definite link between use of dual methods by female sex workers and protection against STI/HIV transmission and unintended pregnancy. Inconsistencies, weak precision, and unconvincing objectivity were reported in the data collection and lack of absolute truthfulness and believability of the responses provided by some of the study participants also emerged.

Consequently, along a spectrum of Good, Fair, and Poor, the overall quality of the study could be rated as Fair.

The additional references provided below should provide readers with the tools to carry out their own detailed critical assessments for comparisons.

- McMaster University Effective Public Health Practice Project (EPHPP). (2010). Quality assessment tool for quantitative studies. Retrieved from http://www.ephpp.ca/PDF/Quality%20Assessment%20Tool_2010_2.pdf

An accompanying dictionary provides explanations of the key items in the tool to guide the rating and scoring process: http://www.ephpp.ca/PDF/QADictionary_dec2009.pdf.

The recommended qualitative research assessment tool together with accompanying guidelines can be accessed at:

- McMaster University, Critical Review Form—Qualitative Studies (Version 2.0): http://www.peelregion.ca/health/library/eidmtools/qualreview_version2_0.pdf
- Guidelines for Critical Review Form: Qualitative Studies (Version 2.0): http://www.peelregion.ca/health/library/eidmtools/qualguidelines_version2_0.pdf

While these are applicable to critical reviews of individual studies, an exemplar of systematic review assessment is also provided later. In the following reflective consideration, a simplified application of the processes involved in implementing EBP is demonstrated using questions to guide the thoughts and interactions among practitioners and students.

Reflective Considerations

Consider the current context of your clinical practice.

Which patient/client or group is the central concern and the incentive for the implementation of EBP?

- Client group of concern: Commercial sex workers in the community; varied ethnic and racial origins; same sex and heterosexual inclinations; varied education backgrounds; varied social and economic circumstances; migrant social status; internet population.

What conditions and related problems and needs do they present?

- Consider the high-risk factors. High incidence of STIs both newly diagnosed as well as long-established and untreated STIs; persistently high transmission rate; relatively higher incidence of

HIV infection. *Additional common, related problems presented*: Risky sexual practices; alcohol, drug, and substance abuse; stigmatization; physical, sexual abuse; poverty; homelessness; and mental health problems such as depression. *Potential challenges encountered in care and service provision*: Possible resource issues; undependable attitudes to uptake of services including STI and HIV testing for early diagnosis and treatment; internet population; the challenges of partner notification and partner management services; inconsistent and erratic compliance to prescribed medication; indifference to health education and advice such as abstention from sexual intercourse during the course of treatment; individuals' recognition of the importance and personal responsibility for consistent and correct use of condoms.

(continues)

Reflective Considerations *(continued)*

What particular treatment intervention, procedure or routine aspects of care raise concerns for the team within the area of practice?

- Consider equity and accessibility of the care and service provision for all members of the community irrespective of social status and financial circumstances; accessible routine STI/HIV testing; robust community pharmacy support services; effective, timely, appropriately targeted health promotion campaigns; adequate supply and accessible and correct use of condoms.

What is/are the shared view(s) about the anticipated outcome(s) for the patients/clients?

- Reduction in the prevalence of STIs and the transmission among the identified high-risk group with appropriate prioritization of support services for young and vulnerable female sex workers and MSM. Integration of services multidisciplinary team collaboration with effective referral system with counseling and psychological support toward reduction in mental health problems associated with abuse, and coercion in sexual relationships.

How practical, realistic, and achievable are these in terms of accessibility of resources and the staffing profile?

- Consider the organizational set up; structure and staffing levels; education and training opportunities that are offered; scope of knowledge and range of expertise; ongoing support and team motivation. Consider joint initiatives; liaison with relevant stakeholders and other support groups including voluntary and non-voluntary organizations working in the area that have already established trust with the client group; police collaboration to work with this client group within the population; involvement of the sex workers and/or their representatives in determining appropriate targeted programs and best ways for the implementation.

What is the team's shared perception of the overall long-term benefits of implementation of EBP in the wider context?

- Consider continuous improvement of sexual and reproductive health among the general population; patient/client empowerment through evidence-based robust sexual health promotion/education

and safer sex practices; provision of substantiated explanations to foster patient/client confidence in the standard and quality of the care and services; partnership and cooperation with the sexual health professional practitioners in all aspects of the care and service provision; informed decision-making and choices; personal involvement of the patient/client in the decisions about own care and treatment interventions.

Readers are encouraged to consider each point carefully within the current context of practice and make appropriate adjustments to the suggestions according to the actuality.

Related Studies for Further Reading

- Balfour, R., & Allen, J. (2014). *A review of the literature on sex workers and social exclusion.* London, U.K.: UCL Institute of Health Equity.
- Erickson, M., Goldenberg, S. M., Ajok, M., Muldoon, K. A., Muzaaya, G., & Shannon, K. (2015). Structural determinants of dual contraceptive use among female sex workers. *International Journal of Gynecology & Obstetrics, 131*(1), 91–95.
- Moore, L., Chersich, M. F., Steen, R., Reza-Paul, S., Dhana, A., Vuylsteke, B., . . . Scorgie, F. (2014). Community empowerment and involvement of female sex workers in targeted sexual and reproductive health interventions in Africa: A systematic review. *Global Health, 10,* 47.
- Ota, E., Wariki, W. M., Mori, R., Hori, N., & Shibuya, K. (2011). Behavioural Interventions to reduce the transmission of HIV infection among sex workers and their clients in high-income countries. *Cochrane Database of Systematic Reviews,* (12), CD006045.
- Steen, R., Wheeler, T., Gorgens, M., Mziray, E., & Dallabetta, G. (2015). Feasible, efficient, and necessary without exception – Working with sex workers interrupts HIV/STI transmission and brings treatment to many in need. *PLoS One, 10*(10), e0121145.
- Wariki, V. M., Ota, E., Mori, R., Koyanagi, A., Hori, N., Shibuya, K. (2012). Behavioural interventions to reduce the transmission of HIV infection among sex workers and their clients in low- and middle- income countries. *Cochrane Database of Systematic Reviews,* (2), CD005272.

In the following section, a simplified examination of a systematic review is presented.

Perusal Activities: Background Reading

Reading relevant research articles, reports, policy documents, and guidelines about a specific issue of clinical interest encourages colleagues to discuss the background material among themselves, especially when a list of the individual readings has been compiled and circulated. Every effort should be made to ensure that the search is as extensive as possible. It is particularly useful to explore a wide range of databases, including national, international, and subject-related educational bibliographic databases and resources.

Importance of Evaluating Evidence to Substantiate Clinical Decision-Making in EBP

An essential requirement for implementing EBP is critical evaluation of the evidence identified for supporting clinical decisions.

Society demands assurance that care and services undergo continuous improvements. Research is prolific in healthcare, but increasingly complex methodologies and designs present additional challenges. Practitioners have the obligation to thoroughly examine and determine the relevance of research findings for clinical application. Distinguishing seminal studies from low-quality studies with misleading findings and claims requires good training and skill development to acquire the appropriate level of efficiency.

Readers are encouraged to access the published paper for detailed information.

- Lopez, L. M., Chen, M., Steiner, M. J., Galo, M. F. (2014). Behavioural interventions for improving condom use dual-method contraceptive use. *Cochrane Database of Systematic Reviews, 1,* CD010915.

Background/Rationale for conducting the review together with a concise description of the clinical issue investigated: protection against HIV/STIs and prevention of unintended pregnancy. The concept of dual-method use is explained in terms of condom use combined with another modern contraceptive method.

The Intervention is clearly explained.

The Methods of defining the criteria in terms of the types of studies, the participants, types of interventions, and outcome measures are comprehensible and provide adequate detail.

The Search Strategies employed for identifying relevant studies are varied, involving electronic searches and other resources, thus indicating adequately extensive literature search.

Study Selection by Inclusion and Exclusion suggests that appropriately meticulous processes were employed, though full details are not presented in the report.

Data Extraction and Management involved two authors for data entry and verifying the accuracy of the study characteristics, risk of bias/quality assessment, and the outcome data.

Risk of Bias Assessment was employed for the included studies.

Assessment of the Quality of Intervention involved application of Borrelli's (2011) framework: "The assessment, monitoring and enhancement of treatment fidelity in public health clinical trials." This framework was used for assessing the design, training of providers, delivery of the intervention, receipt of treatment, and enactment of treatment skills. The reviewers stated their criteria of interest for this review as follows:

- The study design has a curriculum/treatment manual.
- Training: Provider credentials were stipulated; standardized or identical training was used for the intervention.
- Delivery: Adherence to the intervention protocol was assessed.
- Receipt: Participants' understanding and skills for the intervention was assessed.
- Borelli, B. (2011). The assessment, monitoring and enhancement of treatment fidelity in public health clinical trials. *Journal of Public Health Dentistry, 71*(s1), S52–S63.

Critical Evaluation of the Methodological Quality the reviewers applied the principles described by Schulz and Grimes (2002) Higgins and Green (2011), and Campbell, Piaggo, Elbourne, and Altman (2012) for evaluating the quality of the studies involving RCTs.

- Schulz, K. F., & Grimes, D. A. (2002). Allocation concealment in randomised trials: defending against deciphering. *Lancet, 359*(9306), 614–618.
- Higgins, J. P. T., & Green, S. (Eds.). (2011). *Cochrane handbook for systematic reviews of interventions* (Ver. 5.1.0). Retrieved from http://training.cochrane.org/handbook
- Campbell, M. K., Piaggo, G., Elbourne, D. R., & Altman, D. G. (2012), CONSORT 2010 statement: Extension to cluster randomized trials. *British Medical Journal, 345,* e5661.

The recommended tool for evaluating non-randomized controlled trials was also employed.

- Wells, G. A., Shea, B., O'Connell, D., Paterson, J., Welch, V., Losos, M., & Tugwell, P. (2008). *The Newcastle-Ottawa Scale (NOS) for assessing the quality of non-randomised studies in meta-analyses*. Retrieved from http://www.ohri.ca/programs/clinical_epidemiology/oxford.asp

The reviewers reported adequately meticulous application of these for the quality evaluation of studies. Measurement of treatment effect is carefully examined and comparisons reported. In regard to missing data, the reviewers appropriately made direct contact with the relevant researchers.

Data Analysis and synthesis were explained, though not in full detail.

Critical Appraisal of Research for Possible Utilization in Clinical Practice

Burls's (2009) view of critical appraisal suggests careful systematic examination of research studies to assess the significance, integrity, potential benefits, and applicability within a specific professional situation. This forms an essential requirement for evidence-based practice. Indeed, appraisal is a skill that should be definitely acquired by all researchers, reviewers, and evidence-based practitioners.

Principles of Critical Appraisal

To competently carry out critical appraisal of research papers and make appropriate application, it is important to gain a clear insight and understanding of its principles. The main principles are examined below.

- The appraisal should be guided by clearly formulated question(s) that focus on an identified problem/phenomenon or topic. In particular, the topic should represent a significant clinical concern within the area of healthcare provision.
- The appraisal should begin with an extensive search of the literature to identify and retrieve research reports relating to the problem/phenomenon of concern.
- The selection of the papers should be methodical and unbiased to avoid the likelihood of omitting studies with significant findings relevant to the problem.
- The appraiser(s) should methodically examine each of the reports to assess the credibility. Moreover, the reliability, soundness, and accuracy of the findings from the individual studies should be examined.
- The process of synthesizing and consolidating the data and findings from the studies allows for confirming and strengthening the researchers' claims about specific evidence relating to the problem.

The key components of research appraisal are demonstrated in the examples presented here. The intent is to present a concise and simplistic application of critical appraisal. Additional benefit might be gained from exploring other published qualitative research studies conducted within the SRH organization, state, or country in which you currently practice.

Exemplar Qualitative Research Evaluation

- Llewellyn, C., Pollard, A., Miners, A., Richardson, D., Fisher, M., Cairns, J., & Smith, H. (2012). Understanding patient choices for attending sexually transmitted infection testing services: A qualitative study. *Sexually Transmitted Infections, 88*(7), 504–509.

Suggested Questions for Examining Qualitative Research Reports: Example of Application

Examination of the Title of the Study

- Does the study title convey clarity and the essence of the problem/phenomenon investigated or does it lack focus?
- How clear and concise or wordy and ambiguous is the title?
- How much information is conveyed in the formulation of the title?
- In what way does the title convey significance and relevance of the problem to the subject area and clinical specialism?
- What additional useful information does the title provide regarding the target population, the context of the problem, the design of the study?

Title of the Study   The title clear, concise and adequately informative indicating the issue of clinical concern as decisions for attending STI testing services although no particular patient group is specified.

Examination of the Abstract

- How informative and clear is the abstract?
- How clear is the statement of background, main objectives/purpose in indicating what the researcher(s) aimed to learn from the investigation?
- To what extent does the abstract inform about the design, methodology, methods and statistical techniques, the main results, conclusions, and recommendations? In other words, how adequate is the abstract as a useful frame of reference?
- In what way does the abstract inform about internal and external validity of the findings?

Abstract   The abstract is adequately informative and provides concise information about the main objectives/purpose of the research, the methods, results/key findings, and the conclusion.

Questions for Examining the Introduction

- How efficiently has the problem been explained regarding the encumbrance or burden imposed by the problem?

- In accordance with the requirements of the research process, how would you describe the researcher(s') explanation of the significance and implications of the problem/phenomenon within the context of clinical care provision?

- How convincingly has the problem been put in context regarding the environment within which it occurred?

- How pragmatic and achievable were the statement of purpose, aims, and/or objectives (if stated)?

- Do these indicate shortfall(s) or gaps in care provision or discrepancies in procedure guidelines or policy?

- How clear and convincing was the researcher(s') prediction of what they anticipated to achieve from the investigation?

- What contributions did the researcher(s) claim that the findings from the study might make to given aspects of professional practice?

- Did the researcher(s) identify specific shortfalls or gaps in previous studies that needed to be further investigated? Did they indicate their intention to address those in the current study?

- How effectively and realistically did they achieve that intention?

- How candidly did the researcher(s) report on the outcome of that?

- What additional contribution did they claim to have made to the existing professional knowledge?

Introduction The introduction adequately orients the reader to the nature and extent of the clinical problem. A reasonably convincing argument is presented emphasizing the consequences of the impact of the problem—increased sexual health screening, the rise in new diagnoses, and increased demand for access for testing. The need for confidential diagnostic and treatment services also adds to the burden imposed by the problem in terms of provision of the relevant services to meet the patients' needs. The gaps in previous studies are highlighted in terms of lack of qualitative data on patient preferences for STI testing services. Although the findings from this study are considered useful for informing the design of Discrete Choice Experiment, the researchers recognized the potential challenges associated with such future research projects.

- Ryan, M. Watson, V., & Gerard, K. (2008). Practical issues in conducting a discrete choice experiment. In M. Ryan, K. Gerard, & M. Amaya-Amaya (Eds.), *Using discrete choice experiments to value health and health care* (pp. 73–88). Dordrecht, Germany: Springer.

Questions for Examining the Literature Review

- What type of studies did the researcher(s) review?

- How clearly defined is the problem/phenomenon in a theoretical or conceptual framework?

- What evidence in the review indicates that the selection of the studies was carefully planned and guided by well-developed and formally approved set of criteria?

- What is your impression of the scope of the literature search, the amount of studies, and other pertinent materials reviewed?

- How convincingly did the researcher(s) rationalize the relevance of the studies they included in the review?

- How did the researchers explain the significance and usefulness of the literature review for professional practice?

- How convincingly did the researcher(s) argue their perspective on the need to refocus, or ask additional questions for further exploration of the topic to rectify discrepancies in previous studies?

- What is your overall impression of the quality of the review? In what ways did the researcher(s) demonstrate analytical and evaluative skills in their examination of emerging inconsistencies in the methodologies?

The Literature Review In this research report the introduction incorporates the literature review. Therefore, some of the elements in this set of questions may have been addressed in that section. The selection and examination of previous related studies the quality and underpinning conceptual frameworks that also depend on the type of qualitative approach employed probably requires more detail and clarity.

Questions for Examining the Methodology

- How understandable and convincing is the explanation that the research design, decisions, and actions taken in the methodology entirely address problem/phenomenon investigated?

- How applicable were these for exploring the questions to seek answers and solutions to the research problem?

- What clarification did the researchers provide about the characteristics of the target population from which the study participants were selected?

- How convincing are the rationales for selection of the study participants and the total numbers involved in the pilot and the main studies?

- To what extent were the criteria for inclusion and exclusion and the measures to ensure correctness in the selection process strictly applied?

- How plausible is the rationale regarding the suitability of the participants for the type of study and the information gathered about the problem/phenomenon?

- How well-reasoned is the researchers' explanation of the connections between the setting, problem/phenomenon, the characteristics of participants, and the type of information gathered?

- How clear is the researcher's explanation and reasoning regarding the development and testing of the data collection instrument?

- How thorough were the techniques used to test the validity and reliability of the data collection instrument(s)?

- How consistently thorough and accurate was the process of data collection as reported?

- How candidly did the researcher(s) explain complications, if any, that emerged during the development and testing of the data collection instrument(s) and how they dealt with those?

The Methodology A concise argument is presented to justify the choice of study design and the rationale for using focus groups which is pertinent to the investigation conducted. The number of groupings, age range, and relevant social and demographic characteristics are appropriately described and the time frames for the interviews also appropriately explained. The recruitment of participants was reported as eight distinct focus groups identified by quota sampling determined by age, sexual disposition, and gender. A ninth group of overseas students of diverse demographic profiles, plus a tenth group of HIV-positive persons of mixed age range indicates some degree of inconsistency in the recruitment of participants for the focus groups. A table of composition of each focus group provides additional clarification. The settings for the interviews were venues located within the local communities and inevitably some degree of familiarity became evident among the members of specific groups. The focus group sizes comprising eight participants each were apposite and the actual organization of the activities, duration of the discussion sessions, sequence, and content indicate consistency, and the interview questions were pertinent to the problem under investigation.

Questions for Examining the Data Analysis Technique(s)

- How detailed and unambiguous is the researcher(s') explanation of the data analysis techniques?

- How appropriate and applicable were the selected techniques to achieve accuracy in data analysis?

- How clear is the researcher(s') explanation of any coding and categorization systems used in the analysis?

- How do the researcher(s) explain the thoroughness of these tests?

- In what ways did the researchers involve independent validators in these processes?

- To what extent have the researcher(s) effectively used direct quotations from the responses?

- How clearly have the researcher(s) reasoned their use of excerpts from the respondents lived experiences in the narrative accounts and interpretive processes?

- How explicit and unambiguous is the researcher(s') clarification of the emerging themes from the responses?

- How did the researcher(s) substantiate or verify the emerging themes and the related interpretations?

- If a qualitative software package was used to analyze the data, how clear is the researchers' explanation of this?

- What evidence in the report suggests that the researcher(s) carefully examined the suitability of the selected software package for the particular design and type of data?

Data Analysis The applied framework analysis involving a matrix is explained in reasonably simple and comprehensible terms. Certain strengths in the data analysis include the processing of verbatim transcripts and identification of recurring themes that allowed the researchers to make comparisons and contrasts of the major themes that emerged among the groups. To strengthen validity and credibility of the findings, the researchers jointly discussed classification of the supporting quotes and interpretation of the data.

Questions for Examining the Ethical Considerations

- What specific measures were taken by the researcher(s) to safeguard the welfare and fundamental human rights in the best interest of the study participants?

- How convincing is the explanation of the processes that the researcher(s) claim to have fulfilled in their respect of the confidentiality, anonymity, and autonomy of each participant? How clear is the explanation provided to obtain each participant's informed consent?

- What evidence in the report affirms that the researcher(s) adhered strictly to the policy regulations for obtaining access to patients and the premises designated as the study setting(s)?

- In what ways do the researcher(s) demonstrate clear awareness and understanding of the national Data Protection Act?

- What precautionary measures did the researcher(s) claim to have taken to guard against inadvertent harm, criminal act, ill-treatment, or any form of abuse as a direct result of participating in the research study?

- What measures do the researcher(s) report to have taken to address role conflict where the study participants were professional colleagues?

Ethical Considerations The regulation to obtain ethical approval was appropriately met and while measures for ethical considerations such as confidentiality and protection of the individual participant's privacy were not discussed in detail, the researchers mentioned some element of protection in order not to divulge individual's identity by the timing and/or specific tests performed. This section falls short of adequate detail.

Questions for Examining the Data Presentation

- How clearly and comprehensively were the results presented?
- In what way does the format of the presentation of the results make it easy to read, understand, and interpret?
- How well-matched or compatible are the figures, tables, and graphs to specific data sets in terms of accuracy and exactness of the results?
- How clear is the description or narrative presentation of specific data to make sense to the reader?

Data Presentation Appropriate use of tabulation for displaying the group compositions and a table presentation of the sociodemographic detail provides pertinent information. Missing data is also indicated.

Questions for Examining the Discussion of the Findings

- To what extent have the findings from the study been described analytically and in detail in a balanced discussion?
- How well have the researchers demonstrated that the findings derive directly from the responses?
- In their discussion of the findings, how consistently did the researchers make reference to the results from the data analysis?
- How forthright is the researcher(s') account of the limitations that emerged in the course of the study and how they dealt with them?

Discussion of Main Findings The discussion of the findings shows direct reference to the research problem and the questions for exploring the preferences for STI/HIV testing are discussed individually. The researchers present a strong and convincing argument in support of the implications for policy decision-makers and the services provided. The strengths and limitations are highlighted, including apparent inconsistency in the recruitment of the overseas students of diverse backgrounds for focus group nine and the recruitment of HIV-positive persons of varied age range for focus group ten. Some element of bias was reported in terms of limiting the recruitment of participants to current or previous users of the STI testing

services within the past 2 years; exclusion of the population subgroup of Black Caribbean and Black Africans. This undoubtedly constrains generalizability of the findings to the wider population. The full report should be read for more information.

Questions for Examining the Conclusions and Recommendations

- In what ways do the conclusions provide an adequate summary of and reemphasize key findings from the analysis?
- In what ways do the researcher(s) clearly establish that the conclusions directly relate to the results and clearly link to the research problem, questions, theoretical ideas, and their intentions?
- To what extent are the final arguments about the implications and recommendations for clinical practice relevant and practicable?
- How persuasive are the researcher(s') arguments to support the soundness and trustworthiness of their claims?
- In what ways did the researcher(s) suggest that similar future studies could be further improved and carried out more extensively in multiple locations?

Discussion The final discussion shows appropriate application to the wider literature in comparing initiatives to enhance the service provision. The conclusion and recommendations aptly emphasize the need for expansion of the STI/HIV screening and testing services and accessibility of alternative options for the service users. These comments are pertinent, realistic, and noteworthy.

Questions for Examining the Style of Referencing

- In what ways is referencing system recognizable, accurate, and consistent?
- How consistently accurate are the reference citations within the text?
- In what ways do the references conform to the particular reference system employed?
- How complete are the lists of references and bibliography if provided?

References The referencing shows correct and consistent style of in-text referencing and final list of references.

Relevance of Appendices

- How pertinent were the materials enclosed as appendices in the final report?
- Where applicable, how accessible were copies of the instrument for data collection, observational field notes, letters for ethical approval, permission

for access, and participant consent as mentioned by researcher(s)?

- How logically did the researchers put these together in the order in which they appear in the report?

Appendices No appendix was presented.

Suggested Questions for Examining Quantitative Research Reports

The following series of questions and activities provide an appraisal scheme similar to that applied to the qualitative exemplar presented previously. These derive from modifications of various appraisals of research over the years and contain much detail.

Questions for Examining the Research Hypotheses

- In what way is the research problem defined in the form of a hypothesis?
- How concisely and clearly are the hypotheses or hypothesis formulated?
- In what ways do the statements of the hypotheses assert relevant predicted outcomes?
- What was the nature of the prediction?
- How convincing are the researcher(s') reasoning of the hypotheses and how applicable to the quantitative research paradigm or pre-set quantitative principles?
- How clear is the researcher(s') explanation of using quantitative paradigm to guide the conduct of the study?

Questions for Examining the Quantitative Research Design

- What quantitative research design did the researcher(s) employ for the investigating the problem?
- How clearly did the researcher(s) explain how they applied it?
- How detailed was the researchers' description of critical evaluation of the selected design to ascertain its suitability, benefits and potential limitations?
- In what ways does the design fulfill the specific quantitative investigative study?
- What considerations did the researcher(s) take into account in determining that the selected population presented the relevant traits, characteristics, or factors for investigating the research problem and hypothesis?
- What sampling technique was employed for selecting the study and control groups?
- How clearly defined and precise were the criteria for inclusion and exclusion?

- How representative was the sample size to ensure confidence in generalizing the findings?

Questions for Examining the Setting, Instrument(s), and Process of Data Collection

- How clearly do the researcher(s') describe the study setting?
- How convincing is the rationale for the choice of environment?

Questions for Examining the Instrument(s) and Data Collection Process

- What detail did the researcher(s) provide about the type of instrument(s) used for collecting the data in terms of development and pilot testing for validity and reliability?
- How convincing is the explanation about the suitability of the instrument(s) for the type of data collected?
- What information did the researcher(s) provide about the type of data, the process used in collecting them, the timing, and the reactions of study participants to the investigation?
- What kind of refinement, if any, was required following the pilot testing?
- What training was provided to prepare non-researchers involved in the data collection to ensure thoroughness and accuracy in the specific measurements?

Questions for Examining Quantitative Data Analysis and the Results

- How clearly did the researcher(s) explain the method for analyzing the data from each of the hypotheses?
- What statistical technique(s) did the researcher(s) use for the analysis?
- How understandable was the explanation of the statistical techniques?
- How correctly were the statistical measures applied to ensure accuracy of the results?
- How comparable was the analysis of the data obtained from the experimental and the control groups?
- In your opinion, would other tests and measures have been more statistically suitable for investigating the research problem, hypothesis, and type of data?
- If so, which statistical tests, for what reasons and potential benefits?
- How accurate were the tabulations, figures, graphs, and/or charts used to present the data analysis results?
- How simple and clear was the interpretation and conclusions based on the findings?

Questions for Examining the Internal Validity

- Could the changes in the outcome of the study be ascribed to alternative reasons or factors that were not explored in the study?
- Is there any chance that some other factor or extraneous variables unknown to the researcher(s) and therefore unexplored and untested in the current study could have impacted or contributed to the results?
- In other words, could any other factor(s) have influenced the type of findings obtained, the conclusions drawn, and the researcher(s) claims?

Questions for Examining the External Validity

- Did the researchers clearly demonstrate that the findings would be applicable to similar populations of similar age groups and circumstances, functioning in similar environments, and within similar time frames?
- Was there any claim that the findings might be applicable to similar population groups beyond the study participants and beyond the setting within which the study was carried out?
- Is there clear evidence that the random sampling of the study participants was adequately diverse and truly representative of the identified population?
- Were the design, methodology and methods adequately rigorous and clear-cut to have inhibited extraneous and confounding variables?

Questions for Examining the Construct Validity

- Is there clear evidence that the key construct—the speculated or hypothesized observation—was actually detected, clearly observed, and measured in the analysis?
- For example, in the study on oral contraceptive pill-taking behaviors, did the researchers clearly demonstrate that they actually measured "inconsistent and incorrect" patterns of pill taking among the study participants?
- Could they confirm direct link to unintended/unplanned pregnancy?

Reexamination of the Appraisal to Assess the Thoroughness (Evaluation of the Process)

The following challenges are designed for the appraisal/review panel or for multidisciplinary team members to consider as a small group in-house activity. The intent is to review the comments that were documented from the appraisal with a view to confirming that all the key elements have been appropriately addressed.

Reflective Considerations

Review of the thoroughness of the appraisal:

- Has the team thoroughly examined and commented on the strengths and limitations of the study?
- How just and fair were the questions to provide an overall balanced and objective commentary?
- Would the original researchers and practitioners recognize from the appraisal comments the suggestions of how specific areas of strengths and weaknesses could be improved upon in future similar studies?
- Are the suggested areas of improvement and all the recommended alternatives realistically practicable within the context of the research process?
- How practicable are the suggested ideas in relation to the research problem/phenomenon, questions/hypotheses, design, data collection, analysis and interpretation of findings, and the recommendations?
- Regarding the overall impression of the research report, what is the degree of clarity, objectivity, consistency, and thoroughness conveyed in the commentary on specific aspects?
- Does the commentary take account of the rigorousness with consideration of the ethical perspectives, organization of the report, the style of referencing, and compliance to the selected referencing system?

Quality as Objectivity, Scope, and Transparency: Criteria for Quality Evaluation Specific to Quantitative Research Studies

Alternative Quality Evaluation Tools

More recent tools are found to be pragmatic and provide guidelines with methodically structured criteria for the quality evaluation. An example of an alternative tool comprises a set of criteria for evaluating the quality of primary or original research papers (Kmet, Lee, & Cook, 2004). These authors provide an accompanying guide that explains the system of scoring and how the related comments can be analyzed. Their checklist for evaluating the quality of quantitative studies comprises questions devised for both examining and rating the processes employed.

Kmet et al.'s (2004) set of criteria for evaluating the quality of quantitative research studies was designed to assess:

- How clearly formulated and understandable are the research questions/objectives?
- How clearly is the relevance and effectiveness of the study design explained?

- How thorough is the process of sample selection, detailed description of the study participants, and comparison groups who represented the source of information?
- How clear and detailed are the characteristics of the treatment/intervention group and the control groups in experimental studies?
- How clear and detailed is the description of the specific intervention?
- How thorough is the allocation process employed?
- How sound is the explanation of whether blinding of the investigators was achieved?
- How clear is the explanation of whether the interventional process and blinding of subjects were achieved?
- How well defined were the intervention, exposure of the sample groups, and the outcome measures where applicable?
- How exact were the measures for assessing and dealing with incorrect classification?
- How appropriate was the sample size?
- How appropriate and clear is the description of data analysis techniques?
- The degree of accuracy of the statistical processes?
- How clear and detailed is the reporting of the results?
- How were confounding variables or factors that might have affected the outcome of the intervention assessed and controlled?
- How convincing is the discussion of how the conclusions were substantiated or confirmed by the results?

The authors devised a six-column table comprising the question number, the quality criteria, and four columns for scoring the quality valuation against each criterion as follows:

YES   PARTIAL   NO   N/A
(2)   (1)   (0)

By way of an exemplar, a quantitative study by Osterberg et al. (2005) was scored. This study uses a survey perspective. The survey is one of the most widely used methods of gathering data, both in healthcare and other organizations. The researchers are based at the University of California–San Francisco.

1. *How clearly formulated and understandable are the research questions/objectives?*
   QUALITY VALUATION = 2
   After a full explanation, the hypothesis is formulated at the end of the third paragraph, "Grooming is positively related to STIs except for pubic lice that would be reduced by hair removal."

2. *How clearly explained is the relevance and effectiveness of the study design?*
   QUALITY VALUATION = 2

Little evidence is available about the subject area. A survey is appropriate for collecting evidence in a new subject area. A retrospective probability survey of U.S. residents aged 18 to 65 years was used. A questionnaire was designed and is available online. An address-based sampling of the U.S. Postal Service's delivery sequence file was used that is estimated to reach 97% of households. A pre-test survey was done. The survey participant did not know the subject of the survey until after recruitment, nor did the participant see the questions until after he/she had accepted the survey, thereby reducing bias. The survey group used statistical weighting adjustments to correct survey errors such as non-coverage and non-response.

3. *How thorough was the process of sample selection, detailed description of the study participants, and comparison groups who represented the source of information?*
   QUALITY VALUATION = 2
   Demographic factors such as age, sex, and sexual behavior variables such as frequency of sexual activity and number of sexual partners were collected. The study participants were divided into 3 groups, "ever groomers," "extreme groomers" and "high-frequency groomers".

4. *How clear and detailed is the description of the characteristics of the treatment/intervention group and the control groups in experimental studies?*
   QUALITY VALUATION = Not relevant

5. *How clear and detailed the description of the specific intervention?*
   QUALITY VALUATION = Not relevant as a descriptive survey

6. *How thorough is the allocation process employed?*
   QUALITY VALUATION =Not relevant

7. *How clear is the explanation of whether blinding of the investigators was achieved?*
   QUALITY VALUATION = Not relevant

8. *How clear is the explanation of whether the interventional process and blinding of subjects were achieved?*
   QUALITY VALUATION = Not relevant

9. *How well defined were the intervention, exposure of the sample groups, and the outcome measures where applicable?*
   QUALITY VALUATION = 2
   The sample was allocated into groups according to the following outcome measures: "ever groomed," "extreme groomers," and "high frequency groomers." Outcomes variables were considered, such as history of STIs.

10. *How exact were the measures for assessing and dealing with incorrect classification?*
    QUALITY VALUATION = 1

The measures were not specified. Univariable associations between grooming and STI history were investigated by comparing the prevalence of each STI and STI type by grooming status and practices and tested statistically.

11. *How appropriate was the sample size?*
QUALITY VALUATION = 2
7,580 subjects completed the survey out of 14,409 sampled (52.5%).

12. *How appropriate and clear are the description of the techniques of data analysis?*
QUALITY VALUATION = 2
Clear.

13. *How precise was the degree of accuracy of the statistical processes?*
QUALITY VALUATION = 2
Confidence intervals were given for the results. Values of <0.05 were considered statistically significant.

14. *How clear and detailed the reporting of the results?*
QUALITY VALUATION = 2
Clear.

15. *How were confounding variables or factors that might have affected the outcome of the intervention assessed and controlled?*
QUALITY VALUATION = 1
The full characteristics of the sample group such as exposure to other factors that may induce STIs including multiple partners and sexual behavior practices. The number of lifetime partners and age were identified as confounding factors and multivariate regression models were created to measure these associations.

16. *How convincing was the discussion of how the conclusions were substantiated or confirmed by the results?*
QUALITY VALUATION = 2
Various explanations of the results were presented, such as shared use of grooming tools, and the possibility that respondents became groomers after experiencing an STI. The limitations of the study were addressed.

Using Kmet et al.'s (2004) criteria, some of the criteria are not specific to the survey method used in this study. Other appraisal criteria specific to the survey perspective can be found at The Center for Evidence-Based Management (CEBMa) (https://www.cebma.org/).

Similar to the previous example, the authors proposed the following evaluative criteria for assessing the quality of qualitative research using the same system of scoring. Kmet et al.'s (2004) tool for evaluating the quality of qualitative research studies was designed to assess the following:

- How clearly defined and unambiguous the research questions/objectives are.
- How clearly explained the study design and the justification of the relevance and applicability are.
- How clear the explanation regarding the context of the study in terms of the situation-specific circumstances is.
- How comprehensible the linkages demonstrated in the theoretical framework and to specific concepts in the wider body of knowledge are.
- How methodical and clearly discussed the process of participant selection or recruitment is.
- How meticulous the data collection method, clarity of the explanation, and rationales are.
- How accurate and precise the techniques of data analysis are.
- How convincing the explanation of the procedure to confirm trustworthiness is.
- How clear the discussion of how the conclusions were substantiated by the results is.
- How clear the account of researcher reflexivity in terms of personal assumptions, decisions, actions and behavior, and the possible effect on the way the study was conducted is.

Readers are encouraged to identify a qualitative study and make similar application.

Another useful tool/framework proposed by Spencer Ritchie, Lewis, and Dillon, (2003) and Lewis, Spencer, Ritchie, and Dillon (2006) comprises 18 questions for assessing the quality and integrity of published research. This tool can be obtained from the website of the National Institute for Health and Clinical Excellence (NICE) at http://www.publichealth.nice.org.uk.

The structure and content of the framework provides an easily applicable step-by-step guide, and a summary is provided in this chapter. However, readers are urged to access the original work and to acknowledge the full copyright regulations if they decide to adopt it for practical application. The original authors (Lewis et al., 2006; Spencer et al., 2003) explained that the framework is underpinned by four guiding principles, which uphold that research:

- Contributing to advancement of the wider knowledge and understanding about policy, practice, and theory
- Having a recognizable and approved paradigm with a design that is defensible and that can address the questions/challenges of critical evaluation and synthesis
- Embracing qualitative methodology that reflects rigor in terms of thorough and substantiated processes of data collection, analysis, and interpretation
- Providing assertions that are trustworthy with well-substantiated arguments about the practicality of the related evidence

A particular advantage of the framework is that specific quality indicators are also provided to guide the assessment of key elements in the report. These are features that the appraisal teams might want to consider. The original authors acknowledge that the suggested indicators are not necessarily comprehensive. They also acknowledge that teams of practitioners might want to make possible adjustments to meet the assessed needs of the particular area of practice. This would require detailed evaluation of the framework. It is important to read the guiding notes provided by the original authors in relation to that. The framework presents a tabulated format outlining 18 appraisal questions summarized here.

In addition to the indicators, the tabulated format allows for comments on the findings to be documented alongside each appraisal question and related set of indicators. It must be noted that only a brief outline of the key elements construed from the framework is provided in this chapter. Practitioners and other readers are encouraged to explore the authors' original paper to gain better insight of this system of quality evaluation from the detailed content of the framework. A summary of the key components of the 18 questions and related indicators is presented in **Box 2-1**.

To avoid confusion and differing interpretations occurring in an in-house research evaluation exercise, it is important that the members of an appraisal/review team determine their particular perspective on research quality

---

BOX 2-1 Concise Outline of the Appraisal Questions

Findings

1. *How credible are the findings?*
2. *How has knowledge/understanding been extended by the research?*
3. *How well does the evaluation address its original aims and purpose?*
4. *Scope for drawing wider inference—how well is this explained?*
5. *How clear is the basis of evaluative appraisal?*

Design

6. *How defensible is the research design?*

Sample

7. *How well defended is the sample design/target selection of cases/documents?*
8. *Sample composition/case inclusion—how well is the eventual coverage described?*

Data collection

9. *How well was the data collection carried out?*

Analysis

10. *How well has the approach to and formulation of the analysis been conveyed?*
11. *Contexts of data sources—how well are they retained and portrayed?*
12. *How well has diversity of perspective and content been explored?*
13. *How well has detail, depth, and complexity (richness) of the data been conveyed?*

Reporting

14. *How clear are the links between data, interpretation, and conclusions—how well can the route to any conclusions be seen?*
15. *How clear and coherent is the reporting?*

Reflexivity and neutrality

16. *How clear are the assumptions/theoretical perspectives/values that have shaped the form and output of the evaluation?*

Ethics

17. *What evidence is there of attention to ethical issues?*

Auditability

18. *How adequately has the research process been documented?*

Summary of the Quality Indicators

Questions 1–5 address the quality of the findings as follows.

1. Credibility of the findings and conclusions appropriately substantiated by the data; clear stages of analysis and interpretation; findings and conclusion underpinned by plausible reasoning; findings and conclusions reflect additional relevant knowledge and experience; appropriately related to the data and findings from prior research.
2. Contribution to the existing knowledge and understanding—detailed, clear, and adequately substantiated literature review; study aims and design appropriately focused; identified gaps related to policy, professional practice and sound proposition of ideas; effective discussion demonstrating the contribution of prior research to the existing professional knowledge and practice; alternative insights derived from the findings; reasoned discussion highlighting unexplored issues and ideas for future studies.
3. Extent to which the original aims and purpose have been addressed—clear statements of aims/objectives and related rationales; definite linkage of the findings to the statement of purpose and the focus of the investigation; conclusions relatable to the aims of the study; competent discussion of the causes of identified limitations, detailed examination of these in relation to the setting, participant/sampling issues, time constraint.

4. Clarity of the explanation of the scope for wider implications—reasoned discussion of wider application of the findings to population groups beyond the participants of the study; clear description of the background and setting to facilitate applicability; discussion of the findings and recommendations from different viewpoints; evidence from the study verified and confirmed by prior research findings; examination of the constraints for broader suppositions.

5. Examination of the basis of the appraisal—discussion of influences on the evaluation and impact; discussion of the effect produced; clear description of the formal criteria used for the appraisal, its origin, and wider application; discussion of differences in appraisal.

Questions 6–8 address the quality of the research design and the study sample.

6. Description and rationales relating to the type and suitability of the design—the specific components and direct application to the findings; the implications of the potential limitations.

7. Details of the study participants—details of the target population; the selection process and the criteria used; the sample size; appropriateness and related rationales.

8. Description of the sample characteristics—how representative of the population structure, constitution and characteristics; access and process of approaching potential participants; individuals' reasons for declining to participate.

Question 9 addresses the data collection strategy.

9. The thoroughness of the data collection process and the related rationales—the level of competence of the data collector(s); procedure(s) used; the process and quality of the documentation; the type and quality of the information obtained—the scope, detail, and richness of the data; specific influencing factors.

Questions 10–13 address details of the analysis.

10. The detail and clarity of the explanation and rationales for the technique(s) employed for the analysis—the form of the original data; the development of categories or classifications and labels; the use of examples for illustrating concepts in simple terms.

11. The situation and circumstances of the data sources—measures used in stabilizing the setting; measures used to represent the participants' perspectives; origins of written documents; and the systems used for management of the data.

12. Attention to diversity in the sampling—measures employed in dealing with emerging negative case scenarios; outliers, exceptions; discussion of different models; assessment of the impact of influencing factors; highlighting patterns of association or links between dissimilar groups.

13. Extensiveness—the extent of detail and thoroughness conveyed in the depth and richness of the data; terms, concepts, meanings, distinctions, obscurity, inconsistencies and discrepancies in the data; explicit and implicit explanations and influencing factors; patterns of association within the data; helpful and informative textual excerpts.

Questions 14–15 address the quality of the reporting.

14. The reporting—completeness, detail, and clarity of the explanation of the links between data, interpretation, and the conclusions; clear explanation of the original data with use of illustrations; explanation of the data presentation and analysis; the reasoning behind the interpretation and the significance; explanation of how the emerging theories and conclusions link to the original data; how any outliers were dealt with or included in the hypotheses or proposed theories.

15. Clarity of the reporting—explanation to demonstrate the links to the aims and research questions; narrative style and development of themes; signposting for the readers; accessible information for the target audience(s) convincing and substantial summary.

Question 16 addresses reflectivity and objectivity.

16. Clarity of the assumptions that directed the scope of the evaluation—explanation of how the values and viewpoints and ideas of the researcher(s) influenced the development of the methodology; discussion of how the knowledge and experience gained from the research helped to understand and recognize alternative ideas for refining and re-establishing suppositions; forming new ideas, aims, and questions for future studies; discussion of how potential biases and researcher influences were dealt with.

Question 17 addresses the ethical considerations.

17. Measures used for dealing with the ethical issues—regard to the study setting and the participants; the nature of the researcher–participant contacts; processes for dealing with consent, confidentiality, and anonymity; measures for ensuring subsequent participant support as necessary; measures for protecting the participants from harm directly related to the investigative procedures.

Question 18 addresses auditability.

18. Efficient documentation—discussion of the strengths and weaknesses in the methodology and methods; description of adjustments to the research design; explanation and the rationales for any required adjustments to the processes of sampling, data collection, technique of data analysis; reproduction of the related documents—letters, observation templates; framework for management of the data.

Data from Spencer, L., Ritchie, J., Lewis, J., & Dillon, L. (2003) *Quality in qualitative evaluation: A framework for assessing research evidence.* London: National Centre for Social Research; Lewis, J., Spencer, L., Ritchie, J., & Dillon, L. (2006) Appraising quality in qualitative evaluations: approaches and challenges, in J. Popay (Ed.), *Moving beyond effectiveness in evidence synthesis.* London: National Institute for Health and Clinical Excellence.

evaluation. There is no doubt that there are benefits to identification and application of an appropriate evaluation tool with set criteria. Nevertheless, this may also present an additional challenge for the multidisciplinary team. It is important to determine whether the particular appraisal exercise should focus on quantitative or qualitative studies. It is also useful to carefully examine the problem/phenomenon of interest, the questions investigated or the hypotheses tested in previous studies, and the study designs and methods employed.

Conclusion

In broad terms, evidence-based practice represents an approach involving identifying, interpreting, and combining convincing research evidence from seminal studies for making sound judgments to improve care and service provision. It also requires that account be taken of clinician-observed evidence, professional expertise firmly verified by positive outcomes and the expressed needs, preferences, and values of the patient. Society demands high-quality care and service provision that is supported by strong and authentic evidence. This helps to maintain and strengthen public trust with enhanced confidence in the system of healthcare delivery. Nevertheless, despite popular claims about adoption of evidence-based culture in many healthcare organizations, the reality is that many practitioners admit that they are not entirely clear what EBP actually entails.

Different interpretations and rationales for evidence-based practice have been proposed, including those offered by professional regulatory bodies. Nevertheless, these convey common key elements from the principles of EBP. Practitioners need to know and understand what the main components of evidence-based practice involve to make sense of its application within the actuality of clinical practice. However, the difficulty that many practitioners admit to is uncertainty about exactly how to determine best available evidence. Different mechanisms for this have been proposed and it is important for practitioners to know and understand what these entail and how to apply each system correctly. An attempt has been made in this chapter to provide simplified explanations of the rating and classification processes for grading the quality of evidence at different levels.

The processes of searching, selecting, examining, and appraising relevant seminal research studies must be carried out competently. Practitioners must fulfil their professional obligation to acquire the essential knowledge and competencies required for correct and efficient application of these to EBP. It is crucial to keep up-to-date with current research studies in the field of practice and current documents of emerging new policies that guide procedures and interventions. Appropriate training, skills development, required guidance, and support should be offered as necessary to enhance staff confidence and competence for efficient reviewing of the literature as an in-house culture. The process of examining published studies involves logical stages of appraisal. However, potential errors can result in misinterpretation of the findings, and it is important that practitioners are aware of these when appraising research reports.

Various formats of quality evaluation tools have been proposed, two examples of which are discussed in this chapter. Readers are encouraged to explore both the broad/generic research appraisal tools and specific quality evaluation tools to gain more insight and understanding of their effective use. While formal appraisal and evaluative tools may sound useful and convenient, practitioners are reminded about the importance of acknowledging the copyright requirements stipulated by the original authors. Team members should be adequately familiar with and confident to identify and use well-designed formal tools, guidelines, and protocols.

● ● ● **REFERENCES**

Barker, J. (2010). *Evidence-based practice for nurses*. London, United Kingdom: Sage Publications.

Burls, A. (2009). *What is critical appraisal?* London, United Kingdom: Hayward Group Ltd. Retrieved from http://www.whatisseries.co.uk/what-is-critical-appraisal/

Ciliska, D., DiCenso, A., Melnyk, B.M., & Stetler, C. (2005). Using models and strategies for evidence-based practice. In B.M. Melnyk & E. Fineout-Overholt (Eds.), *Evidence-based practice in nursing and healthcare: A guide to best practice* (1st ed., pp. 185–219). Philadelphia, PA: Lippincott Williams & Wilkins.

DiCenso, A., Cullum, N., Ciliska, D., & Guyatt, G. (2005). Introduction to evidence-based nursing. In A. DiCenso, N. Cullum, & D. Ciliska (Eds.), *Evidence-based nursing: A guide to clinical practice* (pp. 3–19). Philadelphia, PA: Elsevier.

Guyatt, G., Cook, D., & Haynes, B. (2004). Evidence-based medicine has come a long way. *BMJ, 329*, 990–991.

Guyatt, G., & Rennie, D. (2002). *Users' guide to the medical literature: A manual for evidence-based clinical practice*. Chicago, IL: American Medical Association Press.

Harris, R.P., Helfand, M., Woolf, S.H., Lohr, K.N., Mulrow, C.D., Teutsch, S.M., & Atkins, D. (2001). Methods Work Group. Third US Preventive Services Task Force. Current methods of the US Preventive Services Task Force: A review of the process. *American Journal of Preventive Medicine, 20*(Suppl. 3), 21–35.

Jordan, Z., Lockwood, C., Aromataris, E., & Munn, Z. (2016). The updated JBI model for evidence-based healthcare. The Joanna Briggs Institute. Retrieved from http://joannabriggs.org/assets/docs/approach/The_JBI_Model_of_Evidence_-_Healthcare-A_Model_Reconsidered.pdf

Kmet, L., Lee, R., & Cook, L. (2004). *Standard quality assessment criteria for evaluating primary research papers from a variety of fields*. Edmonton, Canada: Alberta Heritage Foundation for Medical Research. Retrieved from https://www.biomedcentral.com/content/supplementary/1471-2393-14-52-s2.pdf

Levine, E.R. (2004). Glossary. In A.R. Roberts & K.R. Yeager (Eds.), *Evidence-based practice manual: Research and outcome measures in health and human services* (pp. 971–1007). New York, NY: Oxford University Press.

Lewis J., Spencer L., Ritchie J., & Dillon L. (2006). Appraising quality in qualitative evaluations: Approaches and challenges. In J. Popay (Ed.), *Moving beyond effectiveness in evidence synthesis* pp. 61–72. London, United Kingdom: National Institute for Health and Clinical Excellence.

McKibbon, K.A., & Marks, S. (1998). Searching for the best evidence. Part 1: Where to look. *Evidence Based Nursing, 1*(3), 68–70.

Melnyk, B.M., & Fineout-Overholt, E. (2005). Making the case for evidence-based practice and cultivating a spirit of inquiry. In B.M. Melnyk & E. Fineout-Overholt (Eds.), *Evidence-based practice in nursing and healthcare: A guide to best practice* (1st ed., pp. 3–24). Naylor, C.D., . . . Ricardson, W.S. Philadelphia, PA: Lippincott Williams.

Melnyk, B.M., & Fineout-Overholt, E. (Eds.). (2014). *Evidence-based practice in nursing and healthcare: A guide to best practice* (3rd ed.). Philadelphia, PA: Lippincott Williams & Wilkins.

Osterberg, L., Blaschke, T. (2005). Adherence to Medication. *N Engl J Med.* 2005; *353*(5): 487–497.

Polit, D.F., & Beck, C.T. (2011). *Nursing research: Generating and assessing evidence for nursing practice.* (9th ed.). London, United Kingdom: Wolters Kluwer Health/Lippincott Williams &Wilkins.

Rees, C. (2010). Understanding evidence and its utilisation in nursing practice. In K. Holland (Ed.), *Nursing: Evidence-based practice skills* (pp. 18–38). Oxford, United Kingdom: Oxford University Press.

Rubin, H., & Rubin, J. (2005). *Qualitative interviewing: The art of hearing data* (2nd ed.). London, United Kingdom: Sage.

Rycroft-Malone, J., & Bucknall, T. (2011). *Models and frameworks for implementing evidence-based practice: Linking evidence to action.* London, United Kingdom: John-Wiley & Sons.

Sackett, D.L., Rosenberg, W.M.C., Gray, J.A.M., Haynes, R.B., & Richardson, W.S. (1996). Evidence based medicine: What it is and what it isn't. *BMJ, 312*(7023), 71–72.

Sackett, D.L., Straus, S.E., Richardson, W.S., Rosenberg, W., & Haynes, R.B. (2000). *Evidence-based medicine: How to practice and teach EBM.* Edinburgh, United Kingdom: Churchill Livingstone.

Saks, M., & Allsop, J. (2007). *Researching health: Qualitative, quantitative and mixed methods.* London, United Kingdom: Sage.

Spencer, L., Ritchie, J., Lewis, J., & Dillon, L. (2003). *Quality in qualitative evaluation: A framework for assessing research evidence.* London, United Kingdom: National Centre for Social Research.

● ● ● SUGGESTED FURTHER READING

Altman, D.G., & Bland, J.M. (2005). Treatment allocation by minimization. *BMJ, 330*(7495), 843.

Banks, S. (2012). *Ethics and values in social work* (4th ed.). London, United Kingdom: Palgrave Macmillan.

Beckett, C. (2012). *Values and ethics in social work* (2nd ed.). London, United Kingdom: Sage.

British Association of Social Workers (BASW). (2012). *Code of ethics for social workers.* Retrieved from http://lx.iriss.org.uk /content/code-ethics-social-work-statement-principles

Chambless, D., & Hollon, S. (1998). Defining empirically supportable therapies. *Journal of Consulting and Clinical Psychology, 66*(1), 7–18.

Clark, C.L. (2000). *Social work ethics: Politics, principles and practice.* Basingstoke, United Kingdom: Palgrave Macmillan.

Coughlan, M., Cronin, P., & Ryan, F., (2007). Step-by-step guide to critiquing research. Part 1: quantitative research. *British Journal of Nursing, 16*(11), 658–663.

Cullum, N., Ciliska, D., Haynes, B., & Marks, S. (Eds.). (2008). *Evidence-based nursing: An introduction.* London, United Kingdom: Wiley-Blackwell.

Fineout-Overholt, E., Melnyk, B.M., & Schultz, A. (2005). Transforming health care from the inside out: advancing evidence-based practice in the 21st century. *Journal of Professional Nursing, 21*(6), 335–344.

Guyatt, G.H., Haynes, R.B., Jaeschke, R.Z., Cook, D.J., Green, L., Naylor, C.D., . . . Ricardson, W.S. (2000). Users' guide to the medical literature XXV. Evidence-based medicine: Principles for applying the users guides to patient care. *JAMA, 284*(10), 1290–1296.

Hemingway, P., & Brereton, N. (2009). *What is systematic review?* Kings Hill, United Kingdom: Hayward Group. Retrieved from http://www.bandolier.org.uk/painres/download/whatis /Syst-review.pdf

Higgins, J.P.T., & Altman, D.G. (2008). Assessing Risk of bias in included studies. In J.P.T. Higgins & S. Green (Eds.), *Cochrane handbook for systematic reviews of interventions* (Ver. 5.0.1). Retrieved from www.cochrane-handbook.org.

Higgins, J.P.T., & Green, S. (Eds.). (2008). *Cochrane handbook for systematic reviews of interventions.* Chichester, United Kingdom: John Wiley & Sons Ltd.

Lewis, D.M., & Barnes, C. (1997). Critiquing the research literature. In P. Smith & J. Hunt (Eds.), *Research mindedness in practice: An interactive approach for nursing and health care* (pp. 201–231). Edinburgh, United Kingdom: Churchill.

Lincoln, Y.S., & Guba, E.G. (1985). *Naturalistic inquiry.* Newbury Park, CA: Sage.

National Institute for Health and Care Excellence (NICE). (2005). *Reviewing and grading evidence.* London, United Kingdom: Author.

Polit, D.F., & Beck, C.T. (2008). Translating research evidence into nursing practice: Evidence-based nursing. In D.F. Polit & C.T. Beck (Eds.). *Nursing research: Generating and assessing evidence for nursing practice* (8th ed., pp. 28–54). London, United Kingdom: Lippincott Williams & Wilkins.

Polit, D.F., & Beck, C.T. (2014). *Essentials of nursing research: Appraising evidence for nursing practice.* Philadelphia, PA: Wolters Kluwer/Lippincott Williams & Wilkins.

Ryan-Wenger, N. (1992). Guidelines for critique of a research report. *Heart & Lung, 21*(4), 394–401.

Scottish Intercollegiate Guidelines Network. (2011). *SIGN 50: A guideline developer's handbook.* Edinburgh, United Kingdom: Author.

Wakefield, A. (2014). Searching and critiquing the research literature. *Nursing Standard, 28*(39), 49–57.

Walsh, D., & Downe, S. (2006). Appraising the quality of qualitative research. *Midwifery, 22*(2): 108–119.

World Health Organisation (WHO). (2004). *Selected practice recommendations for contraceptive use.* Geneva, Switzerland: Author.

CHAPTER

3

Systematic Reviews: Consolidating Research Evidence for EBP

THEODORA D. KWANSA

CHAPTER OBJECTIVES

The main objectives of this chapter are to:

- Explore the significance, rationale, and benefits of systematic reviews
- Examine the process of reviewing, condensing, and summarizing research evidence
- Describe the processes of data extraction and abstraction
- Identify the processes of quantitative research synthesis, meta-analysis, and the PRISMA statement
- Explore the approaches to synthesizing qualitative research evidence and the related terminologies
- State the need for systematic reviews, meta-analysis, and qualitative research synthesis

Introduction

This chapter focuses on systematic reviews of multiple studies with similar design(s) and method(s) and combining and condensing the findings for evidence-based support of professional practice. Meta-analysis, which allows for pooling and interpreting emerging concepts to create new theories, is also explored.

The Rationale and Advantages of Systematic Reviews for EBP

Generally, systematic reviews are informative overviews of carefully selected primary research studies that have rigorously applied specific research design(s), methodology, and methods to investigate a clinical problem/phenomenon. This problem/phenomenon and the related review question(s) might relate to the effects of clinical intervention, healthcare policy, or the effectiveness of specific aspects of professional practice. Identifying, compiling, critiquing, summarizing, and condensing the best available evidence and synthesizing these compose the stages of systematic review. As the name suggests, systematic reviews are rigorous in terms of following exact processes, transparent in terms of being applicable to different contexts in actual situations, and repeatable. They provide cumulative evidence from the findings of pertinent studies that policy makers and clinical practitioners can draw on. Thus, systematic reviews can be used to employ evidence-based best practice, designed to achieve positive outcomes and patient satisfaction. Other benefits include helping to inform and direct policy, and clinical decision making, and the development of standards to ensure correct implementation of recommended guidelines.

Hemingway and Brereton (2009) identified specific professionals and stakeholders who may require sound and trustworthy information at varied times, on a considerable range of interventions and aspects of healthcare delivery. Healthcare practitioners—clinicians, nurses, therapists, and healthcare managers—as well as policy makers, patients, and consumer representatives may, at some time or another, seek specific evidence-based information on clinical interventions or aspects of the healthcare policy, such as the effects, practicality, significance, and the relevance of certain aspects of professional practice or a specific treatment. These authors note that systematic reviews help to ease the additional demand on practitioners who may be inundated with several reports and emerging new findings from numerous research studies. Practitioners constantly face the challenge and professional expectation to keep up to date with ongoing advances in scientific techniques and new procedural interventions. Emerging new ideas often involve implementing changes in policy, clinical decisions, and guidelines (Brown et al., 2006; Crombie & Davies, 2009; Petticrew, 2003; Petticrew & Roberts, 2006).

Without a doubt, information from a large amount of research is easier to grasp when condensed in a systematic review (Hemingway & Brereton, 2009). Earlier proponents, including Oxman (1993), maintained that the pooling of several studies yields better assurance, in terms of more comprehensive evidence, about the effectiveness of specific interventions. Systematic reviews allow for determining and confirming consistency in studies that are conducted across different clinical contexts and targeting comparable patient populations. A single independent study, by contrast, may fall short of being generalizable to other population groups.

Systematic reviews have the additional benefit of thoroughness as long as the reviewer(s) use well-designed and approved frameworks. Conducted correctly, systematic reviews can provide a clearer picture of the overall effects, both positive and adverse, of particular clinical interventions. In addition to confirming what is already known, systematic reviews also help to identify the deficits or gaps in professional knowledge and practice and thus provide a guide for future research Brown et al., 2006; Petticrew, 2003; Petticrew & Roberts, 2006). Crombie and Davies (2009) note that a key feature of systematic reviews is the unbiased critical appraisal of all the available relevant studies. A concise summation of the rationales, main benefits, and the significance of systematic reviews is outlined in **Box 3-1**.

BOX 3-1 Summary of the Emphasis on Systematic Reviews for EBP

Provide cumulative evidence from relevant available studies to inform clinical practitioners and policy and decision makers

Provide sound evidence basis for guiding organizational policy decisions on standards of health care and practice

Reveal the impact of specific policy regulations on particular aspects of professional practice

Yield better assurance, more comprehensive and consistent evidence about the effects, practicability, significance, and suitability of specific treatment interventions

Provide a clearer picture with better insight and understanding about the overall outcomes, both positive and adverse, of clinical interventions

Help to identify the deficits or gaps in professional knowledge and practice thus providing a guide to future research and appropriate contexts for particular investigations

(Data from Petticrew, M. (2003). Why certain systematic reviews reach uncertain conclusions. *BMJ*, 326(7392), 756–758; Kitchenham, B. (2004). *Procedures for performing systematic reviews: Joint technical report*. Keel, United Kingdom: Keel University; Petticrew, M., & Roberts, H. (2006). *Systematic reviews in the social sciences: A practical guide.* Malden, MA: Blackwell; Brown, P., Brunnhuber, K., Chalkidou, K., Chalmers, I., Clarke, C., Fenton, M., . . . Young, P. (2006). How to formulate research recommendations. *BMJ*, 333(7572), 804–806.

Despite the above observations, as Petticrew (2003) remarked, systematic reviews are often criticized for not incorporating precise guidance on what indicates evidence of effective or ineffective interventions. However, reviews of healthcare interventions may not yield enough evidence to answer precise questions on the effectiveness or ineffectiveness of specific interventions. Perhaps practitioners might find it less daunting to conduct systematic reviews if they could find review guidelines that state parameters and instructions for applying them to ensure standardization. Arguably, non-systematic review is a quick way to put forth introductory papers on specific opinions on policy and practice. Nonetheless, that process falls short of providing an all-inclusive combination of best available evidence. The general view is that a non-systematic review carried out carelessly and incorrectly can yield serious misrepresentation of detail and cause confusion. Petticrew (2003) examined the reasons for the lack of specific guidance for systematic reviews of social and healthcare interventions. He highlighted Millward, Kelly, and Nutbeam's 2001 work, which showed a limitation in the number of trials in social and health care and reviews involving outcome assessments.

Non-Systematic Reviews Examined

Non-systematic reviews do not necessarily aim to identify all the relevant published studies that applied a specific research design or methodology to investigate a specific clinical problem. Rather than critically appraising and synthesizing the research findings, non-systematic reviews characteristically present a broad discussion of the findings from some studies and substantiate with relevant references. Additionally, non-systematic reviews do not require adherence to an exact and precise review protocol. Consequently, without compliance or application of specific pre-set criteria to the study selection, a non-systematic review might be carried out in a rather haphazard manner. Thus, a non-systematic review may largely represent the reviewer's subjective interpretations based on fixed ideas and lead to distorted conclusions (Sandelowski, 2008). An outline of the principles and essential components of systematic reviews is presented in **Box 3-2**.

Evaluating the Quality of Each Selected Research Study

The process should involve critical examination of each study to assess the methodology for thoroughness and correct application, data analysis techniques, level of detail in the presentation of the research results, degree of accuracy of the measurements, and outcomes/results. Moreover, the process should involve critically examining the methodology for possible replication and generalization of the findings. Some experts recommend blinding the quality assessors to hide the identity of the researchers/authors of the study

BOX 3-2 Key Considerations and Actions in Systematic Reviews

Constructing pertinent review questions: These should be focused, well-defined and unambiguous.

Developing a review protocol: The purpose of this is to outline The process of constructing the review question, the search and retrieval of evidence materials, the eligibility criteria, the study selection, information extraction, quality assessment, synthesis, interpretation, conclusion, and preparation of the review report.

Extensive search of the literature and other relevant sources: The process for locating the pertinent studies should be comprehensive.

Defining and using criteria for selection of eligible studies (inclusion/exclusion criteria): Criteria should be clearly reasoned and applicable to the identified problem/phenomenon and the review questions. The PICO model (**P**atient/**P**opulation/**P**roblem, **I**ntervention, **C**omparison, **O**utcome) may be used and the selection should target full research reports. Experts recommend involvement of at least two reviewers to ascertain consistency in the application of the studies' inclusion/exclusion criteria.

Extracting pertinent details from the reports of the selected studies: The process of data extraction should be consistent. Both electronic and script pro-formas are available.

reports, the institutions, and the particular journals of publication. Subjective preferences in the research report in terms of potential biases should also be given careful consideration.

Initial Preparation

Because systematic reviews involve considerable rigor, preparation is important and should be carefully thought out. It is important to establish what reviews, both previous and current, have been conducted on the particular clinical problem and what review questions were asked.

Another motive for systematic reviews may be obligatory response to a commission. The commissioning body may demand verification of the best available evidence through systematic reviews of such issues as organizational policy, emerging new procedures/treatment interventions, or the prevalence and pattern of spread of an infection. For more detailed information, readers are encouraged to explore both the Cochrane Handbook (Higgins & Green, 2011) and the Centre for Reviews and Dissemination (CRD) publication, *Guidance for Undertaking Reviews in Healthcare* (Centre for Reviews and Dissemination, 2009).

The Need for an Extensive Systematic Review

Readers may find it useful to access the Database of Abstracts of Reviews of Effects (DARE) at www.crd.york.ac.uk/crdweb/. The Cochrane Database of Systematic Reviews (CDSR) at http://www.cochranelibrary.com/cochrane-database-of-systematic-reviews/index.html also provides healthcare researchers and practitioners full and regularly updated texts of systematically reviewed healthcare intervention effects. Policy and protocols also undergo similar high standard review processes conducted by the Cochrane Review Groups in the Cochrane Collaboration system. The U.S. National Library of Medicine (NLM), which is part of the National Institutes of Health (NIH), also produces extensive data on all aspects of medicine and health care, which is accessible at http://www.nlm.nih.gov/.

Other useful sources of systematically reviewed studies include the National Institute for Health and Care Excellence (NICE), the Scottish Intercollegiate Guidelines Network (SIGN), and the Evidence for Policy and Practice Information (EPPI) Centre, which provides reviews of policy and protocols relating to social welfare and social care, health education, health promotion, and public health. The World Health Organization (WHO) is another good source, as it has the reputation of ensuring that its guidelines and recommendations are based on meticulously reviewed research studies, meta-analysis, and meta-synthesis on interventional effects and other forms of substantiated evidence. The Centre for Reviews and Dissemination (2009) provides a detailed guide for systematic review. For copyright reasons, readers are encouraged to explore the CRD document themselves.

Selecting the Team of Reviewers

A carefully selected review team should represent all the disciplines in the particular area of clinical practice. This ensures joint participation in the review and ultimately, shared ownership, support, and cooperation in implementation of EBP. Experts advise that implementation of change should be facilitated by a team of professionals who have the relevant backgrounds of specialism (Lo Biondo-Wood & Haber, 2013). The review team should advise not only practitioners with a range of knowledge and expertise in the clinical specialism, but also in systematic review methods, information retrieval, research, health economics, and statistics.

The Role of a Consultative Committee

The consultative committee represents an advisory group comprising professionals from the healthcare organization, expert researchers, and stakeholders from the public sector(s) (who may be patient representatives and service users). This team of advisers has the responsibility to examine and comment on the review protocol and the final report, and to provide support, clarification, and guidance. In essence, the advisory group ensures that the review is pertinent for meeting the needs of all relevant stakeholders. Therefore, this group should have the authority to examine the feasibility of implementing the recommended guidelines (Gagan & Hewit-Taylor, 2004). It is important that such groups are established prior to commencing the systematic review.

Developing the Review Protocol

Lo Biondo-Wood and Haber (2013) recognize the advantage of putting evidence-based policies, procedures, and guidelines in writing. Public and organizational/administrative dynamics that may potentially hinder the use of research findings should be carefully examined. Appropriate measures should be taken to address these before embarking on the implementation of EBP. Brown, Wickline, Ecoff, and Glaser, (2009) and other authors cite barriers such as inadequate staffing capacity, varied levels of competence, unequal and inadequate management support, neglected research training, and experience. Other limitations include deficient research activities, disinterest and lack of motivation to conduct studies, and poor application of credible findings to clinical practice in certain areas. The tendency to consistently apply unsubstantiated and intuitive practices could lower the standard and quality of care delivery.

The protocol should outline clear, practicable, reasoned, and achievable actions to ensure correct and efficient implementation. An important advantage of developing a protocol is to avoid omissions and inconsistencies that may result in inaccurate conclusions being drawn. In addition, a protocol provides a practical guide to the review process and the intended use for the findings (Crombie & Davies, 2009; Hemingway & Brereton, 2009; Kitchenham, 2004). In reality, while most of the decisions about the systematic review and meta-analysis are incorporated in the protocol, additional decisions may become necessary as the review progresses. The following is a sample protocol derived from existing protocols.

Key Components of the Protocol

The protocol should provide a schedule and venue for the review meetings, specify the processes to be employed in the review, and serve as a guide to deciding on the review question. This helps to refine the question and make clear which intervention is being explored and why.

The protocol should also include an outline of the study selection process. To avoid bias, criteria for inclusion and exclusion should be clearly defined. The protocol should also outline the processes of data extraction and assessment of the quality of the research studies in terms of design and methodology. The technique for data synthesis should be concisely stated together with the strategy for disseminating the findings from the review. Any modifications to these processes should be clearly documented in relation to the review question.

The use of an approved and formal systematic review framework facilitates these processes. While some are produced with accompanying narrative guides or instructions, others are considered relatively self-explanatory and easy to apply. A copy of the review framework should be enclosed separately or incorporated in the protocol (Crombie & Davies, 2009; Hemingway & Brereton, 2009; Kitchenham, 2004). Other key stages are examined here.

Relevance of the PICO(S) Format and Criteria

The process for selecting relevant studies for systematic reviews traditionally considers population, intervention, comparators, and outcome (PICO). Study design has been added to the process to create PICOS.

Application of the PICO(S) Criteria: An Exemplar

The main purpose for the review should be stated, specifying the exact clinical issue that is to be explored. For example:

> To explore the impact of specific campaigns, including sexual health promotion and patient education, sexual health screening, safer sex, and condom usage designed to target young adults between 18–24 years of age in X area(s). The review would cover all clinical settings within the . . . locales and/or geographical areas.

P: Population/Patients or Study Participants Details about the characteristics of the participants should be indicated in the statement or review question. Relevance to the target population should be recognizable such as gender, age range, type of medical condition or specific health problem, degree of severity, and specific status of the problem or condition.

I: Intervention, for example, Specific Medication or Therapeutic Procedure The particular treatment intervention(s) should reflect those specified in the review question. Multiple treatment interventions should be clearly itemized according to relevance to the review. For example:

> Sexual health promotion/education
> Sexual health screening for chlamydia and other STIs
> Promotion of condom use

C: Comparators The nature of the comparators should be explained in terms of the study/control groups or the types of treatment interventions and modes of delivery. For example:

> Comparisons of an intervention group of sexually active young adults who regularly attend sexual health clinics to those who seldom ever or never attend clinics.

> Or,

> Implementation of specific behavior change interventions with guidance and instructions provided in the group context as well as on individual basis.

O: Outcome This relates to the effectiveness of the treatment intervention(s). The outcomes should be recorded as a direct result of the intervention(s) but if not, the compounders or co-interventions that may have been in place should be clearly specified. Additionally, the exact nature of each observed and measured outcome should be clearly recorded. For example:

> *Clear evidence of improvement in the sexual behaviors of the research intervention group.*

> *Clear evidence that increased proportion of the intervention group of young adults demonstrated behaviors indicative of being better informed about and practicing safer sex with fewer sexual risk-taking behaviors.*

Negative outcomes should also be clearly reported and more exact descriptors and terminology specifying the nature of each type of outcome should be stated. The challenge is whether the outcomes were observable, measurable, and recordable to achieve objectivity in each of the selected studies.

S: Study Design A design that allows for objectivity and consistency is likely to have been carefully developed. For example: "*randomized controlled trials*" with appropriate attention to detail. This could prove to be a challenge in some areas of sexual healthcare where empirical quantitative or other seminal studies may be relatively limited.

The above suggestions draw on various guidelines for systematic reviews including Petticrew (2003) and Petticrew and Roberts (2006).

The Literature Search and Retrieval of Published Evidence Materials

Comprehensive systematic search and retrieval of published evidence materials forms an essential requirement in systematic reviews. Documentation provides an audit trail and helps the reviewers, the target audience, and other readers to judge the exhaustiveness of the search. It also allows for determining the extent of inclusion of the range of research studies that were accessed (Kitchenham, 2004).

Determining the time frame over which the search should cover depends on the nature and complexity of the problem/phenomenon under review and on how rapidly that field of clinical practice has undergone progressive development and change. Therefore, the extent to which the particular problem and the related intervention have been investigated could be an influence (Scottish Intercollegiate Guidelines Network [SIGN], 2011). The search for reports on seminal work should lead to identification of empirical studies if the topic has been explored by experienced researchers. Other high-quality studies from both primary and secondary sources may also be identified. An all-inclusive exploration is advantageous to obtain all available pertinent studies on the topic (Crombie & Davies, 2009; Hemingway & Brereton, 2009; Polit & Beck, 2008).

While it is important to consider a varied range of studies, it is crucial to determine whether the studies are directly or indirectly related to the topic. Therefore, in a preliminary search, particular attention should be paid to potential limitations such as publication preferences and other deficiencies that may influence the range of studies published. Because these can influence the selection of studies for reviews, those problems are considered here.

Use of Approved Set of Eligibility Criteria for Objective Selection of the Studies

The stages of study selection outlined here are derived from various sources; in particular, Kitchenham (2004), Hemingway and Brereton (2009), and Higgins and Green (2011).

- Stage one: Abstract selection. Based on the abstracts, studies that are not relevant to the problem are excluded. Studies deemed relevant to the problem of interest are retained.
- Stage two: Population. Studies are examined for relevance of population/patient characteristics.
- Stage three: Intervention. The studies are examined for the nature of the intervention and its delivery. The exact content and mode of delivery should be stipulated. Other facts could include specifying who delivered the intervention and where that intervention took place. Once again, studies that fall short of the specifications are excluded at this stage.
- Stage four: Comparison. This stage examines the comparison and/or control processes and further exclusions carried out as necessary. Comparators should be specifically defined (Hemingway & Brereton, 2009; Kitchenham, 2004).
- Stage five: Expectation. The indicators of the intervention outcome are used to determine the size, nature, and extent and significance of the effects, both positive and adverse, of a specific intervention. The importance of clearly defining the relevant set of outcomes such as measures of mortality and morbidity, quality of life, and specifically related experiences of physical function should be emphasized. In the case of the participants' experiences, the review may involve qualitative studies or a combination of quantitative and qualitative studies. From that assessment, further exclusion is carried out as necessary (Hemingway & Brereton, 2009; Kitchenham, 2004).
- Stage six: Study design. This stage assesses whether the design employed for the investigation in each study accords with the stipulated indicators for those designs. The designs are meticulously examined, followed by more sensitive analysis at the stage of synthesis or integration of findings (Hemingway & Brereton, 2009; Kitchenham, 2004). Robustness of the study design is often the determining factor for

including a study in the review. However, studies of the same design may not necessarily be of the same high standard and quality. A particular caution relates to the risk of omitting studies that have direct relevance within the context of the review if the set criteria were too narrow and/or too rigidly adhered to. However, unrealistically broad criteria that allow for varied interpretations and application could result in poor and/or complicated comparisons and syntheses (Hemingway & Brereton, 2009; Kitchenham, 2004).

At each of these stages, the specific reason for the exclusion should be documented in the appropriate column indicating the nature of the limitation or deficiency (Hemingway & Brereton, 2009; Kitchenham, 2004; SIGN, 2011).

Extracting Pertinent Data

Data extraction is the process of pulling out essential information about the main aspects and key attributes of individual research studies. Because studies of different designs present variations in methodology, the amount and content of data to be extracted is bound to vary. Key considerations for data extraction depend on the purpose of the review and the specific design of the selected research studies. An appropriately devised set of extraction criteria with a clear and methodical system of documentation helps to achieve the desired consistency and accuracy of extraction. Furthermore, the technique for analyzing the data and the data presentation depend on the key issues conveyed in the review question and objectives (Higgins & Green, 2011; Petticrew & Roberts, 2006; Polit & Beck, 2008). A copy of the data extraction form should be included in the review protocol. Because reviews are carried out on several studies, it is pragmatic to use a well-devised purposeful, tested, and approved data extraction form.

Various formats are available, such as the Cochrane Study Selection, Quality Assessment & Data Extraction Form. Two examples of application that may be of interest to readers are the Data Extraction Form for HIV/AIDS Provider Training, and the Quality assessment for Intervention Studies of HIV/AIDS Provider Training. The successive steps in the process of data extraction presented here are applicable to general review purposes. The important thing is for the team of reviewers to critically examine the content then adapt as necessary to suit the particular purpose of the systematic review.

- Identification comprises the reviewer's initials/allocated identification code and the assigned review reference number.
- For each study, the title, author(s), and publication specifics are recorded. The type of systematic review is recorded together with the study designs,

methodology, and techniques of data collection and analysis. Contact with the original authors may be considered for further clarification at the stage of data analysis (National Institute for Health and Clinical Excellence [NICE], 2006; Noyes et al., 2001; Thomas & Harden, 2008).

- Description of the general baseline characteristics, social and economic circumstances directly relating to the setting and context, delivery of the intervention, and the subsequent interpretation and synthesis of the findings is provided. Additionally, the total number of participants and how recruited, and the total number in the treatment intervention and control groups are also recorded (NICE, 2006; Noyes et al., 2001; Thomas & Harden, 2008).
- The type of treatment interventions and co-interventions, related conceptual/theoretical framework and principles, development and mode of delivery, duration, control, and the staff responsible for administering these are stated (NICE, 2006; Noyes et al., 2001; Thomas & Harden, 2008).
- The predicted outcomes, types, how defined, and calculated, the related baseline measurements, subgroups, exclusions, and withdrawals are stated (NICE, 2006; Noyes et al., 2001; Thomas & Harden, 2008).
- Framework approach for establishing the direct relationships between findings and review question(s) should show the key elements extracted.
- Finally, the social and economic implications of the findings, potential impact of change in clinical contexts, health policy, and cost effectiveness are stated (NICE, 2006; Noyes et al., 2001; Thomas & Harden, 2008).

Clearly, the use of an approved framework with a pre-specified set of criteria helps to achieve efficient and well-organized recording of the extracted data (Petticrew & Roberts, 2006; Polit & Beck, 2008). Moreover, standardization increases confidence in the data extraction process (Hemingway & Brereton, 2009). The selected framework or template must be up to standard and easy for the team to use. While certain versions may be useful for introductory purposes, practitioners and educators are urged to explore more comprehensive, formally designed formats and current electronic and updated versions that continue to emerge.

As the team gains more familiarity with the process of data extraction, modification and pilot testing of the identified data extraction forms becomes more practical and achievable. The sample shown in **Box 3-3** can be further adapted: for example, the inclusion and exclusion criteria could be structured to allow for recording indicators relating to the population, the design, the intervention, and the outcomes with an additional column for specifying the elements that justify exclusion (Khan, Kunz, Kleijnen, & Antes, 2011).

BOX 3-3 Simplified Version of Data Extraction Form

Review author's ID or initial: Date:

Code & unique reference number for the study:

Author(s):   Date:

Study title on the research report:

Publication journal: Year / Vol. / Page numbers:

Study type / characteristics:

   Aim:

   Study design: Duration:

   Inclusion: Exclusion:

   Process of randomization / allocation of participants:

   Total number / sample size:

   Intervention group: Control group:

Participant description:

   Age / age range: Gender: Ethnic origin:

Social & economic background:

   Medical diagnosis: Related health problems:

The study setting / context of interventions:

Details of specific intervention(s):

Specific outcomes: How defined: Type of measurement:

1.   ⟵————⟶   1.

2.   ⟵————⟶   2.

Technique(s) of analysis:

Results per sample group:

Findings:

Comments:

Assessment of the Meticulousness of Each Study Design

Because the process of data extraction in systematic reviews and quality assessment of the research studies are linked, these processes tend to be undertaken concurrently.

Assessment of Risk Bias

The strength and truthfulness of the findings from research studies become doubtful when flaws occur in the design. Shortcomings in research design that adversely affect findings may occur in the form of selection, performance, measurement, and attrition biases (Khan et al., 2011). These can be explained as inadequate allocation procedure; dissimilarities in the characteristics of the participant groups; lack of clarity of the blinding process applied to the participants, the care deliverers, and those who assessed the outcomes; and imbalance in the sample sizes caused by unpredicted dropouts or other losses. Further shortfalls may be attributed to inadequate management and lack of clarity of the intention to treat, the related analysis, and how missing data were accounted for. Each predicted bias should be clearly recorded together with the relevant elements of quality assessment (Khan et al., 2011). The impact of specific risk biases may be rated as high, low, or unclear in relation to causing over- or undervaluation and misrepresentation of the true effects of the intervention. To gain a better understanding of this concept, readers are encouraged to explore Higgins & Altman (2008) in the *Cochrane Handbook for Systematic Reviews of Interventions*.

Assessment of the Suitability of the Statistical Techniques and the Degree of Accuracy

The statistical techniques and methods of analyzing data may depend on the adequacy of the sample size. The sample should be appropriately representative of the population in its components, subgroups, strata, and other relevant characteristics (Higgens & Green, 2011; NICE, 2006).

- Assessment of generalizability.
- In the appraisal of findings, two factors are crucial: (1) the study sample should be representative and should characterize the target population, and (2) the findings

should be generalizable to other populations beyond the study population or participants. The study should have been conducted to closely represent standard current practice. Differing views are proposed about assessment of the generalizability of findings from quantitative and qualitative studies, taking account of the specific designs employed (Higgins & Green, 2011).

- Assessment of the quality of the research report.

The research report should be clear and comprehensible. There should be adequate detail on all important aspects addressed in a full quality appraisal to allow for possible replication of the research process. Reporting on a particular criterion should clearly indicate whether it was met or unmet or lacking in clarity.

While some reporting systems only focus on a scoring system, others require the assessors to provide brief statements on specific aspects of the study. In order to deal with the large number of selected studies in systematic reviews, the use of quality assessment checklists has become quite popular.

The more elaborate assessment forms may have all the criteria stated for each key element assessed. Additionally, instructions on exactly how the scoring should be done may accompany the assessment forms. Guidance may also be provided on how to summarize and interpret the overall grade, the aggregate rate, or the total score.

Readers are encouraged to explore different methods before making a choice (Higgins & Green, 2011; NICE, 2006). Suggested sources of additional reading are included in the reference list, and readers are encouraged to explore the National Collaborating Centre for Methods and Tools (NCCMT) Quality assessment tool for quantitative studies (2008). Khan et al. (2011) and Armijo-Olivo, Stiles, Hagen, Biondo, and Cummings's (2012) *Assessment of Study Quality for Systematic Reviews* are also useful.

Tables 3-1 and **3-2** represent simple pro-formas that can be adapted and applied to assessment of quantitative and qualitative research quality in conjunction with data extraction. These should be regarded as rather broad formats that may require adjustments to meet the purpose for the particular review.

Data Abstraction: Relevance in Systematic Review Data Synthesis and Meta-Analysis

Data abstraction is an important process in systematic review and reviewers/meta-analysts should provide a detailed explanation of the process in the full report. Standardized/

Table 3-1	Exemplar of Pro-Forma for Recording Quantitative Research Quality to Accompany the Data Extraction Process			
Key Elements Assessed	**Appraisal Question**	**Quality Criteria/ Quality Status**	**Rating System and/ or Method of Scoring**	**Notes (Quality Implications for the Systematic Review)**
Specific quantitative design: paradigm	Sampling:			
	Allocation concealment			
RCT	Blinding			
CCT	Confounders			
Other				
Unclear				
Study selection				
Risk bias				
Intervention(s)				
Data collection				
Withdrawals/dropouts				
Specific outcomes:				
How defined				
Specific measures				
Statistical techniques of data analysis	Generalizability of the results and findings			
	Internal validity			
	External validity			
The final report				

Data from National Collaborating Centre for Methods and Tools. (2008). *Quality assessment tool for quantitative studies.* Hamilton, ON: McMaster University. (Updated 30 August 2017). Retrieved from http://www.nccmt,ca/knowkedge-repositories/search/14; Khan, K. S., Kunz, R., Kleijnen, J., & Antes, G. (2011). *Systematic reviews to support evidence-based medicine: How to review and apply findings of health care research* (2nd ed.). London, United Kingdom: Hodder Arnold.

Table 3-2	Exemplar of Pro-Forma for Recording Qualitative Research Quality to Accompany the Data Extraction Process				
Key Elements Assessed	**Appraisal Question**	**Quality Indicators**	**The Quality Status (Adequate Inadequate Uncertain)**	**Notes (Quality Implications for the Systematic Review)**	
Specific qualitative design: paradigm					
Risk bias assessment					
Quality of the study interventions					
Specific outcomes:					
How defined					
Specific measures applied					
Specific methods of analysis					
Generalizability					
Quality of the research report					
(Data from Spencer et al. 2006)					

Table 3-3	A Simplified Format for Data Abstraction								
List or Count of Studies	**Date of Abstraction**	**Study Code or Number**	**Author(s)**	**Study Title**	**Year of Publication**	**Inclusion and Exclusion of Studies Based on Defined Criteria and Reasons**	**Specific Key Elements About the Treatment Intervention**	**Quality of Research Design and Methods (Score)**	**Specific Clinical Details**
							Total number of participants *Intervention group *Control group	Techniques of analysis, type and presentation of the results	

formal data abstraction forms can be adopted for use or an original version created, if properly pilot tested. The completed abstraction form should be incorporated in the final report. The information provided in the data abstraction should convincingly show that the selected and included studies are appropriate for synthesizing and combining the results (Grimshaw et al., 2003).

Experts suggest that the process of abstraction be carried out by at least two members of the review team who should work separately. Additionally, they should be blinded to the original authors of the studies and the institutions in which the studies took place. After comparing the abstractions, any discrepancies should be resolved and clearly documented (Grimshaw et al., 2003). Practitioners and systematic reviewers are urged to explore and critically examine selected data abstraction forms.

The scoring systems also vary. Raw figures, risk ratios, and the results from intention-to-treat analyses should all be reported. The latter relates to analysis of participants regardless of whether they received the intervention or not and regardless of what happened later.

An example of a data abstraction form deriving from various sources, including Grimshaw et al. (2003), is provided in **Table 3-3**. This example is intended simply to illustrate possible development of an abstraction format that draws on existing ones. Depending on the type of review and the specific purpose, review teams might prefer to develop a more suitable abstraction format de novo.

- In the column relating to the inclusion and exclusion criteria, the specific factors should be clearly defined with precise statements or scored against benchmarks. The reasons for exclusion should be concisely stated and the degree of diversity or heterogeneity also stated.

- In the column relating to the study design and methods it may be useful to refer to an existing pro-forma for quality appraisal to determine relevant key elements to look for and allocate appropriate scoring for specific study characteristics including, for example, randomization, allocation concealment, blinding, follow-up, analysis of intention-to-treat, sampling technique, sample size, intervention group, control group, baseline characteristics, and observed outcomes against the projected outcomes.

- In relation to the methods, the type(s) of data, techniques of analysis and presentation of the results, the raw data, the effect size—ratios of odds/risks, and other key results should be examined and appropriately scored.

- The impact of heterogeneity among the studies and related subgroup data and sensitivity analysis should be recorded for assessing the impact of the research quality on the results.

- The identified key strengths and the identified key limitations of the study should be stated and the overall quality score recorded.

- In the column relating to specific clinical details, the type of clinical settings, locations, patient characteristics and participant characteristics, age range, gender, and specific problem of clinical/public health interest relating to the study may be indicated.

Data Synthesis Explored

By and large, studies focusing on healthcare interventions essentially quantify the degree and measure of efficacy. Thus, the positive or negative impact of the specific intervention on the outcomes tends to be documented in numerical or statistical formats as summarized and presented by the researcher(s) in their report. Quantitative research studies tend to involve application of comparable processes of data collection and similar techniques in analyzing the data. Moreover, synthesizing quantitative data involves application of approved specific processes and techniques with strict statistical structuring and exactness in documenting the results. Therefore, combining the findings across studies can be achieved meaningfully (Ring, Ritchie, Mandava, & Jepson, 2010). Primary studies included in reviews of quantitative data are likely to be homogenous in their focus on the same topic and application of comparable research design. Importantly, their similarities also include application of comparable methodology in terms of the type of data, the analysis, and the results.

Various approaches have been proposed for identifying and selecting qualitative studies for synthesizing based on the application of a specific set of criteria for inclusion (**Box 3-4**). As Ring et al. (2010) remarked, some approaches applied to the synthesis of qualitative research studies share similarities to the synthesis of quantitative studies, including the search for identifying relevant primary studies, the use of criteria for inclusion and exclusion, and

---

BOX 3-4 Main Assumptions and Rationales for Synthesizing Qualitative Research Evidence

- Synthesizing qualitative research evidence potentially helps to broaden the scope and depth of existing professional knowledge.

- Qualitative research synthesis enables reviewers to create more contemporary concepts and develop new interpretations from the synthesis of available research evidence. This strengthens the basis for ongoing research.

- Apart from gaining deeper insight about the effects of clinical interventions and aspects of healthcare policy, the synthesis may also help to identify issues requiring more in-depth exploration.

- Furthermore, synthesizing research data helps to establish better understanding about specific problems and phenomena encountered in clinical practice.

- The role of qualitative research synthesis in helping determine the factors that enhance or inhibit the effectiveness of specific therapeutic or interventional services is now recognized.

- Synthesis of qualitative research evidence has the potential for generalizing findings in clinical practice and policy decision-making.

Data from Brown, P., Brunnhuber, K., Chalkidou, K., Chalmers, I., Clarke, C., Fenton, M., . . . Young, P. (2006). How to formulate research recommendations. *BMJ, 333*(7572), 804–806; Finfgeld-Connett, D. (2010). Generalisability and transferability of metasynthesis research finding. *Journal of Advanced Nursing, 66*(2), 246–254; Petticrew, M. (2003). Why certain systematic reviews reach uncertain conclusions. *BMJ, 326*(7392), 756–758; Petticrew, M., & Roberts, H. (2006). *Systematic reviews in the social sciences: A practical guide*. Malden, MA: Blackwell.

---

assessment of the quality of the research studies. Nevertheless, the approaches to qualitative research synthesis and the processes involved tend to be more complex, involving multiple interconnected elements, underpinning thoughts, deductions, and reasoning toward the anticipated goals. The findings tend to be presented in various ways and the interpretations also vary rather than reaching a common understanding. Synthesizing primary qualitative research data presents particular challenges (Ring et al., 2010).

Determining an Appropriate Method for Synthesizing Specific Data

Randomized controlled trails (RCT) remain the preferred methodology and are therefore the more commonly used research design for evaluating healthcare interventions. Meta-analysis is the most frequently applied quantitative technique for data synthesis. However, qualitative research synthesis involving narrative process may also be applied as an acceptable alternative if quantification of the data is not considered practicable. Also, RCTs may not be applicable to many systematic review questions on healthcare issues. Moreover, many systematic reviews do not encompass statistical data and, therefore, meta-analysis may not be applicable for combining results from the studies.

The Benefits and Key Elements of Meta-Analysis

Meta-analysis allows for generalizing the findings from related studies to the target population indicated in those studies. Other benefits are that meta-analysis helps to resolve the problem of professionals missing significant findings from high-standard and quality empirical studies. Nevertheless, in determining whether combining the results from multiple research studies would be feasible, account should be taken of the clinical and statistical significance. Meta-analysis is not always possible or necessary (Khan et al., 2011; Sutton & Higgins, 2008).

Summary of Main Arguments for Quantitative Meta-Analysis

- Meta-analysis offers unbiased synthesis of data from carefully selected experimental or other high-quality quantitative studies. The technique allows for integration of multiple studies, including large empirical research and relatively smaller studies that may have been considered as inconclusive.

- The process offers more detailed statistical calculations with precision, which ensures that relatively minor details that may be significant for clinical decisions in treatments can also be identified and taken into account.

- The merging of results from studies with consistently small numbers of participants effectively increases the total sample size and, therefore, improves the statistical power and generalizability of the findings and results.

- The pooled results from larger numbers of patients/clients provide more valid and convincing information about particular clinical problems and the effects of treatment interventions that may not have been extensively investigated. In this case, pooling may also afford greater confidence in the related clinical decisions.

- Rather than simply reporting the odds ratio of occurrence of a condition among the study group comparative to the control group, meta-analysis allows for calculating the risk ratio or relative risk ratio as well. (Khan et al., 2011; Sutton & Higgins, 2008)

Logical Stages of Meta-Analysis

- Because meta-analysis forms a key component of systematic review, the initial stage begins with that.
- Clearly formulated question of clinical significance. This is important because unfocused and broad questions result in ambiguous criteria and inconsistency in the selection of studies.

- Development of a protocol outlining all stages including the technique of combining the results by meta-analysis. Determining which comparable factors, outcome measures, and summary effect measures to be applied should be stated in the protocol.
- Thorough search of the literature and identification of relevant studies.
- Construction and application of eligibility criteria.
- The selection of pertinent studies guided by predetermined set of eligibility criteria. It is important that the operational definitions provided in the research report are carefully noted and a scoring system applied.
- Methodical data extraction to determine comparability of corresponding elements in the selected studies. These include the type of intervention, outcomes, intention-to-treat, and the particular results that can be effectively combined in the meta-analysis.
- Thorough examination of the studies to ensure that pertinent and seminal studies are selected for inclusion while studies with dubious and non-significant results are rejected. The exact quality standards must be defined for deciding which studies to select for meta-analysis:
  - Type of research design/paradigm and thorough critical examination of the conduct of the study. The sampling technique should be examined for the statistical basis for calculating the sample size.
  - Risk bias assessment should be detailed and methodical. Potential systematic errors and the strategies for dealing with them including the system of randomization—allocation/selection bias.
  - The degree of thoroughness in the implementation of the research intervention should be ascertained and there should be planned procedures for dealing with performance bias.
  - Procedures for reporting inconsistencies in the outcome measures and the intervention effects—detection bias.
  - Publication bias can occur in the process of locating and selecting relevant studies for meta-analysis. These may depend on the direction of the results and whether these are statistically significant. Additionally, language and potential interpretation issues can cause publication bias.
  - The statistical techniques employed. Appraisal of the degree of precision applied in the data collection process, the data analysis, and degree of accuracy of the results.
  - Generalizability.
  - The completeness and quality of the research report. (Khan et al., 2011; Sutton & Higgins, 2008)

Amalgamating Research Study Results: Effect Estimates and Weighted Average

Meta-analysis allows for combining the effects from all the relevant studies to calculate the overall mean effect or the summary estimate. Combining effects from a number of studies requires that they are expressed in the same units. An estimation of the effect size represents the extent of the intervention effect. The effect estimates are based on data obtained from the individual studies, and each study produces a different estimate of the magnitude of the intervention effect. While *individual effects* refers to the observed effects in separate studies, *summary effects* refers to the pooling of the effects from each of the studies in a meta-analysis (Khan et al., 2011).

Each study is weighted according to the exactness of the statistical calculation of the sample size. Weighting also takes account of differences in measurement error between studies. Studies that represent more rigorous precision are given weightier effect estimates than those that do not meet the expected level of rigor and precision. The pooled effects observed across the studies are statistically calculated as a weighted average effect. The process allows for determining which studies' results contributed more significantly to the pooled or sum total—the summary effect. The contribution is proportional to the amount of information in the study. The more empirical studies with larger sample sizes attain heavier weighted average when pooled or amalgamated than those with smaller sample sizes (Crombie & Davies, 2009). Further clarification of the weighting process is provided here, together with the combined effect.

The Fixed-Effect Model

This model is based on the assumption that there is one true effect size and that all the included studies estimate the same effect size. Therefore, the combined effect represents that common true effect size. The weight allocated to each study would represent the amount of information generated by that particular study so that the larger studies yielding more information would be more heavily weighted and the relatively smaller studies less weighted (Borenstein, Hedges, & Rothstein, 2007; Khan et al., 2011). This model upholds that consistency persists in all the studies with no variations in the size of treatment effects, thus implying that there is no statistical heterogeneity in the treatment effects among the studies. Any emerging variation occurring within a particular study can be attributed merely to chance. Therefore, the estimated ratios, for example, as calculated in each of the studies would show equivalent values (Borenstein et al., 2007; Polit & Beck, 2008).

Random-Effects Model of Meta-Analysis

This model holds that the estimation of treatment effects could vary between one study and another and that variations can also occur within the same study. Variations in results may be influenced by how vigorous the campaigns, the type and substance of information, and the amount and depth of the education and counseling support provided to the study groups. Other variations in the results may arise from the duration and persistence of the health promotion campaigns targeting different population groups within colleges and places of employment. The random effects model allows for determining the distribution of effects among the various studies. The effect size may be affected depending on how consistently and accurately the outcomes are measured in each study.

The random effects model accepts variations in the results between studies and within studies so that the weighting of studies combines both of these variances. The studies included in the meta-analysis represent random samples of the particular effects. This model aims to estimate the mean of the true effects across the studies; therefore, the combined effects would be calculated to determine the mean in that distribution. The argument is that while large studies present more precise estimates than smaller studies, variations also occur in the effect sizes among these categories of studies. Each effect size represents a separate sample from the population whose mean value is estimated. Therefore, in the allocation of weights, balancing is achieved whereby the larger studies might not overpower and unbalance the analysis and small studies might not be underestimated. In the random effects model, pooling is feasible when the range and size of variations are noticeably diverse and unexplainable with discrete and disparate effect sizes. Individual studies would be found to have yielded differing values or ratios of intervention effects (Borenstein et al., 2007; Crombie & Davies, 2009; Sutton & Higgins, 2008). Understanding the relevance of these models is necessary to enable reviewers to choose the most appropriate model for analyzing selected studies for the systematic review.

Sensitivity Analysis

Sensitivity analysis allows for comparing the findings from given systematic reviews and meta-analyses to determine if these realistically substantiate rigor and validity in the methods applied. The sensitivity tests may help to establish the impact of excluding certain studies categorized as outliers with distinctly divergent results. Thus, the initial process would involve analysis of the findings from all the selected studies that meet the criteria for inclusion (Khan et al., 2011). Following the initial meta-analysis, a repeat process is carried out involving sensitivity testing. In that repeat analysis, those studies that were originally rejected or excluded because of poor or questionable quality and/or lack of detailed reports would be included in order to compare the results. Thus, sensitivity tests afford a means of testing how sensitive the results are to changes in the conduct of the meta-analysis. A further test may involve the intervention effects across the subgroups identified in the selected studies. This may require conducting separate reviews and meta-analyses for subgroups of patients who are likely to respond differently to the treatment intervention because of different preexisting medical conditions or specific characteristics. Thus, sensitivity analysis allows for taking into consideration the ambiguities and lack of confidence created by information that is lost, omitted, or vague and indistinct. More detailed clarification about the related statistical processes of sensitivity analysis can be explored in the *Cochrane Collaboration Handbook* and other texts by various meta-analysts (www.cochrane. org; Higgins & Green, 2011; Khan et al., 2011).

The Relevance of Homogeneity and Heterogeneity

Homogeneity in meta-analysis is based on the assertion that the statistical quantification of the pooled results from the selected research studies should, for practical purposes, represent the combined effect from numerous comparable studies. Many meta-analysts hold the view that it is crucial to ensure that the observed effects from the individual studies are adequately comparable, equivalent, and consistent. This enables the analyst to convincingly assert that the combined estimate of results through meta-analysis realistically produces a true representation across the selected studies (Crombie & Davies, 2009; Deeks, Altman, & Bradburn, 2001).

Heterogeneity is commonly examined and tested for with regard to the range of variation and bias that occurs in the conduct of research studies and their results. Heterogeneity relates to the inevitable occurrence of multiple differences among studies. It is important to explore in what ways the studies differ, identify the specific types of differences, and establish how those differences might influence the effectiveness of a treatment intervention. Examples of diverse factors that may impact on the nature and extent of intervention effect include the type of disease, seriousness of the condition, and the available resources. Other factors include the environment of care delivery, quality of care provided, and the major consequence of the disease or medical condition, such as death or disability of varied durations. Importantly, interpretations from this technique depend to a large extent on the number of studies examined (Higgins, Thompson, Deeks, & Altman, 2003).

Depending on the nature and degree of diversity, the factors may be categorized as clinical, methodological, or statistical heterogeneity. These effectively describe the identified source of the diversity among the studies. Clinical heterogeneity (diversity) refers to patient-related factors. Thus, gender, age, the exact diagnosis and severity of the condition, and other prescribed medications the patients may be using at the time constitute clinical heterogeneity (Higgins et al., 2003; Khan et al., 2011).

Differences in the research treatment interventions in terms of the exact types, dosage, mode(s) of administration, variations in the intensity of the regimen also fall into the category of clinical heterogeneity. Varied definitions of outcomes; the processes employed to detect, record, and measure them; and varied types of clinical settings and available resources have also been classified as clinical heterogeneity (Higgins et al., 2003; Khan et al., 2011).

Methodological heterogeneity refers to diversity in the study designs in terms of how the studies were conducted.

Differences in the clinical trials may occur in the form of crossover or parallel group studies. Variations may occur in the thoroughness of allocation concealment or blinding against detection bias. Varied durations of treatment interventions and analysis of intention-to-treat may also reveal differences among studies. See *Cochrane Handbook for Systematic Reviews of Interventions*: Cochrane Training (http://training.cochrane.org/handbook).

Statistical heterogeneity refers to variations in the treatment effect. Because meta-analysis is applied to estimate the combined effect of numerous studies, it is necessary to carefully examine the treatment effect in the individual studies. To establish statistical heterogeneity, the estimates of the treatment effect in the individual studies are calculated to ascertain that they are adequately comparable to justify a combined estimate of effect (Higgins et al., 2003; Khan et al., 2011). Meta-analysis essentially seeks to combine studies that have yielded similar intervention effect. The intervention effect may yield positive/favorable or negative/unfavorable results. Statistical heterogeneity indicates diversities in the interventions across the studies. These reflect clinical as well as methodological heterogeneity (Polit & Beck, 2008).

Moreover, analysts look for excessive variation in the estimate of the treatment effect. The presence of excessive variation in the observed treatment effects would suggest statistical heterogeneity. In that case, the systematic reviewer may choose not to carry out meta-analysis, as the result could lead to drawing conclusions that are ambiguous and misrepresent the observed effects in the studies (Khan et al., 2011).

Alternative processes of random effects model, subgroup analysis, and meta-regression may be applied. These allow for establishing the reasons for the occurrence of variations in treatment effects in different studies. Brief overviews of these processes are provided.

Meta-Regression and Subgroup Analysis

Calculation of the combined effect size would be questionable and probably lead to inaccurate clinical decisions if wide-ranging heterogeneity across the studies is disregarded. Therefore, it is crucial that review teams and practitioners should ascertain if the treatment effect is likely to vary in different circumstances and in what ways. The disparity in the effects could make the appropriateness of this stage of the meta-analysis questionable and unjustified. Meta-regression allows for examining the types and nature of diversities and the extent to which particular factors influence the intervention outcomes and indeed, the effect size (Polit & Beck, 2008).

Subgroup analysis focuses the meta-analysis on the specific subgroups of participants involved in the studies. In order to avoid errors and drawing ambiguous conclusions, early determination of what groupings will be investigated and analyzed is important. Experts maintain that carrying out subgroup analysis at the later stage of the meta-analysis and after the results have been calculated could create bias in the reporting of the results.

Subgroup analysis may not give clear or full information about how specific variations in the mode of administration of the intervention treatment affected the outcomes (Khan et al., 2011; Noyes et al., 2011). Additionally, subgroup analysis may not reveal or confirm exactly how varied are those observed outcomes among the subgroups from the population studied. Any observed variations could be attributable to particular factors in the characteristics of one subgroup or another. Experts suggest that conclusions from subgroup analysis should be viewed with caution and interpreted tentatively because they derive from subdivisions of studies and contrasts rather than precise scientific statistical tests.

While meta-analysis allows for investigating the extent to which specific study characteristics might be associated with specific intervention effects, meta-regression goes a stage further. For example, meta-analysis could be used for investigating the impact of carefully planned and methodically delivered behavior-change program for one group of study participants and the observed results may show greater degree of effective positive outcome. However, a participant group (a control group) who were not exposed to that behavior-change program would show different outcome effects. This means that two subgroups under investigation may yield different treatment effects in meta-analysis due to certain factors in the study design.

Meta-regression provides a means to identify the specific factors that may have contributed to disparities (Borenstein, Hedges, Higgins, & Rothstein, 2009). However, meta-regression may not be entirely appropriate for assessing differences in treatment effects.

Various processes have been proposed such as determining the relationship between specific factors, study and/or patient characteristics, and the magnitude of effect observed in each study. Nevertheless, systematic reviewers, practitioners, and decision-makers are cautioned that these tests are not entirely flawless. They may have low statistical power and may fall short of revealing all the disparities present in the studies and the results. Meta-regression requires that each study be allocated an appropriate estimated weight. Moreover, careful decision should be made regarding an appropriate effects model that is applicable to meta-regression. Many experts consider the random-effects model to be more appropriate for analyzing variations between studies for the purposes meta-regression (Borenstein et al., 2009).

Summary data incorporates the averages of effect size, severity of disease and length of follow-up. Meta-regression seeks to explore the influence of study characteristics on the size of the effects observed in systematic reviews and/or meta-analysis. However, meta-regression is unable to directly link specific patient factors to the size of treatment effect. Nonetheless, the size of treatment effect may be lost if continuous data with constant/countless number of values were converted to dichotomous data with only two possible values of presence/existence or absence/non-existence. Therefore, regression based on individual patient data may have to be employed to address that limitation (Borenstein et al., 2009).

Reflective Considerations

The following reflective activity can be undertaken on individual basis, in pairs, or in small groups. The summary outline is intended to provide ideas that may serve as directions and/or broad objectives for systematic review teams or colleagues in the multidisciplinary team.

Taking account of the setting, participants, interventions, outcomes, research designs, and methods employed in the studies, carefully reflect on the following:

- Consider the problem of **hospital-acquired infection** and formulate a problem title, questions, and objectives to be explored for systematic review with a view to implementing a feasible intervention in the context of EBP.

- Consider the preliminary stages of literature search and perusal activities.

- Consider the development of a protocol and develop an outline of the key components that should be incorporated for an achievable in-house EBP implementation.

- Consider which members of the multidisciplinary team could effectively participate in the systematic review team.

- Consider which clinical leads could be involved in an advisory committee.

- Discuss the stages of the actual literature review and possible components of a simple format for data extraction and consider a clear format for data abstraction.

- Consider the selection of the pertinent studies; outline the main criteria for inclusion and exclusion.

- Consider the key components of quality appraisal of the selected research studies for classification of the levels of evidence.

- Consider what factors may influence meta-analysis or meta-synthesis of the findings from the included studies.

- Consider the question, "Is the review team confident that combining and meta-analyzing the study results/findings would be pragmatic, meaningful, and consequential for guiding clinical decisions?"

- Consider possible intervention(s) that might be feasible to implement in this scenario.

- Consider what additional steps might be necessary to produce substantial information for drawing conclusions and making recommendations to inform relevant clinical decisions and action plans by the policy/decision-makers.

Reporting and Appraising the Meta-Analysis

The following section considers the importance of detailed reporting of completed meta-analysis. The framework Preferred Reporting Items for Systematic Reviews and Meta-Analysis (PRISMA) is examined here. Practitioners are encouraged to explore and to carefully examine the full PRISMA statement together with the underpinning principles, recommendations, and correct application.

The following key elements derive from the PRISMA checklist and may usefully guide correct development, reporting, and evaluating to finalize completion of in-house systematic review projects and meta-analysis. Detailed, accurate, and transparent reporting is essential if effective judgment is to be made for possible application to evidence-based clinical decision making and care provision.

Box 3-5 presents concise outlines of the main components of the PRISMA frame and draws on the model developed by Moher, Liberati, Tetzlaff, and Altman (2009). Practitioners are encouraged to examine these critically and compare with the original authors' model.

The Role of Narrative Synthesis

Narrative synthesis involves synthesis/integration of evidence relating to effectiveness and other questions in a narrative. The process involves compiling the findings from studies included in a systematic review and summarizing them in textual form (Rodgers et al., 2009). The current recommendation is that all numeric tables presented in systematic reviews should be accompanied by narrative text. Apart from providing an explanation and summary of the main characteristics of the results and findings of the included studies, it also provides an analysis of the variations within and between studies (Noyes, Popay, Pearson, Hannes, & Booth, 2008). An overall judgment of the strength of the evidence should also be stated. Narrative synthesis is necessarily carried out when the studies are found to be overly diverse in terms of clinical and methodological variations to allow for combining the data in meta-analysis. However, some amount of narrative description is necessary to integrate and interpret the evidence. Nevertheless, it is contended that narrative synthesis is not strictly objective but can be potentially subjective compared to the rigor and precision of meta-analysis. To avoid or minimize potential bias, the process should be performed in a strictly methodical manner, detailed and transparent enough to be repeatable, although this could prove to be difficult to achieve (Noyes et al., 2011; Rodgers et al., 2009).

Framework for Narrative Synthesis

Different frameworks have been proposed as a guide for carrying out narrative synthesis and specific formal guidance should be explored. In particular, readers would find it useful to read Popay et al.'s (2006) *Guidance to the Conduct of Narrative Synthesis in Systematic Reviews* and Rodgers et al.'s (2009) *Testing Methodological Guidance on the Conduct of Narrative Synthesis in Systematic Reviews*.

The framework for narrative synthesis comprises four key elements, each of which are addressed by employing particular tools and techniques (Popay et al., 2006). The important thing is to carefully consider which tool would be appropriate for fulfilling the purpose of the review question and the evidence being synthesized.

Transforming Data

Different statistical counts and measurements are used in presenting the data from research studies, and, in quantitative studies, the type of data is predominantly numerical. The initial figures may be in the form of raw data, which may be calculated into summary data or expressed in different statistical figures. In order to enhance the accuracy of the description of the effects, devising a common system of measures to transform the data is necessary. For example, dichotomous data may be converted or transformed into odds ratio, risk ratio, relative risk, and risk difference. Continuous data may be presented in the form of weighted mean difference or standard mean difference. For the purposes of meta-analysis, results from studies may be combined to produce an estimate of effect (Popay et al., 2006; Rodgers et al., 2009). Transforming data helps present results in easy-to-understand ways, and the range of effects from research interventions can be measured and calculated more accurately. This statistical technique is not applicable to narrative synthesis.

Vote-Counting

Vote-counting provides another tool for producing descriptive summary data and involves counting up and calculating the frequency of different types of research results from the studies included in the review. Vote-counting can be used to establish patterns across the studies. In reviews relating to evaluation of intervention effects, vote-counting may be used for tabulating significant and non-significant results (Popay et al., 2006). Thus, this tool is useful for recording findings that may be tabulated according to the direction of the effect. More current techniques of vote-counting continue to be proposed, and the idea of counting and calculating by categories and allocation of weights and scores have emerged as alternative concepts. Despite its potential usefulness, this tool tends to be considered questionable, overly simplistic, and not very informative to provide adequate statistical detail and may not be chosen for high-level synthesis. Nonetheless, some prefer to use it as a way of establishing occurrence or non-occurrence and for counting frequencies. Therefore, it may be useful in supporting specific observations made in the studies.

Similar to the different practices of vote-counting, varied interpretations of the counts have also been proposed.

BOX 3-5 Concise Outline of the Key Elements in the Appraising and Reporting of Meta-Analysis Using the PRISMA Frame

---

PRISMA: The principles and guidelines

Title

This should inform the wider target audience what this evaluation is about. If both systematic review and meta-analysis had been carried out these should be clearly indicated in the title.

Abstract

The abstract should be competently written to convey what the report is about in terms of the focus, context, and the processes involved in the meta-analysis.

Introduction

The introduction should clearly state the rationale and the objectives for the review and meta-analysis if both were performed.

Methods

The required details for this section should include the following:

- Protocol and details of registration if applicable
- Eligibility criteria
- Information sources and databases used and direct contacts with researchers
- Search in terms of full search strategy
- Study selection in terms of the processes of screening and inclusion
- Data collection process in terms of the data extraction, pilot testing, and measures taken to obtain and verify required details from relevant original researchers
- Data items in terms of all the key variables for which data were sought
- Risk of bias in individual studies, assessed and at what levels and how applied to the synthesizing of the data
- Summary measures employed to risk ratio or difference in mean
- Synthesis of results in terms of the detailed methods employed in amalgamating the results of the studies and consistency testing in the meta-analyses
- Risk of bias across studies in terms of selective reporting and publication bias and the potential impact

- Additional analyses in terms of pre-specified methods such as sensitivity analysis, meta-regression, subgroup analysis

Results

- Study selection with use of a flow diagram
- Study characteristics including PICOS, study size, and duration of follow-up and relevant citations
- Risk of bias within studies and outcome level assessment
- Results of individual studies in terms of simple summary data with compliance to the recommended use of forest plot
- Synthesis of results with presentation of the main review results and if meta-analysis done inclusion of the confidence intervals and measures of consistency for each
- Risk of bias across studies with presentation of the results of the assessment or the risk bias
- Additional analysis relating to the presentation of the results of the subgroup analysis, sensitivity analysis, and meta-analysis

Discussion

- Summary of the key findings and the significance and relevance of each main outcome, to the major groups of stakeholders
- Limitations in terms of examining the risk of bias at study and outcome level, biases relating to incomplete study retrieval and reporting bias at the review level
- Conclusion conveying a general interpretation of the results in the context of other evidence and implications for future research

Funding

- Funding should be addressed in terms of the sources for the systematic review, the role of the funders, and envisaged implications for the supply of data.

Readers are encouraged to explore the full document for more detailed information. (Partly draws on Moher et al., 2009)

Modified from Moher, D., Liberati, A., Tetzlaff, J., Altman, D.G., & The Prisma Group. (2009). Preferred reporting items for systematic reviews and meta-analyses: The PRISMA Statement. *PLoS Med*, 6(7), e1000097.

In relation to vote-counting by categories, the interpretation is based on the number of studies in each category so that the category with the highest count of studies is placed topmost. The top category is considered as showing the true size of effect estimate and carrying a higher level of statistical significance as compared to the other categories with a lesser number of studies (Popay et al., 2006; Rodgers et al., 2009). However, this concept is questionable because of equal weighting of studies with dissimilar sample sizes and effect sizes. Contrariwise, the category with the least vote-counts is considered as carrying low statistical significance and is therefore placed at the bottom. Thus, interpretation of results from vote-counting should be considered only tentatively in the synthesis of data.

Table 3-4	Tools and Techniques to Explore Relationships Within and Among Studies
Tool/Technique	**Examples/Notes**
Graphs	Frequency of distribution—# of times a variable appears
	Forest plots—results of individual studies
	Funnel plots—establish biases in smaller studies
Other graphical tools: • Conceptual models • Idea webbing • Concept mapping • Investigator, methodologies, and conceptual triangulation	
Translation	Comparable accounts (reciprocal)
	Opposing accounts (refute translations)
Qualitative case descriptions	Describes differences in statistical findings among studies

Translation of Data

Thematic analysis allows for identifying and analyzing the key concepts and themes that repeatedly occur among several selected studies (Thomas & Harden, 2008). The technique is conventionally used in qualitative research analysis but many researchers also use this in mixed qualitative and quantitative research studies and even in some quantitative studies (Flemming, 2010a). Just as conceptual themes are identified in qualitative research data, the labels applied to specific variables in quantitative research can also be identified as themes or concepts. Therefore, although thematic analysis was originally developed for application to primary qualitative research studies, the data may be converted into frequencies. While this technique involves an inductive process, the conclusions drawn and the conceptual assumptions must derive directly from the research findings (Noyes et al., 2011; Popay et al., 2006; Rodgers et al., 2009).

Some systematic reviewers question the degree of transparency in thematic analysis because it may not be entirely straightforward to determine how the themes and concepts were developed or at what stages of the study. The results of the synthesis involving thematic analysis may not be similar enough to synthesize based on a theory-guided approach. Therefore, to strengthen the transparency of thematic analysis, details of the entire analysis must be clearly and meticulously explained in the researcher's report (noyes et al, 2011; Popay et al., 2006; Rodgers et al., 2009).

Content analysis has been explained as a technique for condensing the amount of content in a text into much reduced content. The textual descriptive data is condensed and structured into fewer categories by applying specific rules and coding system (Popay et al., 2006; Rodgers et al., 2009). In this way, the technique of content analysis serves the purpose of arranging, categorizing, and summarizing the research findings, which should be carried out methodically. The quantitative element of content analysis requires that the data should be converted into frequencies. However,

familiarity with the related theorization and concepts enables the researcher to apply qualitative principles in determining and describing the relevant categories of the key elements in the findings (Flemming, 2010b).

Table 3-4 lists the main tools and techniques that can be used for exploring relationships within and among studies.

Multiple Terminologies and Models of Synthesizing Qualitative Research Evidence

There is an assumption that the different approaches to synthesizing share the common principle of pooling findings from primary qualitative research studies (Finfgeld-Connett, 2010). However, while some approaches focus simply on the process of synthesizing the data, others adopt a wider scope. The latter approaches tend to encompass the essential elements and processes from problem identification to appraisal of the quality of research studies and writing a full report. Some consider the idea of synthesizing the findings from several qualitative research studies as questionable and not possible to achieve. They maintain that the varied methodologies with different theoretical basis that typify qualitative research could present potential flaws in the process of synthesizing. Systematic reviewers and professional practitioners are encouraged to read Barnett-Page and Thomas's (2009) critical review of the methods for the synthesis of qualitative research. Synthesizing and integrating the findings from mixed and varied qualitative methodologies can prove useful for making and supporting clinical decisions (Finfgeld-Connett, 2010).

Alternative Approaches to Qualitative Research Synthesis

The various descriptive terms applied to the different approaches are quite numerous and may prove to be confusing, and as many as 15 have been proposed. Some approve the characteristics of qualitative methodology while others advocate converting qualitative results and findings to quantitative form such as content analysis. However, this practice is considered unnecessary. Some terms are used ambiguously or interchangeably, such as meta-synthesis and meta-study to describe any form of qualitative synthesis. In particular, the use of the term *meta-synthesis* is challenged because it is not specific to qualitative research and often used incorrectly. Experts argue that this depends on the level at which this term is applied, whether the synthesizing or the level of included studies (Dixon-Woods, Agarwal, Jones, Young, & Sutton, 2005). Despite all these considerations, the choice of practice or the process should be guided by the review question, the quantity of relevant studies, and the knowledge and competence within the team for conducting systematic reviews and synthesis of the research findings. A range of practices are explored in **Table 3-5**.

The challenge of qualitative research synthesis in systematic reviews is choosing an approach that will help to produce pertinent conclusions that are convincing. It is crucial that findings from the synthesis are presented in a way that would be easy for policy makers, decision-makers, and practitioners to make sense of and translate into the context of clinical practice.

Table 3-5	Alternative Approaches to Qualitative Research Synthesis
Alternative Approach	**Examples/Notes**
Meta-ethnography (reciprocal translation analysis)	Comparing and synthesizing study results to establish if the same concepts occur in different studies
Grounded theory synthesis (constant comparative method)	Develop concepts from the qualitative data by carrying out simultaneous coding and analyzing Four stages: 1. Comparing occurrences that relate to individual categories 2. Integrating the categories according to their properties 3. Delimiting the emerging theory 4. Reporting in detail
Meta-study	Three phases: 1. Meta-theory 2. Meta-method 3. Meta-data analysis
Critical interpretive synthesis	Draws on meta-ethnography and incorporates elements of grounded theory
Thematic synthesis	Three stages: 1. Developing codes of themes from the word-based findings 2. Organizing the codes into appropriate categories of descriptive themes 3. Producing analytical themes
Textual narrative	Suitable for organizing the studies into homogenous sets
Meta-narrative	Synthesize research findings addressing a variety of theories
Meta-summary	Involves converting qualitative findings into quantitative form and applying statistical techniques for analyzing data
Meta-interpretation	Ultimate goal is to establish meaning through methodical interpretation
Qualitative cross-case analysis	A typical feature of this approach it the use of tables or matrices to summarize the data across qualitative and quantitative research studies
Realist synthesis	Applications of this approach focus on complex social interventions to establish the reasons why these may be successful or unsuccessful in certain contexts
Framework synthesis	Organizes qualitative data using numerical codes for indexing and presents the data in graphs or diagrams
Ecological triangulation	Aims to establish associations between individuals, population groups, behaviors, age, gender, ethnicity, interventions, outcome, environments, and specific settings

The following references provide additional sources for more detail on approaches to synthesizing qualitative research evidence:

- Barnett-Page, E., & Thomas, J. (2009). Methods for the synthesis of qualitative research: A critical review. *BMC Medical Research Methodology, 9, 59.*

- Campbell, R., Pound, P., Morgan, M., Daker-White, G., Britten, N., Pill, R., . . . Donovan, J. (2011). Evaluating meta-ethnography: Systematic analysis and synthesis of qualitative research. *Health Technology Assessment, 15*(43), 1–164.

- Garside, R. (2008). Methods for synthesizing qualitative evidence [Online workshop]. Retrieved from Centre for Knowledge Translation for Disability and Rehabilitation Research (KTDRR) website: at http://www.ktdrr.org./training/workshops/qual/index.html

- Pawson, R., Greenhalgh, T., Harvey, G., & Walshe, K. (2004). *Realist synthesis: An introduction.* Manchester, United Kingdom: ESRC Research Methods Programme. Retrieved from http://www.researchgate.net/publication228855827_Realist_Synthesis_An_Introduction.

- Williams, T. L., & Shaw, R. L. (2016). Synthesising qualitative research: Meta-synthesis in sport and exercise. Routledge Handbook of Qualitative Res Sport and Exercise. Chapter 21. Williams, T. L. & Shaw R. L. Abingdon, United Kingdom: Routledge.

Conclusion

Systematic reviews, meta-analysis, and synthesis of qualitative research evidence are crucial for the implementation of research findings to substantiate all aspects of evidence-based practice. Many healthcare practitioners share the view that systematic reviews are intended to advise, update, and substantiate policy decisions and professional practice. Recommendations to guide professional practice are based on extensive and thoroughly examined evidence from high-quality empirical studies and are therefore considered to be trustworthy for supporting decisions about care and service provision. However, many practitioners are challenged by a deluge of new research evidence, new information, and new additional professional knowledge.

This chapter set out to explore systematic reviews and the synthesizing of quantitative and qualitative research evidence. A range of related methods and processes have been examined including meta-analysis and content analysis applied to quantitative and mixed-method research as well as different approaches to qualitative research synthesis. It is important that the methods selected for exploring, explaining, planning, implementing, and evaluating systematic reviews are carefully selected to produce practical and realistic conclusions and recommendations.

Clearly, efficient implementation of evidence-based practice is crucial and it is important that practitioners adopt EBP with adequate understanding and familiarity with the related concepts, principles, and processes. This practice should be in place for examining all in-house reports from systematic reviews and meta-analysis as well as published complete reports that have relevance to the particular field and area of practice.

The need to pursue appropriate training has become inevitable in contemporary professional practice for acquiring adequate knowledge and insight about systematic reviews linked to evidence-based practice. Review teams and their colleagues in multidisciplinary settings should engage in formally organized and informal reflective activities prior to and following every in-house systematic review project. Therefore, the significance of appropriate preparation and efficient implementation must also receive careful consideration.

● ● ● REFERENCES

Armijo-Olivo, S., Stiles, C. R., Hagen, N. A., Biondo, P. D., Cummings, G. G. (2012). Assessment of study quality for systematic reviews: A comparison of the Cochrane Collaboration Risk of bias tool and the Effective public health practice project quality assessment tool: Methodological Research. *Journal of Evaluation in Clinical Practice, 18*(1), 12–18.

Barnett-Page, E., & Thomas, J. (2009). *Methods for the synthesis of qualitative research: A critical review.* London, United Kingdom: Evidence for Policy and Practice Information and Co-ordinating (EPPI) Centre, Social Science Research Unit.

Borenstein, M., Hedges, L. V., & Rothstein, H. R. (2007). *Meta-analysis: Fixed effect vs. random effects.* Retrieved from https://www.meta-analysis.com/downloads/M-a_f_e_v_r_e_sv.pdf

Borenstein, M., Hedges, L. V., Higgins J. P. T., & Rothstein, H. R. (2009). *Introduction to meta-analysis.* Hoboken, NJ: John Wiley & Sons Ltd.

Brown, P., Brunnhuber, K., Chalkidou, K., Chalmers, I., Clarke, C., Fenton, M., . . . Young, P. (2006). How to formulate research recommendations. *BMJ, 333*(7572), 804–806.

Brown, C. E., Wickline, M. A., Ecoff, L., & Glaser, D. (2009). Nursing practice, knowledge, attitudes and perceived barriers to evidence-based practice at an academic medical centre. *Journal of Advanced Nursing, 65*(2), 371–381.

Centre for Reviews and Dissemination. (2009). *Systematic reviews: CRD's Guidance for undertaking reviews in health care.* York, United Kingdom: Author.

Crombie, I. K., & Davies, H. T. O. (2009). *What is meta-analysis?* London, United Kingdom: Hayward Medical Communications, Hayward Group Ltd.

Deeks, J. J., Altman, D. G., & Bradburn, M. J. (2001). Statistical methods for examining heterogeneity and combining results from several studies in meta-analysis. In M. Egger, G. D. Smith, & D. G.

Altman (Eds.), *Systematic reviews in health care: Meta-analysis in context.* (2nd ed.). London, United Kingdom: BMJ Publishing Group.

Dixon-Woods, M., Agarwal, S., Jones, B., Young, B., & Sutton, A. (2005). Qualitative and quantitative evidence: a review of possible methods. *Journal of Health Services Research & Policy, 10*(1), 45–53.

Finfgeld-Connett, D. (2010). Generalisability and transferability of metasynthesis research finding. *Journal of Advanced Nursing, 66*(2), 246–254.

Flemming, K. (2010a). *The synthesis of qualitative and quantitative research: Its role in producing an evidence base for practice.* London, United Kingdom: Royal College of Nursing.

Flemming, K. (2010b). The synthesis of qualitative and quantitative research: an example of critical interpretive synthesis. *Journal of Advances in Nursing, 66*(1), 201–217.

Gagan, M., & Hewitt-Taylor, J. (2004). The issues of nurses involved in implementing evidence in practice. *British Journal of Nursing, 13*(20), 1216–1220.

Grimshaw, J., McAuley, L., Bero, L.A., Grilli, R., Oxman, A.D., Ramsay, C., . . . Zwarenstein, M. (2003). Systematic reviews of the effectiveness of quality improvement strategies and programs. *Quality & Safety in Health Care, 12*(4), 293–303.

Hemingway, P., & Brereton, N. (2009). *What is systematic review?* Kings Hill, United Kingdom: Hayward Group Ltd.

Higgins, J. P. T., & Altman, D. G. (2008). Assessing risk of bias in included studies. In J.P.T. Higgins & S. Green (Eds.), *Cochrane handbook for systematic reviews of interventions* (Ver. 5.0.0). Retrieved from www.cochrane-handbook.org.

Higgins, J. P. T., & Green, S. (Eds.). (2011). *Cochrane Handbook for systematic reviews of interventions* (Ver. 5.1.0). Retrieved from www.cochrane-handbook.org

Higgins, J. P. T., Thompson, S. G., Deeks, J. J., & Altman, D. G. (2003). Measuring inconsistency in meta-analysis. *BMJ, 327,* 557–560.

Khan, K. S., Kunz, R., Kleijnen, J., & Antes, G. (2011). *Systematic reviews to support evidence-based medicine: How to review and apply findings of health care research* (2nd ed.). London, United Kingdom: Hodder Arnold.

Kitchenham, B. (2004). *Procedures for performing systematic reviews: Joint technical report.* Keel, United Kingdom: Keel University.

Lo Biondo-Wood, G., & Haber, J. (2013). *Nursing research: methods and critical appraisal for evidence-based practice.* (8th ed.). Philadelphia, PA: Elsevier-Mosby.

Millward, L., Kelly, M., & Nutbeam, D. (2001). *Public health intervention research: The evidence.* London, United Kingdom: Health Development Agency.

Moher, D., Liberati, A., Tetzlaff, J., & Altman, D. G. (2009). Preferred reporting items for systematic reviews and meta-analyses: The PRISMA statement. *Open Medicine, 3*(3), 123–130.

National Collaborating Centre for Methods and Tools. (2008). *Quality assessment tool for quantitative studies.* Hamilton, ON: McMaster University. (Updated 30 August 2017). Retrieved from http://www.nccmt,ca/knowkedge-repositories/search/14

National Institute for Health and Clinical Excellence (NICE). (2006). *Methods for development of NICE public health guidance.* London, United Kingdom: Author.

Noyes, J., Booth A., Hannes, K., Harden, A., Harris, J., Lewin, S., & Lockwood, C. (Eds.). (2011). *Supplementary guidance for inclusion of qualitative research in cochrane systematic reviews of interventions.* Cochrane Collaboration Qualitative Methods Group. Retrieved from http://cqrmg.cochrane.org/supplemental-handbook-guidance

Noyes, J., Popay, J., Pearson, A., Hannes, K., & Booth, A. (2008). *Qualitative research and cochrane review.* Chichester, United Kingdom: John Wiley & Sons.

Oxman, A. D. (1993). Meta-statistics: help or hindrance? *ACP Journal Club, 118,* A13. doi:10.7326/ACPJC-1993-118-3-A13

Petticrew, M. (2003). Why certain systematic reviews reach uncertain conclusions. *BMJ, 326*(7392), 756–758.

Petticrew, M., & Roberts, H. (2006). *Systematic reviews in the social sciences: A practical guide.* Malden, MA: Blackwell.

Polit, D.F., & Beck, C.T. (2008). Translating research evidence into nursing practice: Evidence-based nursing. D.F. Polit & C.T. Beck (Eds.), *Nursing research: Generating and assessing evidence for nursing practice* (8th ed., pp. 28–54.) London, United Kingdom: Lippincott Williams & Wilkins.

Popay, J., Roberts, H., Sowden, A., Petticrew, M., Arai, L., Rodgers, M., et al. (2006a). *Guidance on the conduct of Narrative Synthesis in Systematic Reviews: A product from the ESRC Methods Programme.* Retrieved from http://www.lancs.ac.uk/shm/research/nssr/research/dissemination/publications.php

Ring, N., Ritchie, K., Mandava, L., & Jepson, R. (2010). *A guide to synthesising qualitative research for researchers undertaking health technology assessments and systematic reviews.* Retrieved from http://www.healthcareimprovementscotland.org/our_work/technologies_and_medicines/programme_resources/synthesising_research.aspx

Rodgers, M., Sowden, A., Petticrew, M., Arai, L., Roberts, H., Britten, N., & Popay, J. (2009). Testing methodological guidance on the conduct of narrative synthesis reviews: Effectiveness of interventions to promote smoke alarm ownership and function. *Evaluation, 15*(1), 47–71.

Sandelowski, M. (2008). Reading, writing and systematic review. *Journal of Advanced Nursing, 64*(1), 104–110.

Scottish Intercollegiate Guidelines Network (SIGN). (2011). *SIGN 50 A: guideline developer's handbook.* Edinburgh, United Kingdom: Author.

Spencer, L., Ritchie, J., Lewis, J., Dillon, L. (2003). *Quality in qualitative evaluation: A framework for assessing research evidence.* London, United Kingdom: Government Chief Social Researcher's Office.

Sutton, A. J., & Higgins, J. P. (2008). Recent developments in meta-analysis. *Statistics in Medicine, 27,* 625–650.

Thomas, J., & Harden, A. (2008). Methods for the thematic synthesis of qualitative research in systematic reviews. *BMC Medical Research Methodology, 8*(45), 1–10.

● ● ● SUGGESTED FURTHER READING

For additional detailed information, readers may wish to explore other useful sources related to the references listed here. The following may also prove to be useful texts for further reading and additional resources.

Altman, D. (2013). *Systematic reviews: Key principles of their development and reporting.* The Equator Network Workshop. Geneva, Switzerland: World Health Organization.

Doody, C. M., & Doody, O. (2011).Introducing evidence into nursing practice: using the IOWA model. *British Journal of Nursing, 20*(11), 661–664.

Edwards, M., Davies, M., & Edwards, A. (2009). What are the external influences on information exchange and shared decision-making in healthcare consultations: A meta-synthesis of the literature. *Patient Education and Counseling, 75*(1), 37–52.

Flemming, K. (2007).The knowledge base for evidence based nursing: a role for mixed methods research. *Advances in Nursing Science, 30*(1), 41–51.

Garside, R. (2014). Should we appraise the quality of qualitative research reports for systematic reviews, and if so how? *Innovation: The European Journal of Social Science Research, 27*(1), 67–79.

Gough, D. (2007). Weight of evidence: A framework for the appraisal of the quality and relevance of evidence. *Research Papers in Education, 22*(2), 213–228.

Gough, D. A., Oliver, S., & Thomas, J. (2012). *An introduction to systematic reviews.* London, United Kingdom: Sage.

Hannes, K. (2011). Chapter 4; Critical appraisal of qualitative research. In: Noyes, J., Booth, A., Hannes, K., Harden, A., Harris, J., Lewin, S., Lockwood, C. (Editors), *Supplementary Guidance for Inclusion of Qualitative Research in Cochrane Systematic Reviews of Interventions.* Version 1 (Updated August 2011). Cochrane Collaboration Qualitative Methods Group, 2011. Retrieved from: http://methods.cochrane.org/qi/supplemental-handbook-guidance

Harris, R.P., Helfand, M., Woolf, S.H., Lohr, K.N., Mulrow, C.D., Teutsch, S.M., . . . Third US Preventive Services Task Force (2001). (2001). Current methods of the US Preventive Services Task Force: A review of the process. *American Journal of Preventive Medicine, 20*(Suppl. 3), 21–35.

Jesson, J., Matheson, L., Lacey, F. M. (2011). *Doing your literature review: traditional and systematic techniques.* London, United Kingdom: Sage.

Johnston, L. (2005). Critically appraising quantitative evidence. In B.M. Melnyk & E. Fineout Overholt (Eds.), *Evidence-based practice in nursing and healthcare: A guide to best practice.* Philadelphia, PA: Lippincott Williams & Wilkins.

Kolb, S. M. (2012). Grounded theory and the constant comparative method: Valid research strategies for educators. *Journal of Emerging Trends in Educational Research and Policy Studies, 3*(1), 83–86.

Liberati, A., Altman, D.G., Tetzlaff, J., Mulrow, C., Gotzsche, P.C., Ioannidis, J.P.A., . . . Moher, D. (2009). The PRISMA statement for reporting systematic reviews and meta-analyses of studies that evaluate health care interventions: Explanation and elaboration. *PLoS Medicine, 6*(7), e1000100. doi:10.1371/ Journal.pmed.1000100

McCormack, B., Wright, J., Dewar, B., Harvey, G., & Ballantine, K. (2007). A realist synthesis of evidence relating to practice development. *Practice Development in Health Care, 6*(1), 5–24.

Melnyk, B. M., & Fineout-Overholt, E. (Eds.). (2014). *Evidence-based practice in nursing and healthcare: A guide to best practice.* Philadelphia, PA: Lippincott Williams & Wilkins.

Noblit, G. W., & Hare, R. D. (1988). *Meta-ethnography: Synthesizing qualitative studies.* Newbury Park, CA: Sage.

Oliver, S., Rees, R., Clarke-Jones, L., Milne, R., Oakley, A., Gabbay, J., . . . Gyte, G. (2008). A multidimensional conceptual framework for analysing public involvement in health services research. *Health Expectations, 11*(1), 72–84.

Paterson, B.L., Thorne, S.E., Canam, C., & Jillings, C. (2001). *Meta-study of qualitative health research: A practical guide to meta-analysis and meta-synthesis.* Thousand Oaks, CA: Sage.

Popay, J., Roberts, H., Snowden, A., Petticrew, M., Arai, L., Rodgers, M., et al. (2006b). *Guidance on the conduct of narrative synthesis in systematic reviews: Final Report.* Swindon, United Kingdom: ESRC Methods Programme.

Pope, C., Mays, N., & Popay, J. (2007). *Synthesising qualitative and quantitative health evidence: A guide to methods.* Maidenhead, United Kingdom: Open University Press; McGraw-Hill.

Rees, C. (2010). Understanding evidence and its utilisation in nursing practice. In K. Holland (Ed.), *Nursing: Evidence-based practice skills.* Oxford, United Kingdom: Oxford University Press.

Robson, C. (2011). *Real world research* (4th ed.). Chichester, United Kingdom: John Wiley and Sons Ltd.

Rodgers, M., Arai, L., Britten, N., Petticrew, M., Popay, J., Roberts, H., & Sowden, A. (2006). *Narrative synthesis in systematic reviews: An ESRC research methods programmes project.* Retrieved from http://www.lancaster.ac.uk/shm/research/nssr/research/dissemination/publications.php

Roen, K., Arai, L., Roberts, H., & Popay, J. (2006). Extending systematic reviews to include evidence on implementation: Methodological work on a review of community based initiative to prevent injuries. *Social Science & Medicine, 63*(4), 1060–1071.

Sackett, D.L., Richardson, W.S., Rosenberg, W., & Haynes, R.B. (1997). *Evidence-based medicine: How to practice and teach EBM* (1st ed.). London, United Kingdom: Churchill Livingstone.

Sackett, D. L., Straus, S. E., Richardson, W. S., Rosenberg, W., & Haynes, R. B. (2000). *Evidence-based medicine: How to practice and teach EBM* (2nd ed.). Edinburgh, United Kingdom: Churchill Livingstone.

Sandelowski, M., & Barroso, J. (2007). *Handbook for synthesizing qualitative research.* New York, NY: Springer.

Sandelowski, M., Borroso, J., & Voils, C. I. (2007). Using qualitative meta-summary to synthesise qualitative and quantitative descriptive findings. *Research in Nursing & Health, 30*(1), 99–111.

Uman, L. S. (2011). Systematic reviews and meta-analyses. *J Can Acad Child Adolesc Psychiatr.* 20(1): 57-59. *Journal of the Canadian Academy of Child and Adolescent Psychiatry, 20*(1), 57–59.

Webb, C., & Roe, B. H. (2007). *Reviewing research evidence for nursing practice: systematic reviews.* Oxford, United Kingdom: Blackwell.

Weed, M. (2005). Meta-interpretation: A method for the interpretive synthesis of qualitative research. *Qualitative Social Research, 6*(1), 1–17.

Weed, M. A. (2007). A potential method for interpretive synthesis of qualitative research. *International Journal of Social Research Methodology, 11*(1), 13–28.

Wong, G., Greenhalgh, T., & Pawson, R. (2010). Internet-based medical education: A realist review of what works, for whom and in what circumstances. *BMC Medical Education, 10*(12).

Wright, R. W., Brand, R. A., Dunn, W., & Spindler, K. P. (2007). How to write a systematic review. *Clinical Orthopaedics and Related Research, 455*, 23–29.

CHAPTER

4

Evidence-Based Practice: Practical Challenges in the Implementation Process

THEODORA D. KWANSA

CHAPTER OBJECTIVES

The main objectives of this chapter are to:

- Explore ways of determining a realistic in-house sustained culture of evidence-based practice (EBP)
- Examine the need for engendering and maintaining team commitment to EBP
- Examine the process of EBP implementation
- Identify models for EBP implementation and those for evaluating implementation
- Explore potential implementation challenges and possible measures to deal with each

Introduction

The requirement to use credible evidence to substantiate professional decisions and actions in care and service delivery is by no means new. Nevertheless, the professional obligation to adopt evidence-based practice (EBP) principles and have access to appropriate resources to do so cannot be undervalued. Effective leadership, shared ownership, commitment, and accountability are vital if EBP is to be efficiently implemented. Commitment by healthcare practitioners is crucial to avoid mere lip service to EBP implementation. This chapter does not intend to imply that the knowledge, insight, and skills required for EBP are nonexistent among sexual and reproductive healthcare (SRH) professionals. Neither is it intended to imply that an indifferent attitude to the adoption of EBP exists among any particular group of practitioners or among any

healthcare professional disciplines. Nonetheless, varying degrees of commitment occur among different teams of professionals, and their attitudes about the principles and the models likewise may diverge.

Another reality is that rapid staff turnover makes continuity a challenge. New graduates and newly employed staff, and locums who are temporarily employed for training or service, may need help getting up to speed with an organization's EBP policies. This, coupled with increasingly complex patient demands and expectations, justifies the need for constant reviews, updates, and retraining to ensure efficient implementation of EBP.

Continually enhancing and sustaining a culture of EBP is critical, as is constantly reinforcing the team's understanding of what this approach to practice encompasses, in order to maintain the desired high standard of implementation. To do so, the team must feel empowered to communicate and share their views about the implementation process. Including EBP representatives in the multidisciplinary team to engage with team members in exploring their perceptions about EBP can facilitate this kind of open communication. Moreover, appropriate ongoing education and training activities, workshops, and study days keep healthcare professionals up to date with emerging new developments in EBP and systematic reviews. The ideas proposed in this chapter could provide an agenda for periodic in-house exercises to keep the EBP culture active within particular areas of practice.

The intention of this chapter is simply to focus on the practical processes involved in EBP implementation. The scope of this chapter, and indeed this text, does not realistically allow for comprehensive and exhaustive exploration of EBP. However, specific key elements have been adequately explored and reflective considerations have also been incorporated to encourage team deliberations. Practitioners are encouraged to complement these with other, more comprehensive texts.

Concept Clarification and Key Indicators of EBP

Because "evidence-based culture" essentially applies to the entire organization, an attempt to define and confine the concept to any particular part creates gaps that may be confusing and difficult to justify. In practical terms, the cultural initiative occurs at all levels, including the health service organization, hospitals, clinical areas, the multidisciplinary care delivery teams, and individual practitioners. The principal indicators of EBP remain the same, encompassing the following:

- Formulating identified clinical problems into specific and concise questions
- Conducting extensive search to locate and access the best available research and other relevant evidence
- Conducting detailed critique of the evidence materials
- Planning, organizing, and effecting the implementation
- Evaluating the outcome effects by reviewing and conducting necessary clinical audit projects (Thompson, 2012)

Successful achievement of each of these indicators requires unreserved commitment from all stakeholders (management teams, policy makers, clinical leads, multidisciplinary teams, individual practitioners, support agencies, and related organizations), adequate resources, and effective support of practitioners at all levels. It also requires consideration to be given to the environments of care delivery and the environments within which various support services are provided. An exploration of EBP implementation from preparatory activities to post implementation evaluation is presented in the ensuing sections.

Box 4-1 presents a preliminary exercise to ensure that all members of staff gain a clear conception of what EBP actually means and what key elements are involved.

It is crucial to eliminate any strong reservations or even irrational objections that create barriers. The aim is to encourage open-mindedness, which is an absolute prerequisite for conscientious implementation of EBP. Practitioners need to reflect on and construct their personal and professional values about EBP from their knowledge of the background and evolution of the concept. What led to the need for EBP in the first place? A suggested exercise for the team of practitioners is to reflect on the following fundamental reasons and challenges that stirred the need and justification for EBP. These draw on expert views, including Appleby, Walshe, and Ham (1995); McKibbon and Marks (1998); Cullum, Ciliska, Haynes, and Marks (2008); and Belsey (2009).

BOX 4-1 Determining and Defining an In-House Conception of EBP

Suggested Practical Activities (Informal or Formal Workshop 1)

- The suggested activities require team collaboration with active discussions and careful planning to achieve realistic, workable, and beneficial outcomes.
- These will provide a sense of shared ownership of the ideas that emerge, commitment of the staff, readiness, and enthusiasm for participation in the implementation process.
- It is useful to collate and analyze the perceptions, level of comprehension, and what held values about EBP exist among the members of staff.
- One way of obtaining these is to suggest that staff place brief statements of what EBP means to them on the staff notice board in the tea/coffee room or on a particular designated notice board.

What Evidence-Based Practice Means to Me or to Us

- The collation and analysis could be carried out by the EBP working group, comprising representatives of each discipline in the multidisciplinary team.
- The identified common elements can then be outlined and placed on the notice board to inform all staff about the common perceptions and values of EBP that are shared among the team members.
- From that, an intramural concept of EBP formulated from the staff's views can then be devised.

Direct communication and feedback should be maintained at all times.

Reflective Considerations

A professional dilemma and associated potential challenges

- Consider the hypothetical scenario of an identified gap in professional practice. The conviction, assurance, and confidence among the team of practitioners that a particular drug treatment or clinical procedure together with the required/essential education intervention and support would produce best outcomes and satisfaction for patients with an identified health problem.

- Consider that patients, the general public, and the stakeholders also demand and expect the assurance of confidence in the therapeutic procedures employed in the management of the identified health problems.
- Consider the confidence in the objectivity of empirical scientific research studies.
- Consider the benefits of systematic reviews, research quality evaluation, and accumulation of best available evidence from carefully selected studies relating to the particular clinical problem, therapeutic procedure, or drug treatment.
- Consider the resource implications, staffing levels, existing knowledge and expertise, education, training, and support.
- Consider potential barriers, organizational policy regulations, leadership, and commitment.
- Consider the inadequacy of intuitive knowledge developed and passed on from generations of practitioners in a specific field of specialism.
- Consider how such a scenario could be tackled.

Engendering Team Motivation, Preparedness, and Commitment

Effective team leadership and the degree of knowledge, insight, and enthusiasm that leaders convey about EBP, become crucial incentives for the staff, inspiring the team and justifying implementation. Having ascertained the extent of familiarity and what value the practitioners place on EBP, this early stage can identify in-house deficits and needs. The proportion of staff that requires education and training in various forms, including continuing professional development (CPD) can be determined and prioritized.

Although EBP is achievable on an individual basis by independent practitioners, the referral systems in place to achieve holistic care provision create inevitable links with colleagues. Thus, EBP is best embarked on within the context of team collaboration. Rees (2010) cited Dartnell, Hemming, Collier, and Ollenschlaeger's (2008) assertion that clinical guidelines are underpinned by carefully selected evidence that has been translated into action points. Therefore, clinical guidelines essentially serve as suitable options for the autonomous practitioner to competently implement evidence-based procedures and treatment interventions in care provision.

DiCenso, Guyatt, and Ciliska's (2014) evidence-based decision-making framework encompasses the patient's clinical problem, his/her circumstances (as well as cultural and religious values), and his/her expressed particular preferences. It also requires account to be taken of the available healthcare resources, including the level and scope of professional knowledge and expertise in making decisions about care and treatment provision (Melnyk & Fineout-Overholt, 2005, 2014). These authors reemphasize the processes involved in EBP, including assessing the quality of the studies and establishing the relevance to patient care. The application of guidelines and the implementation of recommended findings from published systematic reviews, meta-analyses, and qualitative meta-syntheses should be rigorous in autonomous/independent practice and within the context of team EBP implementation.

Establishing and Maintaining an Intramural EBP Culture

The initial step in the multidisciplinary team context is to engender a culture of EBP that is reflected in the team's endorsement, unanimity, and commitment. Establish an EBP working group to coordinate the consensus ideas for an appropriate model or framework. The working group carefully examines and determines the most appropriate way of interpreting and implementing the EBP principles. Careful consideration should be given to practicability and realism to achieve the most productive and beneficial patient outcomes and satisfaction. Consideration should also be given to productivity/cost effectiveness for the healthcare organization. Success depends on constant support for resources. Convening the working group should take place without delay in the very early stage, with each discipline choosing a delegate to ensure effective two-way support, good coordination, and active dialogues. Every effort should be made to ensure that the views of all team members are given due consideration. **Figure 4-1** presents the essential practical measures of establishing an in-house EBP culture. Team collaboration is vital in this venture.

Establishing Subgroups and Workshop Activities

To complement the team's EBP working group, practitioners with appropriate EBP knowledge and experience should design workshops that critically examine and clarify the rationale, benefits, and other related concepts of EBP. These multidisciplinary subgroups could prove to be an effective and stimulating experiential learning opportunity for newly qualified staff or any staff who may not be entirely familiar with all of what EBP involves in the practical context (e.g., hierarchical rating of research and other evidence, assessing the validity of selected studies). Consulting external experts to design and/or run the workshops when the team has limited collective knowledge of EBP is always a possibility; however, the cost should be carefully considered. These

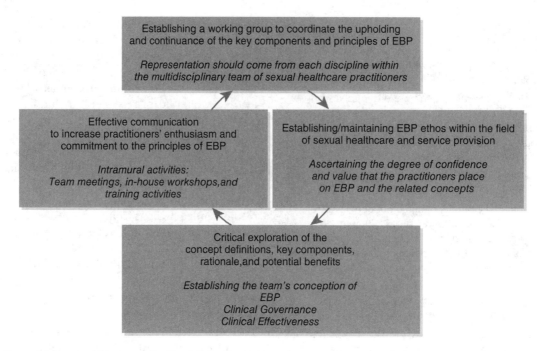

Figure 4-1 Essential Practical Measures for Establishing and Maintaining an Intramural EBP Culture

consultations with staff could inspire team motivation, enthusiasm, and commitment as well as determine its needs.

Identifying and Dealing with Potential Challenges for EBP Implementation

The potential risk in clinical practice is the tendency to be content with existing practices, policies, and procedures simply because they seem to achieve reasonable (though not necessarily best) results. Change can be frustrating and difficult, and the additional demands of research can be quite challenging, which can hinder adoption of and full commitment to EBP in some clinical areas. The easiest and most comfortable action is to perform only sporadic implementation of certain aspects of EBP, thus overlooking essential components of the principles and possibly neglecting a fundamental principle of clinical governance as well as professional accountability.

The challenge, therefore, is for the team of practitioners and indeed the individual in her/his professional capacity to make sense of not only what exactly the concept means, but, also important, the underpinning principles and related rationales. This requires the team of practitioners to determine an agreed-upon description of EBP in practicable terms for their intramural implementation. Should the team decide to adopt or adapt the proposition put forward by previous exponents, it would be appropriate to examine carefully the related copyright regulations and seek appropriate permission and guidance. Of crucial importance, practitioners should bear in mind that there may be organizational or hospital recommendations with which they are required to comply.

Exploration of the literature reveals that not only can the concept be contextualized in many if not all aspects of healthcare (Rees, 2010), but also presents multiple challenges. The rationale for establishing the level of knowledge and personal views inherent within the team is to enhance their motivation for, and cooperation in, effective EBP implementation and to identify and deal with any particular hindrances that may emerge.

Mechanisms for Addressing Specific Challenges to the Implementation of EBP

These activities may be provided at given intervals by the organization or at departmental or unit levels. Healthcare practitioners have a professional obligation to comply with the national and local recommendations. Various interrelated EBP activities are provided at academic institutional, healthcare providers, and/or government organizational levels. These may be in the form of short courses and CPD modules, for example, clinical effectiveness and/or clinical audit project implementation, or indeed EBP. Therefore, where funding support is made available, practitioners should take advantage of the experiential learning opportunities that are necessary for ongoing personal and professional development. **Figure 4-2** presents an overview of the potential challenges that multidisciplinary teams may have to deal with.

The practical exercises outlined here could serve as a preliminary experiential learning activity in an area of practice that involves most if not all members of the multidisciplinary team.

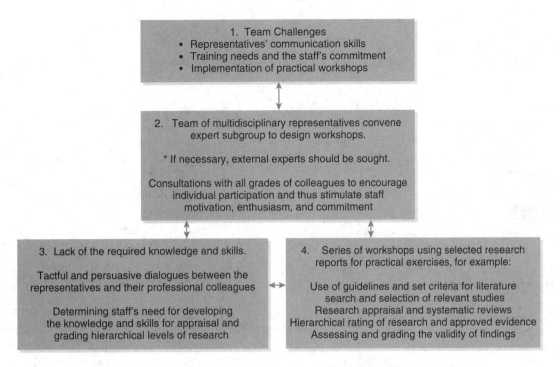

Figure 4-2 Suggested Actions to Deal with the Inevitable Challenges within the Mutlidisciplinary Team

---

Reflective Considerations

- To maintain staff motivation and participation, the identification of the problem of mutual concern should be done transparently to give individuals the opportunity to contribute their ideas.

- A small group of volunteers from each of the professional disciplines could explore the different sources of the literature for relevant research and related evidence material.

- This could be followed by a simple trial run of data extraction and abstraction using the appropriate formal tools or simplified newly developed in-house versions of the tools for the documentation.

- The tabulated findings could then be disseminated to each of the disciplines in the team for perusal as well as placing clearly legible copies on designated staff notice boards.

- Carefully planned group discussions and feedback could prove to be useful follow-up exercises.

Potential Challenges Considered

Craig and Stevens (2012) examine challenges in EBP from three perspectives. First, they postulate the challenge that research evidence bases are not necessarily comprehensive, there are always several unexplored issues in clinical care and various aspects of professional practice. Second, they note that certain evidence bases are dynamic, with a deluge of ongoing research publications. Practitioners can find themselves inundated by the challenge of keeping up to date with new and emerging concepts and theories in various aspects of clinical practice. Third, some research findings may not be directly applicable or generalizable to certain population groups or to particular clinical settings. Therefore, practitioners face the challenges of discretionary choices and correctly determining suitable application to avoid inappropriate translation of findings from various studies into clinical practice. Thus, effectively, the team's knowledge and skills for efficient EBP implementation are challenged as they deal with accessing and translating available research studies. **Box 4-2** outlines the key issues to be considered in the planning, implementation, and evaluation process.

Teams of healthcare professionals are urged to avoid being overambitious and not achieving their desired goal of proper evidence-based practice. Depending on the size of the team and the intramural research expertise it is advisable to focus on a single specific clinical issue at a time. Preliminary considerations are suggested to guide the choice of relevant material and critical appraisal for EBP.

Models for EBP Implementation: Identifying Appropriate Frameworks

Numerous models and frameworks have been developed for EBP implementation. These are generally copyright

> **BOX 4-2 Concise Outline of the Key Considerations in the Planning, Implementation, and Evaluation of EBP**
>
> 1. The particular population group should be clearly identified.
> 2. The specific condition together with the related social context and implications should be carefully examined.
> 3. The precise medication, procedural methods, or aspects of routine care should be identified as the particular concerns that are shared by the multidisciplinary team of caregivers.
> 4. The changes that the team envisages to implement for realization of better outcomes for the patients should reflect the practitioners' consensus initiative, motivation, and assurance.
> 5. The resource implications should be carefully assessed, and it may be useful to establish staff awareness of these issues.
>   a. Achievability of these should be carefully considered.
>   b. Alternative compromises should be considered for putting into place if necessary. This may necessitate a comparison to be made.
>   c. There should be internal discussion to achieve shared ownership by taking account of suggestions by individual staff members.
> 6. The envisioned outcome should be carefully discussed and should be meticulously measured and recorded.

protected and require the permission of the original authors to be adopted or adapted for implementation. Practitioners are encouraged to explore different types of EBP models to determine which model appropriately applies to a specific issue of concern. While this is a useful exercise, practitioners should avoid engaging in overambitious and indiscriminate exploration of every model that has so far been developed. Such actions invariably lead to inundation with indifferent implementation. Superficial EBP implementation, as discovered by Leufer and Cleary-Holdforth (2009), only results in practitioner frustration and inconsistencies in care provision and patient outcomes.

Common Elements in EBP Models

Although key elements of EBP are recognizable in most if not all the models, each also portrays its particular focus and characteristic features. The common recognizable elements that convey similarity in the different models include the following.

- Determining a clinical problem, aspect of care provision, therapeutic intervention, or routine procedure. Essentially, this involves selecting an aspect of clinical care that is deemed to require improvement substantiated by sound evidence.
- Formulating an appropriate question. Many experts advocate basing this on the PICO or PICOS method as previously explained.
- Prioritizing the identified problem/question within the area of clinical care and within the wider context of the healthcare organization.
- Convening an EBP team, which should ideally comprise representation from each of the main stakeholders.
- Conducting extensive search of the literature including relevant documents and reports to identify evidence materials that are pertinent to the identified clinical issue of concern. The skills and expertise among the multidisciplinary team of practitioners should be taken into account. Additionally, the needs of the patient/clients based on the particular health problem, personal and social circumstances, their demands and expectations, and the available healthcare resources should be carefully assessed.
- Selecting the most relevant range of evidence materials.
- Carrying out appropriate rating of the research and other evidence materials and grading the quality of each selected material.
- Conducting critical appraisal and systematically reviewing the selected research studies.
- Judicious pooling, analyzing, and synthesizing of the key findings from the relevant evidence materials.
- Determining and agreeing on approved EBP guidelines/recommendations appropriately substantiated and meticulously documented.
- Confirming the pertinence of the research evidence to the area of clinical practice and the suitability of the findings for application to the provision of patient care.
- Developing specific standards for EBP for the particular healthcare organization.
- Pilot testing of the changes required for the EBP implementation.
- Carrying out careful decision-making and planning based on the positive outcomes achieved from the pilot testing. The aim is to ensure accurate translation and integration of sound and best available evidence into the actuality of professional practice.
- Integrating the EBP within all aspects of the healthcare organization to achieve change toward improvement of care provision and better patient/client outcomes.
- Meticulous and systematic evaluation of the EBP changes, documentation of the processes employed,

and the specific outcomes of the change achieved through the implementation.

- Sustaining ongoing quality improvement measures and monitoring.
- Provision of the required staff education and training. (DiCenso et al., 2014; Levine, 2004; Rees, 2010; Titler, 2008)

Multiple models are summarized here, but exploration of the original works is strongly encouraged to gain better insight about each one.

Overview of Specific Models and Their Key Characteristics

The Stetler Model

Stetler's (2001) model describes five phases as follows.

1. Preparation involves a literature search and identification of relevant research evidence. This requires that the problem be confirmed internally and prioritized to justify the formation of a team and consideration of other related plan of actions prior to embarking on the implementation of evidence-based practice.

2. Validation involves critique and synopsis of the key components of the identified studies in relation to clinical practice. This is accompanied by the logical processes of systematic review, critical appraisal, and rating the quality of each research study.

3. Comparative evaluation/decision-making involves pooling and criteria-based synthesizing of the findings and determining their pertinence to practice.

4. Translation/application involves interpreting the findings into a form that can be applied to clinical practice, determining how specific findings can be used, and implementing an appropriate action plan.

5. Evaluation involves assessment of the implementation process and the extent to which the objectives and goals have been achieved.

The Iowa Model

Titler et al.'s (2001) Iowa model integrates the use of evidence material from varied sources and thus amalgamates research and other forms of best identified evidence. This model addresses EBP from the perspectives of the clinicians as well as the contexts of healthcare organizations and clinical care delivery.

- It requires that clinicians question specific aspects of practice based on their knowledge. Problem-focused prompts are used and supported by thorough search of the relevant literature.

- Where pertinent, high-quality research studies are unavailable or significantly limited, a new and original research study would have to be carried out using appropriately rigorous methodological processes.

- The findings are then integrated with other related best-available evidence to devise EBP guidelines and recommendations for practice.

- The recommendations are compared to the current practice to decide on the justification and feasibility for change.

- The planned process for change involves
  - pilot testing the EBP recommendations and guidelines with a small group of clinicians and patients;
  - revision of the guidelines as appropriate, followed by larger scale implementation;
  - data collection from the outcome of the change regarding the care-providing staff, patients, and administrative staff; and
  - documentation of the stages at which decisions are made and their basis, to determine both whether the problem represents an organizational priority and whether there is strong enough substantive research evidence to warrant a change.

Kitson, Harvey, and McCormack's Multidimensional Framework (1998)

In their involvement in the project, "Promoting Action on Research Implementation in Health Services (PARIHS)," Kitson, Harvey, and McCormack proposed their multidimensional framework, "Enabling the Implementation of Evidence-Based Practice" (1998). The framework presents three key elements focusing on the following:

- The nature of the evidence in terms of the knowledge and information that form the basis of decisions about patient care
- The context in terms of the environment /setting for the implementation of the intended change
- Facilitation in terms of enabling or making things happen

The nature of evidence is described as research, clinical experience, and patient preferences that are classified on a spectrum of low to high. Thus, while low-level research studies are classified as anecdotal and descriptive, at the high end of the spectrum, the evidence is described as empirical, randomized controlled studies. Also on this end are systematic reviews and evidence-based guidelines. In relation to the evidence of clinical experience, the low end of the spectrum comprises inconsistent expert opinions, while strong, consistent consensus views feature at the high end of the spectrum. Patient preferences are classified as no involvement (at the low end of the spectrum) and patient partnerships in care provision (at the high end).

The context classifications focus on three key factors in terms of culture, leadership, and measurement:

1. **Culture**, placed on the low end of the spectrum, would be a task-driven climate with little regard for

the individual practitioner, low morale, and limited continuing professional education and development. The high end of the spectrum would include an effective learning organization, patient-centered approach to care provision, and appreciation of staff and continuing education with ongoing professional development.

2. At the low end of the spectrum, **leadership** is sporadic and undefined, team roles are indeterminate, the organization is ineffective/unproductive, and management is weak/inefficient. At the high end, one would expect clear leadership and roles with effective teams and organizational structures.

3. At the low end of the spectrum, **measurement** via audit feedback, peer performance reviews, and external audits are non-existent. At the high end of the spectrum, routine use of internal measures and audit feedback with peer reviews and external measures is described.

The facilitation process specifies three key factors: role, characteristics, and style.

1. At the low end of the spectrum, facilitation **roles** are inconsistently defined and task-driven with limited time to achieve specific/individual goals, while at the high end, the roles involve external and internal agents, and sustained partnership with a developmental purposefulness. The attributes and skills employed depend on the purpose of the role and include co-counselling and critical reflection skills that require subject/clinical credibility, and flexible management skills.

2. At the low end of the spectrum, **characteristics** are focused on methods in terms of action plans and set of techniques based on audit feedback. The high end of the spectrum describes processes of skill development, involving reflectivity, dialogues, ownership, and realization of potential.

3. The low-end **style** is directive, with a pattern of structured objectives to accomplish tasks, while the high end balances styles that take both tasks and processes into account. (Kitson et al., 1998)

These authors maintain that successful EBP implementation can only be achieved where the these conditions are met at the high end of the spectrums. That means high (strong) evidence (HE), high (well-developed) context (HC), and high (effective) facilitation (HF). Even so, they suggest that HF within a relatively poor context (LC) could achieve a positive outcome. However, implementation is unlikely to succeed with HC but with deficient and ineffective facilitation (LF) (Kitson et al., 1998).

More recent models include Newhouse, Dearholt, Poe, Pugh, and White's (2007) Johns Hopkins EBP model, Tolson, Booth, and Lowndes's (2008) Caledonian development model, and the Reavey and Tavernier's (2008) EBP model

for staff nurses. While these models may incorporate general guidelines and specific instructions for implementation, many authors continue to update and refine their original works, which may be worth exploring.

Evaluating EBP Model Implementation

Evaluating EBP model implementation may prove to be quite complex insofar as implementation itself may have been a multifaceted process. Its evaluation, therefore, may be a prolonged process that has to be conducted logically and meticulously. Melnyk and Fineout-Overholt (2005) demonstrate the importance of evaluation following EBP implementation, maintaining that it should reflect the PICO (problem/ patient/population, intervention/indicator, comparison/comparator, outcome) strategy that formed the basis of the EBP question. Therefore, the measurable outcomes should be evaluated together with other emerging outcomes considered pertinent by the practitioner and the patient. Although optional, some researchers include the time frame for the data collection, duration, or type of study (and thus, PICOT) where that information is required by the project funding organization and relevant stakeholders. The perceived advantage is that this ensures persistent progress of the study to a timely completion.

As part of the overall evaluation of the success of EBP implementation specific aspects include the following:

- Outcome of the treatment intervention (how did it work?)
- Effectiveness of the clinical decision for the particular patients within the context of specific care provision and within the context of identified or specialist professional practice setting
- Whether a particular change was necessary to achieve the expected outcome

If not fully achieved, the factors that may have contributed to the shortfall should be examined by asking the following questions:

- Did the patient adhere to the treatment regimen?
- Was the prescribed dosage of the specific medication adequate?
- Were demographic characteristics of the patient population taken into consideration?
- Did internal policies, procedures, and standards influence any or all aspects of the implementation process?
- Were organizational structure, resource provision, and staff support optimal?
- What leadership styles were used?
- Did the staff have the necessary knowledge, skills, continuing education and professional development, motivation, commitment, morale, and appropriate support to fulfill delegated tasks efficiently?

Various other evaluative models have been proposed that focus on outcome measures. Ingersoll (2005) cited the following examples that readers are urged to explore to compare the different models in terms of structure, components, and application.

- Systems framework model: Doerge, J. B. (2000). Creating an outcomes framework. *Outcomes Management for Nursing Practice, 4*(1), 28–33.
- Input-process-output model: Maljanian, R., Effken, J. A., & Kaerhle, P. I. (2000). Design and Implementation of an outcome measurement model. *Outcomes Management for Nursing Practice, 4,* 19–26.
- Three-dimensional model comprising outcomes measurement and analysis of clinical interventional outcomes (in essence, a multidisciplinary team approach performing measurement and analysis of outcomes): Houston, S., Fleschler, R., & Luquire, R. (2001). Reflections on a decade of outcomes management in women's services. *Journal of Obstetric, Gynecologic, and Neonatal Nursing, 30*(10), 89–97.
- Final outcomes management model: Cho, S-H. (2001). Nurse staffing and adverse patient outcomes: A systems approach. *Nursing Outlook, 49*(2), 78–85.
- Value of care model: Nelson, G., Batalden, P., Plume, S., & Mohr, J. (1996). Improving health care Part 2 – A clinical improvement worksheet and users' manual. *The Joint Commission Journal on Quality Improvement, 22*(8), 531–548.

Each model should perhaps be regarded simply as a prototype rather than blindly adopting the approach. It is always pragmatic to evaluate the content of the selected evidence material critically for practicability within the context of care provision, the staffing profile, and the resource implications. The exemplars should serve as the basis for team discussion during the planning and development of in-house activities, which should derive from expert theorizations. Crucially, any in-house models or guidelines should be thoroughly pilot tested, peer reviewed, audited, and refined as necessary before fully embracing and applying it to practice.

Conclusion

This chapter has explored the practical processes of EBP implementation. The need clearly exists for practitioners to gain adequate familiarity with these processes to embark on EBP implementation with appropriate motivation, commitment, and confidence. Furthermore, practitioners must develop the required professional competence for correct implementation to achieve effective and successful outcomes.

As repeatedly emphasized in this chapter, practitioners are urged to read more comprehensive books written by experts to complement the information gained here. Ongoing education and training opportunities including CPD modules should be incorporated to enhance the knowledge and skills necessary for correct implementation to achieve the desired effective outcomes.

• • • REFERENCES

Appleby, J., Walshe, K., & Ham, C. (1995). Acting on the evidence: A review of clinical effectiveness. Sources of information, dissemination and implementation. (Research Paper No 17). Birmingham, United Kingdom: NAHAT.

Belsey, J. (2009). *What is evidence-based medicine?* London, United Kingdom: Hayward Medical Communications, Hayward Group Ltd.

Craig, V. C., & Stevens, K. R. (2012). Evidence-based practice in nursing. In V.C. Craig & R.L. Smyth, *The evidence-based practice manual for nurses* (3rd ed., pp. 3–23). Oxford, United Kingdom: Churchill Livingstone Elsevier.

Cullum, N., Ciliska, D., Haynes, B., & Marks, S. (Eds.). (2008). *Evidence-based nursing: An introduction.* London, United Kingdom: Wiley-Blackwell.

Dartnell, J., Hemming, M., Collier, J., & Ollenschlaeger, G. (2008). EBN notebook: Putting evidence into context: some advice for guidance writers. *Evidence-Based Nursing, 11*(1), 6–8.

DiCenso, A., Guyatt, G., & Ciliska, D. (2014). *Evidence-based nursing: A guide to clinical practice.* Edinburgh, United Kingdom: Elsevier Health Sciences.

Ingersoll, G. L. (2005). Generating evidence through outcomes management. In: B. M. Melnyk & E. Fineout-Overholt (Eds.), *Evidence-based practice in nursing and healthcare: A guide to best practice* (1st ed.). (pp. 299–332). Philadelphia, PA: Lippincott Williams & Wilkins.

Kitson, A., Harvey, G., & McCormack, B. (1998). Enabling the implementation of evidence based practice: A conceptual framework. *Quality Health Care, 7*(3), 149–158.

Leufer, T., & Cleary-Holdforth, J. (2009). Evidence-based practice improving patient outcomes: *Nursing Standard, 23*(32), 35–39.

Levine, E. R. (2004). Glossary. In A.R. Roberts & K. Yeager, *Evidence-based practice manual: Research and outcome measures in health and human services* (pp. 971–1007). New York, NY: Oxford University Press.

McKibbon, K. A., & Marks S. (1998). Searching for the best evidence. Part 1: Where to look. *Evidence-Based Nursing, 1*(3), 68–70.

Melnyk, B. M., & Fineout-Overholt, E. (Eds.). (2005). *Evidence-based practice in nursing and healthcare: A guide to best practice* (1st ed.). Philadelphia, PA: Lippincott Williams & Wilkins.

Melnyk, B. M., & Fineout-Overholt, E. (Eds.). (2014). *Evidence-based practice in nursing and healthcare: A guide to best practice* (2nd ed.). Philadelphia, PA: Lippincott Williams & Wilkins.

Newhouse, R., Dearholt, S., Poe, S., Pugh, L., & White, K. (2007). *The Johns Hopkins Nursing: Evidence-based practice model and guidelines.* Indianapolis, IN: Sigma Theta Tau.

Reavy, K., & Tavernier, S. (2008). Nurses claiming ownership of their practice: Implementation of an evidence-based practice model and process. *Journal of Continuing Education in Nursing, 39*(4), 166–172.

Rees, C. (2010). Understanding evidence and its utilisation in nursing practice. In K. Holland & C. Rees (Eds.), *Nursing: Evidence-based practice skills* (pp. 18–38). Oxford, United Kingdom: Oxford University Press.

Stetler, C.B. (2001). Updating the Stetler Model of research utilisation to facilitate evidence-based practice. *Nursing Outlook, 49*(6), 272–278.

Thompson, C. (2012). How can we develop an evidence-based culture? In J.V. Craig & R.L. Smyth, *The evidence-based practice manual for nurses* (3rd ed., pp. 323–357.) Oxford, United Kingdom: Churchill Livingstone, Elsevier.

Titler, M. G. (2008). Evidence for evidence based practice implementation. In R.D. Hughes (Ed.), *Patient safety and quality: An evidence-based handbook for nurses.* Chapter 7. Rockville MD: Agency for Healthcare Research and Quality. Retrieved from http://www.ahrq.gov/qual/nurseshdbk/

Titler, M., Kleiber, C., Steelman, V., Rakel, B., Budreau, G., Everett, L., . . . Goode, C.J. (2001). The Iowa Model of evidence-based practice to promote quality care. *Critical Care Nursing Clinics of North America, 13*(4), 497–509.

Tolson, D., Booth, J., & Lowndes, A. (2008). Achieving evidence-based nursing practice: Impact of the Caledonian development model. *Journal of Nursing Management, 16*(6), 682–691.

● ● ● SUGGESTED FURTHER READING

Craig, J.V., & Smyth, R.L. (2012). *The evidence-based practice manual for nurses* (3rd ed.). Oxford, United Kingdom: Churchill Livingston, Elsevier.

II

Applied Reproductive Science; Contemporary Interventions; Accessible Contraception Services

Applied Reproductive System: Scientific Aspects

KEVIN R. SMITH

CHAPTER OBJECTIVES

The main objectives of this chapter are to:

- Provide an overview of human reproductive physiology
- Review current areas of interest and controversy in human reproductive science

Introduction

This chapter reviews key scientific aspects of human reproduction, with particular consideration given to areas that impinge on sexual health and functioning. The focus is upon contemporary issues, concepts, and controversies. Recent research is emphasized, and various academic reviews are noted for the reader who wishes to explore key topics in greater depth. Consulting an adjunct textbook is recommended to the reader who comes to this chapter lacking the essential fundamental knowledge of applied reproductive biology.

The Male Reproductive System

Spermatogenesis

Spermatogenesis, the production of sperm cells, takes place within the coiled seminiferous tubules of the testis. Spermatogonial stem cells divide to produce a prodigious amount of developing sperm cells: the fertile male produces over 2,000 sperm cells per second. The entire process of spermatogenesis, starting with spermatogonial division and concluding with deposition of morphologically complete sperm into the lumen of the coiled seminiferous tubule, takes approximately 10 weeks. These sperm cells are immotile and are conveyed passively to the adjacent ductus epididymis, where they undergo subtle maturation steps required to render them ready for fertilization. Non-ejaculated sperm can be stored in the ductus epididymis for approximately 2–3 weeks. In cases of prolonged abstinence, some storage may also occur in the lower reaches of the vas deferens, to which the ductus epididymis is adjoined. (For reviews and further reading see Carreau, Bouraima-Lelong, & Delalande, 2011; Barratt [1995]; Carreau, Bouraima-Lelong, and Delalande [2011]; Grootegoed et al. [1995]; and Verhoeven [1999].)

Sperm Integrity

The coiled seminiferous tubule is compartmentalized via tight junctions between its composite cells, and is thus to some extent protected from blood-borne cytotoxic and mutagenic molecules. Additionally, there appears to be a particularly high level of mutation repair activity associated with spermatogenesis. Nevertheless, due to the continuous turnover of spermatogonia, sperm cells tend to accumulate mutations as the male ages. Accordingly, a paradigm of elevated risk of transmitting de novo mutations—and hence genetic disorders—to offspring of older men has emerged in recent years. For example, the risk of a 40-year-old man fathering a child with a dominant mutation is approximately the same as the risk of Down syndrome for a child whose mother is 35–40 years. Such paternal age-related mutational risk also applies to polygenic conditions, including autism, schizophrenia, epilepsy, and intellectual disability, with recent literature typically reporting at least a twofold increase in the incidence of such conditions for fathers older than 50 compared with fathers under the age of 30 (Hehir-Kwa et al., 2011; Krishnaswamy et al., 2009; Lynch, 2010; Petersen, Mortensen, & Pedersen, 2011; Reichenberg et al., 2006; Vestergaard, Mork, Madsen, & Olsen, 2005). In this light, a rule on the maximum age for sperm donation would appear prudent. For example, in the United Kingdom the age limit is presently set at 45 years, and at 40 years in the United States, exceptional circumstances notwithstanding.

In recent years, concerns have been raised that sperm counts and, to a lesser extent, sperm quality may be declining compared with historical values (for examples, see Auger, Kuntsmann, Czyglik, & Jouannet, 1995; Carlsen, Giwercman, Keiding, & Skakkeback, 1992; Sharpe, 2010; Swan, Elkin, & Fenster, 2000). The hypothesis here is that the modern environment may impact negatively upon spermatogenesis and semen parameters. For example, pollutants and alleged endocrine disruptors—including dichlorodiphenyltrichloroethane (DDT), polychlorinated biphenyl (PCBs), pesticides, and food additives might exert a subtle toxic effect on testicular cells or other components of the male reproductive tract, especially during fetal development stages (see, for example, Rouiller-Fabre et al., 2009). Lifestyle factors—at least in Westernized nations—such as lack of exercise and obesity might also have a negative impact (Palmer, Bakos, Owens, Setchell, & Lane; Williams et al., 1993). However, data on historical sperm numbers and semen quality extending far enough back in time are sparse and of questionable reliability, making this hypothesis intrinsically difficult to test. Although the issue remains controversial, is seems reasonable to conclude that firm grounds have not been established to support claims that sperm counts or semen quality are in general decline (see for example Bonde, Ramlau-Hamsen, & Olsen, 2011; Olsen, Zhu, & Ramlau-Hansen, 2011; Velde et al., 2010). However, contemporary datasets will prove invaluable for future comparisons between present and future sperm values.

Hormones and Male Reproductive Function

Spermatogenesis is driven by the gonadotrophins follicle stimulating hormone (FSH) and luteinizing hormone (LH). In terms of sex steroid production, LH drives the Leydig cells (located outside the coiled seminiferous tubules) to produce androgens (mainly testosterone). In addition to acting within the coiled seminiferous tubules to drive sperm development, molecules of testosterone enter the bloodstream. Bloodborne testosterone promotes reproductive functionality within the body (e.g., maintenance of sexual morphology) and the brain (e.g., sexual behavior). Testosterone levels are positively correlated with sex drive, with androgen receptors within the brain able to bind and respond to testosterone. However, where testosterone production declines or is eliminated (e.g., iatrogenically), sex drive and male-associated behaviors are not fully eliminated. This apparent paradox is explained by the fact that testosterone acts on the brain during puberty to permanently alter brain function in a masculine direction (see Blakemore, Burnett, & Dahl, 2010; Neave & O'Connor, 2009; Shirtcliff, Dahl, & Pollak, 2009; Sisk & Foster, 2004; Spear, 2000).

Production of Semen

Arousal and ejaculation occur independently of spermatogenesis; the latter operates as a background process, slowly building up reserves of sperm cells. At the peak of sexual excitement, and particularly during mechanical stimulation of the penis, a proportion of these cells are discharged from the epididymis (or lower reaches of the vas deferens) to become mixed with the fluids added by the accessory glands intersecting the tract. This process, termed *emission*, results in the sperm cells becoming suspended in the fluid known as semen (or seminal fluid). The epididymal fluid containing the sperm contributes only about 2% of the volume of semen. Thus, vasectomized men experience no noticeable reduction in the volume of their semen per ejaculate.

The accessory glands that add most of the fluid to form semen are the seminal vesicles (one per vas deferens) and the prostate gland; these structures contract immediately prior to ejaculation to expel their liquid contents. The seminal vesicle provides a thick, mucoid, alkaline fluid making up approximately two-thirds of the semen volume; the prostate secretes a thin, milky, slightly alkaline fluid making up the remaining volume. A typical ejaculate ranges in volume from 2–6 mL, with more frequent ejaculations resulting in diminished volume, and abstinence resulting in higher volumes. Sperm density is typically 100 million sperm per milliliter of semen; levels below 20 million/mL generally equate with substantially impaired fertility, indicating the need for many sperm cells to achieve fertilization. Semen contains a wide mix of molecules, including agents to control the viscosity of the ejaculate, cathelicidins to combat infection, prostaglandins that induce uterine contractions in the recipient female, and a range other molecules, including hormones and growth factors, the functions of which are not fully understood.

Commencing in the early stages of sexual arousal, and continuing until the moment of ejaculation, the paired bulbourethral glands steadily secrete an alkaline fluid into the urethra. This fluid, known as the pre-ejaculate, functions to reduce acidity in the penis (sperm being unable to tolerate low pH environments), and to lubricate the bulbous tip of the penis (the glans penis) to permit foreskin retraction and facilitate vaginal entry. Quantities of pre-ejaculate produced appear to vary significantly and consistently among individual men, reflecting different genetic backgrounds. An important question in the context of human reproductive health is whether the pre-ejaculate contains sperm cells. If so, this would have important implications for sexual behavior, as pregnancy could result in the absence of ejaculation (for example, where a condom was used only immediately prior to ejaculation—a fairly common behavior). Certainly, the standard advice has been that barrier methods of contraception should be deployed prior to any penetrative sexual contact—and of course this advice cannot be faulted for erring on the side of caution, or in terms of avoiding sexually transmitted infections (STIs). However, the numbers of sperm empirically discovered in pre-ejaculatory fluid have been low (Killick, Leary, Trussell, & Guthrie, 2011; Zukerman, Weiss, & Orvieto, 2003), and it thus seems unlikely that pregnancy could arise merely from pre-ejaculatory fluid.

Ejaculation

At the height of sexual arousal, immediately prior to ejaculation, the sperm and fluid contents are mixed and moved along the vasa deferensia by smooth muscle contractions. At this moment, the internal urethral sphincter contracts to avoid retrograde ejaculation (i.e., semen entering the bladder). Ejaculation itself—the expulsion of semen from the penis—is powered mainly by the skeletal musculature associated with the penis. The relevant muscle pairs are located within the abdomen close to the base of the penis and wrapped around the base of the penis. Neurological or muscular conditions can lead to ejaculatory dysfunction, where the penile musculature is unable to forcefully contract to expel the semen, and/or to internal emission problems where the smooth muscle is similarly unable to contract adequately or in a properly coordinated manner.

Semen and Female Immunological Response

Beyond its function as a medium for sperm delivery, there is evidence that semen may contain factors that have physiological effects on the female's body. One such effect is the possible "conditioning" of the female's immune response so as to tolerate the potentially antigenic molecules contributed by the male partner. Following ejaculation, the immune system responds to the presence of foreign proteins from the male (in semen and on the sperm cell surface) in a number of ways, including increased macrophage activity. It is, however, essential that this immune response within the female tract is kept in check, otherwise fertilization would be impossible due to sperm cell destruction; or, if a conceptus was formed, pregnancy would be terminated by immunological attack on the embryo, fetus, or placenta due to the recognition of foreign proteins on the cells of these entities. (The potential of the female tract to react vigorously toward her partner's antigens is evidenced by rare cases of women who are allergic to semen, in whom the result of unprotected sex is severe inflammation of the vulva/vagina, with the possibility of anaphylactic shock.) Normal fertilization and pregnancy is associated with a special immunological tolerance toward potentially antigenic male-contributed proteins. The details of this tolerance have not yet been fully explained; however, there is some evidence that exposure to the semen of one partner may serve as a trigger for immune toleration of proteins from that same male. Indirect evidence comes from the epidemiological observation that preeclampsia, a serious disorder of gestation characterized by proteinuria and high blood pressure, is more common when pregnancy results from a male with whom the woman has not had frequent pre-conception unprotected coitus. Thus, unprotected sex appears to promote immunological tolerance, and the mechanism is triggered by semen exposure (for example, see Sadat, Kalahroudi, and Saberi, 2012). Indeed, this acquired tolerance may be most strongly promoted not by vaginal intercourse but by oral sex (fellatio), especially where the semen is swallowed, suggesting a possible biological role for this sexual practice (Koelman et al., 2000). The male factors assumed responsible for triggering female immunological tolerance to male-contributed antigens appear to be secreted from the prostate gland and seminal vesicle. Candidate factors include transforming growth factor beta (TGF-beta) and other cytokines. These agents are envisaged to interact with the epithelial cells of the lower reaches of the female tract, resulting in activation of cytokines and immune cells that serve to regulate and suppress the potential immune response against male-derived antigens, thus facilitating sperm survival, fertilization and gestation. (See reviews by Robertson [2005], and Rodriguez-Martinez, Kvist, Ernerudh, Sanz, and Calvete [2011].)

Does Semen Play a Role in Mental State?

Several components of semen, including testosterone, estrogen, and prostaglandins, are absorbed through the vaginal epithelium and can be detected in the bloodstream within a few hours of ejaculation, which has led some researchers to hypothesize that these seminal fluid components may have an effect on the mental state of recipient women (Ney, 1986). One study examined this hypothesis among a sample of 293 sexually active college females, condoms usage serving as a proxy for the presence or absence of semen in the reproductive tract, and such usage being compared with depressive symptoms (via the Beck Depression Inventory). Unprotected sex was found to correlate with low depression scores. Among those who used condoms inconsistently, the frequency of condom usage positively correlated with depressive symptoms (Gallup, Burch, & Platek, 2002). Thus, increased exposure to semen appears to correlate with reduced depressive symptoms. However, an alternative explanation exists, namely that females who choose to engage in unprotected sex are either happier with their partners than their condom-using counterparts, or are less depressed for other reasons (e.g., dispositional), with this mental state being the impetus for unprotected sex, as opposed to the converse. Moreover, the Gallup et al. study does not appear to have been replicated and, although interesting and potentially of significant importance in the context of human health, the notion that semen may biochemically alter the recipient's mood remains unproven at present.

The Penis

The penis is composed of erectile tissue sheathed in strong elastic skin. The erect penile tip takes the form of an enlarged glans penis, of significantly greater width than the penile shaft. It has been hypothesized that the glans penis has a protective action during coitus, with the role of absorbing the considerable forces associated with intromission. In a unique and elegant study, Hatzichristou et al. (2003) examined this hypothesis using five volunteer patients scheduled for surgical removal of the glans penis (due to penile carcinoma). During surgery, intrapenile pressure was increased by pumping saline into the erectile tissues, external compressive forces were delivered to the penis effectively mimicking the rigors of coitus, and the resultant pressure changes were recorded. Intrapenile pressures were higher following removal of the glans penis, indicating that the glans penis serves to reduce such pressures during sexual intercourse. Moreover, two of the patients' partners reported pain during sex post-operatively, probably due to the "ramming" action of the end of the rigid shaft of the penis into the vaginal wall, unprotected by the glans penis, suggesting that the protective role of the glans penis during coitus applies to the female as well as to the male (Hatzichristou et al., 2003).

The glans penis has the ability to displace semen out of the vagina by pumping it back along the outside of the penile shaft, as discussed later in this chapter in the context of sperm competition. Such semen removal is contrary to the biological goal of maximizing the likelihood of fertilization, and would thus appear to be maladaptive. It is not so, however, because immediately following ejaculation the penis loses turgor and the glans penis accordingly reduces in size: thus, following ejaculation, penile thrusting does not contribute to sperm loss.

Penile size is notoriously an area of concern among men. Although a number of studies have attempted to establish datasets on penile size, many reports are unreliable due to probable misreporting of sizes by participants, which may be a factor of poor study design. Better quality studies have generally reported an average flaccid length of approximately 3.5 cm and an average erect length of approximately 14.5 cm, with most men being within the range 13–16 cm (Khan, Somani, Lam, & Donat, 2012; Mondaini et al., 2002). Such data are important for a number of purposes, including facilitating clinical reassurance of anxious males as to the normalcy of their penile endowment. Clinical application of such data may relate to counselling in urology and for the purposes of reconstructive surgery; for example, in cases where penile augmentation may be deemed medically necessary or appropriate. Therefore, such data is considered useful before planning any medical/surgical interventions for penile size (see Dillon, Chama, & Honig, 2008).

Erection

Although the processes of erection and ejaculation are closely related during sexual intercourse, ejaculation can occur in the absence of erection. Indeed, each of these sexual responses can exist without the other. Thus, despite their association during coitus, erection and ejaculation are distinct physiological processes. Common to both erection and ejaculation, the pelvic nerve plexus serves as a junction for neural input to the anatomic structures involved. Brain regions that control erection and ejaculation via the spinal cord are part of a larger brain network that regulates overall sexual response. The neurotransmitters dopamine and serotonin both play key roles in the control of erection and ejaculation (see Giuliano, 2011).

At a physical level, penile erection is a hydraulic process. It commences when the arterioles of the penis dilate, allowing a net inflow of blood into the spongiform tissues of the penis, and rigidity increases as expansion of the internal tissues compresses the venous return and thus reduces blood outflow. Arteriole dilation is a consequence of nervous stimulation: sexual arousal (via the brain) and direct sexual contact (locally to the genitalia) lead to the production of cyclic guanosine monophosphate (cGMP) molecules, which in turn act as a signal to the arterioles to induce vasodilation. Nervous stimulation must not cease, because cGMP is continually being broken down by cGMP phosphodiesterase, an enzyme that is always present. A lack of sufficient nervous stimulation will thus lead to failure to produce or maintain an erection; that is, impotence or erectile dysfunction (ED). In the past, ED was frequently treated by injection of a vasodilator into the base of the penis. Such treatment is effective but inconvenient; not only is an injection required, but the resultant erection is immediate and will generally not abate for several hours. Thus, in the past, ED was traded for priapism. In recent years, oral cGMP phosphodiesterase agonists such as sildenafil (Viagra) have become available and have revolutionized the treatment of ED. By inhibiting cGMP phosphodiesterase and thus preventing the breakdown of cGMP, vasodilation and hence erection is facilitated. Unlike the older vasodilator approach, erection is not initiated by the drug treatment alone; sexual excitement is required in order to drive the production of cGMP via nervous stimulation—thus avoiding unwanted erections in inappropriate contexts. Moreover, these new agents are associated with minimal adverse effects (see an interesting review by Tsertsvadze et al., 2009).

The Female Reproductive System

Oogenesis

Prior to ovulation, oocytes are contained within ovarian follicles (one oocyte per follicle). During prenatal life, thousands of primordial follicles are produced, such that the fetal ovary contains over 3 million follicles at its peak. Thereafter, a process of follicular self-destruction, known as atresia, results in the loss of most of these follicles. This process continues throughout the woman's life until the ovary contains no functional follicles, at the time of menopause. Atresia is characterized by the initial development of a small subset of follicles (at a rate of 10–15 follicles per day); prior to puberty all of these follicles fail to develop fully and are lost. During the reproductive years, one follicle per ovarian (monthly) cycle develops fully, resulting in ovulation of a single oocyte. The process of follicular development is under the control of FSH: extra FSH (either for clinical reasons or due to superovulation associated with in vitro fertility [IVF] procedures) results in more than one follicle reaching maturity. Beyond being a mechanism to control numbers of oocytes ovulated, atresia may function as a means to select for the "best" follicles/oocytes. However, this is somewhat speculative, and no clear evidence of a mechanistic basis for such a selection effect exists. Additionally, the surviving oocytes do not represent a perfectly functional population; thus, if such active selection is indeed occurring, it is an imperfect process. The precise factors that control atresia are yet to be explained, and the mechanistic details of follicle/oocyte recruitment and apoptosis presently remain an enigma. (For useful reviews, see Hartshorne , Lyrakou, Hamoda, Oloto, & Ghafari [2009]; Krysko et al. [2008]; and Gougeon [2010]).

The Ovarian Cycle

Although each ovarian cycle lasts (on average) 28 days, the primordial follicle that becomes the ovulatory follicle will have started its maturation several months prior. The exact initiation of follicular maturation is intrinsically difficult to pinpoint, given the microscopic size of primordial follicles and the subtle nature of early changes; thus, it remains unclear as to how long the entire process of oocyte maturation takes. Approximately 3 months prior to ovulation, primordial follicles reach the early antral stage, in which fluid accumulation within the follicle results in a marked increase in size. By day 1–5 of the ovarian cycle, approximately 5 antral follicles exist, one of which will become the dominant (pre-ovulatory) follicle. At 20–25 mm in diameter, this follicle is much larger than its primordial predecessor. The size increase is due to fluid accumulation and multiplication of constituent cells. Ovulation, which typically occurs in most women at a relatively constant 14 ± 2 days prior to the onset of menstrual bleeding, sees the oocyte being released through the ovary wall and into the fimbriated opening (ostium) of the oviduct. Thereafter, the constituent cells of the ruptured follicle undergo dramatic changes as the "damaged" ovarian site is revascularized and remodeled. The overall effect of these changes is to convert the follicle into a corpus luteum, a structure responsible for sex steroid biosynthesis. The corpus luteum develops until approximately midway through the post-ovulatory phase, whereupon it declines, eventually to become the corpus albicans, an inactive structure (**Figure 5-1**).

Hormonal Aspects of Female Reproduction

As mentioned above, follicular/oocyte development is driven by the gonadotrophin FSH. Ovulation is triggered by a surge of the gonadotrophin LH. An additional crucial role for LH is to stimulate the follicular cells such that estradiol and other estrogenic hormones (henceforth referred to collectively as "estrogen") are produced from the ovary. Specifically, LH drives the theca cells (located in the outer region of the follicle) to produce androgens (mainly androstenedione and testosterone), which are then converted to estrogen by the granulosa cells (located in the inner region of the follicle and contacting the oocyte). In addition to acting within the follicle to drive follicular and oocyte development, molecules of estrogen and (non-converted) androgen enter the bloodstream. These blood-borne sex steroids promote reproductive functionality within the body (e.g., maintenance of sexual morphology) and the brain (e.g., sexual behavior). Following ovulation, the corpus luteum produces progesterone, the main function of which (in the non-pregnant woman) is to promote the final maturation of the endometrium in readiness for possible embryo implantation.

The gonadotrophins are released from the anterior pituitary gland in response to stimulation by gonadotrophin releasing hormone (GnRH). The hypothalamus is the source of GnRH, which is released in a pulsatile manner approximately once per hour. Estrogen acts as an inhibitor of GnRH and gonadotrophin release, and the gonadotrophins act on the anterior pituitary to inhibit their own release. Thus, the hormonal axis controlling estrogen production is under negative feedback regulation. However, it is important to note that the hypothalamus is under the control of the brain, and therefore it is mechanistically plausible that mental state may subtly alter GnRH levels, with such alterations thereby affecting levels of the gonadotrophins and sex steroid levels, and thus potentially altering reproductive functioning. For example, in recent years it has become apparent that positive social events (e.g., success in a competitive situation) lead to slightly elevated sex steroid levels, whereas negative events (e.g., failure, reduction in social status) lead to the converse (see, for example, Eisenegger, Haushofer, & Fehr, 2011; Salvador, 2012) Thus, it is possible that environmental cues, mediated through the brain, may alter reproductive functioning. This may help to explain several common observations in the context of reproductive and sexual medical practice, including that reduced fecundity and lack of sexual desire are associated with depression and stress (Campagne, 2006; Li et al., 2011).

The Female Tract During Coitus

From the perspective of fertilization, the preovulatory and periovulatory phases are the crucial times when the female tract functions to facilitate the delivery of sperm to the oocyte. Estrogen stimulation is largely responsible for this functionality. During the preovulatory phase, estrogen levels rise sharply, due to increased secretion from the increasingly developed antral follicles. Sexual arousal during this phase results in the production of vaginal fluid, which functions to lubricate the passageway for the penis. This fluid is the result of exudate from the mucous membrane lining of the vagina and secretion from the Bartholin's glands (greater vestibular glands) lying close to the outer opening of the vagina. The Bartholin's glands are histologically similar to the bulbourethral glands in the male, and arise from the same fetal tissue.

The Physiology of Female Sexual Arousal

Sexual pleasure is of great importance in human sexuality, and the underlying physiological structures and functions

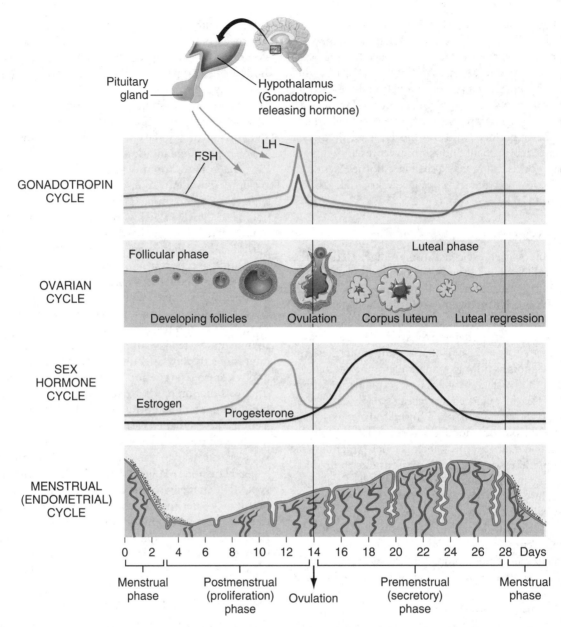

Figure 5-1 Menstrual Cycle: Interconnected Impact of Ovarian, Endometrial, and Pituitary Cycles (Phases of Hormonal Fluctuations and Structural Changes Numbered in Sequence)

are of significant interest. Some aspects in this context remain highly controversial: for example, the existence (or otherwise) of the so-called G-spot, and its anatomy. Other aspects have arguably been underresearched: for example, the anatomy and physiology of the clitoris. Modern imaging technologies, including MRI and ultrasound, have revealed new insights into female sexual anatomy (O'Connell, Sanjeevan, & Hutson, 2005; Puppo, 2011), and the physiology of arousal and penetration. For example, in one recent study ultrasound was performed during coitus, with the female volunteer in the gynecologic position while her partner penetrated her from a standing position. The resultant ultrasound images indicated that the root of the clitoris has a very close relationship with the anterior vaginal wall, with both entities being activated as a single anatomical and

functional unit during thrusting by the penetrating penis. This anatomic relationship might explain the pleasurable sensations associated with the anterior vaginal area, the so-called G-spot (Buisson , Foldes, Jannini, & Mimoun, 2010). Such studies represent the initial phase of a new pathway of research that may reveal fascinating insights into female structure and function during sexual arousal and coitus.

Female Orgasm: Functional?

It has not been reliably demonstrated that female sexual excitement and orgasm have an enhancing effect on fertility, and skepticism surrounds such claims (Levin, 2011). Specific adaptations exist that are suggestive of such a role for female excitement/orgasm, although it is possible that these are vestigial functions only—that is, they may have evolved as adaptations in our pre-human ancestors but now have no clear effects and will eventually be removed by natural selection. As mentioned in the previous section, real-time studies of coitus in human subjects using MRI and ultrasound have cast light on the physical changes within the female tract when coitus occurs (Buisson et al., 2010; Faix, Lapray, Callede, Maubon, & Lanfrey, 2002; Faix, Lapray, Courtieu, Maubon, & Lanfrey, 2001; Schulz, van Andel, Sabelis, & Mooyaart, 1999). In respect of female orgasm, interpretations of such images have suggested that, as orgasm is approached, the cervical region lifts upward and the cervix itself simultaneously dips down towards the tip of the penis, in a process described as "tenting." However, few such studies have been conducted, and it is therefore difficult to draw firm conclusions about whether and to what extent physical changes in the vagina/cervix associated with arousal and orgasm occur to enhance sperm uptake. Issues concerning (1) a possible functional role in terms of enhancing fertilization and (2) its evolutionary origins, have rendered the female orgasm a topic of intense debate among reproductive biologists. Beyond increasing the probability of fertilization from a given instance of coitus, if female orgasm does have a facilitative role in fertilization this may have important implications in terms of "sperm selection." These aspects are discussed later in this chapter.

Semen in the Female Tract

Following ejaculation, substrate proteins from the seminal vesicle are rapidly acted upon by coagulation-promoting enzyme molecules from the prostate gland, such that the liquid semen is coagulated into a gel (coagulum) (Lilja, Oldbring, Rannevik, and Laurell, 1987). The coagulum is hydrophilic and avidly adheres to the vagina and cervix, thus reducing sperm loss through leakage out of the vagina. However, sperm are mechanically trapped and immotile within the gel by binding to semenogelin molecules from the seminal vesicle and zinc ions from the prostate. Trapped sperm must be freed in order to swim into the cervix; slow-acting enzyme molecules from the prostate facilitate this by breaking down the gel matrix (Lilja & Laurell, 1984). This liquefaction process occurs over a period of minutes to more than 1 hour. Individual males exhibit markedly divergent durations of semen coagulation-liquefaction, and sexual behavior (e.g., frequency of ejaculation) causes intra-individual variations in the process (Amelar, 1962; Dunn & Picologlou, 1977).

Cervical Functions Following Sperm Deposition

The cervix sits at the top of the vagina, and is the main site of deposition for semen; hence, this structure is exposed to high numbers of sperm. During the postovulatory phase, due to the presence of high levels of progesterone (secreted by the corpus luteum), the cervical fluid becomes thick, fibrous, and inhospitable to sperm. By contrast, the preovulatory and periovulatory cervix produces a thin, stretchy, highly hydrated fluid in which sperm may swim and thrive. As soon as ejaculation occurs, sperm begin to transit this cervical fluid and enter the uterus; however, many sperm do not immediately pass through the cervical os, and instead become localized in microscopic crypts in the cervical wall. The details of what happens to such sperm en route to the oocyte have been gleaned predominantly from animal studies, and it remains unclear as to what precisely occurs in humans. However, the following descriptive model may be constructed from the available data: sperm within the cervical crypts lose motility and form attachments between their head regions and the crypt surface. Thereafter, at varying periods ranging from minutes to hours or even days, sperm detach from the crypt wall, regain motility and traverse the cervical os to continue their journey toward the upper reaches of the tract. In keeping with this model, the presence of viable sperm has been detected in human cervical fluid up to 5 days post-insemination (Gould, Overstreet, & Hanson, 1984; Mortimer, 1994). Thus, around the time of ovulation, the cervix appears to function as a steady-release mechanism to ensure that relatively steady numbers of sperm reach the ampulla of the oviduct (the site of fertilization) over a protracted period. The benefits of this are likely to be twofold: to maximize the likelihood of fertilization by ensuring that sperm will be present when the oocyte enters the scene, and to ensure that the numbers of sperm reaching the oocyte are low enough to reduce the risk of polyspermy to acceptable levels.

The Role of the Uterus and Oviducts in Sperm Transport

Sperm reaching the oviduct appear to be helped on their journey toward the oocyte by mild peristaltic-like contractions of the uterus. Following estrogen stimulation, and in the absence of progesterone, the myometrium is rendered contractile, and prostaglandins within semen (originating from the seminal vesicles) promote this contractility. Specifically, the prostaglandins appear to promote contraction of the upper part of the uterus at the uterotubular junction, resulting in a negative pressure in the uterus and a mild pumping action of the uterine wall, thus drawing sperm upward into the oviduct (Bygdeman, Gottlieb, Svanborg, & Swahn, 1987; et al., 1987; Karim & Hillier, 1975). Work using modern imaging techniques including sonography has shed further light on this uterine contractility process. Using such techniques, Zervomanolakis et al. (2007) examined the function of the uterus and oviducts to determine whether these structures acted as a sperm pump. Labeled particles (to mimic sperm) were introduced to the vagina during the preovulatory phase and were observed to enter the uterus and oviducts, apparently propelled by peristalsis-like contractions, with the greatest number of particles being directed to the oviduct associated with the ovary containing the mature follicle. Given that such particles were non-motile (unlike sperm), this provides good evidence that the female tract is able to actively pump vaginal contents upward and toward the oocyte. Interestingly, an increase in peristaltic contractions was observed following the administration oxytocin, a hormone associated with female sexual arousal (Zervomanolakis et al., 2007). However, the extent to which such uterine responses may be facilitative for fertilization remains unclear, and more research in this area would be beneficial.

The uterotubular junction functions as an intermittent sphincter, allowing or preventing sperm from accessing the oviduct. Once within the initial region of the oviduct (the isthmus), sperm may form transient attachments with the smooth epithelial lining of the duct, at which point motility is reduced. As with the abovementioned events at the cervix, this process of attachment/slowing may function to maximize steady-stream delivery of sperm to the ampulla, with "dormant" sperm residing in the extensive epithelial folds—although again, much of this perspective has been gained from animal studies, and human details remain to be validated. However, the oviduct is conceptually a very attractive site as a potential storage depot for sperm: in contrast to the lower reaches of the tract (uterus, cervix, vagina), where leukocytes accumulate post-coitus and attack sperm cells (quite possibly including undamaged sperm cells), the oviduct environment is convivial to sperm (Murray & Smith, 1997). It has not been determined with certainty how long human sperm can remain viable within the female reproductive tract. In fact, there may be no single duration figure possible, because genetic and environmental factors affecting both men and women undoubtedly lead to variance in the duration of viable occupation. However, in vitro studies of sperm suggest that 5 days is not unrealistic for sperm deposited shortly prior to ovulation, a number that is supported by research involving human participants (Wilcox, Weinberg, & Baird, 1995). These stored sperm must reside somewhere within the tract, and the isthmus of the oviduct is currently accepted as the most promising reservoir.

Sperm become fully capacitated within the oviduct, due to signaling factors present within the oviduct fluid. Capacitated sperm swim vigorously (a transiently reversible phenomenon known as hyperactivation), bind with the oocyte, and undergo the acrosome reaction, in which enzymes are released from the sperm to facilitate entry into the oocyte. If an oocyte is present in the ampulla, sperm in this region hone in on the oocyte, clearly being attracted to it. The precise nature of the mechanism of attraction remains to be fully elucidated, but appears to involve sensing by the sperm of the subtle temperature gradient (of approximately 2°C) along the oviduct and a chemotactic agent(s) released from the egg. (For a very useful review, see Suarez and Pacey, 2006.)

Sperm Selection in the Female Tract

The current view among most reproductive physiologists, derived from experimental and clinical observations, is that only a small proportion of sperm from the millions ejaculated into the vagina will reach the oviduct (Baker & Bellis, 1993). A typical ejaculate contains around 350 million sperm; numbers of sperm appearing in the oviduct (at around the time of ovulation) in the subsequent hours following ejaculation vary greatly (Williams et al., 1993), but it is likely that the oocyte will typically be exposed to only 200–300 sperm. For a given sperm cell to have any chance of achieving fertilization, it must be healthy enough to traverse the various physical, chemical, and immunological obstacles present throughout the female reproductive tract, from vagina to ampulla (see Foo & Lim, 2008). Moreover, to be successful, a given sperm cell must be on a par, or better than, the millions of other co-ejaculated sperm, in terms of swimming and survival ability. Thus, there exists a *de facto* process of sperm selection, with the "fittest" sperm being most likely to achieve fertilization. Presumably there are adaptive benefits to such selection, in that a weak sperm may also be one that is harboring a genetic defect such as a gross chromosomal aberration or a genetic deficit affecting the process of spermatogenesis. Moreover, there is some evidence that the cervical mucus may act as a barrier to sperm carrying structural genetic abnormalities. Bianchi et al. (2004) carried out in vitro experiments on human cervical mucus to determine whether the mucus can act as a mechanism for the removal of sperm that, despite being morphologically normal, contained chromatin abnormalities. The results obtained indicated that sperm containing higher levels of some forms of DNA structural damage are more likely to be retained by the cervical mucus barrier (Bianchi et al., 2004). Sperm selection within the female tract should act such that, from a mixture of defect-carrying and normal sperm within one ejaculate, fertilization is more likely from the latter sperm. It should also reduce the chances that defects of spermatogenesis are inherited. However, the fact that various genetic defects are frequently transmitted paternally indicates that such selection is far from perfect. Indeed, in many or most cases, genetic defects of a non-structural nature carried by sperm should have no deleterious effects on sperm performance in the female reproductive tract.

Sperm Competition?

Anthropologically, although human reproduction is characterized by lifelong or serial monogamy, the occurrence of extraneous sexual intercourse occurs at a sufficiently high frequency such as to ensure its evolutionary importance. Research surveys have supported this notion. For example, in one study approximately 25% of female college students acknowledged non-monogamy, with approximately one in eight admitting to having sex with two or more males in a 24-hour period (Gallup, Burch, & Mitchell, 2006). Thus, behavioral adaptations may have evolved for males to increase assurance that their genes are indeed the ones transmitted to their chosen (female) partner. However, there is no research to cite in support of this point.

Extrapair Coupling: The Role of Sperm Fitness and Numbers

An additional physiological line of defense may work to assure positive sperm selection. The passive form of sperm selection described would also operate in instances where sperm from two different males came to occupy the same woman's reproductive tract. Suppose a given women has sex with her usual partner on day 12 of her ovarian cycle, and then on day 13 has sex with an extraneous partner. In this case, sperm from both males will be simultaneously present within the woman's reproductive tract, and the sperm from each male is likely to be similarly viable. In such a case, the male who produced sperm of greater "fitness," or in greater numbers, would be more likely to be reproductively successful, in terms of achieving fertilization.

Sperm are the product of intense selection for sperm fitness, and it is therefore unlikely that the outcome of competition between sperm from different healthy partners will generally depend on physiological differences between their sperm. A greater number of sperm would provide a definitive competitive advantage, and non-human primate species that practice frequent polygamy generally have a larger testicular weight (as a percentage of body weight) than do more monogamous primates (Harcourt, Purvis, & Liles, 1995). However, within-species selection for large testes would be strongly moderated by the costs to fitness imposed by maintaining large gonads, especially in view of the high metabolic demands of testicular tissue. In keeping with this evolutionary concept, empirical analysis of human testicular volume (or weight) has demonstrated that, although testis size does positively correlate with the number of sperm ejaculated, there is no evidence of a correlation between testis size and tendency to engage in polygamous sexual behavior (Simmons, Firman, Rhodes, & Peters, 2004).

Physical Removal of Sperm?

In instances where extraneous intercourse had recently occurred, it would be beneficial to the main partner if semen from the extrapair mating were to be removed. In this respect, it has been proposed that the human penis may be structured such as to maximize the displacement of previously deposited semen from the vagina. Results obtained by simulated coitus using artificial penis and vagina models appear to support this contention, and indicate that the coronal ridge (at the base of the glans penis) is the most important morphological feature mediating semen displacement (Gallup et al., 2003). Additionally, sexual behavior may be adjusted as an unconscious means to displace prior semen, and survey-based research has generated findings compatible with this notion. For example, couples who had periods of separation, during which the female partner engaged in extraneous intercourse, often resulted in deeper and more vigorous penile thrusting during subsequent coitus (Gallup et al., 2003; Goetz et al., 2005). However, this field of research is presently limited to a small number of studies, and further research would be required before semen displacement could be accepted as a significant factor in human sperm competition.

Female-Mediated Sperm Flowback and Retention

Another possible form of sperm competition would be active selection of one partner's sperm over the sperm of another partner. For example, in an extrapair coupling with a male of high genetic quality, it would be evolutionarily advantageous to the female if this mate's sperm fertilized her oocyte while her main partner (of lower genetic quality but of proven utility for providing support) brings up the resultant child. Given the aforementioned functionalities of the female tract in terms of storing sperm and preventing or facilitating their journey toward the oocyte, the intriguing possibility exists that the female might be able to (unconsciously) influence the fate of sperm deposited by different males. It would presumably be mechanistically difficult or impossible for the female reproductive tract to differentiate between the sperm of two males when the sperm populations were mixed within her tract. The only plausible way in which the female physiology might be able to select for one set of sperm over another would be to facilitate, or hamper, individual deposits of sperm. In a landmark study using human volunteers, Baker and Bellis (1993) examined sperm loss from the vagina, a process termed *flowback*. They found that flowback occurred in the majority of copulations, with an average of approximately one-third of ejaculated sperm eliminated within 30 minutes following ejaculation. However, in around 1 in 10 copulations, virtually all the sperm were lost through flowback. Sperm appeared to be lost at a lower extent where the woman had experienced an orgasm within 1 minute of the time of ejaculation, suggesting a possible role for female orgasm in sperm retention. The authors proposed the existence of a blow-suck mechanism able to transport the upper vaginal contents into the cervix. Based on the assumption that infidelity is generally associated with a higher rate of orgasm (see Brody, Klapilova, K., & Krejcová, L. 2013; Ellsworth & Bailey, 2013), the implication is that extrapair matings—potentially with genetically desirable males—result in greater sperm uptake and hence a greater probability that the non-partner male fathers a child on whom resources will be expended by the main partner, whose sperm will be subject to a greater degree of flowback (Baker & Bellis, 1993). However, the Baker and Bellis study was of a small scale and does not appear to have been replicated, perhaps due to the intrinsic difficulty of recruiting subjects willing to participate in copulatory experiments involving semen collection, and a great deal of further data on flowback would be required to determine whether the hypothesis of female-mediated sperm selection is valid.

Female Orgasm: Functional Role in Sperm Selection?

Genetically desirable male features include high morphological symmetry (for example, symmetrical facial features). As mentioned earlier in this chapter, it is possible that the female orgasm has a physiological role in facilitating sperm transport and hence maximizing the likelihood of fertilization. Accordingly, the proportion of copulations that are accompanied by female orgasm should positively correlate with the male partner's morphological symmetry. This predicted correlation has been investigated empirically. For example, a questionnaire-based study of 86 sexually active heterosexual couples revealed that women with high-symmetry partners had significantly more (copulatory) female orgasms than did women with partners possessing low symmetry (Thornhill, Gangestad, & Comer, 1995). Subsequent research replicates and supports these findings. For example, in a 2000 study, self-report data from 388 women indicated that women copulating with more attractive men were more likely to experience orgasm than were women who copulated with less attractive men, a correlation that remained significant after statistically controlling for potentially confounding variables (Shackelford et al., 2000). A more recent study explored correlations between female orgasm and various potential markers of male genetic quality, including facial symmetry, and found that more frequent and earlier-timed orgasms occurred in women who copulated with men of apparent high genetic quality (Puts, Welling, Burriss, & Dawood, 2012).

In the context of the apparent correlation between female orgasm and male genetic quality, and in light of the foregoing work on sperm retention by the female reproductive tract, it would be of value to determine whether there is indeed a biological role for the female orgasm in terms of enhancing the likelihood of fertilization. Such a role would be reflective of evolution, in terms of orgasm being an adaptive physiological response. The alternative explanation is that female orgasm is not adaptive but rather has been maintained through evolution simply as a by-product of natural selection on the male physiological apparatus of orgasm associated with ejaculation. These adaptive versus "by-product" explanations have been the subject of vigorous scientific debate. Neither position has been fully tested to date; however, data have emerged that promise to move the debate forward. Zietsch and Santtila (2011) tested one of the central tenets of the by-product explanation, namely that selection pressure on the male orgasm should be transferred to the female genetically, resulting in a positive correlation for orgasmic function in closely related individuals. A questionnaire approach was employed, involving over 10,000 twins and siblings, to examine susceptibility to female orgasm. Significant genetic variation was found for both male and female tendency to orgasm (for a given stimulatory level), as would be expected; however, the researchers found no significant correlation for orgasmic tendency between opposite-sex twins and siblings. This suggests that separate genetic mechanisms control orgasmic tendency/function in males and females.

Therefore, it does not appear that female orgasmic function is strongly co-selected with that of the male, thus challenging the by-product explanation for female orgasm (Zietsch & Santtila, 2011). The notion of female orgasm as being a separate functional entity from the male counterpart is given further support from research that has suggested the female orgasm is a more complex entity than that of the male, and may occur in different forms. For example, King and colleagues reanalyzed historical data on female orgasm and identified four orgasm types from descriptions by over 500 women of their orgasms (King, Belsky, Mah, & Binik, 2011).

Somewhat more contentiously, claims have been made that pleiotropic markers of female orgasm functionality are manifested in measurable female phenotypic traits not directly or obviously connected to reproductive physiology. For example, a survey involving 258 women found a correlation between vaginal orgasm and the prominence of the tubercle of their upper lip (Brody & Costa, 2011). However, such findings would need to be replicated before being fully accepted, due to the inevitable potential presence of survey bias (e.g., the sharpshooter fallacy) associated with isolated correlation surveys of this nature. Moreover, the concept of "vaginal orgasm" is not accepted by most experts in human anatomy (Puppo, 2011).

The claims for a functional, adaptive role for female orgasm in terms of sperm selection are countered by two points. First, although suggestive evidence to support this hypothesis does exist (as discussed), the evidence is mostly indirect and is not of a particularly extensive nature. Second, physiological evidence is either lacking, or may actually serve toward refuting the hypothesis. A particular meta-analysis is of interest here: Levin (2011) examined academic articles relating to sperm transport and function in the human female genital tract in the absence and presence of arousal to orgasm. The conclusion was that the majority of reported evidence indicates that the female orgasm has little or no effective role in the transport of sperm in natural human coitus (Levin, 2011).

Sperm Competition and Hormonal Contraception

There is a limited but growing body of evidence that men and women demonstrate changes in their choice of mate according to the phase of the menstrual cycle. At around the time of ovulation, women tend to display a stronger preference for symmetrical, more masculine and less related men. Ovulating women appear to be more attractive to men, probably through physiological by-products of high estrogen stimulation (as opposed to unconscious female signaling). These cyclical alterations in mate preference are presumably the outcomes of evolutionary pressures, and thus are likely to provide reproductive advantages, in terms of maximizing the chances of ideal mate selection (Gangestad & Thornhill, 2008). Hormonal contraceptives (e.g., the combined contraceptive pill) effectively prevent ovulation and the associated hormonal fluctuations. Evidence has emerged that, by removing the periovulatory change in preferences, hormonal contraception may significantly alter mate choice in both males and females. If this is correct, use of hormonal contraceptives may be associated with altered biological and relationship outcomes. However, this intriguing possibility requires more research before such speculations can be deemed valid (Alvergne & Lummaa, 2010).

Hypoactive Sexual Desire Disorder

Low or absent sexual desire is known as hypoactive sexual desire disorder (HSDD). The condition has only recently been characterized in men (Derogatis et al., 2012), but has been recognized for many years as being more prominent and prevalent among women (Brotto, 2010). The diagnostic category is somewhat controversial, especially in the context of premenopausal women, with claims that HSDD represents an unhelpful form of medicalizing what is often a socially induced and transitory situation (Jutel, 2010). Nevertheless, various medical approaches to the treatment of HSDD have emerged.

Whereas the problem for postmenopausal women lies with the cessation of ovarian sex steroid output, premenopausal women with HSDD in general do not appear to have low levels of sex steroids. For postmenopausal women, administration of estrogenic hormones (i.e., estrogen-replacement therapy) may be effective. However, estrogen-replacement therapy carries side effects and risks. Recent research has indicated that, for both postmenopausal and premenopausal women, androgen therapy can be effective in treating HSSD. This is because androgens such as testosterone bind avidly to androgen receptors within the brain and strongly influence sex drive. (The same process underlies male sex drive; however, it should be noted that androgen levels in men are typically around tenfold higher than in premenopausal women.) Thus, even in premenopausal women, androgen therapy is predicted to enhance sex drive and empirical findings support this notion (Chudakov , Ben Zion, & Belmaker, 2007). Typically, transdermal testosterone patches are employed to deliver a suitable level of androgenic stimulation to positively influence libido while avoiding masculinization. Early results indicate efficacy with minimal side effects, although the positive outcomes reported have not been unequivocal, and longer term studies of side effects are required before androgen therapy could become a mainstream treatment for HSDD (Davis & Braunstein, 2012; Kronawitter et al., 2009; Woodis McLendon, Muzyk, 2012). Even where HSDD may be due to psychological factors (e.g., depression, stress), androgen therapy may be effective (although the psychological causes should also receive direct attention).

Development of the Reproductive Tracts

Genetics of Sex Determination

In humans, male sexual development is initially driven by gene expression from the Y chromosome, with formation of the testes from generalized fetal tissues being the initial morphologically identifiable occurrence. The "default" developmental pathway is female; in other words, in the absence of a Y chromosome, the tissues that would otherwise have developed into the testis instead develop into the ovary. Testicular development is dependent upon the Y-linked testis-determining gene *SRY*; gonadal development in general (for both sexes) is also dependent on several other genes, both X-linked and autosomal. Beginning during fetal life, the testes secrete hormones, required for the development of the male reproductive tract, genitalia, and secondary sexual structures. The Y chromosome, in addition to harboring the *SRY* gene and thus serving as the "master switch" for the male development pathway, also contains genes essential for post-pubertal reproductive functioning; in particular, spermatogenesis. However, the Y chromosome contains relatively few functional genes. The X chromosome, by contrast, contains many more genes, of which only a minority are concerned with sexual development. In evolutionary terms, the Y chromosome is a relic of a distant ancestral autosome that has become 100% male-specific. In comparison, the X chromosome has evolved genes that are of advantage to both sexes. This distinction arises from the fact that, while the Y chromosome is exclusive to males, the X chromosome is possessed by both sexes. (See Schafer and Goodfellow [1996], Kucinskas and Just [2005], and Delbridge and Graves [2007] for useful reviews of the genetics of sexual differentiation.)

Hormonal Aspects

Male and female fetuses remain undifferentiated until the ninth week of development, with primordial ductal and sinal tissues providing the starting material for development of the genitalia and reproductive tracts. Within the *SRY*-induced male developmental pathway, androgenic sex steroids (primarily testosterone), secreted from the Leydig cells of the primordial testicular tissues, drive the development of male genitalia, the male reproductive tract, and masculine body characteristics. Under the influence of testosterone, one pair of ducts, the mesonephric, differentiates to become the key components of the male tract, including the vasa deferentia, ductus epididymides, and seminal vesicles. Testosterone is converted into dihydrotestosterone (DHT) in some target tissues: DHT drives the differentiation of the urogenital sinus to become the prostate and bulbourethral glands. Meanwhile, Sertoli cells, located within the primordial testicular tissue, secrete anti-Müllerian hormone (MSH); this hormone promotes the regression of another pair of ducts, the paramesonephric. In the absence of anti-Müllerian hormone, the paramesonephric ducts differentiate to become the top of the vagina, the uterus, and the oviducts. In the absence of DHT, the urogenital sinus differentiates to become the lower vagina and the Bartholin's and Skene's glands. In terms of development of the external genitalia, DHT drives the genital tubercle to differentiate into the penis; in the absence of DHT the same tissue develops into the clitoris. (See Sajjad [2010] and Stukenborg, Colon, and Soder [2010] for useful reviews.)

Sex-Specific Brain Development

Development of a masculinized brain also occurs under the influence of sex steroids, with sex-specific "neuro-organizational" differences in sexual orientation and gender identity probably being established at this stage. However, because brain differentiation occurs much later *in utero* (i.e., during the first 2 months of pregnancy) than genital/physical differentiation (which occurs during the second half of pregnancy), the two developmental processes are largely independent of one another, and alterations in development (possibly mediated by hormonal signaling) could thus result in transsexuality or altered sexual orientation (Bao & Swaab, 2011; Savic , Garcia-Falgueras, & Swaab, 2010). Although the greatest effects on the brain occur during fetal life, puberty represents another neuro-organizational period, with the possibility that sex hormones may alter behavior. However, the possible role of pubertal hormones in respect to sexual orientation and gender identity is not yet fully understood, and further research in this area is encouraged (Berenbaum & Beltz, 2011).

Conclusion

This chapter has focused on contemporary issues and controversies in the science of human reproduction, with particular emphasis on aspects that affect sexual health and functioning such as sexual arousal, sperm transport, and sperm selection. It should be clear from the foregoing discussion that the science of human reproductive and sexual function comprises a wide range of disciplines, spanning molecular, cellular, physiological, and psychological fields. By the inherent intimate nature of the subject matter, the study of how humans procreate is associated with perhaps more contention than arises in most other scientific fields. Nevertheless, great progress has been made in recent years in terms of advancing our scientific understanding of the underpinning mechanisms and functions, with major implications for medical, nursing, and social practice. Moreover, technical advances such as high-resolution real-time imaging technology, coupled with exponentially increasing molecular genetic knowledge, look set to transform the study of human reproduction over the next several years. Such advances in research may provide data to address the unanswered questions of the scientific controversies associated with human reproduction and sexuality.

● ● ● REFERENCES

Alvergne, A., & Lummaa, V. (2010). Does the contraceptive pill alter mate choice in humans? *Trends in Ecology & Evolution, 25*(3), 171–179.

Amelar, R. D. (1962). Coagulation, liquefaction and viscosity of human semen. *Journal of Urology, 87,* 187–190.

Auger, J., Kunstmann, J. M., Czyglik, F., & Jouannet, P. (1995). Decline in semen quality among fertile men in Paris during the past 20 years. *New England Journal of Medicine, 332*(5), 281–285.

Baker, R. R., & Bellis, M. A. (1993). Human sperm competition–ejaculate manipulation by females and a function for the female orgasm. *Animal Behavior, 46*(5), 887–909.

Bao, A., & Swaab, D. F. (2011). Sexual differentiation of the human brain: Relation to gender identity, sexual orientation and neuropsychiatric disorders. *Frontiers in Neuroendocrinology, 32*(2), 214–226.

Barratt, C. L. R. (1995). Spermatogenesis. In J.G. Grudzinskas & J.L. Yovich (Eds.), *Gametes: The spermatozoon.* (pp. 250-267). Cambridge, United Kingdom: Cambridge University Press.

Berenbaum, S. A., & Beltz, A. M. (2011). Sexual differentiation of human behavior: Effects of prenatal and pubertal organizational hormones. *Frontiers of Neuroendocrinology, 32*(2), 183–200.

Bianchi, P., De Agostini, A., Fournier, J., Guidetti, C., Tarozzi, N., Bizzaro, D., & Manicardi, G. (2004). Human cervical mucus can act in vitro as a selective barrier against spermatozoa carrying fragmented DNA and chromatin structural abnormalities. *Journal of Assisted Reproduction and Genetics, 21*(4), 97–102.

Blakemore, S-J., Burnett, S. & Dahl, R. E. (2010). The role of puberty in developing adolescent brain. *Human Brain Mapping, 31*(6), 926–933.

Bonde, J. P., Ramlau-Hansen, C. H., & Olsen, J. (2011). Trends in sperm counts: The saga continues. *Epidemiology, 22*(5), 617–619.

Brody, S., & Costa, R. M. (2011). Vaginal orgasm is more prevalent among women with a prominent tubercle of the upper lip. *The Journal of Sexual Medicine, 8*(10), 2793–2799.

Brody, S., Klapilova, K., & Krejčová, L. (2013). More frequent vaginal orgasm is associated with experiencing greater excitement from deep vaginal stimulation. *The Journal of Sexual Medicine, 10*(7), 1730–1736.

Brotto, L. A. (2010). The DSM diagnostic criteria for hypoactive sexual desire disorder in women. *Archives of Sexual Behavior, 39*(2), 221–239.

Buisson, O., Foldes, P., Jannini, E., & Mimoun, S. (2010). Coitus as revealed by ultrasound in one volunteer couple. *The Journal of Sexual Medicine, 7*(8), 2750–2754.

Bygdeman, M., Gottlieb, C., Svanborg, K., & Swahn, M. L. (1987). Role of prostaglandins in human reproduction: recent advances. *Advances in Prostaglandin, Thromboxane, and Leukotriene Research, 17B,* 1112–1116.

Campagne, D. M. (2006). Should fertilization treatment start with reducing stress? *Human Reproduction, 21*(7), 1651–1658.

Carlsen, E., Giwercman, A., Keiding, N., & Skakkebaek, N. E. (1992). Evidence for decreasing quality of semen during past 50 years. *BMJ, 305*(6854), 609–613.

Carreau, S., Bouraima-Lelong, H., & Delalande, C. (2011). Estrogens–new players in spermatogenesis. *Reproductive Biology, 11*(3), 174–193.

Chudakov, B., Ben Zion, I. Z., & Belmaker, R. H. (2007). Transdermal testosterone gel application for hypoactive sexual desire disorder in premenopausal women: A controlled pilot study of the effects on the Arizona Sexual Experiences Scale for females and Sexual Function Questionnaire. *The Journal of Sexual Medicine, 4*(1), 204–208.

Davis, S. R., & Braunstein, G. D. (2012). Efficacy and safety of testosterone in the management of hypoactive sexual desire disorder in postmenopausal women. *The Journal of Sexual Medicine, 9*(4), 1134–1148.

Delbridge, M. L., & Graves, J. A. M. (2007). Origin and evolution of spermatogenesis genes on the human sex chromosomes. *Society for Reproduction and Fertility, 65*(Suppl.), 1–17.

Derogatis, L., Rosen, R. C., Goldstein, I., Werneburg, B., Kempthorne-Rawson, J., & Sand, M. (2012). Characterization of hypoactive sexual desire disorder (HSDD) in men. *The Journal of Sexual Medicine, 9*(3), 812–820.

Dillon, B. E., Chama, N. B., & Honig, S. C. (2008). Penile size and penile enlargement surgery: A review. *International Journal of Impotence Research, 20*(5), 519–529.

Dunn, P. F., & Picologlou, B. F. (1977). Variation in human semen viscoelastic properties with respect to time post ejaculation and frequency of ejaculation. *International Journal of Fertility, 22*(4), 217–224.

Eisenegger, C., Haushofer, J., & Fehr, E. (2011). The role of testosterone in social interaction. *Trends in Cognitive Sciences, 15*(6), 263–271.

Ellsworth, R. M., Bailey, D. H. (2013). Human female orgasm as evolved signal: A test of two hypotheses. *Archives of Sexual Behavior, 42*(8), 1545–1554.

Faix, A., Lapray, J. F., Callede, O., Maubon, A., & Lanfrey, K. (2002). Magnetic resonance Imaging (MRI) of sexual intercourse: Second experience in missionary position and initial experience in posterior position. *Journal of Sex & Marital Therapy, 28,* 63–76.

Faix, A., Lapray, J. F., Courtieu, C., Maubon, A., & Lanfrey, K. (2001). Magnetic resonance imaging of sexual intercourse: Initial experience. *Journal of Sex & Marital Therapy, 27*(5), 475–482.

Foo, J. Y. A., & Lim, C. S. (2008). Biofluid mechanics of the human reproductive process: Modelling of the complex interaction and pathway to the oocytes. *Zygote, 16*(4), 343–354.

Gallup, G. G., Jr., Burch, R. L., & Mitchell, T. J. B. (2006). Semen displacement as a sperm competition strategy — Multiple mating, self-semen displacement, and timing of in-pair copulations. *Human Nature, 17*(3), 253–264.

Gallup, G. G. Burch, R. L., Zappieri, M. L., Parvez, R. A., Stockwell, M. L., & Davis, J. A. (2003). The human penis as a semen displacement device. *Evolution and Human Behavior, 24*(4), 277–289.

Gallup, G., Burch, R., & Platek, S. (2002). Does semen have antidepressant properties? *Archives of Sexual Behavior, 31*(3), 289–293.

Gangestad, S. W., & Thornhill, R. (2008). Human oestrus. *Proceedings of the Royal Society of London, Series B, Biological Science, 275*(1638), 991–1000.

Giuliano, F. (2011). Neurophysiology of erection and ejaculation. *The Journal of Sexual Medicine, 8,* 310–315.

Goetz, A. T., Shackelford, T. K., Weekes-Shackelford, A., Euler, H. A., Hoier, S., Schmitt, D. P., & LaMunyon, C. W. (2005). Mate retention, semen displacement, and human sperm competition: A preliminary investigation of tactics to prevent and correct female infidelity. *Personality and Individual Differences, 38*(4), 749–763.

Gougeon, A. (2010). Human ovarian follicular development: From activation of resting follicles to preovulatory maturation. *Annales d'Endocrinologie, 71*(3), 132–143.

Gould, J., Overstreet, J., & Hanson, F. (1984). Assessment of human-sperm function after recovery from the female reproductive-tract. *Biology of Reproduction, 31*(5), 888–894.

Grootegoed, J. A., Baarends, W. M., Hendriksen, P. J. M., Hoogerbrugge, J. W., Slegtenhorsteegdeman, K. E., & Themmen, A. P. N. (1995). Molecular and cellular events in spermatogenesis. *Human Reproduction, 10,* 10–14.

Harcourt, A., Purvis, A., & Liles, L. (1995). Sperm competition—Mating system, net breeding-season, affects testes size of primates. *Functional Ecology, 9*(3), 468–476.

Hartshorne, G. M., Lyrakou, S., Hamoda, H., Oloto, E., & Ghafari, F. (2009). Oogenesis and cell death in human prenatal ovaries: What are the criteria for oocyte selection? *Molecular Human Reproduction, 15*(12), 805–819.

Hatzichristou, D., Tzortzis, V., Hatzimouratidis, K., Apostolidis, A., Moysidis, K., & Panteliou, S. (2003). Protective role of the glans penis during coitus. *International Journal of Impotence Research, 15*(5), 337–342.

Hehir-Kwa, J. Y., Rodriguez-Santiago, B., Vissers, L. E., de Leeuw, N., Pfundt, R., Buitelaar, J. K., . . . Veltman, J.A. (2011). De novo copy number variants associated with intellectual disability have a paternal origin and age bias. *Journal of Medical Genetics, 48*(11), 776–778.

Jutel, A. (2010). Framing disease: The example of female hypoactive sexual desire disorder. *Social Science & Medicine, 70*(7), 1084–1090.

Karim, S. M. M., & Hillier, K. (1975). *Physiological roles and pharmacological actions of prostaglandins in relation to human reproduction.* Ann Arbor, MI: University Park Press.

Khan, S., Somani, B., Lam, W., & Donat, R. (2012). Establishing a reference range for penile length in Caucasian British men: A prospective study of 609 men. *BJU International, 109*(5), 740–744.

Killick, S. R., Leary, C., Trussell, J., & Guthrie, K. A. (2011). Sperm content of pre-ejaculatory fluid. *Human Fertility, 14*(1), 48–52.

King, R., Belsky, J., Mah, K., & Binik, Y. (2011). Are there different types of female orgasm? *Archives of Sexual Behavior, 40*(5), 865–875.

Koelman, C., Coumans, A., Nijman, H., Doxiadis, I., Dekker, G., & Claas, F. (2000). Correlation between oral sex and a low incidence of preeclampsia: A role for soluble HLA in seminal fluid? *Journal of Reproductive Immunology, 46*(2), 155–166.

Krishnaswamy, S., Subramaniam, K., Indran, H., Ramachandran, P., Indran, T., Indran, R., & Aziz, J. A. (2009). Paternal age and common mental disorders. *The World Journal of Biological Psychiatry, 10*(4), 518–523.

Kronawitter, D., Gooren, L. J., Zollver, H., Oppelt, P. G., Beckmann, M. W., Dittrich, R., & Mueller, A. (2009). Effects of transdermal testosterone or oral dydrogesterone on hypoactive sexual desire disorder in transsexual women: Results of a pilot study. *European Journal of Endocrinology, 161*(2), 363–368.

Krysko, D. V., Diez-Fraile, A., Criel, G., Svistunov, A. A., Vandenabeele, P., & D'Herde, K. (2008). Life and death of female gametes during oogenesis and folliculogenesis. *Apoptosis, 13*(9), 1065–1087.

Kucinskas, L., & Just, W. (2005). Human male sex determination and sexual differentiation: Pathways, molecular interactions and genetic disorders. *Medicina, 41*(8), 633–640.

Levin, R. J. (2011). Can the controversy about the putative role of the human female orgasm in sperm transport be settled with our current physiological knowledge of coitus? *The Journal of Sexual Medicine, 8*(6), 1566–1578.

Li, X., Ma, Y., Geng, L., Qin, L., Hu, H., & Li, S. (2011). Baseline psychological stress and ovarian norepinephrine levels negatively affect the outcome of in vitro fertilisation. *Gynecological Endocrinology, 27*(3), 139–143.

Lilja, H., & Laurell, C. (1984). Liquefaction of coagulated human-semen. *Scandinavian Journal of Clinical and Laboratory Investigation, 44*(5), 447–452.

Lilja, H., Oldbring, J., Rannevik, G., & Laurell, C. (1987). Seminal vesicle-secreted proteins and their reactions during gelation and liquefaction of human semen. *JCI, 80(2),* 281–285.

Lynch, M. (2010). Rate, molecular spectrum, and consequences of human mutation. *Proceedings of the National Academy of Sciences, 107*(3), 961–968.

Mondaini, N., Ponchietti, R., Gontero, P., Muir, G., Natali, A., Di Loro, F., . . . Rizzo, M. (2002). Penile length is normal in most men seeking penile lengthening procedures. *International Journal of Impotence Research, 14*(4), 283–286.

Mortimer, D. (1994). *Practical laboratory andrology.* New York, NY: Oxford University Press.

Murray, S., & Smith, T. (1997). Sperm interaction with fallopian tube apical membrane enhances sperm motility and delays capacitation. *Fertility and Sterility, 68*(2), 351–357.

Neave, N., & O'Connor, D. B. (2009). Testosterone and male behaviours. *Psychologist, 22*(1), 28–31.

Ney, P. G. (1986). The intravaginal absorption of male generated hormones and their possible effect on female behavior. *Medical Hypotheses, 20*(2), 221–231.

O'Connell, H., Sanjeevan, K., & Hutson, J. (2005). Anatomy of the clitoris. *Journal of Urology, 174*(4), 1189–1195.

Olsen, J., Zhu, J. L., & Ramlau-Hansen, C. H. (2011). Has fertility declined in recent decades? *Acta Obstetricia et Gynecologica Scandinavica, 90*(2), 129–135.

Palmer, N. O., Bakos, H. W., Owens, J. A., Setchell, B. P., & Lane, M. (2012). Diet and exercise in an obese mouse fed a high-fat diet improve metabolic health and reverse perturbed sperm function. *American Journal of Physiology - Endocrinology and Metabolism, 302*(7), E768–E780.

Petersen, L., Mortensen, P. B., & Pedersen, C. B. (2011). Paternal age at birth of first child and risk of schizophrenia. *American Journal of Psychiatry, 168*(1), 82–88.

Puppo, V. (2011). Anatomy of the clitoris: Revision and clarifications about the anatomical terms for the clitoris proposed (without scientific bases) by Helen O'Connell, Emmanuele Jannini, and Odile Buisson. *ISRN Obstetrics and Gynecology, 2011,* 261464.

Puts, D. A., Welling, L. L. M., Burriss, R. P., & Dawood, K. (2012). Men's masculinity and attractiveness predict their female partners' reported orgasm frequency and timing. *Evolution and Human Behavior, 33*(1), 1–9.

Reichenberg, A., Gross, R., Weiser, M., Bresnahan, M., Silverman, J., Harlap, S., Susser, E. (2006). Advancing paternal age and autism. *Archives of General Psychiatry, 63*(9), 1026–1032.

Robertson, S. (2005). Seminal plasma and male factor signalling in the female reproductive tract. *Cell and Tissue Research, 322*(1), 43–52.

Rodriguez-Martinez, H., Kvist, U., Ernerudh, J., Sanz, L., & Calvete, J. J. (2011). Seminal plasma proteins: What role do they play? *American Journal of Reproductive Immunology, 66,* 11–22.

Rouiller-Fabre, V., Muczynski, V., Lambrot, R., Lecureuil, C., Coffigny, H., Pairault, C.,Moison, D., Angenard,G., Bakalska,M., Courtot,A., Frydman,R., Habert, R., (2009). Ontogenesis of testicular function in humans. *Folia Histochem Cytobiol.* 47(5): S19–S24.

Sadat, Z., Kalahroudi, M. A., & Saberi, F. (2012). The effect of short duration sperm exposure on development of preeclampsia in primigravid women. *Iranian Red Crescent Medical Journal, 14*(1), 20–24.

Sajjad, Y. (2010). Development of the genital ducts and external genitalia in the early human embryo. *Journal of Obstetrics and Gynaecology Research, 36*(5), 929–937.

Salvador, A. (2012). Steroid hormones and some evolutionary-relevant social interactions. *Motivation and Emotion, 36*(1), 74–83.

Savic, I., Garcia-Falgueras, A., & Swaab, D. F. (2010). Sexual differentiation of the human brain in relation to gender identity and sexual orientation. *Progress in Brain Research, 186,* 41–62.

Schafer, A., & Goodfellow, P. (1996). Sex determination in humans. *Bioessays, 18*(12), 955–963.

Schultz, W. W., van Andel, P., Sabelis, I., & Mooyaart, E. (1999). Magnetic resonance imaging of male and female genitals during coitus and female sexual arousal. *BMJ, 319*(7225), 1596–1600.

Shackelford, T., Weekes-Shackelford, V., LeBlanc, G., Bleske, A., Euler, H., & Hoier, S. (2000). Female coital orgasm and male attractiveness. *Human Nature, 11*(3), 299–306.

Sharpe, R. M. (2010). Environmental/lifestyle effects on spermatogenesis. *Philosophical Transactions of the Royal Society B: Biological Sciences, 365*(1546), 1697–1712.

Shirtcliff, E. A., Dahl, R. E., Pollak, S. D. (2009). Pubetal development: Correspondence between hormonal and physical development. *Child Development, 80*(2), 327–337.

Simmons, L., Firman, R., Rhodes, G., & Peters, M. (2004). Human sperm competition: Testis size, sperm production and rates of extrapair copulations. *Animal Behaviour, 68,* 297–302.

Sisk, C. L., & Foster, D. L. (2004). The neural basis of puberty and adolescence. *Nature Neuroscience, 7*(10), 1040–1047.

Spear, L. P. (2000). Adolescent brain and age-related behavioral manifestations. *Neuroscience & Biobehavioral Reviews, 24*(4), 417–463.

Stukenborg, J. B., Colon, E., & Soder, O. (2010). Ontogenesis of testis development and function in humans. *Sexual Development, 4*(4–5),199–212.

Suarez, S., & Pacey, A. (2006). Sperm transport in the female reproductive tract. *Human Reproduction Update, 12*(1), 23–37.

Swan, S. H., Elkin, E. P., & Fenster, L. (2000). The question of declining sperm density revisited: An analysis of 101 studies published 1934–1996. *Environmental Health Perspectives, 108*(10), 961–966.

Thornhill, R., Gangestad, S., & Comer, R. (1995). Human female orgasm and mate fluctuating asymmetry. *Animal Behaviour, 50,* 1601–1615.

Tsertsvadze, A., Fink, H. A., Yazdi, F., MacDonald, R., Bella, A. J., Ansari, M. T., . . . Wilt, T. J. (2009). Oral phosphodiesterase–5 inhibitors and hormonal treatments for erectile dysfunction: a systematic review and meta-analysis. *Annals of Internal Medicine, 151*(9), 650–651.

Velde, E. T., Burdorf, A., Nieschlag, E., Eijkemans, R., Kremer, J. A. M., Roeleveld, N., & Habbema, D. (2010). Is human fecundity declining in Western countries? *Human Reproduction, 25*(6), 1348–1353.

Verhoeven, G. (1999). Spermatogenesis and spermatogenic control: A state of the art. *Verhandelingen–Koninklijke Academie voor Geneeskunde van Belgie, 61*(3), 417–432.

Vestergaard, M., Mork, A., Madsen, K. M., & Olsen, J. (2005). Paternal age and epilepsy in the offspring. *European Journal of Epidemiology, 20*(12), 1003–1005.

Wilcox, A., Weinberg, C., & Baird, D. (1995). Timing of sexual intercourse in relation to ovulation—Effects on the probability of conception, survival of the pregnancy, and sex of the baby. *New England Journal of Medicine, 333*(23), 1517–1521.

Williams, M., Hill, C., Scudamore, I., Dunphy, B., Cooke, I., & Barratt, C. (1993). Sperm numbers and distribution within the human fallopian-tube around ovulation. *Human Reproduction, 8*(12), 2019–2026.

Woodis, C. B., McLendon, A. N., & Muzyk, A. J. (2012). Testosterone supplementation for hypoactive sexual desire disorder in women. *Pharmacotherapy, 32*(1), 38–53.

Zervomanolakis, I., Ott, H. W., Hadziomerovic, D., Mattle, V., Seeber, B. E., Virgolini, I., . . . Wildt, L. (2007). Physiology of upward transport in the human female genital tract. *Reproductive Biomechanics, 1101*, 1–20.

Zietsch, B. P., & Santtila, P. (2011). Genetic analysis of orgasmic function in twins and siblings does not support the by-product theory of female orgasm. *Animal Behaviour, 82*(5), 1097–1101.

Zukerman, Z., Weiss, D. B., & Orvieto, R. (2003). Does preejaculatory penile secretion originating from Cowper's gland contain sperm? *Journal of Assisted Reproduction and Genetics, 20*(4), 157–159.

CHAPTER

6

Sexually Transmitted Infections and Associated Reproductive Tract Infections: Recommended Screening, Care, and Treatment Interventions

THEODORA D. KWANSA AND LINDA A. GRAF

CHAPTER OBJECTIVES

- Clarify the distinction between the terms *STI* and *RTI*
- Explore the range of STIs and RTIs with emphasis on the more prevalent infections with long-term complications
- Examine the clinical manifestations, natural history, associated complications, and course of specific infections
- Examine the emerging trends of evidence-based care and therapeutic interventions and care pathways relating to recommendations and guidelines
- Explore the concepts of empiric treatment and syndromic management of identified STIs
- Explore the various policies and the standards of STI and RTI care provision

Introduction

Sexually transmitted infection (STI) care and treatment guidelines are examined from the perspective of the UK and the U.S. written by two authors with relevant UK and U.S. backgrounds of education and practice. This chapter is written for, targeting mainly, the audiences of U.S. and UK sexual and reproductive health (SRH) practitioners. However, other countries that draw on the recommendations of these countries would also find these applicable. While some treatment regimens may seem repetitive, practitioners should bear in mind that differences may be due to variations in state laws, policy regulations and guidelines. Practitioners are encouraged to carefully examine the similarities and differences in the treatment regimens guided by state and healthcare organizational policies.

This chaper presents UK guidelines on STI treatment and related aspects of care as well as STI screening and treatment in accordance with the recommendations of the U.S. Centers for Disease Control and Prevention (CDC) and the United States Preventative Services Task Force (USPTF).

Sexually transmitted infections are among the most encumbering public health problems in society. Despite the various initiatives to eliminate or reduce the rate of occurrence and spread of the different STIs, transmission rates continue to worsen rather than improve. The main concerns regarding STIs are the potential impact on the sexual health of the general population and, particular social and ethnic groups, as well as the wider social and economic implications. The prevalence and magnitude of the infections are attributable to a variety of factors, including lifestyle behaviors, cultural values and inherent sexual practices, religious beliefs, ethnicity, and socioeconomic circumstances. Other factors include young people's perceptions of sexuality and sexual health, diverse sexual inclinations and sexual-risk taking behaviors, increases of migrant populations. The measures employed to deal with sexual health-related problems vary from country to country and originate at governmental levels in the departments or ministries of health.

The United States (U.S.) has the highest rates of sexually transmitted infections (STIs) of any well-resourced nation in the world (Sammarco, 2017). The U.S. government's Centers for Disease Control (CDC) estimates that there are nearly 20 million new cases of STIs annually in the U.S. Young adults between the ages of 15–24 account for half of these new infections, even though they comprise only 25% of the sexually experienced population. These newly diagnosed STIs account for an estimated $17 billion in healthcare expenditures. Many cases of gonorrhea, chlamydia, and syphilis are either undetected and/or unreported, and additional information on human papilloma virus (HPV), herpes simplex virus (HSV), and trichomoniasis are not routinely reportable to the CDC (CDC, 2015a). Thus, even though such epidemiologic accounts capture only a small fraction of the actual STI burden in the United States, they do provide important insight into the ever-changing scope, distribution, and current trends among these infections CDC, 2016c).

The Centers for Disease Control and Prevention and U.S. Preventive Services Task Force

The U.S. Centers for Disease Control was officially established in 1946 as an outgrowth of the pre-WWII Malaria Control in War Areas (MCWH) organization, which was charged with controlling malaria in and around U.S. military training bases. Over the next 60 years, the CDC, now an official part of the Department of Health and Human Services, expanded its role to include overseeing and protecting the U.S. population from "all infectious diseases, non-communicable diseases, injury and environmental health, health statistics, and occupational health." The primary mission of the CDC is to "(lead) prevention efforts to reduce the burden of preventable and chronic diseases" (CDC, 2015b).

Thus, the CDC is charged with overseeing national health promotion, prevention, treatment, and preparedness by responding to national health emergencies. It is this response to national health emergencies that sets the CDC apart from its peer agencies. It should be noted that currently, the CDC term of preference is *sexually transmitted diseases* or STDs. However, in every day usage, it is widely recognized that the term *sexually transmitted infections* is more precise, and as such, will be used throughout this chapter.

The U.S. Preventive Services Task Force (USPSTF; or the Task Force) was created in 1984 as an independent, volunteer panel of national experts in prevention and evidence-based medicine. The Task Force is charged with "improving the health of all Americans by making evidence-based recommendations about clinical preventative services such as screenings, counseling services, and preventative medications" (USPSTF, 2017). The recommendations of the Task Force are based upon "rigorous review of existing peer-reviewed evidence" with the intention of helping clinicians and patients decide which services are best suited for a patient's needs (USPSTF, 2017). The USPSTF recommendations only apply to persons who have no signs or symptoms of the specific disease or condition under evaluation, and their recommendations only address services offered in the primary care setting. Annually, the USPSTF reports to Congress, identifying critical gaps in evidence-based research related to clinical preventive services, and recommends areas that deserve priority examination. Thus, the USPSTF's focus is on making recommendations for evidence-based screening and preventive measures, and identifying gaps in knowledge in these same areas. The USPSTF is convened and supported by the Agency for Healthcare Research and Quality, a division of the Department of Health and Human Services.

The USPSTF activities serve as a complement to the CDC's epidemiological charge with tracking national health trends and statistics, reviewing curative/restorative disease treatments, and mobilizing urgent responses to public health emergencies. While the CDC and USPSTF recommendations are most often congruent, this is not exclusively the case. This chapter will clarify and discuss these differences where they exist.

State Laws on Mandated STI Reporting

All 50 states in the United States recognize chlamydia, gonorrhea, syphilis, and HIV as *notifiable conditions* (CDC, 2015c). This means that federal law mandates healthcare providers to report new cases of these infections (also referred to as *index patients*) to public health authorities. Reporting typically involves releasing the patient's name to the local health department and noting if the sexual partner was also treated. This information is used to notify and treat the sexual partners of the newly diagnosed patient, and to monitor the prevalence of specific STIs on the community, state, and national levels (CDC, 2008). It is important to note that patient participation in revealing partner contacts must be fully informed and is completely voluntary (CDC, 2008). Currently in the United States, chlamydia is the most common of the notifiable STIs and gonorrhea is second.

Expedited Partner Therapy (EPT) and State Laws

As noted on the CDC website, expedited partner therapy (EPT, also termed *patient-delivered partner therapy* or PDPT) is the clinical practice of treating the sex partners of patients diagnosed with chlamydia or gonorrhea by providing prescriptions or medications to the patient to take to his/her partner *without the healthcare provider first examining the partner* (CDC, 2016a). Clinicians (e.g., physicians, nurse practitioners, physician assistants, pharmacists, public health workers) provide index patients with sufficient medications directly or via prescription for the patient and their partner. EPT is considered one option when facilitating partner treatment, particularly for male partners of women with chlamydia and gonorrhea. As a management strategy, EPT does not replace other strategies such as comprehensive medical management of the individual or provider-assisted referral. Specifically, EPT does not offer sexual partners the opportunity for HIV/STI screening (Brucker & King, 2017). While comprehensive medical management is optimal, it is often not available to patients due to resource limitations. EPT has been shown to be highly effective in decreasing reinfection rates among women when compared with standard partner referrals for examination and treatment (American College of Obstetricians and Gynecologists [ACOG], 2015a; Cramer et al., 2013). EPT has been estimated to save healthcare costs of up to 23% per person, given that only about half of the partners of those diagnosed with an STI come in to the clinic for testing and treatment (Gift, Mohammed, Leichliter, Hogben, & Golden, 2011). Unfortunately, studies suggest that only 10% of U.S. providers regularly use EPT (Rosenfeld, 2014).

In the United States, the legal status of the practice of EPT is dependent on state or territory provisions. EPT is clearly permissible in 39 of the 50 states and the District of Columbia. In another 8 states and Puerto Rico, EPT is potentially allowable with certain restrictions. Only Florida, Kentucky, and West Virginia expressly prohibit EPT (CDC, 2016c). The legislative specifics related to EPT for each of these jurisdictions can be found at the following webpage: http://www.cdc.gov/std/ept/legal/default.htm. The CDC did not assess EPT laws among the various sovereign U.S. tribal nations.

The United Kingdom has instituted a national policy whereby the Department of Health collaborates with the clinical commissioning groups (CCGs), which represent the commissioners of specialist healthcare. That partnership extends to the providers of sexual health services. This ensures appropriate implementation of standardized national policy regulations and recommended guidelines designed for sexual healthcare and services across the country.

The World Health Organization (WHO); various governmental, national, and international organizations such as the British Association for Sexually Transmitted Infections and HIV; and the U.S. CDC and the USPSTF, all endeavor to achieve similar goals. The high-level evidence-based policies, recommendations, general principles, and practice guidelines published by these organizations stipulate required standards for the management of STIs,

HIV, reproductive tract infections (RTIs), and all associated complications. The standards address the therapeutic interventions employed for each of the infections as well as the holistic consequences of each infection.

Other national organizations provide additional support through guidelines and recommendations for managing individuals exposed to STIs to protect the sexual health and welfare of the general public. Within the United Kingdom, the British Association of Sexually Transmitted Infections and HIV (BASHH) published its 2010 and 2014 standards for the management of STIs.

In the United Kingdom, there are nine recommended standards outlining guiding principles that should enable sexual and reproductive healthcare practitioners to provide quality evidence-based care and services for patients who present with different types of STIs. These national standards and guidelines serve to complement the governmental initiative of the Department of Health's National Strategy for Sexual Health and HIV and emphasize ongoing improvements and innovations toward achievement of better prevention, better services, and better sexual health throughout the United Kingdom. The key elements that form the nine standards are the following: principles to guide the care of STI patients/clients; suitably trained staff; clinical assessment procedures; diagnostic procedures and management interventions; regulation and control of information; liaison and cooperation with other services; clinical governance in terms of quality care provision; commitment and answerability; and partnerships with patient representative groups. The Public Health Implementation guidance tools provide supportive systems and procedures for one-to-one interventions advocated by the National Institute for Health and Care Excellence (NICE). Readers are encouraged to explore the relevant documents and the equivalents in the countries in which they practice. It is important to gain the required knowledge, deep insight and understanding, and familiarity with national policy regulations, recommendations, and guidelines.

Concept Clarifications

Sexually Transmitted Infections

The term *sexually transmitted infection* has been extensively employed within the fields of biological and medical sciences since its adoption became widely acknowledged in 1999. The current usage of the term is advocated as a more apt concept that embraces asymptomatic infections, as opposed to the previously used term *sexually transmitted diseases (STDs)* (World Health Organization [WHO], 2003). Sexually transmitted infections are differentiated from reproductive tract infections (RTIs) and characterized by the mode of transmission. Generally, RTIs are associated with more serious long-term complications that affect the health of the individuals.

Reproductive Tract Infections

Reproductive tract infections are distinctive by the specific site or location and manifestation that characteristically occur within the genital tract. While specific RTIs caused by syphilis and gonorrhea are sexually transmitted, other RTIs are classified as non-sexually transmitted. Thus, RTIs encompass three broad categories.

1. **Endogenous infections** comprise microorganisms that are normally present in the female genital tract. While these are not necessarily transmitted and spread from one individual to another, the organisms have the capacity to proliferate, causing symptoms. Typical examples include candidiasis and bacterial vaginosis.

2. **Iatrogenic infections** may originate from internal or external sources through endogenous organisms in the upper vagina or sexually transmitted infective organisms deposited in the vagina and cervix respectively. These can be acquired through internal examinations or invasive medical procedures carried out during pregnancy, labor, or postpartum. The endogenous organisms in the vagina or sexually transmitted organisms in the cervix may be inadvertently introduced into upper genital structures, causing serious damage with complications and ill health. Transvaginal or transcervical procedures may result in infections developing within the uterine cavity and, uterine tubes and extend to structures in the pelvic cavity (WHO, 2003). Other sources of iatrogenic infections may be through indifferent use of contaminated and unsterile instruments and therapeutic equipment; substandard infection control measures during performance of invasive genital tract examinations and procedures; lack of careful hygiene practices; and cultural traditions in which application of appropriate measures of sterilization is nonexistent. A common complication associated with these is pelvic inflammatory disease (PID) (WHO, 2003).

3. **Sexually transmitted infections:** This category represents relatively more common STIs/RTIs in men than in women and generally originates from sexual activities with infected individuals. Examples of specific infections include chancroid and HIV. The actual sites of infection in the female genital structures include the vulva, labia, and lower vagina with manifestations of genital ulcers, such as syphilis, chancroid, and herpes. Genital warts may also develop at these sites. Within the vaginal canal, bacterial vaginosis, candidiasis, and trichomonas may manifest, and infections of gonorrhea, chlamydia, and herpes may occur as cervical manifestations. Within the uterine cavity gonorrhea, chlamydia, and bacterial infections may manifest and may involve the uterine tubes and other pelvic organs (WHO, 2003, 2005).

In the male genital structures, the infections manifest as genital ulcers at the scrotum and penis caused by syphilis, chancroid, and herpes. Genital warts may also develop at those sites. Gonorrheal and chlamydial infections tend to manifest within the urethral canal, epididymis, and the testes (WHO, 2003, 2005).

These categorizations represent the origins of the infections and certain issues of importance should be noted for practical consideration. Because the endogenous STIs are not primarily sexually transmitted, these tend not to be considered in clinical and public health policies and recommended guidelines outlined for STI/RTI care and therapeutic interventions. Moreover, because those conditions are considered as non-sexually transmitted, partner notification and management are absent from care and intervention procedures. Nonetheless, practitioners have an obligation to provide appropriate education, support, and reassurance to all individuals who present with such problems. Another issue of practical importance is that non-sexually transmitted reproductive tract infections are found to be quite common among women of all ages (WHO, 2003, 2005). The clinical manifestations of STIs and RTIs may produce similar symptoms in women. Therefore, practitioners are faced with the challenge of distinguishing between sexually transmitted and non-sexually transmitted RTIs. Correct distinction is crucial to provide the best available effective treatment and education without inadvertently distressing the patient.

Human immunodeficiency virus infection (HIV) is considered an STI. However, it is important to note that this and certain other infections such as hepatitis B and C (HBV and HCV, respectively), which are also considered STIs, do not fall into the classification of reproductive tract infections (WHO, 2003, 2005).

The ensuing sections explore the clinical manifestations and diagnoses of specific STIs. The current therapeutic management, related policy regulations, and the standards that guide implementation of these are appropriately explored. The research underpinning the evidence-based recommendations and guidelines are also considered.

Specific Sexually Transmitted Infections

Chlamydia trachomatis

C. trachomatis first became a reportable infection in the United States in 1986; however, it wasn't until 2000 that all 50 states and the District of Columbia required its reporting (CDC, 2016d). It is the most common reportable bacterial STI in the United States with well over 1 million new cases annually. The high prevalence is due to both increased screening among women and improved methodologies to detect active infection (Brucker & King, 2017). It is estimated that an additional 1.7 million cases of chlamydia remain undiagnosed each year (Beckman, Cassanova, & Chuang, 2014).

Chlamydia trachomatis (Chlamydia) Screening

Current CDC guidelines recommend the following screening regimens using nucleic acid amplification testing (NAAT) via cervical/vaginal/urethral swabs or urine specimen:

- All sexually active females ages 25 and under, either heterosexual or women having sex with women (WSW), should be screened for chlamydia annually (Gorgos & Marrazzo, 2011).

- All sexually active females over the age of 25 who have risk factors (a new sex partner, anonymous sex, more than one sex partner, a sex partner with concurrent sex partners, irregular use of condoms, or a sex partner who has tested positive for an STI) should also be routinely screened.

- All pregnant women should be screened for chlamydia at their first prenatal visit. Pregnant women ages 25 and under should be rescreened during the third trimester. Pregnant women over the age of 25 who have increased risk factors should also be rescreened during the third trimester. Pregnant women with chlamydia should have a test of cure 3–4 weeks after treatment and then be rescreened in 3 months (CDC, 2015d).

- Men having sex with men (MSM) should be screened at least annually for urethral/rectal chlamydia regardless of condom use. Routine oropharyngeal screening for chlamydia is not recommended (Workowski & Bolan, 2015).

- Persons with HIV should be screened for chlamydia at first HIV evaluation and then annually thereafter. More frequent screening may be indicated depending on individual behavioral risks and local prevalence of infection.

- While the prevalence of chlamydia is different in women who have sex with women, the guidelines for screening do not vary with the sex/gender of the partner (King et al., 2015).

- NAATs are not U.S. Food and Drug Administration (FDA) approved for use with oropharyngeal or rectal swab specimens. However, NAATs have been shown to have improved sensitivity and specificity compared to cultures for the detection of chlamydia at rectal and oropharyngeal sites in men and can be used by laboratories that have met all regulatory requirements for an off-label procedure (CDC, 2016d; Workowski & Bolan, 2015).

There is insufficient data at present to recommend routine screening of men. However, screening of sexually active men should be considered in clinical settings where there is a high risk of chlamydia, such as adolescent clinics, correctional facilities, or STI clinics, and in populations with a high burden of infection, such as men having sex with men.

It should be noted that the USPSTF only recommends routine chlamydia screening for sexually active women under the age of 24 and older women who are at increased risk of infection. The USPSTF is in agreement with the CDC that there is insufficient evidence to assess the balance of benefits and harms of routine chlamydia screening in men who are not at an elevated risk (USPSTF, 2014).

Prevalence in the United Kingdom and the Western World

Chlamydia trachomatis—an intracellular gram-negative pathogen—is described as the most pervasive organism that causes STIs in the western world (Medical Foundation for HIV & Sexual Health [MEDFASH]/British Association for Sexual Health and HIV [BASHH], 2014; Mishori, McClaskey, & Winklerprins, 2012; Workowski, Berman, and Centers for Disease Control and Prevention, 2010). Chlamydia is the most common curable STI diagnosed in the United Kingdom; an estimated 5–10% of sexually active women 15–24 years of age and men 20–24 years of age are infected (BASHH, 2008; Nwokolo et al., 2016). Data from 2013 and 2014 indicate a decline in incidence, yet chlamydia remained the most commonly diagnosed STI in the United Kingdom with 206,774 reported cases in 2014 (Public Health England [PHE], 2013, 2015). A similar decreasing trend is observed in the United States, where chlamydia is found to be the most frequently reported infection among young people below 25 years of age (CDC, 2010, 2015a). Readers of this chapter are encouraged to explore and compare the most recent accessible figures in different countries to gain a better idea of the trends in occurrence of this and other STIs both nationally and internationally.

Among the risk factors for chlamydia infection are age (under 25 years), change of sexual partner and/or involvement with a new sexual contact, or more than one sexual partner in the preceding year. Inconsistent and unreliable condom use also constitutes an important risk factor (Paz-Bailey et al., 2005; PHE, 2015; Stonnenberg, 2013). Because the infection is often asymptomatic and remains undetected, interminable transmission among members of the community occurs (Lanjouw et al., 2015). Thus, two-thirds of sexual partners of chlamydia-positive individuals are also found to have acquired the infection (Batteiger et al., 2010a; Lanjouw et al., 2015). The modes of transmission include penetrative sexual intercourse and therefore, mainly vaginal and anal sexual intercourse with a partner who has acquired the infection. However, other modes of infection include oral sex so that oropharyngeal and adult conjunctival infections also occur, while neonatal infections of pneumonia and conjunctivitis tend to be acquired during birth (via passage through the birth vaginal canal) (Batteiger, Tu, et al., 2010).

Of the three strains of *Chlamydia trachomatis* that cause urogenital and extra genital disease in humans, serovars Ab, B, Ba, and C, are found to cause trachoma infection of the eyes and can progress to blindness. These are found to be prevalent in Africa and parts of Asia (Stamm, 2005).

Of particular relevance to this context, *Chlamydia trachomatis* serovars D–K are identified as causing urogenital infection. Associated complications include urethritis, pelvic inflammatory disease (PID; found to occur in 40% of infected women who do not receive treatment), ectopic pregnancy, and tubal-related infertility (Batteiger, Tu, et al., 2010). In males, epididymo-orchitis and sexually acquired reactive arthritis have been identified as common complications of *Chlamydia trachomatis* (Batteiger, Tu, et al., 2010). *Chlamydia trachomatis* serovars L1, L2, and L3 are identified as causing lymphogranuloma venereum (LGV) (Fredlund, Falk, Jurstrand, & Unemo, 2004). It is recommended that the manifestation of lymphogranuloma venereum infections in men who have sex with men requires a rectal specimen for laboratory testing (Ward et al., 2011). However, as Byrne (2010) argues, while occasional reports may have implicated severity of chlamydia-related disease to particular genital serovars (Stevens et al., 2010), more empirical studies with more extensive scope are required to support such observations.

Recent research evidence suggests that after genital infection with *Chlamydia trachomatis*, the individual may develop some degree of protective immunity against the infection (Batteiger, Xu, Johnson, & Rekart, 2010). This is attributed to attenuation of the *Chlamydia trachomatis* bacterium and as a result, the prevalence of the infection within a community may be reduced. Other conjectures are that individuals who receive treatment very early before developing natural immunity might become susceptible to reinfection (Brunham, Pourbohloul, Mak, White, & Rekart, 2005). Another probability is that the concordance rate in couples decreases and the organism load is likely to be lower in those who develop repeat infections (Batteiger, Xu, et al., 2010). Other evidence suggests that while chronic or long-term infection can clear spontaneously without obvious damage to the genital tract, advancing age is associated with improved and higher resistance to the infection (Vicetti Miguel et al., 2013). Both Batteiger, Xu, et al. (2010) and Vicetti Miguel et al. (2013) support Brunham and Rey-Ladino's (2005) observation of the possible implications of these findings for a vaccine against *Chlamydia trachomatis* infection.

Readers may find it useful to explore the original research studies for clearer insight into these findings. It is also worthwhile to explore the medical and legal policies and regulations relating to the procedures employed in obtaining specific specimens from various sites. Also of practical interest concerning different laboratory techniques are the recommendations relating to the techniques of cell culture, enzyme immunoassays (EIAs), and direct fluorescent antibody (DFA) (BASHH, 2008). Public Health England (PHE) (2015) and the British Association for Sexual Health and HIV (BASHH) (MEDFASH/BASHH 2014) recommend the use of more sensitive diagnostic tests such as nucleic acid amplification tests (NAATs). Undoubtedly, apart from the substantiating empirical evidence that underpins the recommendations, the choice of technique employed in different laboratories reflects the technique's sensitivity, specificity, allocated funding, and cost implications.

Characteristic Clinical Signs and Symptoms

An estimated 50% of males who acquire chlamydia infection remain asymptomatic, while approximately 70% of females remain asymptomatic (Dielissen, Teunissen, & Lagro-Janssen, 2013; Lazaro, 2013; Pattman, Sankar, Elawad, Handy, & Price, 2010). The reported symptoms and signs in those who are symptomatic include the following:

Females

- Menstrual abnormalities with postcoital bleeding (PCB), intermenstrual bleeding (IMB)
- Deep dyspareunia
- Low abdominal pain, pelvic pain, and tenderness
- Suspected PID, purulent vaginal discharge
- Mucopurulent cervicitis with or without contact bleeding, inflamed and friable cervix Dielissen et al., 2013; Haggerty & Ness, 2006)

In a differential diagnosis, Lazaro (2013) makes certain specific comparisons to differentiate cervical ectopy from cervicitis. In appearance, cervical ectopy shows a flat red patch all over the cervical os, which may be overexposure of columnar cells that are vulnerable and predictably disposed to infection. Possible causes include biological changes at puberty, the effects of hormones in pregnancy, or the effect of combined oral contraceptive pill (COCP). As a result, the glandular epithelium of the endocervix—which are more vascular—extends over the epithelium of the ectocervix. Cervicitis, on the other hand, shows congestion and swelling and bleeds on contact. While this might be normal, it is more likely to be caused by infections such as chlamydia or gonorrhea (Lazaro, 2013). Other symptoms include frequency of micturition and dysuria, and a coexisting STI such as genital warts (Carey & Beagley, 2010; Haggerty et al., 2010; Lazaro, 2013).

Males

- Urethral discharge
- Dysuria (variable in severity, and therefore could be disregarded by the individual)
- Urethritis, epididymitis, and epididymo-orchitis manifest in sexually active men (Joki-Korpela et al., 2009)
- Asymptomatic rectal infection or anal discharge with anorectal discomfort
- Prostatitis (Wagenlehner, Wiedner, & Naber, 2006)

In both females and males, pharyngeal infections are uncommon and may be asymptomatic (BASHH, 2006; Dielissen et al., 2013; Lazaro, 2013).

Possible Complications

An estimated 10–40% of untreated women who develop PID may have been infected but fail to seek or receive appropriate treatment because they remain asymptomatic or only experience mild or atypical symptoms. Chronic pelvic pain accompanying PID and other associated reproductive complications are reported to increase with recurrent *Chlamydia trachomatis* infection (Paavonen & Eggert-Kruse, 1999). Perihepatitis (Fitz-Hugh-Curtis syndrome) characterized by inflammation of the hepatic capsule with referred pain to the right shoulder may manifest. The combined condition of epididymo-orchitis (Joki-Korpela et al., 2009), adult conjunctivitis, and sexually acquired reactive arthritis (SARA)—Reiter's syndrome—may also manifest, the latter occurring more commonly in men. This is characterized by polyarthritis of the weight-bearing joints (BASHH, 2008; Lazaro, 2013).

Techniques for Diagnosing *Chlamydia trachomatis* Infection

The recommended diagnostic laboratory tests are the NAATs, which are reputed to have high efficacy for sensitivity and specificity (Blatt, Lieberman, Hoover, & Kaufman, 2012; Nwokolo et al., 2016). Of the different types of NAATs techniques, the strand displacement amplification (SDA) and transcription-mediated amplification (TMA) are recommended (Cook, Hutchison, Ostergaard, Braitwaite, & Ness, 2005; Gaydos, Theodore, Dalesio, Wood, & Quinn, 2004). These are endorsed as being highly sensitive and specific for diagnosing genital *Chlamydia trachomatis* infections Scottish Intercollegiate Guidelines Network [SIGN], 2009 (**Figure 6-1**). A third NAAT technique recommended as an alternative to the TMA and SDA is the real-time polymerase chain reaction (rtPCR) (Health Protection Agency [HPA], 2008a; SIGN, 2009). Providing full details of the different NAAT techniques is beyond the scope of this chapter. Therefore, practitioners are encouraged to explore relevant texts regarding recommended diagnostic techniques.

Specimens Obtained

Specimens taken from women who present with characteristic symptoms may comprise endocervical samples taken by speculum examination. Women who present with no symptoms may be offered the option of self-obtained swab from the vulvovaginal area. Some argue that first void urine sample is not recommended due to low sensitivity and the possibility of missed infections in 10–20% of cases. Nonetheless, this was tested by Levett et al. (2008) in their evaluation of three automated nucleic acid amplification systems for detecting chlamydia and gonorrhea infections. Other experts who advocate the use of urine specimen for diagnostic test for *Chlamydia trachomatis* emphasize that the specimen should be first void urine (FVU) or first catch urine (FCU). However, correct instruction is crucial depending on the specific manufacturer's kit regarding how long the individual should hold the urine (1 or 2 hours) before

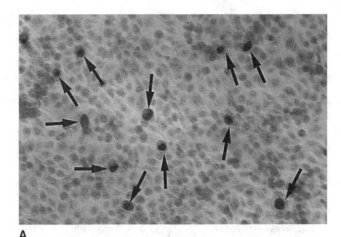

A

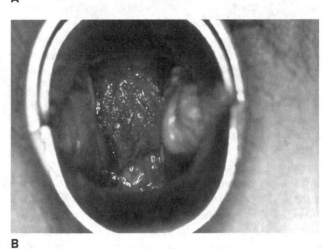

B

Figure 6-1 Chlamydia
(A) CDC/ Dr. E. Arum, Dr. N. Jacobs; **(B)** CDC/ Dr. Lourdes Fraw, Jim Pledger

voiding for the test. Some experts maintain that sensitivity could be reduced to less than 90% with inadequate collection of the urine specimen (BASHH, 2008). Mangin et al. (2012) maintain that when using NAATs the timing of urine sample collection, whether first void or midstream, may not necessarily make any difference. Nonetheless, one must take into account the incubation period and the window period (time from exposure to positive laboratory test identification of the organism). In *Chlamydia trachomatis* infection, possible detection can be made on urine sample tests within the first week post exposure while most likely detection can be made 2 weeks after the last exposure. The period of positive detection with highest accuracy is estimated as 4 weeks after the last exposure (Levett et al., 2008; Mangin et al., 2012).

Correct specimen sample collection is important for testing accuracy. In female patients, cervical or vulvovaginal swabs are more appropriate. Cervical swab collection requires a speculum examination to correctly insert the swab through the os to obtain the required columnar cells from the endocervix. BASHH (2008) substantiates this with evidence from studies that suggest that inadequate cervical specimens reduce NAAT sensitivity. Vulvovaginal swab can be performed by the patient or by the sexual health practitioner. This is also substantiated by evidence from multicenter studies. However, it is also useful to explore more recent studies.

Diagnostic procedures for male patients indicate testing of first void urine and/or urethral swab, both of which are reported to be comparable in effectiveness (BASHH, 2016a). However, urine samples tend to be more favored due to the ease of collection without discomfort. To obtain an adequate specimen, urethral swab collection requires insertion of the swab to a depth of 2–4 cm before being rotated and withdrawn (BASHH, 2016a). Regarding urine sample collection from males, readers may find it useful to read Johnson et al.'s (2002) findings, "Screening Tests to Detect *Chlamydia trachomatis* and *Neisseria gonorrhoeae* Infections." It is important to comply with the manufacturer's instructions that accompany the specific urine specimen collection kit. These instructions should indicate how long the urine should be held in the bladder before providing the sample for the test. There do not appear to be standard laboratory techniques with recommendations for the type of specimens that should be obtained for confirming diagnoses of conjunctival, pharyngeal, and rectal *Chlamydia trachomatis* infections (BASHH, 2016a). The techniques used for testing specimens from these sites vary and may depend on the expertise and resources of the particular laboratory, the policy regulations, evidence-based recommendations, and guidelines. A recommended resource for U.K. practitioners is the BASHH (2016a) *Chlamydia trachomatis UK Testing Guidelines*. Practitioners in other countries are advised to explore similar national guidelines where they practice. It is always useful to make critical comparisons for examples of best practice.

Chlamydia trachomatis Treatment

The CDC recommendations for effective treatment of chlamydia in non-pregnant clients are as follows.

Recommended Non-pregnancy Regimens

- Azithromycin 1 g orally in a single dose preferably administered through onsite, observed therapy to maximize adherence; **or**
- Doxycycline 100 mg orally twice daily for 7 days

Alternate Non-pregnancy Regimens

- Erythromycin base 500 mg orally 4 times a day for 7 days, **or**
- Erythromycin ethylsuccinate 800 mg orally 4 times a day for 7 days, **or**
- Levofloxacin 500 mg orally once a day for 7 days, **or**
- Ofloxacin 300 mg orally twice a day for 7 days

Chlamydia trachomatis Treatment During Pregnancy and for Oral Infections

Doxycycline is contraindicated in the second and third trimesters of pregnancy. Therefore, recommended treatment for chlamydia during pregnancy includes azithromycin or one of the other alternate regimens as listed here. Following treatment, pregnant women should be retested 3–4 weeks after completion of therapy, and then again during the third trimester, as previously noted (Workowski & Bolan, 2015). Given concerns regarding chlamydia persistence following exposure to penicillin-class antibiotics, amoxicillin is now considered an alternative treatment for *C. trachomatis* during pregnancy. Similarly, the increased gastrointestinal side effects of erythromycin can lead to nonadherence with the higher-dose regimen. The lower-dose 14-day erythromycin regimens can be considered if gastrointestinal tolerance is of concern. Erythromycin estolate is contraindicated in pregnancy due to hepatic toxicity.

Available clinical evidence suggests that oropharyngeal chlamydia can be sexually transmitted to genital sites; therefore, oral *C. trachomatis* should be treated with azithromycin or doxycycline. The efficacy of other antimicrobial regimens in the treatment of oropharyngeal chlamydia is unknown at this time.

Recommended Pregnancy Regimens

- Azithromycin 1 g orally in a single dose

Alternate Pregnancy Regimens

- Amoxicillin 500 mg orally three times a day for 7 days, **or**
- Erythromycin base 500 mg orally four times a day for 7 days, **or**
- Erythromycin base 250 mg orally four times a day for 14 days, **or**
- Erythromycin ethylsuccinate 800 mg orally four times a day for 7 days, **or**
- Erythromycin ethylsuccinate 400 mg orally four times a day for 14 days

Management Considerations and Follow-Up

Persons treated for chlamydia should be instructed to abstain from sexual intercourse for 7 days after single-dose therapy or until completion of any 7-day regimen and resolution of symptoms. To minimize reinfection, clients need to be instructed to abstain from sexual intercourse until all of their sex partners have been treated. All persons diagnosed with chlamydia should also be tested for HIV, gonorrhea, and syphilis. It must be noted that retesting to detect client reinfection is distinctly different than test of cure to detect treatment failure. A test-of-cure to detect therapeutic failure 3–4 weeks after completing therapy is not advised for persons treated with the recommended or alternative regimens, unless compliance is in question, symptoms persist, or reinfection is suspected. Additionally, use of NAAT testing at less than 3 weeks after treatment is not recommended, as the continued presence of nonviable organisms can give false positive results. However, a high rate of reinfection has been observed in women and men treated for chlamydia; thus, the CDC does recommend that men and women who have been treated for chlamydia be retested 3 months after treatment, regardless of whether they believe their partners were treated (Workowski & Bolan, 2015). Any person allergic to the recommended treatment regimens should have desensitization instituted and/or be evaluated by an infectious disease specialist.

EPT, where permitted by law, is another means of preventing reinfection by treating partners who may not otherwise be available or have access to treatment. EPT may be given to index clients along with written educational materials for partners concerning information on chlamydia, potential therapy-related allergies and adverse effects, and symptoms suggestive of complications. It must be noted that EPT is not routinely recommended for MSM because of the high risk of other coexisting infections and limited data regarding the effectiveness of the EPT approach in this population.

U.K. Management Recommendations: Information and Advice

Clear advice and guidance is crucial for patients. It is important that all components of the therapeutic interventions, advice, instructions, and health promotion are highly effective, acceptable, comprehensible, and easy to perform. The importance of abstaining from sexual intercourse and oral sex until the treatment regimen is completed by both sexual partners should be emphasized to the patient. For particular medications, such as azithromycin, the patient and partners are advised to wait 7 days following completion of a course of treatment. To encourage adherence to treatment and cooperation with the sexual health professionals, clear explanations should be given to the individual about the infection and the associated long-term potential consequences. The expected benefits and overall outcome of the treatment should be explained to the individual or couple, and additional information leaflets and other forms of written information should be provided (BASHH, 2006, 2016b).

Guidance and Support

All patients/clients who are tested and treated for *Chlamydia trachomatis* should be offered other STI and HIV screening tests, with the explanation that HIV and syphilis tests require repeat testing for high-risk individuals. Furthermore, vaccination against human papilloma virus (HPV) is also offered to those individuals who are not already immune to this virus. In addition to the offer of screening tests, practitioners should emphasize the importance of persuading all the patient's sexual contacts to submit to similar screening tests. The 2012 NHS National Chlamydia Screening Programme Standards is highly recommended as a supportive reference resource. All readers of this chapter should consider this as an example of good practice and compare to programs in other countries.

The key updates to both the 2015 European guidelines (Lanjouw et al., 2015) and the 2015 U.K. guidelines (Nwokolo et al., 2016) are briefly outlined here. However, practitioners are encouraged to read the full documents for more detail on the guidelines and recommendations.

- Point-of-care testing using NAATs
- Providing advice on repeat chlamydia testing
- The adequacy of single-dose azithromycin treatment being considered
- Guidance on treatment of individuals who present with coinfection of chlamydia and gonorrhea
- Guidance on treatment of rectal chlamydia
- Guidance on vertical transmission and management of the neonate

Practitioners in other countries are urged to explore the current national guidelines and make appropriate comparisons for excellence in practice and research.

Emerging Research Relating to Treatment of Genital Tract *Chlamydia trachomatis*

This section outlines the current recommended medication regimens in the United Kingdom. BASHH (2006) cites studies on the use of doxycycline and azithromycin (Horner, 2006; Miller, 2006), as well as the alternative regimens of erythromycin and ofloxacin, which have focused on anti-microbial efficacy. Doxycycline and azithromycin are reported to be the most scrupulously researched (Horner, 2012) and comparative analyses have shown that both medications have >95% efficacy in achieving cure and chlamydia negative on retesting results with NAATs in 2–5 weeks follow-up (Horner, 2006; Miller, 2006). However, a longer period of follow-up reveals 10% chlamydia positive although other claims are reported following differerent treatment regimens. (Horner, 2006, 2012; see also Rank & Yeruva, 2014; Workowski & Berman, 2010; Workowski & Bolan, 2015).

Careful consideration should be given to treatment failure, reinfection, and persistent chlamydial infection. Current recommended regimens in the United Kingdom for first-line treatment in men and women with uncomplicated infection include the following:

- Doxycycline 100 mg orally twice daily for 7 days, or
- Azithromycin 1 g stat administered orally as a single dose (Kong et al., 2014; Lazaro, 2013).

The single dose of azithromycin is recommended for patients who may have difficulty complying with a longer treatment regimen (Lazaro, 2013).

Alternative medications that are recommended include the following:

- Erythromycin 500 mg taken orally twice daily for 10–14 days (Lanjouw et al., 2015), or

- Ofloxacin 200 mg taken orally twice daily for 7 days, otherwise 400 mg may be taken once daily for 7 days (Lazaro, 2013; Wilson, 2011).

Practitioners are encouraged to consider these guidelines as an exemplar.

Special Considerations for Associated Complications and Other Interventions

Intrauterine Device (IUD) or Intrauterine System (IUS) in Situ

A positive chlamydia infection should be treated prior to fitting a patient for an IUD or IUS. Therefore, the test should be carried out as a prefitting screening procedure (Lazaro, 2013). A repeat test should be carried out 6 weeks after completion of the treatment to confirm that the infection has been cleared before the device or system is fitted. If cervicitis with purulent discharge is detected indicating chlamydia or gonorrheal infection in a woman who already has an IUD or IUS in situ, it should be left in place (Lazaro, 2013). Treatment of the infection should be undertaken first as the main concern. Women who present with asymptomatic chlamydia infection while IUD or IUS is in situ should be prescribed an oral dose of azithromycin 1 g stat (Lazaro, 2013).

Pelvic Inflammatory Disease (PID) with IUD in Situ

If a woman who has IUD or IUS in situ presents with PID, the recommendation is to treat the infection while the device or system is left in place. However, if the treatment is ineffective, removal of the device may be considered and further discussion carried out with relevant specialists (Lazaro, 2013). Other complications should be treated accordingly.

Personal Protection Following Treatment and Confirmation of Cure: Test of Cure

NAATs may be performed within a period of 6 weeks for the test of cure following treatment with azithromycin (SIGN, 2009). Repeat testing is recommended 3–12 months or sooner for patients/clients who have undergone treatment if there is a change of sexual partners (SIGN, 2009). Client-centered risk-reduction interventions through one-to-one, face-to-face interactions with counseling support should be provided together with health promotion/ education emphasizing safer sexual practices including condom use. Abstinence during treatment should also be emphasized until previous sexual partners, the index patient, and the current sexual partner have completed the course of treatment and for a period of at least 1 week afterward (SIGN, 2009). The requirement for these may vary due to influencing factors such as age, gender, ethnicity, social circumstances, and sexual orientation; hence the need for client centred interventions (SIGN, 2009).

Enhancing Compliance with Treatment

Apart from encouraging and empowering the individual to ask questions, the sexual health practitioner has a responsibility to provide clear explanation. The following exemplar is based on BASHH & Clinical Effectiveness Group (2014) and the 2015 UK National guideline for the management of infection with *Chlamydia trachomatis* (Nwokolo et al., 2016). The patient should be given information regarding the following:

- What *Chlamydia trachomatis* is and the modes of transmission
- The possibility of having carried the infection for a long period without experiencing any symptoms
- The potential adverse consequences associated with failure to seek medical intervention, delay in treatment, and infections that are never treated
- The importance of encouraging sexual partners to go for assessment and treatment
- What the diagnostic procedures and tests involve in both males and females despite the absence of symptoms in many infected people
- The importance of following the treatment regimen conscientiously, what to do if any of the rare but possible side effects are experienced, and what to do if any treatment dosage is inadvertently forgotten
- Explanation regarding precautions about hormonal contraception and antibiotics
- Explanation of reasons to avoid all practices of sexual intercourse until self and partner have completed the course of treatment and for the specified period after treatment as advised by the clinician, healthcare professional, or qualified pharmacist
- Clear guidance and instruction on correct and conscientious use and handling of condoms

Consideration of Sexual Partners

The recommendation is to offer chlamydia testing to sexual partners and sexual contacts of individuals with confirmed *Chlamydia trachomatis* infection. Chlamydia testing should also be offered to sexual partners of individuals who present with probable clinical signs of *Chlamydia trachomatis* infection even if the diagnosis has not been confirmed (PHE, 20013; SIGN, 2009). Likewise, individuals who have had previous STIs and/or been diagnosed with chlamydia infection in the preceding 12 months should be considered for testing. High-risk groups who should also be offered testing include genitourinary medicine (GUM) sexual health clinic attendees, individuals who practice sexual risk-taking behaviors (e.g., engagement in sexual intercourse with commercial sex workers), and those who have had two or more sexual partners in the previous 12 months. The recommended timing for identifying and notifying previous sexual partners is the preceding 6 months, but if longer than that, the most recent sexual partners should be notified (BASHH, 2006; McClean, Raddcliffe, Sullivan, & Ahmed-Jushuf, 2012). See also https://www.bashh.org/documents/4445.pdf. Partner notification and partner management may be carried out by a sexual health adviser and/or sexual health practitioner who has received the required training and acquired the relevant competencies.

Detection of positive *Chlamydia trachomatis* by NAATs up to 5 weeks after treatment may be attributable to nucleic acid from nonviable organisms. However, it is also found that retesting positive could be attributable to inadequate efficacy of the particular antimicrobial therapy. Reinfection may occur due to sexual intercourse with chlamydia-positive sexual partner who has not completed the prescribed treatment regime, or with a new chlamydia-positive partner who has not received treatment (Walker et al., 2012). Other factors associated with reinfection include younger age group (Lamontagne et al., 2007), numerous sexual partners, frequent changes in sexual partners, and involvement with new and multiple sexual partners. Some sexual partners may be inadvertently missed from treatment due to failed attempts to contact them (Dunne et al., 2008).

Although generally the term *reinfection* refers to recurrence of a particular STI by the same causative organism responsible for the initial infection, Peterman et al. (2006) reported findings of increased rates of new STIs in the year following the original STIs. Therefore, it is important to bear in mind the possibility that the index patient could present with STI(s) again but caused by different rather than the original organisms. In view of these findings, rescreening for STIs should be considered within 6 months of the first STI screening, particularly if the individual falls into any of the aforementioned categories.

The specified period of abstention in relation to a specific medication or other existing condition should be documented in detail. The advice provided and the patient/client's reaction to abstain from oral, genital, and anal sex until completion of the treatment regimen by all sexual partners should also be clearly documented (Lazaro, 2013).

Main Components of Partner Notification and Management

- The recommendation is to discuss partner notification at the time when treatment is being provided.
- The agreed method of partner notification and the outcomes should be clearly documented.

- Full STI screening and HIV testing as well as HPV screening and vaccination if not immune to the virus should be offered.
- Clear explanation should be provided together with the offer of epidemiological treatment for *Chlamydia trachomatis* (Lazaro, 2013). If the individual rejects this he/she should be advised to refrain from sexual intercourse until a negative result is confirmed. However, if the result shows positive *Chlamydia trachomatis* it is important to explain that all the sexual partners who have been exposed to the infection should be offered screening. Furthermore, epidemiological treatment should be offered and clearly documented (Lazaro, 2013, Nwokolo et al., 2016).

Guidelines Regarding Exposure and Cut-Off Periods

The recommendation regarding the "look-back" or "trace-back" period is that it allows for identification of individuals who may have been exposed to and may be at risk of developing chlamydia infection through sexual intercourse with a partner who is chlamydia positive. Within the United Kimgdom, the recommended look-back period is 4 weeks (Lazaro, 2013). However, the period may be extended to 6 months if the index patient is and has been asymptomatic over an indeterminate period of time (which may vary depending on when the last previous sexual intercourse took place) (Lazaro, 2013). The longer period, also arbitrarily determined, allows for identification of sexual partners who should be traced to inform them of their risk. Of equal importance, it allows for offers of clinical assessment and epidemiological treatment for tracing other contacts, and for offering STI testing to all those identified (Nwokolo et al., 2016; Lazaro, 2013). The index patient/client may initiate this process by personally notifying their sexual partner(s) in patient referral, or the healthcare professional practitioner may carry out the notification through the system of provider referral (Nwokolo et al. 2016). The partners and sexual contacts at risk of contracting the infection should be advised to abstain from sexual intercourse with the index patient until negative results are confirmed by laboratory tests (Nwokolo et al. 2016.).

U.K. Policy Regulations to Guide Diagnosis and Treatment

The U.K. National Guideline for the Management of Infection with *Chlamydia trachomatis* (2016) outlines the following:

- All cases involving medicolegal scrutiny should be supported by evidence from NAATs.
- Enzyme immunoassays should be replaced by NAATs.
- Regular updates on how NAATs performs and the outcomes accomplished.
- Epidemiological treatment should be offered to index case contacts.
- Partner notification rates should be carefully recorded for surveillance purposes.

Lymphogranuloma Venereum

Lymphogranuloma venereum (LVG) is a systemic disease caused by one of the three serovars of *Chlamydia trachomatis*—L1, L2, and L3 (Christerson et al., 2010; Fredlund et al., 2004; Stevens et al., 2010). Another variant—L2b—is reported to be transmitted predominantly among men who have sex with men (MSM); however, this strain can also be transmitted by heterosexual men (Peuchant et al., 2011; Verweij et al., 2012). Asymptomatic female carriers and MSM with infections of the rectum and penis are also reported to be a source of transmission in heterosexual relationships (Vall-Mayans, Caballero, & Sanz, 2009).

LVG is also referred to as lymphopathia venereum and lymphogranuloma inguinale. This condition was reportedly rare in developed countries since the mid-1960s. Nevertheless, outbreaks in various European countries since 2003 have revealed particular prevalence among HIV-positive MSM (Peuchant et al., 2011; Rönn & Ward, 2011; Verweij et al., 2012). Within the United Kingdom, increased rates of LGV were reported by Simms et al. (2004) by means of an enhanced surveillance launched by the Health Protection Agency. White, O'Farrell, and Daniels (2013) noted in PHE data that there had been continual increases in the rates of LGV by an estimated 50 cases every quarter-year from 2006 to 2009. Moreover, a sharp increase was reported in the latter part of 2009 and a further increase to a peak of 150 cases per quarter-year was reported in the middle of 2010. From then on, the rate was noted to stabilize at about 80 cases per quarter-year until 2012 (White et al., 2013). **Box 6-1** presents an outline of the information recorded for the surveillance conducted by Simms et al. in 2004.

Clinical Manifestations of LGV

The three stages of lesions are primary lesions, secondary lesions characterized by lymphadenitis or lymphadenopathy, and a tertiary stage characterized by genito-ano-rectal syndrome. The incubation period of 3–30 days following sexual contact may vary depending on whether the genitalia or rectum was the initial site of infection (de Vries, Zingoni, Kreuter, Moi, & White, 2015).

BOX 6-1 Synoptic Outline of the Information Obtained for the LGV Enhanced Surveillance

The reported cases were found to be mainly MSM who were affiliated with large sexual networks. Moreover, >75% were found to have HIV with a coexistent STI such as gonorrhea or coexistent hepatitis C viral (HCV) infection (French, Ison, & MacDonald, 2005).

Initial Lesion

In males, the characteristic initial lesion occurs as a small painless papule or pustule, which may develop into a shallow erosion forming a herpetiform ulcer that may heal spontaneously. Most common sites for these lesions in men are the coronal sulcus, prepuce glans, and scrotum. Rarely, symptoms of urethritis are also experienced (White et al., 2013; de Vries et al., 2015). In recent outbreaks some of the ulcers were described as indurated, with varying degrees of tenderness and lasting for varied durations up to several weeks (White et al., 2013).

In females, the most common sites for LGV lesions tend to be the posterior vaginal wall, fourchette, vulva, or occasionally the posterior cervix uteri. The initial lesions in females are often unapparent and unnoticeable (White et al., 2013). Lesions at sites other than the genital tract have been reported to include the tonsils and extra-genital lymph nodes (White et al., 2013).

Primary LGV: Proctitis

Proctitis was found to be a predominant symptom among MSM in the recent outbreaks of LGV in Europe. The condition manifests within a few weeks of direct transmission via the rectal mucosa and is therefore characterized by severe anorectal pain and bleeding from the rectum. This is accompanied by tenesmus and constipation due to edema of the mucosa and perirectal area (de Vries et al., 2015; Høie, Knudsen, & Gerstoft, 2011; White et al., 2013). Some patients experience fever and malaise (White et al., 2013). Also, while inguinal symptoms (inguinofemoral lymphadenopathy) may not manifest in all cases of LGV proctitis (de Vries et al., 2015; White et al., 2013), proctoscopy and radiology may reveal additional findings that pelvic nodes have been affected (de Vries et al., 2015; Van der Ham & de Vries, 2009).

Pharyngeal LGV cases have been increasingly reported among MSM and the symptoms include ulceration of the mouth and pharynx causing pharyngitis (Dosekun, Edmonds, Stockwell, French, & White, 2013).

Secondary LGV

The second stage of LGV, described as lymphadenopathy, becomes manifest about 10–30 days or even 2–6 weeks following primary lesion appearance (de Vries et al., 2015; White et al., 2013). The strain of *Chlamydia trachomatis* L1-L3 described as lymphotropic can spread through the lymph nodes, causing inflammation and swelling of the nodes and adjacent lymphoid tissues (de Vries et al., 2015; White et al., 2013). The characteristic manifestation occurs as painful lymphadenopathy in the inguinal and femoral lymph nodes. This is frequently found among heterosexual men and is classically unilateral in two-thirds of cases (de Vries et al., 2015; White et al., 2013). A single node or chain of lymph nodes may be affected and the lesions tend to coalesce to form buboes that may rupture to form ulcers that discharge pus and may develop into multiple fistulae (de Vries et al., 2015; White et al., 2013). In about 15–20% of cases bilateral inguinal and femoral lymph node systems are affected but separated by the inguinal ligament to form what is described as the "groove sign" (de Vries et al., 2015; White et al., 2013). Inguinal lymphadenopathy occurring in female patients may affect the rectum, upper vagina, the cervix, and posterior urethra. These drain into the deep iliac or perirectal nodes and may be accompanied by pain in the back and/or abdominal pain, both of which tend to be rather nonspecific (de Vries et al., 2015).

Characteristic symptoms in both genders include myalgia, malaise, chills and fever (de Vries et al., 2015). Systemic dispersion of *Chlamydia trachomatis* is accompanied by arthritis, inflammatory disease of the ocular structures, pulmonary and cardiac problems, aseptic meningitis, and perihepatitis in rare cases (de Vries et al., 2015; White et al., 2013). Most male patients seek medical consultation and are diagnosed at this stage with inguinal lymphadenopathy. However, that is not the case among female patients because manifestation of this lesion occurs less commonly among females, although cervical lymphadenopathy and buboes have been reported (Korhonen, Hiltunen-Back, & Puolakkainen, 2012). In most cases recovery occurs following the second stage.

Tertiary LGV

The tertiary stage is characterized by symptoms affecting the genital, anal, and rectal structures (de Vries et al., 2015; White et al., 2013). Tertiary LGV is referred to as anogenitorectal syndrome (de Vries et al., 2015). Although symptoms that accompany the first two stages are reported to occur less commonly among females, the manifestation of anogenitorectal syndrome in the third stage of LGV is more common among females than males (de Vries et al., 2015). Persistent spread of *Chlamydia trachomatis* inflammation within the anal and genital tissues results in mutilating destruction of the vulva (de Vries et al., 2015; White et al., 2013). Rectal lesions and the accompanying symptoms are found to be more common among MSM and women who habitually indulge in anal-receptive sexual intercourse (Williams & Churchill, 2006).

Proctocolitis is found to be a characteristic symptom of tertiary LGV and, therefore, LGV should be investigated in the diagnosis of proctitis associated with inflammatory bowel disease (de Vries et al., 2015; White et al., 2013). Proctitis is found to be increasingly reported among MSM and may be found to mimic Crohn's disease (Høie et al., 2011; White et al., 2013; Williams & Churchill, 2006). Progressive lymphangitis develops with chronic edema, chronic granulomatous fibrosis with scarring, strictures fistulae developing in the affected area, and chronic ulcerative disease and destruction of the external female genitalia (e.g., LG esthiomene; de Vries et al., 2015; Patel & Gupta, 2011; White et al., 2013). Long-term complications may develop involving destruction of lymph nodes, lymphedema, persistent formation and exudation of pus in the form of suppuration, and pyoderma. Rectal cancer has also been associated with advanced LGV symptoms and the two conditions may be confused; therefore, careful diagnostic investigation is vital (Taylor, Dasari, & McKie, 2011; White et al., 2013).

Diagnosis of LGV

Diagnosis of LGV includes ruling out other STIs such as syphilis as well as genital ulcer disease and inguinal lymphadenopathy. MSM with anorectal syndrome may be diagnosed by clinical signs of genital ulceration, inguinal lymphadenopathy, and proctocolitis. Isolation of *Chlamydia trachomatis* in specimens from the site of infection, histology, and detection of *Chlamydia trachomatis* in infected tissue also aid in the diagnosis. Confirmation of LGV via NAATs is recommended. The diagnosis requires meticulous sexual and clinical history taking, detailed physical examination, careful ruling out of other conditions with similar symptoms, and expert microbiological tests for confirmation. The main procedures in the diagnosis of LGV as outlined by the U.K. national guidelines and the International Union against Sexually Transmitted Infections stipulate the following.

Main Diagnostic Procedures

LGV diagnosis is confirmed by biovar-specific *Chlamydia trachomatis* DNA in swab specimens from the primary lesions of anogenital ulcers. This can also be performed on anorectal swab specimens obtained from the mucosal lining by proctoscopy, a blind swab, or aspirates from buboes (van der Bij et al., 2006). However, culture on bubo aspirate has proved to be problematic. NAATs are reputed to be highly sensitive and specific in detecting LGV DNA from genital and throat swabs, bubo aspirates, lymph node aspirates, biopsy tissue, and urine specimens (White et al., 2013). Rectal swab may be tested for polymorphonuclear leucocytes in predicting LGV proctitis.

Specimens for Laboratory Tests

Because chlamydial organisms are intracellular, it is important that the specimens should contain cellular substance obtained from exudate at the base of the ulcer or rectal mucosa. Aspiration of enlarged lymph nodes or pus from buboes may also be performed (White et al., 2013). For the purposes of NAATs, the recommendation is to extract pus onto the swab and send to the laboratory. In patients with urethritis or inguinal lymphadenopathy, urethral swab or first-catch urine specimens may be collected for testing (White et al., 2013).

Confirmatory Laboratory Tests

To detect *Chlamydia trachomatis* DNA and RNA, polymerase chain reaction (PCR), strand displacement amplification (SDA), or transcription-mediated amplification (TMA) is used (White et al., 2013). These tests are recommended for cervical, urethral, urine, rectal, and pharyngeal specimens due to their high sensitivity and specificity. *Chlamydia trachomatis* positive results are confirmed by real-time PCR for LGV-specific DNA (Alexander, Martin, & Ison, 2008). It is therefore emphasized that detection of LGV DNA should be the only confirmation of the diagnosis and this should be performed on specimens that have tested for positive *Chlamydia trachomatis*. Testing should be performed using NAATs on specimens obtained from symptomatic patients or from a direct sexual contact (White et al., 2013).

Presumptive LGV diagnosis using chlamydia-specific serological assays may be considered if facilities for molecular test are unavailable. High antibody titer in a patient with clinical syndrome of LGV is indicative of diagnosis although low antibody titer does not necessarily indicate absence of LGV infection (van der Snoek et al., 2007). Conversely, a high titer in a patient who does not present the characteristic LGV symptoms does not suggest development of LGV infection (Spaargaren, Fennema, Morre, de Vries, & Coutinho, 2005; van der Bij et al., 2006). Detailed examination of the diagnostic techniques is beyond the scope of this chapter.

Patient Information: Key Elements Addressed

A brief outline of patient information is presented here.

- Inform the patient that LGV is a bacterial infection, which although invasive, can be cured with specific antibiotic treatment. However, if untreated, severe complications can result.
- Provide reassurance that symptoms will abate and clear up within 1–2 weeks of starting antibiotic treatment.
- Advise the patient to avoid unprotected sexual intercourse or refrain from sexual intercourse until he/she and the sexual partner(s) have completed the prescribed antibiotic treatment and the period of follow up (Patel & Gupta, 2011; White et al., 2013).
- Provide clear explanation about the condition and possible long-term effects on the patient's health and that of the partner. Supplement with additional evidence-based written information.

Additional diagnostic considerations may involve testing for other STI causes of genital ulcer diseases such as *Treponema pallidum* (syphilis), *Haemophilus ducreyi* (chancroid), herpes simplex virus (genital herpes), and *Klebsiella granulomatis* (donovanosis). In addition, because gonorrhea, syphilis, and herpes may be associated with proctitis, these should be tested for, as well as HIV and HCV (White et al., 2013).

Recommended Treatment

In this section recommended antimicrobial treatments and alternative treatments are outlined. The key principles are

early diagnosis and treatment; however, prolonged treatment and more than one course of antibiotic treatment may have to be considered.

- Doxycycline 100 mg to be taken orally twice daily for 21 days recommended as first-line treatment, or
- Tetracycline 2 g daily, or
- Minocycline 300 mg stat then 200 mg twice daily (Jayasuriya, 2011; Stamm, 2008)

The second choice of treatment is the following:

- Erythromycin 500 mg orally four times daily for 21 days (Stamm, 2008) or
- Azithromycin 1 g weekly for 3 weeks (White et al., 2013)

The longer treatment regimens are justified because LGV is systemic. Research showed that rectal swabs for *Chlamydia trachomatis* NAATs took 16 days to test negative in LGV proctitis (de Vries et al., 2009). In contrast, in non-LGV chlamydia test undetectable DNA was achieved after 7 days.

HIV-positive patients/clients who develop LGV are recommended to undergo similar treatment regimens as prescribed for HIV-negative persons.

The recommended option for allergy to tetracyclines is to prescribe erythromycin or longer regimen of azithromycin therapy.

Consideration of Sexual Contacts

Consideration to the sexual contacts of patients with LGV infection involves notifying all those with whom the index patient had sexual contact within 4 weeks prior to symptom manifestation. The 2015 CDC guideline stipulates 60 days. However, in asymptomatic LGV patients all those with whom sexual contact occurred in the preceding 3 months should be notified. Contact tracing allows for offers of examination and tests for rectal, cervical, urethral, and pharyngeal infections. Sexual contacts may be provided with the recommended presumptive treatment of doxycycline 100 mg orally twice daily for 7 days or an alternative antibiotic such as azithromycin 1 g orally as a single dose (White et al., 2013).

The recommendation is to follow up all patients with LGV until the symptoms have subsided. In patients with early-stage LGV including proctitis this may take about 1 to 2 weeks. In patients with longer duration of LGV it could take 3 to 6 weeks for symptoms to subside (White et al., 2013). It is possible for asymptomatic LGV patients in early stage to develop symptoms in the first few days of treatment but these settle down relatively quickly. Test of cure is not considered necessary if the recommended treatment regimens have been followed. However, if there is a need to do so this may be timed at 2 weeks following completion of the LGV treatment (de Vries et al., 2009).

Neisseria gonorrhoeae (Gonorrhea)

Gonorrhea is essentially a gram-negative infection caused by the diplococcus *Neisseria gonorrhoeae*, which is contracted by direct inoculation of secretions infected with the organism. The columnar epithelial cells of the mucous membrane linings of the urethra, endocervix, rectum, pharynx, and conjunctiva are the predominant sites of localized infection in uncomplicated gonorrhea. However, the infection can extend along the genital structures, resulting in complications of pelvic inflammatory disease and epididymo-orchitis or manifest as disseminated gonorrhea with bacteremia (Bignell, 2009). The primary mode of transmission is genital-genital, genital-anorectal, orogenital, or oroanal sexual contact, although it could also occur during birth via maternal–child transmission (Bignell, 2005; Hansfield & Sparling, 2005).

Gonorrhea is the second most common reportable infectious disease in the United States. From 1975 through 2009, the United States experienced a marked decline in the rate of gonorrhea; however, since 2009, that rate has increased to 110.7 cases per 100,000 population, with a surge in antibiotic resistance (CDC, 2016d). The major increase in the rate of gonorrhea from 2013–2014 was attributable to men.

Neisseria gonorrhoeae (Gonorrhea) Screening

Current CDC recommendations for gonorrhea screening are as follows:

- All sexually active females ages 25 and under, either heterosexual or WSW, should be screened for gonorrhea annually (Gorgos & Marrazzo, 2011; Workowski & Bolan, 2015).
- All sexually active females over the age of 25 who have risk factors (a new sex partner, anonymous sex, more than one sex partner, a sex partner with concurrent sex partners, irregular use of condoms, or a sex partner who has tested positive for an STI) should also be routinely screened.
- All pregnant women aged 25 and under, or living in an area where gonorrhea is common, should be screened for gonorrhea at their first prenatal visit. Women at increased risk should be rescreened in the third trimester.
- MSM are at high risk for gonorrhea and should be regularly screened at sites of exposure (urethra/rectum/pharynx) regardless of condom use (CDC, 2015d).

As previously noted with chlamydia, the USPSTF only recommends routine gonorrhea screening for sexually active women under the age of 24 and older women who are at increased risk of infection. The USPSTF is in agreement with the CDC that there is insufficient evidence to assess the balance of benefits and harms of routine gonorrhea screening in men who are not at an elevated risk (USPSTF, 2014).

In the United Kingdom Gonorrhea is reported to be the second most prevalent bacterial STI after *Chlamydia trachomatis*, with an incubation period of 2–5 days in most cases (up to 10 days in some). Variations are reported in the degree of virulence and the predisposition to develop systemic dispersal of the disease. Additionally, coinfection with *Chlamydia trachomatis* in females is found to be concomitant with escalated accumulation of gonococcal organisms (Stupiansky et al., 2011).

Relevant epidemiological data compiled in the United Kingdom revealed that a decrease in the prevalence of gonorrhea had been reported over a decade, countering the general increases in the rates of other STIs. Nevertheless, a rise of 6% was reported in 2008–2009, during which period newly diagnosed cases rose from 16,629 in 2008 to 17,385 in 2009 (HPA, 2010b). The highest rates recorded were among young people; 50% of those were under 25 years of age with trends of males 20–24 and females 16–19. Sexual risk-taking behaviors with practices of partying/mixing sexual activities were also additional risk factors. MSM and certain ethnic groups were identified as population subgroups among whom higher prevalence of gonorrhea occurs (HPA, 2008b; Risley et al., 2007).

The trend of gonorrhea infections shows high prevalence among young women in the age group of 20 years (National Institute for Health and Care Excellence [NICE], 2011). Additionally, 40% of women with gonorrhea are found to have a coinfection (Allstaff & Wilson, 2012; Liu et al., 2013; NICE, 2011) with *Chlamydia trachomatis*. However, various experts and researchers have estimated varying figures between 30% – 46% (Liu et al., 2013). The variations depend on the prevalence of these infections among different population groups and ethnic backgrounds in different communities, patient circumstances, and other multiple risk factors (Bignell, 2009; Risley et al., 2007). Particular high-risk groups include commercial sex workers, illicit drug users and MSM. Common sexual risk-taking behaviors involve unprotected sexual intercourse, inconsistent condom use, and multiple and frequent changes of sexual partners (Risley et al., 2007).

Associated Risk Factors

- Age: Young people 15–29 years old, highest risk group under 25 years of age
- Previous STI
- Coexisting STI (HIV coexists in one-third of MSM with gonorrhea, chlamydia in 41% of women and 35% of men with gonorrhea) (Richens, 2011)
- Multiple sexual partners including new sexual partners
- Recent sexual activities during trips to other countries
- Homosexual activities, unprotected anal intercourse, habitual insertive oral sex
- Infrequent condom usage
- Commercial sex work and/or history of drug abuse (Bignell, 2009; Risley et al., 2007)

Characteristic Clinical Symptoms and Signs

Males

A small proportion (10%) of males who develop uncomplicated gonorrhea remain asymptomatic (Bignell & Fitzgerald, 2011). Acute urethral infection in men is characterized by pain and difficulty with micturition in 50% of men but this is not accompanied by urgency or frequency (Bignell & Fitzgerald, 2011). Eighty percent of infected men experience discharge from the urethra, which is initially sparse and mucoid but becomes purulent after 1–2 days (Bignell & Fitzgerald, 2011). Many men who develop rectal infection remain asymptomatic. However, manifestation of acute proctitis is accompanied by anal pruritus with spasm and pain in 7%, involving the anal sphincter (tenesmus) with purulent discharge in 12% of patients, and bleeding may also manifest (Bignell & Fitzgerald, 2011). While pharyngeal infection may be asymptomatic in 90% of men, overt pharyngitis may become manifest (Bignell & Fitzgerald, 2011). Meticulous physical examination may reveal mucopurulent discharge from the urethra, and erythema of the urethral meatus may be evident. Swelling and/or tenderness of the epididymis or clinical evidence indicating balanitis may also be detected (Bignell & Fitzgerald, 2011).

Females

Approximately half of females who develop uncomplicated gonorrheal infection at the endocervix are asymptomatic (Bignell & Fitzgerald, 2011). The rest develop symptoms within 10 days (Richens, 2011).

Vaginal discharge becomes increased or altered in up to 50% of those infected (Bignell & Fitzgerald, 2011). Dysuria is experienced by 12% of those who develop urethral infection; however, in most cases this is not accompanied by urgency or frequency of micturition (Bignell & Fitzgerald, 2011). Intermenstrual bleeding may be noticed and sometimes associated with sexual intercourse. Lower abdominal pain may be accompanied by dyspareunia in up to 25% (Bignell & Fitzgerald, 2011). Those who develop rectal gonorrhea experience symptoms of anal pruritus, spasm, and pain of the anal sphincter (tenesmus) with purulent discharge or bleeding. Similarly to males, pharyngeal infection with gonorrhea may be asymptomatic in >90% of females although pharyngitis may become manifest (Bignell & Fitzgerald, 2011). Meticulous physical examination may reveal mucopurulent endocervical discharge, or readily induced endocervical bleeding. This occurs in less than 50% of the infected females and is not a strong predictive finding (Bignell & Fitzgerald, 2011).

Purulent discharge from the urethra is uncommon but may occur. Pelvic inflammatory disease would be accompanied by abdominal and pelvic tenderness (Bignell & Fitzgerald, 2011).

Diagnosis of Gonorrheal Infection: the Laboratory Tests: Specimens, Culture, and NAATs

Culture

It is suggested that culture could be considered in cases where the patients present with characteristic signs and

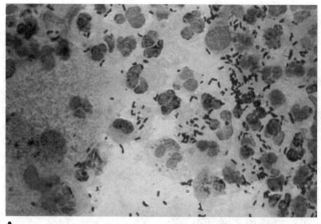

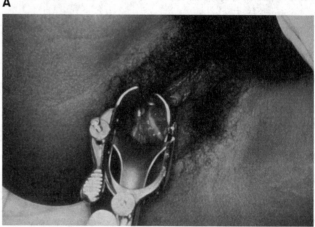

B

Figure 6-2 Gonorrhea
(A) CDC; **(B)** Joe Miller; CDC

symptoms of gonorrhea with or without confirmation (Bignell, 2010) (**Figure 6-2**). This allows for susceptibility test to be carried out together with identification of resistant strains. Some experts recommend gram staining of the endocervical specimen. The characteristic diagnostic finding shows gram-negative diplococci in polymorphonuclear leukocytes (Janda & Knapp 2003). However, efficacy of culture tests on specimens depends on correct and high standard methods of specimen collection and correct medium of transport to the laboratory.

Nucleic Acid Amplification Tests

The Medical Foundation for AIDS & Sexual Health (MEDFASH) endorses NAATs for gonorrhea and *Chlamydia trachomatis* due to the high sensitivity for detecting *Neisseria gonorrhoeae* in different specimens (Bignell, 2010; MEDFASH, 2014). NAATs can detect the presence of relatively low numbers of organisms in the specimens. However, every attempt should be made to avoid inadvertent cross-contamination with unrelated DNA or rRNA, which could give false positive results (Bignell, 2010; MEDFASH, 2014). Despite the high sensitivity and specificity of the techniques it is found that the positive predictive value (PPV) tends to be low in areas where prevalence of the infection is low. That creates a relatively larger proportion of false positives, which is a problem associated with gonorrhea because variations of low prevalence occur among different communities in different geographical areas. Therefore, if the PPV of the single test falls below 90%, the gonorrhea NAATs should be confirmed with a supplementary test. Although culturing of urine specimens for *Neisseria gonorrhoeae* is not recommended (Cook et al., 2005), NAATs can detect *Neisseria gonorrhoeae* in urine specimens (Whiley, Tapsall, & Sloots, 2006).

Turnaround Times

The turnaround time for a test is the time taken in the laboratory (MEDFASH, 2014) for carrying out the tests and the confirmation as necessary. The results must be reported and submitted to the genitourinary physician or the relevant clinician without delay (Bignell, 2010). Recommended turnaround times are 2 working days for initial testing and 3–5 working days for confirmation of a positive result. In the event of delay, a provisional report must be submitted to the clinician. The total amount of time from samples being taken from a patient to the delivery of a full report to the clinician should be within 7 days (Bignell, 2010).

In females, a carefully collected endocervical swab is required for the diagnostic testing, and while the procedure may result in contact bleeding, hyperemia may also be detected during the examination. A specimen of first-void urine may also be used for the diagnostic tests. Microscopy and direct visualization of *Neisseria gonorrhoeae* in urethral discharge and urethral smears from males may confirm the diagnosis in symptomatic men. However, in view of the relatively low sensitivity for detecting the microorganisms in urethral smears in females and asymptomatic rectal infections, diagnostic tests on these sites are not recommended. Furthermore, these tests are considered to be unsuitable for detecting *Neisseria gonorrhoeae* in specimens obtained from the pharynx (Bignell, 2009).

Associated Complications

Disseminated gonococcal infection is a rare complication characterized by symptoms of gonococcal bacteremia, including skin lesions, fever, acute arthritis, arthralgia, and tenosynovitis (Bignell & Fitzgerald, 2011). Other reported complications caused by transluminal spread of *Neisseria gonorrhoeae* via the urethra include epididymo-orchitis and prostatitis in men. In women, pelvic inflammatory disease is the main complication resulting from transluminal spread through the endocervix (Bignell & Fitzgerald, 2011).

U.S. Recommended Treatment and Management of *Neisseria Gonorrhoeae*

Gonorrhea has now developed resistance to sulfonamides, tetracyclines, fluoroquinolones, and penicillin. This resistance leaves ceftriaxone and azithromycin dual therapy (that is, the drugs administered together, preferably on the same day, at the same time, under direct observation) as the only CDC-recommended first-line treatment regimen in the United States (ACOG, 2015b; Workowski & Bolan, 2015). This single-dose treatment regimen improves client compliance and appears effective against pharyngeal infection as well. As many persons infected with gonorrhea are frequently coinfected with chlamydia, this dual-therapy regimen is also approved for use against *C. trachomatis* infection.

Recommended Regimen for Uncomplicated Gonococcal Infections of the Cervix, Urethra, Pharynx, and Rectum

- Ceftriaxone 250 mg IM in a single dose, **plus**
- Azithromycin 1 g orally in a single dose

Alternative Regimens (If Ceftriaxone is not Available or has Limited Efficacy Against Pharyngeal Infection)

- Cefixime 400 mg orally in a single dose, **plus**
- Azithromycin 1 g orally in a single dose

Management Considerations and Follow-Up

All persons treated for gonorrhea should be instructed to abstain from sexual activity for 7 days following treatment and until 7 days after all partners have been treated and any symptoms have resolved. All persons diagnosed with gonorrhea should also be tested for other STIs, including chlamydia, HIV, and syphilis. A test-of-cure is not needed for persons with uncomplicated urogenital or rectal gonorrhea who have received either the recommended or alternative regimens. However, any person with pharyngeal gonorrhea treated with an alternative regimen should return in 14 days for a test-of-cure using either NAAT or culture methods. All positive cultures for test-of-cure should undergo antimicrobial susceptibility testing. Because rates of reinfection caused by failure of sex partners to receive treatment are high, all persons treated for gonorrhea should be retested 3 months after treatment, regardless of whether they believe their partners received treatment. For heterosexual persons with gonorrhea where providers are concerned about partners' access to prompt evaluation and treatment, EPT with cefixime 400 mg and azithromycin 1 g can be dispensed by the patient, public health specialist, or pharmacist as permitted by law (see prior discussion of EPT). Again, EPT should not be considered as a routine strategy for MSM due to the high risk of coexisting infections (particularly HIV) and due to a lack of data on efficacy in this population.

Pregnant women infected with gonorrhea, and persons who are HIV positive with a gonococcal infection should both be treated with the recommended first-line dual therapy regimen of ceftriaxone 250 mg IM in a single dose given simultaneously with azithromycin 1 g orally in a single dose. Pregnant women should be rescreened in

3 months. Any person allergic to the recommended treatment regimens should have desensitization instituted and/or be evaluated by an infectious disease specialist (Workowski & Bolan, 2015).

UK Recommendations: Patient/Client Information, Advice and Support

The explanations that should be provided to the patient are similar to those previously outlined in relation to *Chlamydia trachomatis*. These should encompass clear explanation about the condition, diagnostic investigations, requirements for collecting specimens, the treatment regimen, and potential long-term consequences for personal health and that of sexual partner(s) (Bignell & Fitzgerald, 2011). The importance of avoiding sexual intercourse until completion of the prescribed treatment regimen and further recommended period should always be emphasized and safer sex practices should be encouraged (Bignell & Fitzgerald, 2011).

Partner Notification and Consideration of Other Sexual Contacts

Partner notification by a qualified sexual health adviser should include notification of sexual contacts of male patients with symptomatic urethral infection. The recommendation is that all sexual contacts over the previous 2 weeks, or if longer than that the most recent sexual partner/contact, should be screened for gonorrhea and offered the recommended empirical treatment (Bignell & Fitzgerald, 2011). Similarly, all sexual partners/sexual contacts over the previous 3 months of patients with asymptomatic or infection at other sites of the body should be notified and offered screening and empirical treatment. In both cases, all the relevant sexual partners/sexual contacts should be offered full STI screening and the recommended empirical treatment for gonorrhea and *Chlamydia trachomatis* while awaiting the laboratory test results (Bignell & Fitzgerald, 2011). Thus, the routine screening for concurrent STIs should be clearly explained to gain the cooperation of the patient (Bignell & Fitzgerald, 2011). Depending on the organizational and local policy, the specimen may be obtained before commencement of the antibiotic treatment to test for susceptibility and for identification of resistant strains.

Justification for Offering and Administering Treatment

Microscopic confirmation of the identified intracellular gram-negative diplococci in the smear from the genital tract, *Neisseria gonorrhoeae* positive culture from the infected sites, and positive NAATs for *Neisseria gonorrhoeae* are strong justifications for offering treatment. An auxiliary test should be considered if the positive predictive value is found to be <90% (Bignell & Fitzgerald, 2011; Whiley et al., 2006). Other indications for offering and administering treatment include recent sexual partner or sexual contact of an infected person diagnosed with gonorrhea and epidemiological treatment being offered

following sexual assault (Bignell & Fitzgerald, 2011). In these cases, the individual would have tested positive to gonorrhea, experienced the characteristic symptoms, or would fall into the category of a high-risk group (Bignell & Fitzgerald, 2011).

Recommended Treatment Regimen for Uncomplicated Anogenital Gonorrheal Infection

- Ceftriaxone 500 mg intramuscularly as a stat dose, plus
- Azithromycin 1 g orally as a stat dose

The oral dose of azithromycin is given as cotreatment regardless of the laboratory results and the patient's *Chlamydia trachomatis* infection status (Ison et al., 2004; Newman, Moran, & Workowski, 2007).

Among the range of recommended alternative antimicrobials include cefixime 400 mg orally stat as a single dose, although there have been reports of recurring treatment failures with this antimicrobial agent. Therefore, a pretreatment susceptibility test is recommended (GRASP Steering Group [GRASP], 2009). Spectinomycin is another alternative antimicrobial that may be administered as a single stat dose of 2 g intramuscularly in combination with azithromycin 1 g orally as a single dose. However, this antimicrobial has been reported to have relatively low efficacy and does not adequately eradicate pharyngeal gonorrhea (Bignell & Fitzgerald, 2011; Newman et al., 2007; Tapsall, Ndowa, Lewis, & Unemo, 2009).

Practitioners are encouraged to explore more details of other recommended alternative antimicrobial agents. However, it must be noted that these are not necessarily more efficacious than the recommended antimicrobial treatment with ceftriaxone. Based on reports of diminished susceptibility to cefixime and ceftriaxone (GRASP, 2009) the recommendation is to test for susceptibility as a guide to patient management and for surveillance records. Other alternative treatment regimens should be carefully explored regarding the level of substantive evidence, efficacy, susceptibility, and resistance. The Gonococcal Resistance to Antimicrobials Surveillance Programme (GRASP) scrutinizes and regulates emerging trends of gonococcal antimicrobial drug resistance.

The ongoing problem of *Neisseria gonorrhoeae* resistance and/or diminished sensitivity to many cephalosporins has resulted in the current situation of gonorrhea treatment with multidrug and extended or broad spectrum antimicrobials (Tapsall et al., 2009). Due to the continuous increase in resistance to cephalosporins Chisholm et al. (2010) advocate higher dose cephtriaxone for treatment of gonorrhea. Additionally, these authors advocate the use of azithromycin in combination with cephalosporins regardless of the laboratory test for *Chlamydia trachomatis* infection and maintain that this could limit potential widespread cephalosporin resistance. Research evidence suggests that azithromycin has high efficacy of >98% when given as a single dose of 2 g orally (Bignell &

Garley, 2010). The dilemma seems to be that diminished efficacy of azithromycin 1 g single dose could be as low as 93%. However, the higher dose of 2 g has been reported to be associated with gastrointestinal side effects (GRASP, 2009).

Sathia, Ellis, Phillips, Winston, and Smith (2007) reported eradication of pharyngeal gonococcal infection by combined therapy with azithromycin and cephalosporins. Evidence from in vitro and in vivo research studies have demonstrated synergy in terms of combined effect between azithromycin and cephalosporins (Furuya et al., 2006; Golden, Kerani, Shafii, Whittington, & Holmes, 2009). Nonetheless, drug resistance and treatment failure with azithromycin have also been reported in Europe (Chisholm et al., 2010; Palmer, Young, Winter, & Dave, 2008; Starnino & Stefanelli, 2009). The increasing resistance of *Neisseria gonorrhoeae* to cephalosporins seems to have created various dilemmas with the tendency to resort to higher doses of cephalosporins. Other possible responses include prescribing multi-dose regimens, multi-drug regimens, microbiologically directed treatment, or strengthening research into drug cycling (European Centre for Disease Control [ECDC], 2012).

Recommended Treatment of Gonorrheal Infections

The recommended regimens for gonococcal infection of the pharynx comprise the following:

- Ceftriaxone 500 mg administered intramuscularly as a single dose in combination with a single dose of azithromycin 1 g orally
- Ciprofloxacin 500 mg orally as a single dose
- Ofloxacin 400 mg orally as a single dose

However, it is important that penicillin anaphylaxis, cephalosporin allergy, or fluoroquinolone or azithromycin resistance must be ruled out and susceptibility testing performed (Bignell & Fitzgerald, 2011; Bignell & Unemo, 2013).

Gonococcal Infection with Pelvic Inflammatory Disease (PID)

- Ceftriaxone 500 mg intramuscularly followed by
- Doxycycline 100 mg orally twice daily with
- Metronidazole 400 mg orally twice daily for 14 days (Bignell & Fitzgerald, 2011; Bignell & Unemo, 2013).
- Gonococcal infection with epididymo-orchitis
  - Ceftriaxone 500 mg intramuscularly together with
  - Doxycycline 100 mg orally twice daily for 10–14 days (Bignell & Fitzgerald, 2011; Bignell & Unemo, 2013)

Disseminated Gonococcal Infection (DGI)

The recommended treatment may involve hospitalization.

- Ceftriaxone 1 g intravenously or intramuscularly every 24 hours or

- Cefotaxime 1g intravenously every 8 hours or
- Ciprofloxacin 500 mg intravenously every 12 hours depending on sensitivity test result
- Spectinomycin 2 g intramuscularly may be administered every 12 hours

The recommendation is to continue the treatments for 7 days (Bignell & Fitzgerald, 2011; Bignell & Unemo, 2013). However, oral treatment regimens may be substituted 24–48 hours following the initial parenteral treatment when the symptoms subside. The oral treatments include cefixime 400 mg twice daily or ciprofloxacin 500 mg twice daily or ofloxacin 400 mg twice daily (Bignell & Fitzgerald, 2011; Bignell & Unemo, 2013). In all treatments, accuracy in dosage administration and specified regimens should be closely adhered to.

Test of Cure

Test of cure is recommended due to the persistent cephalosporin resistance and decreased susceptibility to various antimicrobials (Ison, Hussey, Sankar, Evans, & Alexander, 2011). Reports of treatment failures using various cephalosporins indicate that cure and eradication cannot be presumed with all prescribed antimicrobial treatments. The test of cure allows for determining if the patient complied with the prescribed treatment and that symptoms have subsided. It also helps to identify what, if any, adverse reactions the patient may have experienced and to establish through a sexual history if the patient has developed a reinfection. Health promotion and partner notification procedures can be reinforced at this time (Bignell & Fitzgerald, 2011). Test of cure is currently recommended for all patients who undergo treatment for gonorrheal infections. However, there may be situations where selective test of cure has to be the option due to lack of adequate resources. In those situations priority is given to test of cure for patients with persistent symptoms and signs and those with pharyngeal gonococcal infections that fail to cure completely (Bignell & Fitzgerald, 2011; Newman et al., 2007; Sathia et al., 2007). Patients who are treated with alternative antimicrobials or drugs other than recommended first-line antimicrobials, as well as pregnant women, are also considered and prioritized for test of cure (Bignell & Fitzgerald, 2011).

The suggestion for the timing and method of assessing treatment of cure is that for persistent symptoms and signs culture should be performed at least 72 hours following completion of the treatment. In cases of negative culture result NAATs should be carried out 1 week later for increased sensitivity. However, if the patient is asymptomatic NAATs should be carried out if possible, followed by culture. In all cases of positive NAAT results the recommended timing for test of cure is 2 weeks after completion of the antimicrobial treatment. Susceptibility testing is recommended prior to further treatment being prescribed (Hjelmevoll et al., 2011). It is suggested that the presence of infection following treatment could be an indication of recurrent infection rather than failed treatment (Komolafe, Sugunendran, & Corkill, 2004).

There is strong recommendation to report failed cephalosporin treatments. For identifying, confirming, and reporting failed antimicrobial treatments practitioners may find it worthwhile to explore and compare the guidance of their national, WHO global, ECDC, and CDC action/response plans, as listed at the end of this chapter, for additional recommended reading.

The Role of Care Pathway

Another recommendation by MEDFASH requires that a care pathway be prearranged and implemented. This encompasses informing the patient of the laboratory test results, being given the prescribed treatment, and instigation of the partner notification process. The therapeutic management commences without delay and the policy is to ensure that patients/clients using the STI testing services receive their results within 10 days. Promptness in treating patients who are diagnosed positive is emphasized. Additional aspects of care provision, together with the partner notification process, should also be implemented immediately (Bignell, 2010; MEDFASH, 2014).

Treponema pallidum (Syphilis)

Syphilis, a contagious venereal infection caused by *Treponema pallidum*, which are coiled, motile spirochete bacteria, characteristically manifests as a systemic disease (**Figure 6-3**). The prevalence of syphilis is considered as a persistently major problem worldwide. The global estimate of the total number of new cases of syphilis in adults in 2008 was 10.6 million and at any point in 2008 the number of adults infected with syphilis was estimated as 36.4 million (WHO, 2012). Despite the decline in the prevalence of syphilis in developed countries, recent figures indicate resurgence of this STI with increasing rates.

After decades of decline, U.S. cases of syphilis nearly doubled in 2013 with the rate increased among both men and women. This increase in women is of particular concern, as the increase of congenital syphilis has historically followed increases in the rate among women (CDC, 2016d). During 2013–2014, the U.S. rate of congenital syphilis increased 27.5% to 11.6 cases per 100,000 live births. In the United States racial disparities are evident with this infection, with African American women 13.3 times more likely to be infected than white women (Patton, Su, Nelson, & Weinstock, 2014). MSM account for the majority of syphilis cases.

Darkfield examination tests the presence of *T. pallidum* from exudate or tissue samples and is the gold standard for diagnosing early syphilis. A diagnosis of syphilis can be presumed with the required use of two tests: a nontreponemal test such as either the Venereal Disease Research Laboratory (VDRL) or the rapid plasma reagin (RPR),

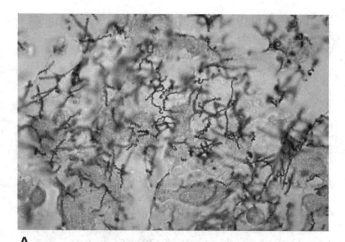

A

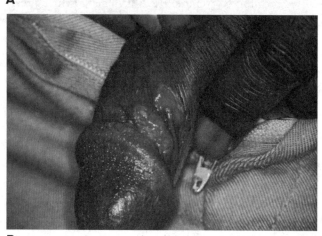

B

Figure 6-3 Syphilis *Treponema Pallidum* Organism and Clinical Manifestation
(A) CDC/Dr. Edwin P. Ewing, Jr.; **(B)** CDC/M. Rein

and a treponemal test. Use of only one type of serologic test is insufficient for diagnosis due to both false positive and false negative results. Thus, persons with a reactive nontreponemal test should always have a confirmatory treponemal test done as follow-up.

Treponema pallidum (Syphilis) Screening in the United States

In the United States, cases of both primary and secondary syphilis are reported together. The CDC recommends the following screening guidelines:

- All pregnant women should be screened at the first prenatal visit, and, if at high risk, retested early in the third trimester, and again at delivery.

- MSM should be tested annually and every 3–6 months if at increased risk.

- Persons with HIV should be screened at first HIV evaluation and then annually. More frequent screening might be appropriate depending on personal behavioral risks and local disease prevalence (CDC, 2015d).

The USPSTF recommends syphilis screening for men and women at increased risk, such as MSM, adults in correctional facilities, paid sex workers, drug users, and pregnant women. Universal screening for syphilis is not recommended for heterosexual men or for non-pregnant females (American Academy of Pediatrics, 2014).

In the United Kingdom, Righarts, Simms, Wallace, Solomou, & Fenton, 2004 reported sporadic outbreaks in various cities across the United Kingdom. In 2007 in the United Kingdom, new diagnoses of infectious syphilis recorded 3,762 cases and the trends in the increase showed that MSM accounted for 73% of those cases (Delvin, 2010; French, 2011; HPA, 2009). More recent figures reveal an apparent decline to 2,911 newly diagnosed cases of syphilis in the United Kingdom in 2010. Of that total, 313 were women while the remainder were men, a greater proportion—60%—being MSM (Delvin, 2016; French, 2011). Reported outbreaks in 2011 indicated that spread of the infection was highest among young heterosexuals (Abu-Rajab & Wallace, 2011; Morgan, Blume, & Carroll, 2011).

The main concerns about the resurgence of this infection relate to its coexistence with HIV and the impact on perinatal morbidity and mortality through maternal–child transmission. Therefore, because the infection is frequently asymptomatic, the recommendation is that screening should be made available to high-risk population groups in special circumstances, including pregnancy and blood donation (French, 2011).

High-Risk Population Groups and Risky Situations

Certain situations, such as poor standards in blood donation, potentially present serious risk of acquiring syphilis and other STIs. Additionally, particular population groups also present heightened susceptibility to acquire various STIs, including syphilis. Therefore, preventive measures and appropriate screening of high-risk groups should be considered a national priority. The following are high-risk groups and associated social circumstances that potentially increase the risk for infection.

- Expectant mothers
- Blood donors
- Newly diagnosed STIs
- Patients/clients with HIV positive diagnosis
- Patients/clients with hepatitis B infection or hepatitis C infection
- Suspected early symptoms of neurosyphilis
- Meningitis
- Unexpected rapid development of uveitis with visual loss
- Unexpected rapid development of otitis with hearing loss
- Men who have sex with men
- Commercial sex workers
- Individuals who practice different forms of risky sexual behaviors (French et al., 2009)

Acquisition of syphilis among MSM has been largely linked to sexual risk-taking behaviors and risky practices such as oral sex. The pattern of outbreaks and acquisition among heterosexual men has been largely linked to risky sexual behaviors among high-risk groups, particularly sex workers, students, and young people. However, the reemergence and increase in congenital syphilis has been linked to the substantial rise in the incidence of infectious syphilis among childbearing women. Hence the recommendation for routine prenatal screening of pregnant women.

Key Considerations in the Prevention and Control of Syphilis

Dean and Fenton (2010) examined the social factors and endeavors that influence prevention and control of HIV/AIDS viral hepatitis and other STIs. The following key measures are considered important in the prevention and control of transmission and acquisition of syphilis.

- Wider accessibility to sexual health/genitourinary clinics
- Availability of unbiased specialist consultations, diagnostic interventions and therapeutic care to all patients/clients regardless of background, and implementation of measures to eliminate nonattendance, delayed diagnosis, and treatment
- Open-mindedness in staff attitudes and nonjudgemental ambiance
- Provision of pertinent sexual health promotion and counseling support
- Availability of alternative referral systems and effective procedures for partner notification and partner management
- Opportunistic screening initiatives in relevant clinics.
- Outreach activities to target high-risk population groups
- Routine prenatal screening for expectant mothers
- Sexual health promotion endeavors (Simms et al., 2005)

Classification of Syphilis: The Progression and Interconnected Stages

The classification of syphilis distinguishes acquired and congenital forms of the condition. The disease is further categorized as early and late syphilis. Early syphilis is characterized by manifestations of primary syphilis, secondary syphilis, and early latent asymptomatic syphilis infection (French et al., 2009; Kingston et al., 2008).

Other classifications identify late latent asymptomatic syphilis and tertiary symptomatic syphilis. In clarifying these, the European Centre for Disease Prevention and Control (ECDC) (2011) distinguishes early syphilis as having been acquired in less than the previous year. The World Health Organization (WHO) on the other hand, distinguishes early syphilis as having been acquired in less than the previous 2 years (WHO, n.d.). Late latent syphilis, according to the ECDC, refers to syphilis acquired longer than the previous 1 year while the WHO distinguishes this as syphilis acquired longer than the previous 2 years (ECDC, 2011; WHO, n.d.). The classification of congenital syphilis distinguishes early and late congenital syphilis. Early congenital syphilis is identified as acquisition occurring in the first 2 years of life. Late congenital syphilis is identified as manifestations of the condition occurring after the first 2 years of life (French et al., 2009).

Primary Syphilis

Primary syphilis appears to have a varied incubation period, lasting an average of 14–21 days, although periods of 9–90 days have been reported (French et al., 2009). The genital and perianal areas are the most commonly affected sites, where a small painless papule appears. This papule forms into an indurated ulcer (chancre) with a margin and produces a clear discharge. Common lesion sites in heterosexual men include the corona sulcus, the glans, inner side of the prepuce, on the shaft, and elsewhere on the external genital structures; balanitis may also be identified (Eccleston, Collins, & Higgins, 2008). However, the commonly affected sites in homosexual men are the anal canal, the mouth, and the genitalia. In women, common lesion sites are the vulva, labia, and cervix (although uncommon). Inguinal lymph node enlargements may manifest but generally this is found to be painless, firm and rubbery, disconnected, and unfixed (Eccleston et al., 2008; French, 2011). A primary lesion at the site of infection may heal within 2–6 weeks (or up to 10 weeks) without the individual being aware of the infection. Other extra-genital lesion sites include the mouth, lips, and hands (Eccleston et al., 2008; French, 2011).

Secondary Syphilis

Secondary syphilis is characterized by bacteremia, during which various systems are affected. This stage manifests 6–8 weeks after primary syphilis (Lautenschlager, 2006), although in approximately one-third of cases this may occur while the primary lesion is still present. This stage may be delayed for quite a few months (French, 2011; French et al., 2009). Multiple systems become affected in the first 2 years. The characteristic lesions affect the skin and mucous membranes and tend to be nonpruritic macules appearing on the trunk and arms. Papular lesions appear on the face the trunk, palms, arms, genitalia, and soles of the feet as a generalized polymorphic rash with widespread painless lymphadenopathy (Baughn & Musher, 2005 French, 2011; French et al., 2009; Lautenschlager, 2006). The skin lesions are usually a mixture of macular and papular formations in the inner sides of the labia and perianal or anal areas. The papules may enlarge and coalesce to form condylomata lata (Parc, Chahed, Patel, & Salmon-Ceron, 2007)—which are large fleshy discs—or they may diminish and disappear spontaneously (French, 2011; French et al.,

2009). Papulosquamous lesions occur when the papules on the palms and soles of the feet undergo scaling (Zetola & Klausner, 2007). Lesions of the mucous membranes tend to be painless, greyish erosions affecting the mucous sides of the lips, cheeks, tongue, pharynx and larynx, the nose, vulva, vagina, glans penis, prepuce, and cervix (French, 2011; French et al., 2009). Systemic symptoms tend to be mild and may include night-time headaches, mild fever, malaise and aches (Baughn, 2005; Lautenschlager, 2006). Uncommon symptoms include patchy alopecia, anterior uveitis, meningitis, glomerulonephritis, and hepatitis (Ghanem et al., 2008; Parc et al., 2007). The majority of patients (80%) progress to the latent asymptomatic stage and remain in that stage permanently while 20% develop an infectious relapse in the ensuing year.

Latent Syphilis

The two classifications of this stage of syphilis are early latent and late latent. In early latent syphilis, the individual has positive serological evidence of *Treponema pallidum* infection but never presents with clinical symptoms. Thus, early latent stage is characterized by asymptomatic syphilis with positive serology of less than 2 years' duration. Late latent syphilis is diagnosed by positive serological tests for 2 years or more but without manifestation of late syphilis symptoms. Kingston et al.'s 2008 concise distinction of early latent and late latent syphilis is worth noting. These authors simply distinguish the period within the first 2 years of latent asymptomatic syphilis as early latent syphilis and the period beyond the first 2 years as late latent syphilis (Kingston et al., BASHH, 2008). However, research evidence reveals that 40% of untreated patients with late *Treponema pallidum* infection present with symptomatic late syphilis.

Symptomatic Late Syphilis

This stage of late symptomatic syphilis (also called tertiary syphilis) is appropriately subclassified as neurological syphilis or symptomatic neurosyphilis, cardiovascular syphilis and gummatous syphilis (BASHH, 2008; Kingston et al., 2008).

Symptomatic Neurosyphilis

Symptomatic neurosyphilis is characterized by meningo-vascular syphilis with signs of acute meningitis. The onset occurs 2 to 7 years after the initial infection and focal arteritis with infarction may manifest depending on the location and the tissues affected. Meningeal inflammation may be associated with papilledema. Early meningovascular syphilis may appear as part of secondary syphilis (Zetola & Klausner 2007). Late meningovascular syphilis is characterized by less acute symptoms but headaches persist with prodrome and symptoms involving the third, sixth, seventh and eighth cranial nerves (Zetola & Klausner, 2007). The characteristic symptoms of late meningovascular syphilis may manifest during a 2–20 year period (French, 2011; French et al., 2009).

Parenchymatous neurosyphilis manifests either as general paresis or tabes dorsalis or rarely as a combined manifestation (Jay, 2006; Zetola & Klausner, 2007). The general paresis may be progressive with cortical neural loss and cerebral atrophy 10–20 years after onset of the primary infection. The characteristic symptoms include hemiparesis irritability, progressively poor cognitive function, moodiness, fatigue, headaches, and tremors while the late symptoms include depression, disorientation, and delusions, with complications of seizures, transient paralysis, and aphasia (Wilcox, 2009). These symptoms may be accompanied by lack of facial expression, dysarthria, tremors of lips and hands with difficulty in writing, optic atrophy with abnormal papillary function, and visual deterioration. Convulsions and emotional instability are additional late complications.

The characteristic features of tabes dorsalis are brought about by degeneration and loss of the dorsal or posterior column of the spinal nerve roots (Jay, 2006; Zetola & Klausner 2007). Thus, paresthesia, increasing sensory ataxia, visual loss, disorder of bladder function, and bowel dysfunction may manifest (Wilcox, 2009). Other signs include impaired sense of position, loss of ankle and knee reflexes, loss of biceps and triceps reflexes, and impaired sense of touch and pain Charcot's joints. Optic atrophy and ocular palsies may also develop.

Cardiovascular Syphilis

Cardiovascular syphilis is characterized by aortitis spreading distally from the root of the aorta. Typical signs are aortic regurgitation, angina with substernal pain, and aortic aneurysm. These signs may manifest over the period 10–40 years following the primary infection (Kingston et al., 2008).

Gummata is characterized by typical inflammatory granulomatous fibrous nodules or plaques. The manifestations of these vary and may be several years (3–12) or even up to 46 years following the primary infection. The sites affected include the skin, mucous membranes, bones, and viscera, though most commonly the skin and bones. Skin lesions generally occur as small groups of firm, painless, necrotic nodules, plaques, or ulcers (French, 2011; French et al., 2009).

The main changes in the 2015 U.K. national guidelines for the management of syphilis include the following:

- Full routine examination and chest x-ray is no longer considered necessary for patients with asymptomatic disease.
- Where benzathine penicillin is suitable, procaine penicillin should be considered as an alternative treatment.
- Procaine penicillin is no longer considered as the preferred treatment, but as an alternative treatment for all stages of syphilis apart from neurosyphilis.
- The duration of the recommended treatment regimen for neurosyphilis is now reduced to 14 days.

- Resistance to macrolide antibiotics restricts their use and therefore are only prescribed when there is no option for a suitable alternative antibiotic.
- A syphilis birth plan has now been developed to guide the team of practitioners and ensure effective communication and high standard of care provision.
- Babies born to mothers who receive treatment for syphilis in the current pregnancy should be carefully assessed and screened for syphilis serology.
- Serology should comprise IgM and non-treponemal titers at birth, at 3 months, then 3-month intervals until clear and negative.
- Screening of untested siblings is recommended when a diagnosis of maternal of congenital syphilis is made.
- Recommendations for minimal follow-up are clearly stipulated.

Diagnostic Procedures: Laboratory Investigations

The diagnosis of syphilis should commence with a detailed history to establish previous screening and diagnosis to determine the current stage of the condition if the patient had been previously diagnosed. This will determine what treatment had been prescribed and establish the serological response to treatment by conducting rapid plasma reagin (RPR) or venereal disease research laboratory (VDRL) tests (French, 2011).

Direct identification of *Treponema pallidum* is crucial for diagnosis. Therefore, dark ground dark-field microscopy is considered the definitive investigative technique for detecting *Treponema pallidum* in primary lesion exudate or tissue (or other direct specimen) (Wheeler, Agarwal, & Goh, 2004). Three specimens collected over 3 consecutive days from early syphilitic lesions should be examined with further specimens obtained for three repeat testings if the initial test result proves (BASHH, 2008; Kingston et al., 2008). Practitioners should confirm this guideline and method of specimen collection in their workplace. Intra-anal and oral specimens are not considered to be suitable for this test (BASHH, 2008; Kingston et al., 2008).

Depending on availability of the required laboratory resources, polymerase chain reaction (PCR) testing may be performed on specimens from oral and other non-urethral lesions (Koek, Bruisten, Dierdrop, Van Dam, & Templeton, 2006). PCR is performed on specimens that could be contaminated by commensal treponems and does not replace dark ground microscopic test. However, while VDRL and RPR are not necessarily specific tor detecting *Treponema pallidum* these tests do, nonetheless, allow for making a presumptive diagnosis of syphilis.

Serological Tests for Primary Syphilis

Serological tests for primary syphilis comprise *Treponema*-specific tests. *Treponema* enzyme immunoassay (EIA) allows for detecting immunoglobulin G (IgG) to determine early syphilis infection or to detect immunoglobulin M (IgM). *Treponema pallidum*-specific tests comprise *Treponema pallidum* hemagglutination assay (TPHA), *Treponama pallidum* passive particle agglutination assay (TPPA), and fluorescent treponemal antibody absorbed test (FTA-abs) (Kingston et al., 2008). These are performed for confirming the diagnosis. No single test should be considered as adequate for diagnosing syphilis due to false positives and potential test limitations. However, the concern is that non-*Treponema* false positive results may be associated with other conditions that are unconnected to syphilis, such as autoimmune disease, older age, and injection drug usage. For that reason, patients who test positive for reactive *Treponema pallidum* should be offered laboratory tests to confirm the diagnosis. Nucleic acid amplification tests are more commonly used for diagnosing syphilis the high degree of sensitivity and specificity that these techniques offer (French, 2011).

Nonspecific Compared to Specific Serological Tests
Nonspecific serological tests commonly used in diagnosing syphilis—RPR and VDRL—can yield positive results 3–5 weeks post infection (French, 2011). The quantitative values allow for determining the disease stage and process. Thus, decreasing titers indicate effective response to the treatment while increasing titers indicate ineffective or failed treatment, or reinfection. A note of caution involves the problem of natural deterioration resulting in decline of the titers in the absence of treatment. Thus, low or negative titers in RPR and VDRL results may be found in patients who are untreated and carrying active syphilis disease (French, 2011). Additionally, false positive results may be produced in reaction to other acute viral infections such as herpes, measles, and mumps. Similarly, false positive results may be detected following certain immunizations, including typhoid, while long-term false positive results may also be associated with autoimmune diseases such as rheumatoid arthritis (French, 2011).

It is recommended that a specimen be collected on the first day of treatment to provide a baseline for monitoring treatment efficacy (Kingston et al., 2008). Repeat screening is recommended following risk of exposure via high-risk sexual behaviors. These include unprotected vaginal, oral, and anal intercourse; multiple sexual partners; anonymous sexual partners and sexual contacts in social sexual networks; commercial sex workers; and sexual partners from areas with high prevalence of syphilis. In such situations, the screening test should be carried out 3 months after exposure to the infection (BASHH, 2008; Kingston et al., 2008). Repeat screening is also recommended following negative result of dark field test on a specimen collected from ulcerative lesions suspected of being syphilis (BASHH, 2008; Kingston et al., 2008).).

Preferred Serological Tests
The EIA tests are currently preferred for detecting *Treponema pallidum* infection and are more commonly used than fluorescent treponemal antibody test (FTA) and TPHA. Moreover, the TPPA is employed in confirming positive EIA tests, which has the benefit of specifically detecting positive *Treponema pallidum* at an early stage of the infection. The TPPA is also found to be relatively easier to establish and employ as routine practice (French, 2011). The technique of combining IgG/IgM and EIA in a composite test supersedes in diagnosing syphilis at an earlier stage at 2–4 weeks of infection (French, 2011). Thus, they provide the only positive serological tests in early syphilis and are found to detect 85–90% positive results in primary syphilis (French, 2011).

Diagnosis of Neurosyphilis: Cerebrospinal Fluid Tests
The recommendation is that cases of suspected neurosyphilis justify detailed neurological examination and lumber puncture for tests on cerebrospinal fluid (CSF). However, the procedure is not carried out as routine although abnormalities in CSF are detectable in early syphilis; secondary syphilis is found to be the stage where CSF tends to yield more positive results. Some STI clinicians hold the view that CSF lumbar puncture should be performed for all patients who have been diagnosed with HIV and syphilis for longer than 2 years to determine if the neurological system has been affected (French, 2011). Abnormally high white cell count in the CSF >5 mm^3 together with abnormally high level of protein exceeding 40 g/L may indicate neurosyphilis (French, 2011; Kingston et al., 2008)) and both treponemal and non-treponemal tests on CSF are effective in diagnosing neurosyphilis. It is suggested that positive CSF VDRL and CSF TPPA tests should be repeated to assess the quantitative values (Kingston et al., 2008). The overall sensitivity of CSF VDRL/RPR may be about 50% with asymptomatic cases showing a range of 10% and symptomatic showing a range of 90% (French, 2011; Kingston et al., 2008). Nevertheless, while positive results of RPR and VDRL in CSF indicate neurosyphilis, negative results in the nonspecific tests but raised white cell count may indicate probable neurosyphilis. Others maintain that serum RPR titer $\geq 1{:}32$ increases the probability of neurosyphilis regardless of the stage of the infection or coexistent HIV infection. Generally, patients with positive treponemal serum tests also have positive EIA or TPPA in the CSF. Negative treponemal test on CSF excludes neurosyphilis. However, while positive result is considered as highly sensitive for neurosyphilis the specificity is considered inadequate (Castro et al., 2006). It is considered that CSF TPHA titer of <320 or TPPA titer of <640 indicates that neurosyphilis is improbable (BASHH, 2008; Kingston et al., 2008).

Diagnosis of Cardiovascular Syphilis
Chest radiography is recommended for patients who have been diagnosed with syphilis for longer than 20 years to screen for asymptomatic cardiovascular syphilis by examining for dilatation at the region of the aortic arch (French, 2011).

Diagnosis of Gummata

The diagnosis of gummata involves meticulous clinical examination and detection of plaques, abnormal nodules, and mutilating wounds/ulcers. Serological tests would confirm positive syphilis and PCR tests on specimens from the nodules would reveal *Treponema pallidum* (BASHH, 2008; Kingston et al., 2008).

Coinfection of HIV and Syphilis

Clinical findings show that in coexisting HIV and syphilis the characteristic ulcers in primary syphilis tend to be multiple, deep, painful, and bigger (Rompalo et al., 2001). The findings also showed coexistent lesions of primary and secondary stages of syphilis in HIV-infected patients along with poor and delayed healing of primary genital ulcers together with secondary syphilitic manifestations (Rompalo et al., 2001). The consequence of syphilis on HIV load and CD4 cell count shows increased viral load and decreased CD4 cell counts. Additionally, syphilis in HIV positive patients tends to be associated with more rapid progression to neurosyphilis, although Wohrl and Geusau (2006) claim that this phenomenon is unlikely in late latent syphilis. Based on the high rates of syphilis and HIV coinfection, it is recommended that all patients with HIV infection be routinely screened for syphilis (French, 2011). The diagnosis and interpretation of treponemal and non-treponemal serological tests for syphilis should be the same in HIV-infected patients as for the general population (Workoski & Berman, 2010).

Key Elements in the Management of Syphilis

The U.S. Perspective

No comparative trials have been done to guide the selection of optimum drug treatments for *T. pallidum* due to its inability to be grown in the laboratory. Thus, parenteral penicillin G has been used for treatment based upon its observed rates of cure. There is little data on non-penicillin regimens. The CDC recommendation for effective treatment of syphilis is as follows:

- *Primary and secondary and early latent syphilis*: Benzathine penicillin G, 2.4 million units IM in a single dose
- *Late latent syphilis or syphilis of unknown duration*: Benzathine penicillin G, 7.2 million units IM **total**, administered in 3 doses of 2.4 million units IM at 1 week intervals
- *Neurosyphilis and ocular syphilis*: Aqueous crystalline penicillin G, 18–24 million units per day administered as 3–4 million units IV every 4 hours or continuous infusion for 10–14 days; an alternative regimen is procaine penicillin G, 2.4 million units IM once daily **plus** probenecid 500 mg orally four times a day, **both** for 10–14 days.

The duration of both the recommended and alternative regimens for neurosyphilis are shorter than the duration of the regimen for latent syphilis. Therefore, benzathine penicillin, 2.4 million units IM once per week for up to 3 weeks, can be considered after completion of the neurosyphilis treatment regimen to provide a similar total duration of therapy. Treatment for pregnant women or for persons infected with HIV is the same as for persons without HIV infection. For persons with a penicillin allergy, consultation with a specialist and desensitization are recommended.

Management Considerations and Follow-Up

The CDC recommends that all persons with primary or secondary syphilis be tested for HIV infection. In areas where HIV infection is high, persons diagnosed with primary or secondary syphilis should be retested for HIV in 3 months if the first test results are negative. While neurosyphilis is possible at any stage of infection, in the absence of clinical signs or symptoms of neurological involvement, routine cerebral spinal fluid (CSF) analysis is not recommended for persons with primary or secondary syphilis.

Follow-up clinical and serologic evaluation should be conducted at 6 and 12 months following treatment. Serologic titers should be compared with the titer at the time of treatment, but definitive criteria for treatment failure have not been established. Failure of nontreponemal titers to decline fourfold within 6–12 months after therapy in primary or secondary syphilis may be indicative of failure. Optimal management of persons who do not have a fourfold decline in titers is unclear. Current recommendations are for these persons to receive additional clinical and serologic follow-up including evaluation for HIV infection. If additional follow-up cannot be ensured, then retreatment is recommended (Workowski & Bolan, 2015). Because treatment failure might be the result of unrecognized central nervous system infection, CSF examination should be considered. Retreatment should consist of weekly benzathine penicillin G 2.4 million units IM for 3 weeks, unless CSF reveals neurosyphilis is present. Given that serologic titers may not decline despite a negative CSF examination and a repeated treatment regimen, while the need for additional therapy or repeat CSF examinations is unclear, it is usually not recommended (Workowski & Bolan, 2015).

The U.K. Recommendations

Multidisciplinary practice is encouraged when considering first- and second-line treatment for syphilis. Patient education regarding treatment and long-term consequences is important, as is emphasis on sexual partner health. Screening for STIs is offered and health promotion regarding sexual risk-taking practices also provided. The patient is advised to avoid any sexual activities until all evidence of syphilitic lesions from the early stage of the infection are fully healed and the result of serology is known following treatment.

Antimicrobial Treatment

Generally parenteral treatment rather than oral medication is preferred as it guarantees bioavailability and supervision.

Kingston et al. (2008) and BASHH (2008) point out the need for substantive clinical data to determine optimal dosages and duration of the treatments. Therefore, laboratory test results, biological probability, expert opinion, clinical proficiency, and case studies serve as the basis for determining the treatment regimens. Treatment should commence immediately after diagnosis to curb infectivity and lessen the risk of progressing to secondary syphilis.

Treatment for Primary, Secondary, and Early Latent Syphilis

- Benzathine penicillin G 2.4 MU administered intramuscularly as a single dose (BASHH, 2008; French, 2007; Kingston et al., 2008; Parkes, Renton, Meheus, & Laukamm-Josten, 2004; Riedner et al., 2005; WHO, n.d.; Workowski & Berman, 2010)
- Procaine penicillin may be prescribed in a dosage of 600,000 units administered intramuscularly, once daily for 10 days (BASHH, 2008; Kingston et al., 2008; Lukehart et al., 2004)

Alternative Treatments for Primary, Secondary, and Early Latent Syphilis

Penicillin allergy should be carefully considered and an alternative treatment prescribed as necessary. Similarly, patients who decline parenteral treatment may receive alternative treatment as follows based on BASHH (2008) guidelines:

- Doxycycline 100 mg orally, twice daily for 14 days (Ghanem, Erbelding, Cheng, & Rompalo, 2006; WHO, n.d.)
- Azithromycin 2 g orally as a single dose or 500 mg orally, daily for 10 days (Riedner et al., 2005)
- Erythromycin 500 mg orally, four times a day for 14 days (BASHH, 2008; Kingston et al., 2008)
- Ceftriaxone 500 mg intramuscularly, daily for 10 days (if patient does not reject parenteral treatment and does not present allergy to penicillin, in which case ceftriaxone is contraindicated) (Stoner, 2007).
- Amoxycillin 500 mg orally four times daily, together with probenecid 500 mg orally four times daily for 14 days (BASHH, 2008; Kingston et al., 2008)

Potential Treatment Side Effect: Jarisch-Herxheimer Reaction

Jarisch-Herxheimer comprises flu-like symptoms of fever, rigors, myalgia, and headache and comes on about 3–12 hours after administration of benzathine penicillin G injection (BASHH, 2008; French et al., 2009; Kingston et al., 2008). It is considered good professional practice to warn patients/clients about reactions they may experience from specific medications. Jarisch-Herxheimer reaction is considered insignificant unless neurological and ophthalmic involvements are detected. The patient is advised to rest and is reassured that symptoms should subside within 24 hours. This condition is found to be uncommon in late syphilis but can prove to be life-threatening if particular locations and structures, such as the coronary ostia, larynx, and nervous system, are affected (Miller et al., 2010). Prednisolone may be prescribed to control the fever, but is not proven to improve the local inflammation (BASHH, 2008; French et al., 2009; Kingston et al., 2008).

Hospitalization is recommended in cases of severe deterioration in early syphilis with cardiovascular and neurological involvement and optic neuritis. To prevent this condition, the following may be undertaken:

- Prednisolone 40–60 mg may be administered intravenously or orally once daily for three days and the anti-treponemal therapy is commenced 24 hours after the first dose of the prednisolone.
- Penicillin allergy may be treated with doxycycline 100 mg orally twice daily for 14 days.
- Other allergic reactions, such as procaine psychosis, procaine mania, and Hoigné syndrome, should be carefully diagnosed to provide the correct treatment. The reaction caused by inadvertent intravenous injection of procaine penicillin is characterized by hallucinations, fear of impending death, and convulsions, manifesting immediately after the injection and lasting about 20 minutes (BASHH, 2008; French et al., 2009; Kingston et al., 2008). Management of this involves calming the patient and providing reassurance.
- The onset of convulsions may be treated with diazepam 10 mg administered rectally, intravenously, or intramuscularly.

It is important to differentiate this from anaphylactic shock commonly caused by penicillin, which should be treated with the following:

- Epinephrine (adrenaline) 1:1,000 administered intramuscularly 0.5 mg in 0.5 mL solution
- Antihistamine – chlorpheniramine 10 mg IM or IV if necessary following the epinephrine
- Hydrocortisone 100 mg administered IM or IV (BASHH, 2008; French et al., 2009; Kingston et al., 2008)

Practitioners may also find it useful and interesting to explore other related descriptions such as antibiomania and antibiotic-induced psychosis to better understand Hoigné syndrome clinical manifestations and management.

Treatment for Late Latent, Cardiovascular, and Gummatous Syphilis

Treatment for late latent syphilis should be carefully planned. Characteristically the patient has positive serology and has had no known negative serology in the preceding 2 years. Physical examination should involve echocardiogram and chest x-ray to rule out aortic valve damage. Depending on the findings, the patient may be referred to a cardiac physician for further investigation. Lumber puncture for CSF examination may be determined by the clinical presentation (Kingston et al., BASHH, 2008). Patients who present as asymptomatic with no clinical signs of neurosyphilis may not have lumbar puncture performed. However, lumber puncture should be performed on patients who present neurological signs and symptoms with ophthalmic involvement and those who present treatment failure and VDRL ≥1:32. The prescribed treatment may be the following:

- Benzathine penicillin G 2.4 MU administered intramuscularly once weekly for three consecutive weeks on day 1, 8, 15 respectively (BASHH, 2008; French, 2007; Kingston et al., 2008; Parkes et al., 2004; WHO, n.d.; Workowski & Berman, 2010)
- Procaine penicillin 600,000 units administered intramuscularly once daily for 17 days (BASHH, 2008; French, 2007; Kingston et al., 2008; Lukehart et al., 2004; Parkes et al., 2004)

Alternative Treatments for Late Latent, Cardiovascular, and Gummatous Syphilis

- Doxycycline 100 mg orally twice daily for 28 days (BASHH, 2008; Kingston et al., 2008; WHO, n.d.)
- Amoxycillin 2 g orally three times daily together with probenecid 500 mg orally four times daily for 28 days (BASHH, 2008; Kingston et al., 2008)

Treatment for Neurosyphilis

The physician should rule out meningovascular and parenchymatous syphilis with general paresis due to meningoencephalitis. A thorough neurological assessment is carried out, including assessment of intracranial pressure. Radiological imaging may be carried out, followed by CSF examination for cell count, total protein, and CSF VDRL/TPPA. Repeat CSF examination is recommended 6 to 12 months following the treatment outlined below.

- Procaine penicillin 1.8–2.4 MU is administered intramuscularly once daily together with
- Probenecid 500 mg orally four times daily for 17 days (Kingston et al., 2008; WHO, n.d.), or
- Benzylpenicillin 18–24 MU daily administered in doses of 3–4 MU intravenously 4 to 6 hourly for 17 days
- Doxycycline 200 mg orally twice daily for 28 days may be prescribed for patients who present with penicillin allergy and for those who decline the parenteral treatment (BASHH, 2008; Kingston et al., 2008)
- Alternative treatments for neurosyphilis as per BASHH (2008) are as follows:
  - Doxycycline 200 mg orally twice daily for 28 days
  - Amoxicillin 2 g orally three times daily together with
  - Probenecid 500 mg orally four times daily for 28 days (Kingston et al., 2008; WHO, n.d.)

- Ceftriaxone 2 g intramuscularly diluted with lidocaine or intravenously diluted with water for 10 to 14 days (BASHH, 2008; Castro et al., 2006; Kingston et al., 2008)

The main alternative non-penicillin antibiotics that have been analyzed include doxycycline, erythromycin, and azithromycin. Erythromycin is found to have minimum effectiveness, and doxycycline may have replaced the earlier use of tetracyclines. However, while the prescribed dosage of 100 mg once or twice daily for 14 days has been found to achieve effectiveness, treatment failure has been reported with this regimen. Azithromycin administered in a single dose of 2 g has been reported to achieve effectiveness that is comparable to benzathine penicillin (Riedner et al., 2005); however, resistance of some *Treponema pallidum* strains (Lukehart et al., 2004) and treatment failure (CDC, 2004) deserves caution. The low prevalence of late syphilis and, undoubtedly, neurosyphilis has been attributed to the effectiveness of the recommended treatments and the role of host immune response. It is estimated that about 60% of untreated syphilis-infected individuals develop host immune response in the early stage of the infection (BASHH, 2008; Kingston et al., 2008; LaFond & Lukehart, 2006).

Some experts consider penicillin desensitization for individuals with penicillin allergy and recommend that appropriate detailed history should be taken (Magpantay, Cardile, Madar, Hsue, & Belnap, 2011; Solensky, 2004). Moreover, there is uncommon possibility that the chancre and other lesions may become more exaggerated. Patient education of this fact would alleviate undue anxiety, provide reassurance, and encourage patients to comply with taking the required antipyretics and nonsteroidal anti-inflammatory medications for those symptoms (French, 2011).

Partner Notification in the Management of Syphilis

A sexual health adviser with partner notification experience should undertake the process from diagnosis through monthly follow-up support until all the relevant processes including surveillance are complete. It is important to carefully estimate the look-back period. This period applies to all sexual contacts, whether condoms were used during intercourse or not. Thus, in primary syphilis the look-back interval should include all sexual partners/sexual contacts since and within the preceding 3 months prior to the onset of symptoms (McClean et al., 2012). Each of the sexual contacts of the individual (index patient) with early syphilis should be offered serological testing on their first clinic attendance then repeated at 6 weeks and 3 months from the last sexual activity with the index patient. The recommendation is to offer epidemiological treatment to particular high-risk contacts and those who may not feel inclined to attend for the repeat syphilis tests.

In secondary and early latent syphilis, all sexual contacts since and within the 2 years prior to the onset of symptoms should be notified (McClean et al., 2012). In latent and late syphilis, the look-back interval for sexual partners and children of female patients should extend to the date of the last known or available negative syphilis serology. If none of these is applicable, the look-back period may be extended to the individual's initial sexual activity if this is realistic (McClean et al., 2012). To take account of congenital syphilis, mothers of patients with late syphilis born outside the United Kingdom in countries where antenatal care is considered to be substandard should also undergo testing for syphilis. Epidemiological treatment is not offered in these cases (McClean et al., 2012).

The contact/notification process should be discussed with the index patient, supervised by the sexual health adviser or healthcare practitioner and details carefully documented. Careful assessment is crucial based on the sexual history risk assessment and particular circumstances. In certain cases it may be considered useful to notify a sexual contact beyond the look-back period/interval and reasons for any omissions should be carefully documented.

Monitoring Response to Syphilis Treatment

Response to treatment is tested by monthly VDRL and IgM serological tests (Allstaff & Wilson, 2012). However, this can be time consuming and variations in results may depend on the pretreatment titer, stage of syphilis, previous syphilis infection, and treatment given. Following treatment for primary and secondary syphilis, serological test results should show a fourfold decrease by 3–6 months after treatment for primary and secondary syphilis (Knaute, Graf, Lautenschlager, Weber, & Bosshard, 2012) and eightfold by 6–12 months (McMillan & Young, 2008). Failed reduction in the VDRL titer or a two-fold increase should indicate the need for more detailed reassessment while rapid decrease in specific IgM indicates successful treatment. In early syphilis patients (following treatment of HIV infection), the specific IgM becomes nonreactive by 3–6 months and in late syphilis becomes nonreactive by 1–1.5 years (Rotty et al., 2010). In cases of reinfection there is a fourfold increase in titer, which is confirmed by testing a second specimen. IgM becomes reactive again after having previously been nonreactive following treatment and this is confirmed by a second specimen (McMillan & Young, 2008). Experts point out that there is no specific microbiological test of cure. Fourfold decreases in VDRL/RPR titers are considered to be significant, but twofold decreases in the titers are not significant (Sato, 2011). Discharge of the patient is only considered when the VDRL result becomes negative or serofast. Results may be sent to the patient's general practitioner or primary care health provider, per patient permission.

Genital Herpes

Genital herpes is a lifelong chronic viral infection. It is caused by herpes simplex virus type 1 (HSV-1) and

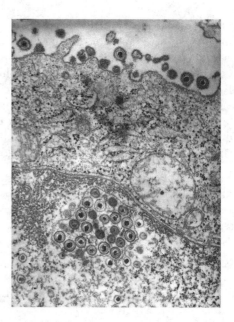

A

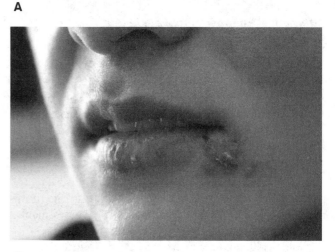

B

Figure 6-4 Herpes Simplex 1 Virus (Oral Herpes)
(A) CDC; **(B)** Dr. Fred Murphy; Sylvia Whitfield; © Cherries/Shutterstock

herpes simplex virus type 2 (HSV-2) (**Figures 6-4** and **6-5**). These viruses are are closely related; however, HSV-1 causes orolabial herpes and HSV-2 causes genital herpes through sexual transmission (BASHH, 2014; Patel et al., 2011). Nonetheless, it is found that both viruses can cause genital herpes (Patel et al., 2011). The majority of cases of recurrent genital herpes are attributed to HSV-2, with millions of people across the world infected (Patel et al., 2011). Acquisition of HSV-1 appears to have evolved from primarily a childhood acquired infection of the oropharynx causing recurrent cold sores, to the manifestation as a STI. Consequently, first episodes of HSV-1 anogenital herpes infections are being diagnosed increasingly among certain population groups. This is now considered as the most common cause of sexually acquired genital ulceration in the United Kingdom (Patel & Gupta, 2011; Ryder, Jin,

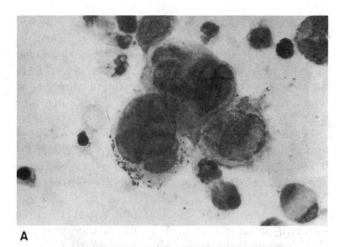

A

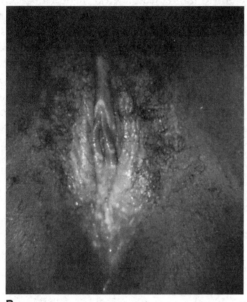

B

Figure 6-5 Herpes Simplex 2 Virus (Genital Herpes)
(A) CDC/Joe Miller; **(B)** CDC/Susan Lindsley

McNulty, Grulich, & Donovan, 2009). Three definitions of HSV-1 and HSV-2 episodes have been identified.

Clinical Manifestations

Initial episode refers to the first manifestation of HSV-1 or HSV-2 and depends on previous exposure to one or the other viral infection. Based on that, specific descriptions are applied to the presence or absence of antibodies. Thus, primary infection refers to the first infection in an individual who did not have preexisting antibodies to either HSV-1 or HSV-2 (Bernstein, Lovett, & Bryson, 1984; Schiffer & Corey, 2009). Non-primary infection refers to first infection in an individual who has preexisting antibodies to either type of HSV. Recurrent episode refers to recurrence of clinical symptoms as a result of reactivation of preexisting latent HSV-1 or HSV-2 (BASHH, 2014).

A cause for clinical concern and a challenge for sexual healthcare practitioners is that many people with HSV-2 infection are asymptomatic and therefore remain undiagnosed. Nonetheless, the organism continues to thrive and is continually shed and deposited in the genital tract. Generally, the incubation period is 5–14 days and the virus passes into the distal axon of the sensory neuron and to the dorsal ganglion where it remains latent. Episodic reactivation is accompanied by passage of the virus into the basal skin layers where the infection may manifest with the characteristic lesions, which may or may not be accompanied by symptoms. HSV-2 is found to recur as frequently as four times during the first year after infection acquisition. A small proportion of those infected may report even more frequent episodes of recurrence during that time (Engelberg, Carrell, Krantz, Corey, & Wald, 2003; Patel et al., 2011).

The clinical manifestation can be quite unpredictable and, as a result, relatively few infected individuals seek medical consultation for appropriate diagnosis, treatment, guidance and support. The estimated prevalence of HSV-2 infection among the U.K. population is 9%, with higher rates occurring among sex workers and among MSM. Consequently, most cases of HSV-2 genital herpes infections are transmitted by individuals who are asymptomatic and not aware that they carry the infection. Thus, they remain a constant source of transmission (Lazaro, 2013). Therefore, management of HSV-2 must extend beyond acute episodes and consider the chronic nature of the infection. Risk of transmission is found to increase during recurrence of lesions, although subclinical viral shedding allows transmission to occur even when no symptoms manifest (Patel et al., 2011). HSV-1 recurrences are comparatively atypical, occurring about once in 18 months. In approximately 4% of patients, these recurrent episodes may be accompanied by severe illness. Nonetheless, subclinical shedding into the genital tract is found to reduce gradually, becoming atypical in HSV-1 as compared to HSV-2 (Engelberg et al., 2003).

Typical Features of Primary HSV-1

In about 80% of individuals with HSV-type specific antibodies, the first episode of viral infection may not be associated with clinical symptoms and therefore goes unnoticed (Bernstein et al., 1984; Schiffer & Corey, 2009). The earliest onset of clinical symptoms of genital herpes usually occurs with the initial infection or may possibly be delayed for some time. Manifestation of symptoms, if they happen in the primary episode, may be more severe than repeat episodes and may last longer (Bernstein et al., 1984 Lazaro, 2013; Schiffer & Corey, 2009). Following the primary infection, the virus enters neighboring ganglia and reactivation occurs sporadically and may or may not be accompanied by symptoms. While replication may be controlled by local lymphocytes, this does not occur. Consequently, viral replication in the dermis results in shedding and continual transmission of the infection Lazaro, 2013; Schiffer, Wald, Selke, Corey, & Magaret, 2011; Wald et al., 2005).

Recognizable Symptoms and Signs

Distinguishing symptoms and signs of infection include eruption of blisters, superficial vesicles that form coalescing ulcerating lesions that increase in size, and tingling sensation with neuropathic pain (Lazaro, 2013; Patel & Gupta, 2011). There may be lymphadenopathy with tenderness in adjacent inguinal lymph nodes usually bilateral in first infections but often unilateral in recurrent episodes (BASHH, 2014; Patel & Gupta, 2011). Associated lymphadenitis is reported in about 30% of HSV infections (BASHH, 2014). Systemic symptoms lasting 5–7 days, although uncommon, include fever, malaise, muscle aches, headaches, and photophobia for a small proportion of patients. Symptoms of erythema and dysuria may be reported, and careful diagnosis should exclude other conditions associated with pain and discomfort on micturition (Lazaro, 2013; Patel & Gupta, 2011). The first episode of HSV may last about 3 weeks without treatment.

Complications

Lesions may be complicated by candida or streptococcal infections. Additionally, auto-inoculation of the adjacent skin and fingers has been reported. Aseptic meningitis and retention of urine due to severe local pain or autonomic neuropathy are occasionally reported (BASHH, 2014; Lazaro, 2013).

Recurrent Episodes

In recurrent episodes, reactivation of latent HSV infection may be asymptomatic or may be preceded by symptoms of itchiness, burning, and stinging at the site of lesion eruption. These prodromal symptoms with tingling and sciatic pain may be mild, occurring about 48 hours preceding lesion eruption, and are found in about half of those affected (Bernstein et al., 1984; Lazaro, 2013; Schiffer & Corey, 2009). The lesions may look similar to nonspecific erythema, erosions, or fissures; however, the site of the infection tends to be smaller than the initial episode and healing occurs more quickly (Lazaro, 2013). Nonetheless, the psychological impact associated with frequent recurrent episodes should be appropriately attended to with counseling and support. Recurrence may be transitory, affecting various parts of the body including the buttocks, perianal area, and thighs (BASHH, 2014; Lazaro, 2013). Recurrence of symptomatic HSV-2 may be associated with more prolonged initial and preceding episodes. The risk of recurrence is further increased when the herpes infection is concurrent with a compromised or impaired immune system. In HIV-positive patients, symptomatic and nonsymptomatic viral shedding is reported to increase. Generally, continuous transmission is associated with asymptomatic viral shedding, which is found to occur in most infected patients (Bernstein et al., 1984; Lazarao, 2013; Patel & Gupta, 2011; Schiffer & Corey, 2009).

Diagnosis

In addition to the characteristic signs and symptoms, findings from detailed history taking and physical examination, virology tests—particularly cell culture and PCR—are performed. The sensitivity of viral culture, which is found to be relatively low, tends to diminish quickly in recurrent HSV lesions that subside and heal. The PCR assays tend to be more sensitive and accurate and are therefore the preferred diagnostic tests (Geretti & Brown, 2005). DNA detection by PCR has higher rates of HSV detection (by 11–71%) as compared to viral culture (BASHH, 2014; Lazaro, 2013). Nonetheless, viral culture isolates are also recommended to determine the type of HSV responsible for the infection. The recommendation is to perform these tests on swabs obtained from the base of the lesions (BASHH, 2014). It is cautioned though, that negative HSV culture or PCR results may not necessarily indicate absence of the infection, but may possibly be due to unpredictable viral shedding (CDC, 2010).

NAATs are reputed to produce similar results and are the preferred diagnostic methods for genital herpes where appropriate facilities are available. While HSV culture continues to be carried out in some organizations, the disadvantage is that this could fall short by about 30% of PCR positive samples, particularly in patients who present with late or mild infection (Lazaro, 2013). Specificity is reported to be nearly 100%, but this is influenced by multiple factors including virus shedding, quality of the specimen, storage of the sample, and how transported to the laboratory (Geretti & Brown, 2005).

Serological Tests

HSV type-specific and non-type-specific antibodies may develop during the immediate several weeks following infection and tend to remain permanently. Detection of HSV-1 IgG or HSV-2 IgG or both in serum sample indicates a previous HSV infection, although it may be difficult to determine how long ago (BASHH, 2014; Patel et al., 2011). While detection of HSV-2 antibodies is usually considered as diagnosis of genital herpes, HSV-1 antibodies do not necessarily differentiate between genital and oropharyngeal infection (BASHH, 2014; Patel et al., 2011). Of crucial importance is accurate interpretation of laboratory test results. Account should be taken of poor predictive values in areas where the prevalence of HSV is consistently low among the populations or patients who are unlikely to acquire genital herpes. The recommendation is to confirm positive HSV-2 antibody results by obtaining a repeat sample for testing or by performing a different assay (BASHH, 2014; Patel et al., 2011; Schiffer & Corey, 2009).

The value of routinely screening general clinic and antenatal patients together with their sexual partners remains debatable and is yet to be widely recognized. However, such screening is useful in counseling the management of asymptomatic partners of patients with genital herpes (BASHH, 2014; Patel et al., 2011).

Positive laboratory-based and clinic-based HSV-2 antibody tests from capillary blood specimens may be available to perform during clinic attendance. The sensitivity for these glycoprotein G type-specific tests for HSV-2 is reported as

80–98%. False negative results are found to be more likely at the early stages of infection; therefore, repeat testing to confirm or diagnose the infection may be indicated if recent acquisition is suspected. Because HSV-2 is almost always sexually acquired, detection of type-specific HSV-2 antibody essentially indicates the presence of anogenital infection. In some U.S. states the recommendation is to consider HSV serologic testing for individuals with multiple sexual partners who attend health care clinics for STI evaluation. It is also recommended that HIV-positive individuals and MSM who fall into the high-risk category for HIV be tested (CDC, 2010). Practitioners are encouraged to explore the current 2015 U.K. national guidelines and the CDC *Sexually Transmitted Diseases Treatment Guidelines* and compare these to the guidelines that underpin the national and organizational practice where they work.

Management

Recommendations for first-episode treatment are based on concerns that newly acquired genital herpes may result in long-term clinical illness, excessive genital ulcerations, and neurological impairment. Prolonged symptoms have been known to establish even after mild manifestation of the first episode. Therefore, the recommendation is to provide anriviral therapy to all patients with first-episode genital herpes. General management encompasses general advice, saline bathing, oral analgesia, and topical anaesthetic agents such as 0.5% lidocaine ointment. Practitioners should be aware of potential sensitization and cautioned about the use of lidocaine (BASHH, 2014; Lazaro, 2013; Patel et al., 2011). The natural history of the infection is not altered by antiviral therapy, and the topical agents tend to be less effective than the oral antiviral medications. Moreover, no great advantage is achieved from using the oral antivirals and the topical agents simultaneously.

Antiviral Therapy

Antiviral drugs should be commenced within 5 days of episode onset and/or while new lesions are developing or persistent systemic symptoms are observed (BASHH, 2014; Lazaro, 2013). Oral doses of acyclovir, valacyclovir, and famciclovir are all reputed to diminish severity and duration of the infection episodes (BASHH, 2014). Intravenous administration is opted for only when the patient is unable to swallow or has been vomiting and unable to tolerate oral medications. The recommended antivirals in the current BASHH guidelines include the following:

- Acyclovir 200 mg orally five times daily for 5 days, or
- Acyclovir 400 orally mg three times daily for 5 days, or
- Valacyclovir 500 mg twice daily for 5 days, or
- Famciclovir 250 mg three times daily for 5 days

There has been no substantive evidence for courses of treatment longer than 5 days. Nonetheless, the patient should be rechecked after 5 days and therapy continued if new lesions appear (BASHH, 2014).

Complications are managed accordingly, and therefore, patients who present with severe constitutional symptoms, inability to take oral antiviral medication, meningism, or retention of urine should be considered for hospitalization. If required, suprapubic (rather than urethral) catheterization should be performed to avoid associated pain and potential risk of iatrogenic ascending infection. After hospital discharge patient should return to the sexual health clinic in 2 to 3 weeks for follow up and full STI screening (Lazaro, 2013). Continue education, and counseling support should continue as necessary.

Patient Involvement in Decisions About the Management of the Recurrent HSV Infections

Based on the frequency of HSV-2 genital lesion recurrence, and severity of the accompanying symptoms, the patient should be involved in infection management decisions. This comprises mainly supportive therapy, episodic treatment, and suppressive therapy (BASHH, 2014). For recurrent episodes, the recommended antiviral treatments should be carefully calculated. However, for patients/clients who present with more serious, frequent, or complicated infections with high risk of transmission, continuous daily regimen of suppressive therapy may be considered as the best option (Patel & Gupta, 2011). Some organizations manage patients with severe viral infectious diseases by hospitalization for intravenous administration of antiviral drug therapy (CDC, 2010).

Recommended Episodic Antiviral Treatment Regimens

- Acyclovir 200 mg five times daily for 5 days, or
- Acyclovir 400 mg three times daily for 3–5 days, or
- Valacyclovir 500 mg twice daily for 5 days, or
- Famciclovir 125 mg twice daily for 5 days (BASHH, 2014)

Patient-initiated antiviral therapy entails giving the patient a prescription for oral treatment as a stand-by for the onset of subsequent episodes. The patient is advised to commence treatment if they recognize signs or symptoms of an impending episode (Lazaro, 2013).

Short Course Regimens

- Acyclovir 800 mg three times daily for 2 days (Wald et al., 2005)
- Famciclovir 1 g twice daily for 1 day (Aoki et al., 2006; Bodsworth, Bloch, & McNulty, 2008)
- Valacyclovir 500 mg twice daily for 3 days (Abudalu, Tyring, Koltun, Bodsworth, & Hamed, 2008)

Suppressive Therapy

The use of antiviral medications may be intended to suppress or curb the frequency and duration of infection recurrence. The main benefit to lessening the frequency of recurrent symptomatic episodes is improvement in the quality of life and the individual's psychological health state. The recommended treatment includes the same types of antiviral medications as used for the therapeutic process (BASHH, 2014; Patel et al., 2011). However, the recommended dosage, schedule, and duration for each treatment differ and these should be carefully noted to avoid errors and adverse effects of treatment. Patients should be provided with clear information about the advantages and disadvantages of suppressive therapy. Decisions are based on the frequency of recurrence, the impact of the inconvenience, and perhaps the cost implications. However, it is worth emphasizing the benefit of reduced episode and it is important for the patient to know that effective suppression is achieved from 5 days into the therapy. In some situations, the cost implication may be an influencing factor on the choice of specific antiviral drug (Lazaro, 2013).

Recommended Regimen for Suppressive Antiviral Therapy

- Acyclovir 400 mg twice daily
- Acyclovir 200 mg four times daily
- Famciclovir 250 twice daily
- Valacyclovir 500 mg once daily (BASHH, 2014)

The main aim of suppressive therapy is to control recurrent episodes of the infection and evidence from earlier studies supports significant reduction in episode frequency in patients receiving suppressive antiviral therapy (Bartlett et al., 2008; Rooney et al., 1993). Therefore, if unexpected recurrences occur whilst on the prescribed antiviral treatment, the daily intake may be increased; for example, from twice daily to three times daily (BASHH, 2014). Choice of treatment may be influenced by the individual's ability to comply with a particular regimen. Discontinuation of suppressive therapy is considered after a maximum period of 1 year, when the frequency of recurrence is reassessed. A minimum period of reassessment may be considered with at least two episodes of recurrence. Very frequent recurrences should indicate the need to restart antiviral treatment (BASHH, 2014; Lazaro, 2013).

Asymptomatic Viral Shedding

Asymptomatic viral shedding occurring in patients with either HSV-1 or HSV-2 genital infections is possible, particularly during the first year following infection and also particularly after HSV-2 infection (BASHH, 2014; Lazaro, 2013). Viral shedding influences the rate of transmission and patients with frequent symptomatic recurrences are also found to present with viral shedding (BASHH, 2014; Lazaro, 2013). Although the HSV shedding diminishes over time, suppressive treatment of acyclovir 400 mg twice daily is recommended to enhance reduction (BASHH, 2014). Acyclovir, famciclovir, and valacyclovir are all reputed to reduce HSV shedding by about 80–90%, and valacyclovir is reported to achieve better suppression of asymptomatic viral shedding than famciclovir (Johnston & Corey, 2016, Wald et al., 2005).

Preventive Measures to Curb Transmission

Condom use is reported to prevent transmission of HSV from males to their female partners by about 50% (Jungmann, 2004). Suppressive therapy is also reported to curb transmission by about 50% (Lazaro, 2013). Evidence varies regarding efficacy of the different antiviral drugs in suppressing viral shedding and transmission. More research is needed to identify the most effective antiviral drug for curbing viral shedding and curtailing transmission.

Significance of Counseling in the Management of HSV Infection

The main counseling aims are to provide accurate evidence-based explanations, support, guidance, and pertinent health promotion. Proper counseling enables the patient to cope with the physical and psychological impact of infection and take appropriate measures to prevent or reduce perinatal transmission. The patient's fears and anxiety may be based on misconceptions about genital herpes, possible severity of clinical manifestations, frequency and gravity of recurrent episodes, possible effect on sexual relationships, risk of transmission to sexual partners, and effect on the ability to have children. Individuals who fail to adjust to the diagnosis and treatment regimens may benefit from referral for more intense counseling (BASHH, 2014; Lazaro, 2013).

Key issues addressed in the counseling intervention are as follows:

- Explain about the source and course of genital herpes infection (BASHH, 2014).
- Explain the natural history of the infection, including the possibility of recurrent episodes, asymptomatic viral shedding, and the consequences of transmission (BASHH, 2014; Lazaro, 2013).
- Teach seropositive patients to recognize symptoms that precede recurrent episodes to avoid ongoing transmission and spread.
- Condom use may help in reducing transmission, but total prevention may not be entirely achievable (BASHH, 2014).
- Explain availability of suppressive antiviral therapy to individuals who present at first episode.
- Give appropriate reassurance that suppressive therapy is effective in curbing recurrent episodes that are accompanied by symptoms (Lazaro, 2013).
- Provide additional reassurance that episodic therapy may help to curb the duration of recurrent infections (BASHH, 2014).

Consideration of Sexual Partners

- Consideration of sexual partners is crucial and all symptomatic index patients together with their sexual partners should be carefully assessed and offered evidence based information, education, and counseling.

- Patients/clients with genital herpes infections should be encouraged to inform current sexual partners about having genital herpes infection and to inform future sexual partners before having sexual contact with them (BASHH, 2014; Lazaro, 2013).
- Explain to patients that, although they may not have symptoms, viral shedding is particularly common in the first 12 months of acquiring HSV-2 infection.
- Individuals with genital herpes infection should be advised to avoid sexual contacts with sexual partners who do not have the infection when lesions or pro-dromal symptoms are experienced (BASHH, 2014).
- Explain that episodic antiviral therapy does not reduce the risk of transmission of genital herpes. Therefore, sexual partners would not be protected from the risk of acquiring the infection (BASHH, 2014; Patel & Gupta, 2011).

Partner Notification

Sexual partners of patients/clients with genital herpes infection should also be advised about their risk of acquiring the infection even though they may not be experiencing any symptoms. Asymptomatic sexual partners of patients with genital herpes infection should be assessed and offered type-specific serologic testing. This may help to reduce anxiety and limit spread of the infection (BASHH, 2014). Although look-back periods are uncertain and difficult to establish, the importance and benefits of partner notification should be explained to all index patients/clients and the process initiated if acceptable to them.

Consideration of HIV-Related Issues

HIV-positive individuals who acquire HSV infection tend to develop more severe and prolonged symptoms with oral, genital, and perianal herpes lesions as well as increased HSV shedding. Additionally, the associated pain may be more severe due to their immunocompromised state. The recommended regimen for daily suppressive therapy involves the same range of antiretroviral therapy as previously mentioned, with carefully calculated dosages (Johnston & Corey, 2016; Patel & Gupta, 2011; Schiffer & Corey, 2009).

Human Papillomavirus (HPV)

Human papillomavirus is the most common sexually transmitted viral infection in the United States. The CDC estimates that 90% of men and 80% of women who are sexually active will be infected with at least one type of HPV at some point in their lives (Chesson, Dunne, & Markowitz, 2014). Half of these infections will be with

a high-risk HPV type (Hariri et al., 2011). In the United States, high-risk HPV types cause approximately 3% of all cancer cases among women and 2% of all cancer cases among men (Jemal et al., 2013). With the advent of the bivalent (Cervarix), quadrivalent (Gardasil), and newly FDA-approved nonvalent (Gardasil-9) vaccines, future reductions in the incidence of HPV types 6, 11, 16, 18, 31, 33, 45, 52, and 58, and their associated sequelae, are anticipated.

There are three HPV vaccines licensed in the United States. The bivalent vaccine targets HPV types 16 and 18 (the strains that account for 66% of all cervical cancers) and is FDA approved for use in females ages 9–26 for the prevention of cervical cancer caused by HPV. The quadrivalent vaccine protects against HPV types 6, 11 (the two strains responsible for 90% of all genital warts), 16, and 18 and is approved for use in both females and males ages 9–26. The nonvalent, newly approved vaccine targets HPV types 6, 11, 16, 18, 31, 33, 45, 52, and 58 (the additional strains being responsible for an additional 15% of cervical cancers) and is also approved for use in females ages 9–26; however, thus far it is only approved for use in males 9–15 years of age (ACOG, 2015c). All of the U.S. HPV vaccines are administered as a 3-dose series of intramuscular injections over a 6-month time period. The second dose is given 1–2 months following the first dose, with the third dose given 6 months after the first dose. Any available HPV vaccine can be used to continue or complete the series, even if different from the original vaccine administered (Jorge & Wright, 2016). While it is ideal for the recommended HPV vaccine series of three injections to be completed prior to a client's sexual debut, vaccination is recommended regardless of sexual activity or HPV exposure (ACOG, 2015c). Even though there is good evidence that receiving even two of the three vaccine doses offers comparable protection, the CDC continues to recommend clients be given all three doses pending more definitive studies. In the United States, the vaccines are not licensed or recommended for use in men or women over the age of 26, nor are they recommended for use in pregnant women (Workowski & Bolan, 2015).

Human papillomavirus (HPV) screening in the United States

Currently, the only approved HPV screening method available in the United States is for detection of active cervical HPV infection. This cervical screening is accomplished by performing a Pap test along with screening for high-risk HPV oncogenic strains (hrHPV cotesting). This cotesting is recommended for women beginning at age 30, and then every 5 years thereafter until age 65. Primary testing using hrHPV as a stand-alone test without the addition of a Pap smear is not recommended. There are no recommended screening methods for other HPV types in women or for men. The CDC and USPSTF recommend women have their first Pap smear for cervical cancer at age 21 regardless of age of sexual initiation or other risk factors. For women ages 21 through 29, Pap testing is recommended every 3 years. Both the CDC and USPSTF do not recommend Pap testing for women before age 21 (CDC, 2016b). For women ages 30 through 65, women should either receive a Pap test every 3 years OR a Pap test plus HPV (cotest) every 5 years. Given the high negative predictive value of cotesting, women who test negative for both HPV and Pap test should not be rescreened for another 5 years.

Anogenital warts caused by the human papilloma virus (HPV) is described as the most frequent STI worldwide that can cause both malignant cancers and benign skin and mucosal tumors (Gross & Pfister, 2004). The microorganism is a double-stranded DNA virus that infests squamous epithelial cells. Anogenital warts manifest as visible lesions of multiple or single papules on the vulva, vagina, cervix, penis, urethra, scrotum, perianal area, and anus (Castle 2008; Doorbar, 2006; Patterson, Smith, & Ozbun, 2005).

Associated symptoms include pruritus, burning, vaginal discharge, and bleeding (Insinga, Dasbach, Elbasha, 2009). Most genital warts (90%) are benign and caused by HPV-6 or HPV-11 (Garland et al., 2007; Lacey, Lowndes, & Shah, 2006). Other strains of HPV—types 16, 18, 31, 33, and 35—are described as carcinogenic (de Villiers, Fauquet, Broker, Bernard, & zur Hausen; International Agency for Research on Cancer [IARC], 2007; Muñoz, Castellsague, de Gonzalez, & Gissmann, 2006). Infrequently, these are detectable in external genital warts as coinfecting organisms alongside HPV-6 and HPV-11. Over 100 HPV genotypes have been identified, 40 of which are found to infect mainly the genital epithelium (McCance, 2004). HPV genotypes are characterized as low risk (noncancerous) or high risk (oncogenic). HPV-6 and HPV-11 are low-risk strains (Garland et al., 2007; Lacey et al., 2006).

Transmission

Transmission of genital HPV occurs mainly via direct skin–skin sexual contact (Sehnal et al., 2012) with an individual who has obvious or subclinical HPV lesions (Winer et al., 2005). Perianal warts are not always acquired through anal sex, but from direct contact with HPV-infected genital secretions that have collected in the perianal area. Transmission may also occur when genital secretions come in contact with minor grazes or abrasions in the skin of the recipient (Burchell, Winer, de Sanjosè, & Franco, 2006; Winer et al., 2003). The organism enters the basal cells of the epithelium and the ensuing replication process initiates in the suprabasal keratinocytes (Snapp & Bienkowska-Haba, 2009). In individuals with poor immune response, the HPV infection may remain latent without visible warts. However, in time lymphocyte infiltration occurs and the lesions regress and disappear spontaneously. One-third of all external visible warts reportedly disappear within 6 months. Immunosuppression is associated with recurrence of HPV infection and reappearance of

visible lesions (Denny et al., 2012). While type-specific protection can be caused by a particular infection there is no evidence to substantiate cross protective immunity. Condom use is reported to be only about 70% effective and therefore unlikely to provide complete protection (Winer et al., 2006). Variations in the incubation period range from 3 weeks to 8 or 9 months with an average of 3 months, although longer periods have been reported (Winer et al., 2005). It is estimated that about 99% of infected people never develop external or visible growths of warts (Woodward & Robinson, 2011). Nevertheless, viral transmission can still occur from such people and as a result it may not be possible to determine the source of an individual's infection (Woodward & Robinson, 2011). Apart from direct genital contacts, transmission can also occur from genital HPV warts to the fingers or vice versa. Clothing and contaminated objects and surfaces have also been reported, though not substantially confirmed as modes of transmission (Gavillon et al., 2010). Other nongenital infections reported include laryngeal warts, causing respiratory papillomatosis and premalignant and malignant oropharyngeal HPV lesions (Lazaro, 2013).

Characteristic manifestations

HPV infection may manifest as latent, subclinical, or clinical, depending on whether the infection is associated with low viral load or high viral load (Moscicki, Ellenberg, Farhat, & Xu, 2004). Prevalence is reported as 30–50% among sexually active adults, most of whom present as subclinical, with less than 10% of infected individuals developing associated lesions. Manifestations include the appearance of lumps or growths, which may be flat papules or pedunculated on the genital mucosa (Sterling, 2004). Genital warts may appear as condylomata accuminata, characterized by cauliflower-like growths, papules, or hyperpigmentation of the skin, and non-keratinized on mucosal surfaces (Juckett & Hartman-Adams, 2010) (**Figure 6-6**). These papules may, however, appear keratotic as a thick, horny layer resembling common warts or seborrheic keratosis. The papules are usually smooth and dome-shaped while the plaques may be macular or slightly raised, flesh colored, and more commonly found on internal surfaces such as the cervix (Sterling, 2004). Although these manifestations are generally asymptomatic, some patients experience discomfort with pruritus, depending on the size and the anatomical location of the warts (Woodward & Robinson, 2011).

Common locations of genital warts include the introitus, under the foreskin of the penis in uncircumcised men, or on the shaft in circumcised men (Lacey et al., 2006). Genital warts may appear in multiple sites: the perineum, perianal skin, vagina, cervix, urethra, scrotum, and intra-anal warts (Sehnal et al., 2012, Sterling, 2004; Woodward & Robinson, 2011). Intra-anal warts are common among individuals who practice anal receptive intercourse (Hernandez et al., 2005), but relatively uncommon among people who do not (Woodward & Robinson, 2011). Nevertheless, as Lazaro

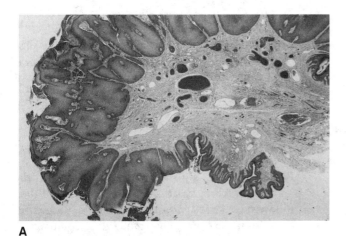

A

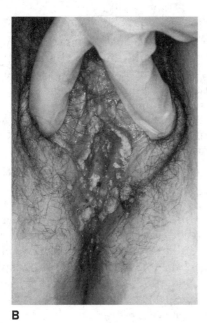

B

Figure 6-6 Genital Warts
(A) © Biophoto Associates/Science Source; **(B)** CDC/Joe Millar

(2013) noted, perianal warts do not develop entirely as a result of anal sexual intercourse. Another causal factor could be HPV-infected genital secretions that might have collected in the perianal area for some time. HPV-6 and HPV-11 may also cause infection at other sites including the conjunctiva, nasal cavity, oral cavity, and larynx. HPV is found to be site specific; therefore auto-inoculation from other sites commonly occurs in infected adults (Woodward & Robinson, 2011).

Factors that Increase the Risk of Genital HPV Infection

The main risk factors include exposure by direct contact with genital warts of an infected person. Therefore, associated risk factors include multiple sexual partners, younger age groups who practice group sexual behaviors, or sexual intercourse with individuals who also have multiple sexual partners (Bosch et al., 2008; Juckett & Hartman-Adams,

2010). Other risk factors are commencement of sexual intercourse at an early age, weakened or compromised immune system, absent or inconsistent use of condoms (Winer et al., 2006), and previous history of STIs. Damaged genital skin, injury, and abrasions may potentially increase the risk of HPV entry.

Possible Associated Complications and the Psychological Impact of HPV Infection

The manifestation of what is perceived as disfiguring growths of HPV warts can create feelings of guilt, anxiety, and low self-esteem in sexual relationships. Additionally, fear of cancer risk and potential infertility can create emotional and psychological problems (Woodhall et al., 2008, 2006). Both premalignant and invasive lesions can coexist and these can develop inside the existing genital warts or lead to misdiagnosis. Warts in the anal canal should be further investigated for *Chlamydia trachomatis, Neisseria gonorrhoeae, Treponema pallidum*, HIV, and HBV (Lacey et al., 2006; Lazaro, 2013).

U.K. Recommendations for Diagnosis of Genital HPV

The diagnosis of genital warts tends to be clinical and is performed by visual inspection. Meticulous inspection is crucial, using a good source of light to carefully examine the lesions. In men, the urethral meatus should be carefully examined by meatoscopy to rule out bleeding from the urethra (BASHH, 2014; Lacey et al., 2006). Additionally, careful examination of the perianal area should include proctoscopy to rule out bleeding from anal canal lesions that may be associated with other infections (Hernandez et al., 2005; Sehnal et al., 2012). Correct differential diagnosis is vital and appropriate rectal specimens should be obtained for the specific laboratory tests. Warts in the anal canal have been associated with penetrative anal sexual intercourse (Hernandez et al., 2005; Sehnal et al., 2012) and related to various infections including chlamydia, gonorrhea, syphilis, and HIV.

In women, similar examination of the perianal area should be performed together with speculum examination of the cervix and vagina to rule out cervical or vaginal lesions. Signs of neoplastic change with bleeding, abnormal pigmentation, and palpable skin lesions or ulceration should be cause for concern (BASHH, 2014; Lacey et al., 2006) and indicate immediate referral for appropriate specialist care (Lacey et al., 2006). Biopsy may be performed under local anaesthetic if necessary to obtain a specimen of tissue cells for histology. This would be determined by suspicious signs of precancer or cancer and if so, colposcopy should be performed (BASHH, 2014).

It is important to consider that not all papules are caused by HPV infection. Careful differential diagnosis is crucial to rule out other lesions such as penile papules, molluscum contagiosum, and seborrheic keratosis (Körber & Dissemond, 2009; Lacey et al., 2006). The uncertainty of HPV DNA typing has led to these methods not being recommended for diagnosing anogenital warts (Lacey et al., 2006; Lazaro, 2013) or other HPV infections. However, the recommendation is to identify and categorize the lesions according to morphology.

Factors affecting ambiguous diagnosis include whether the warts appear pigmented, indurated or fixed; lesion bleeding or ulceration; atypical lesions; failure to respond to treatment; and compromised immune system. Genital maps are useful for illustrating the number, spread, and distribution of lesions, as well as treatment effectiveness for lesion clearing. HPV infections may heal and disappear spontaneously (Lazaro, 2013).

Management of Genital HPV

The treatment of genital warts aims at alleviating the symptoms and wart removal for improved cosmetic effect. Although treatment benefits most patients by effecting warts-free periods, without treatment visible genital warts may evolve with one of three possible outcomes. They may resolve spontaneously in 5–30% of cases at 3 months, persist without change in 20% of cases, or increase in size and number in 50% of cases (CDC, 2015d). While available therapeutic remedies generally reduce genital warts, they may not totally eradicate the HPV infection. It is uncertain whether the reduction in HPV DNA achieved by therapeutic treatment reduces or controls potential transmission (CDC, 2015d).

Human Papillomavirus (HPV) Treatment: United States

Treatment for HPV for both genital warts and precancerous lesions is directed toward macroscopic care. Given that most subclinical genital HPV infections clear spontaneously, specific antiretroviral therapy is not recommended. HPV precancerous lesions should be managed based upon existing guidelines (Workowski & Bolan, 2015). The CDC-recommended treatment regimens for external anogenital warts (warts of the penis, groin, scrotum, vulva, perineum, external anus, and perianus) are guided by the wart size, number, anatomic site, patient preference, cost of treatment, convenience, adverse effects, and provider experience. No one regimen has been proven to be more efficacious than another and no single treatment is ideal for all patients or all warts. Clinicians often use a combination of regimens, both provider and client applied.

Recommended Regimens for HPV External Anogenital Warts

Provider-Administered

- Cryotherapy with liquid nitrogen or cryoprobe, **or**
- Surgical removal either by tangential scissor excision, tangential shave excision, curettage, laser, or electrosurgery, **or**
- Trichloroacetic acid (TCA) or bichloroacetic acid (BCA) 80–90% solution applied once a week

Patient-Applied

- Imiquimod 3.75% or 5% cream (Note: May weaken condoms and vaginal diaphragms): 5% solution is applied at bedtime three times a week for up to 16 weeks. The 3.75% solution is applied at bedtime every night. With both solutions, the treatment area should be washed with soap and water 6–10 hours following application. Appears to be low risk in pregnancy, but data is limited. **or**
- Podofilox 0.5% solution or gel is applied to the anogenital warts twice a day for 3 days and then followed by 4 days without treatment, repeating this cycle for up to four cycles total. Not recommended during pregnancy. **or**
- Sinecatechins 15% ointment (Note: May weaken condoms and vaginal diaphragms) is applied three times daily until complete clearance of warts occurs, but for not more than 16 weeks. Additionally, Sinecatechins is not recommended for use in persons with HIV or during pregnancy.

Human Papillomavirus (HPV) Management Considerations and Follow-Up

Treatment of urethral meatus warts, vaginal and cervical warts, or intra-anal warts is generally accomplished by cryotherapy with liquid nitrogen, surgery, or provider-administered TCA or BCA. For external anogenital warts, follow-up visits should be scheduled to assess treatment response and address any patient medication questions or noted side-effects. It must be noted that podophyllotoxin (Podofilox), podophyllin, and sinecatechins should not be used during pregnancy. Imiquimod appears to be low risk in pregnancy but needs further study (Workowski & Bolan, 2015). Cesarean delivery may be indicated for women with warts obstructing the pelvic outlet or if excessive bleeding from friable tissue is anticipated. Data does not support altered treatment approaches for persons with HIV infection. U.S. cervical cancer screening and follow-up recommendations are evidence-based and largely consistent among all of the major medical organizations (ACOG, American Cancer Society, CDC, and USPSTF). For further information on U.S. cervical cancer screening and follow-up, see http://www.cdc.gov/cancer/cervical/index.htm.

U.K. Recommendations: Patient/client information, education, counseling, and support

Clear and comprehensible evidence-based information should be provided about the infection, how it is transmitted, recommended treatments, and the options available to the individual. Verbal explanations should be complemented by clear and accurate written information (BASHH, 2014). Moreover, a detailed sexual history including previous history of STIs should be obtained and patients offered full STI screening services. This allows for detection of other STIs (BASHH, 2014; Lacey et al., 2006). While the tracing of previous sexual contacts is not considered necessary, assessment of current sexual partners may help in detecting undiagnosed STIs. It also offers the opportunity to provide appropriate recommended management, education, counseling, and support. Where applicable, the patient is encouraged not to interrupt their routine cervical cytology screening.

Key considerations in the planning and implementation of treatment involve personal choices of the patient/client, the nature and accessibility of available resources, and the specialist expertise among the multidisciplinary team of sexual healthcare professionals. Despite the large variety of medications and products available for treatment of warts, no specific brands are entirely ideal for the treatment and eradication of all warts in all patients. Therefore, it is useful to explain about the potential failure of treatment and to raise patient awareness of the possibility of symptom recurrence (BASHH, 2014). However, it is possible that the uncertainties may cause the individual to decline treatment and hope that spontaneous resolution might occur (Woodward & Robinson, 2011).

Standardized treatment protocols or algorithms of the clinical symptoms, specific decisions, actions, and treatment regimens enhance standardization and quality care to achieve effective treatment outcomes. Woodward and Robinson (2011) provide a clear and simplified illustration that practitioners are encouraged to explore and possibly discuss with colleagues in the multidisciplinary team context. Team leaders and members may consider developing an original in-house version rather than adopting a preexisting one. The treatment interventions involve medicinal remedies comprising either cytotoxic drugs or immune stimulants, and physical ablation. The choice of medication may also be guided by the characteristics of the warts, the type, shape, size, how numerous or extensive, the distribution and location of the lesions, and potential adverse effects. Patients may experience itchiness, burning, erosion, and pain (BASHH, 2014; Lacey et al., 2006). Additionally, the risk of scarring and possible change in pigmentation—either hypopigmentation or hyperpigmentation—should be explained to the patient prior to treatment implementation. Clear and accurate supplementary written information outlining the management of treatment reactions or potential adverse effects should be provided (BASHH, 2014; Lacey et al., 2006).

Although uncommon, persistent pain particularly at the site of the treatment, has been reported as well as anal fistulas with pain on defecation. The success or failure of the treatment may depend on the presence or absence of immunosuppression and patient compliance with the prescribed treatment regimen. Because most genital warts respond to treatment within 1 to 6 months, lack of adequate improvement or severe side effects should be indications for change of treatment. Therefore, treatment efficacy should be carefully monitored and reviewed (Woodward & Robinson, 2011).

Recommended Treatment Regimens

Various treatment options should be explained to the patient to allow for personal decision and choice. Treatment regimens involve two classifications: patient-applied regimen and provider-administrated regimen. Unsurprisingly, the option of patient-applied regimens is preferred by most individuals due to the advantage of personal privacy. Compliance is crucial and must be emphasized to the patient. Moreover, competent application of the technique is vital for successful healing. Therefore, it is important to ensure that the individual would be able to identify and access all the genital warts to apply the treatment properly and efficiently. While follow-up visits are not necessarily imperative, they may provide opportunities for addressing patient concerns and questions. It also provides opportunities for the patient to report side effects and allows for evaluation of treatment response.

Effectiveness is crucial in determining specific treatment agents. Podophyllin, podophylotoxin, and trichloroacetic acid are reputed to be effective treatments for soft non-keratinized warts (BASHH, 2014). The choice of treatment for keratinized warts involves ablative methods such as cryotherapy, electro-cautery, or excision. Imiquimod is also reputed to be an effective agent for both keratinized and non-keratinized warts (BASHH, 2014; Lazaro, 2013).

The recommended medications for patient-applied treatment include the following:

- Podophylotoxin in the form of 0.15% cream or 0.5% solution. This antimitotic agent is applied twice daily for 3 days followed by a break of 4 days with no application, then repeated. The solution is recommended for four cycles of application while the cream is recommended for five cycles both under the supervision of medical staff when lesions are greater than 4 cm (BASHH, 2014; Lazaro, 2013). This is not applicable to extra-genital warts (including anal warts) and is contraindicated in pregnancy. Specialist referral is suggested if no treatment effect is observed after the four cycles of treatment (Lazaro, 2013). It is also suggested that treatment should be discontinued if severe adverse effects such as ulceration or soreness occurs. Moreover, unprotected sexual intercourse should be avoided due to potential skin irritation to sexual partners (BASHH, 2014).

- Imiquimod 5% cream is applied alternate nights, three times a week and should be washed off each morning 6–10 hours following application (BASHH, 2014; Gilson, Nathan, Sonnex, Lazaro, & Keirs, 2015; Lazaro, 2013). The full course of imiquimod treatment is 16 weeks. This treatment is suggested for self-application at home by the patient, though not recommended for internal genital warts and is not recommended for use by pregnant women (BASHH, 2014; Lazaro, 2013). Similarly to podophyllotoxin treatment, the patient should be advised to avoid unprotected sexual intercourse due to potential skin irritation of sexual partners and diminished effectiveness of latex condoms (BASHH, 2014; Gilson et al., 2015; Lazaro, 2013).

The use of these treatments requires that the patient be instructed on how to carefully locate the lesions and correctly apply the prescribed agent. For a limited number of relatively small warts, the ablative methods are considered more appropriate irrespective of the type of warts.

Methods of Physical Ablation

- Excision of pedunculated warts and accessible keratinized warts is found to be an effective treatment method that can be repeated as necessary. Nevertheless, some consider ablation to be rather outdated, despite the argument that it offers an immediate and effective option for large lesions (Yanofsky, Patel, & Goldenberg, 2012). An anaesthetic cream is applied, followed by local anesthetic injection prior to excision and hemostasis may be established by electrosurgery or application of silver nitrate (BASHH, 2014; Gilson et al., 2015).

- Cryotherapy with liquid nitrogen or cryoprobe destroys warts by thermal-induced cytolysis with necrosis at the junction of the epidermis and dermis. The procedure involves application of the agent to create a glow of freezing around the lesion, then a freeze-thaw-freeze technique is carried out, followed by a freeze state sustained for 10–30 seconds (BASHH, 2014; Gilson et al., 2015). Appropriate training is required for efficient use of this technique to avoid over- or undertreatment that can result in complications. Pain associated with the application of the liquid nitrogen, necrosis, and possible blistering is commonly reported. Practitioners should comply with health and safety regulations for storage and handling of liquid nitrogen (BASHH, 2014; Gilson et al., 2015).

- Electrosurgery involves burning of the treatment site and surrounding tissue.

- Hyfrecator or electrofulguration can be used to cause superficial burning/charring of the lesion with minimal damage to the dermis. Electrodessication can be performed for deeper penetration of the lesion tissues followed by curettage (BASHH, 2014).

- Monopolar surgery with varied waveforms allows for desiccation, cutting, and coagulation with more precise cut and minimal damage to the healthy tissue around the lesion to aid healing with minimal scarring (BASHH, 2014).

- Laser treatment with use of carbon dioxide is reputed to be an effective method for larger warts located at anatomical sites that are relatively difficult to access for example the urethral meatus or anal canal (BASHH, 2014). This treatment modality may be inaccessible in poorer developing countries due to the relatively expensive cost, required specialist expertise and appropriate staff training. Appropriate evidence-based precautions should be carefully explored and measures taken to protect the staff during all electrosurgical and laser procedures.

Consideration of Sexual Partners

While there are no specific look-back periods for HPV infection due to latency of the infection, there is also no recommendation for partner notification or tracing of sexual contacts (Lazaro, 2013). However, the suggestion is to assess current sexual partners for unobserved genital warts and screen for other STIs. It is also important to the partner HPV infection and genital warts, and course of infection. This may depend on the wishes of the index patient (BASHH, 2014; Lazaro, 2013).

Follow-Up

Practitioners should assess the response to treatment and consider a possible change of treatment if there is a poor response. In essence, where there has been effective response to treatment but appearance of new HPV lesions, the current treatment regimen would be continued (BASHH, 2014; Gilson et al., 2015). However, a change of treatment should be considered if the lesions show less than 50% response to the treatment within 4–5 weeks, or if the patient develops poor tolerance or an adverse reaction. Imiquimod is found to take relatively longer to have the desired observable effect, about 8–12 weeks (BASHH, 2014; Gilson et al., 2015). Relapses have been reported and recommended treatment is employed according to the HPV lesion.

Recommended Treatments for HPV Lesions Located in Specific Anatomical Sites

Intravaginal Warts

Cryotherapy with liquid nitrogen or electrosurgery may be carried out. Trichloroacetic acid (TCA) 80–90% solution is considered suitable for application to warts located at most anatomical sites (BASHH, 2014). As a caustic agent, it causes a severe burning sensation for 5–10 minutes after application and results in necrosis of the tissue cells. A potential adverse effect is ulceration, which may break through into the dermis (Gilson et al., 2015). Therefore, TCA is not recommended for treatment of large volume warts (BASHH, 2014; Gilson et al., 2015). Further, TCA is extremely caustic, with a corroding effect; therefore, petroleum jelly should be applied to protect the surrounding skin of the warts being treated. Additionally, there should always be sodium bicarbonate available to deal with accidental spillage or over-application (BASHH, 2014; Gilson et al., 2015).

Cervical Warts

A frequent associated pathological manifestation that requires specialist consultation and biopsy is cervical intraepithelial neoplasia (CIN). Colposcopy may be considered if there is ambiguity about the diagnosis (Gilson et al., 2015), although routine colposcopy is not recommended for women with genital warts and cervical lesions. Treatment procedures may comprise cryotherapy, electrosurgery, laser ablation, trichloroacetic acid treatment, or excision (BASHH, 2014; Woodward & Robinson, 2011).

Urethral Meatal Warts

The recommended treatments for urethral warts comprise cryotherapy, electrosurgery, or laser ablation. Podophyllotoxin 0.5% or imiquimod 5% may also be considered. Patients who present with lesions that are deeply located within the urethra should be referred to a urologist for surgical ablation under direct vision via meatoscopy (BASHH, 2014; Gilson et al., 2015).

Intra-anal Warts

Cryotherapy, trichloroacetic acid, electrosurgery, or laser ablation may be considered for treating intra-anal warts (Gilson et al., 2015; see also Hernandez et al., 2005; Sehnal et al., 2012).

Additional Considerations

In relation to cervical cytology, the U.K. National Cervical Screening Programme recommends that required screening intervals should remain unchanged in women who develop anogenital warts (BASHH, 2014).

Individuals with an impaired immune system associated with organ transplant and HIV-infected people are reported to be more vulnerable to unsuccessful treatment responses. Moreover, they present with more frequent relapses and may require extended courses of treatment (Gilson et al., 2015). Relatively higher risk of anogenital intraepithelial neoplasia is also noted among this group (BASHH, 2014).

There is no doubt that HPV infection poses a particular challenge in sexual healthcare due to the numerous genotypes that cause complex manifestations of anogenital warts and other associated lesions. While most of the HPV types cause benign lesions, the dread of oncogenic types can cause significant psychological distress for individuals who develop symptomatic HPV with complications. The current 2015 U.K. national guidelines and the European Guidelines on the Management of Anogenital Warts (Gilson et al, 2015) are highly recommended here as further reading for more detailed information.

Trichomonas vaginalis (Trichomoniasis)

Trichomonas vaginalis (*T. vaginalis*), while a sexually transmitted infection, is not nationally reportable. However, *T. vaginalis* parasitic infection is the single most prevalent non-viral STI in the United States. It is estimated that 3.7 million Americans (roughly 3% of the U.S. population) are infected with *T. vaginalis*, more than gonorrhea and chlamydia combined. Despite its common occurrence, *T. vaginalis* has long been considered a "neglected" parasitic infection due to limited knowledge of its sequelae and associated economic burden (Meites, 2013). It is conservatively estimated that direct U.S. medical costs from *T. vaginalis* exceed $24 million annually. Accurate measurement of disease prevalence and cost is limited by the lack of sensitivity in commonly used clinical testing methods (e.g., wet mount) and the vast number of asymptomatic infections (Secour Meites, Starr, & Workowski, 2014).

Disparities are the hallmark of *T. vaginalis*; non-Hispanic black women have the highest rates of infection (13.3%) with approximately 10 times the rate for Mexican-American or non-Hispanic white women (1.8% and 1.3% respectively) (Secour et al., 2014). *T. vaginalis* is more prevalent in women over the age of 40 (11%), STI clinic patients (26%), and incarcerated persons (32%). While the prevalence in MSM is low (Workowski & Bolan, 2015), it is unknown if the rectum can be a reservoir for *T. vaginalis*. In pregnant women *T. vaginalis* is strongly associated with a two- to threefold increased risk of acquiring HIV, premature rupture of the membranes, premature birth, and low birthweight infants. For HIV-positive women *T. vaginalis* increases the risk for PID (Workowski & Bolan, 2015).

T. vaginalis (Trichomoniasis) Screening

Trichomoniasis is most commonly detected by identifying the motile, flagellated parasites during wet mount microscopic examination of genital secretions. This is despite the fact that wet mount sensitivity is only 51–65%. While culture can be considered the gold-standard for detection, it is expensive and time consuming, requiring a return visit for treatment, all of which lead to limited practical application in the clinical setting. The first NAAT test specific for *T. vaginalis* was approved by the FDA in 2011. Other sensitive, rapid point-of-care tests are also available allowing treatment to be provided at the same visit (Secour et al., 2014). Pap tests are not considered diagnostic for trichomoniasis because both false positives and false negatives can occur. The USPSTF has not released any guidelines for screening for trichomoniasis. The CDC screening guidelines are as follows:

- All women (WSW or WSM, or pregnant) seeking care for vaginitis or vaginal discharge should be screened for *T. vaginalis*.
- All HIV-infected women should be screened upon entry into care and then annually thereafter.
- All HIV-infected pregnant women should be screened at their first prenatal visit.
- Screening should be considered for asymptomatic women at high risk for infection.
- Screening in asymptomatic males (MSM or MSW) is currently not recommended as few data are available regarding testing or screening in men.

In the United Kingdom, the prevalence of *Trichomonas vaginalis* among STI and genitourinary clinic attendees is reported as 5,595 and 437 new diagnoses of women and men, respectively. The causative organism *Trichomonas vaginalis* is described as a flagellated protozoan. The usual sites of infection in women involve the vagina, urethra, and the para-urethral glands and in men mainly within the urethra and under the foreskin.

Transmission

Trichomoniasis is almost entirely a STI among adults. It is acquired through sexual intercourse and hence access may occur through the vagina or through the urethra (Lazaro, 2013; Sherrard et al., 2014).

Clinical Manifestations of *Trichomonas vaginalis*

Females

Infected women carry the infection for several months without any symptoms. In fact, 10–50% of women are reported to be asymptomatic (although the vaginal pH may be high), while others may develop only minimal symptoms (Hollman, Coupey, Fox, & Harold, 2010). Symptomatic women may present with malodorous, frothy vaginal discharge with a pH > 4.5 accompanied by vulval irritation and dysuria. These symptoms, however, are not confined to *Trichomonas vaginalis* infection (Hay, 2011; Lazaro, 2013; Sherrard et al., 2014). Occasional additional symptoms may be low abdominal discomfort and ulceration of the vulva (Lazaro, 2013; Sherrard et al., 2014). Clinical examination may reveal signs of vulvitis, vaginitis, and an estimated 70% of infected women may present with vaginal discharge that varies in consistency from thin and scanty to profuse and frothy (Hollman et al., 2010; Lazaro, 2013; Sherrard et al., 2014). The typical discharge is described as homogenous, yellow-green or off-white, and frothy (Hollman et al., 2010), and 2% of the infected women may present with manifestation of cervicitis described as "strawberry cervix" (Lazaro, 2013).

Males

Generally, an estimated 15–50% of infected men remain asymptomatic, while others may develop nongonococcal urethritis (NGU) and dysuria (Hay, 2011; Sherrard et al., 2014). Most infected men are likely to have acquired the infection from their female sexual partners. While 20–60% of infected men present with small or moderate amounts of urethral discharge (Seña et al., 2007; Sherrard et al., 2014), in rare cases copious purulent discharge from the urethra is present and prostatitis has also been occasionally reported. Balanoposthitis is a rare complication (Sherrard et al., 2014).

Complications Associated with *Trichomonas vaginalis* Infection

Evidence shows that *Trichomonas vaginalis* infection is associated with preterm delivery and low birthweight in pregnant women (Mann et al., 2009). However, Stringer et al. (2010) found no association between treatment of *Trichomonas vaginalis* and preterm birth or low birthweight.

Other evidence associates enhanced HIV transmission with *Trichomonas vaginalis* infection and increased risk of *Trichomonas* infection among HIV-positive individuals (McClelland et al., 2007).

Diagnosis of *Trichomonas vaginalis* Infection

Women who present with vaginal discharge, vulvitis, vaginitis, and specific high-risk population groups should be targeted for testing (CDC, 2015d). The latter include women who have frequent changes, new and multiple sexual partners, those with a history of STIs, sex workers, and those who engage in illicit drug use (CDC, 2015d; Hay, 2011). Additionally, women whose cervical cytology reveals *Trichomonas vaginalis* organisms, or whose sexual partners are diagnosed with this infection, should be tested as well as women who present with failed treatment of vaginal discharge, or severe or recurrent symptoms (Sherrard, Donders, White, Jensen, & IUSTI, 2011; Sherrard et al., 2014). Men who have been exposed to this infection through direct sexual contact and individuals who present with constant urethritis should be tested (Sherrard et al., 2014).

Specimens for Laboratory Tests for *Trichomonas vaginalis*

In women, swab from the posterior vaginal fornix obtained at speculum examination, self-taken vaginal swab (the more preferred specimen), or urine specimen are sent for laboratory investigation. In men, urethral specimen or first-void urine may be obtained for culture or microscopic tests. While some argue that urine culture has relatively low sensitivity (Mohamed et al., 2001), others consider the technique to be effective in diagnosing trichomonas in 60–80% of patients (Sherrard et al., 2014).

Diagnostic tests comprise immediate microscopy involving wet preparations of saline and vaginal secretions (Nye, Schwebke, & Body, 2009). Although this is found to have a relatively low sensitivity 51–65% (Hollman et al., 2010), it is nonetheless considered a useful test for visualizing the motile organisms (Nye et al., 2009).

Compared to microscopy, the use of culture for diagnosing *Trichomonas vaginalis* is found to demonstrate greater sensitivity at 75–96% and specificity up to 100% (Huppert et al., 2005; Huppert et al., 2007; Nye et al., 2009). Culture can be performed on vaginal secretions of women suspected to have acquired trichomoniasis but not confirmed by microscopic investigation; it can also be used to diagnose the infection in men (Hobbs et al., 2006; Nye et al., 2009).

Nucleic acid amplification tests are reputed to provide the greatest sensitivity for diagnosing *Trichomonas vaginalis* and are the recommended diagnostic techniques (Nye et al., 2009; Sherrard et al., 2014).

The Recommended Management of *Trichomonas vaginalis*

The key principles of management involve provision of relevant information, support, and encouragement. The course of the infection and the long-term effects on health should be emphasized to the patient and the sexual partner to encourage them to cooperate and comply with the treatment regimens. Moreover, avoidance of sexual intercourse should be emphasized until 1 week after the patient and the sexual partner have fully completed the therapy and at follow-up program (CDC, 2015d; Sherrard et al., 2014). They should also be screened for other concurrent STIs.

Effects of the Antibiotic Treatment
U.S. Recommendations for *T. vaginalis* (Trichomonas) Treatment

Nitroimidazoles are the only category of antimicrobial therapy known to be effective against *T. vaginalis*. Of these medications, metronidazole and tinidazole have FDA approval for both oral and parenteral treatment of this infection. Tinidazole is more expensive, but reaches higher serum and genitourinary concentrations, has a longer half-life (12.5 versus 7.3 hours), has fewer gastrointestinal side effects, and achieves higher cure rates (92–100% versus 84–98%). Thus, tinidazole is equivalent or superior to metronidazole in achieving parasitologic cure (Workowski & Bolan, 2015). The CDC recommendations for effective treatment of trichomoniasis are as follows:

- *Recommended for treating trichomoniasis*: Metronidazole 2 g orally in a single dose **or** tinidazole 2 g orally in a single dose
- *Trichomoniasis in pregnancy*: Metronidazole 2 g orally in a single dose
- *Women with HIV infection*: Metronidazole 500 mg orally twice daily for 7 days
- *Alternate regimen*: Metronidazole 500 mg orally twice a day for 7 days

T. vaginalis Management Considerations and Follow-Up

Persons infected with *T. vaginalis* must abstain from sex until they and their sex partners have completed treatment and any symptoms have resolved. Testing for other STIs—including HIV—should be performed in persons with trichomoniasis. Given the high rate of reinfection among women treated for *T. vaginalis* (17% within 3 months in one study), retesting of all sexually active females within 3 months following initial treatment is recommended regardless of whether they believe that their sex partners were treated. Pregnant women who are HIV positive should also be rescreened 3 months following treatment. Clinicians should counsel all symptomatic pregnant women regarding the potential benefits of treatment and the importance of partner treatment and condom use in the prevention of

sexual transmission. Data are insufficient to recommend routine screening, alternative regimens of longer duration, or retesting in men (Workowski & Bolan, 2015).

U.K. Recommendations

Due to the high incidence of urethral and para-urethral gland involvement, thorough treatment with antibiotics is recommended (Sherrard et al., 2014). Various experts maintain that most nitroimidazole antibiotics provide effective cure when administered as a single oral dose (CDC, 2015d; Sherrard et al., 2011; Sherrard et al., 2014). However, side effects are commonly reported with this treatment. Additionally, although better compliance is achieved with this regimen, higher failure rates are also reported, particularly when sexual partners do not receive the same treatment at the same time (Sherrard et al., 2011).

The recommended treatment regimens are the following:

- Metronidazole 2 g orally is administered as a single dose, or
- Metronidazole 400–500 mg orally, twice daily for 5–7 days (Hay, 2011; Sherrard et al., 2014)

Alternative treatment:

- Tinidazole 2 g orally as a single dose (Hay, 2011; Sherrard et al., 2014)

In both regimens patients should avoid alcohol consumption due to possible adverse effects similar to disulfiram (Antabuse) reaction (CDC, 2015d; Sherrard et al., 2014). Patients are strongly advised to avoid alcoholic drinks throughout the duration of the treatment and for at least 48 hours after metronidazole treatment regimen (Sherrard et al., 2014) or for at least 72 hours after tinidazole treatment regimen (Sherrard et al., 2011; Sherrard et al., 2014).

Allergic reactions should be borne in mind. While hypersensitivity reactions have been reported in patients receiving metronidazole and tinidazole treatments (Sherrard et al., 2014), there seems to be a need for more clarity about true associated allergies. Potential adverse reactions have been described as anaphylaxis, skin rash, pruritus, urticaria, flushing, and fever. However, detailed history should be obtained to confirm true allergy (Sherrard et al., 2014).

Treatment failure has been associated with inadequate treatment, reinfection, or resistance of the organisms to the antibiotic treatment. Kissinger et al. (2008) reported failed response to the 2 g single dose of metronidazole and tinidazole treatment regimens among a significant number of women. Therefore, careful examination of the sexual history is crucial, and it is also important to establish whether the patient complied with the prescribed treatment regimen. It should be noted how well the patient had tolerated the treatment and if vomiting occurred following the oral dose of treatment. Treatment of the sexual partner should also be confirmed (Sherrard et al., 2014). Recent evidence indicates that the single oral dose of 2 g metronidazole does not appear to achieve as adequate effectiveness as 500 mg twice daily for 7 days in HIV-positive patients (Kissinger et al., 2010).

Resistance to the Antibiotic Treatment

Although strong resistance is reported to be rare, weak resistance to metronidazole has been reported. The alternative treatment regimen of tinidazole or increased doses of metronidazole seem to overcome identified resistance (Sherrard et al., 2011). The protocol for nonresponse to the recommended regimen requires that reinfection and nonadherence should first be excluded. The protocol outlines repeat courses of the treatment with higher doses for longer durations. The first course of repeat therapy (Das, Huengsberg, & Shahmanesh, 2005) is followed by a second course of further increased doses (Bosserman, Helms, Mosure, Secor, & Workowski, 2011; Das et al., 2005). A third regimen of still further increased doses (Bosserman et al., 2011; Mammen-Tobin & Wilson, 2005). may be prescribed as necessary, according to the response to the resistance. Where a third regimen is required, the recommendation is to carry out resistance testing to guide the treatment (Bosserman et al., 2011). Practitioners are encouraged to carefully confirm the regimen for each repeat course for successive failed response to treatment.

Management of Sexual Partners

The process of partner management, contact tracing, and treatment is crucial. The patient should be advised about the importance of partner notification to offer them the same treatment to avoid the risk of recurrent infections. These should include current sexual partners and all sexual contacts in the preceding 4 weeks of the manifestation. The full range of STI screening should be performed together with treatment for *Trichomonas vaginalis*. The notification options should be clearly explained and the individual's preference discussed to gain full cooperation (Schwebke & Desmond, 2010).

Recommended management of the male sexual partners who present with urethritis involves STI screening and initial treatment for *Trichomonas vaginalis*. A repeat testing of urethral specimen is suggested prior to administering additional treatment for nongonococcal urethritis. The recommended treatment for male sexual partners of women with failed nitroimidazole treatment comprises the following:

- Metronidazole 400–500 mg twice daily for 7 days, or
- Tinidazole 2 g orally as a single dose (Sherrard et al., 2014)

Follow-Up and Test of Cure

Follow-up and test of cure is recommended for patients whose *Trichomonas vaginalis* infection remains symptomatic and for those who develop recurrent infections (Sherrard et al., 2014). Evidence reveals that an estimated 17% of patients treated for *Trichomonas vaginalis* infection present with repeat infections mainly attributed to reinfection acquired through sexual intercourse with untreated sexual partner(s) (CDC, 2010).

There is no doubt that trichomoniasis can be entirely cured. Nonetheless, problems of reinfections and recurrences that require repeat treatment regimens of increasing dosages of antibiotic therapy present particular challenges in sexual healthcare.

Bacterial Vaginosis (BV)

This polymicrobial syndrome is a condition in which vaginal lactobacilli are replaced by high concentrations of anaerobic bacterial organisms, *Gardnerella vaginalis*, urea plasma, *Mycoplasma hominis* and other bacterial species (Mitchell, Manhart, & Thomas, 2011). Consequently, the pH of the vaginal secretions rises >4.5–6.0 (Sherrard et al., 2014). Bacterial vaginosis (BV) is described as the most predominant cause of abnormal vaginal discharge among women of childbearing age, although menopausal women are also affected (Akinbiyi, Watson, & Feyi-Waboso, 2008; Fang, Zhou, Yang, Diao, & Li, 2007; Koumans et al., 2005). The prevalence varies among different population groups. For example, high prevalence is reported among women in the sub-Saharan African country Uganda. Variations in prevalence within the United Kingdom have been reported among pregnant women attending an antenatal clinic and women undergoing termination of pregnancy (Akinbiyi et al., 2008; Sherrard et al., 2014).

Risk Factors

The risk factors include multiple sexual partners of both sexes, new sexual partners, inconsistent or lack of condom use, douching, and diminished vaginal lactobacilli. It is also reported that women who acquire BV have increased risk of acquiring other STIs such as HIV, *N. gonorrhoeae*, *C. trachomatis*, and HSV-2. They are also at higher risk of developing complications after gynaecological surgery and recurrent bacterial vaginosis.

Clinical Manifestations

The distinguishing signs and symptoms include a typical homogenous thin, white discharge that adheres to and smoothly coats the walls of the vagina and the vestibule. However, BV is not associated with signs of vaginitis, and therefore there would be no associated inflammation with soreness, itchiness, or irritation. The most typical symptom is described as an offensive fishy smell of the vaginal discharge (Hay, 2011). Approximately 50% of women with bacterial vaginosis are asymptomatic.

Potential Complications Associated with Bacterial Vaginosis

While BV is not classified as sexually transmitted, the condition is associated with increased risk of acquiring

STIs, particularly HSV, as well as higher risk of HIV transmission (Atashili, Poole, Mdumbe, Adimora, & Smith, 2008; Nagot et al., 2007). The prevalence of BV is high in women who present with PID, although there is no substantive evidence that confirms that BV causes PID (Ness et al., 2005). An association between BV and transvaginal hysterectomy has been reported (Lazaro, 2013).

Diagnosis of Bacterial Vaginosis

Diagnosis may involve the use of Amsel's clinical criteria, which requires confirmation of three specific signs and symptoms out of four defined criteria.

1. Presence of thin white homogenous vaginal discharge
2. Clue cells on microscopic wet mount examination (vaginal epithelial cells thickly coated with the typical bacteria)
3. Vaginal fluid pH >4.5 (3.5–4.5 normal)
4. Produces a fishy odor on adding alkali: 10% potassium hydroxide (KOH) to vaginal secretions on a slide (Amsel et al., 1983; Landers, Wiesenfeld, Heine, Krohn, & Hillier, 2004)

The Hay/Ison criteria represent another method of diagnosis that involves examination of a gram-stained smear of vaginal discharge (Ison & Hay, 2002). Depending on the morphotypes present, the grading may be described as normal, intermediate, or BV. The criteria comprise:

1. Grade 1 – Morphotypes of lactobacillus predominate (Normal)
2. Grade 2 – Mixed organisms, some lactobacilli and other morphotypes either gardnerella or mobiluncus (Intermediate)
3. Grade 3 – Few or absent lactobacilli but the main morphotypes are *Gardnerella* and *Mobiluncus* (BV) (Hay, 2011; Ison & Hay, 2002).

The Nugent score, which is also based on gram-stained vaginal smear, is the gold standard (Hay, 2011; Nugent, Krohn, & Hillier, 1991). representing a laboratory benchmark for diagnosing BV. This involves estimating the relative concentration of lactobacilli and other types of bacteria in the vaginal smear specimen and allocating scores between 0 and 10 to describe normal, intermediate, or BV. Scores are <4 (normal), 4–6 (intermediate), and >6 (BV) (Hay, 2011; Nugent et al., 1991).

Although new point-of-care tests are effective, these are not widely available, and NAATs for diagnosing BV-associated bacteria are undergoing ongoing development. It is important to bear in mind that coexistence of BV and other causes of abnormal vaginal discharge have been reported. Practitioners are encouraged to confirm the specific microscopic tests recommended in the sexual health organizations where they work.

Necessity for Treatment

- Manifestation of symptoms of BV
- Women undergoing certain surgical procedures

Recommended Treatment Regimens

Administration of prescribed antibiotics with effective anti-anaerobic action is recommended. The treatment aim for symptomatic women is symptom alleviation while also minimizing the risk for other STI acquisition. The recommended treatment regimens comprise the following:

- Metronidazole 400 mg orally twice daily for 5–7 days, or
- Metronidazole 2 g orally as a single dose, or
- Intravaginal metronidazole gel (0.75%) once daily for 5 days, or
- Intravaginal clindamycin cream (2%) once daily for 7 days (CDC, 2015; Sherrard et al., 2014).

Alternative regimens comprise the following:

- Tinidazole 2 g orally as a single dose, or
- Tinidazole 2 g orally once a day for 2 days, or
- Tinidazole 1 g orally once a day for 5 days, or
- Clindamycin 300 mg orally twice daily for 7 days (CDC, 2015; Sherrard, 2014)

Related Research Evidence and Treatment Considerations

Research study evidence has revealed that vaginal clindamycin cream efficacy at 66–83%, and oral metronidazole efficacy at 68–87% are relatively comparable after 4 weeks of treatment (Sherrard et al., 2011). Dosages of oral metronidazole administered in the different studies varied from 400 mg orally twice daily for 5 days to 500 mg orally twice daily for 7 days (Sherrard et al., 2014). This treatment choice justified by the evidence that oral metronidazole is reported to be well tolerated, relatively less expensive, and a well-established treatment regimen. The efficacy of intravaginal metronidazole gel is reported to be comparable to the efficacy of clindamycin cream, although this second option is more costly (Sherrard et al., 2014).

Issues Requiring Caution in the Care Provision

Patients receiving metronidazole treatment should be advised to avoid alcohol intake due to possible adverse effect similar to disulfiram (Antabuse) reaction. Additionally, patients using clindamycin cream or metronidazole gel should be advised to avoid condom use because those agents are reported to contain certain mineral oils that diminish condom efficacy (CDC, 2015; Sherrard et al., 2014). Moreover, although rare, allergy to metronidazole has apparently been reported and for that reason 2% clindamycin cream may be used as an alternative treatment.

Recurrence and Consideration of Sexual Partners

Routine screening and treatment of sexual partners is not considered to be necessary (Mehta, 2012). Neither is a test-of-cure required for those whose symptoms effectively clear up, though evidence indicates that most patients, up to 70%, develop recurrent BV within 3–12 months regardless of the treatment regimen they received. However, there is no evidence to suggest antibiotic resistance (Lazaro, 2013; Sherrard, 2011). Therefore, various studies have investigated measures to curb frequent recurrences of BV (Marcone, Calzolari, & Bertini, 2008; Wilson et al., 2005). Suppressive treatment with 0.75% metronidazole vaginal gel twice daily is reported to reduce recurrence rate (Sobel et al., 2006). Adjuvant vaginal application of probiotics has also been reported to enhance recurrence prevention (Eriksson Carolsson, Forsum, & Larsson, 2005; Marcone et al., 2008; Ya, Reifer, & Miller, 2010).

Suggested episodic or suppressive treatment regimens may involve 4–6 months of treatment (Pattman et al., 2010):

- Metronidazole 400 mg orally twice daily for 3 days at the beginning and end of menstruation
- Metronidazole 2 g orally once a month
- Metronidazole 0.75% intravaginal application twice weekly for 16 weeks (Pattman et al., 2010)

Key Issues Addressed in Patient Information

The patient should be provided clear explanation about the specific treatment regimen, such as the type of antibiotic medication prescribed, how it should be taken, possible adverse effects, and risk of recurrence. Compliance with routine STI screening and testing procedures should reflect the national guidelines.

Etiological Diagnosis and Clinical Diagnosis: Two Conventional Approaches to Diagnosing STIs

In the broader context, an essential aspect of sexual health care involves the use of an etiological approach to diagnosis based on laboratory diagnostic techniques to detect the organisms that cause particular infections. Clinical diagnosis, which involves application of clinical knowledge and expertise, allows for determining the typical symptoms and signs that characterise particular STI/RTI infections and the related impact on health. These are examined here.

Etiological Approach to STI Diagnosis

Generally, it is viewed that etiological diagnosis provides a more reliable basis for treatment decisions regarding specific STIs. The etiological approach offers the benefit of confirming the causative organism (WHO, 2007), which allows for ascertaining the most effective antimicrobials for treatment. The laboratory techniques used provide precide data for calculating correct dosages and treatment schedules. Moreover, they can detect evolving organism strains and identify species specific resistance to antimicrobials as well as level of susceptibility and coexisting microorganisms.

One challenge to the etiological diagnostic approach is that investigative tests must be scientifically validated, approved, and sustainable resource-wise. Laboratory testing requires adequate funding, specialist equipment, and staff competence. Continual emergence of new research findings may require implementation of new investigative techniques. Likewise, new equipment for more sophisticated tests justifies the need for ongoing staff training, appropriate supervision, and enhancement of professional competencies.

Related Practical Considerations

Specimen collection and transportation to laboratories must be efficient to avoid specimen deterioration, causing diagnostic errors. Assuring laboratory resource availability is likewise important. Specific laboratory test results may take time, causing a patient's motivation to decline when returning for results. Consequently, appropriate treatment and necessary repeats testing may be missed. Furthermore, there is a risk of continued infection transmission while waiting for laboratory results.

Ray et al.'s (2009) work provides a worthwhile reading for more insight on these issues. Ghebremichael (2014) also examines syndromic alongside laboratory diagnosis of STIs in clinical settings with limited resources.

Nonetheless, the etiological approach to diagnosis is recognized as a vital component of STI/RTI care and service provision. Etiological diagnostic findings should essentially complement clinical diagnosis.

Clinical Diagnosis and Management

Clinical diagnosis derives from the practitioner's clinical knowledge and expertise to correctly identify specific symptoms and signs that are typical of a particular infection (WHO, 2007). It incorporates thorough physical examination to identify specific clinical signs. However, infections with similar symptoms and/or signs could prove to be difficult to distinguish between, leading to misdiagnosis and inappropriate treatment. Additionally, there may be delay in symptom alleviation, effective treatment, and transmission control. Concurrent onfections are more likely detectable via laboratory diagnostic tests rather than clinical diagnosis. Thus, sole reliance on clinical diagnosis risks missing the presence of an STI that could potentially cause long-term adverse effects or permanent complications. Clinical diagnosis requires professional knowledge, extensive experience, thoroughness in related procedures, and ongoing support for continuing education. The concepts of empirical and epidemiological treatments are briefly examined here.

Epidemiological Treatment

Epidemiological treatment represents the administration of prescribed medication to the named contact(s) of an index patient following exposure to a STI when acquisition of the infection is very likely. This may also depend on the epidemiological trends in terms of endemic/pandemic fluctuations and outbreaks, causing increased infection acquisition risk from sexual partners in the particular area or community. The key factors that influence infection rate of spread include prevalence of the infection, risk of acquisition, and ongoing transmission. These in turn influence the probability that an exposed susceptible person will acquire the infection. The rate of exposure of susceptible sexual partners/sexual contacts to the infection and the time that newly infected partners remain infectious are also influencing factors. Epidemiological treatment is recommended in the management of sexual partners and sexual contacts of index patients with *Chlamydia trachomatis* infection (Lazaro, 2013).

Empirical Treatment

Empirical treatment involves offering and administering treatment to the sexual partner(s) of the index patient with the aim to reduce transmission and spread of infection within the community (Pattishall, Rahman, Jain, & Simon, 2012). In the wider context, empirical treatment aims at curbing spread of the infection among three population groups. The core groups present problems of high rate of change of sexual partners, increased rate of spread, and high frequency of transmission. The rate and extent of spread depend on the rate of transmission between the core group and the bridging group comprising the sexual partners. However, the rate decreases between the sexual partners and the wider general population. Treatment is offered and administered on the first day of clinic attendance prior to availability of confirmatory diagnostic test results or without the relevant laboratory test being performed. Thus, epidemiological treatment essentially takes account of the occurrence, acquisition, and spread of the particular infection rather than treatment based on laboratory test. Experts suggest that treatment should still be made available to the sexual partner/contact even if the person declines to have diagnostic tests performed. That includes those who refuse to have the relevant specimens taken or refuse to personally supply self-taken specimens for the diagnostic investigations (Faricy, Page, Ronic, Rdesinski, & DeVoe, 2012).

Significance of Empirical Treatment

The importance of empirical treatment of identified curable STIs is rationalized in the following ways. Because those infections are highly transmissible, it is highly likely that the sexual partner/contact would contract the infection through sexual intercourse or other sexual activity with the index patient. Many sexual partners may not feel motivated or willing to attend subsequent clinic visits to be treated according to the laboratory test result(s). That initial visit may be the only opportunity for direct interaction with the sexual health practitioner for prompt treatment. Moreover, individuals are more likely to accept the immediate single dose treatment that they perceive to be easily accessible and effective with little or no side effects. Where practical, the partner should be managed by the same provider and in the same sexual healthcare setting as the index patient. If geographical or structural factors make these arrangements difficult, the individual should be referred to an accessible sexual health clinic with similar facilities (BASHH, 2010). The immediate treatment could prove useful in minimizing infection transmission among the high-risk population groups who engage in sexual risk-taking behaviors and constant movements among social or sexual network groups. Health promotion and correct and consistent use of condoms should be continually emphasized and advice given regarding abstinence from sexual intercourse for the stipulated period following the treatment.

The practice of presumptive treatment for specific STIs is also implemented in some sexual healthcare organizations (Steen et al., 2012). Sexual partners who have been exposed to syphilis through sexual intercourse with index patients in primary, secondary, or early latent stages and who are likely to continue sexual activities may be considered for presumptive treatment. This is considered in situations where serological test results are not immediately available and the chances of extended serological investigation to cover the window period cannot be ascertained. In this case the presumptive treatment may involve a single dose of benzathine penicillin administered intramuscularly (Steen et al., 2012).

While some argue about the implications of unnecessary or overtreatment of sexual partners through the system of empirical treatment, the potential benefit in reducing the risk of transmission is worth considering. It sould also be argued that some sexual partners may find it reassuring to be given the prompt empirical treatment at their initial clinic attendance.

A standard letter should be given to the index patient for the sexual partner to take to his/her primary care provider stating his/her recent exposure to STI and the likelihood of having contracted a specific infection. The individual has a right to be provided the recommended empirical treatment, examination, and diagnostic tests.

Syndromic Case Management of STIs/RTIs

This problem-based approach to STI/RTI case management focuses on specific syndromes that comprise a combination of the patient's complaint, reported symptoms, and clinically observed signs (Mitchell, 2004; WHO, 2005, 2007). The recommended treatment is intended to alleviate the STIs that produce the particular syndrome. This approach allows for administering a single-dose treatment and providing pertinent evidence-based information, and sexual health promotion/education, counseling, and support. Nonetheless, total reliance on syndromes alone for diagnosing and treating STIs is considered deficient because certain STIs may occur with or without overt manifestation of symptoms. This argument consistently challenges the rationalization for syndromic case management and opinions vary regarding its use. (See Behets, Miller, and Cohen [2001] and Zemouri et al. [2016].) The general view in current practice is that syndromic case management with empirical treatment and confirmatory etiological diagnosis should be regarded as complementary approaches. The British Association for Sexual Health and HIV (2010) proposes that syndromic case management without diagnostic tests should be avoided whenever possible.

Synoptic Outline of the Potential Benefits of Syndromic Case Management

- It offers a problem-based approach to the clinical diagnosis and treatment by focusing on the symptoms and signs presented by the patient (WHO, 2007).

- It provides an accessible system of integrated care of patients with STIs within various settings at primary healthcare level and involves administration of appropriate treatment and support (Ghebremichael, 2014; Mahmood & Saniotis, 2011).

- Effective use of algorithms or flow charts ensures standardization and consistency in the treatment of specific curable STIs, patient care, and service provision (Mahmood & Saniotis, 2011).

- It allows opportunity for health promotion/education on preventive measures including condom distribution and instruction on correct use (WHO, 2007).

- It is reported to be functionally, substantively effective, particularly for the management of urethral discharge, genital ulcer disease, lower abdominal pain, and pelvic inflammatory disease.

Synoptic Outline of The Potential Limitations of Syndromic Case Management

Various limitations to the syndromic case management approach have been highlighted. For example, Tann et al. (2006) argued the following:

- Similarities in symptoms could lead to inaccuracies and misdiagnosing of infections thus resulting in treatment errors.

- Atypical symptoms could cause confusion and diagnostic errors.

- Concurrent infections could lead to misdiagnosis or missed infections, and inability to diagnose asymptomatic infections could lead to missed and untreated infections.

- The implications of overdiagnosis and overtreatment include potential side effects, drug interactions, and increased financial burden.

Syndromic case management has been used to establish standardization of STI care provision in poorly resourced countries (Ghebremichael, 2014). However, quality care provision underpined by best available evidence is recognized. Various interpretations of syndromic case management and adaptations of best practice algorithms have emerged over the years. Many of these interpretations are based national or internal policy guidelines or relate to sexual healthcare capacity and available resources (Mahmood & Saniotis, 2011).

Some critics consider the use of algorithms for syndromic case management as simplistic mechanisms to allow less qualified healthcare workers to provide STI care. Others may contend, though, that this view disregards the training and supervision provided to carefully screened healthcare staff. A sexual healthcare practitioner must be able to recognize signs and symptoms of different STIs, efficiently perform physical examinations, elicit sensitive and confidential details of a patient's sexual history, and administer the recommended treatments for the particular STI/RTI syndrome while safeguarding patient safety. Provision of appropriate health education, counseling, and ongoing support with appropriate referrals also form significant components of syndromic case management.

Four main STI syndromic case management algorithms are presented in the following sections. Each one is preceded by a brief overview of the identified syndrome or condition. Consider how effectively each of the algorithms can be further adjusted, simplified, or elaborated on as necessary, to achieve more effective standardized, practical application within that particular area of STI clinical practice. These algorithms are meant as illustrations for critical discussion among teams of sexual healthcare practitioners. They do not supersede any existing national or organizational guidelines or models.

Vaginal Discharge

In healthy women, some amount of vaginal discharge is considered normal (Spence & Melville, 2007). Hormonal fluctuations in the menstrual cycle cause pre- and postovulatory changes in cervical mucus secretions (Eschenbach et al., 2000). Other factors also affect the nature and content of the vaginal secretions, such as lactobacilli metabolizing vaginal epithelial glycogen to maintain the pH ≤ 4.5 from production of lactic acid (Eschenbach et al., 2000; Mitchell, 2004). Another factor is the presence of commensal organisms, including *Candida albicans* and *Staphylococcus aureus* that can colonize, resulting in change in the vaginal discharge. Other vaginal inhabitants, such as anaerobes, diphtheroids, coagulase-negative staphylococci, and α-hemolytic streptococci, can also colonize causing change in the vaginal discharge with adverse consequences (CDC, 2015; Faculty of Sexual and Reproductive Healthcare [FSRH], 2012).

Causal Factors of Abnormal Vaginal Discharge

Causal factors of abnormal vaginal discharge are categorized as infective and noninfective. Infective vaginal discharge may be caused by nonsexually transmitted BV and *Candida albicans*, while the sexually transmitted organisms include *Chlamydia trachomatis, Neisseria gonorrhoeae, Trichomonas vaginalis,* and herpes simplex virus (HSV) (Australian Sexual Health Alliance [ASHA], 2015; WHO, n.d.). Other factors associated with vaginal discharge include cervical polyps, malignant lesions in the genital tract, fistulae, retained objects such as tampons and condoms, and allergic reactions (ASHA, 2015; FSRH, 2012).

- Bacterial vaginosis is reported to be the most frequent cause of abnormal vaginal discharge in women of childbearing age (Hay, 2011; Sherrard et al., 2011; NICE, 2014). BV occurs due to the colonization of mixed organisms displacing the lactobacilli and raising the vaginal pH >4.5. Bacterial vaginosis has also been attributed to *Mycoplasma hominis* and *Mobiluncus* species (Hay, 2011; Sherrard et al., 2011). In view of the lack of evidence substantiating that BV is directly caused by sexual activities or intercourse, this is considered an associated factor rather than a true STI (Hay, 2011).

- An estimated 70–90% of cases of vulvo-vaginal candidiasis (VVC) are reportedly caused by *Candida albicans* (Hay, 2011; Saporiti et al., 2001). VVC is also found to be common among women with certain medical conditions or taking an antibiotic therapy, and therefore it is not categorized as an STI (Hay, 2011; Pirotta et al., 2004; Ray, Ray, george, & Swaminathan, 2011).

- *Chlamydia trachomatis,* which is found to be asymptomatic in 70% of infected women (Dielissen et al., 2013; Hay, 2011; Pattman et al., 2010), causes cervicitis and endometritis with postcoital and intermenstrual bleeding, dyspareunia, lower abdominal pain, and dysuria (Carey & Beagley, 2010; Haggerty et al., 2010; Lazaro, 2013).

- *Neisseria gonorrhoeae* infection is an STI that causes abnormal vaginal discharge and lower abdominal pain (Hatterty et al., 2010), although 50% of infected women are found to be asymptomatic (Bignell & Fitzgerald, 2011; Hay, 2011).

- *Trichomonas vaginalis* causes vulvitis, vaginitis, and cervicitis (ectocervix with the appearance of the surface of strawberry) and gives rise to frothy yellow discharge (Hollman et al., 2010; Sherrard et al., 2014).

It is obvious that various factors contribute to changes in the normal vaginal discharge. Apart from the physiological sources of the normal vaginal discharge and in addition to microorganisms, retained objects can cause abnormality in the vaginal discharge (Pushplata, Devyani, Pyari, & Deo, 2014). Douching, which is found to alter the vaginal flora, may also contribute to changes in the characteristics of the vaginal discharge of women who use this as normal practice of personal hygiene (Hay, 2011).

Main Components in the Syndromic Case Management of Vaginal Discharge

The first step after establishing the woman's reason for the clinic visit is to obtain a detailed history (WHO, 2007). The patient's fears, anxieties, and any misconceptions that she may hold will need to be sensitively addressed during the history taking. Sexual history seeks to explore sexual behaviors and activities, the gender and number of sexual partners, and attitude to and practice of condom use. This information is used to assess the individual's risk of exposure to or of contracting STIs. Higher risk is associated with age under 25 years, multiple sexual partners, or change of sexual partner(s) in the preceding 12 months. Of equal importance, the history should establish the characteristics of the vaginal discharge and determine the nature of the patient's symptoms (ASHA, 2015; WHO, 2007). The sexual history taking should be very thorough to establish the causal factor.

Associated risk factors in sexually active young women include the following:

- Multiple sexual partners in the preceding 3 months
- A new sexual partner in the preceding 3 months
- Current sexual partner with STI
- Being a victim of sexual assault
- Use of inappropriate treatment for STIs (ASHA, 2015; FSRH, 2012; WHO, 2007)

Key factors in establishing the characteristics of vaginal discharge include the following:

- Nature of change in the discharge
- Time since onset (or when first noticed)
- Color
- Odor (ASHA, 2015; FSRH, 2012)

It should also be established how the discharge relates to the menstrual cycle, if relevant. Additionally, the texture (thickness, runniness, and stickiness) and occurrences of the increase in amount of discharge—for example, following sexual intercourse (Lazaro, 2013) should be established.

Related symptoms should be explored: itchiness, nature of dyspareunia (superficial or deep), pain at the vulva, pain in the vagina, dysuria, abnormal bleeding related to the menstrual cycle or postcoital, pelvic/abdominal pain, and fever. It is important to establish what medications or agents have been tried for symptom relief (ASHA, 2015; FSRH, 2012).

Physical Examination

A thorough physical examination should encompass vulval inspection for signs of discharge, vulvitis, lesions, ulceration, or other identifiable changes. Speculum examination allows for inspection of the vaginal walls, cervix, retained objects, and the amount, texture, and color of discharge. If symptoms of upper genital tract infection are present, careful abdominal palpation and pelvic examination may be performed by a clinician (ASHA, 2015; FSRH, 2012; NICE, 2013).

While physical examination may not be considered necessary for all cases (for example, BV or candidiasis) (FSRH, 2012; Lazaro, 2013), women should be encouraged to return without delay if the discharge persists or increases despite the prescribed treatment. However, where the woman's risk of STI is minimal and she does not present any symptoms of upper genital tract infection, an examination may not be considered necessary. Thus, a risk assessment is useful. If the woman rejects the offer of a physical examination, a self-taken vulvovaginal swab may be an acceptable option for NAATs investigation. Although urine is not deemed to be a useful specimen for women, this is considered appropriate for male patients.

If vaginal examination is carried out, a specimen obtained from the lateral vaginal walls should be tested to establish candidiasis pH ≤4.5, *Trichomonas vaginalis* pH >4.5, or BV. If testing for STI is considered, endocervical swab should be taken for chlamydia and gonorrhea. HVS is also performed if indicated (FSRH, 2012). Identified key indications for laboratory testing of vaginal discharge include patient at high risk of acquiring STI, poor response to previous STI treatment, post abortion, postpartum, recent IUD insertion, signs and symptoms indicative of PID, uncertainty about the diagnosis (ASHA, 2015). Thus, the detailed helps to establish care and treatment options that are appropriate for symptom alleviation. If the discharge persists, consider empirical or syndromic case treatment administered to low-risk patients, and the importance with follow-up.

Sexual health practitioners are encouraged to know and understand the specific laboratory tests for which they obtain patient specimens and be able to read and interpret the test results. Additionally practitioners should provide the laboratory with appropriately detailed information for accurate testing, which includes the site from which the specimen was collected, the type of infection suspected, failed treatment, or recurrence of signs and symptoms, current or recent insertion of intrauterine device or system, current or recent pregnancy, recent instrumental procedure, or retained object (ASHA, 2015; FSRH, 2012).

Recommended Treatment for Abnormal Vaginal Discharge Syndrome

Syndromic treatment should cover infections characterized by cervicitis and vaginitis, including gonorrhea, *Chlamydia trachomatis*, *Trichomonas vaginalis*, herpes simplex, BV, and candidiasis (**Figure 6-7**).

The recommendation for treatment of patients who present with abnormal vaginal discharge that is malodorous but without itchiness suggests aiming at BV (FSRH, 2012; Lazaro, 2013):

- Metronidazole 400 mg orally twice daily for 5 to 7 days, or
- Metronidazole 2 g orally as a single dose

For patients who present with abnormal vaginal discharge but no offensive odor, the recommendation suggests treating for candidiasis (FSRH, 2012; Lazaro, 2013):

- Fluconazole 150 mg orally as a single dose, or
- Clotrimazole 500 mg PV as a single dose

It is important for practitioners to thoroughly familiarize themselves and keep up to date with local policy regulations and guidelines for STI care and treatment. This includes patient education and support as well as partner/sexual contacts outreach.

Urethral Discharge Syndrome in Men

Urethral discharge syndrome in men encompasses discharge from the urethra with dysuria and meatal inflammation. Sexually active men who present with obvious urethral discharge are frequently found to have acquired gonorrhea and/or chlamydial infection.

Causal Factors of Urethritis in Men

In addition to urethral discharge the patient may complain of a burning sensation and discomfort during micturition. These are often suggestive of sexually acquired urethral infection. The main causal pathogens are *Neisseria gonorrhoeae* and *Chlamydia trachomatis*, although nonspecific urethritis may also be accompanied by similar symptoms (Richens, 2011). While symptomatic gonorrhea manifests within 2–5 days of exposure (Bignell & Fitzgerald, 2011), chlamydia may manifest in 1–2 weeks. It is important to note that although mild cases of infection may be accompanied by urethral discomfort and dysuria, there would be no urethral discharge. Infrequent causes of urethritis include trichomoniasis, herpes simplex virus infection, *Mycoplasma genitalium* infection, *Escherichia coli*, trauma, or other, rarer, causes (Richens, 2011; WHO, 2005).

Diagnostic Investigations

- Specimens of urethral smear and urine should be obtained and tested for gonorrheal and chlamydial infections.
- Gram stain and culture may be performed if the patient had held the urine for 4 hours or longer before voiding.

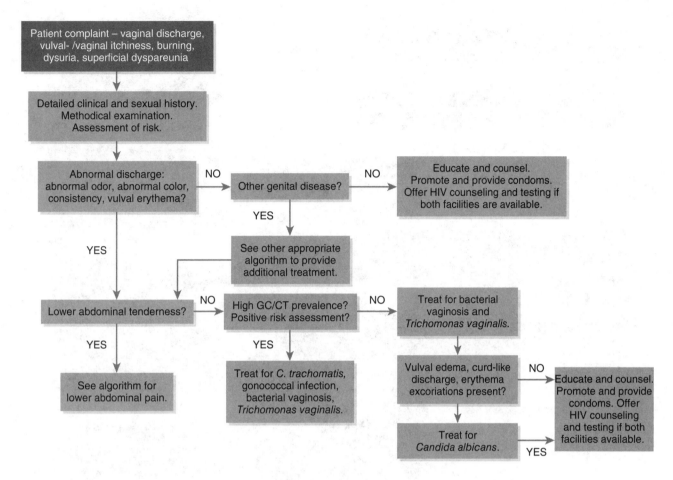

Figure 6-7 Algorithm for Syndromic Case Management of Vaginal Discharge (A Simplified Representation from Varied Sources)

- Treatment should be administered for gonorrhea and chlamydia if urethral gram stain is positive.
- Confirmatory tests should include NAATs performed on the first void urine for gonorrhea and chlamydia (Richens, 2011).

Recommended Syndromic Management of Urethritis in Men

The management of urethritis in men encompasses the following processes. If reliable laboratory facilities are unavailable, the recommended syndromic management should be employed (**Figure 6-8**; Richens, 2011; WHO, 2005). Obtain a detailed clinical and sexual history, then perform a physical examination with careful inspection of the urethral discharge. If necessary, a gentle massage from the base of the penis toward the urethral meatus may be carried out to "milk" the urethra for evidence of discharge (Richens, 2011). If none is obtained due to recent urination, administer empirical treatment if there is evidence that strongly indicates STI (Richens, 2011; WHO, 2005). In organizations that advocate syndromic management, the treatment should cover the main causative pathogens of urethral discharge and dysuria in men, including *Neisseria*

gonorrhoeae and *Chlamydia trachomatis* (Richens, 2011; WHO, 2005). In many centers where syndromic treatment is administered without prior tests, the preferred antimicrobials are the following:

- Ceftriaxone 250 mg intramuscularly stat
- Doxycycline 100 mg orally twice daily for 7 days

In other centers, the antimicrobials administered for *Neisseria gonorrhoeae* and *Chlamydia trachomatis* urethral discharge infections are the following:

- Ciprofloxacin 500 mg intramuscularly stat
- Doxycycline 100 mg orally twice daily for 7 days (Lewis, 2011; Richens, 2011; WHO, 2005)

Prompt treatment has the benefit of symptom relief while also curbing infection transmission. All recent partners should be notified, tested, and given the same treatment. The index patient should be advised to abstain from sexual intercourse until the sexual partner(s) have been tested and treated. If no evidence of gonorrheal infection is detected, azithromycin, doxycycline, or erythromycin may be administered. These are found to be effective against chlamydial infection and other pathogens responsible for

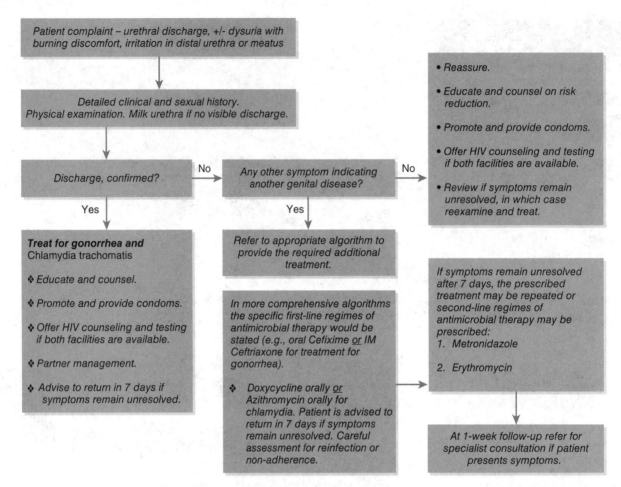

Figure 6-8 Algorithm for Syndromic Case Management of Urethral Discharge in Men (A Simplified Representation from Varied Sources)

nongonococcal urethritis. Possible side effects of doxycycline and erythromycin should be carefully considered and explained to the patient (Richens, 2011; WHO, 2005).

While these regimens are reported to effectively alleviate the symptoms for most patients, some may report persistent symptoms or may present with persistent asymptomatic abnormal discharge and/or smears (Richens, 2011). Where there is an indication, the index patient is carefully reassessed for failed treatment, reinfection, or presence of other causative organisms such as *Trichomonas vaginalis* and *Mycoplasma genitalium* (Richens, 2011).

The decision to repeat, continue, or change the prescribed treatment or await spontaneous resolution should be carefully considered. The patient should be advised and encouraged to return after 7 days if the symptoms remain unresolved (Richens, 2011). Epididymitis is found to be an uncommon complication of untreated urethral infection and should be considered throughout the care and treatment of urethral discharge in men.

Partner management should involve administering similar treatment to all sexual partners in the previous 2 months. This ensures that female sexual partners who are asymptomatic despite infection receive appropriate care, treatment, and support. It is also recommended that female sexual partners be provided with similar treatment and management as prescribed for cervicitis (WHO, 2005).

In the United Kingdom, syndromic treatment without appropriate testing is not deemed to be ideal and may only be considered in certain restricted and justifiable circumstances. In such cases, the recommendation is to obtain specimens for testing before administering antimicrobial treatment (Lazaro, 2013). The recommended empirical treatment administered on the first day of consultation, may comprise the following. For treatment of chlamydiaI Infection:

- Azithromycin 1 g orally as a single dose, or
- Doxycycline orally 100 mg orally twice daily for 7 days

For gonorrheal infection:

- Ceftriaxone 500 mg intramuscularly stat plus azithromycin 1 g orally as a single dose, or
- Cefixime 400 mg orally as a single dose plus azithromycin 1 g orally as a single dose (Bignell & Fitzgerald, 2011)

Patient Information and Partner Considerations

Patients who present with gonorrheal infection require a test of cure following treatment and should be given patient education materials. It is important that partners receive similar information and support. The look-back periods for partners based on the type of infection and manifestation of the urethral symptoms are estimated as follows:

- In symptomatic gonorrheal infections all partners in the previous 2 weeks
- In asymptomatic gonorrheal infections all partners in the previous 3 months
- In symptomatic chlamydial infections, all partners in the previous 4 weeks
- In asymptomatic chlamydial infections, all partners in the previous 6 months (Bignell & Fitzgerald, 2011)

Pelvic Inflammatory Disease (PID)

This section explores the etiology and management of pelvic inflammatory disease (PID). The recommended treatment regimens are evidence based and represent the United Kingdom's exemplar of best practice.

PID comprises varied inflammatory disorders affecting the upper genital tract of females. Sexually active women presenting with lower abdominal pain create a particular challenge in the provision of sexual and reproductive healthcare. Characteristically the mixed manifestations of PID may be associated with any of the common inflammatory disorders including endometritis, salpingitis, tubo-ovarian abscess, parametritis, pelvic peritonitis, and oophoritis (Ross, Judlin, & Jensen, 2014; Ross & McCarthy, 2011; Wiesenfeld et al., 2005). In some cases, the infection originates from the endocervix and ascends into the pelvic cavity (Ross & McCarthy, 2011). Frequently, the inflammatory disorder is caused by common STI micro-organisms, in particular *Neisseria gonorrhoeae* and *Chlamydia trachomatis*, although other multiple mixed organisms may also be present. Various bacterial organisms that habitually thrive in the vagina including streptococci, staphylococci, *E. coli*, and *Haemophilus influenzae* are also found to frequently cause upper genital tract inflammation including endocervical and pelvic infections.

Thus, it is recommended that all women who present with acute PID should have *Chlamydia trachomatis* and *Neisseria gonorrhoeae* testing performed as well as be screened for HIV (Lazaro, 2013). Nonetheless, as Haggerty and Taylor (2011) noted, in up to 70% of patients the etiology remains uncertain and the exact causative organism remains unidentifiable. Evidence suggests that *Mycoplasma genitalium* described as a genital tract microorganism is present in the genital tracts of 15–20% of young females who attend adolescent STI and related clinics in the United States (Huppert et al., 2008). The transmission pattern of this infection among sexual partners substantiates evidence that

Mycoplasma genitalium is a sexually transmissible infection (Thurman et al., 2010; Tosh et al., 2007). Other experts, including Haggerty and Taylor (2011), maintain that there is a convincing connection of *Mycoplasma genitalium* with pelvic inflammatory disease that is unrelated to gonococcal or chlamydial infections (Haggerty & Taylor, 2011; Ross et al., 2014). There is also evidence that implicates the organisms as causing cervicitis, which can progress to endometritis (Gaydos, Maldeis, Hardick, Hardick, & Quinn, 2009; Haggerty 2010; Haggerty & Ness, 2006; McGowin & Anderson-Smits, 2011). Long-term reproductive disorders, including tubal-related infertility (Haggerty et al., 2010; Jaiyeoba & Soper, 2011) with elevated *Mycoplasma genitalium* antibody titers, have also been reported (Haggerty & Taylor, 2011). Furthermore, there is evidence that the organisms can cause resistance to many PID antimicrobial treatment regimens and may be associated with failed response to cephoxitin and doxycycline treatments (Haggerty et al., 2008). The evidence from different sources substantiate that *Mycoplasma genitalium* is a relatively common cause of upper genital tract infection and cervicitis.

Risk Factors Associated with PID

The main PID risk factors are sexual risk-taking behaviors such as young age group, multiple sexual partners, frequent changes with recent new partner within the preceding 3 months, and history of STIs in the patient and/or sexual partner (Ross et al., 2014). Other potential risk factors include termination of pregnancy, insertion of IUD in the preceding 6 weeks, and procedures such as in vitro fertilization and hysterosalpingography (Ross et al., 2014).

Characteristics, Symptoms, and Signs of Pelvic Inflammatory Disease (PID)

The main symptoms of PID include the following:

- Lower abdominal pain, which is typically bilateral
- Deep dyspareunia
- Abnormal vaginal bleeding, which may be inter-menstrual, menorrhagia
- Postcoital vaginal or cervical discharge that may be purulent (Royal College of Obstetricians and Gynaecologists [RCOG], 2009; Ross & McCarthy, 2011)

Identified clinical signs may include the following:

- Fever >38°C with or without general malaise (WHO, 2005; Ross, 2011)
- Bilateral lower abdominal tenderness
- Vaginal examination may reveal adnexal tenderness Cervical motion tenderness on bimanual vaginal examination (CDC, 2015; RCOG, 2009; Ross & McCarthy, 2011)

Differential Diagnosis

In making a differential diagnosis the general view is to relate the details from the history to relevant findings from the clinical examination. Ectopic pregnancy should be carefully ruled out. In this case, the patient presents with a history of amenorrhea. Acute appendicitis in which the pain is typically unilateral and often accompanied by nausea and vomiting is reported in only 50% of patients presenting with PID. Endometriosis is characterized by a history of chronic symptoms related to the menstrual cycle while complications associated with ovarian cyst such as rupture or torsion are characterized by sudden onset. Urinary tract infection (UTI) may be associated with lower abdominal pain, although this is typically accompanied by frequency of micturition and dysuria. Patients who present with functional pain of unknown origin tend to have a prolonged history, and irritable bowel syndrome is characterized by previous history of bowel complaints (Lazaro, 2013; Ross, 2011; Ross et al., 2014; WHO, 2005).

Possible Associated Complications

Opinions vary regarding the management of possible complications. Tubo-ovarian abscesses and pelvic peritonitis are reported to be the main complications of PID (Ross et al., 2014). Apart from the lower abdominal pain and fever, ultrasound scanning may be used to identify the abscess. Right upper quadrant pain associated with perihepatitis (Fitz-Hugh-Curtis syndrome) has been reported in some patients who present with PID. However, in view of limited evidence from clinical trials to substantiate recommendations beyond those for uncomplicated PID, the treatment has involved laparoscopic division of hepatic adhesions (Ross & McCarthy, 2011; Ross et al., 2014). HIV-positive women present with more severe symptoms but respond effectively to the recommended antimicrobial therapy (Mugo et al., 2006). Women who present with PID while having intrauterine contraceptive device in situ require careful consideration regarding removal of the device (Altunyurt, Demir, & Posaci, 2003). The aim is to achieve better treatment outcome symptoms alleviation in the short term. However, the risk of pregnancy must be carefully ruled out and some may consider it appropriate to prescribe emergency contraception as deemed necessary.

Range of Diagnostic investigations for PID

The clinical manifestation of PID may present as symptomatic or asymptomatic. However, signs and symptoms are found to have low specificity and sensitivity and clinical diagnosis of this condition is found to be vague (Jaiyeoba & Soper, 2011). The positive predictive value is estimated at 65–90% compared to laparoscopic diagnosis (Ross et al., 2014).

While positive result of laboratory testing for *Neisseria gonorrhoeae* and *Chlamydia trachomatis* adequately confirms a diagnosis of PID, negative result does not necessarily rule out this diagnosis (CDC, 2015). Raised erythrocyte sedimentation rate (ESR) and raised C-reactive protein also support the diagnosis in terms of assessing PID severity.

This may not be entirely consistent, as normal values may occur in mild and moderate infections (CDC, 2015; Jaiyeoba & Soper, 2011). Moreover, although the absence of pus cells in the endocervix or vagina presents adequate predictive value of 95% for PID diagnosis, the presence of pus cells only presents a predictive value of around 17% (Yudin et al., 2003).

Specialist Investigative Procedures

Laparoscopic examination may be considered as a useful diagnostic procedure for revealing abnormalities that indicate pelvic inflammatory disease. In some women, endometritis may be the only etiologic factor for diagnosing PID, and therefore, endometrial biopsy may be considered for women undergoing laparoscopy. Histology on tissue from endometrial biopsy is considered by some clinicians as the most decisive factor for confirming endometritis in the diagnosis of PID. However, these methods are found to be associated with various limitations and are not routinely employed for diagnosing PID (Ross et al., 2014). Other more sophisticated diagnostic methods have also been described, such as transvaginal sonography or magnetic resonance imaging (MRI), which may reveal thickened uterine tubes filled with fluid and the presence of free fluid in the pelvic cavity with tubo-ovarian involvement. Doppler technique may also show tubal hyperemia (CDC, 2015; Jaiyeoba & Soper, 2011). Nevertheless, these are not routinely employed in many centers due to various resource implications including sustainable funding, equipment, technological support, specialist expertise, training, and supervision.

Main Components of the Management Interventions

The importance of early detection and prompt treatment must be recognized due to the risk of long-term consequences from delayed medical intervention. Ectopic pregnancy, infertility, and persistent pelvic pain have been reported, and because there is no definitive diagnostic criteria, low threshold for empirical treatment of PID is recognized (CDC, 2015; NICE, 2015; Ross & McCarthy, 2011). Current practice advocates that PID should be suspected and prompt empirical treatment offered to any sexually active young woman <25 years of age who presents with bilateral lower abdominal pain and tenderness on vaginal examination. The aim is to prescribe broad-spectrum antibiotic treatment regimens to eliminate both *Neisseria gonorrhoeae* and *Chlamydia trachomatis* (NICE, 2015). It is important, of course, to rule out pregnancy in all cases.

History and Physical Examination

A detailed history should explore the personal medical and surgical history, current medications, and allergy. Key elements in gynecological history should include the menstrual cycle and date of last menstrual period to exclude pregnancy (bearing in mind the risk of ectopic pregnancy), history of previous abortions, abnormal vaginal discharge, and abnormal vaginal bleeding. Sexual history should explore the types of contraception used and history of previous or current STIs (Lazaro, 2013; NICE, 2015). The differential diagnoses as previously outlined should be carefully examined to rule out each condition. Physical examination should encompass abdominal exam, speculum exam, and bimanual exam (Lazaro, 2013; Ross & McCarthy, 2011; Ross et al., 2014).

Clinical Criteria for PID Diagnosis

Cervical motion tenderness, uterine tenderness, and adnexal tenderness may be determinant factors for PID diagnosis. Other criteria include oral temperature 38.3°C (101°F), abnormal vaginal/cervical mucopurulent discharge, abundant white blood cells on saline microscopy of vaginal fluid, elevated erythrocyte sedimentation rate, and elevated level of C-reactive protein. High vaginal swab and endocervical swab should be obtained for laboratory investigations for gonorrhea and chlamydia (CDC, 2015; Gradison, 2012; NICE, 2015).

Laboratory Investigations and Additional Diagnostic Considerations

Pregnancy test should be performed, and UTI should also be excluded (NICE, 2015). STIs should be tested for; in particular, *Neisseria gonorrhoeae* and *Chlamydia tracomatis*. While NAATs should be performed on endocervical and vulvovaginal specimens swab for gonococcal culture test should be sent immediately to the lab prior to commencement of the antimicrobial treatment regimen. This allows for detecting antimicrobial or antibiotic resistance (Lazaro, 2013; NICE, 2015). NAATs may also be performed on first-void urine specimen for *Chlamydia trachomatis*, although urine is not considered to be an ideal specimen to test for this in women. Blood samples should also be obtained for laboratory testing for HIV and syphilis infections (Lazaro, 2013; NICE, 2015).

Factors that Influence Decisions about the Treatment Regimens

As Ross and McCarthy (2011) noted, influencing factors such as cost must be carefully considered regarding the types of antimicrobial drugs available for the treatment. Epidemiology also influences the nature of demand for treatment. Moreover, antimicrobial efficacy may influence the treatment decision. The particular strains of organisms, evidence of antimicrobial sensitivity, and emerging drug resistance in the particular area should also be carefully examined as influencing factors. It is also important to anticipate the severity of the disease when contracted and therefore the dosages of antimicrobial regimens required to achieve effective cure. The possibility of recurrences or reinfections requiring repeat treatments should also be taken into consideration. Personal preferences influenced by tolerance and possible side effects of specific drugs may affect individuals' treatment compliance. It is important to

gain patient cooperation by providing pertinent information, advice and support to encourage compliance with the prescribed treatment regimen.

Practical therapeutic Advice

Depending on the severity of the disease, the patient should be advised to rest and prescribed effective pain relief. Patients diagnosed with mild or moderate PID may be provided outpatient treatment. Explain to patients what PID involves, possible causes, the treatment and possible long-term consequences. Implications for the individual's personal and sexual health and that of the sexual partner should be explained and they should be strongly encouraged to abstain from sexual intercourse. The importance of fulfilling this advice until they have both completed the treatment regimen and follow-up program should be emphasized (CDC, 2015; NICE, 2015; Ross & McCarthy, 2011). For patients who present with severe illness accompanied by fever >38°C, clinical evidence of tubo-ovarian abscess, or clinical evidence of pelvic peritonitis, parenteral IV antimicrobial treatment may be considered (Ross & McCarthy, 2011; Ross et al., 2014).

Key Elements in the Information Provided

The patient should be given information regarding the prescribed antimicrobial treatment and the possible side effects. It should be explained that fertility may not be affected, but do not withhold the risk of potential complications. The patient should be made aware of the potential risk of future infertility, ectopic pregnancy, and chronic pelvic pain (NICE, 2015; Ross & McCarthy, 2011). The risk of possible complications is greater in more severe PID, and repeat episodes also increase the risk of infertility. Therefore, consistent and correct use of barrier contraception should be strongly emphasized and key information should be reinforced by clearly written explanations and guidance (NICE, 2015; Ross & McCarthy, 2011).

The decision for hospital admission may be influenced by the need to administer parenteral treatment, carry out closer observation, perform further investigation, and possible surgical intervention (NICE, 2015; Ross & McCarthy, 2011). Other factors include failed or poor response to oral antimicrobial therapy; PID with severe illness accompanied by nausea, vomiting, and high fever; the patient's inability to tolerate the oral antimicrobial drugs, or poor treatment compliance (NICE, 2015; Ross, 2011; Ross & McCarthy, 2011). Intravenous administration of the antimicrobial drug should be continued for 24 hours after improvement of the clinical signs and symptoms, then changed to oral administration. Although the efficacy of the different antimicrobials has been reported to be comparable, slight adjustments in the recommended dosages may be influenced by organizational regulations. Additionally, while there is no stipulation regarding the duration of the treatment regimens, findings from clinical trials indicate that 10–14 days of treatment produces observable response as anticipated (Ross et al., 2014).

Recommended Evidence-Based Treatment Regimens

The prescribed regimen for outpatient treatment may comprise the following:

- Ceftriaxone 500 mg intramuscularly as a single dose followed by
- Doxycycline 100 mg orally twice daily **plus** metronidazole 400 mg orally twice daily for 14 days (Ness et al., 2005; Ross & McCarthy, 2011), **or**
- Ofloxacin 400 mg orally twice daily for 14 days or levofloxacin 500 mg once daily for 14 days, **plus** metronidazole 400 mg orally twice daily for 14 days (Lazaro, 2013; Ross & McCarthy, 2011)

The benefit of metronidazole in the treatment regimen is to cover for anaerobic bacteria, which play a significant role in severe PID. This treatment can be stopped in patients with mild or moderate PID who are unable to tolerate it (Ross & McCarthy, 2011). Due to increasing quinolone resistance in the United Kingdom, the suggestion is to omit ofloxacin and moxifloxacin from the treatment regimen of those patients who are at high risk of gonococcal PID. These include the patient who presents with clinically severe PID, had sexual contact abroad, or has a sexual partner with gonorrhea. Moreover, it is cautioned that quinolone should be avoided in the empirical treatment regimen for PID in areas where >5% of cases have been attributed to *Neisseria gonorrhoeae* resistant strain (Ross & McCarthy, 2011). The once-daily dosage of levofloxacin may be prescribed as an alternative to ofloxacin (Judlin et al., 2010).

The recommended alternative regimens include the following:

- Ceftriaxone 500 mg intramuscularly as a single dose followed by
- Azithromycin 1 g orally once per week for 2 weeks

Or, if allergy or intolerance is reported use the following:

- Moxifloxacin 400 mg orally once daily for 14 days; this should be used with great caution due to reported risks, including hepatic reactions (Ross & McCarthy, 2011)

Recommended inpatient regimens for PID include the following:

- Ceftriaxone 2 g intravenously daily, **plus**
- Doxycycline 100 mg intravenously twice daily **followed by**
  - Doxycycline 100 mg orally twice daily, **plus**
  - Metronidazole 400 mg orally three times daily for 14 days total (Ross & McCarthy, 2011)

- Clindamycin 900 mg intravenously three times daily, **plus**
- Gentamycin 2 mg/kg loading dose (levels of this drug should be carefully monitored) **followed by**
  - Gentamycin 1.5 mg/kg three times daily (this may be substituted by a single daily dose of 7 g/kg) **followed by *either***
    - Clindamycin 450 mg orally four times daily, **or**
    - Doxycycline 100 mg twice daily, **plus**
    - Metronidazole 400 mg orally twice daily to complete 14 days

Alternative regimens include the following:

- Ofloxacin 400 mg intravenously twice daily, **plus**
- Metronidazole 500 mg intravenously three times daily for 14 days, **or**
- Ciprofloxacin 200 mg intravenously twice daily, **plus**
- Doxycycline 100 mg intravenously or orally twice daily, **plus**
- Metronidazole 500 mg intravenously three times daily for 14 days (Ross & McCarthy, 2011)

Laparoscopy may be performed to drain pelvic abscess.

Management of Sexual Partners and Follow Up

The recommendation is to offer the male sexual partners advice and screening for gonorrhea and chlamydia. The male sexual partner diagnosed with these infections should receive similar treatment at the same time as the index patient. However, if it is not possible to screen for gonorrhoea, antibiotics that are particularly effective against gonorrhea may be administered, such as ceftriaxone 500 mg intramuscularly (Ross & McCarthy, 2011). Additionally, depending on the patient's sexual history, all other recent sexual contacts over the period of 6 months of the onset of symptoms should be traced and offered similar screening (Ross & McCarthy, 2011). Because many cases of gonorrhea may not be caused by *Neisseria gonorrhoeae* or *Chlamydia trachomatis*, the recommendation is to offer male sexual partners empirical treatment with broad-spectrum antibiotics; for example, azithromycin 1 g orally as a single dose (Ross & McCarthy, 2011).

Follow-Up

For patients who presented with clinical symptoms and signs of moderate or severe PID, a review in 72 hours is advocated (Ross & McCarthy, 2011). With effective treatment, considerable improvement in the patient's condition should be apparent. Failed treatment may be dealt with by performing further investigations, administering parenteral antimicrobial treatment, and considering surgical intervention as necessary. Further review may be carried out after 2–4 weeks of the treatment to assess the patient's compliance with the treatment regimen, the extent of response to the treatment, and the progress with partner management (Ross & McCarthy, 2011). Patients who present with persistent infection may be retested for *Neisseria gonorrheae* and *Chlamydia trachomatis* as well as performing antimicrobial resistance test for gonorrhea. Thus, three key elements that should be assessed include the patient's compliance, patterns of recurrence, and re-infection. The ensuing section presents an illustration of the stages employed in the syndromic case management of lower abdominal pain/PID together with the treatment regimen provided (**Figure 6-9**).

The treatment regimens employed in different countries for syndromic management vary in terms of the specific antibiotic drugs and the prescribed dosages. For example, outpatient treatment regimen may comprise the following:

- Ceftriaxone 500 mg intramuscularly as a single dose, **or**
- Cefoxitin 2 g intramuscularly as a single dose with probenecid 1 g orally as a single dose, **followed by**
  - Doxycycline 100 mg orally twice daily, **plus**
    - Metronidazole 400 mg orally twice daily for 14 days
- Ofloxacin 400 mg orally twice daily may be prescribed, **plus**
  - Metronidazole 500 mg orally twice daily for 14 days (Ross et al., 2014)

Levofloxacin 500 mg once daily may be prescribed instead of ofloxacin (Judlin et al., 2010).

Inpatient treatment regimen may comprise the following:

- Cefoxitin 2 g intravenously four times daily, **or**
- Cefotetan 2 g intravenously twice daily, **or**
- Ceftriaxone 1 g intravenously/ intramuscularly once daily plus doxycycline 100 mg intravenously twice daily **followed by**
  - Doxycycline 100 mg orally twice daily, **plus**
    - Metronidazole 400 mg orally twice daily to complete 14 days (Ross et al., 2014)
- Clindamycin 900 mg intravenously three times daily, **plus**
  - Gentamycin 2 mg/kg loading dose followed by 1.5 mg/kg three times daily **followed by** *either*
    - Clindamycin 450 mg orally four times daily, **or**
    - Doxycycline 100 mg orally twice daily to complete 14 days, **plus**
      - Metronidazole 400 mg orally twice daily to complete 14 days (CDC, 2015; Ross, 2011; Ross et al., 2014)

Sexual health practitioners are encouraged to examine the algorithm critically, discuss with colleagues, and make necessary adjustments to enhance its usefulness. Adjustments

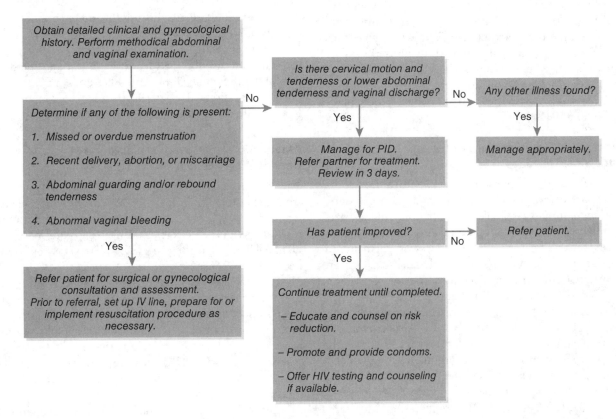

Figure 6-9 Algorithm for Syndromic Case Management of Lower Abdominal Pain in Women (A Simplified Representation)

should reflect staff competenties, allocated funding, and available resources and facilities.

Genital Ulcer Disease

The most frequent etiological factors associated with genital ulcer disease (GUD) are the genital herpes simplex viruses HSV-1 and HSV-2 (BASHH, 2014; Patel et al., 2011). The *Treponema pallidum* of syphilis (Eccleston et al., 2008; French, 2011), *Haemophilus ducreyi* of chancroid (Roett, Mayor, & Uduhiri, 2012), and *Chlamydia trachomatis* LGV serovars L1, L2, and L3 are also implicated. Characteristically, genital, anal, and perianal ulcers tend to be caused by concurrent infectious conditions, particularly herpes and syphilis together (Roett et al., 2012). Genital herpes, syphilis, and chancroid are attributed to high risk of HIV transmission. Moreover, GUD clinical manifestations and disease patterns are atypical in HIV-positive patients (CDC, 2010, 2015; WHO, 2005).

Detailed History

Patient history should establish lesion characteristics, such as appearance, duration of manifestation, recent use of systemic or topical agents, pain, tenderness, and history of similar manifestation. Medical history should include HIV status skin eruptions, allergic reactions, and current medications.

Related issues in the sexual history may include the gender and number of sexual partners, venue where the sexual partners are met, intercourse with commercial sex workers, sexual partners/contacts with symptoms and signs of GUD, and partners with diagnosed HSV or recently diagnosed with syphilis. Key elements relating to travel history include countries visited and venues where sexual risk-taking activities and intercourse took place (Roett et al., 2012).

Characteristic Manifestations of Lesions in Genital Ulcer Disease

Physical exam identifies the presence, nature, and characteristic appearance of genital, anal, and perineal ulcers. Practitioners should assess ulcer distribution, number, size, and tenderness. Lumph nodes should also be examined for enlargement and tenderness. Other necessary elements to include are the skin, mouth, palms of hands, soles of feet, and cardiovascular and neurological systems (Eccleston et al., 2008; French, 2011; Roett et al., 2012).

Depending on the etiologic factor, the ulcers may appear as erosive, pustular, vesicles, or papules, often accompanied by inguinal lymphadenopathy (Eccleston et al., 2008; French, 2011). Herpes lesions tend to be painful grouped vesicles with an erythematous base; and the patients present with fever and malaise accompanied by muscle aches (Cohen & Mayer, 2007; Roett et al., 2012). Syphilis lesions appear as painless indurated ulcers with serous exudate. In more than

70% of cases, there is only a single lesion (French, 2011). Chancroid lesions have the characteristic appearance of single or multiple, nonindurated painful anogenital ulcers with a purulent base (Roett et al., 2012). There is usually contact bleeding, and inguinal lymphadenopathy may be present. This manifestation is usually unilateral (Patel & Gupta, 2011; Roett et al., 2012). Associated complications include ulceration with extensive destruction of the affected tissue, development of inguinal abscess (bubo), and chronic suppurative sinuses (Patel & Gupta, 2011).

Granuloma Inguinale (Donovanosis)

Granuloma inguinale (donovanosis) is a genital ulcerative disease reported to be prevalent in certain developing countries including India, Papua New Guinea, the Caribbean, central Australia, and South Africa (O'Farrell, 2002). The responsible organism is *Klebsiella granulomatis* (previously, *Calymmatobacterium granulomatis*). Secondary bacterial infection can occur and concomitance with other sexually transmitted microorganisms has also been reported (CDC, 2010, 2015; Patel & Gupta, 2011). The characteristic ulcers are slowly progressive, painless ulcerative lesions that develop on the genitals or on the perineum, and there is no regional lymphadenopathy. The lesions are granulomatous, highly vascular, and bleed easily on contact (CDC, 2010, 2015; Roett et al., 2012). Variations in the clinical manifestation are described as hypertrophic, necrotic, and sclerotic (Roett et al., 2012), and extra-genital manifestations can extend to pelvic structures and spread to involve intra-abdominal organs, the mouth, and the bones (Cohen & Mayer, 2012; Patel & Gupta, 2011; Roett et al., 2012). Diagnosis of granuloma inguinale is made by examining cellular material obtained from the lesion and the detection of dark-staining Donovan bodies on biopsy and tissue crush preparation (CDC, 2010, 2015; Patel & Gupta, 2011; Roett et al., 2012).

Diagnostic Tests Covering the Range of Genital Ulcer Disease

The diagnostic laboratory tests include routine swabs taken from the lesions for culture for HSV or polymerase chain reaction test, where facilities are available and if national regulations permit (CDC, 2010, 2015; Patel & Gupta, 2011). The PCR testing in HSV diagnosis is reported to be 96–100% sensitive with specificity of 97–98% (CDC, 2010, 2015; Patel & Gupta, 2011).

Serous fluid from the lesion may be sent for dark-field microscopy or direct fluorescent antibody testing for syphilis if facilities are available. Other syphilis serologic nontreponemal tests may include the venereal disease research laboratory (VDRL) test, rapid plasma reagin test, or treponemal-specific enzyme immunoassay (CDC, 2010, 2015; Patel & Gupta, 2011).

Diagnostic tests for chancroid include microscopy and culture, although the sensitivity of these tests is reported to be rather poor. PCR test may be performed where facilities are available and if national regulations permit (CDC, 2010, 2015; Patel & Gupta, 2011; Roett et al., 2012).

Biopsy of the genital, anal, and perianal ulcers may be considered to detect rare and atypical etiologic factors as causes of the ulcers or in cases of failed response to the prescribed treatment regimen. HIV testing is also recommended for all patients/clients who present with genital, anal, and perianal ulcers if they are not already known to have acquired HIV infection (CDC, 2010, 2015; Patel & Gupta, 2011; Roett et al., 2012).

The patient's personal and sexual history may indicate the necessity to obtain a swab from the lesion for culture or NAATs. This is particularly important for *Chlamydia trachomatis* detection in MSM. Positive result from the *Chlamydia trachomatis* serotesting should be an indication for serovar-specific testing to be carried out for lymphogranuloma venereum (CDC, 2010, 2015; Patel & Gupta, 2011). Genital swabs or bubo aspirate may be obtained for culture for *Chlamydia trachomatis* serovars L1, L2, L3, and/or for direct immunofluorescence or NAATs (Roett et al., 2012; Workowski et al., 2010).

Despite the various diagnostic tests, no pathogenic cause is found in up to 25% of cases of genital ulcer disease (Low et al., 2006). However, it is recommended that sexual partners who have had intercourse with the patient diagnosed with donovanosis within the preceding 60 days prior to the onset of the patient's symptoms should be examined and offered the recommended empirical treatment.

Recommended Syndromic Antibiotic Treatment Regimens

Syndromic management of GUD depends on epidemiological factors; in particular, the prevalence of certain infecting conditions within specified communities. That is, the causative organisms for GUD vary by geographical area and may continually evolve. Differential diagnosis then becomes difficult in areas where there are multiple causative organisms reported.

Moreover, concurrent infections with HIV infection alter the clinical manifestations of GUD. Therefore, once the physical exam confirms GUD, the treatment regimen should target the prevalent etiologic infective organisms and take into account patterns of organism antibiotic sensitivity and resistance (Cohen & Mayer, 2007; Roett et al., 2010; WHO, 2014).

Thus, in areas with a high prevalence of syphilis and chancroid, the principle is to treat patients who present with genital ulcers for both conditions. If granuloma inguinale is also prevalent in that area, treatment for that condition should be incorporated into the therapeutic regimen.

The recommended antibiotic may be administered at the initial clinic visit so that nonreturners would have received therapy during that clinic attendance. Likewise, if lymphogranuloma venereum is also prevalent, the appropriate antibiotic therapy should be incorporated into the treatment regimen (Cohen & Mayer, 2007; Roett et al., 2012).

In this way, a combination of therapies may target syphilis, chancroid, and HSV-2 in a particular country, while in another geographic area patients may require treatment of syphilis, chancroid, HSV-2, and lymphogranuloma venereum. Genital HSV-2 is reportedly the most common cause of GUD in areas where HIV infection is endemic. In those HIV prevalent areas, both HSV-2 and HIV infective organisms frequently occur concurrently, and the atypical genital HSV ulcers are found to persist for longer periods in the HIV-infected patients.

Although there is no specific treatment for HSV-2, antiviral therapy with acyclovir may curtail the duration of active disease and control or decrease transmission (WHO, 2005). In locations where economic constraints create drug shortage or otherwise curtail accessibility, treatment may be reserved for patients with severe HSV-2 or herpes zoster infection. These two infections are high risk factors for HIV transmission (WHO, 2005).

Recommended Syndromic Treatment for Syphilis

- Benzathine penicillin 2.4 million IU intramuscularly as a single dose (divided into two doses and administered at separate sites)

Alternative antibiotic treatment for syphilis:

- Procaine, benzylpenicillin 1.2 million IU intramuscularly once daily for 10 days

Alternative antibiotic treatment for the penicillin allergic:

- Doxycycline 100 mg orally twice daily for 15 days, **or**
- Tetracycline 500 mg orally four times daily for 15 days, **plus**
- Recommended syndromic treatment for chancroid where etiologicaly prevalent:
  - Ciprofloxacin 500 mg orally twice daily for 3 days, **or**
  - Erythromycin 500 mg orally four times daily for 7 days, **or**
  - Azithromycin 1 g orally as a single dose

Alternative antibiotic treatment for chancroid:

- Ceftriaxone 250 mg intramuscularly as a single dose, **plus**
- Recommended syndromic treatment for lymphogranuloma venereum where etiologicaly prevalent:
  - Doxycycline 100 mg orally twice daily for 14 days, **or**
  - Erythromycin 500 mg orally four times daily for 14 days
- Alternative antibiotic treatment for lymphogranuloma venereum:

- Tetracycline 500 mg orally four times daily for 14 days with inclusion of:
- Recommended syndromic treatment for HSV-2:
  ○ Acyclovir 400 mg orally three times daily for 7–10 days
- Recommended syndromic treatment for granuloma inguinale:
  ○ Azithromycin 1 g orally first day and 500 mg once daily, **or**
  ○ Doxycycline 100 mg orally twice daily for 21 days
- Alternative antibiotic treatment for granuloma inguinale:
  ○ Erythromycin 500 mg orally four times daily for 21 days, **or**
  ○ Tetracycline 500 mg orally four times daily for 21 days with inclusion of:
  ○ Recommended syndromic treatment for HSV-2:
  ○ Acyclovir 400 mg orally three times daily for 7–10 days

For penicillin allergy, if not pregnant, doxycycline or tetracycline may be prescribed.
(Roett et al., 2012)

Recommended Syndromic Treatment for Inguinal Buboes

Buboes are painful, tender swollen lymph nodes in the groin (inguinal or femoral) and tend to be fluctuant. Buboes commonly manifest in patients with chancroid or lymphogranuloma venereum. However, they may also be associated with other lower limb or systemic infections. The recommendation is to aspirate the fluctuant lymph nodes through a healthy part of the skin and no attempt should be made to perform incision and drainage or lymph node excision.

Syndromic antibiotic treatment may comprise the following:

- Ciprofloxacin 500 mg orally twice daily for 3 days, **plus**
- Doxycycline 100 mg orally twice daily for 14 days, **or**
- Erythromycin 500 mg orally four times daily for 14 days

Special Considerations in Syndromic Case Management of Gud

Coexisting Genital Ulcer Disease and HIV Infection

Evidence suggests that the natural course and progression of syphilis becomes altered when there is coexisting HIV infection. The characteristic primary and secondary lesions become altered and there is an increased rate of failed or ineffective single-dose penicillin treatment (Roett et al., 2012).

In HIV-infected patients with chancroid, the lesions are found to be more widespread, compound, and destructive in nature and may be accompanied by symptoms of malaise, pyrexia, and chills. Treatment failure is also reported with single-dose antibiotic therapy. In HIV-infected patients with herpes simplex infection, the lesions in HIV-infected patients tend to be compound and persist for longer durations, in contrast to the self-limiting vesicles that manifest in immunocompetent individuals. Thus, antiviral therapy is recommended as early as possible (Patel & Gupta, 2011).

There is no specific difference in the treatment of patients with granuloma inguinale and HIV infection and those who are HIV-negative; the same treatment regimen is recommended in both cases. Administration of carefully calculated aminoglycoside parenterally (gentamicin administered intravenously) may be considered as an additional component of the treatment regimen for granuloma inguinale (Patel & Gupta, 2011). Special consideration is necessary where no improvement is observed despite the treatment and for patients who present with concurrent infections of granuloma inguinale and HIV.

Patients with HSV should be advised on appropriate care of the lesions to keep them clean and dry. The patient should be advised to return in 7 days for review or return without delay if the lesions fail to heal or worsen despite the treatment.

In all cases, the patient should be provided with clear explanations, counseling, and education including consistent condom use and/or abstention from sexual intercourse until the lesions heal completely. Importantly, compliance with the antibiotic treatment regimen should be emphasized. Management of sexual partners is recommended, although the benefit of empiric treatment of asymptomatic individuals has not been adequately substantiated by evidence from randomized controlled trials.

Synoptic Outline of the Management of Genital Ulcer Disease

- Recommended treatment for syphilis and chancroid should be offered.
- Genital herpes treatment should be offered, and treatment of HSV-2 offered in areas where the prevalence of HSV-2 is 30% or higher.
- Taking account of local epidemiological trends, the recommended empiric treatment for granuloma inguinale (donovanosis) should be included with treatment for lymphogranuloma venereum.
- Patient education and support should emphasize the importance of keeping ulcers clean and dry.
- Aspiration of fluctuant glands should be performed by a clinician.
- Education and counseling should be provided with emphasis on compliance with the treatment regimen to reduce the risk of transmission and reinfection.

- Correct and consistent condom usage should be promoted together with supply of condoms.
- Depending on availability of appropriate facilities and resources, HIV serological testing together with counseling support should be offered.
- Patients should be encouraged to return in 7 days if lesions are not completely healed or to return immediately if clinical symptoms worsen.
- Support and assistance should be provided for partner treatment and management. (Partly draws on WHO, 2005.)

Following is an algorithm for syndromic management of genital ulcer disease in males and females (**Figure 6-10**). This can be adapted to incorporate national or local treatment regimens or supplemented by separate boxed dialogues with guidelines for treatment of specific genital ulcers. The recommended empiric treatment should be offered for primary and recurrent HSV infections. If characteristic syphilitic ulcerating lesions are detected, primary syphilis should be suspected even if the initial serologic test result is negative.

Repeat serologic testing is important and should be carried out in 2–4 weeks. If there is doubt about the individual's compliance with the follow-up, the recommended empirical treatment should be offered initially. Similarly, in suspected LGV infection, the recommended empirical treatment should be offered at the initial visit. In all cases of ulcerating STIs, treatment of sexual partners should form an important component of the case management.

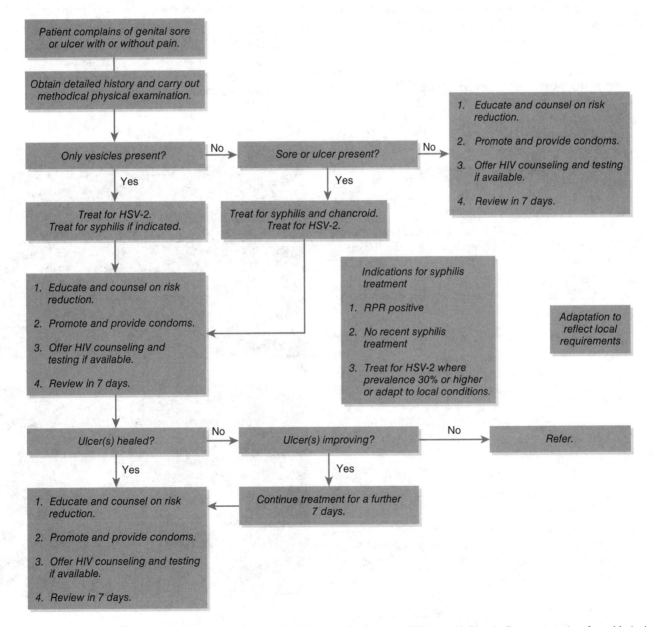

Figure 6-10 Algorithm for the Management of Genital Ulcer Disease in Men and Women (A Simple Representation from Varied Sources)

The Function of Algorithms in Syndromic Management of STI/RTIs

The emergence of syndromic management of STI/RTIs has received mixed opinions over the years. To be successful the format should be functional and reflect optimal efficiency in navigating clearly defined stages of STI/RTI management. It is important that practitioners perceive it as a useful and pragmatic means of implementing a standardized approach to STI/RTI care provision to encourage commitment to its use. Involving practitioners in the development of such algorithms engenders shared ownership, enhanced motivation, correct application, regular evaluations, and updates as appropriate.

Nonetheless, common key elements in the standard syndromic algorithms comprise the patient/client's complaint, physical examination, treatment, health promotion/education, and counseling.

Human Immunodeficiency Virus (HIV)

In the United States in 2011, approximately 16% of the estimated 1.2 million persons infected with HIV were unaware of their infection (Workowski & Bolan, 2015). HIV-positive individuals who are unaware of their sero status are believed to be accountable for 45% of new U.S. infections (Del Rio, 2015). Despite the availability of effective antiretroviral therapy (ART), many cases of HIV infection are not diagnosed until advanced stages. Across the United States, 32% of persons with HIV are diagnosed with AIDS at or within 12 months of their initial HIV diagnosis (Workowski & Bolan, 2015).

The CDC has the following specific recommendations that apply to testing for HIV infection:

- HIV testing must be voluntary and free from any coercion.

- Clients must be notified that HIV screening will be done, unless the person declines (opt-out screening).

- General informed consent for medical care is sufficient to establish informed consent for HIV testing (a separate signed consent specific for HIV testing is not required).

- Use of antigen/antibody combination tests is encouraged (even though results take longer) unless individuals are unlikely to receive their HIV results.

- Providers need to be aware of the possibility of acute HIV infection and perform an antigen/antibody immunoassay or HIV RNA test in conjunction with an antibody test.

- Persons newly diagnosed with HIV need to be supported and informed regarding the importance of receiving prompt care, and the highly effective nature of ART treatment. They need to be immediately referred to a healthcare provider or facility experienced in caring for persons with HIV. (Workowski & Bolan, 2015)

Human Immunodeficiency Virus (HIV) Screening

The CDC recommends the following screening guidelines:

- All women ages 13–64 (opt-out)

- All women who seek evaluation and treatment for STIs

- All pregnant women at their first prenatal visit (opt-out)

- Retest all pregnant women in the third trimester, especially if at high risk (opt-out)

- All men aged 13–64 (opt-out)

- All men who seek evaluation and treatment for STIs

- All MSM at least annually for sexually active MSM with HIV status that is unknown or negative and the client himself or his sex partner(s) has had more than one sex partner since the most recent HIV test (**Figure 6–11**)

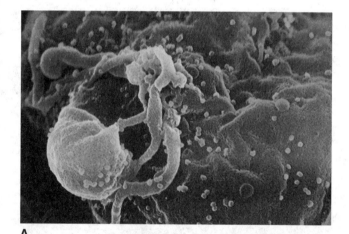

A

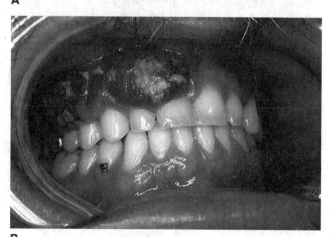

B

Figure 6-11 HIV/AIDS
(A) Cynthia Goldsmith/CDC; **(B)** Sol Silverman, Jr., DDS/CDC

Management and Prevention Considerations

Detailed discussion of the complex management issues for individuals infected with HIV is beyond the scope of this chapter. Interested persons are referred to the U.S. National Institutes of Health (NIH) ART guidelines at http://aidsinfo. nih.gov/guidelines. Two areas of HIV management that healthcare providers need to consider are preexposure prophylaxis (PrEP) and nonoccupational postexposure prophylaxis (nPEP) in limiting HIV transmission.

The U.S. Department of Health and Human Services (DHHS) first recommended the use of nPEP in 2005. While no randomized, placebo-controlled clinical trials of nPEP have been conducted, data relevant to nPEP guidelines is available from perinatal clinical trials, animal models, observational studies of healthcare workers following occupational exposures, and observational and case studies of nPEP use. Data continue to support that "nPEP initiated soon after exposure and continued for 28 days with sufficient medication adherence, can reduce the risk for acquiring HIV infection for nonoccupational exposures" (Centers for Disease Control and Prevention & U.S. Department of Health and Human Services [CDC & DHHS], 2016).

nPEP Guidelines

The CDC summary guidelines for nPEP are as follows:

- Healthcare providers should evaluate persons for nPEP rapidly when care is sought ≤72 hours after a potential nonoccupational exposure that presents a substantial risk for HIV acquisition.

- All persons considered for nPEP should have determination of their HIV infection status by HIV testing, preferably by rapid combined antigen/antibody, or antibody blood tests.

- If rapid HIV blood tests are not available, and nPEP is otherwise indicated, it should be initiated without delay and can be discontinued if the patient is later determined to have HIV infection already or the source is determined to not have HIV infection.

- nPEP is recommended when the source of the body fluids is known to be HIV-positive and the reported exposure presents a substantial risk for transmission.

- nPEP is NOT recommended when the reported exposure presents no substantial risk of HIV transmission.

- nPEP is not recommended when care is sought >72 hours after exposure.

- A case-by-case determination about nPEP is recommended when the HIV infection status of the source of body fluids is unknown and the reported exposure presents a substantial risk for the transmission IF the source DID have HIV infection.

- All persons offered nPEP should be prescribed a 28-day course of a three-drug antiretroviral regimen.

Preferred nPEP Regimen (for otherwise Healthy Adults and Adolescents)

- Tenofovir disoproxil fumarate (Tenofovir DF or TDF) (300 mg) WITH fixed dose emtricitabine (FTC) (200 mg) (Truvada) once daily, **plus**

- Raltegravir (RAL) 400 mg twice daily or Dolutegravir (DTG) 50 mg daily

Alternative nPEP regimen (for otherwise Healthy Adults and Adolescents)

- Tenofovir DF (300 mg) **with** fixed dose emtricitabine (FTC) (200 mg) (Truvada) once daily, **plus**

- Darunavir (DRV) (800 mg as 2,400 m tablets) and ritonavir (RTV) (100 mg) once daily

Additional Considerations

- All persons evaluated for nPEP use should be provided with any additional indicated prevention, treatment, or supportive care for other exposure-related health risks and conditions (other STIs, traumatic injuries, viral hepatitis B or C, or pregnancy).

- All women who are prescribed nPEP should also be offered emergency contraception to prevent pregnancy (Del Rio, 2015).

- All persons who are prescribed nPEP should be re-screened for HIV infection with a fourth-generation HIV antigen and antibody test 3 months after completion of the course of treatment (Del Rio, 2015).

- All persons who report behaviors or situations that place them at risk for frequently recurring HIV exposure (injection drug use [IDU], or sex without condoms) or who report ≥1 course of nPEP in the past year should be provided with risk-reduction counseling and intervention services including consideration of PrEP (CDC & DHHS, 2016).

The three-drug nPEP regimen offers the best evidence-based data for maximal suppression of viral replication; the best likelihood for prevention of acquiring resistant virus compared with a two-drug regimen, and in the event that HIV infection occurred despite nPEP, a three-drug regimen will more likely limit emergence of resistance than a two-drug regimen (CDC & DHHS, 2016). Providers are warned that abacavir sulfate (Ziagen, Epzicom) should **not** be prescribed in any nPEP regimen. Prompt initiation of nPEP does not allow time for testing to see if a patient has the *HLA-B*5701* allele, the presence of which is strongly associated with a potentially fatal hypersensitivity syndrome (CDC & DHHS, 2016).

The CDC first recommended preexposure prophylaxis (PrEP) to be used along with safer sex practices to reduce the risk of sexually acquired HIV-1 in adults at high risk of becoming infected in 2012 (CDC, 2014). To be clinically eligible for PrEP, clients must be documented as being HIV negative; have no signs or symptoms of acute HIV infection; have normal renal function; be on no other contraindicated medications; and have documented hepatitis B virus infection and vaccination status (CDC, 2014). Daily oral PrEP (tenofovir disoproxil fumarate [TDF] 300 mg and emtricitabine [FTC] 200 mg) has been shown to be safe and effective in reducing the risk of sexual HIV acquisition in adults; therefore, the CDC has issued the following recommendations.

PrEP Guidelines for HIV Prevention

The CDC summary guidelines for PrEP are as follows:

- Daily oral PrEP with the fixed dose of TDF 300 mg coformulated with FTC 200 mg (Truvada) is recommended as one prevention option for sexually active adult MSM at substantial risk of acquiring HIV.

- PrEP is recommended as one prevention option for adult heterosexually active men and women who are at substantial risk of HIV acquisition.

- PrEP is recommended as one prevention option for adult injection-drug users (IDU) at substantial risk of HIV acquisition.

- PrEP should be discussed with heterosexually active women and men in HIV-discordant relationships (whose partners are known to have HIV infection) as one of several options to protect the uninfected partner during conception and pregnancy so that an informed decision can be made in awareness of what is known and unknown about the benefits and risks of PrEP for mother and fetus.

- PrEP use periconceptually and during pregnancy is permitted by FDA labeling and perinatal treatment guidelines; however, data on its safety in the developing fetus of these HIV-negative women are limited. Yet, because TDF and FTC are both widely used for the treatment of HIV infection and continued during pregnancies that occur, the data from the use of these antiretroviral medications as used in HIV-infected pregnancies have shown no adverse effect among infants so exposed (CDC, 2014).

- The risks and benefits of PrEP in adolescents should be discussed and carefully weighed within the context of laws and regulations related to healthcare decision-making by minors.

  - The *only* FDA-approved medication regimen recommended for PrEP with all populations specified within the CDC guidelines is the daily TDF 300 mg coformulated with FTC 200 mg (Truvada).

  - TDF alone can be considered as an alternative regimen for IDUs and heterosexually active adults, but not for MSM, among whom its efficacy has not been studied.

- PrEP for coitally timed or other non-continuous daily use is not recommended.

- The time from initiation of daily treatment with PrEP to maximal protection against HIV infection is unknown. Data from exploratory studies suggest maximum intracellular concentrations are reached in the blood following approximately 20 days of oral dosing, in rectal tissue after approximately 7 days, and in cervicovaginal tissues after approximately 20 days. There is no data yet available regarding penile tissue PrEP concentrations to form guidelines for male insertive partners (CDC, 2014).

- The use of other antiretroviral medications for PrEP, either in place of or in addition to TDF/FTC (or TDF), is not recommended (CDC, 2014).

Persons taking PrEP need to be assessed every 3 months for HIV infection, as individuals with incident infection can discontinue taking PrEP. The two-drug PrEP regimen is inadequate treatment for established HIV infection and its continued use may lead to resistance to either or both drugs. Renal function should be assessed at baseline and then monitored every 6 months as persons who develop renal failure do not continue taking PrEP. Lastly, when clinicians prescribe PrEP, patients should be given full access to proven, effective risk-reduction services. Given that clinical trials clearly demonstrated high medication adherence as being critical to the success of PrEP, patients should be encouraged and enabled to use PrEP in combination with these other effective prevention resources (CDC, 2014).

U.S. Barriers to STI Screening and Treatment

In any jurisdiction, if secondary STI prevention efforts are to be effective, then barriers to both symptomatic and asymptomatic screening and prevention need to be eliminated. Recognized barriers can be generalized into three categories: system barriers such as prohibitive legal policies, long clinic wait times, inconvenient facility locations, lack of insurance coverage, or medical providers unaware of or not practicing to accepted care standards (Lechtenberg et al., 2014); social and interpersonal barriers such as fear and stigma attached to STIs or discriminatory attitudes and behavior on the part of healthcare staff; and lastly, knowledge barriers due to low health literacy on the part of individual clients (Hitt, 2010; Leichliter, Sejiler, & Wohlfeiler, 2015; Peterman & Carter, 2016; Seidman, Carlson, Weber, Witt, & Kelly, 2015; Tilson et al., 2004).

The majority of systemic barriers to STI screening and treatment in the United States center around EPT laws, clinic procedures/policies, provider missed opportunities, and issues surrounding payment for services. As previously noted, there are eight states/territories where EPT may be permissible with certain restrictions and three states where EPT is clearly prohibited (**Figure 6-12**). EPT has been proven to be a highly effective means of controlling the spread and reinfection of bacterial STIs, particularly when

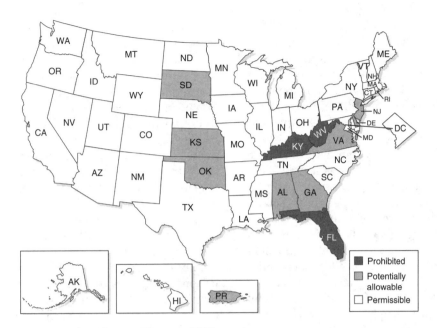

Figure 6-12 Legal Status of Expedited Partner Therapy (EPT)
Reproduced from CDC. (2017). Legal status of Expedited Partner Therapy (EPT). Retrieved from https://www.cdc.gov/std/ept/legal/default.htm

index patients are directly given medication to bring to their partners versus being given written prescriptions that need to be filled (Peterman & Carter, 2016; Workowski & Bolan, 2015). Many U.S. healthcare facilities do not stock or dispense the recommended medications for treating bacterial STIs. Many providers are not aware of the efficacy and legal permissibility of EPT (Arya et al., 2014; Mehringer, Hertz, & DiPaolo, 2014; Reilley et al., 2015). More effort needs to be directed toward encouraging providers to use EPT and for healthcare systems to make receiving treatment directly at the point of service a universal norm for clients (Schillinger, Gorwitz, Rietmeijer, & Golden, 2016).

Healthcare entities can optimize provider use of STI-screening/treatment standards and EPT through timely reminders built in to their electronic medical record systems (EMR). By integrating the CDC and USPSTF recommendations into the EMR, providers are prompted to note if EPT was offered and received or declined, follow-up screening appointments were made, and any active (direct) referrals given (Taylor, Frasure-Williams, Burnett, & Park, 2015). Direct linkage to other medical and social services is key to patient compliance with follow-up screenings and treatment (Carter et al., 2015). Fully integrated EMR systems can also guide practitioners to obtaining a complete and nonmarginalizing sexual history and behavioral risk assessment (Workowski & Bolan, 2015). Fully integrated EMR systems ensure that routing STI screening is offered on an "opt-out" basis (where screenings are presented as a routine part of recommended healthcare and individuals may decline being tested) versus "Opt-in" screening (where a client must specifically ask to be screened). opt-out screening has been shown to be more efficacious in having more individuals receive appropriate STI screening (Chou, 2011). Ultimately, "screening programs work amazingly

well if they are done automatically" (Peterman & Carter, 2016). Making sure that EMR systems are fully congruent with current STI standards is one low-cost, highly effective means for accomplishing this goal.

With the advent of the Affordable Care Act (ACA) in 2014, more individuals are now covered by some form of health insurance than ever before. Even so, an estimated 10.4% of the U.S. population remains uninsured (Smith & Medalia, 2014). Having health insurance coverage does not guarantee that individuals will seek appropriate STI screening and treatment. Fear of discrimination, stigma, and loss of confidentiality often cause delays in seeking out services, particularly among adolescents and young adults—the population at highest risk for STIs (Tilson et al., 2004). The 2014 enactment of the ACA now permits younger clients to remain covered by their parents' health insurance up to age 26.

Unfortunately, in most states, insurance companies are required by law to send policy holders (in this case, the parents of the insured dependent) a written "Explanation of Benefits" (EOB) following every medical encounter. These EOBs clearly verify who was seen and what services were provided, along with the dollar amount that was covered under the insured's plan. Thus, insured dependent young adults wishing to maintain their healthcare privacy need to either pay out of their own pocket, or attempt to find low-cost or free STI services. Access to low-cost and free STI services is extremely limited, particularly in rural areas.

According to the U.S. Department of Health and Human Services (DHHS), only 12% of U.S. adults have proficient health literacy, defined as being able to follow directions on a prescription drug label, adhering to immunization schedules, being able to give two reasons why someone without symptoms should be tested for a disease, or being able to calculate their share of insurance health costs for a year (DHHS, 2008). Patients with low health literacy are often disenfranchised from care, have difficulty navigating healthcare systems, have poor quality of communication (including cultural overlay) with providers, and ultimately poorer health outcomes (McCray, 2005).

The USPSTF recommends intensive behavioral counseling for all sexually active adolescents and for adults who are at an increased risk for sexually transmitted infections (STIs). The USPSTF noted that data was insufficient to recommend behavioral counseling to non-sexually active adolescents or adults who were not at increased risk (LeFevre, 2014). This "intensive" behavioral counseling is defined as 20 minutes to more than 2 hours of contact time providing basic information about STIs and STI transmission, training in pertinent skills such as condom application, role-playing communications with partners about safer-sex, problem solving, and goal setting (LeFevre, 2014). While even brief behavioral counseling has been shown to be effective in young, moderately high-risk heterosexual men and women (Peterman & Carter, 2016), high-risk MSM "do not seem to benefit from behavioral counseling as it is currently construed" (Brookmeyer, Hogben, & Kinsey, 2016). Additionally, persons who use substances in ways other than injection should also be offered adherence support and behavioral counseling regarding STI screening, treatment, and prevention (Del Rio, 2015).

Future Directions in STI Screening and Treatment in the United States

Given that the United States has among the highest rates of STIs among well-resourced nations, there is much work to be done. Research studies focused on decreasing the population burden of STIs in the United States have revealed several areas for improved services as well as other areas in need of further research.

Areas known to be in need of improvement include increased national health literacy (see previous discussion), increased provider and institutional adherence to national guidelines for screening and treatment, national legislation to clearly permit EPT in all jurisdictions and to guarantee insurance coverage of ETP, and efforts to reduce STI-associated stigma (Friedman, Kachur, Noar, & McFarlane, 2016; Leichliter et al., 2015). First and foremost, all healthcare providers need to be thoroughly educated in the basics of taking a comprehensive, non-marginalizing sexual and STI behavioral risk assessment, which should include STI screening. Behavioral risk screenings need to include "The Five P's": partners, practices, prevention of pregnancy, protection from STIs, and past history of STIs (Workowski & Bolan, 2015). Secondly, providers need to be intimately familiar with the CDC/USPSTF guidelines for STI prevention, screening, and treatment, and then be

given regular systemic reminders so that screening/follow-up occurs automatically in all appropriate clients.

Institutional systems demonstrating need of consistent efforts to reduce STIs include U.S. correctional facilities (Bernstein, Chow, Pathela, & Gift, 2016; Workowski & Bolan, 2015). The U.S. has one of the highest incarceration rates in the world, primarily due to the prevalence of illicit drugs. Illicit drug use disproportionately affects impoverished populations and poverty and substance abuse individually and synergistically are risk factors for STIs (Thierry, Marrazzo, & LaMarre, 2004). Multiple studies have found persons entering correctional facilities have high rates of STIs including HIV and viral hepatitis. Many short-term correctional facilities house detainees for less than a year, with up to half of all entrants being released within 48 hours (Workowski & Bolan, 2015). With no national guidelines regarding STI care and management for correctional populations, this is an area where consistent application of screening and treatment could produce major population benefit.

Future research should be directed at examining social media uses for STI awareness, behavior change, and decreasing stigma (Friedman et al., 2016); use of self-collected home-based specimens for mail-in chlamydia and gonorrhea screening (Bernstein et al., 2016); how clinic facility design and placement of universal collection kits impact STI screening (Taylor et al., 2015); if national screening guidelines for trichomoniasis should be added to current CDC recommendations (Hoots et al., 2013; Meites, 2013; Secour et al., 2014); and better data collection on the actual number of new cases of STIs found and effectively treated (versus previously identified cases ineffectively treated or followed-up) along with more detailed costs of various clinic-and non-clinic-based screening programs (Bernstein et al., 2016). These additional findings will assist local, state, and national programs to offer more comprehensive, socially acceptable, efficacious care to help achieve the goal of reduced STI burden in the United States.

Conclusion

Effective clinical practice requires sexual health professional practitioners to demonstrate adequate knowledge and insight about specific STIs. This chapter explored STI clinical manifestations, diagnosis, treatment, partner notification and the required follow-up program, short- and long-term consequences, and related patient anxieties. Adequate knowledge about the etiology, modes of acquisition and transmission, the prevalence and epidemiology of the different STIs is crucial. Practitioners should be able to answer the patients' questions and provide reassurance for their concerns about the symptoms and signs, natural history of the acquired infection, and potential complications.

Patients are more motivated to return to clinic for laboratory test results and further investigation when diagnostic reasoning and procedures are clearly explained. Sexual health practitioners should recognize the guiding principles and standards of STI/RTI treatment to provide a high standard of care. Enhancement of overall care with continuous improvement of services contributes toward better patient outcomes and satisfaction. The choice of antimicrobials and dosage calculations are crucial. Patients should be told the importance of compliance and completion of the prescribed regimens.

Although recommended treatment options for empiric, syndromic, and presumptive therapy are proposed, evidence shows that the concepts and guiding principles together with the related algorithms may vary somewhat in different settings. While some teams or sexual healthcare organizations employ more elaborate versions of algorithms and/or flow charts for their syndromic case managements, others use more concise algorithms. The later formats invariably allow for adjustments to be made to certain aspects at the discretion of the individual practitioner. There is no doubt the type of algorithm developed may be influenced by the national policy and regulations, as well as social and economic circumstances.

Considerations regarding sexual partners and the tracing of sexual contacts should form part of the totality of the sexual healthcare. Of crucial importance is reinforcement of health education/health promotion and reiteration of self-protection from repeat STI acquisition by consistent and correct use of condoms. The benefits of the recommended follow-up program and test of cure, where applicable, should be explained in such a way as to encourage the patient's acceptance of personal responsibility and cooperation.

Practitioners are encouraged to explore the various STI policies and the standards published by the WHO and the BASHH regarding STI and RTI care provision. These could also be compared to the current standards and policies outlined by the CDC. While findings from related research have been considered in this chapter, practitioners are encouraged to continually reflect critically on issues that require further investigation or evaluation through more detailed investigative studies or clinical audit projects. There is clearly a need to ensure that the principles of evidence-based practice consistently thread through all aspects of STI/RTI care provision.

••• REFERENCES

Abudalu, M., Tyring, S., Koltun, W., Bodsworth, N., & Hamed, K. (2008). Single-day patient initiated famciclovir therapy versus 3-day valacyclovir regimen for recurrent genital herpes: A randomised, double-blind, comparative trial. *Clinical Infectious Diseases, 47*(5), 651–658.

Abu-Rajab, K., & Wallace, L. A. (2011). Heterosexual transmission of infectious syphilis in central Scotland, 2009. *International Journal of STD & AIDS, 22*(9), 517–518.

Akinbiyi, A. A., Watson, R., & Feyi-Waboso, P. (2008). Prevalence of *Candida albicans* and bacterial vaginosis in asymptomatic pregnant women in South Yorkshire, United Kingdom: Outcome

of a prospective study. *Archives of Gynecology and Obstetrics, 278*(5), 463–466.

Alexander, S., Martin, I. M., & Ison, C. A. (2008). Comparison of two methods for the diagnosis of lymphogranuloma venereum. *Journal of Medical Microbiology, 57*(8), 962–965

Allstaff, S., & Wilson, J. (2012). The management of sexually transmitted infections in pregnancy. *Obstetrics & Gynecology, 14*(1), 25–32.

Altunyurt, S., Demir, N., & Posaci, C. (2003). A randomised controlled trial of coil removal prior to treatment of pelvic inflammatory disease. *European Journal of Obstetrics & Gynecology and Reproductive Biology, 107*(1), 81–84.

American Academy of Pediatrics (AAP). (2014). Screening for nonviral sexually transmitted infections in adolescents and young adults. *Pediatrics, 134*(1), e302–e311.

American College of Obstetricians and Gynecologists (ACOG). (2015a). ACOG opinion: Expedited partner therapy in the management of gonorrhea and chlamydial infection. Retrieved from http://www.acog.org/Resources-And-Publications/Committee-Opinions/Committee-on-Gynecologic-Practice/Expedited-Partner-Therapy-in-the-Management-of-Gonorrhea-and-Chlamydial-Infection

American College of Obstetricians and Gynecologists (ACOG). (2015b). Committee opinion: Dual therapy for gonococcal infections. *Obstetrics & Gynecology, 126*(5), e95–e99.

American College of Obstetricians and Gynecologists (ACOG). (2015c). Committee opinion: Human Papillomavirus Vaccination. *Obstetrics & Gynecology, 126*(3), e38–e42.

Amsel, R., Totten, P. A., Spiegel, C. A., Chen, K. C., Eschenbach D., & Holmes, K. K. (1983). Nonspecific vaginitis: Diagnostic criteria and microbial and epidemiologic associations. *American Journal of Medicine, 74*(1), 14–22.

Aoki, F. Y., Tyring, S., Diaz-Mitoma, F., Gross, G., Gao, J., & Hamed, K. (2006). Single-day, patient initiated famciclovir therapy for recurrent genital herpes: A randomised, double-blind, placebo-controlled trial. *Clinical Infectious Diseases, 42*(1), 8–13.

Arya, M., Yin Zheng, M., Amspoker, A. B., Kallen, M. A., Street, R. L., Viswanath, K., & Giordano, T. P. (2014). In the routine HIV testing era, primary care physicians in community health centers remain unaware of HIV testing recommendations. *Journal of the International Association of Providers of AIDS Care, 13*(4), 296–299. Retrieved from http://dx.doi.org/10.1177/2325957413517140

Atashili, J., Poole, C., Ndumbe, P. M., Adimora, A. A., & Smith, J. S. (2008). Bacterial vaginosis and HIV acquisition: A meta-analysis of published studies. *AIDS, 22*(12), 1493–1501.

Australian Sexual Health Alliance (ASHA). (2015). Vaginal discharge – Australian STI management guidelines for use in primary care. Retrieved from http://www.sti.guidelines.org.au/syndromes/vaginal-discharge#diagnosis

Bartlett, B. L., Tyring, S. K., Fife, K., Gnann, J. W., Hadala, J. T., Kianifard, F., & Berber, E. (2008). Famciclivir treatment options for patients with frequent outbreaks of recurrent genital herpes: The RELIEF trial. *Journal of Clinical Virology, 43*(2), 190–195.

Batteiger, B. E., Tu, W., Ofner., S., Van Der Pol B., Stothard, D. R., Orr, D. P., . . . Fortenberry (2010). Repeated *Chlamydia trachomatis* genital infections in adolescent women. *The Journal of Infectious Diseases, 201*(1), 42–51.

Batteiger, B. E., Xu, F., Johnson, R. E., & Rekart, M. L. (2010).Protective immunity to *Chlamydia trachomatis* genital infection: evidence from human studies. *The Journal of Infectious Diseases, 201*(2),178–189.

Baughn, R. E., & Musher, D. M. (2005). Secondary syphilitic lesions. *Clinical Microbiology Reviews, 18*(1), 205–216.

Beckman, C. R., Cassanova, R., & Chuang, A. (2014). *Obstetrics and gynecology* (7th ed.). New York, NY: Wolters Kluwer.

Behets, F. M-T. F., Miller, W. C., & Cohen, M. S. (2001). Syndromic treatment of gonococcal and chlamydial infections in women seeking primary care for the genital discharge syndrome: decision-making. *Bulletin of the World Health Organization, 79*(11), 1070–1075.

Bernstein, K. T., Chow, J. M., Pathela, P., & Gift, T. L. (2016). Bacterially sexually transmitted disease screening outside the clinic: Implications for the modern sexually transmitted disease program. *Sexually Transmitted Diseases, 43*(Supp. 1).

Bernstein, D., Lovett, M., & Bryson, Y. (1984). Serologic analysis od first episode nonprimary genital herpes simplex virus infection: Presence of type 2 antibody in acute serum samples. *The American Journal of Medicine, 77*(6), 1055–1060.

Bignell, C. (2009). European (IUSTI/WHO) guideline on the diagnosis and treatment of gonorrhoea in adults. *International Journal of STD & AIDS, 20*(7), 453–457.

Bignell, C., & Fitzgerald, M. (2011). UK national guidelines for the management of gonorrhoea in adults. *International Journal of STD & AIDS, 22*(10), 541–547.

Bignell, C., & Garley, J. (2010). Azithromycin in the treatment of infection with *Neisseria gonorrhoeae*. *Sexually Transmitted Infections, 86*(6), 422–426.

Bignell, C., & Unemo, M., & European STI Guidelines Editorial Board. (2013). 2012 European guideline on the diagnosis and management of gonorrhoea in adults. *International Journal of STD & AIDS, 24*(2), 85–92.

Blatt, A J., Lieberman, J. M., Hoover, D. R., & Kaufman, H. W. (2012). Chlamydia and gonococcal testing during pregnancy in the United States. *American Journal of Obstetrics and Gynecology, 207*(1), 55.e1–55.e8.

Bodsworth, N, Bloch, M., & McNulty, A. (2008). 2-day versus 5-day famcyclovir as treatment of recurrences of genital herpes: Results of the FaST study. *Sexual Health, 5*(3), 219–225.

Bosch, F. X., Burchell, A. N., Schiffman, M., Giuliano, A. R., de Sanjose, S., Bruni, L., . . . Muñoz, N. (2008). Epidemiology and natural history of human papillomavirus infections and type-specific implications in cervical neoplasia. *Vaccine, 26*(10), K1–16.

Bosserman, E. A., Helms, D. J., Mosure, D. J., Secor, W. E., & Workowski, K. A. (2011). Utility of antimicrobial susceptibility testing in *Trichomonas vaginalis*-infected women with clinical treatment failure. *Sexually Transmitted Diseases, 38*(10), 983–987.

British Association for Sexual Health and HIV (BASHH). (2006). *United Kingdom national guideline for the management of genital tract infection with* Chlamydia trachomatis. Retrieved from http://www.bashh.org/guidelines

British Association for Sexual Health and HIV (BASHH). (2008). Guidelines for the management of *Chlamydia trachomatis* genital infection, July 2008. Retrieved from https://www.bashhguidelines. org/current-guidelines/urethritis-and-cervicitis/chlamydia-2015

British Association for Sexual Health and HIV (BASHH). (2010). Chlamydia trachomatis *UK testing guidelines*. Retrieved from https:// www.bashhguidelines.org/current-guidelines/urethritis-and-cervicitis /chlamydia-2015

British Association for Sexual Health and HIV. (2016a). *2015 UK national guideline for the management of infection with* Chlamydia trachomatis. Retrieved from https://www.bashhguidelines .org/current-guidelines/urethritis-and-cervicitis/chlamydia-2015

British Association for Sexual Health and HIV (BASHH). (2016b). A guide to chlamydia. Retrieved from https://www.bashh.org /documents/Chlamydia_PIL_DIGITAL_2016.pdf

British Association for Sexual Health and HIV (BASHH) & Clinical Effectiveness Group. (2014). National guideline for the management of genital herpes. Retrieved from https://www.bashhguidelines. org/current-guidelines/genital-ulceration/anogenital-herpes-2014

Brookmeyer, K. A., Hogben, M., & Kinsey, J. (2016). The role of behavioral counseling in sexually transmitted disease prevention program settings. *Sexually Transmitted Diseases, 43*(Suppl. 1). S102-S112.

Brucker, M. C., & King, T. L. (2017). *Pharmacology for women's health* (2nd ed.). Burlington, MA: Jones and Bartlett.

Brunham, R. C., Pourbohloul, B., Mak, S., White, R., & Rekart, M. L. (2005). The unexpected impact of a *Chlamydia trachomatis* infection control program on susceptibility to reinfection. *The Journal of Infectious Diseases, 192,* 1836–1844.

Brunham, R. C., & Rey-Ladino, J. (2005). Immunology of chlamydia infection: Implications for a *Chlamydia trachomatis* vaccine. *Nature Reviews Immunology, 5*(2), 149–161.

Burchell, A. N., Winer, R. L., de Sanjosé S., & Franco, E. L. (2006). Epidemiology and transmission dynamics of genital HPV infection. *Vaccine, 24*(3 Suppl. 3), 52–61.

Byrne, G. I. (2010). *Chlamydia trachomatis* strains and virulence: Rethinking links to infection prevalence and disease severity. *The Journal of Infectious Diseases, 201*(2), 126–133.

Carey, A. J., & Beagley, K. W. (2010). *Chlamydia trachomatis* a hidden epidemic: Effects on female reproduction and options for treatment. *American Journal of Reproductive Immunology, 63*(6), 576–586.

Carter, M. W., Wu, H., Cohen, S., Hightow-Weidman, L., Lecher, S. L., & Peters, P. J. (2016). Linkage and referral to HIV and other medical and social services: A focused literature review for sexually transmitted disease prevention and control programs. *Sexually Transmitted Diseases, 43*(Supp. 1).

Castle, P. E. (2008). Human papillomavirus genotype 84 infection of the male genitalia: Further evidence for HPV tissue tropism? *The Journal of Infectious Diseases, 197*(5), 776–778.

Castro, R., Prieto, E. S., Águas, M. J., Manata, M. J., Botas, J., Araújo, C., . . . Exposto, Fda L. (2006). *Journal of Clinical Laboratory Analysis, 20*(6), 233–238.

Centers for Disease Control and Prevention (CDC). (2004). Brief report. Azithromycin treatment failures in syphilis infections – San Francisco, California, 2002–2003. *MMWR, 53*(09), 197–198.

Centers for Disease Control and Prevention (CDC). (2008). *Recommendations for partner services programs for HIV infection, syphilis, gonorrhea, and chlamydial infections.* Retrieved from http://www.cdc.gov/mmwr/preview/mmwrhtml/rr5709a1.htm

Centers for Disease Control and Prevention (CDC). (2010). *Sexually transmitted diseases treatment guidelines 2010.* Retrieved from http://www.cdc.gov/std/treatment/2010/pid.htm

Centers for Disease Control and Prevention (CDC). (2014). *Pre-exposure prophylaxis for the prevention of HIV infection in the United States–2014: A clinical practice guideline.* Retrieved from https://www.cdc.gov/hiv/pdf/prepguidelines2014.pdf

Centers for Disease Control and Prevention (CDC). (2015a). *CDC fact sheet: Reported STDs in the United States 2014 national data for chlamydia, gonorrhea, and syphilis.* Retrieved from https://www.cdc.gov/std/stats14/std-trends-508.pdf

Centers for Disease Control and Prevention (CDC). (2015b). *Summary of notifiable diseases and conditions - United States 2013.* Retrieved from http://www.cdc.gov/mmwr/preview/mmwrhtml/mm6253a1.htm

Centers for Disease Control and Prevention (CDC). (2015d). *Screening recommendations referenced in treatment guidelines and original recommendation sources.* Retrieved from http://www.cdc.gov/std/tg2015/screening-recommendations.htm.

Centers for Disease Control and Prevention (CDC). (2016a). *Expedited partner therapy.* Retrieved from http://www.cdc.gov/std/ept/default.htm

Centers for Disease Control and Prevention (CDC). (2016b). Gynecologic cancers: What should I know about screening? Retrieved from http://www.cdc.gov/cancer/cervical/basic_info/screening.htm

Centers for Disease Control and Prevention (CDC). (2016c). *Legal status of expedited partner therapy.* Retrieved from http://www.cdc.gov/std/ept/legal/default.htm

Centers for Disease Control and Prevention (CDC). (2016d). *Sexually transmitted disease surveillance 2014.* Retrieved from http://www.cdc.gov/std/stats/default.htm

Centers for Disease Control and Prevention (CDC) & the U.S. Department of Health and Human Services (DHHS). (2016). *Updated guidelines for antiretroviral postexposure prophylaxis after sexual, injection drug use, or other nonoccupational exposure to HIV-United States, 2016.* Retrieved from http://stacks.cdc.gov/view/cdc/38856

Chesson, H. W., Dunne, E. F., & Markowitz, L. E. (2014). The estimated lifetime probability of acquiring human papillomavirus in the United States. *Sexually Transmitted Diseases, 41*(11), 660–664.

Chisholm, S. A., Mounton, J. W, Lewis, D. A., Nichols, T. A., Ison, C. A., & Livermore, D. M. (2010). Cephalosporin MIC creep among gonococci: time for a pharmacodynamic rethink? *Journal of Antimicrobial Chemotherapy, 65*(10), 2141–2148.

Chou, R. (2011). Routine screening for chronic human immunodeficiency virus infection: Why don't the guidelines agree? *Epidemiologic Reviews, 33,* 7–19.

Christerson, L., de Vries, H. J., de Barbeyrac, B., Gaydos, C. A., Henrich, B., Hoffmann, S., . . . Morré, S. A. (2010). Typing of lumphogranuloma venereum *Chlamydia trachomatis* strains. *Emerging Infectious Diseases, 16*(11), 1777–1779.

Cook, R. L., Hutchison, S. L., Ostergaard, S., Braithwaite, R. S., & Ness, R. B. (2005). Systematic review: Non-invasive testing for *Chlamydia trachomatis* and Neisserria gonorrhoeae. *Annals of Internal Medicine, 142*(11), 914–925.

Cramer, R., Leichliter, J. S., Stenger, M. R., Loosier, P. S., Slive, L., & SSuN Working Group. (2013). The legal aspects of expedited partner therapy practice: Do state laws and policies really matter? *Sexually Transmitted Diseases, 40,* 657–662.

Das, S., Huengsberg, M., & Shahmanesh, M. (2005). Treatment failure of vaginal trichomoniasis in clinical practice. *International Journal of STD & AIDS, 16*(4), 284–286.

Dean, H. D., & Fenton, K. A. (2010). Addressing social determinants on health in the prevention and control of HIV/AIDS viral hepatitis, STIs and tuberculosis. *Public Health Review, 125*(4), 1–5.

Del Rio, C. (2015). Perspective HIV prevention: Integrating biomedical and behavioral interventions. *Topics in Antiviral Medicine, 22*(5), 702–706.

Delvin, D. (2016). *Syphilis.* Retrieved from http://www.netdoctor.co.uk/conditions/sexual-health/a2206/syphilis/

Denny, L. A., Franceschi, S., de Sanjose, S. Heard, I., Moscicki, A. B., & Palefsky, J. (2012). Human papillomavirus, human immunodeficiency virus and immunosuppression. *Vaccine, 30*(5), F168–174.

de Villiers, E. M., Fauquet, C., Broker, T. R., Bernard, H. U., & zur Hausen, H. (2004). Classification of papillomaviruses. *Virology, 324*(1), 17–27.

de Vries, H. J. C., Smelov, V., Middelburg, J. G., Pleijster, J., Speksnijder, A. G., & Morre, S. A. (2009). Delayed microbial cure of lymphogranuloma venereum proctitis with doxycycline treatment. *Clinical Infectious Diseases, 48*(5), e53-e56.

de Vries, H. J. C., Zingoni, A., Kreuter, A., Moi, H., & White, J. A. (2015). 2013 European guideline on the management of lymphogranuloma venereum. *Journal of the European Academy of Dermatology and Venereology, 29,* 1–6. doi:10.1111/jdv.12461

Dielissen, P. W., Teunissen, D. A. M., & Lagro-Janssen, A. L. M. (2013). Chlamydia prevalence in the general population: Is there a sex difference? A systematic review. *BMC Infectious Diseases, 13*(534), 1186–1191.

Doorbar, J. (2006). Molecular biology of human papillomavirus infection and cervical cancer. *Clinical Science, 110*(5), 525–541.

Dosekun, O., Edmonds, S., Stockwell, S., French, P., & White, J. A. (2013). Lymphogranuloma venereum detected from the pharynx in four London men who have sex with men. *International Journal of STD & AIDS, 24*(6), 495–496.

Dunne, E. F., Chapin, J. B., Reitmeijer, C. A., Kent, C. K., Ellen, J. M., Gaydos, C. A., . . . Markowitz, L. E. (2008). Rate and predictors of repeat *Chlamydia trachomatis* infection among men. *Sexually Transmitted Diseases, 35*(11), S40-S44.

European Centre for Disease Prevention and Control (2011) Surveillance Report: Sexually Transmitted Infections in Europe 1990-2009. Stockholm: ECDC.

Eccleston, K., Collins, L., & Higgins, S. P. (2008). Primary syphilis. *International Journal of STD & AIDS, 19*(3), 145–151.

Engelberg, R., Carrell, D., Krantz, E., Corey, L., & Wald, A. (2003). Natural history of genital herpes simplex virus type 1 infection. *Sexually Transmitted Diseases, 30*(2), 174–177.

Eriksson, K., Carlsson, B., Forsum, U., & Larsson, P. G. (2005). A double-blind treatment study of bacterial vaginosis with normal vaginal lactobacilli after an open treatment with vaginal clindamycin ovules. *Acta Dermato-Venereologica, 85*(1), 42–46.

Eschenbach, D. A., Thwin, S. S., Patton, D. L., Hooton, T. M., Stapleton, A. E., Agnew, K., . . . Stamm, W. E. (2000). Influence of the normal menstrual cycle on vaginal tissue, discharge, and microflora. *Clinical Infectious Diseases, 30*(6), 901–907.

European Centre for Disease Control (ECDC). (2012). Response plan to control and manage the threat of multidrug-resistant gonorrhoea in Europe. Stockholm, Sweden: Author.

Faculty of Sexual and Reproductive Healthcare Clinical Guidance. (2012). Management of vaginal discharge in non-genitourinary medicine settings: Clinical Effectiveness Unit. London: Faculty of Sexual and Reproductive Healthcare.

Fang, X., Zhou, Y., Yang, Y., Diao, Y., & Li H. (2007). Prevalence and risk factors of trichomoniasis, bacterial vaginosis and candidiasis for married women of child-bearing age in rural Shandong. *Japanese Journal of Infectious Diseases, 60*(5), 257–261.

Faricy, L., Page, T., Ronic, M., Rdesinski, R., & DeVoe, J. (2012). Patterns of empiric treatment of *Chlamydia trachomatis* infections in underdeveloped populations. *Family Medicine, 44*(6), 408–415.

Fredlund, H., Falk, L., Jurstrand, M., & Unemo, M. (2004). Molecular genetic methods for diagnosis and characterisation of *Chlamydia trachomatis* and *Neisseria gonorrhoeae*: Impact on epidemiological surveillance and interventions. *ACTA Pathologica, Microbiologica Et Immunologica Scandinavia. 112*(11–12), 771–784.

French, P. (2007). Syphilis. *BMJ, 334*(7585), 143–147.

French, P. (2011). Syphilis: Clinical features, diagnosis and management. In K. E. Rogstad (Ed.), *ABC of sexually transmitted infections*, (6th ed., pp. 70–77). Chichester, United Kingdom: Wiley-Blackwell.

French, P., Gomberg, M., Janier, M., Schmidt, B., Van Voorst Vader, P., & Young, H. (2009). IUSTI: 2008 European guidelines on the management of syphilis. *International Journal of STD & AIDS, 20*(5), 300–309.

French, P., Ison, C. A., & MacDonald, N. (2005). Lymphogranuloma venereum in the United Kingdom. *Sexually Transmitted Infections, 81*(2), 97–98.

Friedman, A. L., Kachur, R. E., Noar, S. M., & McFarlane, M. (2016). Health communication and social marketing campaigns for sexually transmitted disease prevention and control: What is the evidence for their effectiveness? *Sexually Transmitted Diseases, 43*(2, Suppl. 1), S83–S101.

Furuya, R., Nakayama, H., Kanayama, A., Saika, T., Iyod, T., Tatewaki, M., . . . Tanaka, M. (2006). In vitro synergistic effects on double combinations of á lactams and azithromycin against clinical isolates of *Neisseria gonorrhoeae. Journal of Infection and Chemotherapy, 12*(4), 172–176.

Garland, S. M., Hernandez-Avila, M., Wheeler, C. M., Perez, G., Harper, D. M., Leodolter, S., . . .Koutsky, L. A. (2007). Quadrivalent vaccine against human papillomavirus to prevent anogenital diseases. *New England Journal of Medicine, 356*(19), 1928–1943.

Gavillon, N., Vervaet, H., Derniaux, E., Terrosi, P., Graesslin, O., & Quereux, C. (2010). How did I contract humanpapillomavirus (HPV)? *Gynécologie Obstetrique & Fertilité, 38*(3), 199–204.

Gaydos, C., Maldeis, N. E., Hardick, A., Hardick, J., & Quinn, T. C. (2009). Mycoplasma genitalium as a contributor to the multiple etiologies of cervicitis in women attending sexually transmitted disease clinics. *Sexually Transmitted Diseases, 36*(10), 598–606.

Gaydos, C. A., Theodore, M., Dalesio, N., Wood, B. J., & Quinn, T. C. (2004). Comparison of three nucleic acid amplification tests for detection of *Chlamydia trachomatis* in urine specimens. *Journal of Clinical Microbiology, 42*(7), 3041–3045.

Geretti, A. M., & Brown, D. W. (2005). National survey of diagnostic services for genital herpes. *Sexually Transmitted Infections, 81*(4), 316–317.

Ghanem, K. G., Erbelding, E. J., Cheng, W. W., & Rompalo, A. M. (2006). Doxycycline compared with benzathine penicillin for the treatment of early syphilis. *Clinical Infectious Diseases, 42*(6), e45–e49.

Ghanem, K. G., Moore, R. D., Rampalo, A. M., Erbelding, E. J., Zenilman, J. M., & Gebo, K. A. (2008). Antiretroviral therapy is associated with reduced serologic failure rates for syphilis among HIV-infected patients. *Clinical Infectious Diseases, 147*(2), 258–265.

Ghebremichael, M. (2014) Syndromic versus laboratory diagnosis of sexually transmitted infections in resource-limited settings. *ISRN AIDS, 2014,* 103452.

Gift, T. L., Mohammed, P., Leichliter, J. L., Hogben, M., & Golden, M. R. (2011). The cost and cost-effectiveness of expedited partner therapy compared with standard partner referral for the treatment of chlamydia and gonorrhea. *Sexually Transmitted Diseases, 38,* 1067–1073.

Gilson, R., Nathan, M., Sonnex, C., Lazaro, N., & Keirs, T. (2015). *UK national guidelines on the management of anogenital warts 2015.* Retrieved from https://www.bashh.org/documents/UK%20national%20guideline%20on%20Warts%202015%20FINAL.pdf

Golden, M., Kerani, R., Shafii, T., Whittington, W., & Holmes, K. (2009). Does azithromycin co-treatment enhance the efficacy of oral cephalosporins for pharyngeal gonorrhoea? Presented at 18th International Society for STD Research (ISSTDR) Conference, London, United Kingdom: June 2009.

Gorgos, L. M., & Marrazzo, J. M. (2011). Sexually transmitted infections among women who have sex with women. *Clinical Infectious Diseases, 53*(S3), S84–S91.

Gradison, M. (2012). Pelvic inflammatory disease. *American Family Physician, 85*(8), 791–796.

GRASP Steering Group. (2009). *The gonococcal resistance to antimicrobials surveillance programme (GRASP), Year 2008 collection.* London, United Kingdom: Health Protection Agency 2009. Retrieved from http://webarchive.nationalarchives.gov.uk/20140714113631/http://www.hpa.org.uk/webc/HPAwebFile/HPAweb_C/1245914960426

Gross, G., & Pfister, H. (2004). Role of human papillomavirus in penile cancer, penile intraepithelial squamous cell neoplasias and in genital warts. *Medical Microbiology and Immunology, 193*(1), 35–44.

Haggerty, C. L. (2008). Evidence for a role of *Mycoplasma genitalium* in pelvic inflammatory disease. *Current Opinion in Infectious Diseases, 21*(1), 65–69.

Haggerty, C. L., Gottlieb, S. L., Taylor, B. D., Low, N., Xu, F., & Ness, R. B. (2010). Risk of sequel after *Chlamydia trachomatis* genital infection in women. *The Journal of Infectious Diseases, 201*(2), 134–155.

Haggerty, C. L., & Ness, R. B. (2006). Epidemiology, pathogenesis and treatment of pelvic inflammatory disease. *Expert Review of Anti-infective Therapy, 4*(2), 235–247.

Haggerty, C. L., & Taylor, B. D. (2011). Mycoplasma genitalium: an emerging cause of pelvic inflammatory disease. *Infectious Diseases in Obstetrics and Gynecology, 2011,* 959818.

Haggerty, C. L., Totten, P. A., Astete, S. G., Lee, S., Hoferka, S. L., Kelsey, S. F., & Ness, R. B. (2008). Failure of cefoxitin and doxycycline to eradicate endometrial *Mycoplasma genitalium* and the consequence for clinical cure of pelvic inflammatory disease. *Sexually Transmitted Infections, 84*(5), 338–342.

Hariri, S., Unger, E. R., Sternberg, M., Dunne, E. F., Swan, D., Patel, S., & Markowitz, L. E. (2011). Prevalence of genital human papillomavirus among females in the United States, the National Health and Nutrition Examination Survey. *The Journal of Infectious Diseases, 204*(4), 566–573.

Hansfield, H. A. H., & Sparling, P. F. (2005). *Neisseria gonorrhoeae.* In G. L. Mandell, J. E. Bennett, & R. Dolin (Eds.), *Principles and practice of infectious diseases* (6th ed., pp. 2514–2529). Philadelphia, PA: Churchill Livingstone.

Hay, P. (2011). Vaginal discharge: Causes diagnosis and treatment. In K. E. Rogstad (Ed.), *ABC of Sexually Transmitted Infections,* (6th ed., pp. 42–47). Chichester: Wiley-Blackwell.

Health Protection Agency (HPA). (2008a). Chlamydia trachomatis *infection testing by Nucleic Acid Amplification Tests (NAATs).* Retrieved from https://www.gov.uk/government/publications/smi-v-37-chlamydia-trachomatis-infection-testing-by-nucleic-acid-amplification-test-naat

Health Protection Agency. (2008b). Data from UK GUM clinics up to 2007 indicates continued increase in diagnoses of STIs. *Health Protection Report* [Serial online], 2(29). HIV/STIs http://www.hpa.org.uk/hpr/archives/2009/news2009.htm

Health Protection Agency (HPA). (2010b). Major step forward in chlamydia screening in 2009/10. *Health Protection Report, 4*(23).

Hernandez, B. Y., McDuffie, K., Xhu, X., Wilkens, L. R., Killeen, J., Kessel, B., . . . Goodman, M. T. (2005). Anal human papillomavirus infection in women and its relationship with cervical infection. *Cancer Epidemiology, Biomarkers & Prevention, 14*(11 Pt. 1), 2550–2556.

Hitt, E. (2010). Young women face barriers to STI testing—Including their own misconceptions. Retrieved from www.Medscape.come/viewarticle/718753

Hjelmevoll, S. O., Olsen, M. E., Ericson Sollid, J. U., Haaheim, H., Melby, K. K., Moi, H., . . . Skogen, V. (2011). Appropriate time for test-of-cure when diagnosing gonorrhoea with a nucleic acid amplification test. *Acta Dermato-Venereologica, 92*(3), 316–319.

Hobbs, M. M., Lapple, D. M., Lawing, L. F., Schwebke, J. R., Cohen, M. S., Swygard, H., . . . Seña, A. C. (2006). Methods for detection of *Trichomonas vaginalis* in the male partners of infeted women: implications for control of trichomoniasis. *Journal of Clinical Microbiology, 44*(11), 3994–3999.

Høie, S., Knudsen, L. S., & Gerstoft, J. (2011). Lymphogranuloma venereum proctitis: A differential diagnosis to inflammatory bowel disease. *Scandinavian Journal of Gastroenterology, 46*(4), 503–510.

Hollman, D., Coupey, S. M., Fox, A. S., & Harold, B. C. (2010). Screening for *Trichomonas vaginalis* in high-risk adolescent females with a new transcription mediated nucleic acid amplification test (NAAT): Associations with ethnicity, symptoms, and prior and current STIs. *Journal of Pediatric & Adolescent Gynecology, 23*(5), 312–316.

Hoots, B. E., Peterman, T. A., Torrone, E. A., Weinstock, H., Meites, E., & Bolan, G. A. (2013). A trich-y question: Should Trichomonas vaginalis infection be reportable? *Sexually Transmitted Diseases, 40*(2), 113–116. doi: 10.1097/OLQ.0b013e31827c08c3

Horner, P. (2006). The case for further treatment studies of uncomplicated genital *Chlamydia trachomatis* infection. *Sexually Transmitted Infections, 82*(4), 340–343.

Horner, P. (2012). Azithromycin antimicrobial resistance and genital *Chlamydia trachomatis* infection: Duration of therapy may be the key to improving efficacy. *Sexually Transmitted Infections, 88*(3), 154–156.

Huppert, J. S., Mortensen, J. E., Reed, J. L., Khan, J. A., Rich, K. D., Miller, W. C., & Hobbs, M. M. (2007). Rapid antigen testing compares favourably with transcription-mediated amplification assay for the detection of *Trichomonas vaginalis* in young women. *Clinical Infectious Diseases, 45*(2), 194–198.

Huppert, J. S., Batteiger, B. E., Braslins, P., Feldman, J. A., Hobbs, M. M., Sankey, H. Z., . . . Wendel, K. A. (2005). Use of an immunochromatographic assay for rapid detection of *Trichomonas vaginalis* in vaginal specimens. *Journal of Clinical Microbiology, 43*(2), 684–687.

Huppert, J. S., Mortensen, J. E., Reed, J. L., Khan, J. A., Rich, K. D., & Hobbs, M. M. (2008). Mycoplasma genitalium detected by transcription-mediated amplification is associated with *Chlamydia trachomatis* in adolescent women. *Sexually Transmitted Diseases, 35*(3), 250–254.

International Agency for Research on Cancer (IARC). (2007). *IARC Monographs on evaluation of carcinogenic risks to humans: Human papillomaviruses* (Vol. 90). Lyon, France: WHO and IARC. Retrieved from https://monographs.iarc.fr/ENG/Monographs/vol90/mono90.pdf

Insinga, R. P., Dasbach, E. J., & Elbasha, E. H. (2009). Epidemiologic natural history and clinical management of human papillomavirus (HPV) disease: A critical and systematic review of the literature in the development of an HPV dynamic transmission model. *BMC Infectious Diseases, 9,* 119.

Ison C. A., Mounton J. W., Jones K., Fenton K. A., Livermore D. M., & North Thames Audit Group. (2004). Which cephalosporin for gonorrhoea? *Sexually Transmitted Infections, 80*(5), 386–388.

Ison, C. A., Hussey, J., Sankar, K. N., Evans, J., & Alexander, S. (2011). Gonorrhoea treatment failures to cefixime and azithromycin in England, 2010. *Euro Surveillance, 16*(14), pii=19833. Available online: http://www.eurosurveillance.org/ViewArticle.aspx?Articled=19833. (Accessed 2014).

Ison, C. A., & Hay, P. E. (2002). Validation of a simplified grading of Gram stained vaginal smears for use in genitourinary medicine clinics. *Sexually Transmitted Infections, 78*(6), 413–415.

Jaiyeoba, O., & Soper, D. E. (2011). A practical approach to the diagnosis of pelvic inflammatory disease. *Infectious Diseases in Obstetrics and Gynecology, 2011,* Article ID 753037. Retrieved from https://www.hindawi.com/journals/idog/2011/753037/

Janda, W. J., & Knapp, J. (2003). Neisseria and Moraxella catarrhalis. In P. R. Murray, E. J. Baron, M. A. Pfaller, J. H. Jorgensen, & R. H. Yolken (Eds.), *Manual of clinical microbiology* (8th ed., 585–608). Washington, DC: American Society Microbiology.

Jay, C. A. (2006). Treatment of neurosyphilis. *Current Treatment Options in Neurology, 8*(3), 185–192.

Jayasuriya, A. (2011). Vaccinations, treatments and post exposure prophylaxis. In K. E. Rogstad (Ed.), *ABC of sexually transmitted infections* (6th ed., pp. 132–140). Chichester, United Kingdom: Wiley-Blackwell.

Jemal, A., Simard, E. P., Dorell, C., Noone, A. M., Markowitz, L. E., Kohler, B., ... Edwards, B. K. (2013). Annual report to the nation on the status of cancer, 1975–2009, featuring the burden and trends of human papillomavirus (HPV)-associated cancers and HPV vaccination coverage levels. *Journal of the National Cancer Institute, 105*(3), 175–201.

Johnson, R. E., Newhall, W. J., Papp, J. R., Knapp, J. S., Black, C. M., Gift, T.L., ... Berman, S. M. (2002). Screening tests to detect *Chlamydia trachomatis* and *Neisseria gonorrhoeae* infections. *MMWR Recommendations* Report, 51(RR-15).

Johnston, C., & Corey, L. (2016). Current concepts for genital herpes simplex virus infection: diagnostics and pathogenesis of genital tract shedding. *Clinical Microbiology Reviews, 29*(1), 149–161.

Joki-Korpela, P., Sahrakorpi, N., Halttunen, M., Surcel, H. M., Paavonen, J., & Tiitinen, A. (2009). The role of *Chlamydia trachomatis* infection in male infertility. *Fertility and Sterility, 91*(4), 1448–1450.

Jorge, S., & Wright, J. D. (2016). Update: HPV prevention. Retrieved from http://contemporaryobgyn.modernmedicine.com /contemporary-obgyn/news/update-hpv-prevention

Juckett, G., & Hartman-Adams, H. (2010). Human papillomavirus: clinical manifestations and prevention. *American Family Physician, 82*(10), 1209–1214.

Judlin, P., Liao, Q., Liu, Z., Reimnitz, P., Hampel, B., & Arvis, P. (2010). Efficacy and safety of moxifloxacin in uncomplicated pelvic inflammatory disease: The MONALISA study. *BJOG: An International Journal of Obstetrics & Gynaecology, 117*(12), 1475–1484.

Jungmann, E. M. (2004). Genital herpes. *American Family Physician, 70*(5), 912–914.

Medical Foundation for HIV & Sexual Health (MEDFASH) and British Association for Sexual Health and HIV (2014) Standards for the management of sexually transmitted infections (STIs). Revised and Updated January 2014.

King, T. L., Brucker, M. C., Kriebs, J. M., Fahey, J. O., Gegor, C. L., & Varney, H. (2015). *Varney's midwifery* (5th ed.). Burlington, MA: Jones and Bartlett.

Kingston, M., French, P., Goh, B., Goold, P., Higgins, S., Sukthankar, A., ... Young, H. (2008). UK national guidelines on the management of syphilis 2008. *International Journal of STD & AIDS, 19*(11), 729–740

Kissinger, P., Mena, L., Levison, J., Clark, R. A., Gatski, M., Henderson, H., ... Martin, D. H. (2010). A randomised treatment trial: single versus 7 day dose of metronidazole for the treatment of *Trichomonas vaginalis* among HIV-infected women. *JAIDS, 55*(5), 565–571.

Kissinger, P., Secor, W. E., Leichliter, J. S., Clark, R. A., Schmidt N., Curtin, E., & Martin, D. H. (2008). Early repeated infections with *Trichomonas vaginalis* among HIV-positive and HIV-negative women *Clinical Infectious Diseases, 46*(7), 994–999.

Knaute, D. F., Graf, N., Lautenschlager, S., Weber, R., & Bosshard, P. P. (2012). Serological response to treatment of syphilis according to disease stage and HIV status. *Clinical Infectious Diseases, 55*(12), 1615–1622.

Koek, A. G., Bruisten, S. M., Dierdrop, M., Van Dam, A. P., & Templeton, K. (2006). Specific and sensitive diagnosis of syphilis using a real-time PCR for treponema pallidum. *Clinical Microbiology and Infection, 12*(12), 1233–1236.

Komolafe, A. J., Sugunendran, H., & Corkill, J. E. (2004). Gonorrhoea: Test of cure for sensitive bacteria? Use of genotyping to disprove treatment failure. *International Journal of STD & AIDS, 15*(3), 212.

Kong, F. Y. S., Tabrizi, S. N., Law, M., Vodstrcil, L. A., Chen, M., Fairley, C. K., ... Hocking, J. S. (2014). Azithromycin versus doxycycline for the treatment of genital chlamydia infection: A meta-analysis of randomized controlled trials. *Clinical Infectious Diseases, 59*(2), 193–205.

Körber, A., & Dissemond, J. (2009). Pearly penile papules. *Canadian Medical Association Journal, 181*(6–7), 397.

Korhonen, S., Hiltunen-Back, E., & Puolakkainen, M. (2012). Genotyping of *Chlamydia trachomatis* in rectal and pharyngeal specimens: identification of LGV genotypes in Finland. *Sexually Transmitted Infections, 88*(6), 465–469.

Lacey, C. J., Lowndes., C. M., & Shah, K. V. (2006). Burden and management of non-cancerous HPV-related conditions HPV6/11 disease. *Vaccine, 24*(3), 35–41.

LaFond, R. E., & Lukehart, S. A. (2006). Biological basis for syphilis. *Clinical Microbiology Reviews, 19*(1), 29–49.

Lamontagne, D. S., Baster, K., Emmett, L., Nichols, T., Randall, S., McLean, L., ... Fenton, K. A. (2007). Incidence and re-infection rates of genital chlamydial infection among women aged 16–24 years attending general practice, family planning and genitourinary medicine clinics in England: A prospective cohort study by the Chlamydia Recall Study Advisory Group. *Sexually Transmitted Infections, 83*(4), 292–303.

Landers, D. V., Wiesenfeld, H. C., Heine, R. P., Krohn, M. A., & Hillier, S. L. (2004). Predictive value of the clinical diagnosis of lower genital tract infection in women. *American Journal of Obstetrics and Gynecology, 190*(4), 1004–1010.

Lanjouw, E., Ouburg, S., de Vries, H. J., Stary, A., Radcliffe, K., & Unemo, M. (2015). 2015 European guideline on the management of *Chlamydia trachomatis* infections. *International Journal of STD & AIDS, 27*(5), 333–348.

Lautenschlager, S. (2006). Cutaneous manifestations of syphilis: recognition and management. *American Journal of Clinical Dermatology, 7*(5), 291–304.

Lazaro, N. (2013). *Sexually transmitted infections in primary care*. London, United Kingdom: RCGP/BASHH. Retrieved from http://www.rcgp.org.uk/clinical-and-research/clinical-resources /sexually-transmitted-infections-in-primary-care.aspx

Lechtenberg, R. J., Samuel, M. C., Bernstein, K. T., Lahiff, M., Olsen, N., & Bauer, H. M. (2014, May). Variation in adherence to treatment guidelines for *Neisseria gonorrhoeae* by clinical practice setting, California, 2009–2011. *Sexually Transmitted Diseases, 41*(5), 338–344.

LeFevre, ML. (2014). Behavioral counseling interventions to prevent sexually transmitted infections: U.S. Preventive Services Task Force recommendation statement. *Annals of Internal Medicine, 161*(12), 894–901.

Leichliter, J. S., Sejiler, N., & Wohlfeiler, D. (2015, March). Sexually transmitted disease prevention policies in the United States: Evidence and opportunities. *Sexually Transmitted Diseases, 43*(2 Suppl. 1), S113–S121.

Levett, P. N., Brandt, K., Olenius, K., Brown, C., Montgomery, K., & Horsman, G. B. (2008). Evaluation of three automated nucleic acid amplification systems for detection of *Chlamydia trachomatis* and *Neisseria gonorrhoeae* in first void urine specimens. *Journal of Clinical Microbiology, 46*(6), 2109–2111.

Lewis, D. A. (2011). Sexual health care in resource poor settings. In K. E. Rogstad (Ed.), *ABC of sexually transmitted infections* (6th ed., pp. 127–131). Chichester, United Kingdom: Wiley-Blackwell.

Liu, B., Roberts, C. L., Clarke, M., Jorm, L., Hunt, J., & Ward, J. (2013). Chlamydia and gonorrhoea infections and the risk of obstetric outcomes: a retrospective cohort study. *Sexually Transmitted Infections, 89*(8), 672–678.

Low, N., Broutet, N., Adu-Sarkodie, Y., Barton, P., Hossain, M., & Hawkes, S. (2006). Global control of sexually transmitted infections. *Lancet, 368*(9551), 2001–2016.

Lukehart, S. A., Godornes, C., Molini, B., Sonnett, P., Hopkins, S., Mulcahy, F., . . . Klausner, J. D. (2004). Macrolide resistance in treponema pallidum in the United States and Ireland. *New England Journal of Medicine, 351*(2), 154–158.

Magpantay, G., Cardile, A. P., Madar, C. S., Hsue, G., & Belnap C. (2011). Antibiotic desensitization therapy in secondary syphilis and listeria infection: Case reports and review of desensitization therapy. *Hawaii Medical Journal, 70*(12), 266–268.

Mahmood, M. A., & Saniotis, A. (2011). Use of syndromic management algorithm for STIs and RTIs management in community settings in Karachi. *Journal of the Pakistan Medical Association, 61*(5), 453–457.

Mammen-Tobin, A., & Wilson, J. D. (2005). Management of metronidazole-resistant *Trichomonas vaginalis* – A new approach. *International Journal of STD & AIDS, 16*(7), 488–490.

Mangin, D., Murdoch, D., Wells, J. E., Coughlan, E., Bagshaw, S., Corwin, P., . . . Toop, L. (2012). *Chlamydia trachomatis* testing sensitivity in midstream compared with first-void urine specimens. *The Annals of Family Medicine, 10*(1), 50–53.

Mann, J. R., McDermott, S., Barnes, T. L., Hardin, J., Bao, H., & Zhou, L. (2009). Trichomonas in pregnancy and mental retardation in children. *Annals of Epidemiology, 19*(12), 891–899.

Marcone, V., Calzolari, E., & Bertini, M. (2008). Effectiveness of vaginal administration of Lactobacillus rhamnosus following conventional metronidazole therapy: How to lower the rate of bacterial vaginosis recurrences. *New Microbiologia, 31*(3), 429–433.

McCance, D. J. (2004). Papillomaviruses. In A. J. Zuchermak, J. E. Banatvala, J. R. Pattison, P. Griffiths & Schoub B. (Eds.), *Principles and practice of clinical virology* (5th ed.). New York, NY: John Wiley & Sons Ltd.

McClean, H., Raddcliffe, K., Sullivan, A. K., & Ahmed-Jushuf, I. (2012). *BASHH statement on partner notification for sexually transmissible infections*. Retrieved from https://www.bashh.org/documents/4445.pdf

McClelland, S. R., Sangaré, L., Hassan, W. M., Lavreys, L., Mandaliya, K., Kiarie, J., . . . Baeten, J. M. (2007). Infection with *Trichomonas vaginalis* increases the risk of HIV–1 acquisition. *Journal of Infectious Diseases, 195*(5), 698–702.

McCray, A. T. (2005). Promoting health literacy. *Journal of the American Medical Informatics Association, 12*(2), 152–163. Retrieved from http://dx.doi.org/10.1197/jamia.M1687

McGowin, C. L., & Anderson-Smits, C. (2011). Mucoplasma genitalium: an emerging cause of sexually transmitted disease in women. *PLOS Pathogens, 7*(5), e1001324.

McMillan, A., & Young, H. (2008). Reactivity in the Venereal Disease Research Laboratory test and the Mercia IgM enzyme immunoassay after treatment of early syphilis. *International Journal of STD & AIDS, 19*(10), 689–693.

Medical Foundation for AIDS & Sexual Health (MEDFASH). (2014). *Standards for the management of sexually transmitted infections (STIs)* (Rev. ed.). Retrieved from http://www.medfash.org.uk/uploads/files/p18dtqli8116261rv19i61rh9n2k4.pdf

Medical Foundation for HIV & Sexual Health (MEDFASH) and British Association for Sexual Health and HIV (BASHH). (2014). *Standards for the management of sexually transmitted infections (STIs)*. Retrieved from http://www.medfash.org.uk/uploads/files/p18dtqli8116261rv19i61rh9n2k4.pdf

Mehringer, M., Hertz, D., & DiPaolo, A. (2014). A qualitative exploration of STI screening practices and barriers among OB-GYNs and family practitioners in the United States. *Value in Health, 17*(3), A162.

Mehta, S. D. (2012). Systematic review of randomised trials of treatment of male sexual partners for improved bacteria vaginosis outcomes in women. *Sexually Transmitted Diseases, 39*(10), 822–830.

Meites, E. (2013). Trichomoniasis: The "neglected" sexually transmitted disease. *Infectious Disease Clinics of North America, 27*(4), 755–764.

Miller, K. E. (2006). Diagnosis and treatment of *Chlamydia trachomatis* infection. *American Family Physician, 73*(8), 1411–1416.

Miller, W. M., Gorini, F., Botelho, G., Moreira, C., Barbora, A. P., Pinto, A. R. S. B., . . . da Costa Nery, J. A. (2010). Jarisch-Herxheimer reaction among syphilis patients in Rio de Janeiro, Brazil. *International Journal of STD & AIDS, 21*(12), 806–809.

Mishori, R., McClaskey, E. L., & Winklerprins, V. J. (2012). *Chlamydia trachomatis* infections: Screening, diagnosis and management. *American Family Physician, 86*(12), 1127–1132.

Mitchell, H. (2004). Vaginal discharge – Causes, diagnosis, and treatment. *BMJ, 328*(7451), 1306–1308

Mitchell, C., Manhart, L. E., & Thomas, K. K. (2011). Effect of sexual activity on vaginal colonization with hydrogen peroxide producing lactobacilli and gardnerella vaginalis. *Sexually Transmitted Diseases, 38*(12), 1137–1144.

Morgan, E., Blume, A., & Carroll, R. (2011). A cluster of infectious syphilis among young heterosexuals in South East Hampshire. *International Journal of STD & AIDS, 22*(9), 512–513.

Moscicki, A. B., Ellenberg, J. H., Farhat, S., & Xu, J. (2004). Persistence of human papillomavirus infection in HIV-infected and -uninfected adolescent girls: Risk factors and differences by phylogenic type. *Journal of Infectious Diseases, 190*(1), 37–45.

Mugo, N. R., Kiehlbauch, J. A., Nguti, R., Meier, A., Gichuhi, J. W., Stamm, W. E., & Cohen, C. R. (2006). Effect of human immunodeficiency virus-1 infection on treatment outcome of acute salpingitis. *Obstetrics and Gynecology, 107*(4), 807–812.

Muñoz, N., Castellsagué, X., de González, A. B., & Gissmann, L. (2006). HPV in the aetiology of human cancer. *Vaccine, 24*(3), S3/1–10.

Nagot, N., Ouedraogo, A., Defer, M. C., Vallo, R., Mayaud, P., & Van de Perre, P. (2007). Association between bacterial vaginosis and Herpes simplex virus type–2 infection: Implications for HIV acquisition studies. *Sexually Transmitted Infections, 83*(5), 365–368.

National Institute for Health and Clinical Excellence (NICE). (2011). Gonorrhoea: Clinical knowledge summaries (CKS) Retrieved from https://cks.nice.org.uk/gonorrhoea

National Institute for Health and Care Excellence (NICE). (2015). Pelvic inflammatory disease: Clinical knowledge summaries (CKS). Retrieved from https://cks.nice.org.uk/pelvic-inflammatory-disease

Ness, R. B., Hillier, S. L., Kip, K. E., Soper, D. E., Stamm, C. A., McGregor, J. A., . . . Richter, H. E. (2005). Bacterial vaginosis and risk of pelvic inflammatory disease. *Obstetrical & Gynecological Survey, 60(2),* 99–100.

Newman, L. M., Moran, J. S., & Workowski, K. A. (2007). Update on the management of gonorrhoea in adults in the United States. *Clinical Infectious Diseases, 44(3),* S84–S101.

Nugent, R. P., Krohn, M. A., & Hillier, S. L. (1991). Reliability if diagnosing bacterial vaginosis is improved by a standardised method of gram stain interpretation. *Journal of Clinical Microbiology, 29(2),* 297–301.

Nwokolo, N. C., Dragovic, B., Patel, S., Tong, C. Y. W., Barker, G., & Radcliffe, K. (2016). UK national guideline for the management of infection with *Chlamydia trachomatis. International Journal of STD & AIDS, 27(4),* 251–267.

Nye, M. B., Schwebke, J. R., & Body B. A. (2009). Comparison of APTIMA *Trichomonas vaginalis* transcription-mediated amplification to wet mount microscopy, culture, and polymerase chain reaction for diagnosis of trichomoniasis in men and women. *American Journal of Obstetrics and Gynecology, 200(2),* 188. e1–188.e7.

O'Farrell, N. (2002). Donovanosis. *Sexually Transmitted Infections, 78(6),* 452–457.

Paavonen, J., & Eggert-Kruse, W. (1999). *Chlamydia trachomatis*: Impact on human reproduction. *Human Reproduction Update, 5(5),* 433–447.

Palmer, H. M., Young, H., Winter, A., & Dave, J. (2008). Emergence and spread of azithromycin-resistant *Neisseria gonorrhoeae* in Scotland. *Journal of Antimicrobial Chemotherapy, 62(3),* 490–494.

Parc, C. E., Chahed, S., Patel, S. V., & Salmon-Ceron, D. (2007). Manifestations and treatment of ocular syphilis during an epidemic in France. *Sexually Transmitted Infections, 34(8),* 553–556.

Parkes, R., Renton, A., Meheus, A., & Laukamm-Josten, U. (2004). Review of current evidence and comparison of guidelines for effective syphilis treatment in Europe. *International Journal of STD & AIDS, 15(2),* 73–88.

Patel, R., Alderson, S., Geretti, A., Nilsen, A., Foley, E., Lautenschlager, S., . . . Moi, H. (2011). European guideline for the management of genital herpes, 2010. *International Journal of STD & AIDS, 22(1),* 1–10.

Patel, R., & Gupta, N. (2011). Genital ulcer disease. In: Rogstad, K. E., ed. *ABC of Sexually Transmitted Infections,* 6th ed. Chichester, United Kingdom: Wiley-Blackwell.

Patterson, N. A., Smith, J. L., & Ozbun, M. A. (2005). Human papillomavirus type 31b infection of human keratinocytes does not require heparin sulphate. *Journal of Virology, 79(11),* 6838–6847.

Pattishall, A. E., Rahman, S. Y., Jain, S., & Simon, H. K. (2012). Empiric treatment of STIs in a pediatric emergency department: Are we making the right decisions? *American Journal of Emergency Medicine, 30(8),* 1588–1590.

Pattman, R., Sankar, N., Elawad, B., Handy, P., & Price, D. A. (Eds.). (2010). *Oxford handbook of genitourinary medicine, HIV and sexual health.* 2nd ed. Oxford, United Kingdom: Oxford University Press.

Patton, M. E., Su J. R., Nelson, R., & Weinstock, H. (2014). Primary and secondary syphilis - United States, 2005–2013. *MMWR, 63(18),* 402–406.

Paz-Bailey, G., Koumans, E.H., Sternberg, M., Pierce, A., Papp, J., Unger, E. R., . . . Markowitz L. E. (2005). Effect of correct and consistent condom use on chlamydial and gonorrhoeal infection among urban adolescents. *Archives of Pediatrics & Adolescent Medicine, 159(6),* 536–542.

Peuchant, O., Baldit, C., Le Roy, C., Trombert-Paolantoni, S., Clerc, M., Bébéar, C., & de Barbeyrac, B. (2011). First case of *Chlamydia trachomatis* L2b proctitis in a woman. *Clin Microbiol Infect.* 17(12): e21–23.

Peterman, T. A., & Carter, M. W. (2016). Effective interventions to reduce sexually transmitted disease: Introduction to the special issue. *Sexually Transmitted Diseases, 43*(Suppl. 1), S1–S2.

Peterman, T. A., Tian, L. H., Metcalf, C. A., Satterwhite, C. L., Malotte, C. K., DeAugustine, N., . . . Douglas, J. M. Jr. (2006). High incidence of new sexually transmitted infections in the year following a sexually transmitted infection: A case for re-screening. *Annals of Internal Medicine, 145(8),* 564–572.

Pirotta, M., Gunn, J., Chondros, P., Grover, S., O'Malley, P., Hurley, S., & Garland, S. (2004). Effect of lactobacillus in preventing post-antibiotic vulvovaginal candidiasis: A randomised controlled trial. *BMJ, 329(7465),* 548.

Public Health England (PHE). (2013). *National chlamydia screening programme.* Retrieved from www.chlamydiascreening.nhs.uk/ps/

Public Health England (PHE). (2015). *Infection report.* Retrieved from https://www.gov.uk/government/collections/sexually-transmitted-infections-stis-surveillance-data-screening-and-management

Pushplata, S., Devyani, M., Pyari, J. S., & Deo, S. (2014) Bizzare foreign objects in the genital tract – Our experience and review of literature. *Open Journal of Obstetrics and Gynecology, 4(7),* 427–431.

Rank, R. G., & Yeruva, L. (2014). Hidden in plain sight: Chlamydial gastrointestinal infection and its relevance to persistence in human genital infection. *Infection and Immunity, 82(4),* 1362–1371.

Ray, K., Muralidhar, S., Bala, M., Kumari, M., Gupta, S. M., & Bhattacharya, M. (2009). Comparative study of reproductive tract infection/sexually transmitted infections in women in Delhi. *International Journal of Infectious Diseases, 13(6),* 352–359.

Ray, A., Ray, S., George, A. T., & Swaminathan, N. (2011). Interventions for prevention and treatment of vulvovaginal candidiasis in women with HIV infection. *The Chochrane Database of Systematic Reviews, 8,* CD008739. doi: 10.1002/14651858.CD008739.pub2

Reilley, B., Leston, J., Tulloch, S., Neel, L., Galope, M., & Taylor, M. (2015). Implementation of national HIV screening recommendations in the Indian Health Service. *Journal of the International Association of Providers of AIDS Care, 14(4),* 291–294. Retrieved from http://dx.doi.org/10.1177/2325957415570744

Richens J. (2011). Main presentations of sexually transmitted infections in male patients. In K. E. Rogstad (Ed.), *ABC of sexually transmitted infections,* (6th ed., pp. 29–34). Chichester, United Kingdom: Wiley-Blackwell.

Riedner, G., Rusizoka, M., Todd, J., Maboko, L., Hoelscher, M., Mmbando, D., . . . Hayes, R. (2005). Single dose azithromycin versus penicillin G benzathine for the treatment of early syphilis. *New England Journal of Medicine, 353*(12), 1236–1244.

Righarts, A. A., Simms, I., Wallace, L., Solomou, M., & Fenton, K. A. (2004). Syphilis surveillance and epidemiology in the United Kingdom. *Euro Surveillance, 9*(12), 21–25.

Risley, C.L., Ward, H., Choudhry, B., Bishop, C. J., Fenton, K. A., Spratt, B.G., . . . Ghani, A. C. (2007). Geographical and demographic clustering of gonorrhoea in London. *Sexually Transmitted Infections, 83*(6), 481–487.

Roett, M. A., Mayor, M. T., & Uduhiri, K. A. (2012). Diagnosis and management of genital ulcers. *Am Fam Physician 85*(3): 254–262.

Rompalo, A. M., Lawlor, J., Seaman, P., Quinn, T. C., Zenilman, J. M., & Hook, E. W. (2001). Modification of syphilitic genital ulcer manifestations by co-existent HIV infection. *Sexually Transmitted Diseases, 28*(8), 448–454.

Rönn, M. M., & Ward, H. (2011). The association between lymphogranuloma venereum and HIV among men who have sex with men: systematic review and meta-analysis. *BMC Infectious Diseases, 11*, 70.

Rooney, J. F., Straus, S. E., Mannix, M. L., Wohlenberg, C. R., Alling, E. W., Dumois, J. A., & Notkins, A. L. (1993). Oral acyclovir to suppress frequently recurrent herpes labialis: A double-blind placebo-controlled trial. *Annals of Internal Medicine, 118*(4), 268–272.

Rosenfeld, E. A. (2014). Exploratory research on healthcare provider's perspectives on expedited partner therapy to treat patients with chlamydia (Doctoral dissertation). Retrieved from d-scholarship.pitt.edu/22565/.

Ross, J. D. C. (2011). Pelvic inflammatory disease and pelvic pain. In K. E. Rogstad (Ed.), *ABC of sexually transmitted infections* (6th ed., pp. 49–52). Chichester, United Kingdom: Wiley Blackwell.

Ross, J., Judlin, P., & Jensen, J. (2014). 2012 European guideline for the management of pelvic inflammatory disease. *International Journal of STD & AIDS, 25*(1), 1–7.

Ross, J. D. C., & McCarthy, G. (2011). *UK National guideline for the management of pelvic inflammatory disease.* Retrieved from http://www.bashh.org/documents/3572.pdf (Last accessed March 2014).

Rotty, J., Anderson, D., Garcia, M., Diaz, J., Van de Waarsenburg, S., Howard, T., . . . Hoy, J. (2010). Preliminary assessment of treponema pallidum-specific IgM antibody detection and a new rapid point-of-care assay for the diagnosis of syphilis in human immunodeficiency virus–1-infected patients. *International Journal of STD & AIDS, 21*(11), 758–764.

Royal College of Obstetricians and Gynaecologists (RCOG). (2009). *Pelvic inflammatory disease.* Green Top Guidelines, Number: 32 London, United Kingdom: RCOG Press. Retrieved from https://www.bashh.org/documents/3572.pdf

Ryder, N., Jin, F., McNulty, A. M., Grulich, A. E., & Donovan, B. (2009). Increasing role of herpes simplex virus type 1 in first-episode anogenital herpes in heterosexual women and younger men who have sex with men, 1992–2006. *Sexually Transmitted Infections, 85*(6), 416–419.

Sammarco, A. (2017). *Women's health issues across the life cycle: A quality of life perspective.* Burlington, MA: Jones and Bartlett.

Saporiti, A. M., Gómez, D., Levalle, S., Galeano, M., Davel, G., Vivot, W., & Rodero, L. (2001). Vaginal candidiasis: Etiology and sensitivity profile to antifungal agents in clinical use. *Revista Argentina de Microbiologia, 33*(4), 217–222.

Sathia, L., Ellis, B., Phillips, S., Winston, A., & Smith, A. (2007). Pharyngeal gonorrhoea—Is dual therapy the way forward? *International Journal of STD & AIDS, 18*(9), 647–648.

Sato, N. S. (2011). Serologic response to treatment in syphilis. In N. S. Sato (Ed.), *Syphilis recognition, description and diagnosis* (pp. 109–122). Vienna, Austria: InTech Open. Retrieved from https://www.intechopen.com/books/syphilis-recognition-description-and-diagnosis

Schiffer, J. T., & Corey, L. (2009). New concepts in understanding genital herpes. *Current Infectious Disease Reports, 11*(6), 457–464.

Schiffer, J. T., Wald, A., Selke, S., Corey, L., & Magaret, A. (2011). The kinetics of mucosal herpes simplex virus-2 infection in humans: evidence for rapid viral-host interactions. *Journal of Infectious Diseases, 204*(4), 554–561.

Schillinger, J. A., Gorwitz, R., Rietmeijer, C., & Golden, M. R. (2016). The expedited partner therapy continuum: A conceptual framework to guide programmatic efforts to increase partner treatment. *Sexually Transmitted Diseases, 43*(2 Suppl. 1), S63–S75. http://dx.doi.org/10.1097/OLQ.0000000000000399

Secour, W. E., Meites, E., Starr, M. C., & Workowski, K. A. (2014). Neglected parasitic infections in the United States: Trichomoniasis. *The American Journal of tropical Medicine and Hygiene, 90*(5), 800–804. Retrieved from http://dx.doi.org/10.4269/ajtmh.13-0723

Schwebke, J. R., & Desmond, R. A. (2010). A randomised controlled trial of partner notification methods for prevention of trichomoniasis in women. *Sexually Transmitted Diseases, 37*(6), 392–396.

Scottish Intercollegiate Guidelines Network (SIGN). (2009). Management of genital *Chlamydia trachomatis* infection: A national clinical guideline. Edinburgh, United Kingdom: Author.

Sehnal, B., Driák, D., Neumannová, H., Kolařik, D., Menzlová, E., & Sláma, J. (2012). Prevalence of anal human papillomavirus infection among women and its relation to cervical HPV infection. *Czech Gynecology, 77*(3), 210–214.

Seidman, D., Carlson, K., Weber, S., Witt, J., & Kelly, P. J. (2015). United States family planning providers' knowledge of and attitudes toward preexposure prophylaxis for HIV prevention: A national survey. *Contraception, 93*, 463–469. Retrieved from http://dx.doi.org/10.1016/j.contraception.2015.12.018

Seña, A. C., Miller, W. C., Hobbs, M. M., Schwebke, J. R., Leone, P. A., Swygard, H., . . . Cohen, M. S. (2007). Trichomonas vaginalis infection in male sexual partners: implications for diagnosis, treatment, and prevention. *Clinical Infectious Diseases, 44*(1), 13–22.

Sherrard, J., Donders, G., White, D., Jensen, J. S., IUSTI. (2011). European (IUSTI/WHO) guideline on the management of vaginal discharge, 2011. *International Journal of STD & AIDS, 22*(8), 421–429.

Sherrard, J., Ison, C., Moody, J., Wainwright, E., Wilson, J., & Sullivan, A. (2014). United Kingdom national guideline on the management of Trichomonas Vaginalis 2014. International Journal of STD & AIDS, 25(8), 541–549.

Simms, I., Fenton, K. A., Ashton, M., Turner, K. M., Crawley-Boevey E. E., Gorton, R., . . . Solomou, (2005). Re-emergence of syphilis in the UK: The new epidemic phases. *Sexually Transmitted Diseases, 32*(4), 220–226.

Simms, I., McDonald, N., Ison, C., Alexander, S., Lowndes, C. M., & Fenton, K. A. (2004). Enhanced surveillance of lymphogranuloma venereum (LGV) begins in England. *Euro Surveillance, 8*(41), pii. 2565.

Smith, J. C., & Medalia, C. (2014). *Health insurance coverage in the United States: 2014.* Retrieved from https://www.census.gov/content/dam/Census/library/publications/2015/demo/p60-253.pdf

Snapp, M., & Bienkowska-Haba, M. (2009). Viral entry mechanisms: Human papilloma virus and a long journey from extracellular matrix to the nucleus. *The FEBS Journal, 276*(24), 7206–7216.

Sobel, J. D., Ferris, D., Schwebke, J., Nyirjesy, P., Wiesenfeld, H. C., Peipert, J., Soper, D., Ohmit, S. E., & Hillier, S. L. (2006). Suppressive antibacterial therapy with 0.70% metronidazole vaginal gel to prevent recurrent bacterial vaginosis, *American Journal of Obstetrics and Gynecology, 194*(5), 1283–1289.

Solensky, R. (2004). Drug desensitization. *Immunology and Allergy Clinics of North America, 24*(3), 425.

Spaargaren, J., Fennema, H. S. Morre, S. A., de Vries, H. J., & Coutinho, R. A. (2005). New lymphogranoloma venereum *Chlamydia trachomatis* variant, Amsterdam. *Emerging Infectious Diseases, 11*(7), 1090–1092.

Spence, D., & Melville, C. (2007). Vaginal discharge. *BMJ, 335*(7630), 1147–1151.

Stamm, W. E. (2005). Chlamydial diseases. In G. L. Mandell, J. E. Bennell, & R. Dolin (Eds.), *Principles and practice of infectious diseases* (6th ed., pp. 2236-2256). Philadelphia, PA: Elsevier.

Stamm, W. E. (2008). Lymphogranuloma venereum. In K. K. Holmes, P. F. Sparling, W. E. Stamm, P. Piot, J. N. Wasserheit, L. Corey, . . . D. H. Watts (Eds.), *Sexually transmitted diseases* (4th ed., pp. 595–606). New York, NY: McGraw-Hill, pp. 595–606.

Starnino, S., Stefanelli, P., & *Neisseria Gonorrhoeae* Italian Study Group. (2009). Azithromycin-resistant *Neisseria gonorrhoeae* strains recently isolated in Italy. *Journal of Antimicrobial Chemotherapy, 63*(6), 1200–1204.

Stonnenberg, P., Clifton, S., Beddows, S., Field, N., Soldan, K., Tanton, C., . . . Johnson, A. M. (2013). Prevalence, risk factors, and uptake of interventions for sexually transmitted infections in Britain: Findings from the National Surveys of Sexual Attitudes and lifestyles (NATSAL). *Lancet, 382*(9907), 1795–1806.

Steen, R., Chersich, M., Gerbase, A., Neilsen, G., Wendland, A., Ndowa, F., . . . de Vlas, S. J. (2012). Periodic presumptive treatment of curable sexually transmitted infections among sex workers: A systematic review. *AIDS., 26*(4), 437–445.

Sterling, J. C. (2004). Viral infections. In T. Burns, S. Breathnach, N. Cox, & C. Griffiths (Eds.), *Rook's textbook of dermatology,* (7th ed., pp. 1–83). Oxford, United Kingdom: Blackwell Science Ltd.

Stevens, M., Twin, J., Fairley, C., Donovan, C., Tan, S., Garland, S., & Tabrizi, S. (2010). Development and evaluation of an ompA quantitative real-time PCR assay for *Chlamydia trachomatis* serovar determination. *Journal of Clinical Microbiology, 48*(6), 2060–2065.

Stoner, B. P. (2007). Current controversies in the management of adult syphilis. *Clinical Infectious Diseases, 44(3),* S130–S146.

Stringer, E., Read, J. S., Hoffman, I., Valentine, M., Aboud, S., & Goldenberg, R. L. (2010). Treatment of trichomoniasis in pregnancy in Sub-Saharan Africa does not appear to be associated with low birthweight or preterm birth. *South African Medical Journal, 100*(1), 58–64.

Stupiansky, N.W., Van Der Pol, B., Williams, J. A., Weaver, B., Taylor, S. E., & Forlenberry, J.D. (2011). Coinfection with chlamydia in women associated with high gonococcal organism loads, which potentially increase transmission: The National Institute of Incident Gonococcal infection in adolescent women. *Sexually Transmitted Diseases, 38*(8), 750–754.

Tann, C. J., Mpairwe, H., Morison, L., Nassimu, K., Hughes, P., Omara, M., . . . Elliot, A. M. (2006). Lack of effectiveness of syndromic management in targeting vaginal infections in pregnancy in Entebbe, Uganda. *Sexually Transmitted Infections, 82*(4), 285–289.

Tapsall, J. W., Ndowa, F., Lewis, D. A., & Unemo, M. (2009). Meeting the public health challenge of multidrug- and extensively drug-resistant *Neisseria gonorrhoeae. Expert Review of Anti-infective Therapy, 7*(7), 821–834.

Taylor, G., Dasari, B. V. M., & McKie, L. (2011). Lymphogranuloma vanareum (LGV) proctitis mimicking rectal cancer. *Colorectal Disease, 13,* e63–e64.

Taylor, M. M., Frasure-Williams, J., Burnett, P., & Park, I. U. (2015). Interventions to improve sexually transmitted disease screening in clinic-based settings. *Sexually Transmitted Diseases, 43*(2 Suppl. 1), S28–S41.

Thierry, J., Marrazzo, J., & LaMarre, M. (2004). Barriers to infectious disease prevention among women. *Emerging Infectious Diseases, 10*(11). Retrieved from http://dx.doi.org/10.3201/eid1011.040622_07

Thurman, A. R., Musatovova, O., Purdue, S., Shain, R. N., Baseman, J. G., & Baseman, J. B. (2010). Mycoplasma genitalium symptoms, concordance and treatment in high-risk sexual dyads. *International Journal of STD & AIDS, 21*(3), 177–183.

Tilson, E. C., Sanchez, V., Ford, C. L., Smurzynski, M., Leone, P. A., Fox, K. K., . . . Miller, W. C. (2004). Barriers to asymptomatic screening and other STD services for adolescents and young adults: Focus group discussions. *BMC Public Health, 4,* 21.

Tosh, A. K., Van Der Pol, B., Fortenberry, J. D., Williams, J. A., Katz, B. P., Batteiger, B. E., & Orr, D. P. (2007). Mycoplasma genitalium among adolescent women and their partners. *Journal of Adolescent Health, 40*(5), 412–417.

U.S. Department of Health and Human Services (DHHS). (2008). *America's health literacy: Why we need accessible health information.* Retrieved from Health.gov/communication/literacy/issuebrief/

U.S. Preventive Service Task Force (USPSTF). (2014). *Chlamydia and gonorrhea: Screening.* Retrieved from https://www.uspreventiveservicestaskforce.org/Page/Document/UpdateSummaryFinal/chlamydia-and-gonorrhea-screening

U.S. Preventive Services Task Force (USPSTF). (2017). About the USPSTF. Retrieved from http://www.uspreventiveservicestaskforce.org/Page/Name/about-the-uspstf

Vall-Mayans, M., Caballero, E., & Sanz, B. (2009). The emergence of lymphogranuloma venereum in Europe. *Lancet, 374*(9686), 356.

van der Bij, A. K., Spaargaren, J., Morré, S. A., Fennema, H. S., Mindel, A., Coutinho, R. A., & de Vries, H. J. (2006). Diagnostic and clinical implications of anorectal lymphogranuloma venereum in men who have sex with men: A retrospective case control study. *Clinical Infectious Diseases, 42*(2), 186–194.

van der Bij, A.K., Spaargaren, J., Morre, S. A., Servaas, A. M., Fennema, H. S. A., Mindel, A., . . . de Vries, H. J. (2006). Diagnostic and clinical implications of anorectal lymphogranuloma venereum in men who have sex with men: A retrospective case-control study. *Clinical Infectious Diseases, 42(2), 186–194.*

Van der Ham, R., & de Vries, H. J. (2009). Lymphogranuloma venereum: where do we stand? Clinical recommendation actions. *Drugs of Today (Barc), 45(3), 39–43.*

Verweij, S. P., Ouburg, S., de Vries, H., Morre, S. A., van Ginkel, C. J., Bos, H., & Sebens, F. W. (2012). The first case record of a female patient with bubonic lymphogranuloma venereum (LGV) serovariant L2b. *Sexually Transmitted Infections, 88(5), 346–347.*

Vicetti Miguel, R. D., Harvey, A. S. K., LaFramboise, W. A., Reighard, S. D., Matthews, D. B., & Cherpes, T. L. (2013). Human female genital tract infection by the obligate intracellular bacterium *Chlamydia trachomatis* elicits robust type 2 immunity. *PLoS ONE, 8(3),* e58565. doi: 10.1371/journal.pone.0058565

Wagenlehner, F. M., Wiedner, W., & Naber, K. G. (2006). Chlamydial Infections in urology. *World Journal of Urology, 24(1), 4–12.*

Wald, A., Langenberg, A. G. M., Krantz, E., Douglas, J. M., Handsfield, H. H., DiCarlo, R. P., et al. (2005). The relationship between condom use and herpes simplex virus acquisition. *Annals of Internal Medicine, 143(10), 707–713.*

Walker, J., Fairley, C., Bradshaw, C., Tabrizi, S., Chen, M., Twin, J., . . . Hocking, J. S. (2012). *Chlamydia trachomatis* incidence and reinfection among young women – behavioural and microbiological characteristics. *PLoS One, 7(5),* e37778.

Ward, H., MacDonald, N., Ronn, M., Dean, G., Pallawela, S., Sullivan, A., . . . Ison, C. (2011). Lymphogranuloma venereum in the UK: is there evidence for rectal to rectal transmission? Results of a multicentre case control study. *Sexually Transmitted Infections, 87(1),* A40–A40.

Wheeler, H. L., Agarwal, S., & Goh, B. T. (2004). Dark ground microscopy of treponemal serological tests in the diagnosis of early syphilis. *Sexually Transmitted Infections, 80(5), 411–414.*

Whiley, D. M., Tapsall, J. W., & Sloots, T. P. (2006). Nucleic acid amplification testing for *Neisseria gonorrhoeae*: An on-going challenge. *Journal of Molecular Diagnostics, 8(1), 3–15.*

White, J., O'Farell, N., & Daniels, D. (2013). UK national guideline for the management of lymphogranuloma venereum: Clinical Effectiveness Group of the British Association for Sexual Health and HIV (CEG/BASHH) Guideline Development Group. *International Journal of STD & AIDS, 24(8), 593–601.*

Wiesenfeld, H. C., Sweet, R. L., Ness, R. B., Krohn, M. A., Amortegui, A. J., & Hillier, S. L. (2005). Comparison of acute and subclinical pelvic inflammatory disease. *Sexually Transmitted Diseases, 32(7), 400–405.*

Wilcox, R. D. (2009). The challenge of neurosyphilis in HIV. *HIV Clinician, 21(3),* 1, 5–6.

Williams, D. & Churchill, D. (2006). Ulcerative proctitis in men who have sex with men: an emerging outbreak. *BMJ, 332(7533),* 99–100.

Wilson, J. (2011). Sexually transmitted infections and HIV in pregnancy. In K. E. Rogstad (Ed.), *ABC of sexually transmitted infections* (6th ed., pp. 59–63). Chichester, United Kingdom: Wiley Blackwell.

Wilson, J. D., Shann, S. M., Brady, S. K., Mammen-Tobin, A. G., Evans, A. L., & Lee, R. A. (2005). Recurrent bacterial vaginosis: The use of maintenance acidic vaginal gel following treatment. *International Journal of STD & AIDS, 16(11), 736–738.*

Winer, R. L., Lee, S. K., Hughes, J. P., Adam, D. E., Kiviat, N. B., & Koutsky, L. A. (2003). Genital human papillomavirus infection: Incidence and risk factors in a cohort of female university students. *American Journal of Epidemiology, 157(3), 218–226.*

Winer, R. L., Kiviat, N. B., Hughes, J. P., Adam, D. E., Lee, S. K., Kuypers, J. M., & Koutsky, L. A. (2005). Development and duration of human papillomavirus lesions after initial infection. *Journal of Infectious Diseases, 191(5), 731–738.*

Winer, R. L., Hughes, J. P., Feng, Q., O'Rilley, S., Kiviat, N. B., Holmes, K. K., & Koutsky, L. A. (2006). Condom use and the risk of genital human papillomavirus infection in young women. *New England Journal of Medicine, 354(25), 2645–2654.*

Wöhrl, S., & Geusau, A. (2006). Neurosyphilis is unlikely in patients with late latent syphilis and a negative blood VDRL test. *Acta Demato-Venereologica, 86(4), 335–339.*

Woodhall, S., Ramsey, T., Cai, C., Crouch, S., Jit, M., Birks, Y., . . . Lacey, C. J. (2008). Estimation of the impact of genital warts on health-related quality of life. *Sexually Transmitted Infections, 84(3), 161–166.*

Woodhall, S. C., Jit, M., Soldan, K., Kinghorn, G., Gilson, R., Nathan, M., . . . Lacey, C. J. (2011). The impact of genital warts: Loss of quality of life and cost of treatment in eight sexual health clinics in the UK. *Sexually Transmitted Infections, 87(6), 458–463.*

Woodward, C.L.N., & Robinson, A. (2011). Genital growths and infestations. In K. E. Rogstad (Ed.), *ABC of sexually transmitted infections* (6th ed., pp. 78–83). Chichester, United Kingdom: Wiley Blackwell.

Workowski, K. A., Berman, S., & Centers for Disease Control and Prevention. (2010). Sexually transmitted diseases treatment guidelines 2010. *MMWR Recommendations and Reports, 59* (RR–12).

Workowski, K. A., & Bolan, G. A. (2015). Sexually transmitted disease treatment guidelines, 2015. *MMWR, Morbid Mortal 64(3).* Retrieved from www.CDC.gov/std/tg2015/tg-2015-print.pdf.

World Health Organization (WHO). (n.d.). *New guidelines for the treatment of Treponema pallidum (syphilis).* Retrieved from http://www.who.int.reproductivehealth/publications/rtis/syphilis-treatment-guidelines/en/

World Health Organization (WHO). (n.d.). *New guidelines for the treatment of Neisseria gonorrhoea.* Retrieved from http://www.who.int/reproductivehealth/publicatons/rtis/gonorrhoea-treatment-guidelines/en/

World Health Organization (WHO). (n.d.). *New guidelines for the treatment of Chlamydia trachomatis.* Retrieved from http://www.who.int/reproductivehealth/publications/rtis/chlamydia-treatment-guidelines/en/

World Health Organization (WHO). (n.d.). *New guidelines for the treatment of Genital Herpes Simplex Virus.* Retrieved from http://www.who.int.reproductivehealth/publications/rtis/genital-HSV-treatment-guidelines/en/

World Health Organization (WHO). (2003). *Guidelines for the management of sexually transmitted infections.* Geneva, Switzerland: Author.

World Health Organization (WHO). (2005). *Sexually transmitted and other reproductive tract infections: A guide to essential practice.* Geneva, Switzerland: Author.

World Health Organization (WHO). (2007). *The WHO strategic approach to strengthening sexual and reproductive health policies and programmes.* Geneva, Switzerland: Author. Retrieved from http://www.who.int/reproductivehealth/topics/countries/strategic_approach/en/

World Health Organization. (WHO). (2012). *Prevention and control of viral hepatitis infection: Framework for global action.* Geneva, Switzerland: Author.

World Health Organization (WHO). (2012). *Global incidence and prevalence of selected curable sexually transmitted infections.* Geneva, Switzerland: Author.

Ya, W., Reifer, C., & Miller, L. E. (2010). Efficacy of vaginal probiotic capsules for recurrent bacterial vaginosis: A double-blind, randomised, placebo-controlled study. *American Journal of Obstetrics and Gynecology, 203*(2), 120–126.

Yanofsky, V. R., Patel, R. V., & Goldenberg, G. (2012). Genital warts. *The Journal of Clinical and Aesthetic Dermatology, 5*(6), 25–36.

Yudin, M. H., Hillier, S. L., Wiesenfeld, H. C., Krohn, M. A., Amortegui, A. A., & Sweet, R. L. (2003). Vaginal polymorphonuclear leucocytes and bacterial vaginosis as markers for histologic endometritis among women without symptoms of pelvic inflammatory disease. *American Journal of Obstetrics and Gynecology, 188*(2), 318–323.

Zemouri, C., Wi, T. E., Kiarie, J., Seuc, A., Mogasale, V., Latif, A., & Broutet, N. (2016). The performance of the vaginal discharge syndrome management in treating vaginal and cervical infection: A systematic review and meta-analysis. *PLoS ONE, 11*(10), e0163365, 1–21.

Zetola, N. M., & Klausner, J. D. (2007). Siphilis and HIV infection: An update. *Clinical Infectious Diseases, 44*(9), 1222–1228.

• • • RECOMMENDED READING

Alexander, S., Martin, I. M., & Ison, C. A. (2007). Confirming the *Chlamydia trachomatis* status of referred rectal specimens. *Sexually Transmitted Infections, 83*(4), 327–329.

Armstrong, N., & Donaldson, C. (2005). The economics of sexual health. London, United Kingdom: The Family Planning Association. Retrieved from www.fpa.org.uk/sites/default/files/economics-of-sexual-health.pdf

Beachmann, L. H., Johnson, R. E., Cheng, H., Markowitz, L., Papp, J. R., Palella, F. J. Jr., & Hook, E. W. 3rd. (2010). Nucleic acid amplification tests for diagnosis of *Neisseria gonorrhoeae* and *Chlamydia trachomatis* rectal infections. *Journal of Clinical Microbiology, 48*(5), 1827–1832.

Blower, S. M., and Farmer, P. (2003) Predicting the public health impact of antiretrovirals: preventing HIV in developing countries. *AIDScience* 3(11). Retrieved from http://aidscience.org/Articles/AIDScience033.asp

Bosu, W. (1999). Syndromic management of sexually transmitted diseases: Is it rational or scientific? *Tropical Medicine & International Health, 4*(2), 114–119.

British Association for Sexual Health and HIV (BASHH) and Clinical Effectiveness Group. (2006). *National guideline for the management of bacterial vaginosis.* Retrieved from http://www.bashh.org/documents/62/62.pdf

British Association for Sexual Health and HIV (BASHH) publications on various STIs.

Brown, Z. A., Wald, A., Morrow, R. A., Selke, S., Zeh, J., & Corey, L. (2003). Effect of serologic status and Caesarean section delivery on transmission rates of herpes simplex virus from mother to infant. *JAMA, 289*(2), 203–209.

Cagliano, V., Baan, R., Straif, K., Grosse, Y., Secretan, B., & El Ghissassi, F. (2005). Carcinogenecity of human papilloma viruses. *The Lancet Oncology, 6*(4), 204

Carne, C. A. (1997). Epidemiological treatment and tests of cure in gonogoccal infection: Evidence for value. *Genitourinary Medicine, 73*(1), 12–15.

Clark, R. A., Theall, K. P., & Kissinger, P. (2006). Consideration for empiric *Trichomonas vaginalis* treatment among selected high-risk HIV-infected female populations with concurrent *Neisseria gonorrhoea* or *Chlamydia trachomatis* cervical infections. *Sexually Transmitted Diseases, 33*(2), 124–125.

Clark, J. L., Lescano, A. G., Konda, K. A., Leon, S. R., Jones, F. R., Klausner, J. D., . . . Caceres, C. F. (2009). Syndromic management and STI control in Urban Peru. *PLoS ONE, 4*(9), e7201.

Delpech, V., Martin, I. M., Hughes, G., Nichols, T., James, L., & Ison, C. A. (2009). Epidemiology and clinical presentation of gonorrhoea in England and Wales: Findings from the Gonococcal Resistance to Antimicrobials Surveillance Programme 2001–2006. *Sexually Transmitted Infections, 85*(5), 317–321.

Department of Health. (2013). *Framework for sexual health improvement in England.* London, United Kingdom: Author.

de Vries, H. J. C., Morré S. A., White, J. A., & Moi, H. (2010). IUSTI 2010 European guideline on the management of lymphogranuloma venereum. *International Journal of STD & AIDS, 21*(8), 533–536.

Faculty of Sexual and Reproductive Healthcare (FSRH). (2012). *Management of vaginal discharge in non-genitourinary medicine settings.* Retrieved from https://www.bashh.org/documents/4264.pdf

Foxman, B., Muraglia, R., Dietz, J. P., Sobel, J. D., & Wagner, J. (2013). Prevalence of recurrent vulvovaginal candidiasis in European countries and the United States: Results from an internet panel survey. *Journal of Lower Genital Tract Disease, 17*(3), 340–345.

Galvin, S. R., & Cohen, M. S. (2004). The role of sexually transmitted diseases in HIV transmission. *Nature Reviews Microbiology, 2*(1), 33–42.

Gaydos, C. A., Cartright, C. P., Colaninno, P., Welsch, J., Ho, S. Y., Webb, E. M., . . . Robinson, J. (2010). Performance of the Abbott Real time CT/NG for detection of *Chlamydia trachomatis* and *Neisseria gonorrhoeae. Journal of Clinical Microbiology, 48*(9), 3236–3243.

Health Protection Agency (HPA). (2010). *Epidemic of lymphogranuloma venereum (LGV) in men who have sex with men in the UK.* Retrieved from https://www.guideline.gov/summaries/downloadcontent/ngc-10066?contentType=pdf

Health Protection Agency (HPA). (2011). *Trends in STI diagnoses and rates of STIs by age and by ethnic group.* London, United Kingdom: HIV and STI Department, Health Protection Agency.

Health Protection Agency (HPA). (2012). *National chlamydia screening programme standards.* 6th ed. London, United Kingdom: Author.

Holmes, K. K., Sparling, P. F., Stamm, W. E., Piot, P., Wasserheit, J. N., Corey, L., . . . Watts, D. H. (2008). *Sexually transmitted diseases* (4th ed). New York, NY: McGraw-Hill.

Huang, W., Gaydos, C. A., Barnes, M. R., Jett-Goheen, M., & Blake, D. R. (2013). Comparative effectiveness of rapid point-of-care test for detection of *Chlamydia trachomatis* among women in a clinical setting. *Sexually Transmitted Infections, 89*(2), 108–114.

Janier, M., Hegyi, V., Dupin, N., Unemo, M., Tiplica, G. S., Potočnik, M., . . . Patel, R. 2014 European guideline on the management of syphilis. *Journal of the European Academy of Dermatology and Venereology, 28*(12), 1581–1593. doi: 10.1111/jdv.12734

Jit, M., Chapman R., Hughes, O., & Choi, Y. H. (2011). Comparing bivalent and quadrivalent human papillomavirus vaccines: Economic evaluation based on transmission model. *BMJ, 343,* d5775.

Jordan, R. G., Engstrom, J. L., Marfell, J. A., & Farley, C. L. (2014). *Prenatal and postnatal care: A woman centered approach.* Ames, IA: Wiley Blackwell.

Knott, L. *Professional reference: Gonorrhoea.* Retrieved from https://patient.info/doctor/gonorrhoea-pro

Karim, Q. A., Karim, S. S. A., Frohlich, J. A., Grobler, A.C., Baxter, C., Mansoor, L. E., . . . Taylor, D. (2010). Effectiveness and safety of tenofovir gel, an antiretroviral microbicide for the prevention of HIV infection in women. *Science, 329*(5996), 1168–1174.

Kingston, M., French, P., Higgins, S., McQuillan, O., Sukthankar, A., Scott, C., . . . Sullivan, A. (2016). UK national guidelines on the management of syphilis 2015. *International Journal of STD & AIDS, 27*(6), 421–426.

Kong, F. Y. S., & Hocking, J. S. (2015). Treatment challenges for urogenital and anorectal *Chlamydia trachomatis. BMC Infectious Diseases, 15*(1), 293.

Kuomans, E. H., Sternberg, M., Bruce, C., McQuillan, G., Kendrick, J., Sutton, M., & Markowitz, L. E. (2007). The prevalence of bacterial vaginosis in the United States, 2001–Associations with symptoms, sexual behaviours, and reproductive health. *Sexually Transmitted Diseases, 34*(11), 864–869.

Lowndes, C. M., & Hughes, G. (2010). Epidemiology of STIs: UK. *Medicine, 38*(5), 211–215.

Marra, C. M., Maxwell, C. L., Smith, S. L., Lukehart, S. A., Rompalo A. M., Eaton, M., . . . Barnett, S. H. (2004). Cerebrospinal fluid abnormalities in patients with syphilis: association with clinical and laboratory features. *Journal of Infectious Diseases, 189*(3), 369–376.

Morré, S. A., Spaargaren, J., Fennema, J. S., de Vries, H. J.C., Coutinho, R. A., & Pena, A. S. (2005). Real-time polymerase chain reaction to diagnose lymphogranuloma venereum. *Emerging Infectious Diseases, 11*(8), 1311–1312.

Msuya, S. E., Uriyo, J., Stray-Pedersen, B., Sam, N. E., & Mbizvo, E. M. (2009). The effectiveness of syndromic approach in managing vaginal infections among pregnant women in northern Tanzania. *East African Journal of Public Health, 6*(3), 263–267.

National Cancer Institute (NCI). (2016). Human papillomavirus (HPV) vaccines. Retrieved from www.cancer.gov/about-cancer/causes-prevention/risk/infectious-agents/hpv-vaccine-fact-sheet

National Health Service Scotland. (2011). Improving sexual health services in Scotland: Integration and innovation November 2011. Edinburgh, United Kingdom: Healthcare Improvement Scotland.

Ng, Lai-King, & Martin, I. E. (2005). Laboratory diagnosis of *Neisseria gonorrhoeae. Canadian Journal of Infectious Diseases and Medical Microbiology, 16*(1), 15–25.

Ratnam, S. (2005). The laboratory diagnosis of syphilis. *Canadian Journal of Infectious Diseases and Medical Microbiology, 16*(1), 45–51.

Royal Pharmaceutical Society. *Sexual health toolkit.* Retrieved from https://www.rpharms.com/resources/toolkits/sexual-health-toolkit

Savage, E. J., Marsh, K., Duffell, S., Ison, C. A., Zaman, A., & Hughes, G. (2012). Rapid increase in gonorrhoea and syphilis diagnoses in England. *Euro Surveillance 17*(29), pii=20224. Available online: www.eurosurveillance.org/images/dynamic/EE/V17N29/art20224.pdf (accessed August 14, 2017).

Schachter, J., McCormack, W. M., Chernesky, M. A., Martin, D. H., Van Der Pol, B., Rice, P. A., . . . Chow, J. M. (2003). Vaginal swabs are appropriate specimens for diagnosis of genital tract infection with *Chlamydia trachomatis. Journal of Clinical Microbiology, 41*(8), 3784–3789.

Schaeffer, A., & Henrich, B. (2008). Rapid detection of *Chlamydia trachomatis* and typing of the lymphogranuloma venereum associated L-serovars by TaqMan PCR. *BMC Infectious Diseases, 8*(56), 1–10.

Scheinfeld, N., & Lehman, D. S. (2006). An evidence-based review of medical and surgical treatments of genital warts. *Dermatology Online Journal, 12*(3), 5.

Schwebke, J. R., & Desmond, R. (2007). A randomised trial of metronidazole in asymptomatic bacterial vaginosis to prevent the acquisition of sexually transmitted diseases. *American Journal of Obstetrics and Gynecology, 196*(6), 517 e1–6.

Sebitloane, H. M., Moodley, J., & Esterhuizen, T. M. (2011). Pathogenic lower genital tract organisms in HIV-infected and uninfected women, and their association with postpartum infectious morbidity. *South African Medical Journal, 101*(7), 466–469.

Shrivastava, S. R. B. L., Shrivastava, P. S., & Ramasamy, J. (2014). Utility of syndromic approach in the management of sexually transmitted infections: public health perspective. *Journal of Coastal Life Medicine, 2*(1), 7–13.

Singh, S., Bell, G., & Talbot, M. (2007). The characterization of recent syphilis outbreak in Sheffield, UK, and an evaluation of contact tracing as a method of control. *Sexually Transmitted Infections, 83*(3), 193–199.

Steen, R., Wi T. E., Kamali, A., & Ndowa, F. (2009). Control of sexually transmitted infections and prevention of HIV transmission: Mending a fractured paradigm. *Bulletin of the World Health Organization, 87*(11), 858–865.

Sobel, J. D. (2013). Vulvovaginal candidosis. *Lancet, 369*(9577), 1961–1971.

Tsai, C. H., Lee, T. C., Chang, H. L., Tang, L. H., Chiang, C. C., & Chen, K. T. (2008). The cost effectiveness of syndromic management for male sexually transmitted disease patients with urethral discharge symptoms and genital ulcer disease in Taiwan. *Sexually Transmitted Infections, 84*(5), 400–404.

The Regulation and Quality Improvement Authority. (2013). *Review of specialist sexual health services in Northern Ireland. October 2013.* Belfast, Northern Ireland: The Regulation and Quality Improvement Authority.

UNAIDS. (1998). *The public health approach to STD control.* UNAIDS Technical Update. Retrieved from www.who.int/hiv/pub/sti/en/stdcontrol_en.pdf

Unemo, M., Ballard, R., Ison, C., Lewis, D., Ndowa, F., & Peeling, R. (Eds.) (2013). *Laboratory diagnosis of sexually transmitted infections, including human immunodeficiency virus.* Geneva, Switzerland: WHO.

Vickerman, P., Watts, C., Alary, M., Mabey, D., & Peeling, R. W. (2003). Sensitivity requirements for the point of care diagnosis of chlamysia trachomatis and *Neisseria gonorrhoeae* in women. *Sexually Transmitted Infections, 79*(5), 363–367.

Wang, Q., Yang, P., Zhong, M., & Wang, G. (2003). Validation of diagnostic algorithyms for syndromic management of sexually transmitted diseases. *Chinese Medical Journal, 116*(2), 181–186.

Ward, H., Martin, I., MacDonald, N., Alexander, S., Simms, I., Fenton, K., . . . Corey, L. (2007). Lymphogranuloma venereum in the United Kingdom. *Clinical Infectious Diseases, 44*(1), 26–32.

World Health Organization (WHO). (2007). Global strategy for the prevention and control of sexually transmitted infections. Retrieved from http://www.who.int/reproductivehealth/publications/rtis/9789241563475/en/

Zetola, N. M., Angelman, J., Jensen, T. P., & Klausner, J. D. (2007). Syphilis in the United States: An update for clinicians with an emphasis on HIV coinfection. *Mayo Clinic Proceedings, 82*(9), 1091–1102.

CHAPTER

7

HIV/AIDS: Contemporary Interventions

FRED STEPHEN SARFO

Introduction

There is a brighter hope for patients living with human immunodeficiency virus (HIV) infection today than there was 3 decades ago, when the infection was first described. Mortality and morbidity from HIV infection have significantly improved with the advent of antiretroviral therapy (ART). This achievement has largely been driven by the tremendous advancement in our knowledge of the pathobiology of the human immunodeficiency virus, which led to the introduction of highly potent and effective ART for lifelong treatment of this once fatal disease. This chapter reviews the pathogenesis of HIV infection leading to clinical disease and focuses on ART use mainly in resource-limited settings, where nearly 80%

of HIV-infected patients reside. A discussion of the current 2013 World Health Organization (WHO) guidelines for use of ART in these settings forms the core of this text.

Epidemiology

Since the beginning of the epidemic, almost 70 million people have been infected with the HIV and about 35 million people have died of acquired immunodeficiency syndrome (AIDS) since the clinical syndrome was first described in 1981 (UNAIDS, 2013). HIV, initially referred to as either the lymphadenopathy-associated virus (LAV) or the human T-cell lymphotropic virus type III (HTLV-III) was first identified as the causative agent of AIDS in 1983 (Barre-Sinoussi et al., 1983). The predominant route of HIV transmission is through unprotected sexual intercourse (>75%); followed by vertical transmission from mother to baby, during pregnancy, at birth, or through breastfeeding (5–10%); and to a lesser extent via the parenteral route (<2%) (through injection drug use and/or injection/transfusion of contaminated blood products). Certain sexual activities carry a higher risk of infection than others; for example, unprotected anal sex carries a greater risk of infection than either vaginal (Seidlin, Vogler, Lee, Lee, & Dubin, 1993) or oral sex (Coates & Collins, 1998). It is also apparent that the presence of other sexually transmitted infections (STIs) significantly increases the risk of HIV infection.

Globally, an estimated 35.3 (32.2–38.8) million people were living with HIV in 2012 (UNAIDS, 2013), compared to 26.2 million in 1999, according to epidemiological data from UNAIDS/WHO. In spite of intensive research efforts and the massive roll-out of treatment interventions, HIV/AIDS continues to pose the most serious infectious disease challenge to public health. Sub-Saharan Africa (SSA) remains most severely affected, with nearly 1 in every 20 adults (4.9%) living with HIV and accounting for 69% of the people living with HIV worldwide (UNAIDS, 2013).

In fact, 61% and 90% of all HIV infections in women and children respectively occur in SSA. Indeed, in SSA approximately 1.2 million (1.1–1.3 million) of the global total of 1.6 million (1.4–1.9 million) deaths in 2012 were attributable to HIV/AIDS, accounting for 72% of all HIV/AIDS-related mortality worldwide (UNAIDS, 2013).

Within the SSA region, the eastern and southern African countries are the most devastated, with an average national prevalence ranging from 15–35% of populations affected (**Figure 7-1**). However, like the trend globally, the prevalence of HIV infection (percentage of persons infected with HIV) is stabilizing, although the number of persons living with HIV

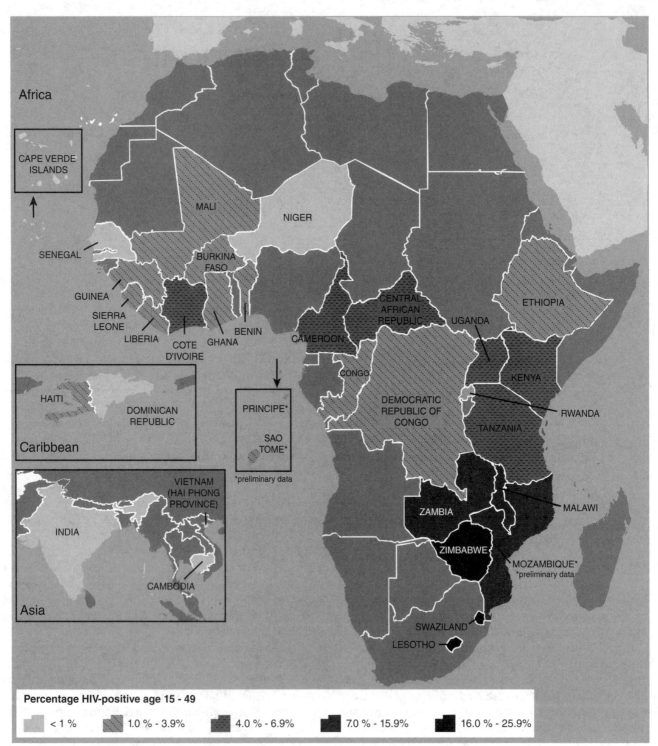

Figure 7-1 National HIV Prevalence Map, 2010

Reproduced from The DHS Program. (2010). National HIV prevalence. Retrieved from http://dhsprogram.com/What-We-Do/GIS-Map-Gallery.cfm

continues to increase mainly due to an increasing number of newly acquired and diagnosed infections (albeit, at a reduced rate), longer survival times—which is a corollary of ART introduction—and the unprecedented expansion of ART in Africa and other developing countries. For instance, the number of new infections in 2012 in SSA was 1.6 million compared with 2.2 million in 2001. An estimated 5.2 million people in low- and middle-income countries were receiving life-saving ART by end of 2009, representing an increase of 1.2 million people or 30% over the number receiving such treatment 12 months earlier. Furthermore, the number of people on ART increased by 1.6 million in 2012, the biggest increase in one year to date, and at the end of 2012, 9.7 million people in low- and middle-income countries were on ART.

In SSA, nearly 37% (34–40%) of people eligible for treatment were accessing antiretroviral (ARV) drugs by December 2009 and this unprecedented roll-out of ART has translated into an estimated 320,000 (or 20%) fewer AIDS-related deaths in 2009 than in 2004. Four out of five people newly put on treatment live in SSA. Over the last decade, ART scale-up in low- and middle-income countries has saved an estimated 4.2 million lives. Clearly, the current data demonstrate that investments in the HIV response has started to yield fruitful dividends in reducing discrimination and stigma, helping people access information and services to reduce their risk of HIV infection and delivering the treatment, care, and support that will extend and improve the lives of people living with HIV.

Prevalence of HIV/AIDS in the United States

Despite the decline in incidence of HIV infections in the United States since the 1980s, the incidence of newly infected people seems to persist around 50,000 each year. This shows over two-thirds reduction from the estimated 130,000 during the climax of the epidemic. Therefore, the significance of HIV testing is emphasized and the current policy is that among the U.S. population groups routine testing is recommended for all persons 13–64 years of age. Nevertheless, among those infected 16% do not know their HIV infection status, while as many as 32% are diagnosed in advanced stage of their illness (Centers for Disease Control and Prevention [CDC], 2013). The public health burden of HIV infection encompasses the persistently high prevalence rates and widespread transmission.

High-Risk Factors

According the Centers for Disease Control and Prevention's (CDC) most recent estimates, 1.2 million people in the United States are reported to be currently living with HIV, and the number is continually increasing. Nevertheless, although an estimated 86% are diagnosed, approximately 14% remain unaware that they have acquired the infection (CDC, 2015c). There are high-risk factors that have been identified as increasing the vulnerability of certain subgroups to HIV infection. Among these factors

are social and economic consequences, demographic factors, and risky lifestyle and behaviors. The impact of low educational status, stigma, and discrimination presents additional contributing factors to an individual's risk and vulnerability to HIV infection. In relation to transmission rates, men who have sex with men (MSM) are reported to present the highest number of new HIV infections regardless of race and ethnic background. Other high-risk groups include African American heterosexual women. In relation to other ethno-racial subgroups, African Americans present more newly diagnosed HIV infections as compared to the population subgroup of Latinos. The geographical/regional differences in the number of new HIV diagnoses shows that per 100,000 of the U.S. population, the South presents 18.5; Northeast, 14.2; West, 11.2; and the Midwest, 8.2. However, a decrease in newly diagnosed HIV infections was reported in the Northeast and South, while the rates of new diagnosis stabilized in the Midwest and West during the period 2010 through 2014 (CDC, 2015b).

The CDC (2016b) cautions that despite the apparent stable levels of HIV infections in recent years, persistent increase in the number of people living with HIV infection will result in undesirable consequences. The CDC urges for preventive endeavors, testing, care, and treatment interventions to be intensified and constantly and actively directed to those population subgroups who are identified to be at highest risk.

HIV Infection and Disease Progression

HIV Structure

HIV is a retrovirus, meaning its genetic information is stored in the form of ribonucleic acid (RNA) instead of deoxyribonucleic acid (DNA) and the virus therefore requires reverse transcription in order to replicate. HIV belongs to a sub-family of lentiviruses, which include the simian immunodeficiency virus (SIV) in monkeys, feline immunodeficiency virus (FIV) in cats, and related viruses in sheep, goats, and horses. These retroviruses are characterized by the lengthy time period between infection of the host and clinical manifestation of symptoms. Two strains of HIV have been identified—HIV-1 and HIV-2—the latter was identified 2 years after HIV-1 (Clavel et al., 1986). HIV-1 is derived from the SIV of the chimpanzee *Pan troglodytes*, while HIV-2, which is quite dissimilar, is genetically closer to the virus derived from the sooty mangabey (*Cercocebus atys*). HIV-2 is associated with a slower and more benign disease course, is more difficult to transmit via sexual and parenteral routes than HIV-1, and is endemic in West Africa. However, HIV-1 is the major cause of AIDS worldwide and even in West Africa.

HIV-1 is further divided into three groups, group M (main group, >98%), group O (outlier, <1%), and group N (new, <1%). Group M is responsible for the majority of infections worldwide and is further subcategorized into recognized phylogenetic subtypes or clades. There are also recombinants, which contain a mix of subtypes.

HIV-1 viral particles are roughly spherical in shape and approximately 100 nm in diameter. A double layer of lipoprotein membrane, known as the viral envelope, surrounds the virus. There are proteins embedded in the membrane, which form glycoprotein spikes. Each spike is composed of glycoprotein (gp) 120 and transmembrane gp41. The virus needs gp120 to attach to the host cell. The HIV matrix proteins consisting of the p17 protein, lie anchored to the viral envelope, and encompasses the viral core. The viral core or capsid, contains the viral protein p24, which surrounds two single strands of HIV-1 RNA and the enzymes required for viral replication, including reverse transcriptase, integrase, and protease.

HIV Replication Cycle

The CD4 surface receptor is the primary target for HIV entry into the host cell. CD4 is present in approximately 60% of T-cell helper lymphocytes, T-cell precursors, monocytes and macrophages, eosinophils, dendritic cells, and microglial cells of the central nervous system (CNS). However, in addition to CD4, human coreceptors (CCR5 and CXCR4) also located on the host cell surface are necessary for viral entry.

An understanding of the basic virology of HIV helps to appreciate how antiretroviral therapies work in suppressing virus replication. HIV replication can be divided into 6 stages: attachment/uncoating, reverse transcription, integration, transcription, translation, and assembly/release, as schematically illustrated in **Figure 7-2** and described below.

Attachment/uncoating In this stage, the HIV gp120 binds to the CD4 surface receptor of the host cell. This binding process activates certain proteins on the cell's surface that allow contents of the HIV particle to be released into the cell.

Reverse transcription The genetic information stored in the RNA of HIV must be reverse transcribed into proviral HIV DNA in order for the virus to replicate. This process is mediated by the viral reverse transcriptase enzyme, which utilizes host deoxynucleotide triphosphates (dNTPs) in the cytoplasm of the host target cell.

Integration The viral DNA is then transported into the host cell nucleus and integrated into the host cell genome (facilitated by integrase enzyme). The newly incorporated viral DNA is now a provirus and the cell is permanently infected.

Transcription The host cell creates new viral RNA molecules, using the provirus DNA as a template.

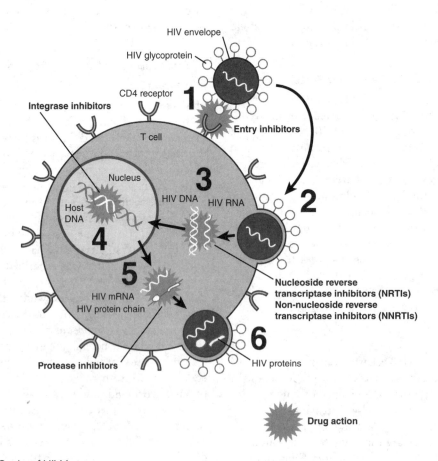

Figure 7-2 The Life Cycle of HIV-1

Reproduced with permission from David Spach, MD, and Mountain West AIDS Education and Training Center. Retrieved from http://www.hivwebstudy.org/cases/initial-evaluation/acute-primary-hiv-infection

Translation The messenger RNA (mRNA) is transported out of the cell nucleus. It contains code that is translated into polyproteins (long-chain amino acids), which form the enzymes and protein components of new virus particles.

Assembly/release All the components needed to create new virus particles migrate toward the cell surface and assemble into a new viral bud. These buds are cut by the protease enzyme and are released as new virus particles.

Natural History of HIV Infection

The natural history of HIV infection refers to disease progression in the absence of antiretroviral treatment and can be described in three phases: primary or acute infection, latent or asymptomatic infection, and symptomatic infection.

Primary infection is the period from initial infection with HIV to the development of an antibody response (seroconversion) and typically lasts between 1 to 3 months. It is characterized by a surge in plasma viremia due to unrestrained viral replication, with plasma viral loads (pVL) reaching over 100 million copies/mL in the absence of any detectable adaptive immune response (Embretson et al., 1993; Pantaleo & Fauci, 1996). Following seroconversion, there is a marked decline in the number of CD4 T lymphocytes as a result of both destruction by HIV and migration to peripheral lymph tissue. During this period, patients may develop a generalized rash, sore throat, and swollen lymph glands, which are frequently misdiagnosed as flu because no HIV-specific antibodies are detectable during this early phase of infection. Although higher pVL during primary infection are not directly indicative of disease progression, they are linked to the severity of these initial symptoms. Certainly, it has been observed that individuals presenting with more severe symptoms during acute infection tend to have poorer long-term clinical outcomes and progress more rapidly to AIDS (Keet et al., 1993; Vanhems et al., 1998).

An immune response capable of controlling viral replication develops over the following weeks, which is evidenced by a diminution of the high pVL. This coincides with a concurrent increase in the CD4 count, although levels rarely reestablish to preinfection values in the absence of ART. The high plasma viremia during the primary infection stage makes patients highly infectious; hence, accurate early diagnosis of acute HIV infection is important, as infection of sexual partners can potentially be prevented.

Latent infection refers to the time period in which equilibrium is established between rate of viral replication and the host immune response. This is often referred to as the viral "set point" where the level of viral RNA remains constant (Feinberg, 1996; Henrard et al., 1995) and is a strong predictor of the speed of HIV disease progression following infection (Mellors et al., 1996). In the absence of antiretroviral treatment, this period of clinical latency can last for 8–10 years or more (Enger et al., 1996; Hessol et al., 1990), and during this period many infected individuals do not present with any clinical symptoms of the disease. However, the term *latency* is misleading, giving the high turnover of virus (up to 10^{10} new virions per day) and the relentless daily destruction of CD4 cells (Perelson, Neumann, Markowitz, Leonard, & Ho, 1996).

A number of host factors have been identified to influence the time spent in clinical latency, including gender (Farzadegan et al., 1998), age (Carre et al., 1994), viral fitness, and genetic predisposition (CCR5-Δ32 deletion) (Huang et al., 1996).

Symptomatic infection eventually occurs in the presence of high viral replication and consequent destruction of the immune system. Although the immune system has the capacity to regenerate, it is not unlimited, and HIV finally overcomes the immune response. Indeed, once CD4 counts fall to below 200/μL, the immune system is sufficiently compromised and patients are at significant risk of contracting many AIDS-defining illnesses, including a number of opportunistic infections (e.g., tuberculosis) and certain neoplasms (e.g., Kaposi's sarcoma). Above 200/μL, most AIDS-defining illnesses are rare events. Without antiretroviral treatment, most patients with symptomatic infection will eventually succumb within 2–3 years.

Non-AIDS-defining events

Deaths in the era of combined antiretroviral treatment (cART) have largely been due to AIDS-defining clinical events. However, the dynamics of mortality are believed to be changing in industrialized countries, with non-AIDS-defining clinical events assuming greater importance as causes of death as patients live longer on potent antiretroviral medications (Deeks & Phillips, 2009; Mocroft et al., 2010). Non-AIDS-defining events are classified as cardiovascular, renal, hepatic, or non-AIDS-defining malignancies that are likely to have an impact on morbidity and mortality (CDC, 1992). The diagnosis of a non-AIDS clinical event was defined using established Division of AIDS (DAIDS) tables for Grading Severity of Adult Adverse Experiences (DAIDS AE Grading Table). The conditions classified under the DAIDS AE Grading Table include cerebrovascular accident (stroke), cerebral/subarachnoid hemorrhage, myocardial infarction, coronary artery disease, congestive cardiac failure, endstage renal disease, renal failure, cirrhosis of the liver, esophageal varices, hepatic failure, hepatic coma, hepatic encephalopathy, intestinal adenocarcinoma/lymphoma, penile carcinoma, small-cell lung carcinoma, malignant melanoma, hepatocellular carcinoma, squamous cell carcinoma, and squamous cell carcinoma of the anus (Division of AIDS & NIAID, 2004).

It was initially thought that the premature development of non-AIDS conditions during HIV infection was attributable to the metabolic complications of cART and other drug-related toxicities. Evidence from the Data collection of Adverse events of anti-HIV Drugs (DAD) study involving nearly 23,000 HIV-infected patients showed that each additional year of ART use was associated with a 26%

increased risk from myocardial infarction (Friis-Møller et al., 2003); most of this risk was attributable to protease inhibitor use and dyslipidemia. However, additional analyses of the DAD study as well as data from the SMART trial have highlighted the impact of immune suppression on the occurrence of these non-AIDS events. The underlying mechanisms by which HIV-related immune depletion may promote non-AIDS diseases are beginning to be unraveled. Essentially, immune activation—which is a hallmark of HIV infection—appears important in the pathogenesis of viral replication and CD4-cell depletion. Indeed, many of the inflammatory biomarkers that are elevated during HIV infection are also associated with risk for cardiovascular events and certain cancers as well as progression of renal disease. In addition, coinfection with other viruses such as human papillomavirus (HPV), hepatitis B (HBV), and hepatitis C (HCV), in the setting of long-standing impaired immune function may favor a pro-oncogenic state or contribute to the progression of end-organ diseases.

Reflective Considerations

With what we know about the life cycle of HIV, what do you think is hindering the eradication or cure of this infection from human hosts?

Care Interventions and Treatment

HIV Testing

The laboratory diagnosis of an HIV infection is normally made indirectly by measurement of virus-specific antibodies (Gürtler, 1996), with most screening tests based on the enzyme linked immunosorbent assay (ELISA) principle. HIV infection may also be diagnosed through detection of the virus using branch chain DNA, PCR, and GenProbe, detecting either intracellular proviral complementary DNA (cDNA) in leukocytes or extracellular HIV-1 RNA in the cell-free compartment. However, this approach to viral detection is only relevant in certain situations, such as suspected primary infection or to test babies born to HIV-infected mothers in resource-endowed settings.

In all cases, HIV infection can only be confirmed/ diagnosed by a reactive (positive) result followed by at least one confirmatory test result. HIV infection should never be diagnosed (or reported to the patient) on the basis of a single reactive screening assay alone. Whereas qualitative testing for viral genome/virus-specific antibodies serves as a marker of infection, the quantitative detection of HIV RNA in plasma (in copies per milliliter of plasma) and the CD4 T-lymphocyte count (number of cells per microliter of blood) are key prognostic indicators of a patient's viral burden/infectivity status and immunological function,

and are routinely used to guide clinical and therapeutic management of HIV-infected patients. HIV RNA is commonly measured by commercially available RT-PCR kits, and has a detection limit of 50 copies/mL; hence, in current practice, patients with a pVL below or equal to this value are referred to as "undetectable" and described as being virologically suppressed.

Clinical and Laboratory Staging of HIV Disease

In developing countries, the WHO staging system that includes clinical, laboratory, and combined clinical /laboratory classifications is used to stage HIV/AIDS in adults and adolescents, as shown in **Table 7-1**. The clinical markers fall into four stages of prognostic significance and this forms the basis of the WHO clinical staging. In resource-limited settings this staging system, which has proven reliable in predicting morbidity and mortality, is used to classify clients according their level of immunosuppression, to help prompt clinicians to look out for other disease features when one is present in a stage, and to decide when to start cART.

Combination Antiretroviral Therapy (cART)

Combination antiretroviral therapy (cART) involves the simultaneous administration of 3 or more antiretroviral drugs. Currently there are more than 20 antiretroviral medications from 6 different drug classes, including: the nucleoside/nucleotide reverse transcriptase inhibitors (NRTIs), non-nucleoside reverse transcriptase inhibitors (NNRTIs), protease inhibitors (PI), entry/fusion inhibitors (FIs), CCR5 antagonists, and integrase strand transfer inhibitors (INSTIs). These drugs target different stages in the HIV life cycle. In addition, there are several novel and experimental antiretroviral drugs at various stages of development.

Nucleoside/Nucleotide Reverse Transcriptase Inhibitors (NRTIs)

Blockade of the viral reverse transcriptase enzyme was the first attempt to inhibit the HIV life cycle, and in 1987 the first antiretroviral, zidovudine (AZT), was licensed for treatment of HIV infection. The NRTIs act as competitive inhibitors of reverse transcriptase. The NRTIs interfere with reverse transcription by disrupting new pro viral DNA construction, which ultimately halts the HIV replication process.

The overall tolerability of NRTIs is fairly good, with initial side effects being easy to manage. The pill burden is low compared with other drug classes (once-daily dosing is sufficient for most NRTIs), which reduces the potential for non-adherence (Claxton, Cramer, & Pierce, 2001). There is also a reduced risk of drug interactions, as NRTIs predominantly undergo renal excretion and are less likely to interact with drugs metabolized hepatically. Despite these potential advantages, NRTIs are associated with long-term safety problems, including mitochondrial toxicity caused by their inhibition of mitochondrial DNA polymerase-γ (Côté et al., 2002).

Table 7-1	The Revised WHO Clinical Staging of HIV/AIDS for Adults and Adolescents	
Clinical Stage	**Clinical Conditions**	
1^0 HIV Infection	Acute retroviral syndrome	
1	Asymptomatic	
	Persistent generalized lymphadenopathy	
2	Moderate unexplained weight loss <10% of presumed or measured body weight	Recurrent oral ulcerations
	Recurrent upper respiratory tract infections	Papular pruritic eruptions
	Herpes zoster	Seborrheic dermatitis
	Angular cheilitis	Fungal nail infections of fingers
3	***A presumptive diagnosis can be made on the basis of clinical signs or simple investigation**	****A diagnostic confirmatory test is necessary**
	Severe weight loss >10% of presumed or measured body weight	Unexplained anaemia (<8g/dl), and or neutropenia (<500/mm^3)
	Unexplained diarrhea for >1 month	Unexplained thrombocytopenia (<50,000/mm^3) for >1month
	Unexplained persistent fever (intermittent or constant)	
	Oral candidiasis	
	Oral hairy leukoplakia	
	Pulmonary tuberculosis diagnosed within the last 2 years	
	Severe presumed bacterial infections (e.g., pneumonia, empyema, meningitis, bone and joint infection)	
	Acute necrotizing ulcerative stomatitis, gingivitis, or periodontitis	
4	HIV wasting syndrome	****A diagnostic confirmatory test is necessary**
	Pneumocystis pneumonia	Extrapulmonary cryptococcosis
	Recurrent severe or radiological bacterial pneumonia	Disseminated non-TB mycobacterial infection
	Chronic herpes simplex infection (orolabial, genital, or anorectal) >1 month	Progressive multifocal leukoencephalopathy (PML)
	Esophageal candidiasis	Candida of trachea, bronchi, or lungs
	Extrapulmonary tuberculosis	Cryptosporidiosis
	Kaposi sarcoma	Isosporidiosis
	CNS toxoplasmosis	Visceral herpes simplex infection
	HIV encephalopathy	Visceral leishmaniasis
		Invasive cervical carcinoma
		Lymphoma (cerebral or B cell non-Hodgkin)
		Recurrent non-typhoidal salmonella sepsis
		Any disseminated mycosis such as histoplasmosis, coccidiomycosis, or penicilliosis
		Cytomegalovirus (CMV) infection (retinitis or of any organ other than liver, spleen, or lymph nodes)

Data from WHO. (2007). *WHO case definitions of HIV for surveillance and revised clnical staging and immunological classification of HIV-related disease in adults and children.* Geneva: Author.

Two NRTIs remain an integral part of cART and are combined with either an NNRTI or a ritonavir-boosted PI. There are currently seven NRTIs available:

- Zidovudine (AZT)
- Didanosine (ddI)
- Stavudine (d4T)
- Lamivudine (3TC)
- Tenofovir (TDF)
- Abacavir (ABC)
- Emtricitabine (FTC)

Extensive data support the inclusion of 3TC and/or FTC as one of the two integral NRTIs Arribas et al., 2008; Gallant et al., 2006; Smith et al., 2009). Single-pill formulations containing two or more NRTIs are also licensed to further simplify treatment regimens. Combinations include AZT + 3TC (Combivir), ABC + 3TC (Kivexa), TDF + FTC (Truvada), and 3TC + AZT + ABC (Trizivir).

Non-nucleoside Reverse Transcriptase Inhibitors (NNRTIs)

The NNRTIs, which include efavirenz (EFV), nevirapine (NVP), and delavirdine (DLV), also possess a high affinity for the enzyme reverse transcriptase. However, they function somewhat differently from NRTIs in that they prevent reverse transcriptase enzyme from converting RNA to DNA, thus disrupting viral replication.

EFV can cause mild central nervous system (CNS) manifestations, including dizziness, somnolence, impaired concentration, and nightmares, and is best taken at night. However, these effects are usually transient, only occurring during the initial 2 to 4 weeks of therapy, although they can persist in approximately one-fifth of patients (Arendt, de Nocker, von Giesen, & Nolting, 2007; Lochet et al., 2003). NVP can provide an alternative to EFV in pregnant women or patients with baseline mental health disorders. However, NVP is known to cause elevation of liver enzymes in up to 16% of patients, which can result in severe hepatotoxicity, and must be administered under specific CD4 criteria. Women with good immune status—particularly those with CD4 >350/mm^3—appear to be more prone to this effect. DLV is rarely prescribed due to its high pill burden and inconvenient schedule, and is not licensed in Europe or Africa.

Overall, the NNRTIs are well tolerated and have relatively long half-lives, permitting simple dosing. Their one major drawback, however, is the low genetic barrier to resistance, in which single amino acid substitutions are sufficient to confer NNRTI cross-resistance (Antinori et al., 2002), necessitating a swift but decisive change in treatment regimens. In addition, a risk of drug–drug interactions with NNRTIs is high, as both EFV and NVP are metabolized by the CYP450 system and cause induction (NVP) or both induction and inhibition (EFV) of CYP3A4 and CYP2B6 and can therefore impact the metabolism of concurrent drugs (Smith, DiCenzo, & Morse, 2001).

Second-generation NNRTIs Due to the genetic frailty and potential for cross-resistance, a second generation of NNRTIs, including etravirine (ETV) and rilpivirine (RPV), was developed. These second-generation NNRTIs have a somewhat different mechanism of action than first-generation NNRTIs in that they can adapt to changes in the NNRTI-binding pocket by binding in at least two conformationally distinct modes. Overall the second-generation NNRTIs have a better resistance profile and therefore are recommended for treatment-experienced adults on a multidrug regimen.

Protease Inhibitors (PI)

The first protease inhibitor, saquinavir (SQV), was introduced in December 1995. Since then, the PIs have remained an essential component of cART, particularly among treatment-experienced patients. The PIs target the HIV protease enzyme, responsible for cleaving large HIV precursor proteins into infectious viral particles that are able to bud through the host cell membrane (during the assemble/release phase of the HIV life cycle). The drugs mimic peptides and prevent protease from binding to viral polyproteins. As a result, the virus cannot mature and non-infectious viral particles are produced.

These drugs are prone to variable pharmacokinetics and extensive drug–drug interactions when given in combination or with other concomitant medications. Boosting a PI with RTV increases drug exposure and/or prolongs the elimination half-life, allowing for a reduction in pill burden and dosing frequency, which in turn improves patient adherence and limits the development of resistance.

The RTV-boosted PIs recommended for initial treatment in naïve patients include atazanavir (ATV), lopinavir (LPV), amprenavir (APV; administered as the pro-drug fosamprenavir [FPV]) and SQV. In addition, boosted darunavir (DRV), which is active against multidrug resistant strains of HIV-1 and shown to be superior to LPV in patients with HIV RNA >100,000 copies/mL, was approved for initial treatment in early 2009. Boosted PIs have a higher genetic barrier to resistance and exhibit improved immunological responses compared to NNRTIs (Riddler et al., 2008). However, most PIs (excluding ATV) are commonly associated with undesirable effects on lipid metabolism, including hyperlipidemia (an increase in total and low density [LDL] cholesterol and triglyceride levels, which poses an increased cardiovascular risk) and lipodystrophy (redistribution of body fat, often with fat wasting at the extremities and around the face, and fat deposition around the trunk).

Entry Inhibitors

For treatment-experienced patients harboring resistance virus and those failing multiple regimens, antiretroviral drug combinations have become increasingly complex and in recent years new and more potent agents have been introduced that possess activity against both wild-type and resistant strains.

Inhibition of viral entry is a promising target for therapeutic intervention, because neither NRTIs/ NNRTIs nor PIs prevent viral entry. In theory, all stages of viral entry can be inhibited, including, attachment or binding to the CD4 receptor, binding to coreceptors, and fusion of the virus and host membranes. Hence, entry inhibitors can be divided into three classes: *attachment inhibitors, coreceptor antagonists,* and *fusion inhibitors.*

Attachment Inhibitors

These agents interfere with the interaction between the HIV glycoprotein gp120 and the CD4 receptor, which is the first step toward viral entry into the target cell. Attachment inhibitors are a very heterogeneous class because sites on the CD4 receptor as well as the binding site for gp120 can be blocked; both are currently being investigated.

Coreceptor Antagonists

In addition to the CD4 receptor, HIV also requires co-receptors to gain entry into a target cell. Coreceptor antagonists block either CCR5 or CXCR4 in a similar way to endogenous chemokines, whose structure they partially resemble. The CCR5 antagonists, in particular, are in the later stages of development. Maraviroc (MVC) is the first licensed coreceptor (CCR5 receptor) antagonist and was approved in August 2007.

Fusion Inhibitors

Enfuvirtide (T-20) is the only fusion inhibitor approved for clinical use, although other compounds of this class are currently in development. T-20 binds to an intermediated structure of the gp41 protein to ultimately prevent fusion of HIV with the target cell.

Integrase Inhibitors

The viral enzyme integrase, which is encoded by the HIV pol gene, is involved in the integration of viral DNA into the host genome, rendering it a key pharmacological target. Moreover, the enzyme is unlikely to be present in human cells. Integration of viral DNA is a stepwise process, all of which can be theoretically inhibited. Raltegravir (RAL) is the first integrase inhibitor to be licensed by the Food and Drug Administration (FDA) in 2007. The drug specifically inhibits the strand transfer step in the integration process, by preventing the docking and irreversible binding of the hydroxyl ends of viral DNA to the phosphodiesterase bridges of the host DNA. An additional integrase inhibitor, elvitegravir (Shimura et al., 2008), also a strand transfer inhibitor, is in the late stages of clinical development, but has yet to be approved.

More recently, dolutegravir, a novel second integrase strand transfer inhibitor has been added to the arsenal of anti-HIV therapeutics. Dolutegravir has demonstrated superior or non-inferior efficacy in both treatment-naïve as well as treatment-experienced individuals (Raffi et al., 2015; Walmsley et al., 2013). Dolutegravir has superior resistance profile, can be taken as a convenient once-daily dosing, and has a low propensity for drug–drug interactions.

In summary, over the past 30 years, tremendous strides have been made in antiretroviral drug development. Data from the MOTIVATE (maravaroc), BENCHMARK (raltegravir), TORO (T-20), and DUET (etravirine) studies have shown clear benefit of adding a fully active drug to an existing optimized regimen in multidrug-experienced patients. Therefore, it is hoped that with access to these additional classes, patients with extensive multidrug resistance can realistically achieve the same virologic and immunologic responses seen in naïve patients. However, these novel antiretroviral drug classes are expensive and though available in resource-endowed settings are not accessible to the majority of people living with HIV in resource-limited settings.

Initiating First-Line Combination Antiretroviral Therapy

Goals of Treatment

Eradication of HIV infection is currently not achievable with the available ART even though a potent combination of ARTs may be suppressing plasma viral load below the limits of detection. The primary reason is that a pool of latently infected CD4 T cells is established during the earliest stages of acute infection and persists with a long half-life, despite prolonged suppression of plasma viremia (**Box 7-1**).

HIV suppression with ART may also decrease inflammation and immune activation thought to contribute to higher rates of cardiovascular and other end-organ damage reported in HIV-infected cohorts.

Achievement of these treatment goals requires a balance of competing considerations such that providers and patients must collaborate to define individualized strategies to achieve treatment goals as is feasible within the settings. Careful consideration should be given to the selection of an initial combination regimen. If available, pretreatment genotype resistance testing should be used to guide the selection of the most optimal initial ARV regimen and ensure treatment adherence.

When to Start

One of the most crucial decisions is when to initiate ART, as this can influence a patient's long-term response to treatment. Most of the early treatment guidelines (in particular the 2002 WHO guidelines) recommended that treatment be delayed until the CD4 cell count had fallen below 200 cells/μL, because the risk of opportunistic diseases is higher at this threshold. However, over time treatments have improved and the number of treatment options available has increased. In 2010, the WHO reviewed its guidelines and recommended that all adolescents and adults, including pregnant women,

---

BOX 7-1 Goals of Antiretroviral Therapy

1. Reduce HIV-associated morbidity and prolong the duration and quality of survival
2. Restore and preserve immunologic function
3. Maximally and durably suppress plasma HIV viral load
4. Prevent HIV transmission

with HIV infection and CD4 counts of ≤350 cells/mm^3 should start ART, regardless of the presence or absence of clinical symptoms. Those with severe or advanced clinical disease (i.e., WHO clinical stage 3 or 4) should start ART irrespective of their CD4 cell count (WHO, 2010). This recommendation was based on moderate-quality evidence from randomized controlled trials (Emery et al., 2008; Severe et al., 2010) and observational studies (Sterne et al., 2009; Wong et al., 2007) showing that initiating ART at or below the 350 cells/mm^3 threshold was associated with reduction in mortality, disease progression (including tuberculosis), vertical transmission, and serious adverse events (**Table 7-2**).

Asymptomatic patients with CD4 counts >500 cells/mm^3 have a low short-term risk of disease progression; thus, it is recommended that treatment in these subjects should be deferred in the majority of cases. The question of whether to initiate ART in asymptomatic patients with CD4 counts >350 cells/mm^3 (and even >500 cells/μL) has been uncertain. However, a systematic review of evidence from observational studies and randomized controlled trials reporting morbidity, mortality, and virological and immunological outcomes has shown that initiating ART at CD4 >350 cells/mm^3 reduced the risk of progression to AIDS and/or death, tuberculosis, development of non-AIDS defining events, and increased likelihood of immune recovery (Clouse et al., 2013; Lima et al., 2015; Young et al., 2012). Hence, in the most recent 2013 WHO guidelines, initiation of ART is recommended in

all individuals with HIV infection with a CD4 count >350 cells and ≤500 cells/mm^3 regardless of WHO clinical stage. Indeed, previous concerns with respect to starting therapy early had been based on the toxicity risks (for example, metabolic complications) associated with long-term ART. However, because simpler, less toxic, and more tolerated agents are now available, as well as an increased number of options in the case of virologic failure, early initiation of therapy is becoming an increasingly viable consideration at least in resource-endowed settings. Importantly, results from two recently reported randomized clinical trials (RCTs)—The Strategic Timing of Antiretroviral Treatment (START) trial and the Early Antiretroviral Treatment and/or Early Isoniazid Prophylaxis Against Tuberculosis in HIV-infected Adults (TEMPRANO) trial—have provided definitive support for early initiation of ART at CD4 threshold >500 cells/mm^3 compared with <350 cells/mm^3 (TEMPRANO ANRS 12136 Study Group 2015; Lundgren et al., 2015).

Reflective Considerations

What do you think will be the merits and demerits of initiating ART at CD4 >500 cells/mm^3 in asymptomatic HIV-infected patients in SSA?

Table 7-2	Summary of the 2013 WHO Recommendations on When to Start ART in Adults, Adolescents, Pregnant and Breastfeeding Women, and Children
Population	**Recommendation**
Adults and adolescents (≥10 years)	**Initiate ART if CD4 cell count >500 cells/mm^3.** • **As a priority**, initiate ART in all individuals with severe/advanced HIV disease (WHO clinical stage 3 or 4) or CD4 count ≤350 cells/mm^3. **Initiate ART regardless of WHO clinical stage and CD4 cell count:** • Active tuberculosis • HBV coinfection with severe chronic liver disease • Pregnant and breastfeeding women with HIV • HIV-positive individual in a serodiscordant partnership (to reduce HIV transmission risk)
Children ≥5 years old	**Initiate ART if CD4 cell count >500 cells/mm^3.** • **As a priority**, initiate ART in all children with severe/advanced HIV disease (WHO clinical stage 3 or 4) or CD4 count ≤350 cells/mm^3. **Initiate ART regardless of CD4 cell count:** • WHO clinical stage 3 or 4 • Active tuberculosis
Children 1–5 years old[#]	**Initiate ART in all regardless of WHO clinical stage and CD4 cell count.** • **As a priority**, initiate ART in all HIV-infected children 1–2 years old or with severe/advanced HIV disease (WHO clinical stage 3 or 4) or with CD4 count ≤750 cells/mm^3 or <25%, whichever is lower.
Infants <1 year old[#]	**Initiate ART in all infants regardless of WHO clinical stage and CD4 cell count.**
[#] **Initiate ART in all HIV-infected children below 18 months of age with presumptive clinical diagnosis of HIV infection.**	

Data from WHO. (2015). Guideline on when to start antiretroviral therapy and on pre-exposure prophylaxis for HIV. Geneva: Author.

It is also recommended that ART be initiated regardless of CD4 cell count under the following circumstances:

- *Treating active tuberculosis (TB) disease*: Active TB disease refers to TB infection in which the person has symptoms and clinical disease as opposed to latent TB infection, in which a person has TB infection but is asymptomatic. The WHO recommends starting ART in all people with HIV and active TB regardless of CD4 cell count, and that TB treatment should be started first, followed by ART, as soon as possible afterwards (and within the first 8 weeks).

- *HIV and HBV coinfection with evidence of severe chronic liver disease*: Patients with HIV/HBV coinfection have accelerated liver fibrosis progression with increased risk of cirrhosis and hepatocellular carcinoma, higher rates of liver-related mortality, and decreased ARV response. In view of this evidence, the WHO recommends that in HIV patients with HBV coinfection, ART should be initiated in all individuals with CD4 ≤ 500 cells/mm^3 and regardless of CD4 cell count in the presence of severe chronic liver disease. Severe chronic liver disease includes cirrhosis and end-stage liver disease and is categorized into compensated and decompensated stages. Decompensated cirrhosis refers to the development of clinically evident complications of portal hypertension (ascites, variceal bleeding, and hepatic encephalopathy) or liver insufficiency (jaundice). There is, however, insufficient evidence to support the initiation of ART in all HBV/HIV coinfected individuals, particularly those with CD4 >500 cells/mm^3 without evidence of liver disease. The challenge in many resource-limited countries is that most HIV patients are unaware of their HBV status due to absence of routine screening, and there is limited access to costly diagnostic investigations for staging liver disease.

- *HIV-positive partners in HIV-serodiscordant couples*: Evidence from observational studies together with one randomized controlled trial—the HPTN 052 study—has shown that ART can greatly reduce transmission of HIV to a sexual partner. In the HPTN 052 study, ART used in combination with condoms and counseling reduced HIV transmission by 96.4% providing evidence to support the use of ART to prevent HIV transmission among HIV serodiscordant couples (Cohen et al., 2011). In HIV-serodiscordant couples one of the sexual partners is HIV-positive and the other in HIV-negative. Hence, it is currently recommended to initiate ART for treatment and prevention in serodiscordant couples to the sexual partner with HIV, regardless of CD4 count.

Emerging evidence also suggest that ART may delay, prevent, or reverse some non-AIDS-defining complications such as HIV-associated kidney disease, liver disease, cardiovascular disease (CVD), neurologic complications and malignancies as discussed here:

- *HIV-associated nephropathy (HIVAN)*: HIVAN is the most common cause of chronic kidney disease in HIV-infected individuals that may lead to end-stage kidney disease. The pathogenesis of HIVAN is linked with involvement of renal injury due to ongoing viral replication and can occur at any CD4 count, whereas HIVAN is uncommon in virologically suppressed patients. ART in patients with HIVAN has been associated with both preserved renal function and prolonged survival. Thus, ART should be initiated in patients with HIVAN regardless of CD4 count.

Factors Influencing Response to cART

An individual's response to ART is dependent on many confounding variables, which relate to the patient or "host," the virus, and the drug(s) administered. Thus, treatment failure can occur due to physiological, pathological, genetic, and behavioral factors, and pharmacologically, due to poor pharmacokinetics, drug interactions, a lack of treatment efficacy, or the development of viral resistance; all of which are explored further in the following sections.

Viral Factors

Drug Resistance Treatment failure is often indicated by a high pVL in a patient on ART and it implies that the virus has acquired resistance to a particular drug or a whole drug class (cross-resistance). Resistance occurs when viruses acquire mutations that render them slightly different from the original wild-type population. The development of resistance in HIV is rather ubiquitous because of the rapid and error-prone replication process, as the reverse transcriptase enzyme does not contain a DNA proofreading stage like other retroviruses (Martinez-Picado & Martinez, 2008). Specifically, mutations that confer drug resistance accumulate when viral replication occurs in the presence of selective pressure from antiretrovirals and/or immune response. The potential for selection of drug-resistant strains is, therefore, substantially higher in the presence of suboptimal antiretroviral concentrations, when the replicative capacity of the virus becomes greater. For this reason, effective monitoring of antiretroviral concentrations may be a viable tool for evaluating or predicting the risk of resistance in patients, particularly those with high pVL and/or suspected adherence issues.

However, many drug-resistant mutations that emerge during antiretroviral treatment have a detrimental effect on viral fitness and replication. In general, mutations conferring resistance to the NRTIs and NNRTIs do not reduce viral fitness to the same extent as those conferring resistance to the PIs. In the era of cART, the transmission of resistant strains is an emerging problem that has clear implications for long-term treatment options. As a result, in resource-endowed settings, newly diagnosed patients are screened for resistant strains prior to initiation of therapy.

Pharmacological Factors

Pharmacological factors that may incur therapeutic failure include poor drug pharmacokinetics, inadequate potency and a low genetic barrier to resistance, unfavorable toxicity profiles, and poor penetration of antiretrovirals into viral sanctuary sites.

Pharmacokinetics Pharmacokinetics is the area of pharmacology that describes the **A**bsorption, **D**istribution, **M**etabolism, and **E**limination (ADME) of drugs by physiological systems in the body. In the field of HIV, acquiring and maintaining antiretroviral concentrations within the systemic circulation is essential in ensuring that therapeutic drug concentrations reach their local receptor site (i.e., within CD4+ cells) in order to exert the desired pharmacological response.

Most significantly, the NNRTIs and PIs have well-defined pharmacokinetic/pharmacodynamic (PK/PD) and pharmacokinetic/toxicity relationships in which systemic (plasma) drug levels have been shown to correlate with observed virologic response, or to independently predict the risk of treatment failure/success or toxicity. Thus, the key to selecting an optimal dose for a drug is to balance the relationship between antiretroviral pharmacokinetics (systemic exposure or a single concentration) and drug response (beneficial and/or adverse), and to design strategies to optimize response and tolerability while avoiding unwanted toxicity.

Furthermore, it is essential that antiretroviral concentrations remain above a so-called minimum effective concentration (MEC)—in order to ensure adequate potency and avoid viral rebound or development of resistance. On the other hand, concentrations must not be so high as to cause unwanted toxicity. These concentration-based therapeutic cut-offs (MEC) that are well defined for most NNRTIs and PIs (La Porte et al., 2006)—are utilized in both prospective and observational pharmacokinetic studies, and in routine therapeutic drug monitoring (TDM) in resource-endowed settings. When evaluated alongside virological (pVL) and immunological (CD4 counts) markers, they may aid in the interpretation of an individual's response to therapy, enabling physicians to make more rational or evidence-based decisions regarding dose adjustment in case of sub-therapeutic concentrations or an unsuppressed pVL. Nevertheless, these values serve only as estimates, and because they are derived primarily from accumulated pharmacokinetic data obtained from controlled trials, they may not reflect real-life clinical situations, such as the effects of drug interactions, coinfections, or pregnancy, as well as differences in age, race, and disease status upon overall drug exposure. Indeed, in reality, there is higher inter and intra-individual variation in antiretroviral plasma concentrations, even in patients receiving equivalent dose (Back et al., 2002). The foundations for such an effect is not fully understood, although it is possible that pharmacokinetic factors, such as differences in drug absorption, metabolism, and distribution, along with external patient or host influences (as will be discussed) could contribute to the underlying variability in antiretroviral concentrations seen in HIV-infected patients.

All antiretrovirals, with the exception of T-20, are administered orally; thus, in order to reach the systemic circulation and be distributed throughout the body, they must be absorbed through the enterocytes and the gut wall. The rate and extent of drug absorption is highly dependent upon an agent's physicochemical properties, such as its lipophilicity and its solubility, but may also be regulated by gastrointestinal motility, and gastric and gastrointestinal pH and blood flow which, in turn, can be affected by food (mainly fat) intake, pregnancy, disease states, and circadian differences. Most antiretrovirals excluding NRTIs, which are eliminated renally, are ultimately eliminated via urine or bile. Internal oxidative reactions and passage through the liver subject the drugs to "first-pass metabolism," resulting in significantly reduced drug oral bioavailability (the fraction of unchanged orally administered drug reaching systemic circulation).

What to Start With

Achieving viral suppression requires the use of ARV regimens with at least two, and preferably three, active drugs from two or more drug classes. Viral load reduction to undetectable limits in an ART-naïve patient usually occurs within the first 12–24 weeks of therapy. Virologic success is predicted by a high potency of ARV regimens, excellent adherence to treatment regimen, low baseline viremia, higher baseline CD4 count (>200 cells/mm^3), and rapid reduction of viremia in response to treatment.

The 2010 WHO ART guidelines recommended that ART in treatment-naïve adults should initially consist of an NNRTI (either NVP or EFV) plus two NRTIs, one of which should be 3TC (or FTC) and the other, AZT or TDF (**Box 7-2**). Emphasis was also placed on the importance of avoiding d4T in first-line regimens because of its well-known mitochondrial toxicity. In practices, the phasing out of d4T as the preferred option in first-line ART has been variable, with some countries making more substantial progress than others. Thus, the recommended regimens in the 2013 WHO guidelines are those with better toxicity profiles than d4T but were considered comparable in terms of efficacy. Furthermore, the new guidelines promote simplification of ART delivery by reducing the number of preferred first-line regimens and focusing on regimens that may be used across a range of populations.

Hence:

- The preferred first-line regimen currently is TDF plus 3TC (or FTC) plus EFV, a combination that is available as a once-daily, fixed dose combination and offers good potential for harmonizing treatment across different populations.

- DF/FTC or TDF/3TC are the preferred NRTI backbone for people coinfected with HIV and HBV and

---

BOX 7-2 Indications for Initiating ART According to the HHS PANEL Guidelines 2012

Indications for initiating ART in treatment-naïve patients

ART is recommended for all HIV-infected individuals. The strength of this recommendation varies on the basis of pretreatment CD4 cell count:

CD4 count <350 cells/mm^3 (AI)

CD4 count 350–500 cells/mm^3 (AIII)

CD4 count >500 cells/mm^3 (BIII)

Regardless of CD4 count, initiation of ART is strongly recommended for individuals with the following conditions:

- Pregnancy (AI)
- History of an AIDS-defining illness (AI)
- HIV-associated nephropathy (HIVAN) (AII)
- HIV/hepatitis B virus (HBV) coinfection (AII)

*Rating of recommendations: **A** = **strong; B** = **moderate; C** = **optional***
*Rating of evidence: **I** = **data from randomized controlled trials; II** = **data from well-designed nonrandomized trials or** observational cohort studies with long-term clinical outcomes; III** = **expert opinion***

Data from Panel on antiretroviral guidelines for adults and adolescents. (2016). Guidelines for the use of antiretroviral agents in HIV-1-infected adults and adolescents. Department of Health and Human Services. Retrieved from https://aidsinfo.nih.gov/contentfiles/lvguidelines /AdultandAdolescentGL.pdf

---

can be used among people coinfected with TB and among pregnant women.

- EFV is the preferred NNRTI for people with HIV and TB (pharmacological compatibility with TB drugs) and HIV and HBV coinfection (less risk of hepatic toxicity) and can be used among pregnant women, including those in the first trimester (**Table 7-3**).

In most developing countries, EFV has replaced NVP as the preferred NNRTI due to higher incidence of skin rash and hepatotoxicity with NVP. Specifically a systematic review has shown that patients on NVP are twice as likely as those receiving EFV to discontinue treatment because of adverse events (Shubber et al., 2013). Concerns still remain about the use of NVP in women with CD4 >250 cells/mm^3. Hence, NVP should be used cautiously in pregnant women and women who might be pregnant, given the apparent elevated risk of NVP-associated toxicity. Even though the U.S. Food and Drug Administration and European Medicines Agency advise against the use of EFV in the first trimester of pregnancy and women of child-bearing potential due to the potential for birth defects, the British HIV Association has recently changed its recommendation to allow EFV to be used in the first trimester. This has stemmed from data from the Antiretroviral Pregnancy Registry and meta-analysis that suggested an estimated prevalence of birth defects among children born to women on EFV of 0.07% was comparable to estimates of 0.02–0.20% in the general population in the USA (U.S. Department of Health and Human Services, 2012).

The 2012 British HIV Association (BHIVA) guidelines recommend for treatment-naïve patients a combination of three or more antiretroviral agents: an NNRTI or a RTV-boosted PI in combination with a dual NRTI backbone (preferably containing either FTC or 3TC). These recommendations are summarized in **Table 7-4** (BHIVA, 2012). Because ART is lifelong, it is crucial that initial drug regimens are tailored toward an individual patient's needs, taking into account any concurrent illnesses and concomitant medications, in order to achieve the maximum potency and tolerability, and avoid long-term complications and possible drug interactions.

Reflective Considerations

Does the limited repertoire of first-line ART in resource-limited settings compromise treatment outcomes compared with resource-endowed settings?

Laboratory Testing for Initial Assessment and Monitoring While on ART

A number of laboratory tests are important for initial evaluation of HIV-infected patients upon entry into care, during follow-up if ART has not been initiated, and prior to and after initiation or modification of therapy to assess virologic and immunologic efficacy of ART (see Table 7-4 for WHO-recommended testing). Equally important, patients

Table 7-3	First-Line ART Regimens for Adults, Pregnant and Breastfeeding Women, and Children (2013).	
First-line ART	**Preferred first-line regimens**	**Alternative first-line regimens[1,2]**
Adults (including pregnant and breastfeeding women and adults with TB and HBV coinfection)	TDF + 3TC (or FTC) + EFV	AZT + 3TC + EFV AZT + 3TC + NVP TDF + 3TC (or FTC)+ NVP
Adolescents (10 to 19 years) ≥35 kg	TDF + 3TC (or FTC) + EFV	AZT + 3TC + EFV AZT + 3TC + NVP TDF + 3TC (or FTC) + NVP ABC + 3TC + EFV (or NVP)
Children 3 years to less than 10 years and adolescents <35 kg	ABC + 3TC + EFV	ABC + 3TC + NVP AZT + 3TC + EFV AZT + 3TC + NVP TDF + 3TC (or FTC) + EFV TDF + 3TC (or FTC) + NVP
Children <3 years	ABC or AZT + 3TC + LPV/r	ABC + 3TC + NVP AZT + 3TC + NVP

[1] For adolescents, using d4T as an option in first-line treatment should be discontinued and restricted to special cases in which other ARV drugs cannot be used and to the shortest time possible, with close monitoring. In children, d4T use should be restricted to the situations in which there is suspected or confirmed toxicity to AZT and lack of access to ABC or TDF.

[2] ABC or boosted PIs (ATV/r, DRV/r, LPV/r) can be used in special circumstances.

Data from WHO. (2013). First-line ART for pregnant and breastfeeding women and ARV drugs for their infants. Retrieved from http://www.who .int/hiv/pub/guidelines/arv2013/art/artpregnantwomen/en/; WHO. (2013). *Consolidated guidelines on the use of antiretroviral drugs for treating and preventing HIV infection: Recommendations for a public health approach.* Geneva: Author.

should be monitored for laboratory abnormalities that may be associated with ARV drugs. Two surrogate markers are used routinely to assess the immune function and level of HIV viremia: CD4 T-cell count (CD4 count) and plasma HIV RNA (viral load). Baseline resistance testing should ideally be used to guide selection of an ARV regimen in both ART-naïve and ART-experienced patients. A viral tropism assay should be performed prior to initiation of a CCR5 antagonist; and HLA-B*5701 testing should be performed prior to initiation of abacavir to avert possible ABC hypersensitivity reaction. Suffice to say that aside from CD4 cell count testing and routine hematobiochemistries, in most resource limited settings, viral load, resistance, viral tropism assays, and HLA-B*5701 screening are not routinely available to guide management decisions.

CD4 T-cell Count

The CD4 T-cell count serves as the major laboratory indicator of immune function in patients with HIV infection. The CD4 count is one of the most critical determinants of the decision to initiate ART and/or prophylaxis against opportunistic infections. It is also used for monitoring therapeutic response. An adequate CD4 response for most patients on therapy is defined as an increase in CD4 count in the range of 50–150 cells/mm^3 per year, generally with an accelerated response in the first 3 months. Subsequent increases in patients with good virologic control show an average increase of approximately 50–100 cells/mm^3 per year for the subsequent years until a

steady state level is reached (Kaufmann et al., 2003). The CD4 cell count response to ART varies widely, but a poor CD4 response is rarely an indication for modifying a virologically suppressive ARV regimen. In general, CD4 counts should be monitored every 3–4 months to determine when to start ART in untreated patients, assess immunologic response to ART, and assess the need for initiation or discontinuation of prophylaxis for opportunistic infections. Among patients on ART with virologic suppression, CD4 counts should be assessed every 6–12 months.

Plasma HIV RNA Testing

Plasma HIV RNA (viral load) should be measured in all patients at baseline and on a regular basis thereafter, especially in patients who are on treatment, because viral load is the most important indicator of response to ART and is an important predictor of clinical progression. Optimal viral suppression is generally defined as a viral load persistently below the level of detection (<20–75 copies/mL, depending on the assay used). However, isolated "blips" (viral loads transiently detectable at low levels, typically <400 copies/mL) are not uncommon in successfully treated patients and are not thought to represent viral replication or to predict virologic failure (Havlir et al., 2001). For most individuals who are adherent to their ARV regimens and who do not harbor resistance mutations to the prescribed drugs, viral suppression is generally achieved in 12–24 weeks, after which viral load should be monitored every 3–4 months or as clinically indicated. The capacity for

Table 7-4	WHO Recommended Laboratory Tests for HIV Screening and Monitoring	
Phase of HIV Management	**Recommended**	**Desirable (if feasible)**
HIV diagnosis	HIV serology CD4 cell count TB Screening	• HBV (HBsAg) serology[1] • HCV serology • Cryptococcus antigen if CD4 ≤100 cells/µL[2] • Screening for sexually transmitted infections • Assessment for major non-communicable chronic diseases and comorbidities[3]
Follow-up before ART	CD4 cell count (every 6–12 months)	
ART initiation	CD4 cell count	• Hemoglobin test for AZT[4] • Pregnancy test • Blood pressure measurement • Urine dipsticks for glycosuria and eGFR and serum creatinine for TDF[5] • Alanine transaminase for NVP[6]
Receiving ART	CD4 cell count (every 6 months) HIV viral load (at 6 months after initiating ART and every 12 months thereafter)	Urine dipstick for glycosuria and serum creatinine for TDF[3]
Treatment failure	CD4 cell count HIV viral load	HBV (HBsAg) serology (before switching ART regimen if this testing was not done or if the result was negative at baseline)

[1]If feasible, HBsAg testing should be performed to identify people with HIV and HBV coinfection and who therefore should initiate TDF-containing ART.

[2]Can be considered only in settings with a high prevalence of cryptococcal antigenemia (>3%).

[3]Consider assessing the presence of chronic conditions that can influence ART management such as hypertension and other cardiovascular diseases, diabetes, and tuberculosis.

[4]Among children and adults with a high risk of adverse events associated with AZT (low CD4 or low BMI).

[5]Among people with a high risk of adverse events associated with TDF: underlying renal disease, older age group, low body mass index (BMI), diabetes mellitus, hypertension, and concomitant use of a boosted PI or potential nephrotoxic drugs.

[6]Among people with a high risk of adverse events associated with NVP, such as being ART-naïve, women with HIV with a CD4 count >250 cells/mm[3], and HCV coinfection. However, liver enzymes have low predictive value for monitoring NVP toxicity.

Reproduced from WHO. (2013). Consolidated ARV guidelines 2013. Laboratory monitoring before and after initiating ART. Retrieved from http://www.who.int/hiv/pub/guidelines/arv2013/art/artmonitoring/en/

routine virologic monitoring in most SSA countries and other resource-limited settings is sorely inadequate.

Treatment Failures

Treatment failure on ART can be clinical, immunological, or virologic, as well as a toxicity-limiting continuation of an ARV regimen (see **Table 7-5**).

Clinical Failure

Clinical failure refers to a new or recurrent clinical event indicating severe immunodeficiency (WHO clinical stage 4 condition—refer to Table 7-1) after 6 months of effective treatment. Some stage 3 clinical conditions such as tuberculosis and other severe bacterial infections may indicate treatment failure; however, clinical treatment failure conditions should be distinguished from immune reconstitution inflammatory syndrome (IRIS).

IRIS is a spectrum of clinical signs and symptoms thought to be associated with immune recovery brought about by a response to ART. This phenomenon occurs among 10–30% of people initiating ART, usually within 4–8 weeks after initiating therapy. Two major clinical presentations are recognized: paradoxical IRIS, in which an opportunistic infection or tumor diagnosed before ART initially responds to treatment but then deteriorates after ART starts; or unmasking IRIS, in which initiating ART triggers disease that was not clinically apparent before ART. Hence, the diagnosis of IRIS is considered only when

Table 7-5	WHO Definitions of Clinical, Immunological, and Virological Failure for the Decision to Switch ART Regimens	
Failure	**Definition**	**Comments**
Clinical failure	**Adults and adolescents** New or recurrent clinical event indicating severe immunodeficiency (WHO clinical stage 4 condition) after 6 months of effective treatment **Children** New or recurrent clinical event indicating advanced or severe immunodeficiency (WHO clinical 3 or 4 clinical condition with exception of TB) after 6 months of effective treatment	The condition must be differentiated from immune reconstitution inflammatory syndrome occurring after initiating ART. For adults, certain WHO clinical stage 3 conditions (PTB and severe bacterial infections) may indicate treatment failure.
Immunological failure	**Adults and adolescents** CD4 count falls to the baseline (or below) Or Persistent CD4 levels below 100 cells/mm^3 **Children** Younger than 5 years Persistent CD4 levels below 200 cells/mm^3 or <10% Older than 5 years Persistent CD4 levels below 100 cells/mm^3	Without concomitant or recent infection to cause a transient decline in the CD4 cell count.
Virological failure	Persistent viral load above 1,000 copies/mL based on two consecutive viral load measurements after 3 months, with adherence support	The optimal threshold for defining virological failure and the need for switching ART regimen has not been determined. An individual must be taking ART for at least 6 months before it can be determined that a regimen has failed. Assessment of viral load using Dried Blood Spot and point-of-care technologies should use a higher threshold.

Reproduced from WHO. (2013). Consolidated ARV guidelines 2013. WHO definitions of clinical, immunological and virological failure for the decision to switch ART regimens. Retrieved from http://www.who.int/hiv/pub/guidelines/arv2013/intro/tables/en/

the presentation cannot be explained by a new infection, expected course of a known infection, or drug toxicity. The clinical spectrum of IRIS is diverse and has been reported for many different infections, tumors, and non-infectious conditions such as tuberculosis, cryptococcosis, Kaposi's sarcoma, and herpes zoster. This is what makes the diagnosis of IRIS and differentiation from clinical failure difficult particularly in resource-limited settings where diagnostic facilities are limiting. IRIS is generally self-limiting and interruption of ART is rarely indicated. Because IRIS is associated with a low CD4 cell count at ART initiation, presence of disseminated opportunistic infections or tumors, and a shorter duration of therapy for opportunistic infections before ART initiation, measures to reduce its development include earlier HIV diagnosis and initiation of ART before a decline to below 200 CD4 cells/mm^3; improved screening for opportunistic infections before ART, especially TB and *Cryptococcus*; and optimal management of opportunistic infection before initiating ART.

Immunologic Failure

Immunologic failure can be defined as the failure to achieve and maintain an adequate CD4 response despite virologic suppression. Although no accepted specific definition exists, the WHO has focused its definition on an inability to increase CD4 counts above pretherapy levels by >50 or 100 cells/mm^3 after 1 year of therapy. Other studies have focused on patients who fail to increase CD4 counts above a specific threshold (e.g., >350 or 500 cells/mm^3) over a specific period of time (e.g., 4–7 years) (Engsig et al., 2014; Moore & Keruly, 2007; also see the guidelines accesible at AIDS *info,* http://aidsinfo.nih.gov/guidelines). A persistently low CD4 count while on suppressive ART is associated with a small, but appreciable, risk of AIDS- and non-AIDS-related morbidity and mortality. There is no consensus on when and how to treat immunologic failure. However, given the risk of clinical events, it is reasonable to focus on patients with CD4 counts

<200 cells/mm³. Suggested strategies include adding a new drug to an existing regimen, changing the regimen to another (e.g., from NNRTI-based to PI-based or an immune-based therapy), but all these have not resulted in clear virologic or immunologic benefit.

The current WHO guidelines on immunological and clinical monitoring for treatment failure have a poor sensitivity and lower positive predictive value for identifying virological failure in adults (Rawizza et al., 2011). The implication is that many patients identified with immunological failure may in fact be adequately suppressed virologically and risk being misclassified as having treatment failure and switched unnecessarily to second-line therapy.

Virologic Failure

Virologic failure is defined as an inability to achieve and maintain suppression of viral replication (to an HIV RNA level <200 copies/mL). Persistent HIV RNA levels >200 copies/mL, particularly >500 copies/mL, often are associated with evidence of viral evolution and drug-resistance mutation accumulation and should be distinguished from viremic "blips" in which viral suppression is followed by a detectable HIV RNA level and then subsequent return to undetectable levels. The optimal threshold for defining virological failure and for switching ART regimens has not been established; however, the WHO has set a cut-off value of 1,000 copies/mL. The WHO has now recommended viral load monitoring as the preferred approach to diagnose and confirm ARV treatment failure; however, its widespread implementation within many resource-constrained countries will require substantial support as governments are saddled with the increasing cost of initiating ART for more patients and procuring expensive second-line ARTs. Hence, two strategies for viral-load monitoring are proposed (**Figure 7-3**), namely, routine viral-load monitoring every 6–12 months to enable earlier and more accurate detection of treatment failure, or a targeted viral-load monitoring strategy to confirm failure suspected on clinical or immunological criteria. Data are needed on which of these approaches would be feasible and implementable in resource-constrained settings.

There are multiple reasons for virologic failure, including patient, ARV regimen, and provider characteristics. Data from older patient cohorts suggested that suboptimal adherence and drug intolerance/toxicity accounted for 28–40% of virologic failure and regimen discontinuations (d'Arminio Monforte et al., 2000; Mocroft et al., 2001), whereas more recent data suggest either preexisting (transmitted) drug resistance or suboptimal adherence (Paredes et al., 2010) as the most common reasons for virologic failure. It is crucial to identify the reasons for virologic failure because the approaches to subsequent therapy differ substantially. Thus, the care provider should explore issues of patient adherence, medication intolerance, pharmacokinetic issues, and suspected drug resistance. Samples for resistance testing

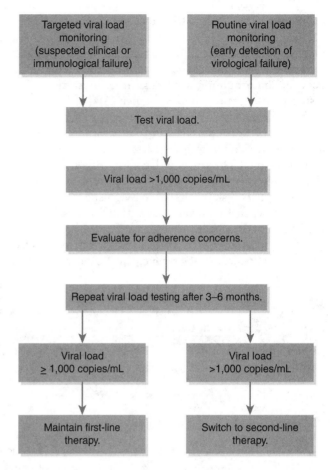

Figure 7-3 Proposed WHO Viral Load Testing Strategies to Detect or Confirm Treatment Failure and Switch ART Regimen in Adults, Adolescents, and Children
Reproduced from WHO. (2013). *Consolidated guidelines on the use of antiretroviral drugs for treating and preventing HIV infection: Recommendations for a public health approach.* Retrieved from http://apps.who.int/iris/bitstream/10665/85321/1/9789241505727_eng.pdf

should be obtained while the patient is taking the failing regimen or within 4 weeks after regimen discontinuation if the plasma HIV RNA level is >500 copies/mL. In interpreting drug resistance results, careful consideration is given to the patient's prior treatment history and prior resistance test results. Upon confirming virologic failure, it is generally recommended that the regimen be changed as soon as possible to avoid progressive accumulation of resistance mutations. Ideally, a new ARV regimen should contain at least two, and preferably three, fully active drugs based on drug treatment history, resistance testing, or new mechanistic class.

ART-Associated Adverse Effects

Adverse effects are among the most commonly cited reasons for switching or discontinuing therapy as well as for medication non-adherence. Indeed, all known antiretroviral drugs have adverse effects and rates of these events among patients enrolled in randomized trials appear to be declining with use of newer ARV regimens. Predisposing risk factors for these adverse effects is determined by individual demographic, genetic, comorbidities, and drug–drug interactions. For instance, compared with men, women (ART-naïve women with CD4 counts >250 cells/mm^3) appear to have a higher propensity for developing Stevens-Johnson syndrome, rashes, and hepatotoxicity from NVP (Bersoff-Matcha et al., 2001) and also have higher rates of lactic acidosis from NRTIs (Bolhaar & Karstaedt, 2007). Predisposition to abacavir hypersensitivity rash is determined by genetic factors, while comorbidities such as alcoholism and chronic viral hepatitis may increase the risk for hepatotoxicity.

Careful consideration is therefore required in the selection of an individual's ARV regimen and further monitoring necessary for prevention and or early detection of adverse effects. The overarching goal of ART should be its safety in addition to its virologic and immunologic efficacy. Hence, delaying substitutions or switches when there are severe adverse drug effects may cause harm and may affect adherence, leading to drug resistance and treatment failure. When drug interruptions are required, such as for severe and life-threatening adverse events related to toxicity, it is important to consider the various half-lives of ARV drugs. For instance, when NNRTIs must be discontinued, a staggered approach should be used by prolonging the use of the NRTI backbone for 2 to 3 weeks. Alternatively, the NNRTI could be temporarily substituted with a boosted PI. **Table 7-6** summarizes the toxicities associated with commonly used first- and second-line ARV drugs used in sub-Saharan African countries.

Table 7-6	Types of Toxicities Associated with Commonly Used First- and Second-Line ARV Drugs in Developing Countries		
ARV Drug	**Major Types of Toxicity**	**Risk Factors**	**Suggested Management**
ABC	Hypersensitivity reaction	Presence of HLA-B*5701	If ABC is being used in first-line ART, substitute with TDF or AZT or d4T.
			If ABC is being used in second-line ART, substitute with TDF.
AZT	Anemia	Baseline anemia or neutropenia	If AZT is being used in first-line ART, substitute with TDF or ABC.
	Neutropenia	CD4 count <200 cells/mm^3	If AZT is being used in second-line ART, substitute with d4T.
	Myopathy	BMI >25 (or body weight >75 kg)	
	Lipoatrophy or lipodystrophy	Prolonged exposure to nucleoside analogues	
	Lactic acidosis or severe hepatomegaly with steatosis		
d4T	Peripheral neuropathy, lipoatrophy, or lipodystrophy	Older age	If d4T is being used in first-line ART, substitute with TDF or AZT or ABC.
	Lactic acidosis or severe hepatomegaly with steatosis, acute pancreatitis	CD4 count ≤200 cells/mm^3	If d4T is being used in second-line ART (after TDF or ABC are used in first-line ART), substitute with AZT.
		Concomitant use of isoniazid or ddI	
		BMI >25 (or body weight >75 kg)	
		Prolonged exposure to nucleoside analogues	
TDF	Tubular renal dysfunction, Fanconi syndrome	Underlying renal disease	If TDF is being used in second-line ART (after d4T + AZT use in first-line ART), substitute with ABC or ddI.
	Decreases in bone mineral density	Older age	
		BMI <18.5 (or body weight <50 kg)	Use alternative drug for hepatitis B treatment (such as entecavir).
	Lactic acidosis or severe hepatomegaly with steatosis	Untreated diabetes mellitus	
		Untreated hypertension	
	Exacerbation of hepatitis B (hepatic flares)	Concomitant use of nephrotoxic drugs or a boosted PI	
		History of osteomalacia and pathological fracture	
		Risk factors for osteoporosis or bone loss	
		Prolonged exposure to nucleoside analogues	
		Obesity	
		Discontinuation of TDF due to toxicity	

ARV Drug	Major Types of Toxicity	Risk Factors	Suggested Management
NVP	Hepatotoxicity Severe skin rash and hypersensitivity reaction (Stevens-Johnson syndrome)	Underlying hepatic disease HBV and HCV coinfection Concomitant use of hepatotoxic drugs CD4 >250 cells/mm^3 in women CD4 >400 cells/mm^3 for men First month of therapy (if lead-in dose is not used) Risk factors unknown	EFV. If the person cannot tolerate either NNRTI, use boosted PIs.
EFV	Persistent central nervous system toxicity (such as abnormal dreams, depression, or mental confusion) Convulsions Hepatotoxicity Hypersensitivity reaction, Stevens-Johnson syndrome Potential risk for neural tube defects (very low risk in humans) Male gynecomastia	Depression or other mental disorder (previous or baseline) Daytime dosing History of seizure Underlying hepatic disease HBV and HCV coinfection Concomitant use of hepatotoxic drug Risk factors unknown	NVP. If the person cannot tolerate either NNRTI, use boosted PIs.
LPV/r	Electrocardiographic abnormalities (PR and QT interval prolongation, torsades de pointes) QT interval prolongation Hepatotoxicity Pancreatitis Risk of prematurity, lipoatrophy or metabolic syndrome, dyslipidemia or severe diarrhea	People with preexisting conduction system disease Concomitant use of other drugs that may prolong the PR interval Congenital long QT syndrome Hypokalemia Concomitant use of drugs that may prolong the QT interval Underlying hepatic disease HBV and HCV coinfection Concomitant use of hepatotoxic drugs Advanced HIV disease Risk factors unknown	If LPV/r is used in first-line ART for children, use an age-appropriate NNRTI (NVP for children younger than 3 years and EFV for children 3 years and older). ATV can be used for children older than 6 years. If LPV/r is used in second-line ART for adults, use ATV/r or DRV/r. If boosted PIs are contraindicated and the person has failed on treatment with NNRTI in first-line ART, consider integrase inhibitors.

Modified from WHO. (2013). Consolidated ARV guidelines 2013. Types of toxicities associated with first-, second- and third-line ARV drugs. Retrieved from http://www.who.int/hiv/pub/guidelines/arv2013/intro/tables/en/

Second-Line ART

Second-line therapy is required after failure of a first-line ART. Because first-line ART in programs in resource-limited settings is based on an NNRTI, PI-based regimens are recommended for second-line therapy. Thus, using a boosted PI plus a two-NRTI combination is recommended as the preferred strategy for second-line treatment in adults, adolescents, and also children for whom NNRTI-containing regimens were used in first-line ART. In children using a PI-based regimen for first-line ART, switching to NNRTI or maintaining the PI regimen is recommended according to age. See **Table 7-7** for WHO guidelines of second-line ART regimens.

Third-line ART

As ART program mature, patients on second-line ART may fail therapy, warranting a sequencing of third-line therapy. Evidence from cohort studies has shown a high mortality among people for whom second-line ART had failed. Thus it is recommended that national program should develop policies for third-line ART and that these regimens should include new drugs with minimal risk of cross-resistance to previously used regimens, such as integrase inhibitors and second-generation NNRTIs and PIs. The high-cost of third-line therapy is real and it is recognized that financial constraints will limit widespread adoption of third-line regimens. Hence, patients on failing second-line regimen

Table 7-7	Preferred Second-Line ART Regimens for Adults, Adolescents, Pregnant Women, and Children		
Second-Line ART		**Preferred Regimens**	**Alternative Regimens**
Adults and adolescents (≥10 years), including pregnant and breastfeeding women		AZT + 3TC + LPV/r [1] AZT + 3TC + ATV/r [1]	TDF + 3TC (or FTC) + ATV/r TDF + 3TC (or FTC) + LPV/r
Children	If a NNRTI-based first-line regimen was used	ABC + 3TC + LPV/r [2]	ABC + 3TC + LPV/r [2] TDF + 3TC (or FTC) + LPV/r [2]
	If a PI-based first-line regimen was used — <3 years	No change from first line regimen in use [3]	AZT (or ABC) + 3TC + NVP
	3 years to <10 years	AZT (or ABC) + 3TC +EFV	ABC (or TDF) + 3TC + NVP

[1] DRV/r can be used as an alternative PI and SQV/r in special situations; neither is currently available as heat-stable fixed-dose combination, but a DRV + RTV heat-stable fixed-dose combination is currently in development.

[2] ATV/r can be used as an alternative to LPV/r for children older than 6 years.

[3] Unless failure is caused by lack of adherence resulting from palatability of LPV/r.

Reproduced from WHO. (2013). Consolidated ARV guidelines 2013. Summary of preferred second-line ART regimens for adults, adolescents, pregnant women and children. Retrieved from http://www.who.int/hiv/pub/guidelines/arv2013/intro/tables/en/

with no new ARV options are recommended to continue with the tolerated regimen.

Overview of U.S. CDC Initiatives for Prevention, Care, and Treatment

Ongoing improvements in preventive, care, and treatment interventions have brought about substantial reduction in AIDS-related morbidity and mortality, with longer life expectancy. This is largely attributed to advancements in highly effective ART, which effectively lowers viral load and risk of transmission as well as preserving the health of individuals living with HIV (CDC, 2015a; 2016b). Therefore, several ongoing initiatives are aimed at determining best evidence-based approaches to deal with the burden of HIV/AIDS prevalence, widespread transmission, and associated consequences in society. These developments have transformed the U.S. policy and approach to HIV prevention and care. Nevertheless, the CDC cautions that without appropriate care and medication the probable prognosis of HIV infection could be progression to AIDS and premature death. Current estimates show that approximately 13,000 AIDS victims die each year in the United States (CDC 2015c; 2016a).

The U.S. National HIV/AIDS strategy (2010) outlines a number of explicit goals pertaining to early HIV diagnosis with effective care interventions. The key aims emphasize increasing the following:

- The number of HIV-positive individuals aware of their infection status to 90%
- The proportion of newly diagnosed patients who are linked to care within 3 months to 85%
- The proportion of HIV-diagnosed individuals who maintain effective viral suppression, in particular, the population sub-groups of gay and bisexual men, African Americans, and Latinos

Appropriate preventive interventions and care are hoped to significantly reduce new HIV infections in the United States. This is the core and fundamental element inherent in the National HIV/AIDS Strategy.

High-Impact HIV Prevention: An Initiative Exemplifying Evidence-Based Practice

High-impact HIV prevention emphasizes the implementation of combinations of scientifically proven, cost-effective, scalable/accessible interventions intended to target the right populations in the right geographical areas. Therefore, all Americans at risk for HIV infection, including gay and bisexual men, transgender women and men, injecting drug users, ethnic communities, women, and youths should benefit from this initiative. Moreover, the approach is designed to maximize the impact of HIV prevention endeavors toward accomplishing the goals of the National HIV/AIDS Strategy (NHAS). Particular consideration should be given to the social circumstances, community, and financial and structural factors that create the vulnerability and risk for particular groups. The strategies that are verified and endorsed for high-impact HIV prevention are clearly stipulated (Box 7-3).

The U.S. HIV/AIDS Care Continuum: An Examplar of Excellence in HIV Care and Services

The HIV/AIDS care continuum initiative, also described as a model of HIV treatment cascade, represents an exemplary approach comprising specified sequences of care to which HIV-infected individuals are exposed from the initial stage of diagnosis. The spectrum of care is progressive and aimed at achieving viral suppression with HIV medication for improved health, low viral load, and reduced risk of transmission.

Sequence of the HIV Care Continuum

The HIV care continuum comprises specific stages from the initial diagnosis to the eventual achievement of viral suppression:

- Diagnosed with HIV infection.
- Linked to care (attended healthcare provider within 3 months of positive HIV diagnosis). Taking account of the differences in monitoring the continuum, linkage to care may be calculated as engaged in care or retained in care. This allows for calculating the percentage of people diagnosed with HIV in a particular calendar year who had one or more recorded viral load or CD4+ test within 3 months of diagnosis (CDC, 2014a).
- Engaged or retained in care (received the recommended care for HIV infection).
- Prescribed ART to control HIV infection.
- Virally suppressed (HIV viral load at minimal level).

Prevalence-based HIV care continuum represents each stage of the continuum as a percentage of total number of people living with HIV. The prevalence percentages include the estimates of both HIV diagnosed and undiagnosed—infected but unaware. Moreover, prevalence-based care continuum can provide information about care continuum for the general population of Americans as well as monitoring outcomes among the broader population groups. Thus, the percentages of diagnosed, linked to care, engaged in care, prescribed ART, and viral suppression are calculated for these purposes.

The diagnosis-based HIV care continuum represents the percentage of the HIV-diagnosed people calculated to be at each stage in terms of percentage—linked to care, retained in care, prescribed ART, and viral suppression. Moreover, this calculation can also be applied to separate population subgroups for implementation of appropriate interventions to achieve better health outcomes. The data required for calculating the prevalence-based and diagnosis-based HIV care continuum are obtained from two main sources explored in the following paragraphs.

The National HIV Surveillance System (NHSS)

The NHSS involves all U.S. states, territories, and the District of Columbia, obtaining information on people who are diagnosed and people who have died from HIV. The required details include race/ethnicity, age, and mode of transmission. The information is reported to the CDC by state and local health departments. However, variations occur in the surveillance systems of different states and data from the states and the District of Columbia may also provide complete laboratory reporting. For more information on the current status of the national surveillance system see Cohen, Gray, Ocfemia, Johnson, and Hall (2013).

The Medical Monitoring Project (MMP)

The Medical Monitoring Project provides information on the experiences of people receiving HIV care and the outcomes of their treatment. The details show the number of HIV patients in different stages of care:

- Receiving care
- Prescribed ART
- Achieved viral suppression

The data are reported to the CDC by sample states, cities, and Puerto Rico. Based on these, the MMP data are weighted to be to be nationally representative.

While the CDC has drawn on the best available data to develop the HIV care continuum. It acknowledges that there is no single best way to develop such a continuum.

Variations occur in care continuums depending on the purpose for which each was developed, differences in data sources, and differences in the calculation of progression along the continuum (**Table 7-8**).

Application to Monitoring of Progress and Needs Identification

The information obtained from each stage of the continuum is used by the CDC to establish what proportion of HIV-infected people are in each stage. Federal and state entities can then identify deficits in care provision and determine appropriate interventions to improve patient outcomes all along the continuum. Nationally, the care continuum data are used to prioritize and target resources and for monitoring purposes. Locally compiled data can also be used to determine required improvements and

Table 7-8	A Simplified Synoptic Outline of the Data Sources for Calculating the Stages of the Continuum	
Stages of Progression	**The Data Sources Defined and Synopsized**	
HIV prevalence	• Prevalence-based care continuum Estimates of total number of people living with HIV—diagnosed and undiagnosed Statistical computation utilizing NHSS Data from all U.S. states and D.C. (Represents denominator for prevalence-based continuum)	• Diagnosis-based care continuum
Diagnosed with HIV infection	• Number of people living with HIV and have been diagnosed Calculated as part of the prevalence estimate	• NHSS data used to calculate number of people currently diagnosed and living with HIV (Represents denominator for diagnosis-based continuum)
Linked to care	• Percentage of people diagnosed with HIV in a given calendar year Had one or more recorded viral load or CD4+ test within 3 months of diagnosis Utilizes NHSS data from states and D.C. that encompasses full laboratory reporting Use of different denominator (one calendar year) therefore not comparable to the calculation of other stages on the continuum; presented differently on the care continuum	
Engaged or retained in care	• MMP data used; calculation of percentage of people living with HIV who attended at least one HIV medical care visit in the observed year of the survey's sampling period NHSS data from the states and D.C. that encompass full laboratory reporting used to estimate those "in care" calculated as the percentage of persons diagnosed who had at least one documented viral load or CD4+ test within the observed year, and "retained in care" calculated as persons diagnosed who had two or more documented viral load or CD4+ tests performed at least 3 months apart in the observed year	
Prescribed ART	• MMP data used; estimation of number and percentage of people receiving medical care Have documented ART prescription in their medical records in the observed year	
Viral suppression	MMP or NHSS data from the states and D.C. encompassing full laboratory reporting Used to estimate percentage of persons with most recent viral load, less than 200 copies/mL in the observed year	

Data from CDC. (2014). Understanding the HIV care continuum. Retrieved from https://www.cdc.gov/hiv/pdf/dhap_continuum.pdf

how to best implement them with appropriate resource allocation.

CDC's Policies Toward Improving Stages of the HIV Care Continuum

- Direct funding of health departments and community-based organizations (CBOs)—intended to support communities with the greatest encumbrance of HIV to subsidize more testing, linkage to care, uptake, and adherence/compliance with the prescribed treatment within community settings.

- Technical assistance to enable states and CBOs to develop appropriate tools and interventions for HIV prevention and purposefully tailored HIV care continuum designed to meet the needs of the particular community.

- Authorized and advocated use of surveillance data to identify persons out of care, and to relink and reengage them in the HIV care continuum.

- Endorsement and support of ongoing research and development of evidence-based behavioral studies and organizational interventions to encourage HIV-infected persons to persevere with their care and medications.

- Recommendation of guidelines for healthcare providers on service provision including HIV testing, care, treatment, and prevention.

- Instituting educational campaigns advocating integration of simple prevention principles and practices into routine care for persons living with HIV infection. (CDC, 2014b)

For more information on the U.S. exemplar of HIV policy on care continuum and prevention, see CDC (2014a, 2016b).

HIV/AIDS: Implications of the Burden—WHO and Affiliated Nations

HIV/AIDS is a pandemic with social, cultural and, economic implications. Therefore, the World Health Organization and various national HIV/AIDS programs have drawn up documents on policy, guidelines and regulations on the governance of HIV/AIDS across countries. The overarching objective of these national policies on HIV/AIDS is to provide a framework for leadership and coordination of a national multisectoral response to the HIV/AIDS pandemic. This includes formulation, by all sectors, of appropriate interventions that will effectively prevent the transmission of HIV/AIDS and other sexually transmitted infections, protect and support vulnerable groups, and mitigate the social and economic impact of HIV/AIDS. Provision is also made for a framework for strengthening the capacity of institutions, communities, and individuals in all sectors to arrest the spread of the pandemic.

It remains imperative that the prevention and control of the HIV/AIDS epidemic continue to depend on effective community-based prevention, care, and support interventions. Hence, local government councils are pivotal for involving and coordinating public and private sectors, non-governmental organizations (NGOs), and faith groups in planning and implementing HIV interventions, particularly community-based interventions. This approach is essential for preventing further HIV/AIDS transmission through blood and blood product safety, promotion of safer sex practices (including monogamy, abstinence, non-penetrative sex, and consistent condom use), early and effective treatment of STIs in health facilities that target high-risk groups, and early diagnosis of HIV infection through voluntary testing and counseling. Pre-test and post-test counseling may encourage those who are HIV-negative to avoid high-risk behaviors and encourage HIV-positive patients to receive treatment and avoid virus transmission.

In many developing countries, governments collaborate with donor agencies to provide leadership in assuring availability of antiretroviral medications and medications for opportunistic infection treatment. Governments should be at the forefront of fund-raising activities, budgeting, and mobilizing resources for HIV/AIDS management. Strong and sustained political commitment, leadership, and accountability at all levels are necessary for national HIV/AIDS programs. Additionally, many countries have enacted laws to address legal and ethical HIV/AIDS-related issues and to establish a multisector response to HIV/AIDS management. Policy makers and governments in resource-limited countries have tough decisions to make in the coming years, namely ensuring that patients living HIV/AIDS are provided with an expanded repertoire of ARV sufficient to meet the needs of growing numbers of ART-naïve as well as ART-experienced patients failing therapy.

Conclusion

That ART has reduced morbidity and mortality from HIV infection cannot be overemphasized. This intervention has made HIV a manageable chronic infectious disease for which, although there is no cure at present, patients on ART are expected to have a near-normal life expectancy. In sub-Saharan Africa, ART roll-out has been phenomenal and is administered using a limited repertoire of ARV drugs. As these programs mature, more patients will require second- or third-line medications—which at the moment are expensive and not accessible to the majority of patients who might need them. The hope is that in the coming years the cost of ARVs and the means of monitoring treatment response—namely, viral loads—will continue to decline, giving more patients access to these life-saving medications and the most sensitive means of determining treatment efficacy in resource-constrained settings.

• • • **REFERENCES**

Antinori, A., Zaccarelli, M., Cingolani, A., Forbici, F., Rizzo, M. G., Trotta, M. P., ... Perno, C. F. (2002). Cross-resistance among non-nucleoside reverse transcriptase inhibitors limits recycling efavirenz after nevirapine failure. *AIDS Research and Human Retroviruses, 18*(12), 835–838.

Arasteh, K., Rieger, A., Yeni, P., Pozniak, A., Boogaerts, G., van Heeswijk, R., et al. (2009). Short-term randomised proof-of-principle trial of TMC278 in patients with HIV type-1 who have previously failed antiretroviral therapy. *Antiviral Therapy, 14*(5), 713–722.

Arendt, G., de Nocker, D., von Giesen, H. J., & Nolting, T. (2007). Neuropsychiatric side effects of efavirenz therapy. *Expert Opinion on Drug Safety, 6*(2), 147–154.

Arribas, J. R., Pozniak, A. L., Gallant, J. E., DeJesus E., Gazzard, B., Campo, R. E., ... Cheng, A. K. (2008). Tenofovir disoproxil fumarate, emtricitabine, and efavirenz compared with Zidovudine/Lamivudine and efavirenz in treatment-naïve patients: 144-week analysis. *JAIDS, 47*, 74–78.

Back, D., Gatti, G., Fletcher, C., Garaffo, R., Haubrich, R., Hoetelmans, R., Kurowski, M., Luber, A., Merry, C., Perno, C. F. (2002). Therapeutic drug monitoring in HIV infection: current status and future directions. *AIDS, 16* (Suppl 1): S5–37.

Baeten, J. M., Strick, L. B., Lucchetti, A., Whittington, W. A., Sanchez, J., Coombs, R. W., ... Celum, C. (2008). Herpes simplex virus suppression therapy decreases plasma and genital HIV-1 levels in HSV-2/HIV-1 Co-infected women: a randomised, placebo-controlled, cross-over trial. *The Journal of Infectious Diseases, 198*(12), 1804–1808.

Barre-Sinoussi, F., Chermann, J. C., Rey, F., Nugeyre, M. T., Chamaret, S., Gruest, J., ... Montagnier, L. (1983). Isolation of a T-lymphotropic retrovirus from a patient at risk for acquired immune deficiency syndrome (AIDS). *Science, 220*(4599), 868–871.

Bersoff-Matcha, S. J., Miller, W. C., Aberg, J. A., van Der Horst, C., Hamrick, Jr, H. J., Powderly, W. G. & Mundy, L. M. (2001) Sex differences in nevirapine rash. *Clinical Infectious Diseases, 32*(1): 124–129.

Bolhaar, M. G., & Karstaedt, A. S. (2007). A high incidence of lactic acidosis and symptomatic hyperlactatemia in women receiving highly active antiretroviral therapy in Soweto, South Africa. *Clinical Infectious Diseases, 45*(2), 254-260.

British HIV Association (BHIVA). (2012). *BHIVA guidelines for the treatment of HIV-1 positive adults with antiretroviral therapy 2012. Retrieved from* www.bhiva.org/HIV-1-treatment-guidelines.aspx

Carré, N., Deveau, C., Belanger, F., Boufassa, F., Persoz, A., Jadand, C., ... Bucquet, D. (1994). Effect of age and exposure group on the onset of AIDS in heterosexual and homosexual HIV-infected patients. SEROCO Study Group. *AIDS, 8*(6), 797–802.

Centers for Disease Control and Prevention (CDC). (1992). 1993 revised classification system for HIV infection and expanded surveillance case definition for AIDS among adolescents and adults. *MMWR, Recommendations and Reports, 41*,1–19.

Centers for Disease Control and Prevention (2014a). Understanding the HIV Care Continuum National Center for HIV AIDS, Viral Hepatitis, STD, and TB Prevention Division of HIV/AIDS Prevention.

Centers for Disease Control and Prevention. (2014b). Vital signs: HIV diagnosis, care, and treatment among persons living with HIV. United States 2011. *MMWR (CDC). 63*(47), 1113–1117.

Centers for Disease Control and Prevention (2015a). HIV PREVENTION IN THE UNITED STATES: New Opportunities, New Expectations. Centers for Disease Control and Prevention. National Center for HIV/AIDS, Viral Hepatitis, STD, and TB Prevention. Division of HIV/AIDS Prevention.

Centers for Disease Control and Prevention (CDC). (2015b). *HIV Surveillance Report, 2014;* Vol. 26. http://www.cdc.gov/hiv/library/reports/surveillance/. Published November 2015. (Accessed August 19, 2017)

Centers for Disease Control and Prevention (CDC). (2015c). Prevalence of diagnosed and undiagnosed HIV infection – United States, 2008-2012. *CDC MMR Weekly, 64*(24), 657–662. Retrieved from http://stacks.cdc.gov/view/cdc/31699

Centers for Disease Control and Prevention (CDC). (2016a) *CDC fact sheet: Today's HIV/AIDS epidemic. Retrieved from* https://www.cdc.gov/nchhstp/newsroom/docs/factsheets/today-sepidemic-508.pdf

Centers for Disease Control and Prevention. (2016b). *Today's HIV/AIDS epidemic.* Retrieved from https://npin.cdc.gov/publication/todays-hivaids-epidemic.

Clavel, F., Guétard, D., Brun-Vézinet, F., Chamaret, S., Rey, M. A., Santos-Ferreira, M. O., ... Rouzioux, C. (1986). Isolation of a new human retrovirus from West African patients with AIDS. *Science, 233*(4761), 343–346.

Claxton, A. J., Cramer, J., & Pierce, C. (2001). A systematic review of the associations between dose regimens and medication compliance. *Clinical Therapeutics, 23*,1296–1310.

Clouse, K., Pettifor, A., Maskew, M., Bassett, J., Van Rie, A., Gay, C., ... Fox, M. P. (2013). Initiating ART when presenting with higher CD4 counts results in reduced loss to follow-up in a resource-limited setting *AIDS, 27*(4), 645–650.

Coates, T. J., & Collins, C. (1998). Preventing HIV infection. *Scientific American, 279*(1), 96–87.

Cohen, M. S., Chen, Y. Q., McCauley, M., Gamble, T., Hosseini-pour, M. C., Kumarasamy, N., ... HPTN 052 Study Team. (2011). Prevention of HIV-1 infection with early antiretroviral therapy. *New England Journal of Medicine, 365*, 493–505.

Cohen, S. M., Gray, K. M., Ocfemia, M. C. B., Johnson, A., & Hall, H. I. (2013). The status of the national HIV surveillance system, United States, 2013. *Reports, 129*(4): 335–341.

Cooper, D. A., Heera, J., Goodrich, J., Tawadrous, M., Saag, M., Dejesus, E., ... Mayer, H. (2010). Maraviroc versus efavirenz, both in combination with Zidovudine-lamivudine, for the treatment of antiretroviral-naïve subjects with CCR5-tropic HIV-1 infection. *The Journal of Infectious Diseases, 201*(6), 803–813.

Côté, H. C., Brumme, Z.L., Craib, K. J., Alexander, C. S., Wynhoven, B., Ting L., ... Montaner, J. S. (2002). Changes in mitochondrial DNA as a marker of nucleoside toxicity in HIV-infected patients. *New England Journal of Medicine, 346*(11), 811–820.

d'Arminio Monforte, A., Lepri, A. C., Rezza, G, Pezzotti, P., Antinori, A., Phillips, A. N., ... Moroni, M. (2000). Insights into reasons for discontinuation of the first highly active antiretroviral therapy (HAART) regimen in a cohort of antiretroviral naïve patients. I.CO.N.A. Study Group. Italian Cohort of Antiretroviral-naïve patients. *AIDS, 14(5),* 499–507.

Das, K., Clark, A. D., Lewis, P. J., Heeres, J., de Jonge, M. R., Koymans, L. M. H., ... Arnold, E. (2004). Roles of conformational and position adaptability in structure-based design of TMC 125-R165335 (Etravirine) and related non-nucleoside reverse transcriptase inhibitors that are highly potent and effective against wild-type and drug-resistant HIV-1 variants. *Journal of Medicinal Chemistry, 47,* 2550–2560.

Deeks, S. G. & Phillips, A. N. (2009). HIV infection, antiretroviral treatment, ageing and non-AIDS related morbidity. *BMJ, 338,* a3172.

Department of Health and Human Services. (2012). Recommendations for use of antiretroviral drugs in pregnant HIV-1-infected women for maternal and interventions to reduce perinatal HIV transmission in the United States. Retrieved from https://aidsinfo.nih.gov/guidelines/html/3/perinatal/0

Division of AIDS & NIAID. (2004). *Division of AIDS table for grading severity of adult adverse experiences.* Rockville, MD: National Institute of Allergy and Infect Diseases.

Drumright, L. N., & Colfax, G. N. (2009). HIV risk and prevention for non-injection substance users. In K. H. Mayer & H. F. Pizer (Eds.), *HIV prevention: A comprehensive approach* (pp. 340–375). London, United Kingdom: Academic Press/Elsevier.

Dunne, E. F., Whitehead, S., Sternberg M., Thepamnuay, S., Leelawiwat, W., McNicholl, J. M., et al. (2008). Suppressive Acyclovir therapy reduces HIV cervicovaginal shedding in HIV- and HSV-2-infected women, Chiang Rai, Thailand. *JAIDS, 49(1),* 77–83.

El-Sadr, W. M., Lundgren, J., Neaton, J. D., Gordin, F., Abrams, D., Arduino, R. C., ... Rappoport, C. (2006). CD4+ count–guided interruption of antiretroviral treatment. *New England Journal of Medicine, 355,* 2283–2296.

Embretson, J., Zupancic, M., Ribas, J. L., Burke, A., Racz, P., Tenner-Racz, K., & Haase, A. T. (1993). Massive covert infection of helper T lymphocytes and macrophages by HIV during the incubations period of AIDS. *Nature, 362(6418),* 359–362.

Emery, S., Neuhaus, J. A., Phillips, A. N., Babiker, A., Cohen, C. J., Gatell, J. M., ... Wood, R. (2008). Major clinical outcomes in antiretroviral therapy (ART)-naïve participants and those not receiving ART at baseline in the SMART study. *The Journal of Infectious Diseases, 197,* 1133–1144.

Enger, C., Graham, N., Peng, N., Chmjel, J. S., Kingsley, L. A., Detels, R. & Munoz, A. (1996). Survival from early, intermediate, and late stages of HIV infection. *JAMA, 275(17),* 1329–1334.

Engsig, F. N., Zangerle, R., Katsarou, O., Dabis, F., Reiss, P., Gill, J., ... Fätkenheuer, G. (2014). Long-term mortality in HIV-positive individuals virally suppressed for >3 years with incomplete CD4 recovery. *Clinical Infectious Diseases, 58(9),* 1312–1321.

Fagard, C., Colin, C., Charpentier, C., Rami, A., Jacomet, C., Yeni, P., ... ANRS 139 TRIO Trial Group. (2012). Long-term efficacy and safety of Raltegravir, Etravirine, and Darunavir/Ritonavir in treatment-experienced patients: weeks 96 results from the ANRS 139 TRIO trial. *JAIDS, 59,* 489–493.

Farzadegan, H., Hoover, D. R., Astemborski, J., Lyles, C. M., Margolick, J. B., Markham, R. B., . . . Vlahov, D. (1998). Sex differences in HIV-1 viral load and progression to AIDS. *Lancet, 352(9139),* 1510–1514.

Feinberg, M. B. (1996). Changing the natural history of HIV disease. *Lancet, 348(9022),* 239–246.

Finzi, D., Hermankova, M., Pierson, T., Carruth, L. M., Buck, C., Chaisson, R. E., ... Siliciano, R. E. (1997). Identification of a reservoir for HIV-1 in patients on highly active antiretroviral therapy. *Science, 278(5341),* 1295–1300.

Friis-Møller, N., Sabin, C. A., Weber, R., d'Arminio Monteforte, A., El-Sadr, W. M., Reiss, P., ... DAD Study Group. (2003). Combination antiretroviral therapy and the risk of myocardial infarction. *New England Journal of Medicine, 349,* 1993–2003. [Erratum in *(2004). New England Journal of Medicine, 350,* 955.

Fuller, C. M., Ford, C., & Rudolf, A. (2009). Injection drug use and HIV: Past and future considerations for HIV prevention and interventions. In K. H. Mayer & H. F. Pizer (Eds.), *HIV prevention: A comprehensive approach* (pp. 305–339). London, United Kingdom: Academic Press/Elsevier.

Gallant, J. E., DeJesus, E., Arribas, J. R., Pozniak, A. L., Gazzard, B., Campo, R. E., ... Study 934 Group. (2006). Tenofovir, D. F., emtricitabine, and efavirenz vs. zidovudine, lamivudine, and efavirenz for HIV. *New England Journal of Medicine, 354(3),* 251–260.

Gürtler, L. (1996). Difficulties and strategies of HIV diagnosis. *Lancet, 348(9021),* 176–179.

Havlir, D. V., Bassett, R., Levitan, D., Gilbert, P., Tebas, P., Collier, A. C., ... Wong, J. K. (2001). Prevalence and predictive value of intermittent viremia with combination HIV therapy. *JAMA, 286(2),* 171–179.

Henrard, D. R., Daar, E., Farzadegan, H., Clark S. J., Phillips, J., Shaw, G. M., & Busch, M. P. (1995). Virologic and immunologic characterisation of symptomatic and asymptomatic primary HIV-1 infection. *JAIDS, 9(3),* 305–310.

Hessol, N. A., Byers, R. H., Lifson, A. R., O'Malley, P. M., Cannon, L., Barnhart, J. L., et al. (1990). Relationship between AIDS latency period and AIDS survival time in homosexual and bisexual men. *JAIDS, 3(11),* 1078–1085.

Hope, T. J., & Trono, D. (2000). Structure, expression, and regulation of the HIV genome. *Cell., 100,* 587–597.

Huang, Y., Paxton, W. A., Wolinsky, S. M., Neuman, A. U., Zhang, L., He, T., ... Koup, R. A. (1996). The role of a mutant CCR5 allele in HIV-1 transmission and disease progression. *Nature Medicine, 2(11),* 1240–1243.

Katlama, C., Haubrich, R., Lalezari, J., Lazzarin, A., Madruga, J. V., Molina, J. M., ... DUET-1, DUET-2 Study Groups. (2009). Efficacy and safety of Etravirine in treatment-experienced, HIV-1 patients: Pooled 48-week analysis of two randomised, controlled trials. *AIDS, 23,* 2289–2300.

Kaufmann, G. R., Perrin, L., Pantaleo, G., Opravil, M., Furrer, H., Telenti, A., ... Swiss HIV Cohort Study Group. (2003). CD4 T-lymphocyte recovery in individuals with advanced HIV-1 infection receiving potent antiretroviral therapy for 4 years: The SWISS HIV Cohort Study. *Archives of Internal Medicine, 163(18),* 2187–2195.

Keet, I. P., Krijnen, P., Koot, M., Lange, J. M., Miedema, F., Goudsmit, J., Coutinho, R. A. (1993). Predictors of rapid progression to AIDS in HIV-1 seroconverters. *AIDS, 7(1),* 51–57.

Keiser, O., Fellay, J., Opravil, M., Hirsch, H. H., Hirschel, B., Bernasconi, E., ... Swiss HIV Cohort Study. (2007). Adverse events to antiretrovirals in the Swiss HIV Cohort Study: Effect on mortality and treatment modification. *Antiviral Therapy, 12*(8), 1157–1164.

La Porte, C. J. L., Back, D. J., Blaschke, T., Boucher, C. A. B., Fletcher, C. V., Flexner, C., ..., & Burger D. M. (2006). Updated guidelines to perform therapeutic drug monitoring for antiretroviral agents. *Antiviral Therapy, 3*, 4–12.

Landovitz, R. J., Angel, J. B., Hoffmann, C., Horst, H., Opravil, M., Long, J., ..., & Fätkenheuer G. (2008). Phase II study of vicriviroc versus efavirenz (both with Zidovudine/Lamivudine) in treatment-naïve subjects with HIV-1 infection. *The Journal of Infectious Diseases, 198*(8), 1113–1132.

Lima, V. D., Reuter, A., Harrigan, P. R., Lourenço, L., William, C., Hull, M., ... Montaner, J. S. G. (2015). Initiation of antiretroviral therapy at high CD4$^+$ cell counts is associated with positive treatment outcomes. *AIDS, 29*(14), 1871–1882.

Lochet, P., Peyriere, H., Lotthe, A., Mauboussin, J. M., Delmas, B., & Reynes, J. (2003). Long-term assessment of neuropsychiatric adverse reactions associated with efavirenz. *HIV Medicine, 4*(1), 62–66.

Lundgren, J. D., Babiker, A. G., Gordin, F., Emery, S., Grund, B., Sharma, S., ... Neaton, J. D. (2015). Initiation of antiretroviral therapy in early asymptomatic HIV infection. *New England Journal of Medicine, 373*(9), 795–807.

Martinez-Picado, J., & Martinez, M. A. (2008). HIV-1 reverse transcriptase inhibitor resistance mutations and fitness: A view from the clinic and ex-vivo. *Virus Research, 134*(1-2), 104–123.

Martinez-Picado, J., Savara, A. V., Sutton, L., & D'Aquila, R. T. (1999). Replicative fitness of protease inhibitor-resistant mutants of human immunodeficiency virus type 1. *Journal of Virology, 73*(5), 3744–3752.

Mellors, J. W., Rinaldo, C. R. Jr, Gupta, P., White, R. M., Todd, J. A., & Kingsley, L. A. (1996). Prognosis in HIV-1 infection predicted by the quantity of virus in plasma. *Science, 272*(5265), 1167–1170.

Mocroft, A., Reiss, P., Gasiorowski, J., Ledergerber, B., Kowalska, J., Chiesi, A., ... EuroSIDA Study Group. (2010). Serious fatal and nonfatal Non-AIDS-defining illnesses in Europe. *JAIDS, 55*, 262–270.

Mocroft, A., Youle ,M., Moore, A., Sabin, C. A., Madge, S., Lepri, A. C., ... Phillips, A. N. (2001). Reasons for modification and discontinuation of antiretrovirals: Results from a single treatment centre. *AIDS, 15*(2),185–194.

Moore, R. D., & Keruly, J. C. (2007). CD4+ cell count 6 years after commencement of highly active antiretroviral in persons with sustained virologic suppression. *Clinical Infectious Diseases, 44*(3), 441–446.

National HIV/AIDS Strategy for the United States. (July 2010) https://www.obamawhitehouse.archives.gov/sites/default/files/uploads/NHAS.pdf

Pantaleo, G. & Fauci, A. S. (1996). Immunopathogenesis of HIV infection. *Annual Review of Microbiology, 50*, 825–854.

Parades, R., Lalama, C. M., Ribaudo, H. J., Schackman, B. R., Shikuma, C., Giguel, F., ... AIDS Clinical Trials Group (ACTG) A5095 Study Team. (2010). Pre-existing minority drug-resistant HIV-1 variants, adherence and risk of antiretroviral treatment failure. *The Journal of Infectious Diseases, 201*(5). 662–671.

Perelson, A. S., Neumann, A. U., Markowitz, M., Leonard, J. M., & Ho, D. D. (1996). HIV-1 dynamics in vivo: virion clearance rate, infected cell life-span, and viral generation time. *Science, 271*(5255), 1582–1586.

Raffi, F., Rachlis, A., Brinson, C., Arasteh, K., Gorgolas, M, Brennan, C., ... Walmsley, S. (2015). Dolutegravir efficacy at 48 weeks in key subgroups of treatment-naïve HIV-infected individuals in three randomized trials. *AIDS, 29*(2), 167–174.

Rawizza, H., Chaplin, B., Meloni, S. T., Eisen, G., Rao, T., Sankale, J. L., ... Kanki, P. J. (2011). Immunologic criteria are poor predictors of virologic outcome: Implications for HIV treatment monitoring in resource-limited settings. *Clinical Infectious Diseases, 53*, 1283–1290.

Reynes, J., Arasteh, K., Clotet, B., Cohen, C., Cooper, D. A., Delfraissy, J. F., ... Saigo, M. P. (2007). TORO: Ninety-six-week virologic and immunologic response and safety evaluation of Enfuvirtide with an optimised background of antiretrovirals. *AIDS Patient Care and STDs, 21*(8), 533–543.

Riddler, S. A., Haubrich, R., DiRienzo, A. G., Peeples, L., Powderly, W. G., Klingman, K. L., ... AIDS Clinical Trials Group Study A5142 Team. (2008). Class-sparing regimens for initial treatment of HIV-1 infection. *New England Journal of Medicine, 358*, 2095–2106.

Sarfo, F. S., Sarfo, M. A., Kasim, A., Phillips, R., Booth, M., & Chadwick, D. (2014). The long-term effectiveness of first-line NNRTI-based antiretroviral therapy in Ghana. *Journal of Antimicrobial Chemotherapy, 69*(1): 254–261.

Sarfo, F. S., Sarfo, M. A., Norman, B., Phillips, R., Bedu-Addo, G., & Chadwick, D. (2014). Risk of deaths, AIDS-defining and Non-AIDS defining events among Ghanaians on long-term combinations antiretroviral therapy. *PLoS One, 9, e10. 9:e10*

Sax, P. E., DeJesus, E., Mills, A., Zolopa, A., Cohen, C., Wohl, D., ... GS-US-236-0102 Study Team. (2012). Co-formulated elvitegravir, cobicistat, emtricitabine, and Tenofovir versus coformulated efavirenz, Emtricitabine, and tenofovir for initial treatment of HIV-1 infection: A randomised, double-blind, phase 3 trial, analysis of results after 48 weeks. *Lancet, 379*(9835), 2439–2448.

Seidlin, M., Vogler, M., Lee, E., Lee, Y. S., & Dubin, N. (1993). Heterosexual transmission of HIV in a cohort of couples in New York City. *AIDS, 7*(9), 1247–1254.

Severe, P., Juste, M. A., Ambroise, A., Eliacin, L., Marchand, C., Apollon, S., ... Fitzgerald, D. W. (2010). Early versus standard antiretroviral therapy for HIV-infected adults in Haiti. *New England Journal of Medicine, 363*, 257–265.

Shimura, K., Kodama, E., Sakagami, Y., Matsuzaki, Y., Watanabe, W., Yamataka, K., ... Matsuoka, M. (2008). Broad antiretroviral activity and resistance rofile of the novel human immunodeficiency virus Integrase inhibitor elvitegravir (JTK-303/GS-9137). *Journal of Virology, 82*(2), 764–774.

Shubber, Z., Calmy, A., Andrieux-Meyer, I., Vitoria, M., Renaud-Thery, F., Shaffer, N., ... Ford, N. (2013). Adverse events associated with nevirapine and efavirenz-based first-line antiretroviral therapy: A systematic review and meta-analysis. *AIDS, 27*, 1403–1412.

Smith, P. F., DiCenzo, R., & Morse, G. D. (2001). Clinical pharmacokinetics of non-nucleoside reverse transcriptase inhibitors. *Clinical Pharmacokinetics, 40*(12), 893–805.

Smith, K. Y., Patel, P., Fine, D., Bellos, N., Sloan, L., Lackey, P., … HEAT Study Team. (2009). Randomised, double-blind, placebo-matched, multicenter trial of abacavir/lamivudine or tenofovir/emtricitabine with lopinavir/ritonavir for initial HIV treatment. *AIDS, 23*(12), 1547–1556.

Steigbigel, R. T., Cooper, D. A., Kumar, P. N., Eron, J. E., Schechter, M., Markowitz, M., … BENCHMARK Study Teams. (2008). Raltegravir with optimised background therapy for resistant HIV-1 infection. *New England Journal of Medicine, 359*(4), 339–354.

Sterne, J. A., May, M., Costagliola, D., de Wolf, F., Phillips, A. N., Harris, R., … Cole, S. R. (2009). Timing of initiation of antiretroviral therapy in AIDS-free HIV-1-infected patients: A collaborative analysis of 18 HIV cohort studies. *Lancet, 373,*1352–1363.

Stevenson, M. (2003). HIV-1 pathogenesis. *Nature Medicine, 9*(7), 853–860.

TEMPRANO ANRS 12136 Study Group. A trial of early antiretrovirals and isoniazid preventive therapy in Africa. *New England Journal of Medicine, 373*(9), 808–822.

UNAIDS. (2013). *UNAIDS global report 2013.* Retrieved from http://www.unaids.org/en/media/unaids/contentassets/documents/epidemiology/2013/gr2013/UNAIDS_Global_Report_2013_en.pdf

Vanhems, P., Lambert, J., Cooper, D. A., Perrin, L., Carr, A., Hirschel, B., et al. (1998). Severity and prognosis of acute human immunodeficiency virus type 1 illness: A dose-response relationship. *Clinical Infectious Diseases, 26*(2), 323–329.

Walmsley, S. L., Antela, A., Clumeck, N., Duiculescu, D., Eberhard, A., Gutierrez, F., … SINGLE Investigators. (2013). Dolutegravir plus abacavir-lamivudine for the treatment of HIV-1 infection. *New England Journal of Medicine, 369*(19),1807–1818.

Wilkin, A., Pozniak, A. L., Morales-Ramorez, J., Lupo, S. H., Santoscopy, M., Grinsztejn, B., … TMC278-C204 Study Group. (2012). Long-term efficacy, safety, and tolerability of rilpivirine (RPV, TMC278) in HIV type 1-infected antiretroviral-naïve patients: Week 192 results from a phase IIb randomised trial. *AIDS Research and Human Retroviruses, 28*(5), 437–446.

Wong, K. H., Chan, K. C., Cheng, K. L., Chan, W. K., Kam, K. M., & Lees, S. S. (2007). Establishing CD4 thresholds for highly active antiretroviral therapy initiation in a cohort of HIV-infected adult Chinese in Hong Kong. *AIDS Patient Care and STDs, 21,* 106–115.

World Health Organization (WHO). (2010). Antiretroviral therapy for HIV infection in adults and adolescents, recommendations for a public health approach 2010 revision. Retrieved from http://www.who.int/hiv/pub/arv/adult2010/en/

Young, J., Psichogiou, M., Meyer, L., Ayayi, S., Grabar, S., Raffi F., Bucher, H. (2012). CD4 cell count and the risk of AIDS or death in HIV-infected adults on combination antiretroviral therapy with a suppressed viral load: A longitudinal cohort study from COHERE. *PLoS Med, 9*(3), e1001194.

Zukerman, R. A., Lucchetti, A., Whittington, W. L., Sanchez, J., Coombs, R. W., Zuñiga, R., … Celum, C. (2007).Herpes simplex virus (HSV) suppression with valacyclovir reduces rectal and blood plasma HIV-1 levels in HIV-1/HSV-2-seropositive men: A randomised, double-blind, placebo-controlled cross-over trial. *The Journal of Infectious Diseases, 196*(10), 1500–1508.

● ● ● **SUGGESTED FURTHER READING**

AIDS*info. Guidelines for the use of antiretroviral agents in HIV-1-infected adults and adolescents. Retrieved from* https://aidsinfo.nih.gov/guidelines/html/1/adults-and-adolecent-arv/0

CHAPTER

8

Contraception in a Changing World

ELIZABETH D. KENNEDY

Introduction

The terms *contraception, family planning*, and *birth control* are used interchangeably worldwide when referring to the intentional prevention of conception/pregnancy through the use of various devices, agents, drugs, sexual practices, or surgical procedures. These concepts refer to any of the following:

- Intentional prevention of sperm from reaching the ovum
- Inhibiting ovulation deliberately
- Intentional prevention of fertilization of an ovum or implantation of a fertilized ovum
- Intentionally destroying/killing sperm
- Intentional prevention of the sperm from entering the seminal fluid
- Deliberately preventing conception by using natural methods of sexual practices to achieve family planning/birth control

Family planning services should be easily accessible to all sexually active people, which includes being locally available and culturally acceptable to the relevant community and population. Contraception/family planning helps to safeguard the well-being and autonomy of women, enabling them to support the health and development of their communities.

Family planning care and provision includes support, referral to a sexual reproductive health counselor, encouragement to make informed decisions, and referral to a specialist clinician for methods requiring surgical procedures or as otherwise needed.

Evidence suggests that women who have more than four children have an increased risk of maternal mortality (Parnell, 1989; Zimicki, 1989). Family planning enables women to limit the size of their families if they wish to do so, and prevent unintended pregnancies of older women, who experience increased risk for developing pregnancy-related and other health problems. Moreover, accessible contraceptive services help delay pregnancies in adolescents and young girls who are at increased risk of health problems and death from early child bearing.

This chapter explores the different methods of contraception and uses case study scenarios to showcase clinician–patient interactions.

Brief Overview of the Unmet Need for Contraception/Family Planning

An estimated 225 million women in developing countries may wish to prevent conception but are not using any methods of contraception (World Health Organization [WHO], 2015). Yet, contraception use and family planning can strengthen a woman's right to determine how many children she wants to have and to space her pregnancies. Contraception and family planning also reduce the overall need for abortions, and specifically the complications associated with unsafe methods of abortion. Finally, family planning and contraception use reduces the overall incidence of maternal and infant deaths (Chola, McGee, Tugendhaft, Buchmann, & Hofman, 2015; Stover & Ross, 2010; see also **Box 8-1**, which explains the advantages of contraception usage).

BOX 8-1 Advantages of Contraception Use/Family Planning

- Preventing pregnancy-related health risks
- Reducing infant mortality from closely spaced and ill-timed pregnancies and births
- Helping prevent transmission of HIV and other STIs
- Reducing risk of unintended pregnancies among women living with HIV, leading to fewer infected children and orphans
- Empowering people and enhancing education to enable them to make informed choices about their sexual and reproductive health
- Family planning presents opportunities for women to pursue their education or paid employment
- Reducing adolescent pregnancies and related consequences: preterm, low birthweight, neonatal mortality
- Family planning helps unsustainable population growth with negative impact on economy and the environment

---

BOX 8-2 Reasons for Neglect of Contraception Use and Unmet Need for Family Planning

- Limited choice of methods
- Limited access to contraception particularly among young people, poorer population subgroups, and unmarried people
- Fear of potential side effects
- Cultural and religious opposition
- Poor quality of available services
- User and provider bias
- Gender-based barriers (WHO, 2015)

Reproduced from WHO. (2017). Family planning/contraception. Fact sheet no. 351. Retrieved from http://www.who.int/mediacentre/factsheets/fs351/en/

Although contraceptive use continues to increase in various parts of the world, such as Asia and Latin America, use is still relatively low in sub-Saharan Africa. Globally, a slight increase was reported in contraception use from 54–57.4% in 2014. The proportion of women 15–45 years of age who reported using modern methods of contraception in different regions during 2008–2014 showed:

- Africa: 23.6–27.6%
- Asia: 60.9–61.6%
- Latin America and the Caribbean: 66.7–67.0% (WHO, 2015)

The use of contraception by men is reported to be relatively low and the available methods are limited to male condoms and sterilization/vasectomy.

Global Unmet Need for Contraception

The unmet need for contraception remains considerably high and is mainly due to the constantly growing population with a shortage of family planning (FP) services. In Africa, 23.2% of women of reproductive age have an unmet need for modern contraception (Sedgh & Hussain, 2014). In Asia, and in Latin America and the Caribbean, the unmet need is 10.9% and 10.4%, respectively (United Nations Department of Economic and Social Affairs [UNDESA], 2013. **Box 8-2.**)

Sedgh and Hussain (2014) examined the reasons for non-use of contraception despite the unmet need in developing countries, while Bradley, Croft, Fishel, and Westoff's (2012) analytical studies provide additional insights for informed policy choices, as well as the skills and resources required for high-quality demographic and health surveys.

The World Health Organization (WHO) continues to promote developments in family planning services in the following ways:

- Evidence-based guidelines on contraceptive methods
- Developing quality standards
- Providing essential contraceptive commodities with guidance for introducing, adopting, and implementing the tools to meet identified needs
- Developing new methods to increase contraceptive choices for men and women (WHO, 2015)

Contraception, Sex, and Choice

It is important for providers to remember that contraception is a choice, and this choice lies with the patient. The provider's job is to explain the options available so that the patient has full knowledge of what she can obtain, where she can obtain it, how effective it will be, how she will use it, and what effects it might have on her body.

Obtaining contraception is difficult for some patients. To ask for contraception, a patient needs to recognize herself as a sexually active mature woman. This can be challenging for younger women, particularly when society and the media present sexual activity as exciting and adult, concentrating on the glamorous aspects such as romance, fun, love, trust, and hope. These emotions are exciting and exhilarating. Who needs to think about the boring, tedious facts about contraception and relationships when you are being loved and cherished so much? Who wants to think about pregnancy, termination, and infection when sex is so wonderful?

Young people may get bored by constant exhortations to use condoms and other contraception to prevent sexually transmitted infections (STIs) and pregnancy. Adolescents, in particular, feel immune to consequences and engage in risky behavior. They are often ill-prepared to deal with the potential outcomes of STI acquisition or pregnancy. Globally, sex is used to manipulate human beings. It is a currency in the case of prostitution; a commodity in media and advertising; a profitable product in the porn industry; a form of power and domination in abusive relationships; and a weapon of war when mass rapes occur.

In the United Kingdom, and most first world countries, people can access contraception easily and in some cases it is provided free of charge. In these countries, patients are educated about contraception and can access it if they so choose, allowing them to make positive choices about reproduction. Unfortunately, in other parts of the world, contraception is not available and women are not so empowered to access it. There may be no nearby clinics, or women may lack education, money, or employment to gain independence. There may be a cultural imperative to have children no matter what the cost to the woman.

This chapter started by stating that contraception is a choice, but choice means different things to different people in different parts of the world and at different stages of their lives. Health professionals must treat every case individually and "walk with the patient" to find out what is best suited to her life.

Planning Contraceptive and Sexual Health Services

Within each district there should be a system for planning and organizing sexual healthcare services with consultation from health authorities, community partnerships, and religious groups. Service provision should be a joint effort with community and hospital specialist services, obstetric and gynecological services, public health centers, nursing and other health-related schools, voluntary agencies, and retail outlets. Services should be located near population centers, schools, and public transportation routes. These services should be open at convenient times and accessible to everyone. The target population is everyone who is sexually active, who is considering engaging in sexual activity, or who has been sexually active in the past. However, special efforts should be made to attract young people, minorities, and vulnerable groups such as the homeless, drug and alcohol users, learning disability patients, patients with mental health problems, and sex workers.

Good access to a clinic is an essential part of contraceptive uptake and includes extended hours with weekend or evening hours, good transportation access, and drop-in services that people can access without appointments. If there is an appointment system, ensure it is linked so that the patient needs only to phone one number to get an appointment. Web-based appointment systems are available in some areas, through which patients can email or text for their appointments. If you do have an appointment system, try

to ensure a low "Did Not Attend" rate by texting reminders to patients prior to the appointment time. Consider specialized clinics for subgroups such as young people, psychosexual patients, menopausal women, and patients with learning difficulties. Clinic and surgery times can be advertised by posters and leaflets and in phone directories, newspapers and libraries. Websites and sexual health applications for smart phones can also be brought into service. It is useful to link with as many organizations as possible so that people can be signposted to services that they require. Therefore, connecting with and having information about pharmacies and school nursing services is important.

As with many health services, it is important to maximize capacity by improving and modernizing. This may mean increasing the nursing role in clinics, reducing unnecessary follow up, shorter consultation times, targeting clients following risk assessments, and focusing on specific client groups. If possible, there should be choice of clinic/surgery and access times, choice of staff, and of course, full choice of contraception. In the United Kingdom, over 59% of women access their general practitioner (GP) for contraception. Retail services such as pharmacies are used by 41% of men to access condoms. However, 21% of women and 45% of men who are sexually active report no use of any service (French et al., 2009).

When contraceptive care is provided through the patient's primary provider, the practitioner has the opportunity ask about smoking, alcohol, and domestic abuse; check on weight, diet, and the possibility of eating disorders; check on the individual's current place of residence and circumstances regarding housing, boarding, and lodging, or shelter; check on cervical smear status; and advise about the availability of emergency contraception. Services can be improved by the active participation of patients through focus groups, open clinic days, patient interviews, patient satisfaction surveys, and the use of volunteers in the department.

Within groups of targeted patients, it is often useful to have specific clinics:

- **Learning disability:** The use of specialized nurses who work with clients who have learning disabilities is very comforting to the patients. Confidentiality should be maintained, but it is important to interact with parents, carers, and guardians. Care must be taken to use patient-education materials that are easily understood.

- **Young people:** They should be involved in the organization of the clinic, making sure the services are open at appropriate times, that staff are young-people friendly and non-judgemental, clinics are easy to access, and that a walk-in option is offered. It is useful to partner with other community groups that work with young people.

- **Minorities:** It is important to take cultural issues into account. Patients from some cultures and religions do not feel comfortable with certain types of contraception or with irregular bleeding patterns. It is important to have access to patient information in their own language and to have interpreters available who are not members of their own families. Females should have access to a female healthcare professional.

- **Homeless:** One difficulty in working with the homeless population is that sexual health is not seen as a priority. The homeless often have more pressing needs, such as food, shelter, and safety. Alcohol and drug use are common issues in this client group and need to be treated sensitively by appropriate health workers. If patients do not have a home, then they cannot keep supplies of contraception easily and do not receive appointment reminders for the clinics. Certain types of contraception—mainly long-acting, reversible contraception (LARC) methods such as IUDs, IUSs, or implants—can be more useful.

- **Sex workers:** It is important to build up trust with sex workers, as this is a particularly vulnerable group. Patients may struggle with drug or alcohol problems as well as violent and abusive relationships. Patient safety is important. Sex workers cannot work when they bleed, so it is important to have an awareness of contraception which will suit.

Training

Training is a very important aspect of sexual and reproductive healthcare (SRH) services. Both theoretical and practical training are provided for health professionals. Other professionals who may have an interest in sexual and reproductive health such as school nurses, physiotherapists, pharmacists, teachers, social workers, youth workers, and addiction specialists can be offered training in conjunction with health promotion. All reception staff should be specifically trained in dealing sensitively with requests and in being nonjudgmental.

The Contraceptive Consultation

The contraceptive consultation is very different from that in many other areas of medical care in that the provider does not seek out what the patient feels is wrong with her, yet does need to determine what the patient wants. It is best to use an informal approach with a patient focus. Some practitioners may need to include presenting complaint and history of presenting complaint in patient notes.

A good contraceptive consultation will involve greeting the patient in an open and friendly way, for the provider to introduce themselves and wear a name badge if appropriate. The provider should always smile and remember that the patient has chosen to come to the clinic and that this interaction can make a huge difference to the way she feels about herself and about her sexual behavior. Providers should try to have an open approach to the patient's thoughts and feelings, which can be reflected in a variety of ways, including the support staff, waiting room set up, the way patients are called to the consultation room, and

the way providers position themselves in the consultation room (Clutterbuck, 2005).

Contraceptive clinic staff, or those who deal with contraception, should be trained in confidentiality, of course, but above all they must be pleasant, friendly, and polite to the patient. This may sound obvious, but in many areas of health, the patient is looked upon as a distraction to the real work of training, research, or management. Once again, go back to the premise that contraception is a choice.

The waiting room should be clean and non-intimidating. Try not to have the chairs in rows, but group them around tables. Have up-to-date information on the walls and make sure it is targeted at all patients, not just one group (Guillebaud, 2012). The way the patient is called also contributes to the atmosphere. If possible, the provider should collect the patient from the waiting room, introduce themselves as they walk back to the consulting room, and treat the patient as an equal. Providers should always be respectful and polite (even if the patient is not) and remember that it is unprofessional to reflect personal feelings when with a patient.

Once the patient is in the consulting room, the provider should situate themselves at a 90° angle from the patient rather than positioning a desk between them (Glasier & Gebbie, 2008). If the patient has brought anyone in with her, the provider should establish who it is and ask the patient if she wants the person present throughout the consultation and/or examination, as personal questions must be asked. If there is a trainee present, the provider should ensure the patient is aware of who it is, what their role is, and allow the patient the choice and courtesy of refusing to have an extra person listening to or running the consultation. This should be done prior to the trainee entering the room, as it is more difficult for patients to say "no" when the trainee is present.

Accompanying Persons

If the patient brings a young child, it may be due to logistical problems with babysitters, but may also be a strategy to avoid staying too long or getting too involved with the discussion. A young child can be distracting. If the provider senses there is more that the patient wishes to discuss, he/she should arrange for the patient to come back without the child.

If a husband or partner asks to be present during the consultation, it may be because both parties wish to find out about contraception. However, providers must be aware of signs of control or underlying irritation or anger. The provider can always ask the extra person to leave by saying that there are some things that must be discussed privately or suggesting that an examination is needed and it would be best for the other person to wait in the waiting room.

If the patient is an adolescent or young woman, her mother or, more rarely, her father may come in to the consultation. Again, providers must be aware that the consultation may not be entirely truthful and should ask the other party to leave if they sense there is any concealment of answers. This is particularly relevant if the father or father figure is the person accompanying the patient.

Some young people like to bring their friends in to the consultation—again, this may be supportive and gives the patient some courage—but some young people can be bullied and coerced, so patients should always be seen alone, at least for part of the consultation. Providers can simply state that this is normal practice. These nuances in the consultation are sometimes difficult to pick up, but the easiest way to learn these skills is for practitioners to listen to a more experienced practitioner consult and then request that practitioner sit in and "review" an initial consultation.

Language

If the patient and provider speak different languages, then a holistic "choice" consultation is much more difficult. Interpreters should be available via a language line or a similar system. These services may need to be booked in advance, so the patient may need to make another appointment. It is extremely difficult to have a friend or family member acting as interpreter in contraceptive consultations when some of the questions will be about menstruation and sex. If there is an interpreter in the room with the patient, the interpreter must be comfortable with the questions and should not already know the patient personally. This can occur in smaller geographic locations.

Even if the patient and provider speak the same language, contraceptive consultations may be difficult, as the health practitioner may use different words for the anatomy and sex practices. It is important to check from time to time to see if the patient understands what is meant and to change the language to a less formal version if needed. Again, this should be done without undermining the patient or embarrassing the provider. It is a good idea for the provider to ask the patient to explain back what she understands.

How to Take a Contraceptive History

Once the patient is in the room, the provider should introduce her/himself again and ask, "How can I help you today?" or "What can I do to help you?" The provider needs to let the patient explain in her own words why she has come and give the patient their full attention without looking through notes or fiddling with computer settings. Doing so is disrespectful to the patient.

Once it is clear what the patient wants to talk about, the provider can be more directive in the way they collect information. Each provider has their own way of collecting a history. What follows are some suggestions for what to say to a patient:

- "You are here to see about birth control pills [implant, coil, etc.], but can I ask you some basic questions first?"
- "Are you a healthy person, or do you go to your own doctor a lot?"

Then, the provider should ask specifically about migraines with aura, cardiovascular disease (heart disease and stroke), liver problems, diabetes, epilepsy, venous thromboembolism (blood clots), hyperlipidemia, and breast cancer: "Are you on any tablets/inhalers/creams that are prescribed by your doctor or that you buy regularly from the pharmacy?"

Then ask specifically about any herbal remedies, especially St. John's Wort, and about allergies: "Are you allergic to anything?" Rarely, people are allergic to lactose, more commonly latex.

- "Now can I ask a bit about your sexual history?"

It is important to find out here about whether the patient has a partner, is at risk of sexually transmitted infections, and when they last had sexual intercourse. Useful questions may be:

- "Do you have a partner just now?"
- "How long have you been with him (or her)?"
- "When did you last have sex?"
- "What are you using just now for contraception?"

It is also imperative to ask in this section:

- "Have you ever had any problems having sex?"
- "Is having sex sore?"
- "Is it difficult for you to have sex?"
- "Have you ever been forced into something you did not want to do?"

Asking these questions can bring out any concerns about pain with sex—dyspareunia, vaginismus, non-consummation, and erectile problems. It can also open the door for discussion about abuse, assault, and gender-based violence. This might not mean the patient wishes to discuss any of these issues today but can give them the chance of returning to discuss then in the future because the provider has opened the consultation up and given them the "permission" to seek further help.

- "Can I just check if you are a smoker?"
- "Do you have any worries about the amount of alcohol you drink?"
- "Have you ever taken any drugs?"

The last question can be opened out—most people will recognize this is asking about illegal drug taking. If there are any concerns about drug use, then a bloodborne virus history and risk assessment should be taken.

- "Now can I check when your last period was?"
- "Was this a normal period?"

The timing of periods and type of menstruation is very important in taking a contraceptive history. It is necessary to rule out pregnancy and to help with choice of contraception. For example, if a woman says her periods are heavy and/or painful, then it is good to consider contraception that would give the gynecological benefit of shortening or lightening her periods or, in fact, cause amenorrhea.

- "Have you had any pregnancies?"
- "Any miscarriages or terminations?"

During this part of the history the provider can find out when her pregnancies were, how she was delivered, and how she feels about being pregnant again. It can also be a way of checking her reaction to a termination—even if this was many years in the past.

- "Are you up to date with your Pap smears?"

The schedule for cervical smear will likely be different depending in the country in which the provider practices. Information about when the patient had her last smear test can be found on some computer systems or by getting in touch with the patient's primary care provider.

- "OK, we are finished with the basic history. Can we now check your blood pressure, your weight, and your height?"

Blood pressure (BP) is necessary as a baseline measurement for a lot of contraceptive methods, and height and weight are vital to check the patient's body mass index (BMI).

There may be many other things that come out during history taking and basic examination that need to be investigated further. The patient may have a chronic disease, be taking medication, she may be a smoker or be overweight. Information on what type of contraception suits a patient who has medical problems or concerns is found in the United Kingdom Medical Eligibility Criteria (Faculty of Sexual and Reproductive Healthcare [FSRH]. 2016), an evidence-based resource available on www.fsrh.org.

Patients may have issues such as mood swings or physical symptoms around their period and it is important to recognize premenstrual syndrome (PMS) and to be informed and treat it professionally. Many women will have come to expect that their symptoms due to their period are something they must put up with or indeed, have not been taken seriously by other practitioners when they presented with symptoms.

As mentioned, the provider may pick up issues with a past termination of pregnancy and should try not to ignore a catch in the voice or the welling up of tears in haste to get the patient through the clinic. Instead, the provider can say, "You seem really upset talking about this; do you want to talk more about it now?" Sometimes the provider may be the first practitioner who has ever asked or wanted to know about the patient's distress. This is important, as unresolved and unrecognized feelings have a huge impact on the patient's interpretation of her future sexual life and their use of contraception.

After the relevant information is obtained, it is time to talk about choice of contraception (Box 8-3).

All these methods have benefits, side effects, and risks. In a good contraceptive consultation, the patient should be

---

BOX 8-3 Types of Contraception

1. Irreversible and very effective: Sterilization—male and female
2. Reversible, long-acting, and very effective: Injectable, implant, IUD, and IUS
3. Reversible, short-acting, and effective: Combined hormonal contraception—pill, patch, and ring; progestogen-only pill
4. Reversible, short-acting, and efficacy dependent on user: Condoms—male and female; diaphragms and caps; fertility awareness; coitus interruptus
5. Emergency contraception

---

encouraged to explain what she needs, and then the "best fit" contraceptive should be offered. All methods of contraception have extensive literature and evidence-based information available. The best and most up-to-date information is on various websites, including those of the Centers for Disease Control and Prevention (CDC), WHO, American Congress of Obstetricians and Gynecologists (ACOG), U.S. Department of Health and Human Services (DHHS), and the National Health Service (NHS) of the United Kingdom.

Counseling for Contraception

"I don't really know what to do."

There are a few patients who are not sure of the type of contraception they wish to use and it is important to have an open discussion with them. To help them decide a good starter question is "How would you feel about becoming pregnant?" If the answer is "It would be a disaster," then the barrier methods and fertility awareness would be best avoided, as these have the highest failure rates if not used properly.

The practitioners should then enquire, "Are you good at remembering to take pills? Do you think you would be quite forgetful?" Again, if the answer is, "I would probably forget to take pills," then perhaps look at the long-acting reversible types of contraception.

Another good question is, "How do you feel about hormones?" Some women prefer no extraneous hormones as they feel this causes mood swings, bloating, headaches, and other problems. Many patients have tried several types of contraception in the past and have not felt comfortable with any type due to side effects. The practitioner should try to find out a bit more about these beliefs, as the availability of a hormone method gives more choice. However, if that is not an option, intrauterine devices (IUD), condoms, female condoms, fertility awareness, sterilization, and diaphragms should be discussed.

Always remember to include information about condoms and emergency contraception.

The following is a case study reflecting the author's experience with a patient seeking contraception options.

Case Study 8-1

Ms. A, 26 years old with one previous unsuccessful pregnancy, attended an integrated sexual and reproductive health (SRH) clinic. She is on a progestogen-only pill (POP), Micronor®. She gives a history of two episodes of severe abdominal pain since she started on this pill 6 months ago. One episode occurred following 2 months of amenorrhea and the other occurred quite recently during sex. She is worried about this as she had an ectopic pregnancy in the past and was hospitalized. She has some difficulty remembering to take the POP within its 3-hour window. We discussed her options. Combined hormonal contraception is not appropriate due to her migraines with aura. She does not want the Nexplanon as she has a friend who had this in and had "nothing but trouble with it." This is a common and interesting dilemma when counseling patients, as although what has happened to their friends will not be transferrable automatically to them, it is difficult to put this in a positive light once they believe that one method is "nothing but trouble." She does not want an IUD because she was told when she had her ectopic that she should never use an IUD because they "cause" ectopic pregnancies. This again is a common misconception that if a pregnancy occurs with the IUD in situ then there is a higher chance it will be ectopic due to the anti-fertilization effect of the IUD. However, the chances of getting pregnant at all with an IUD in situ are very low as the effectiveness of IUDs are very high, and you have a greater chance of an ectopic pregnancy if you are not using any contraception. However, these misconceptions are very difficult to shift if a patient has been counseled erroneously in the past and so an IUD—and an IUS—was not acceptable to her. I spent some time explaining that an IUS was completely different to an IUD but her feeling was she did not want "anything inside" her.

She wanted reliable contraception as she had just started a new job and did not want to be pregnant, so condoms alone were not appropriate. She was also not keen on the injection. We therefore discussed using Cerazette. This progestogen-only pill has an anovulatory effect and therefore would help control what I felt were ovarian cysts, and has a 12-hour window which may make it easier for her to remember to take.

Counseling for the Combined Oral Contraceptive Pill

"I want to start 'the pill'"

The practitioner should first be sure that the patient has made a choice and wants to start combined-hormonal

method/progestogen-only pill contraception. She may not know about many different types of contraception and asking to start the pill may simply be a way to find out what is available.

There are two types of contraception pills available—the combined oral contraceptive pill and the progestogen-only pill. There are also currently three methods of taking combined hormonal contraception available in the United States and United Kingdom—the pill, which is taken daily; the patch, which is used weekly; and the ring, which is used monthly.

The following schema might be an appropriate model for counseling a patient to take a combined oral contraceptive.

Tips for Counseling the Patient

1. *This is presented as if the practitioner is talking to the patient.*
   a. The pill is a mixture of two female hormones.
   b. It works by stopping you from producing an egg each month—"You know how each month one of your ovaries produces an egg; it travels down the fallopian tube into the uterus, and if it meets a sperm you get pregnant, and if it doesn't you have your period. The pill kind of puts your ovaries to sleep and stops the eggs from being produced. However, you will still get what seems like a period every month."
   c. You take one pill every day for 3 weeks–21 days—then you take nothing for one week—7 days—then you are back on the next packet of the pill again for the next 3 weeks. Some "pill" packets have 7 placebo or "sugar" pills so that you just keep taking pills each day
   d. It is a very safe drug—about 20 million women have been on it.
   e. It is very effective—about 99.9%.
   f. As well as preventing pregnancy, it will regulate your periods, making them light and very predictable. In some people, it may lessen symptoms of PMS.
   g. It also helps to prevent ovarian and uterine cancer, breast cysts, and pelvic infection.
   h. The pill is a drug and can have some side effects—you may get some headaches, feel a bit sick, have some abdominal bloating, get a bit of breast tenderness or mood swings. However, if you do, any effects pass within 2–3 weeks. If you are still getting side effects after this, it may be that you need a change of pill. Remember, there are about 30 different types of pill, so just because one doesn't suit you, don't give up on them all.
   i. The pill also has some risks; the two main ones are blood clots in the veins of the legs and breast cancer.

Blood Clots—These affect about 10 women in every 10,000. They are more common if you are very overweight, have varicose veins, are immobile, or if it runs in your family.

Breast Cancer—All hormonal methods of contraception can be associated with breast cancer, but will not increase your risk substantially. (I find the easiest way to think about this is to imagine 1,000 women aged 45 in a big room; none of them have ever taken the pill but 10 of them will get breast cancer. Now imagine another room with 1,000 women aged 45 in it. All of them have either been on the pill in the past or are still on it; 11 of these women will get breast cancer.)

j. Now, show a pill packet to the patient.

k. You may start the pill on the first day of your next period. If you start it on that day, it will be effective from that day on, providing you remember to take it regularly. However, you may prefer to start the pill now, use condoms for one week and return for a pregnancy test in 3 weeks.

l. If you want to be protected against any sexually transmitted disease you will have to continue using condoms.

m. Find a time of day to remember to take the pill; morning, lunchtime, or bedtime. Try to stick to that time, as it will be easier to remember if you get into a habit of taking it regularly then. Some women prefer to put a reminder on their mobile phone.

n. Say your next period starts on a Monday (or you are asked to start the pill today, Monday), you start the pill on Monday night, (tonight) then take one on Tuesday, (tomorrow night) then Wednesday, (the next night) and so on, right round the pack and you will finish this pack on Sunday.

o. Then you will have your week off the pill and you will bleed during this week. Perhaps only for a few days—Tues to Fri—then you start your next pill packet the following Monday.

p. If you are using the pill in an extended use pattern, you simply finish the pill packet on Sunday and start the new packet the very next day- in this example, Monday. You will have no period.

q. You always start your new pill packet on the same day of the week.

NB:

   i. Always make sure the patient has written information to confirm what has been said.

   ii. Always ask at the end of the consultation if they have understood and do a quick check of what they are going to do.

   iii. Remind them the pill only works if you take it properly.

   iv. Ask them if they have heard anything about the pill that worries them.

   v. Make sure they know to contact you if there are any problems.

   vi. Give them a time to return for review.

2. The pill does not put weight on you. The pill can make your appetite increase and you can feel hungry, but you can control this and watch what you eat. If you feel continually uncomfortable or bloated on the pill, come back to discuss it further.

3. If bleeding like a period (breakthrough bleeding) does occur, particularly when you are on your first packet, then keep taking the pills. This is a common side effect and usually settles down. (Remember if this symptom continues, check how the patient is taking the pills, note any absorption issues, and remember to check swabs for possible infection and a smear if appropriate).

4. Missed pills.
You can miss one pill in each packet without any worries about contraceptive effectiveness. However, try not to miss any. If you miss more than one pill, please get in touch with the clinic for further advice.

   If you vomit less than 2 hours after you have taken the pill it is best to use condoms for the next 7 days or until the end of the vomiting illness and then for the next 7 days. Diarrhea is not so important unless it is severe.

   Further information about missed combined hormonal contraception is provided in the next section.

5. It is quite safe to have sex during the 7 pill-free days providing you go back onto your next packet when you should.

6. Even if your "period" has not stopped or for any other reason NEVER START YOUR NEXT PACKET LATE. This is because you have been off the active pill for 7 days and the ovaries are beginning to waken up and may produce an egg. If you are worried, then start your next packet at the correct time and contact us for advice.

   If you do not have a bleed during the pill-free week or placebo pill week then start your pill on the day that you normally do and contact us.

7. There is no effect on a pregnancy if the pill is continued inadvertently. There is a 2% fetal abnormality rate in all pregnancies and being on the pill "by mistake" does not increase that risk.

8. You can continue taking the pill up to age 50 if you are a non-smoker and have no other risk factors such as diabetes or heart disease.

9. You should, however, stop taking the pill at age 35 if you are a smoker.

10. There is no need to "take a break" from the pill. The pill does not "build up in your system"—about a quarter of women who take breaks from the pill end up with unwanted conceptions.

    However, if you do want to take a break that is OK provided we can help find a suitable effective alternative.

11. When you are on the pill we will check periodically to make sure it is still the right choice for you. The main things we check are:

    * BP every year
    * BMI
    * Any change in/new headaches?
    * Any change in personal or family history that may affect the pill.

12. The pill does not affect fertility. It may be a bit delayed when the pill is stopped but there is no long-term effect, and you are as fertile after stopping the pill as you were when you started it—remembering that you will be older when you stop and fertility decreases as you age.

13. Start the pill at 21 days postpartum if you are not breastfeeding. If breastfeeding, other types of contraception may be best.

14. Periods can be postponed by running two or more packets of the active pill together. This is quite safe. Then the normal 7-day break is taken.

15. Using the pill does not delay menopause although it can sometimes mask some of the signs.

16. If the pill is stopped before surgery, make sure you have adequate alternative protection—for example, use Depo-Provera®.

    The pill should be stopped only for major surgery, when the patient is to be on the table for more than 30 minutes, and for any leg surgery.

17. We shall always advise you about stopping smoking when we see you!

18. And we shall ask if you would like condoms.
    All information given orally should be backed up by patient literature. Patient information leaflets are included in all the manufacturers, packets of pills.

Counseling for the Patch

"I want to find out more about the patch."

The patch is a type of combined hormonal contraception and as such, the information to be given to the patient is very similar to that of the pill. The benefits, and risks, efficacy, and side effects are the same.

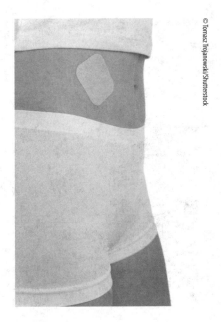

Figure 8-1 Contraceptive Patch

A patient would be advised to start the patch in the same way (presented as if addressing the patient)—If you start between days 1 and 5 of your cycle (day 1 being the first day of bleeding) then you can rely on the patch without needing any extra contraception. Alternatively, you can start it on any day in the cycle provided you are reasonably sure you are not pregnant, use condoms or abstain for 7 days, and check a pregnancy test in 3 weeks if appropriate.

The patch is used in the same cyclical way as the pill. Use a new patch weekly for 3 weeks then have a patch-free week.

The patch can be placed anywhere on the body apart from near breast tissue. You can place it on the skin of the abdomen, back, upper arms or thighs. Try to place it in a position where it is covered with clothing and always put it on a clean, non-greasy area of skin (**Figure 8-1**). It is best to cover the patch for a few seconds with your hand to "seal" the edges. Rotate the patch around various areas on the body to prevent skin irritation.

Will the patch come off? The patch stays on very well whether you are swimming, using a hot tub, or any other activity where you are in water. However, always check the position of patch after drying yourself and do not rub the area too briskly.

Counseling for the Ring

"I want to find out more about the ring."

The ring is also a type of combined hormonal contraception (CHC) and patients should receive information similar to that for the pill or patch. The benefits, risks, efficacy, and side effects are the same.

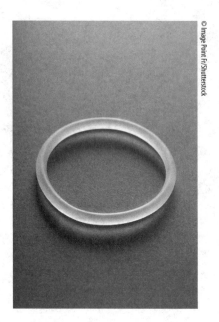

© Image Point Fr/Shutterstock

Figure 8-2 Contraceptive Ring

However, the ring has a smaller total amount of hormone in it compared to the patch or pill and may be suited to women who have had previous hormonal side effects (**Figure 8-2**).

A patient would be advised to start the ring in the same way as any CHC—If you start between days 1 and 5 of your cycle (day 1 being the first day of bleeding) then you can rely on the ring without needing any extra contraception. Alternatively, you can start it on any day in the cycle provided you are reasonably sure you are not pregnant, use condoms or abstain for 7 days, and check a pregnancy test in 3 weeks if appropriate.

The ring is used in the same cyclical way as the pill. Insert a ring into the vagina, leave it there for 3 weeks, and then remove.

How do I use the ring? The ring is made of a very soft flexible material that, when inserted into the vagina, is completely comfortable to use and you are not aware of it. It is held in the vagina by the natural tension of the muscles and does not fall out. One size fits all and it does not have to be fitted by a health professional. If you are comfortable touching your genital area then it is simple to put in, just "fold" it and insert into the vagina like a tampon. It will find its own place to "sit" and does not need to be placed in a particular position. When it is time to remove the ring—after 3 weeks—simply put your index finger into the vagina and hook it out. It cannot get lost inside you.

What if it falls out? This would be really unusual, and you would usually be aware of it. It may come out if you are constipated during a bowel motion but otherwise it is held by the muscles of the pelvis. It is not affected by sex and your partner does not feel it because it is so soft. However, if you wish, it can be removed for sex and replaced afterward. The only time you may bleed with it is on the very first time of use, if you start at the time of your period. Otherwise, it is out of the vagina when you bleed. Occasionally, there is an increase in vaginal discharge while using the ring. This is nothing to worry about.

Minimizing Pregnancy Risk with Missed Combined Hormonal Contraceptives

All CHC inhibit ovulation and maintain anovulation by working on the hypothalamic-pituitary-ovarian axis to reduce luteinizing hormone (LH) and follicle-stimulating hormone (FSH).

Evidence suggests that taking CHC for 7 days prevents ovulation, but further evidence suggests that missing only 4 pills may result in some follicular activity and the possibility of ovulation. Therefore, guidelines for a missed pill or incorrect use of CHC are stricter, and the risk of pregnancy is higher when there are missed pills/incorrect use at the beginning or end of a three-week cycle.

- CHC pill: A missed pill is any pill that has been completely forgotten and more than 24 hours have passed since the pill was due—that is, 48 hours since the last pill was taken. If one pill is missed in that packet then the patient can be reassured and advised to take the forgotten pill as soon as possible, continue the rest of the pills in the packet as normal and no extra precautions or emergency contraception is necessary.

- CHC patch: A patch can remain detached for 48 hours if it has been worn for 7 consecutive days beforehand and no extra or emergency contraception is required.

- CHC ring: If the ring has been used correctly for 7 days, it can be left out of the vagina for 48 hours without any decrease in contraceptive efficacy or need for extra or emergency contraception.

If there are longer time frames without the use of contraception, the following rules should apply:

- CHC pill: If two or more pills have been missed—that is, more than 72 hours since last pill—the patient is advised to take the most recent missed pill as soon as possible, take the remaining pills at the usual time, and use condoms or abstain for 7 days.

- CHC patch: If a patch has been detached more than 48 hours (apart from at the patch-free interval) a new patch should be used and condoms or abstaining should be advised for the next 7 days.

- CHC ring: If a ring has been left out of the vagina for more than 48 hours (apart from at the ring-free interval) a new ring should be inserted and condoms or abstaining should be advised for the next 7 days.

To minimize the risk of pregnancy more effectively, it is necessary to break down the times of missing pills or non-use of patch or ring into weeks one, two, and three of the cycle. Although this is the ideal scenario, bear in mind that patients do not usually know exactly when pills have been missed in the packet. However, the following applies for pills (FSRH, 2012):

- Week 1 (pills 1–7): Advise emergency contraception if unprotected sexual intercourse (UPSI) has taken place. Condoms or abstinence for the next week is advised.

- Week 2 (pills 8–14): There is no indication for emergency contraception providing the pills in the preceding 7 days have been taken correctly and consistently. Condoms or abstinence for the next week is advised.

- Week 3 (pills 15–21): Omit the pill-free interval by finishing the current pack. Start the new pack on the following day. Again, condoms or abstinence for the next week is advised.

For Patches

The patch can be worn for 9 days without affecting contraceptive efficacy. Thereafter, the same advice as the missed pills should be followed—consider emergency contraception if UPSI has taken place and use condoms for the next 7 days.

The patch-free interval can be extended up to 48 hours—a 9-day patch free interval—without affecting the efficacy. Thereafter, the same advice as for the missed pills should be followed according to whether the extension of use occurred in the first, second, or third week. In the first and second week, if the patch has been used for longer than 9 days then use condoms for 7 days until a new patch has been on for this length of time. If the extension of use has been in the third week, then the patch-free week should be omitted, with condom use or abstinence for 7 days.

For Rings

The ring can be worn for 4 weeks without affecting contraceptive efficacy. A ring-free week can then be taken, and condoms or abstinence for 7 days is recommended. Alternatively, a new ring can be inserted immediately and no ring-free week taken. However, condom use or abstinence is advised.

The ring-free interval can be extended by 48 hours before extra contraceptive precautions or emergency contraception is required.

Extended Use of CHC

Traditional cyclical regimens were developed in the 1960s when the contraceptive pill was developed. It was thought that a regular monthly period might be reassuring for women and be considered more natural. However, the bleeding is simply a withdrawal bleed, not an actual period, and there is considerable discussion about whether this is necessary. The stopping and starting of CHC monthly is the major user failure time of the method.

Several CHCs are now available to be used continuously for several months or with a shorter pill-free Jacobson et al. 2012.

The advantages of an extended regimen are that the cycle with bleeding and perhaps side effects, particularly of mood swings, can be abolished. The patient can be advised to take the pill and keep taking it until she experiences some bleeding. She should then stop for 4 or 7 days to let the endometrium settle, then restart. The woman is therefore controlling her own cycle, which is assumed to benefit acceptance and adherence. Women will have different "natural" cycles; some women will be able to take CHC for 9 or 10 months without any breakthrough bleeding, while others will only be able to manage 2 or 3 months. If a woman continues this extended use, the bleeding pattern will eventually settle and bleeding can occur, at the woman's control, two to three times per year. Many women do this already, on their own volition, and it is encouraging to see that it is now accepted practice. It may be difficult at first for some women to believe that this way of taking the CHC is safe and effective. However, during counseling, it might be useful for the provider to explain that until 100–150 years ago most women were often pregnant or breastfeeding for the majority of their reproductive life. This meant that they did not have regular periods. Therefore, regular periods (or interim bleeding) is a product of the 20th century that we have now moved away from.

Case Study 8-2

Ms. B is a 19-year-old woman who presents to the Sexual and Reproductive Health clinic. She is currently taking oral contraceptive pills—ethinyl estradiol and levonorgestrel (Microgynon®ª)—which she obtained from her primary care provider (PCP) 2 years ago. She is good at taking the pill and not forgetful. She complains about her moods, which she feels are worsening over the past year. She also feels she has put on weight and feels bloated in the last year.

I explored other areas of potential problem in her life. She denied any feelings of depression and feels her life is going quite well. She has a boyfriend and is a freshman in college (i.e., first year at University). However, she is now living away from home, cooking for herself, and drinking far more alcohol than she did previously at home. She feels these suggestions may be relevant, but still thinks the pill is probably the root cause of her problems. We talked about long-acting reversible methods (LARCs), but she expressed that she wanted to be in control of her bleeding pattern and was already using the pill in an extended way to reduce the amount of bleeding episodes per year. She had stopped using condoms now that she had a long-term boyfriend and they both had been "checked" for STIs and did not want to return to barrier methods.

I suggested a different type of pill, and she agreed to try this. Although there is very little evidence about different types of pills helping different symptoms, some pills containing a different dose of estrogen or a

Continued

different type of progestogen can suit different women in a much better way. Of course, her symptoms may not be particularly related to the pill. However, Gedarel[b] 30/150 contains the same amount of estrogen (none of her symptoms could be said to be estrogen related) and a different type of progestogen (desorgestrel not levonorgestrel). Desorgestrel is thought to be a more female-friendly progestogen and is not derived directly from testosterone, so can perhaps help with premenstrual symptoms. I advised Ms. B to start the new medication immediately, as she was in the middle of her packet. She would not need to use any extra precautions against pregnancy as she had not missed any pills, was at day 10 in her packet, and was going to continue the new contraceptive pill for another 21 days without a break.

[a]Microgynon® is a form of contraceptive available in the United Kingdom, composed of 30 micrograms ethinyl estradiol and 150 micrograms levonorgestrel. Although this brand is not sold in the United States, similar formulations are available under other brand names (e.g., Alesse, Nordette).

[b]Gedarel 30/150® is a form of contraceptive available in the United Kingdom, composed of 30 micrograms ethinyl estradiol and 150 micrograms desorgestrel. Although this brand is not sold in the United States, similar formulations are available under other brand names (e.g., Mircette®, Desogen®).

Case Study 8-3

Ms. C is a 15-year-old patient who attended the young people's clinic. She came in and asked for "the pill." I thought it was appropriate to discuss all methods with her as some patients ask for "the pill" because this is the only contraceptive method they know about. However, she was adamant that she wanted to start on the pill. She had no contraindications, and I explained how to take it. I asked her how she would remember to take it regularly, and she said she would put a reminder on her phone, or ask her mother to remind her. Her mother was aware of her sexual activity and she was not at any specific risk, having had two partners in the past, both her own age. I gave her ethinyl estradiol and levonorgestrel (Rigevidon®[a]) and asked her to return in 6 weeks. She returned in 4 weeks, saying that she kept forgetting to take the pill and she was bleeding every day. I found she was living half the week with her father and half the week with her mother, and kept leaving her pill in the other house. I did offer her a *Chlamydia trachomatis* test, which had been negative previously and was negative again. I felt her bleeding was as a result of non-absorption and therefore discussed the patch. She seemed interested in this idea; she felt once weekly was better for her than once daily. I asked her to start this immediately, use condoms for 7 days, and return in 3 weeks for a pregnancy test. I happened to see her 3 weeks later; her pregnancy test was negative and she had had no more bleeding.

[a]Rigevidon® is a form of contraceptive available in the United Kingdom, composed of 30 micrograms ethinyl estradiol and 150 micrograms levonorgestrel. Although this brand is not sold in the United States, similar formulations are available under other brand names (e.g., Alesse®, Nordette®).

Case Study 8-4

Mrs. D is 45 years old and has had five pregnancies with three live births and two miscarriages. She has been on the pill for about 20 years and is settled on it. She presented for a repeat prescription. Her BP was normal and she is a non-smoker. Her periods are light and almost nonexistent. She is on 30 micrograms ethinyl estradiol and 150 micrograms levonorgestrel (Microgynon®) at present. We discussed her thoughts about the future. I told her she can stay on the combined oral contraception (COC) until she is 50–52 years old, the natural age of menopause. We also discussed menopausal symptoms and the fact that the pill might mask some of these. Menopause is difficult to diagnose in women who are on the pill, and Mrs. D has several choices about what to do:

- Continue on the COC until she is 50–52, then stop and use condoms. If she has no spontaneous periods over this time, she can stop using condoms after 1 year. If she does have bleeding, she will have to continue using condoms for 1 year after the last bleeding episode.
- Have her follicle stimulating hormone (FSH) level checked after she has stopped the pill sometime over the age of 50; she should be off the pill for at least 1 month before doing this. If she has two levels of FSH, 6 weeks apart, both greater than 30 IU/L, then she will need to use contraception for another year.
- Change to a progestogen-only method of contraception and continue until age 55 when she can stop contraception. She may have menopausal symptoms if she stops the combined pill.
- Change onto a long-acting reversible contraception, such as levonorgestrel-releasing intrauterine system (Mirena®). This can be used for contraception, control of menstruation, and hormone replacement therapy (HRT).

She decided to stay on the COC at present, and after discussion, we reduced the estrogen content in her COC to 20 mcg, as this is a sufficient amount to provide contraception in women over 40. I gave her ethinyl estradiol and desorgestrel (Gedarel 20/150®).

Counseling for the Progestogen-Only Pill

"I want to start the progestogen-only pill."

The progestogen-only pill is a niche pill. It is very useful for women who cannot tolerate estrogen for any reason. This includes women over 35 who are smokers, women who have migraine with aura or who have had a venous thromboembolism, women who are breastfeeding; women with high BMI, and women who have other cardiovascular problems such as diabetes or arterial disease.

The progestogen-only pill (POP) enables couples to have a choice of contraception without imposing unnecessary restriction for use.

How can practitioners counsel someone wishing to start this pill? In the following scenario, the patient is going to start the POP having been on the COC previously. She is mid-cycle just now and has been using condoms because she developed migraine with aura and was advised not to take the COC again.

Tips for Counseling the Patient

A script for giving information to the patient follows:

As the name suggests, this pill only contains one hormone: progestogen. Progesterone is one of the female hormones found in your body, and progestin-only pills mimic this hormone to prevent pregnancy. This pill works by thickening the cervical mucus and creating an almost solid barrier that the sperm cannot swim through. Some types of this sort of pill stop the eggs from being produced in the ovary—and if there are no eggs you cannot become pregnant. They also thin and dry up the lining of the uterus [endometrium], which makes it impossible for anything to settle and grow there.

This is a pill you take every single day. There are no gaps between packets; just take a pill every day. It is best to take this pill at **exactly** the same time every day. Some of these pills have a "3-hour window," and one [Cerazette®, a desogestrel-only brand sold in the United Kingdom] has a "12-hour window." The 3-hour window means that if you normally take your pill at 6 p.m. every night and you forget it one night until after 9 p.m., then you will have to use extra precautions. The 12-hour window means you have a full 12 hours in which to remember to take your pill before needing to use condoms or abstain from intercourse.

However, you only need to use these extra precautions for 2 days, not 7 days like the standard pill. So, if you do forget to take a pill, you need to take the one you missed as soon as you remember, take the next one at the correct time, and use condoms or do not have sex for 2 days.

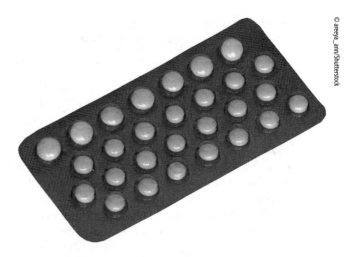

Figure 8-3 Progestogen-Only Pills

The progestogen-only pill used to be called the "mini pill," but don't be confused by that title. It may have fewer hormones in it, but it is just as effective as the standard pill and is safer for you to take due to your other medical conditions.

So, I'm going to show you the packet now. As you can see, there are 28 pills in the packet. I'm going to suggest you start the packet just now and take a pill today or tomorrow—depending on what time of day you feel would be good for you to take it (**Figure 8-3**).

If you start it tonight at 6 pm, then remember not to rely on it for 2 days and use condoms or don't have sex. You can then keep taking it at the same time of day right round the packet, following all the names of the days until the packet is finished. As you are starting it in the middle of a cycle, you might want to take a pregnancy test in 3 weeks' time if you have any worries.

You then start the next packet the following day; don't leave any gap.

You will find that bleeding will usually occur at the end of one packet or at the beginning of the next packet. The bleeding will not be as predictable as on the combined hormonal contraception and it might stop altogether. Don't worry about this. As I was telling you at the beginning, this pill dries up and thins the uterine lining, so bleeding might be regular and light, go away entirely, or become irregular and unpredictable. The longer you stay on this type of pill, the more likely it is that bleeding will disappear. Providing you have taken all your pills properly, this is nothing to worry about.

However, you may like to take a pregnancy test to ensure you are not pregnant from time to time if you have concerns.

As this pill contains only the one hormone, you will find that it does not have many side effects and is safe for most women to take. The reason it is not started as standard in many cases is due to the regularity of pill taking and the irregularity of bleeding. However, as with all hormones, some women find it may cause weight changes, mood swings, bloating, headaches, and breast tenderness. We have no evidence in any of the drug trials to support this, but some women are very sensitive to any hormonal changes in their body. If you find there are any side effects which you find intolerable, please come back to see us. We usually find that any minor, bearable side effects settle down within 3 months.

If you are sick and vomit within 2 hours of taking this pill, it will not get absorbed properly, and you should take another one. Remember to use extra precautions for 2 days after the vomiting illness settles.

There are very few drugs that affect this pill, mainly ones to treat epilepsy, tuberculosis, and HIV. If you have worries about any drug you are on interfering with the pill, then please check with us.

Do you want some condoms in case you miss any of your pills?

Case Study 8-5

Ms. E is 28 years old, G1P1, and is 42 days postpartum. She has had no bleeding since delivery. She is breastfeeding on demand but is worried about becoming pregnant again as her delivery was traumatic. We discussed the delivery and agreed to refer her back to the obstetrician to talk about her fears and concerns. She has not had sex since delivery. As she is breastfeeding on demand, amenorrheic, and her baby is less than 6 months old, the lactational amenorrhea method (LAM) can be discussed. This method, providing the three above criteria are used, is 98% effective. However, Ms. E feels that she wants something more reliable. The combined hormonal contraceptive may affect the production of breast milk. Progestogen-only methods do not affect breast milk taste or production, so a progestogen-only pill, implant, IUS, IUD, or injectable may all be suitable, and of course all LARC methods are more reliable. After discussion about all methods, Ms. E decides on a POP, which she will use alongside the LAM and this will give her confidence in controlling her fertility.

Case Study 8-6

Ms. F is 24 years old and has been on a COC pill since she became sexually active at 18 years old. Over the past 2 years, she has developed headaches, which at first she put down to stress and then to eye strain as she was finishing her degree studies. However, last week she woke up and found she could not see properly out of her right eye. She described this feeling as a black area in the middle of her eye; she could see round it, but if she stared straight ahead, she was "blind" in that eye. The feeling passed after 20 minutes, but then she developed a severe headache. She took painkillers for this, lay down, and eventually the headache went away. She felt weak and unfocused for the rest of the day. She saw her primary care provider (PCP), as she was concerned about these symptoms. Her PCP felt this was a migraine with aura and advised her to stop the COC. The risk of ischemic stroke is increased in women who have migraine with aura and who take the COC. Although it is a very small absolute risk, the consequences of a stroke in a healthy young woman can be catastrophic, so stopping the COC is justified (MacGregor, 1999). Ms. F is a good pill taker and was happy to know she could take the progestogen-only pill, which would continue her effective contraception without the risk of a medical complication. She did not want to consider any other method at present as she is in a regular relationship, so does not wish to use condoms. She felt that a LARC method would not be appropriate until she has thought further about her health and options.

Counseling for Progestogen-Only Injection

"I want to start the injection."

The contraceptive injection is an extremely useful method of contraception that has fallen slightly out of favor recently. It is another progestogen-only method, and this means that it has the usual progestogen-only (PO) mode of action, comprising the following:

- Prevention of ovulation (this can be variable depending on what PO method is used)
- Thickening of the cervical mucus
- Thinning of the endometrium

The contraceptive injection is usually given in the gluteal muscle every 3 months. It has fallen out of favor due to some suggestion that it may cause osteopenia while the patient remains on the drug, theoretically leading to osteoporosis and risk of fracture (Harel et al., 2010). The commercial name of the progestogen-only injection (depot medroxyprogesterone acetate or DMPA) usually used in the United Kingdom and United States is Depo-Provera®.

In this scenario, we have a 25-year-old patient who has tried the combined pill and finds herself forgetful on it, wants something more effective than condoms, but is not keen either on other forms of CHC or of the very long-acting reversible (vLARC) methods such as the implant or the intrauterine devices.

In general, no drugs affect the efficacy of the contraceptive injection. This is particularly useful as the injection can be used as effective contraception for women who are on enzyme-inducing medication.

As there may be a very rare anaphylactic reaction with injectable contraception, it is advisable to have emergency equipment available and ask the patient to stay in the waiting room for 10–15 minutes after her first injection.

There is no guidance for bone density and dual-energy X- ray absorptiometry (DEXA) bone scanning. A useful rule of thumb may be to scan if a woman has been on the injection for 5 years with complete amenorrhea, but there is no need for a baseline scan before a woman starts the injection.

Due to the concern about injectable contraception and osteoporosis (National Institute for Health and Clinical Excellence [NICE], 2013). The advice is to avoid using it in women under 18 (before peak bone mineral density [BMD] is reached) and also avoid using it in the 5 years preceding natural menopause (i.e., between 45 and 50 years of age). However, with counseling, and provided all other methods of contraception have been considered and DMPA is found to be the most appropriate, it can be used even in these age groups. It is advised to review the risk factors and reasons for staying on the injectable contraception every 2 years.

There is a new formulation of progestogen-only injection available in the United States, United Kingdom, and some other countries. This is a subcutaneous single-dose, pre-filled, self-administered injection that is used every 13 weeks. It contains 104 mg of medroxyprogesterone acetate, which is bioequivalent of the standard progestogen-only injection. The risks and benefits are the same, with ease of use and avoidance of clinic visits being the main advantages.

Tips for Counseling the Patient

The injection contains one hormone, progestogen.

It is quite a large dose of this hormone and needs to be given every 3 months—usually into the big muscle of the buttock. **Figure 8-4** illustrates a progesterone injection being administered. It works by stopping your body from producing an egg. It also thins and dries up the uterine lining, and usually, after the first 3 months, your periods stop. During those first 3 months, your periods will be irregular and unpredictable, although you may be lucky and they will disappear completely quite soon.

The injection is very effective in preventing pregnancy and is very safe, as it only contains one hormone so there is lower risk of things like breast cancer and blood clots. It does have some side effects, and the main one is weight change. About one-third of the women we give this to will lose about 3 kg (7 lb), one-third will stay the same weight, and one-third will put on 3 kg (7 lb). We cannot predict who this will happen to, but remember, it is only 3 kg (7 lb); the injection will not cause you to lose or gain any more weight than that.

It also might have affect your mood—some women are very sensitive to progestogen and while it might help premenstrual syndrome (PMS) in certain women, it may have the opposite effect in others. Again, we cannot predict who this may happen to.

Once you have the injection, any benefits and side effects will last for 3 months. We cannot remove it from your system, so you should be aware of this.

There has been some recent research suggesting that the injection, because it is a high dose of one of the female hormones, cancels out another hormone in your body, which leads to a thinning of your bones. This is not a severe problem and does not lead to broken bones or fractures. However, we always ask a few more questions so that we can be sure you are not at risk.

- Are you a smoker? This probably causes more thinning of the bones than any medication.
- Do you have a family history of bone thinning? This condition tends to be inherited and can cause problems especially as you get older.
- Are you worried about the amount you drink? Too much alcohol is associated with a decrease in bone thickness and a poorer diet.
- Have you ever been on long-term steroid treatment? This can include treatment for asthma in the past, including inhalers.
- Have you ever suffered from conditions causing poor absorption of food, such as celiac disease or inflammatory bowel conditions?

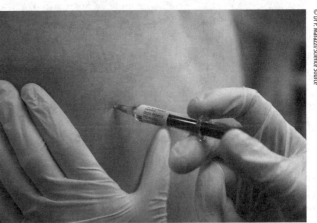

Figure 8-4 A progesterone only injection being administered

- Have you ever had an eating disorder such as anorexia nervosa?
- What is your diet like? Do you eat items such as milk, cheese, yogurt, and eggs?

We usually give out a diet sheet to encourage you to eat and drink items that have more calcium (National Osteoporosis Society, 2016).

We can start the injections with you any time; today would be fine, if you are reasonably sure you are not pregnant, but remember that the injection will not be properly in your system for 7 days, so use condoms or don't have sex for that time. Then it is probably a good idea to have a pregnancy test in 3 weeks' time.

You should come back in 12 weeks for your next injection—I'll give you the date just now. If you can return 12 weeks from today, that would be best. However, we can give the injection up to 2 weeks early or 2 weeks late without you losing the contraceptive effect of it. Don't come any later than 14 weeks from today, as we then may not be able to give you your injection if you have had sex and are at risk of pregnancy.

There are no commonly used drugs that affect the efficacy of the injection but please contact us if you are worried. Do you want some condoms for the first 7 days?

Case Study 8-7

Ms. G is 15 years old. She has been having sex since she was 13 and has had six partners in the last year. A contraceptive implant was inserted in her right arm when she was 14 years old, but she has had continuing problems with it over the last year. She complains of unpredictable and annoying irregular bleeding. She was given "the pill" by her PCP, but she has not found it useful and feels she has become moodier.

We discussed her options. She does not feel she can take the pill regularly and this is borne out on further discussion when she reveals that she has been missing more pills than she has been taking since first prescribed the pill to help with her bleeding. She does not wish to use the IUD/IUS, and she grimaced with horror when the method of insertion was described: "I'm definitely not having *that* inside me!" She does use condoms when she remembers, but alcohol is often involved when she does have sex, and so again, this is not a reliable method. She has heard of the injection and says her older cousin is on it with benefit. She is a thin girl who smokes about 10 cigarettes per day. Her diet is not good, but she says she likes yogurt and cheese. She has no history of osteoporosis in her family and has no past use of steroid medication. She is interested in trying the

---

DMPA injection. Her implant was removed and DMPA given in the left gluteal area. She has since attended for 3 more injections, her irregular bleeding has stopped, she has been in a regular relationship for the past 6 months, and she has reduced her alcohol intake. She will be reviewed every 2 years to determine whether this method of contraception is still right for her.

Counseling for Contraceptive Implant

"I want to get the rod in."

The contraceptive implant is a matchstick-size flexible rod containing 68 mg of etonogestrel that is inserted into the upper, inner non-dominant arm 8–10 cm from the medial epicondyle.

It has recently been redesigned and now comes with a new applicator that was developed to help prevent excessively deep insertions of the implant. It also now comes with 15 mg of barium sulphate, which enables it to be seen on straight X-ray. The commercial name in the United States and United Kingdom is Nexplanon® (**Figure 8-5**).

Enzyme-inducing drugs have an effect on the implant, so if a patient is on any of these drugs long-term—for epilepsy, for instance—then another method of contraception should be advised. In the short term, condoms or abstinence is suitable. There is no link with the implant and osteopenia. There is also no link with the implant and any adverse outcome of an unexpected pregnancy.

As with DMPA, emergency equipment should be available in the event of a rare anaphylactic reaction or vasovagal shock due to needle phobia. Anyone who inserts and removes implants should have appropriate training in the procedure. Some implants inserted incorrectly or by inadequately trained practitioners are too deep for conventional removal. Patients with these implants should be referred to a specialist center for removal where they can be located using ultrasound. The new inserter applicator has been designed to stop this from happening in the future.

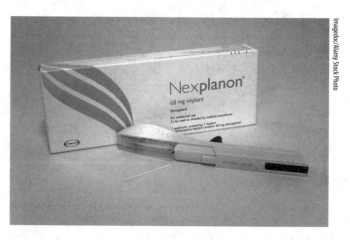

Figure 8-5 Nexplanon®

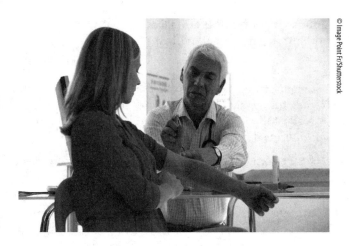

Figure 8-6 Contraceptive Implant

Tips for Counseling the Patient

The rod or implant is a tiny flexible match-stick-sized device that is placed under the skin of your arm (**Figure 8-6**). It slides under your skin using a special applicator and I always put on some local anesthetic first, which makes it pain free. However, getting the local anesthetic can cause some nipping and burning until the area starts to go numb.

The implant is more effective than sterilization and lasts for 3 years, although it can be removed at any time if you don't like or want it anymore. It is completely reversible, and once it is removed your fertility is back to normal in less than a day. However, we would ask you to think about this, and if you are unsure that you can keep the implant in for more than 3 months, then maybe think about another method.

The implant contains a small dose of hormone called progestogen, which gets released gradually over the 3 years and stops your ovary from releasing an egg. It has very few side effects, but some women may notice their skin or hair gets greasier or drier, and some women notice weight changes. The main reason women have problems with this method of contraception is that your bleeding becomes irregular. We cannot predict how that will affect you. In some women, the bleeding will stop completely for the 3 years; in others, it might stop initially and then return. Other women may have irregular light episodes of bleeding throughout the 3 years. Some women will continue with their normal cycle.

In some women, however, the implant can make bleeding more frequent and often heavier. This does not mean the implant is not working, it just means it is not controlling your uterine lining and

making it thin enough. We can often help this side effect by giving you a course of pills to take or even an injection. However, if you find this side effect intolerable, then we will of course remove your implant.

Here is a model of how the implant will feel in the arm. [These models are available from the drug company that produces the implant—at this time, Merck & Co.]

The implant is very easy to put in, and afterward you can feel it in the arm but not see it. It is also very easy to remove and I put in some local anesthetic injection, put a little nick right at the end of the implant, and it just pushes out of your arm. Then if you want another one, I can put a new one in through the same cut. After I put an implant in, I ask you to keep a bandage on your arm for 24 hours to keep the area clean and dry and to prevent any bruising. Then I ask you to keep it covered until the area is healed and until the steristrips, if used, come off.

We can put an implant in for you today if you are reasonably sure you are not pregnant, although it will not take full effect for 7 days and we ask you to use condoms or abstain from sex during this time. Then I should advise having a pregnancy test in 3 weeks' time if there are any concerns about potential risk of pregnancy.

There are no commonly used drugs that affect the efficacy of the implant but contact us if you are concerned.

We do not need to see you again, after insertion, for 3 years, and it is your responsibility to remember the date that your implant stops working. We shall give you a card with the date for replacement on it for your safe keeping. However, if you have any problem with the method, then please come to see us for advice.

Do you want any condoms?

Case Study 8-8

Ms. H is 13 years old. She attends the clinic with 3 friends; an older boy and two girls. She states loudly in the waiting room that she is there to get the "rod" fitted,

Continued

as are her two girlfriends. Her "gay best friend" is here to give them all moral support. Luckily, there are three practitioners on for that clinic, and the three girls are able to be taken into different consulting rooms. Once alone, Ms. H presents very differently and seems quiet and subdued. She was offered the opportunity to have her friends in with her, at least for part of the consultation, but declined. History taking was difficult and monosyllabic at first, but we determined that Ms. H has never had any sexual contact with anybody. She seemed relieved to tell me this and the atmosphere in the room improved. She told me she has ADHD and gets "hyper" sometimes. She goes to "parties" on weekend, usually in a friend's house, where alcohol is consumed. A full child-protection history was taken, and there was no evidence of any inappropriate or worrying episodes. She fulfills the criteria of being able to give informed consent for contraceptive advice and treatment. Her friends are all the same age, she attends school regularly, she lives with her mother and little brother, and she never "gets drunk." We discussed contraception and sexual behavior, and she will think about talking to her mother at a later date. She was introduced to a young people's support worker and has arranged to meet up with this worker on a regular basis.

One of her friends, who attended with her, was sexually active and at risk of pregnancy.

Case Study 8-9

Ms. I is 14 years old and has had two episodes of sex. After the second episode, she went to a pharmacy for emergency contraception and had a prolonged episode of bleeding, which finished the day before yesterday. She has had no sex for over 3 weeks and a pregnancy test was negative. A self-taken vulvovaginal swab was taken for testing for *Chlamydia trachomatis* and *Neisseria gonorrhoea*. She was aware of the implant, as several girls of her acquaintance had one. Some of these girls felt the implant was excellent, but one had problems with it. Ms. I wished to go ahead with the implant today. She has not been able to tell her mother about her sexual activity, but has spoken to an aunt who thinks it would be a good idea for her to get contraception. After further counseling, a contraceptive implant was inserted in her right arm (she is left-handed). She was asked to keep note of any bleeding, advised to telephone for the result of her swab, and given condoms. She thinks she will be able to keep her implant insertion and sexual activity "secret" from her mother, whom she thinks would not understand. She asked that her PCP (GP) should not be informed about the procedure.

Counseling for Intrauterine Device (IUD) and Intrauterine System (IUS)

"I want an IUD (coil)."

It is important for sexual healthcare providers to be properly trained for intrauterine device insertion and removal.

The following guidance should be considered for intrauterine device insertion:

- Perform an STI risk assessment on all women before device insertion.
- If the patient is under age 25, or has had more than one partner in the past 6 months, test for chlamydia and gonorrhea.
- Do not insert intrauterine device until STI results are returned, unless the patient is at high risk for pregnancy.
- Prophylactic antibiotics are not necessary in women with prosthetic heart valves or to protect against bacterial endocarditis.
- Perform a bimanual examination to determine shape and size of the uterus before device insertion.
- Emergency equipment including oxygen (FSRH 2015b), if available, should always be near at hand when IUD/IUS insertions are taking place.
- Measure pulse and blood pressure before and after insertion.
- Always have a trained assistant present during device insertions.
- Occasionally, there is a reaction to instrumentation, which can take the form of a collapse, vasovagal reaction, seizure, or anaphylaxis. Algorithms that advise what to do in an emergency situation should be displayed in all consulting rooms.

The following is a scenario about a patient who wishes to use an IUD for contraception. She is 34 years old and has had two pregnancies. She has heard about the IUD and wishes long-term contraception. However, she does not really know about the two types of intrauterine contraception, so she wishes to hear the good and bad points of both.

Tips for Counseling the Patient

There are two types of intrauterine contraception—one is copper and the other is hormone based.

I'll show you the two types and you can see what I mean. [Always have a copper intrauterine device (Cu IUD) and a levonorgestrel intrauterine system (LNG-IUS) available to show the woman. It is useful also to have a small plastic model of a uterus so that you can demonstrate insertion. These are available from the pharmaceutical companies who supply the devices.]

The copper IUD is T shaped, and the type that has copper wire coiled around its leg only lasts for 5 years; the one that has copper around its leg and its arms usually lasts for 10 years (**Figure 8-7**).

The Cu IUD contains no hormones and is an excellent method of contraception—almost as good as female sterilization, and better in some cases. The way it works is to prevent fertilization by killing sperm. Sperm swimming up the cervical canal into the uterus [demonstrate where the cervical canal and the uterus are on the model] die when they encounter the hostile environment created by the copper IUD. This is not harmful to you or anything else—only sperm. However, as you know, there are millions of sperm per ejaculate, and the Cu IUD has to have a lot of copper to kill every one.

It is put in like this [demonstrate with an out-of-date Cu IUD and the model uterus]; it is small and flexible and it's very simple to place it in the uterus.

You will lie on the examination table for insertion; the procedure can be uncomfortable, but is not usually painful. You should take a non-steroidal anti-inflammatory (NSAID) before the procedure, although I often use an anesthetic gel (Instillagel®ᵃ) and frequently more anesthetic if the patient needs it. [Note: I do not usually explain completely about the cervical block procedure unless the patient requests this, as the idea of a needle going into the cervix makes some women very nervous and squeamish (**Figure 8-8**). However, I do use this method at the first sign of any pain and discomfort for the patient. Always explain to the patient that she has control and the procedure can be stopped at any time if she wishes.]

There will always be someone else with you. This will usually be a healthcare assistant who will talk to you and keep your mind off the procedure so that you don't feel too tense.

The side effects of the Cu IUD are obviously not hormonal, but they are connected to where it sits in the body. Just because it is there and sitting in your uterus, you may get increased crampy pain before your period. The period will come at the normal time, but perhaps be heavier and longer than your usual cycle. Instead of your period lasting for 5 days, it may last for 7 or 8 days, and the bleeding will be heavier, especially at the beginning of the period. However, this will settle with time. You will find the first period after insertion will definitely be heavier than normal.

There is a slight risk that your uterus will not accept the Cu IUD and will push it out again. This usually happens at insertion or slightly afterward. We always advise that you check your own strings to make sure that if this does happen, you are aware of it and do not rely on the device for contraception. There is also a slight risk that the Cu IUD will push its way into and perhaps through the uterine muscle wall, and this will require a small operation for removal. You will usually be aware of this as it will cause you some pain, and again, you will not be able to feel your IUD strings. This is very rare, but is important, as again, the Cu IUD will not be working as a contraceptive if this happens.

Remember that the Cu IUD does not cause infection. It is a sterile device and is inserted in clean circumstances. If you are unlucky enough to get an infection, then it may have already been in your uterus and the IUD has made it more

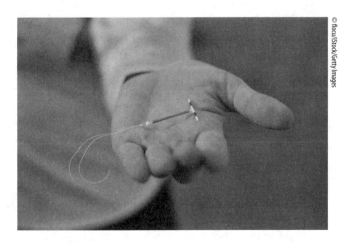

Figure 8-7 IUD

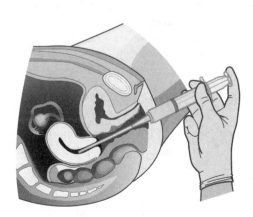

Figure 8-8 Syringe with 2% Mepivacaine Anaesthetic Gel'

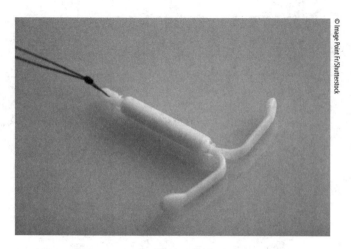

Figure 8-9 IUS

noticeable. The other thing to remember is that these infections are often sexually transmitted, and so if you do have a new partner, use condoms until you have both been checked for any sexually transmitted infection.

The LNG-IUS (Mirena®) is the same shape as some of the Cu IUDs (**Figure 8-9**). However, that is where the similarity ends, as it acts in a completely different way. It contains a progestogen hormone on the leg of the system rather than copper. This progestogen hormone, called levonorgestrel, sits inside the uterus and is continually "leaking out" over the course of 5 years, thinning and drying up the uterine lining and making it impossible for anything to settle there. It also works by preventing ovulation—although not always—and thickening up the mucus at the cervix, making it very difficult for the sperm to penetrate the uterus.

The procedure for insertion is exactly the same—I'll demonstrate on the model—and the way we do the procedure is unchanged. The Mirena® device is an extremely effective method of contraception—more effective than female sterilization, and it lasts for 5 years.

It is hormonal and does have some side effects, as you would expect from any hormonal method. However, it is a very low-dose hormone—equivalent to less than 2 progestogen-only pills per week—so the side effects are minimal.

Some people will complain of greasiness or dryness of the skin and hair and it may cause mild acne in some women. There is no evidence that it causes

weight gain or mood swings, and one of the things we use Mirena® for is to treat PMS. Again though, you must be aware that some women are very sensitive to any change in hormone level and may experience more side effects.

The main change that women find with Mirena® is the change in bleeding pattern, which can be quite unpredictable over the first 3 months. The bleeding might settle and disappear or it may continue relatively regularly, or it may become irregular and lighter. Very rarely does it become heavier, but some women have brownish discharge every day until the endometrium (uterine lining) settles and dries up. The good news is that in most women this happens within 3 to 6 months of insertion and then there is regular light bleeding lasting about 1 day per month or no bleeding at all.

As you can see, Mirena® useful in treating women who have heavy periods, and we often use it to treat this symptom whether or not women have the need for contraception. We also use Mirena® as part of hormone replacement therapy during menopause. It is extremely useful in this situation, as it gives a low-dose option to women who have symptoms.

When we insert either of these devices, we prefer you not to be pregnant. This is because any foreign body in the womb can disrupt pregnancy, making it inappropriate to insert a device. The Cu IUD can, of course, be used as emergency contraception and can be inserted up to 5 days after an episode of unprotected sex or inserted up to day 19 of a 28-day cycle.

A Cu IUD is effective immediately after insertion, but a Mirena® takes 7 days to be effective, and condoms or abstinence is advised. After insertion, we would usually advise you not to have sex for 3–4 days to let any discomfort settle, and we would advise you to use condoms up to 7 days after insertion to reduce any risk of infection.

It is also a good idea not to use tampons until about 6 weeks after insertion. We are probably being overly cautious here, and if you use them and remove them carefully, there should be no problems. Cramping pain is common after insertion and therefore taking a regular pain killer (such as ibuprofen) for 24 hours is useful.

Fertility returns to normal immediately after removal of either the Cu IUD or the LNG-IUS. The devices are very easy to remove—they just fold up on themselves and slip out of the uterus when we pull gently on the strings. [Demonstrate if possible on the model.]

We always ask you to return for review about 6 weeks after an intrauterine procedure. This is to make sure you are not having any problems, and we like to check the IUD/IUS strings to make sure the device is in the correct place. If you are having any worries or concerns, however, remember you can return at any time.

It is your responsibility to remember how long your Cu IUD or Mirena® lasts, and we shall give you a card to remind you, which you should keep in a safe place.

ªInstillagel® is a product comprising lidocaine hydrochloride, chlorhexidine digluconate, methyl hydroxybenzoate, and propyl hydroxybenzoate that is sold in the United Kingdom. It is not available in the United States.

Case Study 8-10

Ms. J is 20 years old and suffers from systemic lupus erythematosus (SLE) with antiphospholipid antibodies. She has had this condition for 6 years. She is in a relationship of 15 months and has been using condoms for contraception. She has had a pregnancy scare and wants something more effective, as she does not want a pregnancy and also feels her medical condition would deteriorate if this were to happen. Patients with SLE who have antiphospholipid antibodies are at increased risk of ischemic heart disease, stroke, and venous thromboembolism, and this limits the options for safe and effective contraception. The option of a copper IUD was fully discussed with Ms. J, who agreed it would be appropriate. She has always had normal, regular, light periods. She is a G0P0 and was apprehensive about the procedure. Insertion of an IUD is usually straightforward in a nulliparous patient, but there is often an increased degree of uterine cramping afterward. Ms. J was advised to take her normal analgesia—which she takes intermittently for joint pain—before the appointment and to continue on this regularly for 3 days after insertion. The procedure was uneventful, and Ms. J coped well with her anxiety. A check at 6 weeks was normal, and there have been no further problems.

Case Study 8-11

Mrs. K is 33 years old. She has two children and has Crohn's disease. She had an abnormal cervical smear result 3 years ago and had colposcopy and some laser treatment. Her deliveries were both cesarean sections due to failure to progress and were complicated by a flare-up of her inflammatory bowel disease and a temporary colostomy. Her disease is well controlled just now, and her last delivery was 5 years ago. She has been using a progestogen-only pill but is concerned that this may not always be absorbed correctly. She has been advised not to use CHC due to a family history of breast cancer. She would like to use IUS as she has heavy periods and has a friend who has found this an excellent method. We discussed her options and an IUS would be suitable. She was advised that if it was impossible to insert an IUS due to her previous colposcopy and section deliveries, that DMPA or an implant would also be suitable. She was asked to return for a fitting appointment after having had something to eat and taken analgesia about 1 hour beforehand. She was asked to continue on the POP. At the insertion visit, further counseling was undertaken and the patient's BP and weight taken for baseline comparison. Before insertion, an internal examination was carried out to determine the position of her uterus, which revealed a small, closed, retroverted cervix and an anteverted mobile, normal-sized uterus. The IUS pack containing a speculum, sponge forceps, Allis forceps (some inserters prefer to use a tenaculum), and a plastic uterine sound was opened. The vulval area was lubricated with an antiseptic solution. The speculum was inserted and the cervix visualized. A very tiny external os was noted. Some local anesthetic was inserted using a quill, which was used in this case not only for anesthesia but also to try to open up the cervical canal. This was quite successful and a size 1/2 Hegar was inserted to about 5 cm. The patient found this uncomfortable and a cervical block was then used. This consisted of 2% mepivacaine, 1 mL inserted into the body of the cervix at 12 o'clock, 3 o'clock, 6 o'clock, and 9 o'clock using a dental syringe and needle. We then waited 3 minutes for this to take effect. While waiting, we discussed the patient's children, her job, and her vacation plans for this year. It is useful to be able to have a conversation about unrelated things when doing an IUS/IUD fit of any kind, as this reduces anxiety and the procedure is less painful. It is also imperative to have an assistant with the IUS/IUD fitter at all times. This helps clinically, and is essential during emergency events, but also reduces apprehension on the part of the patient and makes the procedure easier and more "normal." After this wait, a 3/4 Hegar dilator was inserted to 7.5 cm, the normal sound was also inserted to check correct diameter and length, and a Mirena® was inserted. The uterus was resounded and the patient's BP was checked. The procedure was uneventful and the patient felt well afterward.

Case Study 8-12

Mrs. L, age 43, presented to the clinic requesting an IUD removal and IUS insertion. She had come to this decision due to her heavy periods. She has had the IUD in for 3 years and her periods, although regular and occurring every 4 weeks, last for about 2 weeks each month. She has had 5 pregnancies—5 pregnancies with only 2 live births—and has been married for 18 years. She has been advised, as she is coming for an IUD/IUS change, not to have sex in the preceding week. This is to ensure against the chance of an "iatrogenic" pregnancy when the IUD is removed and an IUS for whatever reason—spasm of cervical canal, vasovagal reaction, pain—cannot be inserted. This would mean that if she had had intercourse in the last week, there may still be live sperm in the genital tract that could fertilize an ovum without the inhibitory effect of an IUD. She feels an intrauterine method suits her well but would like the extra benefits of a Mirena®. Unfortunately, on examination, no strings can be seen or felt. After an ultrasound examination, the IUD is seen to be in situ. A pack is opened and the vulva is "cleaned." (Note: It is most important, though, not to say, "I'm just giving you a little clean down here," or "We're just washing the vulva." This is because the vulva and vagina are self-cleansing organs and it is inappropriate of us clinically to say they need to be "cleaned." Patients should be discouraged from initiating any ill-advised cleansing routines. It is best to just say, "I'm just using this fluid to lubricate the area and make it easier for the speculum to go in.") Once the speculum is inserted and cervix visualized, the search for IUD threads can begin. It is useful to use an Allis forceps or a tenaculum to steady the cervix and to sound the canal and uterus with a plastic sound first. Doing this often enables the practitioner to "feel" the IUD/IUS as a roughness against the sound, which then enables the device to be "visualized" more easily before removal. If you have the facilities for removal under ultrasound control, this would be the gold standard. However, this technology is not available in all areas. Sometimes it is a question of getting the light right and the strings can just be seen. Sometimes the use of anesthetic (Instillagel®) can be useful as the strings can uncurl from the cervix after a little of the gel has been inserted then allowed to drain. String/thread retrievers—plastic rods with notches cut into them—can be inserted a little way into the cervix and twisted clockwise or counter-clockwise to see if the strings get trapped in one of the notches and the device can then be withdrawn. Unfortunately, because of the notches, these devices are quite sharp and can often cause some trauma of the cervix and subsequent bleeding can make the procedure more difficult. One of the easiest and most successful ways to remove an IUD/IUS with "lost" strings is to use "crocodile" or "alligator" forceps (**Figure 8-10**). These are long-handled devices with a small "bite" at the end, which can be inserted into the slightly opened canal to allow capture of the strings or the end of the device so it can be removed. Once the device is removed, it is important to insert the plastic sound into the canal and uterus to keep the canal patent. If this is not done, the canal can go into spasm due to the effects of the procedure and a new IUD/IUS cannot be inserted. Once the new device is out of its packaging, the sound can be withdrawn, the length measured, and the new IUS inserted.

Counseling on Barrier Methods and Fertility Awareness

"I don't like hormones; they don't agree with me."

Methods of contraception that do not have any hormones in them are:

- Intrauterine device
- Male condoms
- Female condoms
- Diaphragms
- Caps
- Fertility awareness

Male condoms are a very common method of contraception, and often women will say, "I think I'll just use condoms for a while and give my body a break."

Most people think they know how to use condoms and would be embarrassed to say otherwise. Men and women should know that condoms come in a variety of sizes (trim, regular, large, king-size), flavors, textures (robs, dots), and types (cooling, warming, glow in the dark). There are also hypoallergenic silicone-based condoms to prevent reactions in latex-allergic individuals. Encourage patients to experiment to find the condoms they most like.

Condoms can be used with a variety of lubricants, but ensure the patient knows to use a water-based lubricant that is safe to be used with condoms. Oil-based preparations—which include many vaginal infection treatments such as clotrimazole cream—as well as petroleum jelly, suntan oil, and lipstick, can damage latex condoms and make them more prone to splitting.

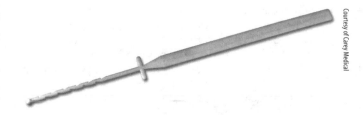

Courtesy of Carey Medical

Figure 8-10 Alligator Forceps Thread Retriever

If a patient states that she wants to use condoms, try to have a demonstrator available. These are obtained from condom manufacturers.

Tips for Counseling the Patient: Male Condoms

Always check that condoms are manufactured to the product-specific safety standard, for example, U.S. FDA standards or U.K./European product-specific safety standard ("Kite marked"), and make sure that they are within the expiration date.

Open the packet carefully, pushing the condom to one side to avoid tearing it when the packet opens. Don't open the packet with scissors or with your teeth. Make sure that when you take the condom out of the packet, it is the right way up. Most condoms are packed rolled up and it is important not to try to unroll them "inside out."

Hold the tip of the condom to squeeze the air out. This is important because if there is air in the tip, the condom may burst with extra pressure when your partner ejaculates (**Figure 8-11**). Condoms should be put on before any penile contact with the vulva or vagina is made, as there is sometimes a leakage of fluid—a pre-ejaculate—that contains sperm.

Place the condom on the top of an erect penis. Roll the condom down the shaft using the sides of your fingers. Avoid using your nails and avoid jewelry snagging on the condom. Once climax has been reached and the penis is flaccid, hold the end of the condom on the penis as you withdraw so that the condom is not inadvertently retained in the vagina.

Dispose of the condom properly—wrap it up and put it in the trash/bin. Do not flush it down toilet, as this will block drains and perhaps end up on beaches.

The condom will protect against most sexually transmitted infections and help prevent pregnancy up to 95% of the time. This means that if sex occurs with a condom 100 times, there will likely be five pregnancies.

"Can I see the female condom?"

Not many patients ask to use the female condom, but it is another useful method and is within the female's control. Again, have a female condom available with a demonstrator if possible (**Figure 8-12**). A good demonstrator is available from www.pasante.com.

Tips for Counseling the Patient: Female Condoms

This condom is bigger than the male condom, but is easy to use and covers the whole of the inside of the vagina and even some of the vulvar skin. It is well lubricated and easy to put inside you. The smaller inner ring is squeezed together and gently pushed into the vagina where it stays in place with the natural tone of the vaginal muscles. The larger ring hangs outside the vagina. The penis has to be guided into the opening of the female condom.

Most people find it comfortable to wear and it can be inserted before penetrative sex takes place provided the woman does not have to walk around too much. Like the male condom, it should be removed carefully after sex and disposed of properly.

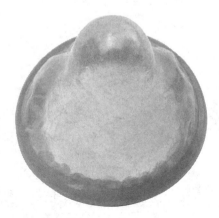

Figure 8-11 Male Condom

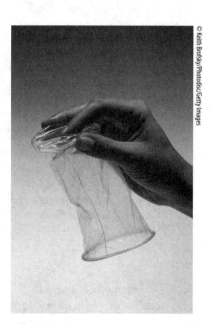

Figure 8-12 Female Condom

There are several misconceptions with the female condom, but it is important to advise patients of the following:

- It does not make a noise during sex.
- It is as effective as the male condom at preventing pregnancy and perhaps more effective at preventing sexually transmitted infection due to its larger size.
- Like the male condom, it can be used for oral sex.
- It can be used during menstruation.

Counseling for Caps and Diaphragms

Caps and diaphragms are female barriers that are used in different ways. The cervical cap fits over the cervix and is held there by suction, while the diaphragm is fitted into the vaginal vault and remains there partly by vaginal muscular tension and partly by its integral design containing a flexible rim.

Case Study 8-13

Mr. A is 18 years. old and presented for a sexual health screen. He has no symptoms but feels he wants a "check-up." He has recently started seeing a girl with whom he would like to have a relationship but he has not had sex as yet with her. He has had three previous sexual partners, all "one-night stands." His screen was carried out with a urine test for *Chlamydia trachomatis/ Neisseria gonorrhoeae* and a blood test for syphilis and HIV. He was asked about contraception, and he says he uses condoms "when he can." On further questioning, he tells you that when he tries to put a condom on he either loses his erection, keeps his erection but the condom falls off, or that he comes so quickly it "is not worth using protection because I don't get anywhere near her." He does appear to have a rather anxious personality and this appears to be reflected in his sexual functioning. A condom demonstration is given and he is encouraged to practice his technique on the model. A variety of condoms are given to him to look at and he says he would like to try the trim condoms and the delay condoms. He is given some of these types and others to use. He also takes some female condoms, as we discussed whether the use of female condoms by his partner would take some of his performance anxiety away. He is encouraged to come back to the clinic to get more condoms or discuss things further and is given the details of the psychosexual clinic. He will, of course, phone for his STI screening results later.

The female barrier methods provide both physical and chemical barrier to sperm, as both devices are used with spermicide. Both devices are made of latex, although there are silicone diaphragms and caps available for men or women with allergies. These silicone diaphragms look good, feel comfortable, and may lead to a renaissance of use in the future. There have been some studies looking at the use of microbicide-impregnated diaphragms to help stop the spread of HIV; study results are inconclusive, but the idea is encouraging Frezieres, Walsh, Kilbourne-Brook, & Coffey, 2012).

Spermicides should contain nonoxynol-9 and are available in several forms (gel, sponge, foam, suppository, liquid).

Female barriers may have some protective effect against STIs and cervical cancer. However, nonoxynol-9 may cause abrasions of the vaginal epithelium, and therefore, diaphragms and caps are not recommended for use in couples with a high risk of HIV/AIDS.

Tips for Counseling the Patient

It is good to have a diaphragm, cap, and anatomical demonstrator available. Explain the differences between a cap and a diaphragm and that each woman needs to be individually assessed and fitted for these methods (see **Figure 8-13** for the diaphragm and **Figure 8-14** for the cap). There is, however, a new diaphragm on the market that allows women who are within a certain size range to buy and use without further examination. Advise that there may be some issues with allergy, pelvic floor tone, and some concerns about a slight increase in urinary tract infections in susceptible women.

Explain that the devices should be used with spermicide and demonstrate that a cap should have some put inside it and then smeared over the entire outside surface. A diaphragm should have two stripes of spermicide on both sides and some smeared around the entire rim of the device. Make sure the patient is clear on the efficacy rate (95% effective if used perfectly). Make sure the woman is comfortable touching her genitals.

Demonstrate how the diaphragm and cap work and where they fit in a model. Explain that the patient should not leave this method in for longer than 30 hours, as the

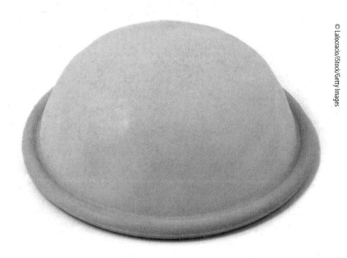

Figure 8-13 Diaphragm

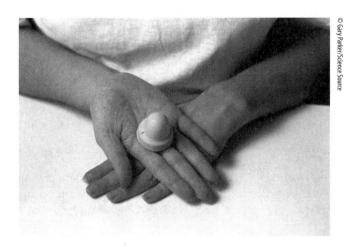

© Gary Parker/Science Source

Figure 8-14 Cap

risk of toxic shock increases. Advise that the method should be left in place for at least 6 hours after intercourse and that if the method is inserted and intercourse does not occur within the first three hours then extra spermicide should be used. If intercourse occurs more than once, then extra spermicide should be used on each occasion, inserted with an applicator and being careful not to dislodge the diaphragm or cap.

The patient should then be asked to undress so that the method can be fitted. For a diaphragm, measure the length of the vagina from the posterior fornix to the pubic symphysis with the examining fingers. Remember that the vagina balloons during intercourse and even if the diaphragm fits well in the consulting room there is no perfect fit in real life and that is why spermicide is also advised. The appropriate size diaphragm can then be fitted. This is easy to do if the practitioner knows the length of her fingers and can compare this to the required size for the diaphragm.

The patient should be asked to remove the diaphragm and put it back in again by herself. Pamphlets with diaphragms may also be useful. Many women find it impossible to fit their own diaphragms in the supine position and need to stand or crouch for optimum insertion potential. Examine the patient again to ensure it is in the correct place. The patient should be advised how to ensure the diaphragm or cap is in the correct place by examining herself and ensuring that she can feel the cervix (like a nose with one nostril) and that it is completely covered by the device.

A similar scenario is used to fit caps, although some women who have "difficult" cervix positions cannot use caps. These include acutely retroverted or anteverted cervixes, a very long vagina, a cervix which is very flat or very wide or any other anatomical problem. If the barrier is not in the correct place, remove it and let the patient try again.

Sometimes, the patient is too nervous to do this in the consulting room and the vagina becomes tighter and it is more difficult to insert the barrier. Advise the patient to go

home and practice, perhaps in the bath, where the warm water relaxes things and allows more confidence.

Even if the woman is happy inserting and removing the barrier method, advise that it should not be relied on completely for 2 to 3 weeks. Condoms or another method can be used until the patient returns to the clinic, wearing the diaphragm or cap to ensure it is in the correct place. Advise the patient that the method cannot get lost inside her.

Supply the patient with diaphragm or cap, spermicide, applicator, and condoms. Ensure the patient is aware of emergency contraception should she forget to use the method or it is inserted incorrectly. Advise that the patient should come back for a recheck of size if she loses or gains 3–4 kg (7 lbs) of weight. She should also be refitted for a diaphragm or cap after giving birth via vaginal delivery.

There is no definite time limit to the use of the individual diaphragm or cap but the woman should be aware to check for any tears, rips, holes, or cracks in the fabric and return if she has any concerns. A discoloration or slight distortion of the diaphragm or cap will not make any difference to the efficacy. As with other latex barriers such as condoms, it is important not to use oil-based lubricants, as they may weaken the latex.

There is no recognized training for a professional to fit female barrier methods, but anyone undertaking fitting should do so within their own recognized competencies.

Counseling for Fertility Awareness

Fertility awareness is fundamental to family planning; it requires a woman to identify the signs and symptoms of fertility throughout her reproductive cycle and to use that awareness to control conception (FSRH, 2015a).

Many women use the techniques of fertility awareness to become pregnant. It is important for the practitioner to understand each patient's feelings about her own fertility. Many women are confused about their menstrual cycle and are unaware of the physiology that causes fertility and their monthly periods. This lack of understanding can cause anxiety for women who do not know when in their cycle they are

---

Case Study 8-14

Mrs. M is 49 years old and presents requesting a "cap." She has used pills in the past but feel they make her moody and is using condoms at present. She does not have any problems with menopausal symptoms or with her periods and wants something simple and non-hormonal to use as a change to condom. Caps and diaphragms are discussed and an examination is undertaken. She has a long vagina and her cervix is retroverted. It is felt that a cap may be difficult to use and a diaphragm is therefore fitted. A size 90 is inserted and the patient can remove it then replace it

Continued

herself. She is given spermicide gel, applicator, and a box of emergency contraception (levonorgestrel, sold in the United Kingdom as Levonelle® and in the United States as Plan B®) as well as some condoms. She is asked to come back in 2 weeks with the diaphragm in for a check and to "practice" with it until then—putting it in, keeping it in for at least 6 hours, removing it, and in fact, carrying out all her normal activities with the diaphragm in to ensure it is comfortable. She returns in 3 weeks. You ask if a trainee can come and sit in with her while the consultation is being carried out as diaphragm use is rare in this area. She refuses, however, and says that she does not like the diaphragm, it is messy, she forgets to use it, and she now has a urinary tract infection (UTI). She does not want to use a cap and feels she now wants to try something hormonal. She is counseled for and fitted with an IUS.

Case Study 8-15

Ms. N is 34 years old and has used a diaphragm for the last 3 years. She finds it easy to use and likes the fact it is in her control and she does not need to take hormones. She has three children and has come in for a refit of her diaphragm, as she is 8 weeks postpartum. A size 85 diaphragm is fitted and she has previously used this size, so there is no change. She is breastfeeding but is advised that she can use emergency contraception should she have any concerns. She continues to use spermicide and is very happy with this method.

---

able to become pregnant (whether they are attempting to become pregnant or trying to avoid it). Fertility awareness takes between 3 and 6 months to learn effectively.

As many indicators of fertility as possible should be monitored, and the symptothermal method is the most reliable (Clubb & Knight, 1996). Fertility awareness and natural family planning includes:

- Measuring basal (waking) body temperature
- Identifying cervical mucus symptoms
- Identifying changes in the cervix
- Recording cycle lengths and using calendar calculations
- Other minor indicators of fertility

Temperature

Temperature should be taken immediately on waking with a specific fertility thermometer. It can be taken orally, vaginally, or rectally. The basal temperature increases by about 0.2°C following ovulation due to secretion of progesterone from the corpus luteum. This higher level is maintained until the next period.

Cervical Mucus

Cervical glands (or crypts) produce mucus that changes in consistency during the menstrual cycle. At the time of ovulation, the discharge is typically wetter and more slippery than the mucus at other times of the cycle. Fingertip testing shows that this mucus is profuse, thin, transparent, and stretchy and is often described as being like raw egg white.

Cervical Changes

At ovulation the cervix is higher, feels shorter, and is open and wet. A woman can examine herself to determine the normal position of her cervix and how it changes when she ovulates.

Calendar Calculations

A calculation based on past cycle lengths can be used to back up the cervical and mucus changes. Ovulation occurs 12–16 days before the next menstruation regardless of cycle length; calculations can be done on the basis of the last six cycles.

The longest and shortest cycles are noted over the last six cycles. Three days are allowed for the viability of the sperm and 2 days for the life of the ovum, taking into account that ovulation might occur on any of 5 days in each cycle.

The calculation is:

Shortest Day (S) minus 20 = Last infertile day of the pre-ovulatory phase

Longest Day (L) minus 10 = Last fertile day

For example: Shortest cycle 27 and Longest cycle 30, so S = 27 and L = 30

Therefore: S − 20 = 7 and L − 10 = 20

This means the last infertile day is day 7 and the last fertile day is day 20. To avoid conception, this couple was recommended to avoid intercourse between days 8 and 20 inclusive. Using the calendar method by itself can give rise to long periods of perhaps unnecessary abstinence, and therefore the full symptothermal methods are advised.

Minor Symptoms

Minor symptoms of ovulation include abdominal cramping and breast pain or tingling due to high estrogen levels. The cramping can be distinguished from the heavy fullness that commences in the second part of the cycle and lasts until menstruation and is a progesterone effect. Libido often increases at the time of ovulation—nature's way of encouraging intercourse at a time most likely for procreation. Premenstrual syndrome, with its associated bloating and emotional lability, signifies a time of low or null fertility.

Fertility awareness is an effective method of contraception if used consistently and committedly by both partners. It is especially effective if taught and supported by a natural family planning teacher. It makes couples aware of their bodies and natural cycles, does not use any chemicals or physical devices, and there are no side effects. It is acceptable to all faiths and cultures. It may not be so useful to women who do not have periods, and takes longer to use and understand if the patient has irregular periods, after stopping hormonal contraception, postnatally, during breastfeeding, after having a termination or miscarriage, or when approaching menopause.

Lactational Amenorrhea Method (LAM)

This method of fertility awareness is only effective if all of the following conditions are met:

- The patient is fully (or almost fully) breastfeeding and not giving the baby any other liquid or solid food
- The baby is less than 6 months old
- The patient is amenorrheic

If all the above points apply, the method is 98% effective. "Almost fully breastfeeding" means the mother is giving no more than a teaspoonful or two of other foods/liquids. Frequent suckling is important to maintain infertility during lactation.

Counseling for Coitus Interruptus

The common name for this contraception method is "withdrawal," as the penis is withdrawn from the vagina before ejaculation. Efficacy is difficult to measure and figures are variable, ranging from 60% to 80%. Efficacy often depends on the skill of the couple and the frequency of sex.

Couples should be counseled that there are sperm present in the pre-ejaculate (which may account for the failure rate) and that spermicide use can increase efficacy. When used effectively and consistently, this method appears to have as good a contraceptive effect as condom use. There are better and more effective methods, but most people accept it as a practical contraceptive solution, and most couples have used this method at some time in their sexual career.

Counseling for Emergency Contraception

"I think I might need emergency contraception; can you tell me what I can use?"

There are three types of emergency contraception currently available in the United States and United Kingdom. Emergency contraception does not cause an abortion; rather, it inhibits or delays ovulation. In some cases, it prevents fertilization if ovulation has already occurred. The methods are the following:

- Progestin-only pill
- Ulipristal acetate
- Copper IUD

Taking a patient's sexual history is paramount in this type of consultation. The practitioner must ask the following questions::

- When was the last episode of sexual contact?
- Have there been any other episodes in this cycle?
- When was her last menstrual period? (from this, you can work out what day of the cycle she is in)
- Was the sexual contact a new partner? (make a risk assessment about STI screening)
- What sort of contraception she has been using?
- General health, past medical history, and family history

It is important to tell the patient the efficacies of all three methods.

While the following presents the U.S. example, practitioners in the United Kingdom and other countries are strongly encouraged to carefully familiarize themselves with the specific product that is licensed for use in their SRH organization.

Case Study 8-16

Mr. A (32 years old) and **Ms. B** (30 years old) are in a committed relationship. They have one child, age 2 years. They have been trying for another pregnancy since the birth of the first child.

Ms. B has heavy, irregular periods. They were referred to a fertility awareness teacher, and following symptothermal charting, it was apparent that Ms. B had late ovulations. The couple had been focusing on having sex on day 14, but Ms. B was ovulating on day 20–23 of her cycle. When they timed intercourse to suit the ovulation, Ms. B became pregnant on the second cycle.

Mr. and Mrs. C, both aged 40, have had five children. Three of these deliveries have been by cesarean section. In her last pregnancy, Mrs. C was advised that she should not have any more children due to high blood pressure and the effects of the surgery. They have never used any formal contraception and are interested in fertility awareness. The fertility awareness teacher spent many visits with them, organizing the symptothermal charts and explaining about fertility. Mrs. C states that her mother had an early menopause, and although her periods are regular at present, this adds an extra complication her fertility awareness for the future. However, the couple are eventually competent and happy to use the method in the knowledge that it may not be for too long, given Mrs. C's family history.

Ms. D is 4 months postpartum and is fully breastfeeding. She has broken up with the father of her child but has developed a new relationship. She wants to use fertility awareness as she "does not like using hormones." She was advised about the use of condoms for prevention of infection and counseled about lactational amenorrhea method. She is happy to use condoms and the LAM in the meantime and will continue to learn about symptothermal testing for the future.

Progestin-Only Pill

The progestin-only pill is available in the United States as Plan B One Step®, Plan B®, Take Action™, Next Choice One Dose™, My Way™, and After Pill™. These products contain the hormone levonorgestrel and are most effective within 72 hours following unprotected sex or suspected contraceptive failure. The mode of action depends on when during the menstrual cycle it is taken, but it can inhibit, delay, or prevent ovulation; or prevent fertilization from occurring.

In the United Kingdom, the available form of progestin-only pill, Levonelle®, contains 1,500 mg of levonorgestrel and is licensed up to 3 days after unprotected sex. Efficacy rates are 96% effective within the first 24 hours, dropping to 85% effective 24–48 hours post-intercourse, and then to 58% effective from 48–72 hours. All the U.S. listed products are available over the counter, except Plan B®, which is available behind the pharmacy counter to women 17 years and over. It is a very safe drug and the only FDA-noted contraindication is known or suspected pregnancy. Side effects, although mild, include headache, abdominal pain, fatigue, nausea, dizziness, and breast pain. Patients should be counseled as follows:

- Consult your PCP or SRH practitioner if you vomit within 2 hours of taking an emergency contraceptive pill.

- This pill may bring on your next period earlier or later and it could be lighter or heavier.

- Please return for a pregnancy test in 3 weeks if your period has not come or is very different from usual.

- If there is risk of STI acquisition, please return in 2 weeks for testing.

- It is a good idea to think about future contraception. Have you decided what you might like to try?

If the patient has decided on a method, it is best to counsel her for a "quick start" if possible. The term *quick starting* has been adopted to describe starting contraception at the time a woman requests it, rather than waiting for the next menstrual cycle. Condoms and barrier methods can be started at any time, but quick starting is outside the terms of the product license for hormonal contraceptives and the LNG-IUS, and is not in line with the instructions for some copper-bearing intrauterine devices (C IUDs) (FSRH, 2015c).

Any CHC, POP, or implant can be commenced immediately and the advice is to use condoms for 7 days and to take a pregnancy test in 3 weeks. The same can be done for the patient requesting a DMPA injection but it is advised that this should not be done as a first-line "quick start" due to the potential problems with a possible pregnancy.

The emergency pill should be given to the patient with some water while the practitioner is in the consulting room and the time given, day of cycle, and time since unprotected sex should all be noted. It is also useful to note what the efficacy is, depending on the time of presentation after sex.

Emergency IUD

It is most important to offer the IUD to every patient who presents for emergency contraception because it is the only method that is virtually 100% effective against conception (**Figure 8-15**). Counseling and device insertion are the same as described earlier in this chapter. However, women requesting the IUD for emergency contraception should also be counseled as follows:

- We cannot absolutely guarantee 100% efficacy.

- Once inserted, the IUD can be used as long-term contraception or we can remove it at your next period if you prefer a different form of contraception.

- If the patient has been with a new partner, give prophylactic antibiotics—especially azithromycin 1 g—when the IUD is fitted to try to ensure no infection of the upper genital tract.

- The IUD can be inserted up to 5 days after unprotected sex or up to day 19 of a 28-day cycle. Therefore, there is usually no need for a sudden decision to be made about the fitting of an IUD.

This author's practice is often to counsel the patient about all types of contraception, give out the most suitable oral hormonal method, and invite her to return at a suitable time for insertion of IUD.

If it is possible to insert the IUD at the time of first consultation, that might be preferable, but sometimes it is not possible if the patient is in a rush or if the correct staff or equipment are not available in the clinic. The reason for offering and giving hormonal emergency contraception before an interval fitting of an emergency IUD is that the patient may not return for an IUD or it may prove technically impossible to fit an IUD with a particular patient.

Many emergency contraception requests are from nulliparous patients and young patients. The IUD is very straightforward in many nulliparous patients; the fact of nulliparity should not dissuade patients from choosing an IUD. In young patients, however, IUD discussion can be

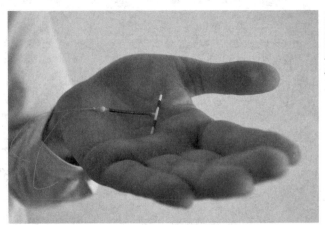

Figure 8-15 Copper IUD

© flocu/iStock/Getty Images

time consuming, as internal examination and speculum use must also be explained. It is better in most cases to involve a parent or guardian, although younger women may not want to discuss their sexual activity with a parent.

Ulipristal Acetate

Ulipristal acetate is available by prescription only under the brand name Ella®. Similar to progestin-only pills, it works by inhibiting ovulation (Rosato, Farris, & Bastianelli, 2015). It is most effective within 120 hours (5 days) of unprotected sexual intercourse or contraceptive failure. Efficacy rates remain at 96% at the fifth day. Ulipristal may be particularly suitable to young women, as efficacy is extended over a longer period and it does not involve internal examination or IUD insertion. As with progestin-only pills it is a safe drug and the only contraindication is known or suspected pregnancy.

Counseling is as follows:

- This form of emergency contraception is effective for up to 5 days after unprotected sex.
- If 1,000 women at risk of pregnancy were to take ulipristal acetate, there would be 5 pregnancies.
- It is very safe, although there are some rare side effects such as nausea and dizziness. If you were to vomit within 2 to 3 hours of taking the tablet, we would advise you to speak to us in case you need a further dose.
- It works by interfering with ovulation, sometimes stopping or delaying it.
- It only works as emergency contraception and does not give you any further protection should you have more unprotected sex.
- If you are going to start or continue any hormonal contraception, you will have to use extra precautions, for example condoms, or abstain for the next 2 weeks.
- Some drugs will interact with ulipristal, including certain drugs you can buy over the counter. It is important that we know about any medications you are taking.
- This tablet can alter your bleeding pattern, so if your period does not come at the expected time, or is lighter or heavier than normal, please take a pregnancy test 3 weeks after the unprotected sex (Prabakar & Webb, 2012).

All three methods of emergency contraception should be discussed with and offered to the patient. However, progestin-only pills are currently more widely available in the United States and the United Kingdom.

If the patient has had one episode of unprotected sex less than 72 hours ago:

- The IUD is the most effective method.

- Ulipristal acetate and levonorgestrel are both effective. Ulipristal has some evidence suggesting it is more effective than levonorgestrel and specifically it seems more effective around the time of ovulation (Brache et al., 2010). However, as has already been discussed, progestin-only pills are more widely available. Ulipristal will not disturb an implanted pregnancy, so if the episode of unprotected sex has been within the last 72 hours, then this can be used.

If the patient has had one episode of unprotected sex 72–120 hours ago:

- The IUD is the most effective method, but ulipristal acetate (Plan B® [United States] or Levonelle® [United Kingdom]) is also licensed for this time period; it may be used and may have some effect, but efficacy is not guaranteed.

If the patient has had one episode of unprotected sex more than 120 hours ago:

- If the expected date of ovulation was 5 days ago (or fewer than 5 days), then an IUD can be fitted (due to its anti-implantation effect). So, in a 28-day cycle, if the episode of unprotected sex was on days 1–19, then an IUD can be fitted even if the patient does not present until more than 120 hours after the actual episode of unprotected sex.

If there has been more than one episode of unprotected sex in this cycle, then:

- An IUD can be used up to 5 days after the last episode of unprotected intercourse or up to day 19 of a 28-day cycle.
- Ulipristal can be used if all the episodes of unprotected intercourse were within the past 5 days.

If a patient presents more than once in the same cycle requesting emergency contraception, then:

- Ulipristal acetate can be used, and this is supported by the WHO.
- Patients should always be informed about STI testing and offered the opportunity to return for a screen in 2 weeks and 12 weeks for blood-borne virus checks.

Case Study 8-17

Ms. O is 28 years old and is studying in the United Kingdom. She has two children who are both at home with her family in Uganda. Her husband has come over to the United Kingdom for a visit; she had sex with him 2 days ago and used a condom, which split. She is HIV positive, as is her husband, and she is on antiretroviral treatment,

Continued

which controls her disease. You look at the website www.hiv-druginteractions.org to check what is advised. Antiretroviral drugs have the potential to either decrease or increase the bioavailability of steroid hormones in hormonal contraceptives. There is limited data, but interactions can potentially alter the safety and effectiveness of both the contraceptive and the antiretroviral drug. After discussion of all the options, Ms. O decides to have a copper IUD fitted as emergency contraception, as this is the most effective and safest method for her. She does not want the possibility of becoming pregnant when she is studying. However, she does not want to use the IUD long term as she is worried about potential heavy periods and the effect that they may have on her health. Therefore, at the same time as the IUD was inserted, she was given an injection of DMPA. She had used this before with good effect but she had let it lapse as she did not think she would need it while studying here. Although this is not ideal, given the small risk of pregnancy and the effects of DMPA, it was felt to be pragmatically the correct decision. She was strongly advised to have a pregnancy test in 3 weeks. The pregnancy test was negative.

Case Study 8-18

Ms. P is 16 years old and attended the clinic 48 hours after having unprotected sex. Her last period was 19 days ago and you find out she attended another clinic 5 days ago following unprotected sexual intercourse (UPSI) and was given "the new tablet." After some investigation, you find she was given ulipristal acetate (Ella®) 5 days ago, mid cycle, having presented following UPSI 94 hours previously. Her periods are regular and she has been with her partner for 2 months. She is advised about an IUD, but she does not want this, and so you suggest Plan B® (United States); Levonelle® (United Kingdom). It is not advised to give ulipristal more than once in a cycle, but levonorgestrel can be used. It is difficult to give a measure of efficacy given this history. Discussion about a long-term method of contraception was undertaken and she decided to have a contraceptive implant inserted. Luckily, this could be done at the same time in this consultation. She was advised that the contraceptive implant would not be effective for 7 days and advised to use condoms. She was advised to come back in 3 weeks for a pregnancy test and to have a *Chlamydia trachomatis* test (advice was also given to ask her partner to attend). She presented in 3 weeks and both tests were negative. She will continue with the subdermal implant. Her partner still has not presented for testing.

Counseling for Sterilization

"I want to be sterilized."

Both male and female sterilization are popular and common procedures. Many patients see the operations as a complete solution to their fertility, but there is a failure rate with both operations. The purpose of this section is to look at what counseling is necessary for both types of procedure.

It is important to remember there are effective alternatives to sterilization; in particular, LARC methods.

Tips for Counseling the Patient

Sterilization is a permanent way of preventing pregnancy and involves having an operation. For women, the method is called tubal ligation or tubal occlusion; for men it is called vasectomy (**Figure 8-16**). If you are in a long-term relationship, you need to consider both methods and decide which one is best for you as a couple.

Vasectomy carries less risk than tubal ligation of getting pregnant again or of complications. Vasectomy is usually done under local anesthetic, while tubal occlusion is usually done in hospital under general anesthesia (although you will usually leave the hospital the same day).

You must keep using contraception right up to the operation and for some time afterward, either until after your first period or until you have a negative sperm test. It is not a good idea to have a tubal ligation at the same time as a cesarean section, or immediately after giving birth or having an abortion. You may regret it later.

You can have tubal ligation or a vasectomy if you are sure that you do not want more children or that you will never want children. If you have a partner, you should discuss and agree together which option suits you best as a couple. Your doctor or nurse can talk to you about your choices and help you to come to a decision. Some couples,

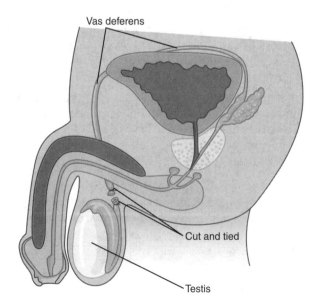

Figure 8-16 Male Sterilization

for example, choose vasectomy rather than tubal ligation because the operation is less risky and there is less chance of getting pregnant again.

Research has shown that you are more likely to have regrets later on if you are under 30 or if you do not have children already. You need to be very sure about your decision and that you fully understand what it will mean. No one can force you to have the operation if you do not want to.

Sterilization fails if the tubes that have been cut (ligation) or blocked (occlusion) as part of the operation join up later. You can get pregnant immediately or at any time (even several years) after a failed operation. There is less chance of a pregnancy after a vasectomy. A pregnancy results for only 1 in every 2,000 men who have been given the all-clear (that is, after tests have confirmed there are no sperm in their semen) after a vasectomy. It seems that the longer it is since your vasectomy, the lower the risk that your partner will get pregnant.

For all methods of tubal ligation or occlusion, there will be around 1 pregnancy in every 200 procedures that are carried out. Over a period of 10 years, 2 or 3 out of every 1,000 tubal occlusions done with Filshie clips resulted in pregnancy (Royal College of Obstetricians and Gynaecologists [RCOG], 2004a, 2004b; **Figure 8-17**).

The main risk after a vasectomy is that your partner gets pregnant because you stop using contraception too soon after the operation; that is, before you have been told that it is safe to do so or before you have had a negative sperm test. If you get pregnant after a tubal occlusion, there is a chance that the pregnancy will develop in the fallopian tube rather than in the womb. This is called an ectopic pregnancy.

All sterilization operations are meant to be permanent. The chances of an operation to reverse it being successful vary a great deal. There is no guarantee of success. The best chances of successfully reversing a tubal occlusion seem to be when clips or rings have been used and when the reversal is done by microsurgery.

A few women develop complications during or after the operation. Your surgeon should tell you more about these risks. All operations carry some risk, but the risk of serious complications is low. You are most at risk of complications if you have had abdominal surgery before or if you are very overweight. Most complications are minor and can be dealt with during the operation. Some, however, such as injuries to the bowel, bladder, or blood vessels, can be more serious and as a result of them some women may need to have a laparotomy (which involves making an opening in your abdomen through either a bikini line or a midline cut). Bowel injuries are rare but they can be very serious.

There is no evidence that having a tubal ligation/occlusion causes problems that would mean you need a hysterectomy. There is no evidence that having a tubal occlusion affects your sex drive.

If you were on the contraceptive pill before your tubal ligation your periods may become heavier again, compared to the withdrawal bleed you had while taking the pill. This is quite normal.

Research shows that if you are over 30 years old when you have a tubal occlusion, it is not linked to getting heavier or irregular periods (Harlow, Missmer, Cramer, & Barbieri, 2002; Peterson et al., 2000; see also Sadatmahelleh, Ziaei, Kazemnejad, & Mohamadi, 2016). There is little evidence about how having a tubal occlusion affects your periods if you have the operation when you are under 30.

To find out whether your vasectomy has been successful, you will be asked to give at least one semen sample, at least 8 weeks after the operation. Exactly how and when these tests are done will vary from area to area.

If there are no sperm in your semen, the test result is negative. You should usually be told that you can stop using contraception.

If you still have sperm in your semen, you should be given another test. You must wait until you get a negative test before you stop using contraception.

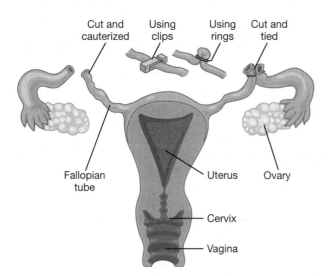

Figure 8-17 Female Sterilization

A few men continue to have small numbers of sperm in their semen, but these sperm do not move (they are known as "non-motile" sperm). It is not always clear whether this means you could make your partner pregnant. If you are one of these men, your doctor will discuss your options with you.

See **Box 8-4** for a discussion of the risks of vasectomies.

Counseling for Postnatal Contraception

"I've just had a baby and want contraception."

This is an important time to discuss future contraception, but it is also useful to discuss contraception in the antenatal period to give the patient more time to reach a decision.

During the consultation, the practitioner should create opportunities for women and/or their partners to raise issues relating to postnatal sexual problems, body image, and mental and emotional well-being. Health professionals should allow opportunities for time alone with women in the antenatal and postnatal period, and should know how and where to access information and support for individuals affected by domestic violence. Postnatal depression is a common problem and again this can be enquired about at a postnatal contraceptive consultation.

Assessment of Contraceptive Needs

Health professionals should find opportunities during both the antenatal and postnatal period to discuss all methods

---

Case Study 8-19

Mrs. Q is 37 years old and wants a sterilization procedure. She is very overweight and her BMI is 40. She has had four pregnancies and has been married for 10 years. She is referred to the gynecology outpatient department, but sterilization is deferred on account of her weight. She is asked to lose weight before the operation. Her husband does not want to go for a vasectomy and she is distraught about this outcome. Eventually, an IUS is inserted with some difficulty. She is initially happy with this method but feels her moods suffer with hormonal intervention and she is not happy with the irregular bleeding. She is referred again to the hospital and a sterilization procedure is carried out—with some postoperative complications mainly due to her weight. The IUS is removed at the procedure. However, 8 months after the procedure you see her again. She is complaining of heavy painful periods and asks for the IUS again. "I really felt good on that." An IUS is again inserted and you have not seen her again.

Case Study 8-20

Mr. B is 44 years old and had a vasectomy when he was 25 years old at the request, he says, of his wife at that time. They had one son and they did not want any more children so that she could concentrate on her career. They broke up shortly after the operation was performed, and Mr. B spent 10 years without a partner. He then met another woman, whom he married. She wanted to have children and he paid privately for the vasectomy to be reversed. The reversal operation was not successful. She has now left him and is pregnant with another man. He has many psychosexual concerns and a huge burden of regret that a vasectomy operation was done so early in his life.
This case study has been included to highlight the regret factor. However, the majority of men who have vasectomy have no further problems.

> **BOX 8-4 Vasectomy: What Are the Risks?**
>
> - There is no evidence that having a vasectomy affects your sex drive.
> - As an operation, it carries less risk than tubal occlusion does for women.
> - Having a vasectomy does not increase the risk of getting testicular cancer or heart disease. Current research suggests that having a vasectomy does not increase the risk of getting prostate cancer (Harvard Health Publications, 2016).
> - Some men get pain in one or both testicles after a vasectomy. It can happen immediately or some time (even a few months) after the operation. It may be occasional or it may be quite frequent. Some men find the pain continues over time; this is known as chronic pain. For most men, however, any pain is quite mild and they do not need further help for it (RCOG, 2004b).
>
> Reproduced from Royal College of Obstetricians and Gynaecologists.(2004). Sterilisation for women and men: What you need to know. Retrieved from https://www.rcog.org.uk/globalassets/documents/patients/patient-information-leaflets/gynaecology/sterilisation-for-women-and-men.pdf

of contraception. Health professionals should assess a woman's postpartum contraceptive needs by taking account of her personal beliefs/preferences, cultural practices, sexual activity, breastfeeding pattern, menstruation, medical, and social factors. The benefits of long-acting reversible contraception (LARC) methods in terms of efficacy should be highlighted to all postpartum women.

Considerations for Breastfeeding Women

Women can be informed that available evidence suggests that use of progestin-only contraception while breastfeeding does not affect breastmilk volume and that there is currently insufficient evidence to prove whether combined hormonal contraception (CHC) affects breastmilk volume. Women can also be informed that progestogen-only contraception has been shown to have no effect on infant growth.

Women may be advised that if they are <6 months postpartum, amenorrheic, and fully breastfeeding, the lactational amenorrhea method is over 98% effective in preventing pregnancy. Women using LAM should be advised that the risk of pregnancy is increased if the frequency of breastfeeding decreases (stopping night feeds, supplementary feeding, use of pacifiers), when menstruation returns or when >6 months postpartum (**Box 8-5**).

BOX 8-5 How to Advise Women on Starting Specific Methods Postpartum

- Women can be advised that contraception is not required before day 21 postpartum.

- If starting a hormonal method on or before day 21, there is no need for additional contraception.

- If starting a hormonal method after day 21, clinicians should be reasonably sure that the woman is not pregnant or at risk of pregnancy and should advise that she avoids sex or uses additional contraception for the first 7 days of use (2 days for the progestogen-only pill), unless fully meeting LAM criteria.

- CHC should not be commenced before day 21 due to the increased risk of thrombosis.

- Non-breastfeeding women may start CHC from day 21 postpartum.

- Breastfeeding women should avoid CHC in the first 6 weeks postpartum as there is insufficient evidence to prove the safety of CHC use while establishing breastfeeding.

- Use of CHC between 6 weeks and 6 months should not be recommended in fully breastfeeding women unless other methods are not acceptable or available. In partially or token breastfeeding women the benefits of CHC use may outweigh the risks.

- Postpartum women (breastfeeding and non-breastfeeding) can start the POP at any time postpartum.

- Non-breastfeeding women can start a progestogen-only injectable method at any time postpartum.

- Breastfeeding women should not start a progestogen-only injectable method before day 21 unless the risk of subsequent pregnancy is high.

- Women should be advised that troublesome bleeding can occur with use of depot medroxyprogesterone acetate (DMPA) in the early puerperium.

- If more convenient, breastfeeding and non-breastfeeding women can choose to have a progestogen-only implant inserted before day 21, although this is outside the product license for Contraceptive implant.

- Unless a copper-bearing intrauterine device can be inserted within the first 48 hours postpartum (breastfeeding and non-breastfeeding women), insertion should be delayed until day 28 onward. No additional contraception is required.

- A levonorgestrel-releasing intrauterine system (LNG-IUS) can be inserted from day 28 postpartum (breastfeeding and non-breastfeeding women). Women should avoid sex or use additional contraception for 7 days after insertion unless fully meeting LAM criteria.

- Women who choose a diaphragm or cervical cap should be advised to wait at least 6 weeks postpartum before attending for assessment of size requirement.

- Women and men considering sterilization should be informed of the permanence of the procedure; about the risks, benefits, and failure rates associated with sterilization; and about other methods of contraception including LARC.

- Women can be advised that unprotected sexual intercourse or contraceptive failure before day 21 postpartum is not an indication for emergency contraception.

- Women can be advised that progestogen-only emergency contraception can be used from day 21 onward and the emergency Cu IUD from day 28 onward (FSRH, 2009).

Data from Faculty of Sexual and Reproductive Healthcare (FSRH). (2017). *FSRH guideline: Contraception after pregnancy. London,* United Kingdom: Author.

Case Study 8-21

Ms. R is 25 years old and is an insulin-dependent diabetic. She is 6 weeks postpartum. She has had a difficult but successful pregnancy and wants to have short-term contraception before she has another pregnancy. She is not breastfeeding and has used the CHC in the past. She has none of the diabetic complications, particularly vascular disease, and is happy to use the COC again for another year as she feels she will then be ready for another pregnancy.

Case Study 8-22

Ms. S telephones you in a panic. She is 2 weeks postpartum and had sex last night without using any contraception. She wonders if she needs emergency contraception. As she is less than 3 weeks postpartum you are able to reassure her that emergency contraception is not necessary just now. You take the opportunity of asking her what she plans to do in the future for contraception and counsel her on her options. She is healthy but unsure what to use so after discussion you send out some literature about different methods. She attends 6 weeks later for an IUS insertion.

Counseling for Contraception and Perimenopause

"I think I might be going through menopause and I want to know what to do about contraception."

Advice about contraception varies with age and circumstances, but no method of contraception is specifically contraindicated due to age alone.

Combined Hormonal Contraception

Women with cardiovascular disease, stroke, or migraine with aura should be advised against the use of CHC. Practitioners who are prescribing CHC to women aged over 40 years may wish to consider a pill with <30 mcg ethinyl estradiol as a suitable first choice. Hypertension may increase the risk of stroke and myocardial infarction (MI) in those using COC. Blood pressure should be checked before and at least 6 months after initiating a woman over 40 years old on CHC and monitored at least annually thereafter.

Progestin-Only Contraception

- Women can be informed that there is no conclusive evidence of a link between progestin-only methods and breast cancer.
- Progestogen-only methods may help to alleviate dysmenorrhea.
- Women should be advised that altered bleeding patterns are common with use of progestogen-only contraception (POC).
- Women should be advised that the LNG-IUS can be used for the treatment of heavy menstrual bleeding once pathology has been excluded.
- Women should be informed that the progestogen-only injectable is associated with a small loss of BMD, which usually recovers after discontinuation.
- Women who wish to continue using DMPA (Depo-Provera®) should be reviewed every 2 years

to assess the benefits and potential risks. Users of DMPA should be supported in their choice of whether or not to continue using DMPA up to a maximum recommended age of 50 years.

- Women can be advised that although the data are limited, POC does not appear to increase the risk of stroke or MI, and there is little or no increase in venous thromboembolism risk.
- Caution is required when prescribing DMPA to women with cardiovascular risk factors due to the effects of progestogens on lipids.

Non-Hormonal Methods of Contraception

- Women should be informed that spotting, heavier or prolonged bleeding, and pain are common in the first 3–6 months of copper-bearing intrauterine device use.
- Men and women can be advised that when used consistently and correctly, male condoms and female condoms are, respectively, up to 98% and 95% effective at preventing pregnancy.
- Women can be advised that when used consistently and correctly with spermicide, diaphragm and caps are, respectively, estimated to be between 92% and 96% effective at preventing pregnancy.
- When using lubricant with latex condoms, a non-oil-based preparation is recommended.

Emergency Contraception and Sexually Transmitted Infections

- Women should be made aware of the different types of emergency contraception available including when they can be used and how they can be accessed.
- Men and women should be advised that the use of condoms can reduce the risk of acquiring and transmitting sexually transmitted infections.

Stopping Contraception

- Women using non-hormonal methods of contraception can be advised to stop contraception after 1 year of amenorrhea if aged over 50 years, 2 years if the woman is aged less than 50 years.
- After counseling (about declining fertility, risks associated with insertion, and contraceptive efficacy), women who have a Cu IUD containing ≥300 mm² copper, inserted at or over the age of 40 years, can retain the device until the menopause or until contraception is no longer required.
- Women who continue to use their IUD until contraception is no longer required should be advised to return to have the device removed.

- Women using exogenous hormones should be advised that amenorrhea is not a reliable indicator of ovarian failure.

- In women using contraceptive hormones, follicle-stimulating hormone (FSH) levels may be used to help diagnose menopause, but should be restricted to women over the age of 50 years and to those using progestogen-only methods.

- FSH is not a reliable indicator of ovarian failure in women using combined hormones, even if measured during the hormone-free interval.

- Women over the age of 50 years who are amenorrheic and wish to stop POC can have their FSH levels checked. If the level is ≥30 IU/L the FSH should be repeated after 6 weeks. If the second FSH level is ≥30 IU/L contraception can be stopped after 1 year.

- Women who have their LNG-IUS inserted for contraception at the age of 45 years or over can use the device for 7 years (off license) or if amenorrheic until the menopause, after which the device should be removed.

Hormone Replacement Therapy and Contraception

- Women using hormone replacement therapy (HRT) should be advised not to rely on this as contraception.

- Women can be advised that a progestogen-only pill can be used with HRT to provide effective contraception but the HRT must include progestogen in addition to estrogen.

- Women using estrogen replacement therapy may use the LNG-IUS to provide endometrial protection. When used as the progestogen component of HRT, the LNG-IUS should be changed no later than 5 years after insertion (the license states 4 years), irrespective of age at insertion. (FSRH, 2010.)

Case Study 8-23

Ms. T is 50 years old and has been using CHC all her life. She has no children but is in a long-term relationship. She has had very sparse bleeding in her pill-free interval for the past year. She wants to know when she can stop contraception. You advise her that you cannot tell this when she is on a CHC, and she can either stop the CHC and use condoms or stop and use the POP. She opts to stop and use condoms. She returns in 4 weeks and you check her FSH and then in 6 weeks' time for another blood test. Both levels are over 30 IU/L. You advise her to continue using condoms for 1 year and then she can discontinue contraception. After 6 months she returns to see you due to her menopausal symptoms. She has had no bleeding but she has insomnia, hot flushes/ hot flashes, night sweats, and pain with sex. She feels awful and begs you to put her back on the pill. After discussion about the benefits and risks of hormone replacement therapy (HRT), she decides to try a combined continuous hormone replacement therapy (CCT HRT). She is warned that there might be some irregular bleeding for the first 6 months. She reattends in 3 months for review. Her symptoms have disappeared; she had slight spotting for 1 month and pain-free sex. She continues on CCT HRT. Although this type of HRT is not specifically contraceptive, it does have a daily dose of progestogen in it equivalent to the progestogen-only pill (POP). Ms. T can use this off-label to provide the contraception she needs for the 6 months or so until she can be reassured she is at no risk of pregnancy. She may, of course, continue to use condoms if this is more reassuring for her.

Case Study 8-24

Ms. U is 53 years old and is on a POP. She is happy on this and has no periods. She has a few menopausal symptoms, which she can cope with. She is advised to stay on the POP until she is 55 years old then stop, which she is happy to do.

Case Study 8-25

Mrs. V is 51 years old. She is married and her husband has a vasectomy. She has embarked on an affair with an old college friend and does not know what to do. She feels no emotional attachment to her husband, but her children are still in school, and she does not want any disruption at home. She feels deeply in love with her old friend but deeply guilty. It is suggested that she perhaps needs to discuss some of her feelings with a counselor, but as a healthcare practitioner, you need to ensure her safety. It would be advisable to discuss the risks of STI and for both partners to be tested. As her new partner does not have a vasectomy, she is at risk of possible pregnancy. She wishes to use a contraceptive that her husband will not be aware of—"we never have sex now anyway." She has heavy, regular periods and is starting to have some menopausal symptoms. An IUS is suggested and is acceptable. This can be explained to her husband as treatment for her gynecological symptoms but is also a contraceptive.

It is important for healthcare practitioners to be non-judgmental, show no possible prejudices or discriminatory behavior, and always to conduct themselves in a professional manner.

Counseling for Contraception for Young People

"I have just started having sex with my boyfriend and I want to be safe."

Legal and Ethical Framework

Whether in United Kingdom or United States, practitioners may wish to inform a young person of the state and federal law in relation to sexual activity. A clinician should assess a young person's competence to consent to treatment by their ability to understand information provided, to weigh up the risks and benefits, and to express their own wishes. Competence to consent to treatment should be assessed and documented at each visit where relevant (e.g., for under-16-year-olds). Health professionals may wish to use checklists to assess competence and risk when providing contraceptive advice or treatment to young people.

Young people should always be made aware of the confidentiality policies for the service they are attending, including the circumstances in which confidentiality may need to be breached.

All sexual and reproductive healthcare services should have a named person identified as the local lead for child protection. All staff involved in contraceptive services for young people should receive appropriate training to alert them to the possibility of exploitation or coercion. Staff should know who they can contact for advice and how to act on child protection issues in accordance with local policy and procedures.

Contraceptive Options for Young People

Young people should be informed about all methods of contraception, highlighting the benefits of long-acting, reversible contraception (LARC), and should be advised to return for follow-up within 3 months of starting hormonal contraception. This allows side effects or other concerns to be addressed and helps ensure correct use of the method. Young people should be encouraged to return at any time if they develop problems with contraception.

Age alone should not limit contraceptive choices, including intrauterine methods. Young people should be made aware of the types of emergency contraception available, when they can be used, and how they can be accessed.

Even if presenting for EC within 72 hours of unprotected sexual intercourse, women of all ages should be offered the copper-bearing intrauterine device or advised how they can access it. See **Box 8-6** for tips on addressing young people's concerns regarding contraceptive use.

BOX 8-6 Addressing Young People's Health Concerns and Risks

- **Weight gain**: Young people may be advised that there is no evidence of weight gain with combined hormonal contraception (CHC) use. Weight gain can occur with depot medroxyprogesterone acetate (DMPA or Depo-Provera®) use, but there is little evidence of a causal association between other progestogen-only methods and weight gain.

- **Acne**: Young people may be advised that combined oral contraception (COC) use can improve acne. Young women whose acne fails to improve with COC may wish to consider switching to a COC containing a less androgenic progestogen or one with higher estrogen content. The progestogen-only implant may be associated with improvement, worsening, or onset of acne.

- **Mood changes and depression**: Young people may be advised that hormonal contraception may be associated with mood changes but there is no evidence that hormonal contraceptives cause depression.

- **Fertility**: Individuals should be advised that there is no delay in return of fertility following discontinuation of the progestogen-only pill or CHC, intrauterine contraception, or the progestogen-only implant. There can, however, be a delay of up to 1 year in the return of fertility after discontinuation of DMPA.

- **Bleeding patterns and dysmenorrhea**: Individuals should be informed that altered bleeding patterns can occur with hormonal contraception use. Primary dysmenorrhea may improve with use of CHC.

- **Bone health**: Young people should be informed that use of the progestogen-only injectable contraceptive (DMPA) is associated with a small loss of bone mineral density, which is usually recovered after discontinuation. DMPA can be used in women under the age of 18 years after consideration of other methods. Women who wish to continue using DMPA should be reviewed every 2 years to reassess the benefits and risks.

- **Thrombosis**: Young people may be informed that although the risk of venous thromboembolism is increased with CHC, the absolute risk is very small.

- **Cancer**: Young people may be advised that COC use is not associated with an overall increased risk of cancer. Rather, COC use reduces the risk of ovarian cancer and the protective benefit continues for 15 or more years after stopping. Any increase in breast cancer with hormonal contraception use is likely to be small and to reduce after stopping. However, there may be a very small increase in the risk of cervical cancer with prolonged COC use.

- **Sexually transmitted infections and young people**: The correct and consistent use of condoms should be advised to reduce the risk of transmission of sexually transmitted infections (STIs). When advising condom use, young people should be informed about correct use of condoms and lubricants, different sizes, types and shapes of condoms, and how to access further supplies, STI screening, and EC. STI risk assessment should be made and testing offered as appropriate, taking window periods into consideration.

Reproduced from Faculty of Sexual and Reproductive Healthcare. (March 2010). Contraceptive choices for young people: Clinical effectiveness unit. Retrieved from https://www.fsrh.org/standards-and-guidance/documents/cec-ceu-guidance-young-people-mar-2010/

Case Study 8-26

This study is historical and is presented in a different format, but like the others is a true but anonymized case.

I first saw Ashleigh about 8 years ago. She had presented to the Young People's Clinic nurse requesting emergency hormonal contraceptive pills. At this time, she was just 13 years old, and the nurse felt she wanted some support.

Ashleigh was a small, thin girl with long, dark hair highlighted with blonde, who sat curled up in one of our chairs. She looked up at me nervously when I came in. I explained who I was and said that the nurse had asked me to see her. She made eye contact again but she didn't say anything. I said I wondered how I could help her.

She looked up and said, "I'm here for the morning-after pill. The nurse said I had to see you first." I said, "That's right, I like to see all the patients about your age and have a chat with them about having sex, about who they are having sex with, and to see if they want to have sex. Do you mind if I ask you some questions?"

"No—on you go," she said.

"Can you tell me when you had sex?"

"Last night about 9 o'clock."

"Is this your first time?"

"No—I"ve been having sex since I turned 13."

"So, how many partners have you had?"

"Three now, this lad is the fourth."

"And do you quite like having sex?"

"It's OK; mostly I've been drinking."

"Do you ever get forced into it?"

"No, it's what they want, and I don't mind. We use condoms, but this one burst."

"What ages are your partners?"

"They are all in my class at school."

I asked her about drinking. "Do you ever feel you drink too much?"

"Yes, sometimes when I go to parties but I'm never 'out of it.' I'd not sleep with just anyone."

"Can you talk to your Mum?"

"No, she'd go ballistic; she's got problems of her own anyway."

"Anyone else you are close to?"

"Well, I can talk to my big cousin; she is 19, and she's OK about things."

I wondered to myself why this patient had started her sexual life so young and what she was looking for by having sex. So I tried again.

"How do you feel having sex; do you enjoy it?"

Continued

She thought a bit. "I don't really FEEL anything, it's not sore like if that's what you mean."

I was concerned about Ashleigh, yet she was competent, seemed to understand what she was doing, and could talk to an adult (but not her mother). "OK," I said, "let's see about the emergency pill." I thought about an emergency IUD but discarded this idea without discussing it with Ashleigh. Why? Perhaps it was her "youngness"—her child-like behavior expressed in the way she was sitting. However, I justified this to myself as the emergency hormonal contraceptive (EHC) was less traumatic and it was less than 24 hours since she had sex.

We talked about EHC, I explained how it worked and how effective it was, I then got some water and watched her take the first tablet. Although we now are able to give EHC as a single dose, 8 years ago we had to give two tablets to be taken 12 hours apart. I impressed on Ashleigh how important it was to take the other tablet in 12 hours and to return if her period didn't come when expected. I asked her about a regular form of contraception but she said she didn't want to go on the pill.

"What about some other method?"

"No, it's alright."

"Well, I'll give you a leaflet. What about condoms?"

"I got some from the other woman." (she meant the nurse.)

"Do you know about the types of infection you can get from having sex?"

"Yeah, we got it at school."

I asked her to come back and speak to one of the nurses but by this time her eyes had completely glazed over and I knew it was time to finish. I gave her information about the young women's groups and hoped she would attend.

I didn't see Ashleigh again until she was just over 14 years. Again, I was asked to see her at the Young People's Clinic. My usual opening: "Hi, my name is Liz Kennedy; I'm one of the doctors here. I don't know if you remember me but I saw you about a year ago. What can I help you with today?"

She smiled a bit at me and seemed to remember.

"I need the morning-after pill."

We went through her story. She had now been going out with Rick, a boy in the year above her at school, for 3 months.

"He is really nice," she said.

"Any other partners?" I enquired.

"No, just him. I haven't been with anyone else for ages."

"Remember when you were here the last time, you told me about other boys you had been with—what happened?"

"I stopped all that, didn't really like it anyway."

So, we went over the emergency contraception again. I asked her about a more regular contraception.

"Well, I've heard the pill makes you fat."

We talked about that misapprehension, but still she didn't want anything but condoms. I discussed DMPA, but she was not keen on needles. I suggested she go for a check-up at the general sexual health clinic and offered to make her an appointment. She said she would make one herself. Again, at that time, 7 years ago, we had no integration of service and no ability to do STI testing in a community setting.

I was happier at that consultation, we had gone over things again, she now seemed to be in a good relationship but she was still 14 and at risk of pregnancy and STI. I found out she had been attending a support group for young women run by some youth workers I knew.

About 10 months later, one of the nurses brought in a set of notes to me.

"I'm a bit worried about this girl—she has been in for emergency contraception 6 times in the last 6 months and I can't get her to consider doing anything safer."

It was Ashleigh.

"Do you think she will come and talk to me?"

She managed to avoid me for a few weeks but eventually, one Monday, I saw her.

She had changed. Her hair was short and spiky; she had piercings and looked about 20 years old. She looked sullen and unhappy.

I explained that we didn't know the long-term effects of using EHC frequently and while we didn't think there were any problems about using a high dose of hormone regularly we didn't know for sure. She considered that. "Yeah, the nurses have said that but it always seems easier just to use condoms and get the pills when I need them."

She was not with Rick anymore. "He dumped me."

She had several other short-term partners. She usually used condoms but not always. She seemed to be drinking heavily at weekends. "But I'm never on the game."

"Can you still talk to your big cousin?"

"Yes, but I don't see her so much now. My mum got bad depression and started drinking and kicked me out. She couldn't cope with me going out so much. I stay with my Gran now but she lives on the other side of the city."

"Do you speak to your Gran?"

"Yes sometimes, she doesn't mind me going out at night."

"So how about thinking of the pill, or the injection, or something else?"

"Wel, OK—I guess I could try the pill."

We went on to a full history; I checked her weight and blood pressure and counseled her about taking the pill. She was a smoker and we talked about smoking and health problems.

Again, the concern with weight: "I won't put weight on, will I?"

She went away with condoms, 3 months' supply of the pill, and a promise to talk to her cousin and maybe her Gran. I asked her again to remember about STIs and offered to make her an appointment, which she declined.

Ashleigh came back to see us in 6 weeks. She complained that she was bleeding all the time and had put on weight. I was concerned about the bleeding. She was at risk of STI, especially chlamydia. She seemed to be taking her pill correctly.

"Tell me what is happening."

"Oh, I'm bleeding all the time, and it's sore when I have sex."

She had not made the sexual health clinic appointment I had suggested at a previous visit. We talked about STIs and that chlamydia was very common; I told her we couldn't test her in this clinic and made her an appointment at the sexual health clinic.

Two months later, Ashleigh returned. Her bleeding had stopped shortly after her last visit so she didn't go to her appointment at the clinic.

She didn't reckon she needed the pill anymore as she was not seeing anyone. So she stopped it. As she had now had no period for 2 months a friend had thought she should come in for a pregnancy test. The test was positive.

She was 15 years old.

"I can't cope with a baby."

We went through her options and counseled her about the process of a termination of pregnancy. She was quite composed and seemed to understand her choices and what she was going to do. She decided to try DMPA after the termination was over.

The following practice applies to the U.K. context. The United States does not have pregnancy termination laws that support this process.

I made her appointment at the termination unit, gave her all the necessary documents, and arranged for her to come back 2 weeks after the termination to see how she was and to find out how the DMPA was suiting her.

Some time later, I received a letter from the hospital stating that she had been for her termination and they had given her an injection of DMPA before she left the ward. The letter also said she had been tested for chlamydia—standard procedure—and found to be positive. She had been given antibiotic treatment. She was planning to attend our young people's clinic for further contraception.

Ashleigh returned eventually. She wanted emergency contraception again. She didn't like the DMPA—it had made her bleed and put on weight. She didn't reckon she needed contraception anyway as "I'm not with anyone." However, she had had sex last night with a boy she knew, didn't use condoms, and was by now not protected by the DMPA.

We talked again mainly about the emergency pill, future contraception, and risk of STI. We talked about herself and how she felt.

"OK," she said.

She thought it might be a good idea to start on the pill again and get another STI check. I thought it might be a better idea if she thought about the implant, which was now available, but she "didn't want anything inside her."

Continued

She went away after taking the emergency pill, getting a 3-month supply of a different sort of pill, and a card to remind her to phone the sexual health clinic.

I felt dispirited; I wondered how Ashleigh was really feeling. Her life was so full of difficulties. She had had a termination and an STI. Her mother was still depressed, and she was staying with her Gran. She had changed schools as she had not been attending her old school, but she didn't like her new school. Her attempts at finding love had not worked. Her life seemed blighted before it had really started.

However, much to my delight, she stayed on the pill. We saw her three times for more pills and then lost touch with her.

I then saw Ashleigh when she was 17. She came in to our new clinic for subdermal rod insertion. She had been seen by one of the nurses in the clinic, who had made out notes for her, counseled her about the implant, and arranged for her to see me for insertion.

I remembered her straight away and she recognized me. During the procedure, she chatted about herself. She had continued on the pill, attending her GP for it as she felt she had "grown out of" the Young People's Clinic.

"It's full of kids."

She had gone to college to sit some exams and was now going to start a nursing course—hence the reason she wanted a reliable long-term contraceptive.

"I'm really pleased to see you again." I told her. "I was always so worried about you when you were younger and I saw you at the Young People's Clinic. What changed?"

She shook her head.

"I don't really know. I was dead stupid back then wasn't I?"

So, that's Ashleigh's story. No answers, but loads of questions.
Why had she taken all these risks?
Why had she been unable to act on information and advice?
Would she be permanently damaged by her experiences as a young teenager?
Could we have done anything different?
Perhaps if she had a more stable background—
Perhaps if she had more self-esteem—
Perhaps if we had been able to offer more integrated care—
We now have a more integrated service offering contraception and STI services in one clinic. We have more stringent child protection guidelines; the United Kingdom has a new Sexual Offences Act. We offer services for all ages including termination services, "office" gynecology, psychosexual medicine, all STI screening, treatment and partner notification, and full range of contraceptives. Support is offered for other issues affecting relationships such as domestic abuse and alcohol counseling. Men and women attend and we hope we are on our way to take the stigma out of sexual issues.

Would this have changed the course of Ashleigh's journey?
Would it help those who follow?
What was the problem with Ashleigh's sexual life? She seemed to understand what she was doing and sometimes even seemed to enjoy it. She was making informed choices—yet there was a feeling of unease. Was she making these choices because she didn't know or couldn't think of any others? Was this due to lack of education, lack of employment, poverty, lack of engagement, or fulfilment with life?

Currently, I still see girls like Ashleigh. We have a better Sexual Health Service and more choices of contraception. Young people's sexual health is a priority for us, but the poverty is not in our services—the poverty is in the lack of true choices and opportunities for young people.

Counseling for Psychosexual Problems

"I have pain having sex—what can I do?"

"I have loss of sex drive—I think it's my pill. Can you change it, please?"

There are many causes of sexual pain, including sexually transmitted infections due to *Chlamydia trachomatis*, *Trichomonas vaginalis*, *Neisseria gonorrhoeae*, herpes simplex; or vaginal infections such as bacterial vaginosis and candidiasis. Other causes of sexual pain are vulvovaginal atrophy caused by lack of estrogen (urogenital atrophy), chemical irritation ("too clean" syndrome), vulvodynia, vaginismus, and skin conditions such as lichen sclerosis. The treatment of these conditions are specific antibiotics, antivirals, and antifungals for the infections, and local or systemic hormone replacement therapy (HRT) for vulvovaginal atrophy. Local anesthetics, antidepressants, physiotherapy for vulvodynia, and genital skin care advice (remove soaps and wipes, avoid conditioners and bleached products) are options for the patients who are being too clean/too cruel to their vulva. However, there are many patients who do not respond to these straightforward measures for helping with pain. These patients may be experiencing psychological distress that is expressed as pain with sex.

The complaint of lack of libido or loss of libido with oral contraception—or any type of contraception—is also common. It is easy to blame a contraception for a change in feeling and hope that an easy change of tablet/method might be a magic wand in bringing desire back to a relationship. It is often impossible in a short consultation to discuss all possible reasons for loss of libido, and it may be initially better to change the method as requested. However, it may be possible to ask about lifestyle and relationship. What has changed since libido was good? Are there different workloads, financial problems, perceived lack of support from the partner or partners family? Do children (or the lack of them) play a part in the dissatisfaction? Pointers and reflections can be offered and the patient might like to think about the issues and return for a further appointment (Skrine, 1997). All psychosexual issues are different, just as all patients and relationships are different. Generalization is impossible, so psychosexual issues are best discussed using scenarios (Skrine & Montford, 2001).

Case Study 8-27

Mrs W came into the room looking quite angry, I thought. Well dressed as if for work in an office. Quite disapproving. Severe. Her hair was tied back and she wore dark-rimmed glasses.

This was reflected in her words at first: "I don't know why I've been asked to complete this form. I don't really want to be at this clinic." The form was for an audit I'm doing; I reassured her and said she did not have to complete it. She went on, "I really don't like coming to this clinic; there are men in the waiting room."

I spent the first few minutes trying to settle her, put her a bit more at ease. I explained the different clinics that were going on. I thought, *Why am I trying to keep this woman so happy?*

"So, what can I do to help?"

"I've got this discharge, it has been there for years, they have taken swabs and said everything is fine. I don't know what is wrong. I can't have sex either, it's too sore."

I began to see this patient's façade slipping a bit, and she seemed more gentle and not so cross.

"What's it like?"

She misunderstood me. "The discharge is white and sometimes clear; sometimes it is there and sometimes not. I want to be normal again."

"What's normal for you?" I tried again.

"I freeze every time he comes near me; we've been married for 15 years. I have three girls and was a single Mum for 10 years. He came along and brought them up; I just want to be me now."

She told me her story—her first marriage broke up when her girls were young. She held herself together for the sake of the children. Then she met Dave. "Sex was good at first. Everything has been fine, you know, but for the past 5 years, we haven't had sex. We don't live together now, he just wants me to be happy and so he has moved out. He stays with me every weekend and we share a bed but every time he comes near me I just freeze. I can't let him near me. He doesn't want to pressure me; we are great friends. I just don't like to think about sex any more."

I'm a bit puzzled—I don't really know what to say.

More story followed: "Dave has struggled with depression for all his life. His father was schizophrenic; he was always worried he would have that. Sometimes he was high and happy, most of the time he was depressed—he couldn't do anything, just sat for days in his pajamas staring at the wall. Given antidepressants by doctor but these made him flat, and he complained he couldn't feel anything. Had to give up his job, then retrained as a support worker for young people and now is much better. Still gets depressed but can sit by himself in his own flat and doesn't feel he is bothering anyone. He refuses to take any more medication.

My three girls have left home now, live in New Zealand, the United States, and Ireland. I miss them; I don't have the same relationship with them that I had with my mother. My mother died about 8 years ago after a long illness—Alzheimer's."

"How did you cope with that?"

"Just had to. I was the one here—my brother was in Canada and he was useless, he said he wanted to remember her as she was. It would be great to have that choice, but I had to cope."

Continued

"Sounds like that is what you have done all your life."

She paused. "I suppose I have had to rely on myself a lot. But now I am by myself, I want to do something for me. I thought things would get easier as I got older, but they are so difficult. There's nothing." Tears were in her eyes now. I felt sad for her.

We held the silence for a bit, and then I asked her how she would like things to be. She said Dave was much more stable now, "and even his bad days aren't so bad. I would like us to be a couple again."

"I wonder if it would help if I examined you again," I said. "I know you have had all the swabs and everything is negative, but sometimes an examination of the area that is hurting you can let us see where the pain is. Pain in your life often shows up as pain in your body, and if part of the pain is sexual and private, it often comes in the private areas of the body."

She agreed to examination and went behind the screen. The severe lady who had come in to the consulting room had disappeared, and the atmosphere was much better.

Examination started fairly easily; she had definite atrophic changes in the vulva. She said "I hope you don't need to use the spec . . . thing, it was really sore when I was here to see the nurse for the swabs."

I said I was just going to examine her with my fingers to feel how everything was. She put her hand out and touched my hand.

"I'm frightened of having sex again. He kept pushing me away when he was depressed, even when he was happy, I knew he was going to get depressed again really soon and would reject me. I had to care for my Mum, protect my girls, and pretend that nothing was wrong. But I have always loved him and just want to be with him properly." Tears started.

In the end I did not examine her. She got dressed and came back to sit down.

We talked about what she was frightened of—pain, rejection, emptiness. We talked about her barriers of being busy, always coping, never letting her guard down. I said when she came in to the consulting room at first I was a bit nervous of her; she looked so confident and seemed cross with everything. She smiled a bit at this and agreed. The atmosphere now was quite friendly.

We talked about her sex drive and I said everyone has a sex drive but everyone chooses their own way to use it. She could pick up her sex drive and use it again if that was now what she wanted. The answer was in herself; she had her libido previously, and she could choose to have it again.

We also talked about HRT and lubrication to help with any difficulty and about menopausal changes. She decided to use local estrogen and I wrote to her PCP (GP) to ask for a lubricant.

I asked her to come back if she felt she wanted to talk again, but I haven't seen her since.

Case Study 8-28

Miss X was a patient I was asked to see by one of the nurses in our department.

She had had treatment for herpes simplex virus (HSV) 2 years ago, but had come back with pain again. She did not want to be examined. She also felt her contraception wasn't working well and made her depressed and moody. She cried constantly during the consultation and my colleague felt out of her depth.

She presented as a student in jeans, top, and scarf. Slightly overweight, mild acne, black hair tied back. She seemed nervous and tense.

"What can I do to help you today?" I asked

The tears came immediately. "I want to feel normal again, I want sex to be natural, he is so good, but I am only 23 and don't want to go on like this, he'll leave me if I don't get this sorted, I have to force myself to do it, it's so sore—whenever he touches me. I don't want to do it, it should be natural but it's not, everyone else is OK, why has this happened to me?" She cried and cried—unhappy, messy tears.

The storm of tears and grief was quite overwhelming. I offered the box of tissues and sat quietly for a little while. I noticed that I didn't touch this patient—sometimes I put my arm round someone or pat their hand . . . but not with this patient. I wondered why.

I tried to find something to say that would match the emotion. "You seem sad about this," didn't seem to fit so I said, "That was quite overwhelming for me, so it must be completely awful for you to have so much grief."

She looked at me and nodded.

She then was able to tell me her story. She had her first sex with a partner when she was 18. She had just left home to come to college. From her first episode of sex, she got herpes. "It was awful—the nurse said it was the worst case she had ever seen." She had to be admitted to hospital and was catheterized. She was away from home and was sore, lonely, ashamed, and guilty.

She got treatment and counseling about HSV. She gradually felt better about it and although she got recurrences, it was OK and she could cope.

She met her current partner, Barry, about a year afterward, and for the first 6 months, it was fine. She told him about her herpes and they both read up about it. He said that he had had cold sores in the past, so it didn't bother him. Sex was good, she said; she enjoyed it and life was going well. She was at college, had a part time job, was close to her family and had a nice boyfriend.

Then she started going off sex. It was sore and Barry didn't want to hurt her, sometimes she felt she had a discharge, sometimes she felt she had a recurrence of HSV. She was also having problems with her contraception, she felt "woozy" with one type of pill, another made her skin worse. She wondered if the pill caused loss of sex drive. She had been counseled on various other forms of contraception but wanted to stay on pill as it made her periods better. Eventually she found that Gedarel 30/150® was good.

She told me that she had always had painful periods, used to have to stay off school and go to bed. She also said that she couldn't use tampons and one time had been given a pessary for "thrush" and felt sick at the thought of using it. She has not had a cervical smear because she didn't like the thought of it.

I wondered if I could examine her but she refused, saying she had a stomach upset and did not feel clean. "I hate being touched, you know."

"You know that's funny, as I didn't feel it was right to touch you when you were crying. You must put out vibes."

She agreed and looked quite pleased.

I was a bit stymied—was this control, defense, power? I had to find out more, so I said: "What happened the last time you had sex?"

"Well, we were in bed, and I said to Barry it would be OK. We hadn't done it for a long time and I knew he wanted to."

"Were you ready to have sex—does he touch you first?"

"Oh no, I don't like that. I don't touch myself you know, it's sore."

"Did you feel excited or wet?" I pressed. I found I really wanted to know what happened during sex with this patient.

She started to cry again. "He doesn't come inside me. I can't let him, I feel ashamed and guilty, and I know it's not natural, but I just can't do it."

Eventually I found she was masturbating him and there was no penetration. There had never been any penetration except the first time she had ever had sex, with her first partner—"and look what happened then."

She couldn't let Barry touch her and she had never been orgasmic, couldn't masturbate. I now understood where the feeling of being overwhelmed came from. This seemed a huge problem, one which she was overcome by.

"This is awful for you; it seems so unfair that sex, which is supposed to be good and fun and awesome has turned out to be so devastating."

She nodded.

We had some discussion then about her feelings about the herpes, her distaste about that area of her body, her lack of orgasm. She explained that she had never been very confident about her body, she felt overweight and ugly, but then she met this lovely boy when she arrived at college, he made her feel so good. . . . "Then I got herpes. He left me, just texted me a few times."

The feeling again was of sadness but also of anger, and I found I was angry with this "lovely boy."

"You know, I've never met this boy but I'm so angry with him. How do *you* feel about him?"

"I bloody hate him."—bit of a smile through the tears.

I handed her the tissues and touched her hand.

Case Study 8-29

Ms. Y stood up when I called her in from the waiting room. She moved quickly and was stick thin. She wore leggings and a tight-fitting T shirt; her hair was blonde with dark roots, and she had a tattoo on her neck.

You note, I had already made a bit of a judgment.

I noticed from her notes that she had been to see us three times recently complaining of discharge; swabs were always taken, and on two occasions she had been positive for bacterial vaginosis (BV), treated with metronidazole, and given advice about the use of acidic gels. She had also been counseled about genital skin care and advised to use emulsifying ointment and avoid conditioners and soaps.

She sat down and she complained about her discharge again and finally said that, "Really, I've come because sex is sore and I'm fed up."

The way she told me sounded as if she was really sad about it . . . or was it anger or irritation?

"That sounds upsetting for you."

"Yes, I really liked sex. I've always enjoyed it but now I can't be bothered any more."

I wondered out loud why this had happened.

"Well, it's not very nice being smelly down there all the time. I'm so dry as well, it's like sandpaper."

"Is that what happens? Has none of the treatment helped?"

"Well it helps a bit, but it always comes back and I'm just fed up now." A flash of anger. "Every time he comes back, we have sex and this happens again. I hate having sex now."

"Comes back . . . Does he work away from home?"

"No, I get angry with him and we fall out and then I throw him out."

"That doesn't sound a very easy way to live—is that the way things have always been between you two?"

"No, it was great at first. We had our two kids, a boy and a girl, and then I got pregnant again last year. He didn't want it, said we had two children and couldn't afford any more. I kind of agreed, always said we'd just have two children, went for a termination."

"Was it OK?"

"No, it was awful. The nurses were nice and all, but he never came with me, went away to his work that day. I had to get my mother to look after the kids; he never even asked me how it went. Won't say anything about it now. Seems like it never happened for him. Now every time we fight, every time we have a drink it's always about that."

"Does anyone else know?"

"No, just you and my doctor. Told my Mum I was going in for an operation to help my periods. They put a coil in." I looked at her; she looked so defeated, sad, angry, and unhappy.

"What do you want to happen now?"

She looked into space. "I want this coil out, I want to have sex again and enjoy it, and I want us to be together again. I feel dried up and dead inside." A cry of misery and a kind of sob in her voice. She looked desolate, dry eyed.

"You look empty and so sad, I feel sad as well. . . . Do you think your man feels like this, too?"

She shrugged and seemed to focus again.

"So, what can I do?" she said.

"I think you know what you want to do; is it possible for you to do it?"

She thought for a bit, "I'll away home and try to speak to him without a drink so I don't get angry. Perhaps that will make things better."

I agreed and the consultation ended. No examination done.

I checked her notes again before writing this, and she had her IUS removed 2 weeks ago.

How to Bring These Cases of Sexual Problems Together

- **Mrs. W** was so busy holding herself together that her libido was squeezed out and replaced with pain.
- **Miss X** was betrayed by sex and scared of her pain.
- **Ms. Y** had her choice removed, and her pain and loss of libido reflected this.

With respect to desire and arousal, sex drive decreases as men and women age, but women are two to three times more likely to be affected. In younger patients, desire triggers arousal, but in older patients or those who have had sexual difficulties in the past, desire follows arousal. Patients often have to be "taught" how to have sex. A patient may have to make a conscious decision to allow herself to be aroused before any desire for sex or enjoyment is found.

Contraception is involved in these patient's cases, but is not the major factor in addressing their problem. However, it was in a sexual health clinic that they presented, so it is important for any health professional to look at the patient as a whole person and not as a symptom or a case.

Counseling for Contraception Following Termination of Pregnancy

"I've just had a termination; what can I do for future contraception?"

Ideally, the patient who has decided to have a termination should have been given the opportunity to think about all suitable methods before the termination procedure is carried out. After the decision to terminate a pregnancy has been made, the next question should be what to use for contraception in the future.

Termination of pregnancy is not a simple decision emotionally, and it is important to help the patient avoid being in that situation again. Pregnancy, fertility, termination, and decisions surrounding this are fraught with problems. It can be a hugely emotional situation for a woman to realize she is pregnant and does not want to be. She may be in a stable relationship and not wish another child for personal or economic reasons. She may have started in a new relationship and does not want to have a child so soon. She may be in a bad or abusive relationship and does not want to have a child with this man.

Again, as with many areas associated with women's fertility and control of that fertility, people have strong opinions about what is right and what is wrong. If a practitioner feels that termination of pregnancy does not fit within their moral code, it is essential to refer the patient to a practitioner who is able to accept that option. The Royal College of Obstetricians and Gynaecologists (RCOG) and the American Congress of Obstetricians and Gynecologists (ACOG) have produced guidance on this topic that includes the following principles:

- Healthcare staff caring for women requesting abortion should identify those who require more support in the decision-making process.
- Pathways to additional support, including counseling and social services, should be available.
- Women should be given information about the different methods of abortion appropriate to gestation, the potential adverse effects and complications, and their clinical implications.
- Where possible, women should be given the abortion method of their choice.

Termination of pregnancy in the United States and United Kingdom is complicated and is generally dictated by state laws and professional guidelines. Practitioners must check local laws to review both duties and options in counseling and making recommendations for women wishing termination.

Guidelines suggest that methods of contraception can and should be started immediately after termination. An IUD or IUS can be inserted immediately; CHC methods and POP can be started immediately, as can a contraceptive implant or DMPA. Starting regimens:

- CHC: Up to and including day 5 post abortion (day 1 for estradiol valerate/dienogest pill). At any other time, if it is reasonably certain she is not pregnant, but use extra precautions for 7 days.
- DMPA (Depo Provera®): Initiate on day of surgical or second part of medical abortion or immediately following miscarriage: No additional contraception is required. If started >5 days after abortion or miscarriage, additional contraception is required for 7 days.
- POP: Initiate on the day of surgical abortion or second part of medical abortion or immediately following miscarriage. POPs initiated >5 days after surgical abortion or second part of medical abortion or miscarriage require extra precautions for 48 hours.
- Implants (Nexplanon®): Can be inserted up to day 5 following surgical abortion, second part of medical abortion or miscarriage. No additional contraception is required. If inserted beyond 5 days after abortion or miscarriage, then additional contraception is required for 7 days.
- IUD/IUS: Ideally insert at the time of a first- or second-trimester surgical abortion for immediate contraceptive effect. Following medical or surgical abortion, ideally insert within the first 48 hours or delay until 4 weeks postpartum. However, waiting until 4 or more weeks post-termination may put women at risk of pregnancy. After counseling and when intrauterine contraception is the preferred method, it can be inserted by an experienced clinician at any time post-abortion if there is no concern that the pregnancy is ongoing.
- Condoms and other barrier methods should be used immediately.

Case Study 8-30

Ms. Z is 21 and planning to finish college and apply to enter the Diplomatic Corps. She has recently started seeing a new partner of 2 months and become pregnant. She has not been using any form of contraception. Her new boyfriend is going to be studying abroad for the next year. She decides on a termination even though "she always thought she wouldn't" and opts for an implant. She was counseled for this in her pre-termination consultation. The implant is then inserted before she has been discharged, following a medical termination.

Case Study 8-31

Ms. AA is 33 years old and has recently found that she is pregnant. She was always told she couldn't become pregnant as she has polycystic ovarian syndrome, and she has never used contraception. She is shocked and distressed, as she has no regular partner and never wanted any children. She is counseled for an IUS in her pre-termination consultation and an appointment is made for her to attend the clinic on the day of her termination for insertion. She is happy to go ahead and the insertion is uneventful and straightforward. However, she reattends after 3 weeks and requests removal. She now feels she has made the wrong decision although has had full counseling beforehand. The IUS is removed and further counseling is offered and accepted.

Contraception Service Provision in the United States

This section presents an overview of the magnitude of demand for contraceptive services, types, and role of the healthcare providers.

Reported figures show that there were almost 3 million unintended pregnancies in the United States during 2008–2011 (Finer & Zolna, 2016). By the age of 45 years, more than half of all American women will have experienced unintended pregnancy, and 3 in 10 will have had an abortion (Jones & Kavanaugh, 2011). In 2013, the records revealed 67 million U.S. women of reproductive age 13–44 years. More than half (38 million) were in need of contraceptive services and supplies in terms of being sexually active with the possibility of becoming pregnant, though not pregnant and did not wish to conceive (Frost, Frohwirth, & Zolna, 2015).

The Need for Publicly Funded Services

Of the 30 million women in need of contraceptive services in 2013, 20 million required publicly funded services and supplies because of their low-income status (below 250% of the federal poverty level). That applied to 15.3 million women (77%); another 4.7 million (23%) also required publicly funded services because they were below the age of 20 years (Frost et al., 2015).

A steady increase in the need for contraceptive services has been transpiring since 2000, and Medicaid is reported as bearing 75% of the total expenditures, while states bear 12% and Title X bears 10%. The other sources reported are maternal and child health block grants, social services block grants, with Temporary Assistance for Needy Families (TANF) bearing 3% of the funding expenditure (Sonfield & Gold, 2012). A safety-net health center that provides contraceptive services represents a site that offers contraceptive services to the general public and uses public funds, including Medicaid, to provide free or reduced-fee services to some clients.

Provider agencies include public health departments, Planned Parenthood affiliates, hospitals, community health centers, and other independent organizations. Some of these centers specialize in the provision of contraceptive services while others offer contraceptive care within the context of comprehensive primary care (Frost, Zolna, & Frohwirth, 2013). Contraceptive needs are generally provided for within Planned Parenthood centers, health department clinics, federally qualified health centers, and hospital outpatient clinics.

The Title X family planning program represents the only dedicated source of federal funding for family planning services. This system advocates high quality, culturally sensitive family planning services and other preventive health care. The services are offered confidentially to low-income, underinsured, and uninsured individuals who may not otherwise get access to the comprehensive family planning services that they need. Title X is the only federal program that funds the family planning program, as public services not paid for under Medicaid and private insurance. State, county, and local health departments make up the majority (53%) of Title X service providers. Hospitals, family planning councils and Planned Parenthood affiliates, federally qualified health centers, and other private, non-profit organizations make up the rest of the Title X network (National Family Planning and Reproductive Health Association [NFPRHA], 2016).

Reported Impact of U.S. Family Planning Services

In 2013, publicly funded family planning services were reported to have avoided 2 million unintended pregnancies, which could have resulted in numerous unintended births and nearly 700,000 abortions (Frost et al., 2013). In 2010, STI testing services provided as part of publicly funded family planning consultations prevented 99,000 chlamydia infections and 16,000 gonorrhea infections (Frost et al., 2013; Frost, Sonfield, Zolna, & Finer, **Figure 8-18**).

CDC: Recommended Strategies to Prevent Unintended Pregnancies

The CDC strategies to prevent unintended pregnancies aimed to remove avoidable medical hindrances to the use of

Effectiveness of Family Planning Methods

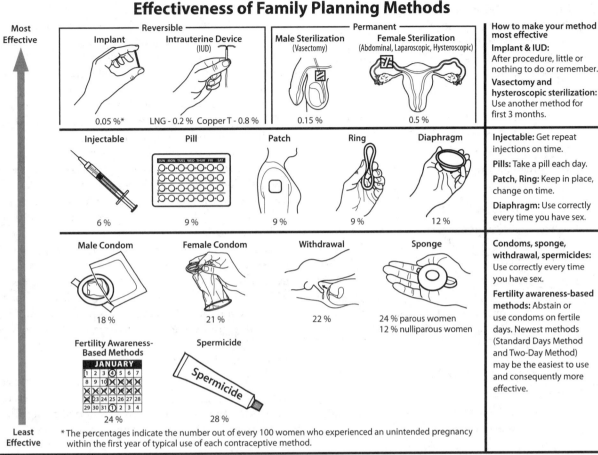

* The percentages indicate the number out of every 100 women who experienced an unintended pregnancy within the first year of typical use of each contraceptive method.

CS 242797

CONDOMS SHOULD ALWAYS BE USED TO REDUCE THE RISK OF SEXUALLY TRANSMITTED INFECTIONS.

Other Methods of Contraception

Lactational Amenorrhea Method: LAM is a highly effective, temporary method of contraception.

Emergency Contraception: Emergency contraceptive pills or a copper IUD after unprotected intercourse substantially reduces risk of pregnancy.

Adapted from World Health Organization (WHO) Department of Reproductive Health and Research, Johns Hopkins Bloomberg School of Public Health/Center for Communication Programs (CCP). Knowledge for health project. Family planning: a global handbook for providers (2011 update). Baltimore, MD; Geneva, Switzerland: CCP and WHO; 2011; and Trussell J. Contraceptive failure in the United States. Contraception 2011;83:397–404.

Figure 8-18 Effectiveness of Family Planning Methods
Reproduced from CDC. (n.d.). Effectiveness of family planning methods. Retrieved from https://www.cdc.gov/reproductivehealth/unintendedpregnancy/pdf/contraceptive_methods_508.pdf

contraception. Moreover, these aimed at encouraging women and men who are likely to get unintended pregnancies to decide on and select appropriate contraceptive methods that they can use correctly and consistently to achieve effective pregnancy prevention.

The U.S. Selected Practice Recommendations (U.S. SPR) for Contraceptive Use 2013 (American Congress of Obstetricians and Gynecologists [ACOG], 2013; Curtis et al., 2016) provides evidence-based guidance that addresses routine yet quite complex management issues relating to commencement and use of specific contraceptive methods. The recommendations include the timing when women can commence to use contraceptive methods and what physical examinations and laboratory tests may be required before commencement of a particular method. Also included are recommendations on appropriate follow-up visits/consultations and how to address

contraceptive method side effects. The American Congress of Obstetricians and Gynecologists (ACOG) endorses the U.S. SPR and encourages its fellows to use the document *Understanding and Using the U.S. Selected Practice Recommendations for Contraceptive Use 2013* (ACOG, 2013).

The U.S. Medical Eligibility Criteria (U.S. MEC) for Contraceptive Use 2010 focuses on guidance about who can safely use specific methods of contraception. Thus, the U.S. MEC provides recommendations specifically to guide safe contraceptive methods for women with certain medical conditions such as hypertension and diabetes, and characteristics such as age, parity, and smoking status. Healthcare providers use these documents together with CDC provider tools including summary charts, U.S. MEC Wheel, and mobile tools to access this guidance (Centers for Diseases Control and Prevention [CDC], 2010).

The CDC Contraceptive Guidance for Healthcare Providers (June 17, 2015)

The CDC published comprehensive recommendations for provision of family planning services. These comprise the following:

- Providing contraception to enable women and men plan and space births, prevent unintended pregnancies, and reduce the number of abortions.
- Offering pregnancy testing and counseling services.
- Supporting clients with a desire to achieve conception.
- Providing basic infertility services.
- Providing preconception health services to improve outcomes for the infant and mother and improve the health of women, their infants, and men.
- Providing sexually transmitted disease (STD) screening and treatment services to prevent potential complications that could lead to tubal infertility and improve the sexual health of women and men, and the health of their infants.

The recommendations emphasize the importance of the following:

- Defining the essential or core set of family planning services for women and men
- Describing the contraceptive services provision, and other related clinical services, adolescent services, and performance of quality improvement
- Encouraging the use of family planning visits to provide selected preventive health services for women, in accordance with the recommendations for women issued by the Institute of Medicine (IOM) and adopted by the Department of Health and Human Services

Five Key Stages in Contraceptive Service Provision

- Establishing and maintaining rapport
- Obtaining clinical and social information
- Work interactively: select most effective medically appropriate method
- Physical assessment, when warranted
- Provide method, instructions, follow-up plan; confirm understanding

Clinicians are required to discuss all methods that can be used safely and correctly by the patient. Physical examination should be limited and blood pressure evaluation should be carried out before commencement of hormonal contraceptives, or pelvic examination before insertion of an intrauterine device; weight monitoring may also be useful. Documentation of the contraception consultation should record the patient's understanding of the use, benefits, risks, and individualized follow-up plan. All patients, including adolescents, lesbian, gay, bisexual or transgender, patients with disabilities, or those with limited English proficiency should receive high-quality care in a tolerant and non-judgmental atmosphere. The CDC advocates advanced provision of emergency contraception because no test reliably verifies cessation of fertility. Therefore, it is practical to consider contraceptive use until menopause or until the age of 50–55 years.

Family physicians are considered uniquely suited to deliver an all-encompassing family planning service to patients of all ages (Frost, 2013). Clinicians are challenged to apply evidence-based expert professional knowledge on how to achieve or prevent pregnancy and treat STIs. They also have professional responsibility to offer the safest and most effective options available for patients with various medical conditions, social circumstances, adherence problems, and financial barriers to care. These stages should be implemented together with a tiered approach to counseling that begins with the most effective methods. Some key elements of contraceptive counseling are briefly outlined here. Rational communication and task-oriented communication are briefly considered in relation to contraceptive counseling.

Rational Communication in Counseling

Rational communication is defined as interpersonal interactions that contribute to forming a positive therapeutic relationship between the provider and the patient. The underlying principles relate to the inherent ethical value of positive interpersonal interactions and evidence that links positive patient–provider communication with improved health outcomes.

Rational communication involves the following:

- Developing close personal relationship toward fostering a therapeutic relationship: Should avoid dismissing concerns expressed by the patient
- Building trusts Should involve respectfully addressing the patient's concerns about contraceptive methods. There should be no pressuring of women to use a specific method.
- Optimizing decision-making dynamics: Includes incorporating aspects of shared decision making and focusing on patient preferences for the merits of given contraceptive methods. It should not convey assumptions that efficacy is the only or most important merit to consider. The practitioner should avoid using self-disclosure as a means of directing a patient to a specific method (Dehlendorf, Krajewski, & Borrero, 2014).

Task-Oriented Communication in Counseling

Task-oriented communication, on the other hand, is defined as conveying essential information about diagnosis and treatment options and plans. The underlying principle is the evidence linking provision of information with improved health outcomes. This approach involves offering adequate evidence-based counseling about side effects, but the process should not arouse concerns about the potential for side effects that have not been substantiated by any association with a given method. Additionally, this involves anticipating and addressing barriers to consistent and correct contraceptive use and the practitioner should not fail to consider possible limitations in understanding health-related terms and figures about contraceptive efficacy. Task-oriented communication should also take into account advance provision of emergency contraception to all sexually active women. The practitioner should not create barriers to switching methods if a patient is dissatisfied; instead, he or she should address misconceptions of low susceptibility to pregnancy and abstract concepts such as percentages or relative risks should not be used when communicating about risks and effectiveness. Counseling about dual protection for women at risk of STIs should include consideration of self-efficacy for negotiating condom use. Consideration should be given to protective coercion and offering harm-reduction strategies (Dehlendorf et al., 2014).

Disparities emerge in contraceptive counseling, perhaps unintentionally, but it is crucial that practitioners develop awareness of personal biases in order to make a conscious effort to overcome or curb the potential impact on professional behavior. The practitioner should not assume that suppressing deliberate and calculated stereotyping automatically eliminates the potential effect of consistently biased and limited health communication.

Additional Guidance: Sources for Healthcare Providers

Services to be offered during a family planning clinic visit:

- High quality, evidence-based family planning services in accordance with recommendations of the CDC and the U.S. Office of Population Affairs 2014.

Best ways to initiate and manage specific contraceptive methods:

- *U.S. Selected Practice Recommendations for Contraceptive Use, 2013* adapted from the *World Health Organization Selected Practice Recommendations for Contraceptive Use, 2nd edition.*

Contraceptive methods recommended as safe for women with specific characteristics and medical conditions:

- *U.S. Medical Eligibility Criteria 2nd edition for Contraceptive Use, 2010.* Update for use during postpartum period, and for those with, or at high risk of, human immunodeficiency virus infection.

Treatment recommended as appropriate for persons who have or are at high risk of sexually transmitted infections:

- *CDC Sexually Transmitted Diseases Treatment Guidelines, 2015* (Updated for drug resistance patterns).

Information available for patients who are considering various contraceptive options:

- CDC Patient Resource on Contraception.

The CDC's contraceptive guidance for healthcare providers 2015 covers the following:

- The U.S. Medical Eligibility Criteria for Contraceptive Use 2010 (current revised version 2016)
- The U.S. Selected Practice Recommendations for Contraceptive Use 2013 (current version 2016)
- How to use the U.S. MEC and the U.S. SPR
- Providing quality family planning services
- CDC contraceptive methods guidance: Slide sets for healthcare providers
- Social media tools

A useful illustration showing the effectiveness of each of the 15 current methods of contraception is the CDC (2013) chart showing an adaptation developed from the WHO Department of Reproductive Health and Research and other sources. This would prove useful for clinical teaching of students as well as patient information. Additionally, practitioners are encouraged to carefully examine the CDC recommendations and guidance on the different methods of contraception. In relation to this, Curtis, Tepper, Jamieson, and Marchbanks (2013) conducted a systematic review to ascertain the extent of need and scope for the adaptation. They examined the scientific evidence and healthcare professionals met together to discuss translation of the evidence into recommendations. Practitioners in the United States should be clear about the extent to which the state in which they are currently employed may have interpreted and translated specific recommendations for practical application. Differences in state legislations and regulations may influence these in terms of specific clinical procedures for implementation of specific family planning methods.

Conclusion

Contraception is a choice that has a major impact on the lives of virtually everyone. It is important for personal and political reasons. It is important for economic reasons both worldwide and within the family. It is a hugely personal choice, but one that is facilitated by healthcare professionals. It is our duty to give the best and most complete information and counseling we can so that this choice can be respected. Contraception service provision in the United States has been explored to provide practitioners some insight of the recommendations and guidelines for relevant healthcare providers. The impact of need for contraception and family planning and the trends in uptake should be continually explored together with appropriate clinical audits and evaluative studies.

• • • REFERENCES

American Congress of Obstetricians and Gynecologists (ACOG). (2013). Committee opinion No. 577: Understanding and using the U.S. Selected Practice Recommendations for Contraceptive Use, 2013. *Obstetrics and Gynecology, 122*(5), 1132–1133.

Brache, V., Cochon, L., Jessam, C., Maldonado, R., Salvatierra, A. M., Levy, D. P., . . . Croxatto, H. B. (2010). Immediate pre-ovulatory administration of 30 mg uliprital acetate significantly delays follicular rupture. *Human Reproduction, 25*(9), 2256–2263.

Bradley, S. E. K., Croft, T. N., Fishel, J. D., & Westoff, C. F. (2012). *Revising unmet need for family planning.* DHS Analytical Studies, No. 25. Calverton, MD: ICF International.

Centers for Disease Control and Prevention (CDC). (2010). U.S. medical eligibility criteria for contraceptive use (US MEC), 2010. *MMWR Recommendations and Reports, 59*(RR-4), 1–86.

Centers for Disease Control and Prevention (CDC). (2013). Effectiveness of contraceptive methods. Retrieved from www.cdc.gov/reproductivehealth/unintendedpregnancy/pdf/contraceptive_methods_508.pdf

Centers for Disease Control and Prevention (CDC). (2016). U.S. Medical eligibility criteria for contraceptive use. *MMWR Recommendations and Reports, 65*(RR-3), 1–103.

Chola, L., McGee, S., Tugendhaft, A., Buchmann, E., & Hofman, K. (2015). Scaling up family planning to reduce maternal and child mortality: The potential costs and benefits of modern contraceptive use in South Africa. *PLoS ONE, 10*(6), e0130077. doi:10.1371/journal.pone.0130077.

Clubb, E. & Knight, J. (1996). *Fertility: Fertility awareness and natural family planning* (3rd ed.). Exeter, United Kingdom, David & Charles.

Clutterbuck, D. (2005). *Sexually transmitted infections and HIV.* London, United Kingdom: Mosby | Elsevier.

Curtis, K. M., Jatlaoui, T. C., Tepper, N. K., Zapata, L. B., Horton, L. G., Jamieson, D. J., & Whiteman, M. K. (2016). U.S. selected practice recommendations for contraceptive use, 2016. MMWR *Recommendations and Reports 65*(4), 1–66.

Curtis, K. M., Tepper, N. K., Jamieson, D. J., & Marchbanks, P. A. (2013). Adaptation of the World Health Organization's selected practice recommendations for contraceptive use for the United States. *Contraception, 87*(5), 513–516.

Dehlendorf, C., Krajewski, C., & Borrero, S. (2014). Contraceptive counselling: Best practices to ensure quality communication and enable effective contraceptive use. *Clinical Obstetrics and Gynecology, 57*(4), 659–673.

Faculty of Sexual and Reproductive Healthcare (FSRH). (2009). Clinical Effectiveness Unit. *CEU guidance postnatal sexual and reproductive health.* London, United Kingdom: Author.

Faculty of Sexual and Reproductive Healthcare (FSRH). (2010). *CEU guidance contraception for women aged over 40 years.* London, United Kingdom: Author.

Faculty of Sexual and Reproductive Healthcare (FSRH). (2015a). *CEU guidance fertility awareness methods.* London, United Kingdom: Author.

Faculty of Sexual and Reproductive Healthcare (FSRH). (2015b). *CEU guidance intrauterine contraception.* London, United Kingdom: Author.

Faculty of Sexual and Reproductive Healthcare (FSRH). (2015c). *Guideline: Quick starting contraception after UPA.* London, United Kingdom: Author.

Faculty of Sexual Health and Reproductive Healthcare (FSRH). (2016). UK Medical Eligibility Criteria for Contraceptive Use (UKMEC). London, United Kingdom: Author.

Finer, L. B., & Zolna, M. R. (2016). Declines in unintended pregnancies in the United States 2008-2011. *New England Journal of Medicine, 374,* 843–852.

French, R. S., Mercer, C. H., Johnson, A. M., Fenton, K. A., Erens, B., & Wellings, K. (2009). Men and women's use of contraceptive services in Britain: Findings from the second National Survey of Sexual Attitudes and Lifestyles. *The Journal of Family Planning and Reproductive Health Care, 35,* 9–14.

Frezieres, R. G., Walsh, T., Kilbourne-Brook, M., & Coffey, P. S. (2012). Couples' acceptability of the SILCS diaphragm for microbicide delivery. *Contraception, 85*(1), 99–107.

Frost, J. J. (2013). *U.S. women's use of sexual and reproductive health services: Trends, sources of care and factors associated with use 1995-2010.* New York, NY: Guttmacher Institute.

Frost, J. J., Frohwirth, L., & Zolna, M. R. (2015). *Contraceptive needs and services, 2013 update.* New York, NY: Guttmacher Institute. Retrieved from https://www.guttmacher.org/sites/default/files/pdfs/pubs/win/contraceptive-needs-2013.pdf

Frost, J. J., Sonfield, A., Zolna, M. R., & Finer, L. B. (2014). Return on investment: A fuller assessment of the benefits and cost savings of the U.S. publicly funded family planning program. *Milbank Quarterly, 92*(4), 696–749.

Frost, J. J., Zolna, M. R., Frohwirth, L. (2013). *Contraceptive needs & services 2010.* New York: Guttmacher Institute. Retrieved from https://www.guttmacher.org/sites/default/files/report_pdf/contraceptive-needs-2010.pdf

Glasier, A., & Gebbie, A. (2008). *Handbook of family planning and reproductive healthcare* (5th ed.). London, United Kingdom: Churchill Livingstone.

Guillebaud, J. (2012). *Contraception, your questions answered.* (6th ed.). London, United Kingdom: Churchill Livingstone.

Harel, Z., Johnson, C. C., Gold, M. A., Cromer, B., Peterson, E., Burkman, R., . . . Bachrach, L. K. Recovery of bone mineral density in adolescents following the use of depot medroxyprogesterone acetate contraceptive injections. *Contraception, 81*(4), 281–291.

Harlow, B. L., Missmer, S. A., Cramer, D. W., & Barbieri, R. L. (2002). Does tubal sterilization influence the subsequent risk of menorrhagia and dysmenorrhea? *Fertility and Sterility, 77*(4), 754–760.

Harvard Health Publications. (2016). *2017 Annual report on prostate diseases.* Cambridge, MA: Harvard Health Publications.

Jacobson, J, Likis, F, Murphy, P. (2012) "Extended and continuous combined contraceptive regimens for menstrual suppression." *Journal Of Midwifery & Women's Health.* November 57(6):585–659.

Jones, R. K., & Kavanaugh, M. L. (2011). Changes in abortion rates between 2000 & 2008 and lifetime incidence of abortion. *Obstetrics and Gynecology, 117*(6), 1358–1366.

MacGregor, A. (1999). *Managing migraine in primary care.* Malden, MA: Blackwell Science.

National Family Planning and Reproductive Health Association (NFPRHA). (2016). Title X. Retrieved from https://www.nationalfamilyplanning.org/title_x

National Institute for Health and Clinical Excellence (NICE). (2005). Long-acting reversible contraception: The effective and appropriate use of long-acting reversible contraception. Retrieved from https://www.nice.org.uk/guidance/cg30/evidence/full-guideline-194840605

National Osteoporosis Society (UK). (2016). *A balanced diet for bones*. Retrieved from https://nos.org.uk/about-osteoporosis/prevention-are-you-at-risk/a-balanced-diet-for-bones/

Parnell, A. M. (Ed.). (1989). *Contraceptive use and Controlled fertility: Health issues for women and children background papers*. Committee on Population, National Research Council (US). Washington, DC: National Academic Press (US). Retrieved from http://www.nap.edu/catalog/1422.html

Peterson, H. B., Jeng, G., Folger, S. G., Hillis, S. A., Marchbanks, P. A., Wilcox, L. S.; U.S. Collaborative Review of Sterilization Working Group. (2000). The risk of menstrual abnormalities after tubal sterilization. *New England Journal of Medicine, 343*(23), 1681–1687.

Prabakar, I., & Webb, A. (2012). Emergency contraception. *British Medical Journal, 344*, e1492.

Rosato, E., Farris, M., & Bastianelli, C. (2015). Mechanism of action of ulipristal acetate for emergency contraception: A systematic review. *Frontiers in Pharmacology, 6*, 315. doi: 10.3389fphar.2015.00315

Royal College of Obstetricians and Gynaecologists (RCOG). (2004a). *Male and female sterilisation*. London, United Kingdom: RCOG Press.

Royal College of Obstetricians and Gynaecologists. (RCOG). (2004b). Sterilisation for women and men: What you need to know. Retrieved from https://www.rcog.org.uk/globalassets/documents/patients/patient-information-leaflets/gynaecology/sterilisation-for-women-and-men.pdf

Sadatmahalleh, S. J., Ziaei, S., Kazemnejad, A., & Mohamadi, E. (2016). Menstrual pattern following tubal ligation: A historical cohort study. *International Journal of Fertility and Sterility, 9*(4), 477–482.

Sedgh, G., & Hussain, R. (2014). Reasons for contraceptive non-use among women having unmet need for contraception in developing countries. *Studies in Family Planning, 45*(2), 151–169.

Skrine, R. (1997). *Blocks and freedoms in sexual life: Handbook in psychosexual medicine*. Boca Raton, FL: CRC Press.

Skrine, R., & Montford, H. (2001). *Psychosexual medicine: An introduction* (2nd ed.). Boca Raton, FL: CRC Press.

Sonfield, A., & Gold, R. B. (2012). *Public funding for family planning, sterilization and abortion services, FY1980-2010*. New York, NY: Guttmacher Institute. Retrieved from http://www.guttmacher.org/pubs/Public-Funding-FP-2010.pdf

Stover, J., & Ross, J. (2010). How increased contraceptive use has reduced maternal mortality. *Maternal and Child Health Journal, 14*(5), 687–695.

United Nations Department of Economic and Social Affairs (UNDESA). (2013). *World contraceptive patterns 2013*. Retrieved from http://www.un.org/en/development/desa/population/publications/family/contraceptive-wallchart-2013.shtml

World Health Organisation (WHO). (2014). *Ensuring human rights in the provision of contraceptive information and services: Guidance and recommendations*. Geneva, Switzerland: Author. Retrieved from http://www.who.int/reproductivehealth/publications/family_planning/human-rights-contraception/en/

World Health Organisation (WHO). (2015). *Family planning/contraception*. Retrieved from http://who.int/mediacentre/factsheets/fs351/en

Zimicki, S. (1989) The relationship between fertility and maternal mortality. In A. M. Parnell (Ed.), *Contraceptive use and controlled fertility: Health issues for women and children*, 1–47. Washington, DC: National Academic Press. Retrieved from https://www.ncbi.nlm.nih.gov/books/NBK235085/

● ● ● **SUGGESTED FURTHER READING**

Cleary, T. P., Tepper, N. K., Cwiak, C., Whiteman, M. K., Jamieson, D. J., Marchbanks, P. A., & Curtis, K. M. (2013). Pregnancies after hysteroscopic sterilization: A systematic review. *Contraception, 87*(5), 539–548.

> *According to these authors, female sterilization is the second most common form of contraception used in the United States. Alternative approaches to female sterilization including hysteroscopic methods have been approved in the United States since 2002. However, little is known about the occurrence and timing of pregnancies after these procedures.*

The new UK Medical Eligibility for Criteria (UK MEC): What has changed? [Editorial]. (2016). *Journal of Family Planning & Reproductive Health Care, 42*(2), 81–82.

Tepper, N. K., Goldberg, H. I., Bernal, M. I. V., Rivera, B., Frey, M. T., Malave, C., … Jamieson, M. D. (2016). Estimating contraceptive needs and increasing access to contraception in response to the Zika Virus disease outbreak—Puerto Rico. *MMWR, 65*(12), 311–314.

> *The Zika virus is described as a flavivirus transmitted primarily by Aedes species mosquitoes. Increasing evidence links zika virus infection during pregnancy to damaging pregnancy and birth outcomes including pregnancy loss, intrauterine growth restriction, eye defects, congenital brain abnormalities, and other fetal abnormalities. The virus has also been determined to be sexually transmitted.*

Faculty of Sexual and Reproductive Healthcare (FSRH). (2012). CEU guidance combined hormonal contraception. London, United Kingdom: Author.

Tepper, N. K., Curtis, K. M., Nanda, K., & Jamieson, D. J. (2016). Safety of intrauterine devices among women with HIV: A systematic review. *Contraception, 94*(6), 713–724.

Tepper, N. K., Steenland, M. W., Marchbanks, P. A., & Curtis, K. M. (2013). Hemoglobin measurement prior to initiating copper intrauterine devices: a systematic review. *Contraception, 87*(5), 639–644.

> *These authors maintain that women using copper IUDs frequently experience bleeding abnormalities. Therefore, their systematic review was conducted to evaluate the evidence regarding whether haemoglobin levels should be measured prior to copper IUD insertion.*

Tepper, N. K., Steenland, M. W., Marchbanks, P. A., & Curtis, K. M. (2013). Laboratory screening prior to initiating contraception: A systematic review. *Contraception, 87*(5), 645–649.

> *Certain contraceptive methods may increase the risk of adverse events for women with certain medical conditions. These include diabetes, hyperlipidemia, liver disease, cervical cancer, sexually transmitted infections (STIs), and human immunodeficiency virus (HIV). The review was conducted to evaluate the evidence regarding health outcomes among women with and without laboratory testing to identify certain medical conditions prior to initiating contraceptives.*

The U.S. Selected Practice Recommendations (U.S. SPR) for contraceptive use, 2016.

Practitioners' attention is drawn to the updated recommendations in the 2016 version of the U.S. SPR, which was launched following the 2013 version. The current 2016 version stipulates the importance of carefully advising the woman regarding appropriate timing to recommence using regular contraception following emergency contraceptive pills.

Advice should also be given regarding abstention from sexual intercourse or use of barrier methods after restarting regular contraception and if necessary, having a pregnancy test performed if no withdrawal bleed had occurred within 3 weeks.

Additional new recommendations relate to the administration of medications to ease IUD insertion.

The full details are provided in the:

U.S. SPR for Contraceptive Use, 2016. *Morbidity and Mortality Weekly Report Recom Rep.* 2016 Jul 29. 65(4);1–66.

Practitioners are strongly urged to ascertain the correct details as translated into practice in their internal policy regulations and procedure guidelines.

It is also worthwhile to examine the American Congress of Obstetrics and Gynecologists (ACOG) endorsement of the U.S. SPR and Congress guidance for its fellows: "Understanding and using the U.S. Selected Practice Recommendations (U.S. SPR) for Contraceptive Use, 2013" together with the more current version launched by ACOG.

Also issued by ACOG is a comprehensive and culturally appropriate reproductive life planning to avoid unintended pregnancy. This document examines the cultural and economic barriers to preventing unintended pregnancy. For more details see the full document: "Reproductive Life Planning to Reduce Unintended Pregnancy"

ACOG Committee Opinion #654—Reproductive life Planning to Reduce Unintended Pregnancy.

Practitioners are urged to explore the external resources of recommendations and guidelines provided in relation to this topical issue. Centers for Disease Control and Prevention. Reproductive life plan tool for health professionals. Retrieved from www.beforeandbeyond.org/

United Kingdom Medical Eligibility Criteria for Contraceptive Use. The new UK Medical Eligibility for Criteria (UK MEC): April 2016.

US AID Health Policy Initiative. How contraceptive use affects maternal mortality. Dec 2008. US Agency for International Development (USAID).

● ● ● **ADDITIONAL SOURCES OF REFERENCE**

www.mhra.gov.uk

www.nos.org.uk

www.e-lfh.org.uk

P
A
R
T

III

Support Services in Sexual and Reproductive Health Care

CHAPTER

9

Sexually Transmitted Infections and HIV: Requirements for Surveillance Systems, Policy Regulations, Control, and Prevention

THEODORA D. KWANSA

Introduction

Measures to deal with sexual health–related problems vary from country to country and originate at all governmental levels. The United Kingdom's exemplar of excellence is its national policy of collaboration between the Department of Health and commissioning organizations to address the complex challenge of sexual healthcare and service provision. The aim of this collaboration is to ensure appropriate implementation of standardized national policy regulations and recommended guidelines. Major governmental and national organizations collaborate with the World Health Organization (WHO) in striving toward a common goal in control and prevention initiatives for sexually transmitted infections (STIs) and human immunodeficiency virus (HIV). Examples of participant organizations include the British Association for Sexually Transmitted Infections and HIV (BASHH) and the Centers for Disease Control and Prevention (CDC) in the United States.

Magnitude of the STI and RTI Burden: Associated Consequences

Certain serious STIs and reproductive tract infections (RTIs), along with associated life-threatening maternal and natal consequences, increase the national economic burden due to the impact of morbidity and mortality. Actual health problems vary from painful, disfiguring lesions and psychological distress to moderately acute ill-health. Direct consequences may manifest as impairment of the reproductive capacity and deterioration of quality of life.

Evidence of specific consequences includes the following:

- Men with *Neisseria gonorrhoeae* infection experience pain during micturition, while women may develop acute or persistent low abdominal pain (Bignell & Unemo, 2013; Workowski & Bolan, 2015).

- Individuals with untreated *Treponema pallidum* infection may not initially experience symptoms or any discomfort, although later in life cardiovascular, neurological, and/or bone diseases may manifest (Workowski & Bolan, 2015).

- The physical impact of chancroid is described as debilitating, painful ulcers if an individual with immunocompromised status does not receive treatment within a few days of manifestation (Lewis, 2003).

- Genital herpes, which is characterized by recurrence with considerable discomfort and psychosexual anguish, can hamper quality of life, particularly among young people (Bernstein et al., 2013).

Various researchers also maintain that certain STIs, such as herpes simplex virus 2 (HSV-2) and syphilis, can increase acquisition and replication of HIV as well as promote vertical mother-to-child transmission (Ferreira et al., 2011). Furthermore, some STIs can lead to serious reproductive tract infections and damage, resulting in complications such as infertility (Ward & Rönn, 2010; World Health Organization [WHO], 2015).

An additional significant direct consequence of acute or severe STIs and RTIs is the impact on perinatal and neonatal morbidity and mortality rates due to prenatal exposure or vertical transmission (Allstaff & Wilson, 2012; WHO, 2013). Overall fetal and neonatal morbidity as direct consequences of acute or severe STIs/RTIs may include congenital abnormalities or malformations, prematurity, low birth weight, sepsis, pneumonia, and conjunctivitis (Rours et al., 2011; WHO, 2013). Syphilis in pregnancy alone is reported to account for an estimated 305,000 fetal, perinatal, and neonatal deaths every year. *Chlamydia trachomatis* affects the morbidity and mortality of 215,000 babies annually with complications of congenital abnormalities, prematurity, and low birth weight (Rours et al., 2011; WHO, 2013).

Association Between Particular STIs and HIV Infection

Evidence of the association between certain STIs and HIV also implicates increased vulnerability among particular high-risk groups, thereby imposing further economic burden. Therefore, implementation of measures to reduce the prevalence and spread of STIs among those identified groups should be a national priority. High-risk groups include commercial sex workers and individuals who are likely to have multiple sexual partners. The overall economic impact of the prevalence and spread of these infections includes direct and indirect financial losses through work days lost due to illness, long-term debilitating illnesses, and in some cases death. Whether treatment and control of STIs also achieves prevention of HIV infections by reducing prevalence and transmission rate remains a contentious assumption.

Evidence indicates that STIs associated with inflammation and genital ulceration such as syphilis, chancroid, and herpes increase susceptibility to contracting HIV infection (Corey et al. 2004). As such, when interventions for curbing the prevalence and frequency of diagnosis of new STI cases within a community are devised and implemented, account should be taken of the STI–HIV transmission connection. Increased susceptibility to HIV infection in those with ulcerative genital lesions occurs when the inflammatory and ulcerative cells of the genitalia attract an increased amount of activated CD4 cells (T-cells from the immune system), thus creating a build-up of cells that are readily susceptible to HIV infection (Corey, Wald, Celum, & Quinn, 2004; WHO, 2013). Research reveals that STIs associated with inflammatory disorders of the genitalia triggered by the immune system include gonorrhea, chlamydia, and trichomoniasis. Various other STIs are associated with both inflammatory and ulcerative damage to genital structures (Corey et al., 2004). As Ferreira et al. (2011) explain, STIs can increase HIV-1 replication (copying and reproducing increasing amount of HIV-carrying cells) in the genital tract of females through inflammatory processes in the genital epithelial cells. These authors maintain that the buildup of HIV-1 replication enhances sexual and vertical maternal–child transmission of HIV (Ferreira et al., 2011). Therefore, unprotected sexual intercourse between infected and uninfected partners with any of the above conditions creates a particularly high-risk cofactor effect Centers for Disease Control and Prevention [CDC], 2015; WHO, 2007).

Prevalence of STIs Among Different Populations and Subgroups

World Health Organization (WHO) data from 2008 revealed that approximately 498 million new cases of curable STIs occur annually on a global level (WHO, 2012). These curable infections are mainly syphilis, gonorrhea, chlamydia, and trichomoniasis. These STIs occur mainly in men and women between 15 and 49 years of age and are found to be more prevalent in south and southeast Asia, followed by sub-Saharan Africa and Latin America (WHO, 2012). Furthermore, there are many other viral STIs including HIV, HSV, human papillomavirus (HPV), and the hepatitis B virus (HBV). HSV-2 is recorded as the primary cause of genital ulcers among 30–80% of women and among 10–50% of men (WHO, 2012). The prevalence among women was further broken down:

- 20–40% among women in central and South America (WHO, 2012)

- 10–30% in the developing countries of Asia (WHO, 2012)

- 19% among people of 14–49 years of age in the United States (Kenyon, Buyze, & Colebunders, 2014; Weinstock, Berman, & Cates, 2004; WHO, 2012)

Admittedly, these figures may not represent an entirely clear picture of the global STI prevalence. Nevertheless, they do somewhat reveal a pattern of the prevalence in different countries and a regional portrayal of the predominance of specific STIs. The WHO's most recently published figures (WHO, 2013) reveal the rate of STI acquisition globally is 1 million persons daily. For additional information, Newman et al.'s (2013) global estimates and surveillance data on syphilis in pregnancy is recommended.

Clearly the magnitude STI infection has a significant global impact. The estimate of illnesses from chlamydia, gonorrhea, syphilis, and trichomoniasis is 500 million annually (WHO, 2012). Chlamydia and gonorrhea are identified as the major causes of pelvic inflammatory disease (PID), which is associated with infertility and unfavorable pregnancy outcomes (WHO, 2013). Other STI infections rates also give cause for concern at all levels, including individual, community, population, governmental, and political. Recent estimated figures show that more than 530 million people worldwide are infected with HSV-2, while more than 290 million women are infected with HPV (WHO, 2013). HSV-2 infection rates are significant due to the potential association of this infection with enhanced risk of HIV acquisition (Looker, Garnett, & Schmid, 2008; UNAIDS, 2010). Consistent evidence confirms that the presence of specific STIs exacerbates susceptibility to the acquisition and spread of HIV (Galvin & Cohen, 2004; Steen, Kamali, & Ndowa, 2009; WHO, 2007).

Regarding long-term complications and the related consequences, HPV is reported as causing an estimated 530,000 new cases of cervical cancer each year. It is also attributed to an estimated mortality of 275,000 each year with more than 85% of cervical cancer deaths occurring in developing countries (WHO, 2012, 2013). HBV infection, which can be acquired via sexual transmission as well as through needle sharing and blood transfusion, is also associated with transmission from mother to baby. Other key consequences of HBV infection are an estimated 350 million cases of chronic liver disease each year and an estimated 1 million deaths per year, mainly as a result of cirrhosis of the liver and hepatocellular carcinoma (Kenyon et al., 2014; WHO, 2012).

While certain STI infections can more than triple the risk of HIV acquisition, most cases of infection are asymptomatic. In addition, the magnitude and complexity of the burden imposed by STIs is further enhanced by emerging drug resistance. Certain STI microorganisms have consistently evolved to resist specific antimicrobial medications, thus creating a significant hindrance to the reduction of STI impact across the world (WHO, 2013). It can be seen from this brief overview that surveillance is crucial to curb the prevalence and continuous transmission of STIs and HIV infection.

Risk Factors Influencing Acquisition and Rate of Transmission of STIs and HIV

Among the key factors that influence the prevalence, acquisition, and transmission of STIs are low social and economic deprivation as well as certain cultural and risky lifestyles and behaviors. Disparities in different regions and communities may be associated with influx and movement of migrants and commercial sex workers (Low et al., 2006). Iatrogenic STI/RTIs may occur for any of the following reasons: healthcare organizations with inadequate policy regulations, guidelines, and procedures on infection prevention and control; poor hygiene precautions; inadequate education and training of the sexual healthcare practitioners; limited resources; inappropriate equipment; and insufficient supply of sterile instruments for performing specific procedures correctly. In particular, postpartum and postabortion gynecological examinations and treatment procedures performed incorrectly in such unsafe conditions can result in serious life-threatening iatrogenic infections (WHO, 2005b). Endogenous yeast infections occur worldwide and may be associated with environmental factors and poor hygiene conditions, although specific hormonal disorders could also be a factor (WHO, 2005b, 2007).

Significance of Control and Prevention of STIs and HIV

The broad concept of infection prevention and control should be explored separately for more detailed consideration. This section focuses on the significance of measures for curbing the prevalence and spread of STIs in relation to the frequency of new diagnoses and associated complications. Sexual healthcare practitioners should be well informed about preventative methods and routine assessment programs. It is important that the interventions at different levels—individual patients, patient partners, community networks, and the general population—achieve beneficial outcomes. Therefore, staff development programs should explore the theories supporting specific prevention methods (e.g., behavior change interventions, motivational interviewing, and biomedical interventions).

Because a previous chapter explores HIV/AIDS, every effort is made to avoid unnecessary repetition here. However, control and prevention of STIs unavoidably linked to HIV prevention and therefore it seems appropriate to examine interrelated strategies. The terms *control* and *prevention* are sometimes used interchangeably, but clear definition is necessary to achieve effective outcomes for both prevention and control measures. Steen et al. (2009) define control of STIs in terms of measures to reduce the prevalence and incidence in the wider context by employing varied collaborative and interactive interventions. Thus, it is necessary to assess how widespread or common specific STIs are and the rate or frequency of occurrence of each type of infection within the particular population. Control of STIs is recognized as a public health concern that has to be prioritized and addressed collaboratively from different levels. The priority is to restrict and reduce the rate of new infection transmission and new diagnoses and ultimately reduce the overall social and economic burden imposed by outbreaks of STI infections. These authors define prevention in terms of precaution and prophylactic measures against STI acquisition and spread (Steen et al., 2009). Prevention is further examined later.

The infection control methods employed depend on the type of STIs, the prevalence, and whether a particular infection or combination of infections is at an epidemic phase. The type of population, communities, sexual partnerships, the descriptions and characteristics of sexual networks within the communities, and the general population are crucial factors that influence STI spread (Doherty, Padian, Marlow, & Aral, 2005). As Steen et al. (2009) maintain, a comprehensive STI control involves focused and directed community-based interventions together with promoting, supporting, and making appropriate facilities available. It also involves clinical services with capacity to provide sustainable essential resources and substantiated information with appropriate details to guide further plans and actions and underpin recommended treatment procedures. Person-to-person transmission and the spread of STI and HIV infection within a community is influenced by various factors such as the type of organism, how virulent, how easily transmissible, how easily spread, and how long the infection persists (Steen et al., 2009). It is necessary to take these factors into account when devising and implementing infection control interventions. The interconnections among individuals, partnerships and sexual network formations, communities, and the wider population are recognized in terms of characteristic sexual behaviors, health seeking, and social activities within the networks (Doherty et al., 2005; Gallo, Macaluso, et al., 2012; Steen et al., 2009).

Manhart and Holmes (2005) demonstrated the importance of recognizing a distinction between individual-level and population-level interventions and recognizing the impact of sexual networks on these interventions. These authors maintain that intermediate-level interventions are needed and that maternal–child partnerships should not be overlooked.

Control and prevention of STIs and HIV also calls for control and prevention of the high rates of unplanned pregnancies and abortions. The Medical Foundation for AIDS & Sexual Health emphasizes the importance of health promotion and education in fostering young people's awareness of how to protect themselves from STIs and prevent unplanned pregnancies (Christophers, Mann, & Lowbury, 2008).

To target control globally, the WHO works with countries to recognize the importance of establishing effective STI services. Emphasis is placed on STI case management and counseling, syphilis testing and treatment with particular attention to women during pregnancy, and hepatitis B and HPV vaccination (WHO, 2013). Moreover, the WHO endorses enhancement of STI prevention in its recommendation to integrate STI services into conventional healthcare systems and services. It also urges for effective countrywide sexual health promotion, and advocates assessment of the STI burden in order to ensure effective monitoring and appropriate actions on emerging concerns such as antimicrobial resistance. Furthermore, the WHO supports and reinforces advancements in new knowledge, expertise, and, improvements of STI prevention procedures and techniques. To that end, the WHO advocates ongoing research studies such as point-of-care diagnostic tests and encourages scientific advancements toward the development of more effective drugs for treating gonorrhea, research for vaccines against preventable STIs, and other biomedical interventions (WHO, 2013).

Key Elements in National and Community Endeavors in STI Control

Worldwide recognition of STIs prevalence evolved from acknowledgement of the HIV/AIDS epidemic. Various experts substantiate that reduction in HIV transmission is achievable through adequate control of STIs (Steen et al., 2009). However, this can only be realistically achieved if the problem is recognized as a public health concern and dealt with through implementation of appropriate public health initiatives. Key interventions must aim to reduce the prevalence and the incidence of outbreaks. Therefore, primary prevention is crucial and encompasses detailed sexual history together with provision of pertinent evidence-based information that is topical, comprehensible, timely, and targeting the right population groups in the right environments.

Program managers for STI infection control at national and organizational levels should include representatives from healthcare providers, relevant stakeholders, and sexual health professional practitioners. The program should emphasize the importance of raising public awareness of the overall potential benefits of the national and community vaccination and screening programs and STI prevention and control endeavors. Shared responsibility and accountability among all stakeholders ensures improvement on STI epidemiology and associated morbidity and mortality consequences. Various studies and clinical audits continue to substantiate the benefits of and social and economic advantages of improved quality of health for the general population (Brook & Family Planning Association [FPA], 2013). STI prevention and control campaigns and education about vaccination and screening programs should be guided by relevant experts, national regulations, and the principles of safe practice. Practitioners should have ongoing training that incorporates updates in required competencies in STI infection prevention and control (Steen et al., 2009).

A particular challenge of STI/RTI prevention and control is that many individuals who acquire STIs remain asymptomatic while others are reluctant to seek medical intervention. Additionally, for various personal reasons, individuals may not feel confident about the notifying their sexual partner. It may be that inherent misconceptions influence ignorance about STIs, the causal factors, associated symptoms and signs, and the potential consequences of delayed treatment or untreated infections. In poorer countries constrained by economic challenges, the prescribed treatment available to STI/RTI patients may be inadequate or fail to achieve desired patient outcomes (Steen et al., 2009; WHO, 2008).

The following section examines STI and HIV surveillance, control, and monitoring, with an overview of worldwide, European, and U.K. initiatives. Readers may find it useful to explore and make comparisons with surveillance systems employed in parts of the United States, and particular developing countries in which individuals have personal and professional interest. In respect of copyright regulations, only a broad overview is presented here without direct reproductions of WHO or UNAIDS documents. Instead, readers are encouraged to explore the original documents as cited in the reference list and the additional recommended readings at the end of this chapter. The original documents provide detailed information and more complete data with the essential recommendations, stipulated requirements, and principles that guide particular interventions in clinical practice. These are underpinned by carefully examined research findings and the levels of evidence are also clearly indicated. Crucially, it is important for professional practitioners to explore and gain familiarity with the national policies, regulations, and guidelines for the country in which they are employed.

Surveillance of STIs and HIV

Surveillance of STIs and HIV/AIDS involves methodically gathering and organizing specific data through the health service organizations and recurrent surveys. The data are analyzed to provide evidence for policy decisions, healthcare planning, and research (CDC, 2015; European Centre for Disease Prevention and Control [ECDC], 2013; UNAIDS/ WHO, 2012). The rationalization for STI surveillance as a shared public health concern and worldwide initiative will be examined.

Standardization of STI surveillance is necessary to achieve effective control. There is a need for private sector involvement to carry out national guidelines and regulations STI surveillance. However, indifferent political support and limited resources (including financial hardships, lack of required expertise for accurate statistical calculations, and lack of appropriate laboratory technology) hamper efforts. Moreover, asymptomatic infections create inconsistencies in diagnoses, and prejudices and aversion toward high-risk population groups also hinder the endeavors to establish regular and effective surveillance programs (WHO/UNAIDS, 2013).

The main goals of STI surveillance are to determine the scale of infections, the prevalence and spread within different communities and among different subgroups, and the consequences and trends over time. This information enables organizational decision-makers to plan and facilitate regular monitoring and evaluation of STI control and related interventions as well as to determine the resources required for the provision of STI care and services. The relevant experts are also able to investigate and determine specific etiologies—the causative microorganisms and antimicrobial resistances—based on the substantive data (WHO/UNAIDS, 2013). The following sections examine the different levels of STI/HIV surveillance and control.

The Global Perspective on STIs and HIV Surveillance

Global surveillance of HIV, AIDS, and STIs has been a joint undertaking by the WHO and UNAIDS. Their working group organizes and standardizes the systems for carrying out compilation of high quality surveillance data, which is used to inform decisions and appropriate planning of HIV, AIDS, and STI services in different parts of the world. Effective surveillance enables policy makers to facilitate implementation of evidence-based public health interventions, and to closely monitor and regulate the conduct of appropriate evaluation projects (UNAIDS/ WHO, 2012; WHO/UNAIDS, 2013). Therefore, the working group operates at global, regional, and national levels. Relevant professional specialists and consultants are involved to provide guidance and practical advice on specific matters. These experts are in the best position to make predictions about prevalence, related risk behaviors of the organisms, and associated mortality. This information is used to substantiate the recommendations for monitoring and controlling the prevalence and spread of the infections among hard-to-reach populations (WHO/ UNAIDS, 2013).

The joint working group identifies best practice from around the globe and develops recommendations and guidelines for designing, implementing, and evaluating national surveillance systems. Some countries may need training resources and possible funding to implement and maintain STI surveillance (WHO/UNAIDS, 2013). Research and development endeavors focus on emerging problems relating to HIV prevalence, monitoring antiretroviral resistance, and exploring alternative methods of laboratory tests using different specimens and alternative samples (WHO/UNAIDS, 2013).

The European Surveillance System (TESSy)

The following presents a brief overview of the surveillance systems employed to control STIs and HIV infection. The European Surveillance System (TESSy) is a database into which the required details for each STI are entered. The TESSy system provides a mechanism to ensure surveillance data can be compared to similar data submitted by other countries. These data are then analyzed and interpreted to help determine epidemiology, identify high-risk groups, and track outbreaks. The amount of detail required about specific infections may vary. However, the E.U. version represents a comprehensive set of variables that form the basis for enhanced surveillance. It is beyond the scope of this chapter to present the total required details for the surveillance. The E.Ul. and U.K. surveillance mechanisms are examined here.

Reported Figures from Surveillance of Identified STIs: The E.U. Context

Apart from the global surveillance undertaken by the WHO and UNAIDS, the European Centre for Disease Prevention and Control (ECDC) also undertakes responsibility for coordinating enhanced surveillance of STIs and has been doing so since 2009. The ECDC compiles surveillance reports comprising instances, occurrences, and epidemiological characteristics of specific reportable infections. The STIs under regular surveillance include chlamydia, gonorrhea, syphilis, congenital syphilis, and lymphogranuloma venereum (ECDC, 2013). Each E.U. country (within the European Union and European Economic Area) must submit information that the European Commission requires and has deemed accessible. The following section presents brief overviews of EU surveillance of specific STIs.

Evidence from the E.U. Surveillance of Chlamydia trachomatis Infection

The published ECDC data spanning 1990 to 2011 revealed that chlamydia was the most commonly reported STI in Europe. In 2011, the number of reported diagnoses of chlamydia infection was 346, 911 among 25 E.U./E.E.A. countries with a rate of 175 per 100,000 population (ECDC, 2013). Gender comparison showed higher rates of infection among women—203 per 100,000—than among men—145 per 100,000 (ECDC, 2013). Additionally, 73% (three-fourths) of all diagnoses were reported among young people between the ages of 15 and 24 years (ECDC, 2013). Despite these numbers, exact figures are presumed to be greater, although exact figures are difficult to determine due to different testing techniques and missing data on extent and type of surveillance systems employed.

It was noted that the U.K. chlamydia testing and screening, for example, seem to show greater focus on the population of young people and an apparent gender difference (ECDC, 2013). Another finding from the European surveillance is that apparent increases in chlamydia infection rates in different European countries may be attributable to factors such as more advanced diagnostic techniques, more effective and presumably more extensive screening programs, and better surveillance mechanisms (ECDC, 2013). Apparent low figures on the other hand, are considered attributable to limited diagnostic facilities and less advanced and less accurate diagnostic techniques, rather than actual reduction in prevalence (ECDC, 2013).

Evidence from the E.U. Surveillance of Gonorrhea Infections

The surveillance figures reported by 28 E.U./E.E.A. states in 2011 revealed that 39,179 gonorrhea infections were diagnosed, indicating an overall rate of 12.6 per 100,000 population. The infection rate showed a gender difference of three times higher among men than among women—21.2 per 100,000 versus 7.6 per 100,000 (ECDC, 2013). The difference in age range showed that 42% of all gonorrhea infections were reported among young people between the ages of 15 to 24 years. One-third of the total reported gonorrhea infections in 2011, 33%, were found to occur among men having sex with men (MSM) and between 2010 and 2011 a rise by 20% or more was reported

by different countries among this population subgroup (ECDC, 2013).

Evidence from the E.U. Surveillance of Syphilis Infections

Surveillance figures in 2011 revealed that 29 E.U./E.E.A. countries reported a total of 20,004 syphilis infections, showing a rate of 4.9 per 100,000 population. This infection was also found to occur three times more frequently among men than among women—7.5 per 100,000 versus 1.9 per 100,000. While an age range difference in the reported infections in 2011 showed more diagnoses among young people between 15 and 24 years, most diagnoses were made on people over the age of 25 years. MSM were found to account for 42% of the total number of syphilis infections (ECDC, 2013). Between 2010 and 2011 the syphilis infection rates were reported by 14 countries to show rising figures and 6 countries reported a 20% or more rise in their syphilis infection diagnoses (ECDC, 2013).

Evidence from the E.U. Surveillance of Congenital Syphilis

The European surveillance of congenital syphilis revealed that 88 diagnoses were reported by 23 countries in 2011, while 11 countries reported no diagnoses (ECDC, 2013). A total number of 3,203 congenital syphilis diagnoses were reported by 24 countries during the period spanning from 1990–2011 (ECDC, 2013). Although the figures show a fall in the number of cases since 2000, and that current rates have steadied (ECDC, 2013), the evidence among different E.U./E.E.A. countries varies. It seems that the countries with the highest number of reported congenital syphilis cases have not seen similar substantial reductions. However, the impact of screening programs employed during the antenatal period is being explored (ECDC, 2013).

Evidence from the E.U. Surveillance of Lymphogranuloma Venereum (LGV) Infection

In 2011, the number of LGV diagnoses reported across the E.U./E.E.A. countries was 697 (ECDC, 2013). Over the period spanning 2000–2011, the total number of LGV diagnoses reported by 8 E.U./E.E.A. countries including the United Kingdom and Ireland was 2,024 (ECDC, 2013). Among those diagnosed with LGV for whom the mode of transmission had been determined, 99% were reported to be MSM and 88% had been confirmed as HIV positive (ECDC, 2013). Although an increase in the number of diagnoses had been reported in 2010, these were reported to have steadied in 2011. The ensuing section examines the U.K. context of HIV/AIDS and STI surveillance.

The U.K. Context of HIV/AIDS and STI Surveillance: Brief Contextual Overview

The U.K. figures on STIs are compiled mainly from the diagnoses of infections at genitourinary medicine (GUM) clinics. However, it must be noted that chlamydia diagnoses occur in a variety of community settings, while HIV and AIDS diagnostic data are compiled from multiple surveillance reports across the United Kingdom (http://www.hpa.org.uk).

In the previous system for compiling STI statistical data, figures were compiled by GUM clinics and submitted to the Health Protection Agency (HPA) (currently Public Health England [PHE]) for collation and analysis. The process allowed for determination of emerging STI rates monitoring diagnostic trends, and determining which high-risk population groups were particularly vulnerable to specific STIs. While that policy was mandatory for all GUM clinics, it was paper-based and is currently substituted by an electronic system. The modern system, referred to as the Genitourinary Medicine Clinic Activity Dataset (GUMCAD) compiles specific information from patients who attend GUM clinics. This dataset organizes the statistical figures based on the areas of residence, age, sexual inclination, ethnic population groups, and country of birth for all patients who attend GUM clinics across the United Kingdom. The system allows for errors in data coding submitted by any GUM clinic to be rectified and it also allows for more accurate comparisons.

The HPA's (2010a) statistical data revealed that, despite apparent disparities, the geographical pattern showed consistent increases in the STI rates in urban areas. The main concentrations were notable among high-risk population groups, who presented characteristic vulnerability to social deprivation. The main increases are considered attributable to the current use of more sophisticated and sensitive tests over the past couple of decades (Health Protection Agency [HPA], 2010a). However, other contributory factors that have been reported include the expansion of chlamydia screening services to community settings with increased uptake of services. These have improved accessibility for chlamydia screening for young people and young adults with increased diagnoses through the National Chlamydia Screening Programmes (NCSP). Lifestyle behaviors in terms of risky sexual activities result in poor sexual health among young adults in heterosexual relationships and among MSM and contributed to the reported increase in STI rates (HPA, 2010a).

The published figures spanning from 2008–2009 revealed that there was an increase of 3% new cases of STIs diagnosed at GUM clinics and community-based settings across the United Kingdom (from 470,701 to 482,896) (HPA, 2010b). The trend in new cases of infection was mainly linked to increased rates in chlamydia by 7%, from 203,773 to 217,570, while new diagnosis of gonorrhea increased by 6%, from 16,451 to 17,385 (HPA, 2010b). New diagnosis of genital herpes increased by 5%, from 28,807 to 30,126, while new cases of genital warts lingered around −0.3%, around 91,503 and 91,257 (HPA, 2010b). A slight decrease in new diagnosis of syphilis by −1%, from 3,309 to 3,273, was noted while new cases

of nonspecific genital infections decreased by −3%, from 96,153 to 93,456 (HPA, 2010b). A continuous increase was noted in the total number of people living with HIV in the United Kingdom, 83,000 at the end of 2008, and of that figure more than 27% were apparently unaware of their HIV infection status (HPA, 2010b). Diagnosis of new HIV cases in 2008 showed a slight decrease from the preceding years (7,298). Transmission through heterosexual relationships had increased from previous years, and there was a continuous high rate of increase persisted among MSM (HPA, 2010b). The ensuing sections explore the U.K. HIV/AIDS and STI surveillance and monitoring systems.

Required Information for Monitoring and Surveillance of HIV and AIDs in the United Kingdom

For notification purposes, clinicians and laboratories throughout the United Kingdom are required to report first diagnoses of HIV infections, first AIDS diagnoses, and associated deaths. These data form the basis of monitoring patterns of new diagnoses. Geographical risk factors and morbidity and mortality consequences are also documented (HPA, 2013; Public Health England [PHE], 2014). Ostensibly, the data compiled from HIV diagnoses may be affected by testing arrangements, migration trends, and variations in reporting mechanisms. Diagnoses may not necessarily reflect the incidence of infection in terms of the true rate of acquisition among the particular population (HPA, 2013; PHE, 2014).

Recent Infection Testing Algorithm (RITA) is a mechanism to monitor the rate or frequency of diagnoses that is combined with epidemiological data to determine how recently an individual may have acquired HIV infection and whether it occurred within the 6 months prior to diagnosis. Current figures show that 60% of individuals diagnosed with HIV are also tested to determine the time frame of infection acquisition (HPA, 2013). However, frequency of diagnoses does not accurately represent actual incidence due to the high demand by recently exposed people (recent sexual contacts of HIV-positive persons) for HIV testing. The results can be useful for partner notification arrangements. The classification of "late diagnosis" refers to individuals who have CD4 counts of ≤350 cells/mm^3 (HPA, 2013) within 91 days of diagnosis confirmation. It indicates a projected mortality risk ten times higher within 1 year as compared to individuals who had early and timely diagnoses (HPA, 2013). Diagnosed HIV prevalence refers to the proportion of people in the age group of 15–59 years who are diagnosed and receiving treatment for HIV infection in the total population of the same age group. Thus, a diagnosed prevalence of 2 per 1,000 population reflects a need to reviewing the HIV testing policy and extend the settings beyond GUM clinics (HPA, 2013; PHE, 2014).

In the United Kingdom, the HIV and AIDS Reporting System (HARS) formally collects demographic details of clinic ID, gender, date of birth, age group, year of first attendance, and ethnic origin. Additionally, clinical data are collected, including latest CD4 cell count, latest viral load, and antiretroviral therapy (ART). The information helps determine how many people access HIV-related services in National Health Service Organizations in England, Wales, and Northern Ireland annually. Moreover, specific details can be used to link up the records of patients who access care at different sites (HPA, 2013).

Quality-of-care indicators—such as immediate HIV testing, care provided without delay, and successful treatment—are used to evaluate clinical care (and care outcomes) provided to HIV-positive patients. Laboratory results should show a viral load of <50 copies/mL following 1 year of commencement of treatment. The immunology response should show CD4 count of ≥350 cells/mm³ following a minimum of 1 year of care (HPA, 2013; PHE, 2014). Studies and in-depth analysis are ongoing.

Undiagnosed HIV infection is assessed through the following surveys:

- GUM clinics target high-risk populations to measure undetected prevalence, to determine the extent of individuals missed or overlooked in HIV testing.

- Pregnant women are surveyed to measure HIV prevalence in pregnancy and the extent to which diagnosis is made before or during pregnancy.

- A survey on injecting drug users (IDUs) measures the prevalence of HIV, hepatitis B, and hepatitis C among those IDUs who access HIV facilities records risk-taking behaviors. (HPA, 2013; PHE, 2014)

The overall numbers of people living with HIV infection is estimated by combining the number of individuals who have diagnosed HIV infection with the projected number of individuals who have undiagnosed HIV infection.

The GUMCADv2 System of STI/HIV Surveillance Data Collection and Processing

Data sources for STI surveillance have changed over the past few years. The current system, the Genitourinary Medicine Clinic Activity Dataset (GUMCADv2), requires more detailed patient information, including area of residence, to help calculate infection rates and testing frequency in specific geographical areas.

The reports submitted by those services other than GUM clinics are expected to record numbers and rates of selected STI diagnoses, screening, patient flow, performance monitoring, data completion, and quality. Data submission is due quarterly and must reach the HPA (currently PHE) within 6 weeks of the end of the quarter (HPA, 2013; PHE, 2014).

The following reflective considerations examine the key elements in the recommended principles, with questions to encourage group deliberation among sexual health practitioners in the multidisciplinary team.

Reflective Considerations: Key Factors in STI Control and Surveillance

- **Key factors that should be considered in STI control and surveillance**
  - In terms of feasibility, what factors should be taken into account for all the sites providing sexual health care and services to achieve consistency in the implementation and reporting of STI surveillance?
  - In what ways can the organization incorporate surveillance while aiming to achieve the desired consistency? (Consider the routine procedures and the pro-forma for documentation.)
  - To ensure application of standard surveillance procedures in all the sites across the sexual healthcare organization, what should be specified in the guidelines? (Consider accurate data collection and recording, staff training, consistent definitions of key elements, related terminology and concepts, accurate analysis and interpretation of the data, the timing and duration in terms of time frame.)
  - In regard to confidentiality, what measures should be taken to safeguard patient confidentiality of the STI surveillance data? (Consider national and organizational policies and regulations, the legal implications, nonconsensual disclosure, the justification for sharing patient details for the purpose of maintaining high quality care. Consider anonymity, privacy, and data storage.)
  - In keeping all relevant staff and stakeholders informed, what measures should be taken into consideration? (Consider the timing and alternative modes of providing adequate information to all concerned in the surveillance.)

The following sections examine the main components of STI surveillance including case-reporting, prevalence assessments, etiologic and syndromic diagnoses, and antimicrobial resistance monitoring.

Case Reporting

Case reporting is a process through which individuals with STIs are identified by clinics or laboratories (often identified by case number only) and reported to the relevant public health authority.

Universal Case Reporting

Universal case reporting requires that each healthcare facility documents and reports all cases of STI infections. This process is used in countries across the globe and the data compiled helps determine the extent of demand for particular services by patients with STIs. However, the information cannot be used to determine the size of the STI problem in a country's general population, due to infrequent and irregular accessing of the services, economic scarcities, and constraining social and cultural influences (Lowndes & Fenton, 2004; UNAIDS/WHO, 2012). Alternative tracking methods such as case finding, screening, and prevalence assessments, are more useful in generalizing data to the greater population (UNAIDS/WHO, 2012). It is recommended that universal case reporting be incorporated into other existing reporting procedures and include age, gender, diagnosis, marital status, education, occupation, and area of residence (Lowndes & Fenton, 2004; UNAIDS/WHO, 2012).

The advantage of universal case reporting is its applicability to both syndromic and etiologic reporting. The information illuminates the extent of STI burden and infection trends. In addition, information can be used to design appropriate STI services (Lowndes & Fenton, 2004; UNAIDS/WHO, 2012). Drawbacks include unpredictable and inconsistent healthcare-seeking behaviors associated with less detection and infrequent reporting of STIs. In those sites where laboratory provision and expertise is inaccessible, syndromic case reporting is employed, which focuses on urethral discharge in men and nonvesicular genital ulcer disease in both men and women. Information is used to monitor STI incidence trends (Lowndes & Fenton, 2004; UNAIDS/WHO, 2012). However, universal case reporting may also involve etiologic case reporting. This is feasible in countries where scientific technology, specialist expertise, and funding support are constantly sustainable. Testing for *Treponema pallidum* microorganism for syphilis infection and *Neisseria gonorrhoeae* for gonorrheal infection is stipulated for etiologic case-reporting (UNAIDS/WHO, 2012). To gain more insight, readers may wish to refer to the original 1999 version of the UNAIDS/WHO, Guidelines for STIs surveillance.

Mandatory Universal Case Reporting

Mandatory universal case reporting has been a long-standing practice requiring all GUM clinics to report every STI diagnosed within the clinic (including chlamydia, gonorrhea, syphilis, congenital syphilis, genital herpes, genital warts, and trichomonas infection) (Lowndes & Fenton, 2004; ECDC, 2013). Gender, age group, sexual orientation, and particular geographic area must all be recorded. While all syphilis and gonorrhea infections must be confirmed by GUM clinics, a considerable number of *Chlamydia trachomatis* infections are diagnosed at nonclinical test settings within the community, which would allow these cases to go unreported. However, the diagnosis must be confirmed by laboratory tests (ECDC, 2013).

Voluntary Universal Case Reporting

Voluntary universal case reporting applies to chlamydia and LGV infections, which must be confirmed

by laboratory test. Full details are compiled and an aggregate format of the data is submitted in the report. In specifying the key elements already mentioned, LGV infection reporting involves more in-depth details for enhanced surveillance (ECDC, 2013; Lowndes & Fenton, 2004; Simms et al., 2004).

Case Finding: An Essential Component of Case Reporting

The case finding process involves routine testing on particular population groups at high risk of contracting STIs, such as all pregnant women, young people, and commercial sex workers. This routine testing might be carried out in family planning clinics and maternal child clinics. Case finding ensures that individuals who may be vulnerable to infections exposure have the opportunity for examination and STI testing. Additionally, case finding allows for tracing sexual contacts so that both individuals can be offered appropriate treatment, guidance, and counseling support (UNAIDS/WHO, 2012). The following section presents a brief contextual overview of case finding through screening programs.

Screening programs allow asymptomatic community members to be tested and examined for STIs outside of healthcare facilities. Often, specific high-risk groups are targeted, such as young people, commercial sex workers, injection drug users, travelers, and people living with HIV infection (Lowndes & Fenton, 2004; M'ikanatha, Lynfield, Van Beneden, & de Valk, 2013; UNAIDS/WHO, 2012). It is recommended that identified cases of infections be reported to public health authorities through established STI surveillance systems (Steen et al., 2009; UNAIDS/WHO, 2012). *Chlamydia trachomatis, Neisseria gonorrhoeae, Trichomonas vaginalis,* candidiasis, and bacterial vaginosis are the infections identified for screening (M'ikanatha et al., 2013; Steen et al., 2009; UNAIDS/WHO, 2012).

There is no substantiating evidence for prenatal screening of asymptomatic women for gonorrhea, *Trichomonas vaginalis,* bacterial vaginosis, and herpes (using type-specific antibody testing for HSV-1 and HSV2) (UNAIDS/WHO, 2012). Case finding and case management using the syndromic approach to treatment, together with interventions for targeted high-risk groups, are recognized as important arrangements (Lowndes & Fenton, 2004; M'ikanatha et al., 2013; Steen et al., 2009). In circumstances such as specific infection outbreaks, targeted mass treatment as indicated by population need and urgency may be considered (Lowndes & Fenton, 2004; M'ikanatha et al., 2013).

Syphilis screening can also be performed at sentinel sites for case reporting, and these programs target the high-risk population groups for data collection (Bremer, Marcus, & Hamouda, 2012; Savage et al., 2012). Thus, pregnant women under 24 years of age attending antenatal clinics and commercial sex workers attending STI/GUM clinics are screened for syphilis. Collected data should adequately correspond to the sample size of each target group attending the specific clinics or screening facilities (UNAIDS/WHO, 2012). Recognition of recent increases in STI rates supports the rationalization of screening vulnerable groups as a measure toward controlling STIs. This has been demonstrated as indicated in the surveillance reports by Bremer et al. (2012) in Germany and Savage et al. (2012) in the United Kingdom. Sexual health practitioners may find it useful to explore the original full texts for more detailed information and more insight about the broad topic of screening and case finding in STI surveillance. Specific screening programs are considered later in this chapter.

Case Definitions in STI Case Reporting for Surveillance

Case definitions in STI case reporting involve a set of pre-specified clinical or laboratory criteria that characterize an infection or disease (UNAIDS/WHO, 2012). Correct surveillance reporting requires clearly defined, consistent, and standardized definitions of STI characteristics (Lowndes & Fenton, 2004). This allows for ease of data comparison across different areas of care and service provision (UNAIDS/WHO, 2012).

Case definitions may be used for syndromic diagnosis for urethral discharge in men and genital ulcer disease in both men and women (UNAIDS/WHO, 2012). The clinical criteria for syndromic case definitions of urethral discharge in men comprise discharge from the urethral meatus even without manual expression and dysuria in some cases (Holmes et al., 2008; Richens, 2011; UNAIDS/WHO, 2012). The main causative organisms are *Neisseria gonorrhoeae* and *Chlamydia trachomatis*, but *Mycoplasma genitalium* and *Trichomonas vaginalis* have also been identified as causing urethral discharge in men (Holmes et al., 2008; Lazaro, 2013; UNAIDS/WHO, 2012).

The following criteria are sued for syndrome diagnosis of genital ulcer disease: in men, a skin ulcer on the penis, scrotum, or rectum; in women, an ulcer on the labia, vagina, cervix, and rectum. Organisms involved are *Treponema pallidum* for syphilis and *Haemophilus ducreyi* for chancroid. However, *Chlamydia trachomatis* strains L1, L2, L3, which cause lymphogranuloma venereum, also cause other infectious conditions. These organisms—identified as *Klebsiella granulomatis*—are implicated as causing granuloma inguinale as well as HSV-1, HSV-2 of genital herpes, and genital ulcer disease (Roett, Mayor, & Uduhiri, 2012; UNAIDS/WHO, 2012).

Etiologic case definitions should be precise enough to ensure accuracy and consistency standardized case reporting STI surveillance throughout each country. As previously explained, this is achievable if laboratory resources are available as part of the existing health service system (Lowndes & Fenton, 2004) with efficient technology and specialist expertise for accurate diagnoses. Thus, for etiologic case definitions for gonorrheal infections, the definitions for consistent surveillance are as follows:

Probable classification indicates gram-negative intracellular diplococci in a specimen obtained from the urethra, the rectum, or the endocervix (UNAIDS/WHO, 2012).

Confirmed classification indicates oxidase-positive by culture, gram-negative intracellular diplococci confirmed with specific species-confirmatory techniques, or detection of the specific DNA for *Neisseria gonorrhoeae*. These must be confirmed by accurate nucleic acid amplification tests (NAATs) on specimens obtained from the endocervix, urethra, rectum, or pharynx (UNAIDS/WHO, 2012). Specific etiologic case definitions stipulated for primary, secondary, and latent syphilis are outlined below.

For primary syphilis, the stipulated criteria are ailment accompanied by ulcers and a reactive treponemal or nontreponemal serologic test.

For secondary syphilis, the stipulated criteria are mucocutaneous lesions and a reactive treponemal or nontreponemal serologic test. These represent the classification of probable syphilis infection. However, the classification of confirmed syphilis infection is characterized by *Treponema pallidum* in clinical specimens detected by dark-field microscopy, direct fluorescent antibody test for *Treponema pallidum* (DFA-TP), nucleic acid test, or comparable techniques (WHO/UNAIDS 2013).

For latent syphilis probable classification applies to cases showing no clinical signs or symptoms and not previously diagnosed. The laboratory criteria for syphilis -treponemal-positive serology (*Treponema pallidum* hemagglutination assay [TPHA] or rapid treponemal test) apply. These should be confirmed by nontreponemal test (venereal disease research laboratory [VDRL] or rapid plasma reagin test [RPR]) without titration (WHO/UNAIDS 2013).

For previously diagnosed patients with latent syphilis, the stipulated laboratory criteria of syphilis-treponemal-positive serology (TPHA) or rapid treponemal test apply. This should be confirmed by nontreponemal test RPR with titration showing a rise of fourfold or more from the latest nontreponemal test titer (WHO/UNAIDS 2013).

Early latent syphilis refers to infection acquired within the preceding 24 months and late latent syphilis refers to existing infection of more than two years (WHO/UNAIDS 2013). Readers are urged to explore other expert texts for more details.

Various versions of case definitions by clinical criteria and laboratory criteria have been employed in different countries. Some adopt particular preferred versions as tools for standard surveillance. The E.U. versions of case definitions clearly outline the required data elements for each of the identified infections and the classifications are as follows:

- *Possible case* indicates N/A.
- *Probable case* applies to case definitions that meet the clinical criteria together with associated epidemiological criteria.

- *Confirmed case* applies to case definitions that meet the laboratory criteria. (ECDC, 2013)

The 2011 Surveillance Report on STIs in Europe (ECDC, 2013) provides more information and insight on case definitions.

Data Elements in Case Reporting for STI Surveillance

To develop an accurate representation of STI distribution among the general population, specific data elements should be documented (UNAIDS/WHO, 2012) based on the type of surveillance and intention for conducting it. These data elements include age, gender, education background, occupation, and place of residence. Clinical details include diagnosis, treatment, previous STIs, behaviors and attitude to the use of condoms, sexual orientation, and sexual partners (UNAIDS/WHO, 2012). Moreover, to achieve more informed uses, data elements can be applied to different age groups, specified by intervals of 5 years (UNAIDS/WHO, 2012).

Analysis of the information may help to identify and monitor different groups' vulnerability to specific STIs and associated sexual health risks and to guide needs assessment for support and specific services.

HIV and AIDS Reporting System (HARS)

HIV and AIDS Reporting System (HARS) is a dataset for collecting information on patients diagnosed with HIV infection who access HIV outpatient care.

Benefits of HARS

The main purpose of HARS is to guide surveillance and help make informed policy decisions in response to HIV-related matters. Moreover, the information is to guide implementation and evaluation of preventive endeavors and initiatives. The output data scrutiny and monitoring of the numbers of new diagnoses of HIV infections, numbers of individuals living with diagnosed HIV infections, incidence of new infections, and associated risk factors (Chau, Brown, & Delpech, 2014; HPA, 2013; PHE, 2014).

Other purposes of HARS include monitoring the quality of care provided in the relevant HIV care facilities.

Sentinel-Site Case Reporting

Sentinel-site case reporting involves identification of a sample of healthcare and service providing facilities referred to as sentinel sites. Examples of sentinel sites include antenatal clinics and GUM/STI clinics. Case reporting data are collected from these sites and are used to determine the size and extent of STIs trends over given periods of time.

One of the main objectives is to record and report all cases of STIs and any particular sexual health or related problems identified at the sentinel sites (UNAIDS/WHO, 2012). Some countries may choose to incorporate additional data elements on demographic, social, cultural factors, and partner notifications, thus helping to provide a broader and more in-depth scope of information.

The information from sentinel sites can be combined with universal case reporting data to get a clearer picture of a country's STI problem and the associated challenges. In that way, sentinel case reporting enhances consistent, complete, and high-quality STI surveillance. As Lowndes and Fenton (2004) point out, the specifying of data elements together with the use of sentinel and enhanced surveillance systems for complementing universal and laboratory case data has advantages. It offers greater insight about the European context of STI spread and the different causal factors and it also guides appropriate responsiveness within the public health context. These authors recognize the impact of ongoing changes in the epidemiology of STIs and emerging new diagnostic techniques on surveillance and monitoring systems. Groseclose, Samuel, Chow, and Weinsotck's (2013) chapter—"Surveillance for Sexually Transmitted Diseases" is highly recommended for more in-depth clarification.

Standardization of sentinel case reporting is better achieved where there is an established national HIV/AIDS and STI control program (Lowndes & Fenton, 2004). It is important that the same case report form is used at all sentinel sites to ensure that the required information is collected methodically and recorded correctly.

The report form should be clearly structured and indicate the required core data elements. Any additional useful data elements should be clearly outlined (Lowndes & Fenton, 2004). Crucially, the form should be uncomplicated and staff should be trained on a regular basis (Lowndes & Fenton, 2004). Regular supervision of the sentinel sites should be conducted from the level of the national HIV/AIDS and STI control. This allows for thorough monitoring of the data collection process and the quality of data collected (Lowndes & Fenton, 2004). Relevant ethical and legal considerations should form part of the regulations and should require safeguarding an individual's anonymity and confidentiality by omitting personally identifiable details (Lowndes & Fenton, 2004; M'ikanatha et al., 2013).

An important advantage of the combined universal and sentinel case reporting is that implemented together, the two mechanisms provide complementary benefits (Lowdes & Fenton, 2004). While universal case reporting provides basic estimates of incidence and prevalence, sentinel case reporting provides additional essential data on the epidemiology and clinical detail about the targeted subgroups (cases) in the wider population. Therefore, it is more beneficial for both systems to be implemented concurrently and reported through the integrated disease surveillance (IDS) system (M'ikanatha et al., 2013). The case reporting of syphilis survey at sentinel sites requires that data be collected from routine clinical examinations and screening. Prevalence can be calculated from the demographic details of the high-risk groups and from the data on all tested patients.

Reflective Considerations: Sentinel-Site Case Reporting

- *The principles of sentinel-site case reporting*
  - *Before exploring more details about sentinel-site case reporting, discuss among colleagues what factors should be taken into account in identifying appropriate clinics to participate as sentinel case-reporting sites for STI surveillance.*
  - *If your clinical area already or currently functions in that capacity, compare the characteristics of that area with the recommended criteria for determining appropriate sites as sentinel case-reporting sites for STI surveillance. (Careful examination of the essential requirements for sentinel-site case reporting is crucial.)*
  - *Discuss the strengths of that clinical area as an efficient sentinel case-reporting site and carefully examine any existing limitations or shortfalls.*
  - *Furthermore, consider how the identified shortfalls could be improved to achieve excellence in sentinel-site case reporting for STI surveillance.*
  - *If your area of clinical practice does not currently participate in sentinel-site case reporting for STI surveillance, discuss the potential strengths and potential limitations of the practice to be considered a sentinel site.*
  - *Consider possible improvements that could improve capacity for becoming a sentinel site for STI surveillance.*

Role and Functions of Laboratories in STI and HIV/AIDS Surveillance

Laboratory-based data provide essential supplementary data to the processes and the case reports developed on the surveillance systems (Department of Health Social Services and Public Safety [DHSSPS], 2011). The laboratory-based data provide information about specific STIs: the causative organisms, how they evolve, and how they respond/react to recommended antimicrobials. In relation to syphilis and HIV surveillance, the laboratory case report may indicate the stage of infection.

The key benefits of laboratory-based case report in STI surveillance as reported by Rietmeijer et al. (2009) emphasize the advantages of collaboration in the sentinel laboratory surveillance. They argue that the information from laboratory data and case reports can be usefully applied in the development, implementation, and evaluation of STI preventive initiatives, policies, and programs. Effective comparisons can also be made and the emergence of similar data may encourage collaboration between local laboratories. Lowndes and Fenton (2004) note that apart from confirming the diagnosis of specific infections based on the symptoms presented by patients, laboratory-based surveillance has the additional benefit of helping to diagnose infections in asymptomatic patients. Taking account of symptomatic versus asymptomatic STIs, the positive and negative results from laboratory tests have been used to calculate the prevalence of infections such as chlamydia and gonorrhea among identified population groups. Furthermore, the microbiological data from laboratory-based surveillance are used to assess the scale and the spread of STIs within the general population (Groseclose et al., 2013; Lowndes & Fenton 2004).

Experts maintain that the most sensitive tests to identify specific infections should be used to enhance screening programs for high-risk groups and further improve detection of asymptomatic and undiagnosed STIs (M'ikanatha et al., 2013; UNAIDS/WHO, 2012). They also emphasize the importance of techniques that accurately detect specific microorganisms rather than serological analyzes, which although appropriate, could prove to be quite complicated to interpret, leading to potential errors. Examples include the complex serological tests for syphilis and HSV-2 (UNAIDS/WHO 2012; M'ikanatha et al., 2013; UNAIDS/WHO, 2012). Nucleic acid amplification tests (NAATs) are considered more sensitive techniques. However, the need for appropriate equipment, highly trained technicians, and specialist supervision may create a hindrance in some countries (Lowndes & Fenton, 2004; M'ikanatha et al., 2013; UNAIDS/WHO, 2012).

Alternative STI testing include rapid diagnostic tests (RDTs), which are less complicated and relatively less costly. Compared to laboratory tests for treponemal organism, sensitivity levels are 85–99% with specificity of 93–100% (Peeling, 2009, 2011; UNAIDS/WHO, 2012). However, experts caution against the use of treponemal RDTs in high-prevalence areas with previously treated patients. Unfortunately, rapid tests for other STIs such as chlamydial, gonococcal, and trichomonal infections are relatively expensive. Moreover, they involve quite complicated techniques that may be less sensitive and therefore probably not realistically feasible for low-income countries with high prevalence of these infections (UNAIDS/WHO, 2012).

HIV/AIDS Surveillance in the United States

In the United States, although the incidence of HIV infections has declined since it peaked in the epidemic of the 1980s, diagnoses of new cases are reported to persist around 40,000–50,000 each year (CDC, 2017; Hall et al., 2008). The HIV diagnosis data represent estimates from all states ane the District of Columbia, as well as six U.S. dependencies. However, statistical calculation of the rates does not include these dependent areas. The National HIV Surveillance System (NHSS) provides the source of data and related information used for tracking the HIV/AIDS epidemic. The surveillance is performed by the relevant health departments. In the surveillance system HIV/AIDS collectively represents three classifications of diagnoses: (1) diagnosis of HIV infection without AIDS, (2) diagnosis of HIV infection followed later by diagnosis of AIDS, and (3) diagnosis of HIV infection concurrently with AIDS (CDC, 2017; Hall et al. 2008).

The suppliers of data include the Centers for Disease Control and Prevention and the National Center for HIV/AIDS, Viral Hepatitis, STD and TB Prevention (CDC/NCHHSTP). The surveillance events take place annually and the surveyed populations comprise all 50 states, the District of Columbia, U.S.-dependent nations; independent nations that have free association with the United States report HIV/AIDS data to the CDC. In most states, surveillance activities involve four main participant sources: hospitals, physicians, public and private clinics, and specific medical records systems such as death certificates. Data collection involves use of standardized confidential case reports sent to the CDC electronically without the individuals' personal identifiable details. For adjustments to the estimated data on HIV infection and AIDS, a maximum likelihood statistical procedure is employed to account for differences in reporting delays among characteristics such as demographic and vital status. Furthermore, HIV/AIDS surveillance data are updated annually. Frequent modifications have been made to the case definitions of HIV and AIDS since 1985, which affects interpretation of data. To assess trends in AIDS cases, deaths, and prevalence it is considered more appropriate to use case definitions that are adjusted for reporting delays and presented by year of diagnosis rather than the rates by year of report (CDC, 2013a).

The following reflective considerations are intended to encourage colleagues to critically examine the factors that may influence the conduct and accuracy of laboratory tests and ultimately impact surveillance of antimicrobial resistance (AMR).

Reflective Considerations: The Role of Laboratories in STI Surveillance

- *Consideration of the role of laboratories in STI surveillance*
  - *For the purposes of conducting useful diagnostic laboratory tests for STI and/or HIV surveillance, consider the reportable or notifiable cases and associated factors that should be selected for regular surveillance and monitoring. (Concentrate on case selection for surveillance.)*
  - *In regard to feasibility, discuss what level and systems of surveillance would be more effective and informative for the Department of Public Health to respond to.*
  - *Consider what expectations each group has of the other. (For example, what does the*

laboratory team expect the clinical staff to do to help them conduct the specific STI tests efficiently and vice versa? Consider the quality of the required specimens for specific tests, the viability of specific specimens.)

- *Consider the adequacy of current knowledge and skill levels within the laboratory and clinical sector to perform the respective roles and responsibilities by critically examining the STI and HIV control, surveillance, monitoring, and prevention.*
- *Identify the knowledge and skills deficits in each area.*
- *Critically discuss the training needs identified by the group that should be fulfilled for the staff in each sector. (This would inevitably have resource implications. Therefore, consider what resources should be taken into account.)*
- *As appropriate, consider relevant professional regulations and related ethical and legal issues.*
- *Finally, consider what laboratory-based case reporting involves, the key components for the purposes of STI and HIV surveillance, and the implications for low-income countries.*

Monitoring of Antimicrobial Resistance (AMR) in STI Surveillance

Antimicrobial resistance (AMR) creates a particular hindrance in the treatment of microorganisms that cause certain STIs—particularly *Neisseria gonorrhoeae* (Lewis, 2010), but also *Treponema pallidum* and *Haemophilus ducreyi*. Various studies have revealed that gonorrheal pathogens or isolates have consistently evolved into strains that exhibit resistance to different antimicrobials (Tapsall, Ndowa, Lewis, & Unemo, 2009). The rapid increase in antimicrobial resistance in recent years has reduced available treatment options. The multiple problems of decreased susceptibility of gonorrhea to oral and injectable cephalosporins, as well as antimicrobial resistance, has resulted in gonorrhea being described as a multidrug-resistant microorganism.

The importance of antimicrobial surveillance and monitoring of antimicrobial resistance is recognized globally (UNAIDS/WHO, 2012) and internationally within the E.U. and E.E.A. (Cole et al., 2011), in the United States (Kirkcaldy, Kidd, Weinstock, Papp, & Bolan, 2013), in the United Kingdom (Delpech et al., 2009; HPA, 2011a) and in various other countries. Undoubtedly, due to the increasing resistance of *Neisseria gonorrhoeae* to the recommended cephalosporin treatments, there is a need to continue monitoring the antimicrobial resistance of this organism.

Antimicrobial resistance and susceptibility monitoring involves extensive scientific investigation of the potency of specific antimicrobial agents in hindering the growth of sexually transmitted organisms. Varying strengths of the specific antimicrobial agent are used on the organisms to determine the lowest potency that inhibits the particular organism's growth. Thus, antimicrobial susceptibility information for infective organisms such as *Neisseria gonorrhoeae* isolates should be indicated in the laboratory-based case reports. Organism isolates reacting to specific antimicrobial agents are classified as sensitive, intermediate, or resistant. Additionally, observed resistance to cephalosporins has been reported by Tapsall et al. (2009), Barry and Klausner (2009), and Golparian, Hellmark, Fredlnd, and Unemo (2010). Others have observed resistance to specific cephalosporins such as cefixime and azithromycin (Ison & Alexander, 2011; Ison, Hussey, Sankar, Evans, & Alexander, 2011), cefixime (Unemo, Golparian, Syversen, Vestrheim, & Moi, 2010), ciprofloxacin (Koedijk, van Veen, de Neeling, Linde, & van der Sande, 2010), and azithromycin (Bignell & Garley, 2010). These and many other similar findings indicate the growing resistance of *Neisseria gonorrhoeae* to a variety of antimicrobial agents (Hughes, Nichols, & Ison, 2011; Unemo & Nicholas, 2012). Therefore, continuous global surveillance and monitoring is strongly urged. *Treponema pallidum, Haemophilus ducreyi*, and the HSV-2 viral organism are also monitored for antimicrobial resistance in laboratories with the required expertise and funding (UNAIDS/WHO, 2012).

The role of national reference laboratories is vital in conducting antimicrobial resistance surveys and susceptibility monitoring. Therefore, strict selection of adequately equipped laboratories staffed with appropriately qualified and efficient technicians and supervised by expert scientists with the relevant knowledge and background is advocated by all relevant stakeholders. In organizations where these are not available the required laboratory service may have to be sought from another area as necessary (UNAIDS/WHO, 2012).

Prevalence Assessment and Monitoring

Prevalence assessment involves ascertaining the frequency of occurrence of an infection or disease and the associated factors within a community. Essentially, prevalence assessment surveys are conducted to establish the prevalence of STIs among the general population, detect the vulnerable groups, and determine the trends based on specific characteristics. Thus, the assessment can be carried out on the entire population or local communities or on identified subgroups within the communities. The process involves cross-sectional surveys to calculate the number or proportion of people in the general population who have acquired the infection or disease (UNAIDS/WHO, 2012).

Comparisons can then be made with other communities to determine the differences in frequency of infection or disease acquisition. In monitoring STI trends within the population and communities, the prevalence assessment data can serve additional purposes. The demographic data from prevalence assessments can be utilized to gain better insight and understanding about what factors make some groups in the general population more at risk of contracting particular infections. Thus, although variations may be noted, the key data elements tend to be the same as for case reporting (UNAIDS/ WHO, 2012). The identification of population subgroups for prevalence assessment surveys may be based on the particular country's typical population. Examples of subgroups include commercial sex workers, MSM, IDUs, patients who attend STI clinics and antenatal clinics, and migrant population groups. Clients of the commercial sex workers may also be targeted as medium-risk subgroups (UNAIDS/WHO, 2012).

Prevalence assessment surveys are conducted at 3- to 5-year intervals and may be in the form of national projects to investigate seroprevalence among the general population. The seroprevalence surveys for syphilis generally take place in the form of screening at antenatal clinics and within the context of blood transfusion services. However, prevalence assessment surveys may also be conducted in the form of separate or unconnected projects at the levels of sexual care provision and may be combined with STI and/or HIV behavioral surveys (UNAIDS/WHO, 2012). Evidence suggests that in countries with adequate data, reduction in the prevalence of HIV among young people is revealed where this is combined with changes in sexual behavior. Readers of this chapter are encouraged to explore the 2010 paper by the International Group on Analysis of Trends in HIV prevalence and behaviors in young people in countries most affected by HIV.

Practical Application of Prevalence Assessments

In addition to uses such as estimating the countrywide prevalence of STIs, the data allow for calculating the relative prevalence of symptomatic versus asymptomatic STIs among the population. Another purpose of prevalence assessment is to plan and implement efficient and useful interventions, evaluate the impact of the interventional programs nationally or even internationally, and determine the required resources and funding (UNAIDS/WHO, 2012).

Prevalence Assessment Surveys Linked to Healthcare-Seeking Behavior: Integrated Biological and Behavioral Surveys

Combined behavioral and prevalence assessment surveys, or integrated biological and behavioral surveys (IBBSs), involve data collection for linking high-risk and healthcare-seeking behavior to acquisition of STIs and HIV. The main objectives and purposes of this concept include assessment of prevalence in terms of how commonly infections occur among the population surveyed. It also helps in identifying subgroups within the wider population considered at high risk of infection exposure and to determine individual patterns of healthcare-seeking behavior (UNAIDS/WHO, 2012). This may reveal the timing for seeking healthcare intervention and where people choose to go to seek diagnosis, advice, and guidance. Moreover, combined prevalence and healthcare-seeking behavior allows practitioners to assess the impact of preventive programs. The information is useful for guiding policy decisions, planning supplementary facilities to enhance existing services, and provide funding and required resources to meet other identified needs. Essentially, this concept is considered more economical in the long term.

Data elements are similar to those previously outlined and additional information may depend on the type of population subgroup and the particular context. Nonetheless, elements to assess risk behaviors should be consistent. For example:

- Number of sexual partners over the preceding 3–12 months
- Number of new sexual partners in the recent 3 months
- Condom use in the most recent sexual intercourse with someone other than the usual sexual partner
- Alcohol/drug use in the recent 12 months
- Giving or receiving reward for sexual intercourse in the recent 12 months (UNAIDS/WHO, 2012)

Readers may wish to explore the full document for more detailed information.

Enhanced Surveillance

Enhanced surveillance of STIs relates to more detailed and advanced-level surveillance, which essentially involves a wider scope of components with more extensive data elements reported. The additional data elements depend on specific factors relating to the particular STI. For example, this was demonstrated in relation to the enhanced surveillance of primary, secondary and early latent stage syphilis (DHSSPS, 2011) as well as lymphogranoloma venereum (LGV) (DHSSPS, 2011; Simms, 2004). To provide the additional data elements for these enhanced surveillance events, GUM clinicians collected and reported extensive data on demographic, clinical, and risk factors for submission to the relevant public health authorities. Anonymity and confidentiality were strongly emphasized in the processes of data collection and case reporting.

The aim of the enhanced surveillance system is to produce detailed comprehensive information from the large amount of data collected (Lowndes & Fenton, 2004; M'ikanatha et al., 2013; Rietmeijer et al., 2009). In this surveillance system, the emphasis is consistently on the quality of the data (UNAIDS/WHO, 2012). The scope of the data collected from the all-encompassing elements allows for detailed epidemiological analysis of disaggregated data at patient level (Hargreaves et al., 2010; Slater, Sadler, Cassell, Horner, & Low, 2007). In this way, the report presents analysis of each data element separately. Generally, enhanced surveillance of STIs is characteristically perceived as being in-depth, extensive, and of high quality. Hargreaves et al.'s 2010 report on enhanced surveillance conducted in England in 2008 is highly recommended as an exemplar of good practice. Other

applications of enhanced surveillance have been reported by Field et al. (2010) and Delpech et al. (2009).

Evaluation and Monitoring of the Surveillance Systems

To establish the effectiveness of surveillance systems, a formal systematic examination of all the different stages is required. It is important to determine the extent to which the set goals are fulfilled. It is also crucial to examine the impact of the current surveillance and monitoring systems such as the impact on specific aspects of STI and HIV control and service provision. Therefore, usage of data should also be evaluated (CDC, 2014; Burke, Harris, & Swinson, 2006; Kent, 2007; Rietmeijer et al., 2009; UNAIDS/WHO, 2013; CDC 2013c).

The initial stage of STI surveillance evaluation involves examining and evaluating processes, such as case reporting, etiologic and syndromic diagnoses, prevalence assessment, and antimicrobial resistance monitoring to determine shortfalls and limitations, and to eliminate redundancies. Furthermore, the evaluation should involve detailed examination of organizational structure and staff capabilities (Rietmeijer et al., 2009; UNAIDS/WHO, 2012), communication, the data collection instruments, methods data transfer, analysis, and information circulation and distribution. Additionally, the reporting and feedback mechanisms and the frequency of these events should be evaluated together with appraisal of the quality maintenance process for the surveillance system (UNAIDS/WHO, 2012).

While the value of dissemination of surveillance data and relevant reports is generally acknowledged, Kent (2007) examines the cost implications and usefulness of the surveillance process. Data dissemination involves the following: stakeholders receive annual reports detailing infection rates, geographical trends, demographic profiles, and prevalence data on populations. Surveillance data may be presented in consumer-facing fact sheets displayed at health department offices and clinics.

Newsletters with summary reports are produced for clinicians and laboratory staff and these may include patient management policy updates. Press releases indicating STIs trends and related disease burden may be produced for public campaigns and appropriate summary data placed on the website (UNAIDS/WHO, 2012). Educational charts and posters reflecting surveillance data may be produced. Feedback from healthcare providers and participating organizations process review and surveillance system improvement (Burke et al., 2006; Rietmeijer et al., 2009; UNAIDS/WHO, 2012).

Monitoring the surveillance system involves determining how many and which sites fail to submit full reports in a timely manner. Delayed report submissions (or missing data) can hinder accurate data compilation for a whole region or an entire healthcare organization. Thus, reporting completeness refers to submission from every participating site by the specified submission date (Rietmeijer et al., 2009; UNAIDS/WHO, 2012). There is no doubt that evaluation and monitoring of STI surveillance systems could prove to be extensive and time consuming, and the above overview is by no means exhaustive. Of crucial importance is thoroughness in the process, accurate collection of data and related information, and efficient reporting to ensure evidence-based improvement of the surveillance systems toward better care and service provision.

Practitioners may wish to split this reflective considerations activity into small parts. The main objective is that by the end of this exercise, practitioners should have gained reasonable insight into what STI surveillance and monitoring involve.

Reflective Considerations: Evaluation of STI Surveillance and Control

- **Consideration of evaluation of STI surveillance and control**
  - To begin with, examine each of the related terms: surveillance, monitoring, evaluation, dissemination.
  - Consider the purposes and potential usefulness for performing evaluation of surveillance systems at the organizational level.
  - Examine the importance of evaluating national surveillance systems.
  - What should be the preliminary considerations? Think of the set goals and the extent to which specific goals have or are being fulfilled.
  - Working together in a group, how would you illustrate a cycle of processes, events, or actions for evaluating STI surveillance and monitoring?
  - Think about the main components of STI surveillance and how these should be organized in a logical sequence from the beginning to completion of the evaluation project.
  - Develop a list of indicators for evaluating each component that you have identified to be included in the evaluation.
  - Consider the specific population groups, the type of data collected, specific data elements, and the ethical implications relating to the organizational policy guidelines on confidentiality, privacy, and anonymity.
  - Consider standardization of data entry and storage.
  - Consider how data are transferred between the levels of administration.
  - Consider the professional level and background of identified staff delegated the duty of collecting the required data and how accurately they perform this task.
  - Consider assessment of the quality of data and the stipulated types of documentation.
  - Consider who analyzes the data, the level of statistical expertise, techniques used, clarity of tabulations, and the related reports.
  - Consider what data would be required for antimicrobial monitoring and why this is significant in STI surveillance. (Discuss practical examples that you are familiar with.)
- **Following the reflective evaluation of each component:**
  - Consider what enhancement or improvement is required for particular components.
  - Consider how any duplications in the surveillance systems could be effectively addressed without creating a limitation in the surveillance mechanism.
  - Consider identified gaps and what could be done to meet each shortfall.
  - Consider which components have not contributed any useful information toward planning and improvement of care and service provision and how these limitations could be addressed by adjustments or completely omitting that element without creating any gaps in the particular surveillance system.
  - Critically examine what the concept of monitoring involves within the STI surveillance system.
  - Consider what monitoring of the entire system of surveillance entails and the usefulness of that process.
- **Final stage of the evaluation of the STI surveillance: Team development of a pragmatic plan for enhancing subsequent surveillance**
  - Consider how the planning and implementation of STI/HIV control and prevention could be prioritized.
  - Consider how an informative evaluation report should be structured and developed for dissemination and how frequently this may be required.
  - Consider which stakeholders should be included in the dissemination of the report and justify why each of the identified parties should be included.
  - Consider the importance of feedback, what modes and formats this should comprise, and who should provide feedback and to whom.

The ensuing section explores measures to deal with the combined burden of STIs and the persistently high rates of unintended and unwanted pregnancy and abortions among adolescent girls.

Practical Preventive Initiatives: Maintaining the Recommended Principles

Prevention involves precautionary and protective methods of prophylactic measures to safeguard individuals, groups, and communities from the risk of STI occurrence, spread, and transmission (Steen et al., 2009). The Joint United Nations Programme on HIV/AIDS (WHO/UNAIDS), explain prevention as a means of improving the health status of the population by prioritizing programs that focus on this goal. They recommend the following strategies:

- Primary prevention activities (promotion of safer sexual behavior, condom provision) alongside National AIDS programs

- Accessible, acceptable, and effective case management of persons with STDs through public and private healthcare systems, including first-level health care using simple algorithms based on syndromic diagnosis

- STD prevention and care services in maternal and child health, antenatal, and family planning services

- Acceptable and effective STD care services to populations identified as being particularly vulnerable to infection with STDs, including HIV

- Early STD healthcare-seeking behavior together with education related to sexual behavior (ECDC, 2013; WHO/UNAIDS, 2013)

Guidance on clinical prevention and control of STIs and diseases emphasize certain key interventions particularly aimed at individuals at risk of acquiring the infections. These interventions include meticulous risk assessment, education, and counseling on how individuals can avert or protect themselves from acquiring STDs through uptake of prevention supportive services, safer sexual practices, and behavior change.

The CDC also recommends pre-exposure vaccination to curb vaccine-preventable STIs, as well as correct screening to identify individuals with asymptomatic and symptomatic STIs. Also of importance is efficient and successful diagnosis, treatment, and follow-up of infected individuals, together with assessment, treatment, and counseling of their sexual partners (CDC, 2015). In addition, some sexual healthcare organizations implement retesting as a preventive measure. The California Department of Public Health (CDPH, 2011) notes research evidence that reveals 20% of females become reinfected within 6 months of their initial diagnosis and treatment of chlamydia and gonorrhea. Reproductive complications of reinfection include PID, ectopic pregnancy, and infertility. Therefore, an exemplar of best practice is a policy of retesting for these STIs at 3 months following treatment, supported by a recall system, education, and counseling. Additionally, opportunistic retesting is recommended at subsequent clinic visits during the 12 months following treatment (CDPH, 2011). Practitioners are strongly advised to explore the full details of this program as presented by CDPH.

The main factors influencing individuals' risk of infection are cultural values, religious beliefs, demographic profiles, and geographical placement. Further larger structures such as political and legal systems, healthcare organizational structure, and related systems of service provision influence this risk (Steen et al., 2009). The potential consequences of STIs and RTIs—including PID, infertility, ectopic pregnancy, abortion, fetal loss, miscarriage, preterm labor, congenital infection, and perinatal morbidity and mortality—increase the burden on society. Therefore, there is a strong and justifiable need to raise public awareness regarding the importance of infection and disease prevention and control.

STI Transmission Dynamics

Research, mathematical constructs are used to determine STI transmission dynamics, which help practitioners understand transmission patterns among sexual networks. Transmission dynamics refer to the dispersion of different infections within and between specific core groups as well as the bridging population subgroups that comprise their sexual partners. From the groups, infection is further dispersed among the general population and may lead to episodes of epidemics. Pattern observed in epidemics shows high-risk core groups of social networks as representing the highest incidence of transmission of the specific microorganism (Aral & Blanchard, 2012 ; Youm, 2010). Transmission then moves to their sexual partners, representing a lower-risk bridge population. Further transmission among and between the core and bridging groups, expands transmission dynamics to the general population. In such scenarios, the regular sexual partners in long-term relationships have increased vulnerability to STI exposure, thus perpetuating the typical transmission dynamics of the specific microorganism (Frost, 2007; Youm, 2010). Essentially, the concept of transmission dynamics denotes population prevalence and spread, duration of infectivity, and the structures and nature of sexual contacts—factors that influence variations in susceptibility and infectivity (Aral & Blanchard, 2011).

As Doherty et al. (2005) had previously noted, STI transmission dynamics produce varied impacts at different levels. These levels include individuals, sexual partnerships, mother–child, community, and the wider population. Doherty et al. also held the view that transmission dynamics depend on the type of STI organism, the habitual practice of socialization, and mixing of contacts for sexual intercourse among the networks. They described sexual networks within specific structural contexts that facilitate links among individuals, which create STI transmission routes (Doherty et al., 2005). Therefore, rather than being a chance occurrence, the formation of networks and the susceptibility to contracting and spreading STIs depends on multiple factors (individual, relationship, demographic, cultural, and geographic factors), extending to health service organization, economic, legal, and political situations. Consequently, individuals' sexual practices within the sexual networks and their healthcare-seeking behaviors significantly impact STI transmission. In effect, those core groups protract epidemic episodes of STIs and they remain as the principal source of recurrent periodic transmission in the general population (Doherty et al., 2005).

By examining STI transmission dynamics, experts can estimate the expected number of secondary cases caused by a single index case in a population of susceptible people. Four key factors apply in this calculation: the degree of infectivity, the degree of transmissibility, how long the infectivity persists, and the frequency of change in sexual partners (Frost, 2007; Youm, 2010). While some pathogens are found to be highly infectious, the duration of infectivity may be relatively short, such as *Haemophilus ducreyi*. Other organisms, such as HIV and herpes simplex virus type-2 (HSV-2), are categorized as low infectivity but persisting for longer duration. *Neisseria gonorrhoeae*, *Chlamydia trachomatis*, and *Treponema pallidum* are categorized as intermediate infectivity and duration (Youm, 2010). Epidemics are influenced by the responsiveness between the community the particular population, and the specific pathogen. Therefore, all related factors should be taken into consideration in planning appropriate preventive programs. For that reason diverse risk factors, including individuals' susceptibility to contracting the infections, particular sexual practices, and the health-seeking behaviors of the different groups should be carefully examined. Moreover, lack of adequate sexual healthcare services with limited accessibility to the required facilities, poor education, and the extent of illiteracy among the general population should be carefully examined (Aral & Blanchard, 2012).

Interventions for STI prevention and control should be geared to the specific infection during the periods of epidemic outbreaks. Thus, the virulence of the infection in terms of what proportion of the population exposed to the infection develop symptoms, how quickly the infection spreads, and the overall health consequences should be carefully considered. The duration of infectivity and how long the epidemic persists may also be indicative of the virulence of the infective organism (Youm, 2010). Evidently, infections that are easily transmissible but producing few or no symptoms, such as *Chlamydia trachomatis*, could spread widely among the general population. The actual rates are found to be higher among those people who engage in unprotected sexual intercourse (Youm, 2010).

In contrast, infections that are highly transmissible and produce symptoms tend to be treated quickly, thus curbing the spread among the sexual contacts at risk of contracting the infection. The timing of treatment implementation to restrain disease virulence while strengthening control and preventive interventions for reduction of risky sexual behaviors is crucial. Appropriate actions aim to restrict disease transmission to very low rates among the general population, even though high transmission rates may persist among the high-risk core groups (Aral & Blanchard, 2012).

Endeavors Toward Curbing Ongoing Transmission and Spread of STIs

This section considers the significance of STI transmission prevention and is followed by examination of practical interventions. Initiatives should aim at curbing transmission and treating sexual contacts, while also preventing reinfection. A nonthreatening ambiance in care and service provision environments enables patients to discuss personal problems in confidence, receive appropriate advice regarding STI infections, and take preventive measures (Brook et al., 2013). Accurate STI and RTI education ensures that patients make informed decisions about their care and treatment. Information on sexual health services—availability, accessibility and function—should be made available to the general public. Additionally, an individuals' motivation may be enhanced if they understand the personal gain from accessing sexual health services. Successful communication campaigns are crucial for provision of effective guidance and support to vulnerable population groups. Health promotion and education on teen pregnancy should emphasize respect and responsibility, delay in commencement of sexual activities, and avoidance of multiple and concurrent sexual partners. Interventions to prevent STIs, RTIs, pre- and early teenage pregnancy should be implemented in a nonjudgmental manner (Clutterbuck et al., 2012).

There is a need for specific services for population subgroups with high-risk sexual practices and behaviors including adolescents, male and female sex workers, military personnel, long-distance truck drivers, and prisoners. These should form important components of the general care and support services that can be accessed on a flexible basis. Moreover, an all-embracing STI case management program should be implemented to include prevention and care of neonatal conjunctivitis and congenital syphilis. The importance of early detection and treatment should be emphasized to promote uptake of STI screening programs at the prescribed intervals. Condom promotion programs should comprise carefully organized activities that coordinate supply and distribution of condoms (Clutterbuck et al., 2012). Conscientious compliance with infection prevention and control regulations together with appropriate high standard measures are the key issues to consider in primary prevention of STIs. The ensuing sections examine primary prevention together with the related practical actions.

Primary Prevention: Interventions and Supportive Services

It is important that patients (and the general public) receive correct evidence-based information about the safety and efficacy of prevention methods. This includes appropriate instruction on correct application of specific products and the opportunity for supervised practice. A brief overview of the preventative interventions and supportive services employed in primary prevention of STIs is presented in this section. Condom use which is considered primary preventative measure is examined first, followed by sexual history-taking incorporating sexual health promotion. The related ethical implications of social marketing are examined and the relevance of social cognitive theory in the facilitation of health communication, health promotion, and education is also explored.

Individuals who contract STIs should be provided with early and effective diagnosis, treatment, and counseling. Asymptomatic individuals who are identified early are able to receive confirmatory diagnosis and treatment (Kingsberg & Janata, 2007).

Assessment, diagnosis, treatment of sexual partners of individuals with STIs should be made available (Kingsberg, 2006; Kingsberg & Janata, 2007). Of equal importance, members of the general public should have the assurance that pre-exposure vaccination programs for high-risk population groups can be accessed (British Association for Sexual Health and HIV [BASHH], 2010, 2014). Furthermore, health promotion/education and counseling support should be provided for high-risk and vulnerable groups (such as young people) and should incorporate guidance on evidence-based recommendations for lifestyle and behavior changes, such as safer sex practices. It should be made clear that these services are crucial components of sexual health care and are available to other relevant groups. Staff should be competent in detailed sexual history-taking and should follow evidence-based techniques to ensure early detection and treatment of symptoms of RTIs and STIs (Brook et al., 2013). Efficiency in care and service provision requires that there should be a well-structured and purposeful referral system in place that allows for provision of care, support, and advice by appropriately qualified staff.

Condom Supply as a Fundamental STI Primary Preventive Measure: Related Evidence

Condom availability is crucial and it is important that patients are provided with accurate instructions on consistent and correct use, as it is important to avoid problems such as slipping off or accidental breaking (Grimely, Annang, Houser, & Chen, 2005). Various studies have examined the experiences of patients/clients regarding problems and errors with condom use (Crosby et al., 2007; Warner et al.,

2008). Such mishaps undoubtedly defeat the purpose of condoms as a protective and preventive measure for STI transmission, especially to an uninfected contact (Holmes, Levine, & Weaver, 2004; Warner et al., 2004). When used correctly, condoms ensure secondary prevention of STI and HIV transmission from an infected person to their sexual contacts. Warner et al. (2004) emphasize the importance of assessing the infection status of the sexual partner.

Investigations of the effectiveness of condom use for STI protection and enhancing prevention have resulted in mixed findings and various factors have been identified as influencing condom use effectiveness. Holmes et al. (2004) focused on primary prevention by examining condom effectiveness in preventing STIs. Effective reduction in the transmission of gonorrhea and chlamydia was also reported by Warner et al. (2004). Similarly, Niccolai, Rowhani-Rahbar, Jenkins, Green, & Dunne, (2005) investigation, which focused on condom use in preventing *Chlamydia trachomatis* infection, showed reduction of transmission. Nevertheless, Warner et al. (2004) pointed out that the infection status of the partner should be assessed where the intention is to determine the measurement effect of condom use for reducing STIs. This seems to be logical in order to get a clear picture of the measure of effectiveness.

In considering the research findings, other investigators note importance of variations in the methods of investigation, frequency of sexual intercourse, consistency of usage, and the method employed to measure consistency (Noar, Cole, & Carlyle, 2006; Warner, Stone, Macaluso, Buehler, & Austin, 2006). Weller and Davis-Beaty's (2007) review of condom effectiveness revealed a range of 35–94% reduction in HIV transmission among heterosexual males who consistently used male latex condoms. Condom use is also found to be effective in preventing other STIs, as well as unplanned and unwanted pregnancies (Gallo, Grimes, Lopez, & Schulz, 2006). Koss, Dunne, and Warner's (2009) investigation of condom use and the risk of syphilis is worth exploring to gain a clearer picture of the extent of the reported effectiveness.

Apart from promotion of condom use (Kerrigan et al., 2006; Rehle et al., 2010; Shisana et al., 2009), practical considerations in primary prevention of STIs should incorporate sexual health screening and clinic attendance early in pregnancy. Screening for syphilis and effective treatment of women with reactive test results should be considered (Peeling & Ye, 2004; WHO, 2005a), together with screening and treatment of husbands/partners. Emergency contraception service should be available for rape victims, and presumptive STI treatment and postexposure HIV prophylaxis should also be readily accessible to high-risk groups.

It is important that sexual partners be offered appropriate treatment when the source of RTI is suspected to be sexually transmitted. Treatment should incorporate evidence-based counseling by a qualified counselor or experienced sexual health practitioner with counseling qualification. Symptomatic STI/RTI management with use of syndromic flowcharts or laboratory-based diagnosis is found to be effective in helping to maintain policy and recommended guidance. Intensive treatment of upper genital tract infections should be provided following abortion or childbirth to prevent PID and to avoid permanent damage to the woman's fertility (WHO, 2005b).

Significance of Sexual History: An Essential Component of Primary Prevention of STIs

Ideally, professional sexual healthcare practitioners are in the best position to introduce primary prevention measures during consultations at initial clinic attendance. Meticulous sexual history-taking provides an opportunity to identify and assess sexual risk-taking behaviors and practices and to assess the individual's risk of contracting and spreading infections. Therefore, assessment of sexual risk-taking practices forms an imperative element in the routine standardized sexual health promotion intervention and is incorporated in the pro-formas for taking the sexual history. It is important to critically examine and select an effective technique that meets the requirement of a comprehensive sexual history-taking (Brook & FPA, 2013; Clutterbuck, 2004; Kingsberg, 2006).

Main Functions and Purposes of Sexual History-Taking

Sexual history-taking is a key principle in STI screening and care provision. Competent technique with tactful questioning, open-ended questions, comprehensible language, and familiar words that convey the norm, combined with warmth and eye contact will put the patient at ease. In addition, patients should receive an explanation of the significance, purpose, and benefits of having a sexual history taken (Clutterbuck, 2004; Brook et al., 2013). Organizations should incorporate policies to require appropriate training for interviewers and provide arrangements for communication issues (e.g., language or sign-language interpreters, as applicable) (Brook & FPA, 2013). The process of sexual history-taking should foster empowerment in the patient to make informed decisions, but at no time should the patient feel directed or coerced. There should be a clear distinction between counseling and interviewing and the use of open-ended questions allows the patient/client to explain personal experiences relating to their specific concern about STIs.

Sexual history-taking should begin with the main complaint, followed by the patient's general health, current or recent medication, specific allergies, history of previous STIs, habits or practices of condom use, history of substance abuse, HIV risk factors, and current status of relevant partners. This information should be linked to the history of HIV testing (BASHH, 2010, 2014; Brook et al., 2013; Clutterbuck, 2004). In exploring past and current sexual practices, the gender, number of the sexual partners, and the most recent exposure, it is also important to establish information about the new sexual partners. This information will help to determine the patient's current STI risk and to develop an appropriate plan for risk reduction and STI prevention.

Because most STIs are not accompanied by symptoms, it is important to explore sexual risk-taking behaviors that can be associated with specific symptoms. General characteristic symptoms of STIs that should be explored include discharge from the genital tract or anus, burning sensation during micturition, itchiness, blisters, ulceration of the genital skin with or without pain, genital warts, rash (on the body, palms, or soles of the feet), lower abdominal pain, and painful intercourse (Clutterbuck, 2004; Kingsberg & Janata, 2007).

Detailed Sexual History: Compliance with Stipulated Policy Regulations and Guidelines

Practitioners are strongly encouraged to explore and comply with relevant policy guidelines and recommendations regarding detailed sexual history-taking within their employing SRH organization. Compliance with stipulated requirements of U.S. Health Insurance Portability and Accountability Act (HIPAA) is crucial, and training programs are offered to staff.

Environment of Sexual History-Taking: The Ambience, Sense of Privacy, and Confidentiality

The atmosphere for sexual history-taking should be warm, hospitable, and conducive to confidential discussion. There should be a feeling of reassurance, trust, and openness to encourage individuals to share intimate and sensitive information about their recent sexual partners. Patients may need to divulge personal experience with the use of specific techniques, products, or materials (Brook & FPA, 2013). The aim is to reassure and empower the individual to divulge symptoms of embarrassing yet distressing genital lesions, ulcers, abnormal discharge, or mutilation of the genitalia associated with severe inflammation and tissue damage. Request for a clinician of a particular gender should be given consideration and chaperoning should be provided for intimate physical examination. The policy of the clinic for safeguarding privacy and confidentiality should be placed in full view and should be reinforced to give continual assurance (Brook & FPA, 2013).

Rationales for Specific Key Elements in the Sexual Health History

The main components of the history relate to sexual behavior, attitudes, and personal preventive actions. Thus, the presence or absence of symptoms and the reason for attending the clinic should be confirmed to ensure that no unreported symptoms are missed. The patient/client should feel confident to disclose and discuss personal concerns relating to possible exposure to a partner's STI (Kingsberg, 2006). Information regarding the most recent sexual contact should include the date and gender of the sexual contact or partner (to identify MSM) and offer hepatitis screening and vaccination. The sites of exposure or intercourse and whether a condom was used allow the practitioner to determine which sites should be sampled for laboratory tests

(Barry, Kent, Philips, & Klausner, 2010; Hunte, Alcaide, & Castro, 2010; Javanbakth et al., 2012; Koedijk et al., 2012). Additional history is obtained to establish the number of sexual contacts in the past 3 months to explore the history of risky sexual activities within the specific look-back period (McLean, Radcliffe, Sullivan, & Ahmed-Jushuf, 2013). This may help determine which sexual contact may have transmitted the STI. Suspected STIs or STI symptoms observed in the most recent sexual contact(s) or partner(s) should also be discussed to instigate partner notification for diagnostic testing, treatment, and support. Because infection transmission can occur during the STI window period, this information is useful to determine the need for preventive measures such as postexposure HIV prophylaxis or emergency contraception (Brook et al., 2013).

For individuals who have not experienced symptoms but present for STI screening (Brook et al., 2013), previous STI(s), risk of bloodborne viral transmission and acquisition, and vaccination history should be explored to guide interpretation of previous syphilis infection and positive serology (Ahmed & French, 2013; French, 2011). Sexual history from females should explore last menstrual period, use of contraception, and cervical cytology. All patients should be asked their preferred method for being informed about specific test results. It is important to establish each patient's competency (regarding protection of children and other vulnerable patients). History of gender-related violence, alcohol abuse, and use of recreational drugs may be required by some organizations or reporting authorities.

Sexual history from symptomatic females attending for STI tests should explore all the previous details as well as obstetric and gynecological history, medical and surgical history, current medication, and allergic drug reactions. The latter is useful to determine medications that may affect STI management, possible drug interactions with STI treatments, and sexual performance problems associated with particular medications. The history from symptomatic males attending for STI tests should also explore all of the details as for asymptomatic patients/clients (Brook & FPA, 2013; Kingsberg & Janata, 2007).

The history taken from female patients attending integrated clinics for STIs and contraception explores more in-depth additional information about the current contraceptive method being used and any problems experienced. In addition, history takers should explore unfulfilled needs, risk of pregnancy, changes in the menstrual cycle with mood swings, abnormal bleeding, problems of sexual performance, smoking habits, family history, and HPV vaccination. The additional in-depth information obtained from men should include contraception and the type used by the female sexual partner. Unfamiliar urinary tract symptoms and unfulfilled sexual needs and performance should be carefully and sensitively discussed (Brook & FPA, 2013; Kingsberg & Janata, 2007).

As full requirements for a comprehensive sexual history are beyond the scope of this chapter, practitioners are encouraged to read the guidelines for sexual history-taking by Brook and FPA (2013). The CDC 2015 guidelines should also be explored by practitioners in the United States for comparison.

The following technique for exploring sexual history, based on the five "Ps", is found to produce useful and practical clinical information (CDC, 2015). Arguably, the nature of information explored would depend on the individual's gender, and it is important to maintain the individual's confidence by ensuring that the questions are pertinent to him/her.

- Partners: Explores information about preferred gender, number of partners, concurrence and/or frequency of change of sexual partners. In the practice of shared partners, it is useful to determine how recently any of the sexual partners had intercourse with other persons.
- Prevention: Explores pregnancy prevention measures taken by the individual. This issue should be explored sensitively and nonjudgmentally.
- Protection: Explores STI and HIV protective measures undertaken by the individual.
- Practices: Explores sexual practices (which helps the practitioner determine potential risks). This area includes vaginal, anal, and oral sex, and condom use.
- Past history: Explores past history of STIs in both the patient and his/her partners. Other questions explore the individual's risk to HIV and sexually transmitted viral hepatitis B and C. Thus, questions about the practice of drug injection either personally or by a sexual partner are also tactfully explored and the individual is encouraged to add further information that she/he considers as pertinent (CDC, 2015).

Client-Centered STI/HIV Prevention and Counseling

Individually tailored STI/HIV prevention and counseling is advocated as part of the sexual history. Practitioners should consider use of visual aids and demonstration tools to teach correct methods of handling and application of prevention tools (e.g., condoms) Individual sessions may be supplemented by small group discussion and education sessions.

Most, if not all, sexual healthcare professional practitioners apply their national, organizational, or departmental guides or pro-formas for sexual history-taking. This ensures that all members of staff apply the same structure and sequence in obtaining detailed, carefully organized, and pertinent information. However, in practices where these are not provided, a multidisciplinary team may consider developing local or in-house pro-formas. In-service education and study days with role plays or simulation provide useful opportunities for training exercises for newly qualified or newly employed staff. These training activities enable the practitioners to further develop the required knowledge and skills for implementing effective history-taking techniques. Internal reviews and discussion about emerging issues and shortfalls in the existing history-taking practice is crucial. This may lead to development of new guidelines, reviewed recommendations, and change in organizational policies based on findings from systematic reviews and examples of best practice. Similar to the United Kingdom's training program for sexual history-taking, the CDC has an established program STD/HIV Prevention Training Centers (https://www.cdc.gov/std/training/default.htm). The role of health promotion in relation to STI primary prevention is considered in the ensuing section.

Role of Health Promotion and Health Education in STI Primary Prevention

Readers are reminded that the topics of health promotion and education have been addressed more comprehensively in a separate chapter. This section only considers the application of health promotion and education within the context of practical interventions aimed at self-protection and curbing the ongoing transmission and spread of STIs and HIV infection. Health promotion and health education targeting individuals, communities, social groups, specific high-risk groups, and the wider society should be carefully planned, effective, acceptable, and persuasive. Cultural sensitivity should be a key consideration in the provision of information and the mode of delivery. It is important to raise the general public's awareness regarding the advantages of sexual health promotion. The Medical Foundation for AIDS & Sexual Health (MEDFASH, 2010) emphasizes the need for people to be made aware of how they can protect themselves from STIs and unplanned pregnancy. The PHE (2013) recognizes that, apart from prevention of infection and associated diseases, health promotion and health education provide other functions. Additional key functions aim at encouraging and facilitating better sexual health in the broader sense by embracing the related issues of sexuality, sexual relationships, and individuals' sexual rights.

On an individual basis, health promotion can begin during the initial consultation and may form part of the process of the sexual history-taking. Individualized health promotion has the advantages of focusing on personal needs and current health related problem. The aim is to empower the individual to take control over the factors that impact his/her health, while recognizing personal values, cultural and religious influences, social and financial circumstances, and other environmental factors (World Conference on Social Determinants of Health; WHO, 2011). Health promotion should address not just the concern about the physical problem of STIs and related disease but also the individual's emotional, mental, and social well-being. Patients will benefit from evidence-based information on the importance of and personal benefits to protective measures.

Involvement of the individual in making choices and decisions may increase motivation and encourage them to accept personal responsibility for avoiding risky sexual behaviors and using appropriate protective STI measures. Application of carefully identified health promotion theories

may help to foster behavior change and encourage the individual to consider the relevant guidance and support provided by the professional practitioners. Individuals should feel empowered to take personal control of their health and to cultivate the self-confidence to change their circumstances, such as by negotiating condom use with a sexual partner(s) or contact(s). Adolescents may be additionally motivated to self-protect against unwanted or unplanned pregnancy (Conner & Norman, 2005). The Health belief model suggests that perception of personal susceptibility to STI and pregnancy increases the motivation of an adolescent girl or young woman to negotiate and implement self-protection measures. These may involve consistent and correct use of condoms, seeking guidance and support with choosing appropriate contraception method, or making a personal decision to delay sexual intercourse (Conner & Norman, 2005).

Health promotion specialists play an important role and should be experts who are well informed about topics of community and public concern. They should possess insight and expertise relevance to the target group, community, or the general public. Communication campaigns, condom promotion, guidance, and instruction should be dealt with efficiently. Recognition of the social and cultural diversities, the varied moral ethical and religious values and principles that influence sexual behaviors and practices is equally crucial (Steen et al., 2009).

Behavioral Strategies Employed Toward Prevention of STIs and HIV

In this chapter, findings relating to the application of health promotion and health education are considered in the context of STI prevention interventions. Thus, reference is made to the health belief model (HBM) (Haggart, 2000; Janz & Becker, 1984), the theory of reasoned action (TRA) (Ajzen & Fishbein, 1980; Fishbein & Ajzen, 2005), the theory of planned behavior (TPB) (Ajzen, 1988; Naidoo & Wills, 2000) and the transtheoretical model (TTM) as examined by Taylor et al. (2006).

Coates, Ritchter, & Carceres, (2009) explain behavioral strategies as facilitations and support systems to encourage behavior modification in individuals and social groups. These may be achieved through various learning processes of information and instruction, inducement and reinforcement, peer-led with development of competence and capability, and the influences of community values and expectations. These authors consider behavioral strategies to include delaying initial sexual intercourse, abstinence, monogamy, reducing the number of sexual partners, consistent use of condoms, HIV testing and counseling, uptake and consistent use of biomedical facilities, compliance with harm-reducing measures, and low substance abuse (Coates et al., 2009).

Aral (2011) noted that most of the evidence concerning the efficacy of behavioral interventions is based on self-reported outcomes of change in behavior. Subjectivity in reporting and inconsistencies in study designs and methodologies indicate that greater reliance should be placed on STI and HIV incidence as outcome measures. Padian et al. (2010) found that using HIV incidence as the outcome measure for behavioral interventions revealed them to be nonefficacious. Nonetheless, evidence from STI incidence as outcome measure revealed that the interventions were obviously efficacious (Wetmore, Manhart, & Wasserheit, 2010). Earlier reports by Stoneburner and Low-Beer (2004) and Slutkin et al. (2006) indicated that reductions in HIV incidence could be ascribed to or associated with modification in sexual behavior. Various prevention endeavors have been launched as national programs for populations, subgroups, or individuals and various studies have been carried out (Crepaz et al., 2009; Marks, Gardner, Craw, & Crepaz, 2010). These have led to programs such as condom use, STI and HIV testing, referral systems, partner notification and management, and counseling and support systems being made available in many countries. Crepaz et al.'s 2009 study revealed that while most HIV-diagnosed MSM protect their sexual partners from HIV infection and themselves from other STIs, many others fail to do so based on perceived status of infectiousness.

Aral (2011) noted that many studies concentrated on separate behavior risks and specific interventions rather than considering interrelated or multi-factorial complex problems. For example, commencement of condom use and multiple or frequent changes of sexual partners should be examined as potentially interconnected factors. Risky behaviors such as alcohol and substance abuse and injecting drug use among high-risk sexual partners being associated with reduced inhibition and indifferent attitude to condom use could be more extensively explored. Additionally, consistent unprotected sexual intercourse could be explored at the same time. Studies should be designed to investigate the complex interrelation of risky behaviors, preventive measures, biomedical circumstances, and interventions (Aral, 2011).

Implementation of behavioral interventions depends on the particular methods and the target audience. Some interventions are designed for implementation at group levels such as schools or population subgroups of young people (Kirby, 2007). However, some interventions target individuals and the suggestion is to take into consideration that an individual's risk of contracting an STI may not entirely depend on their own lifestyle and sexual behavior. Crucially, the risk to the individual may depend on the sexual practices and lifestyle behaviors of the sexual partners, who may not be monogamous (Aral & Leichliter 2010). It may depend on whether or not the partner has STI infection. An individual's risk for contracting and spreading STI may be influenced by partner's behavior, sexual network links and activities, and the rate of STI transmission among the population (Aral & Leichliter, 2010). Therefore, behavioral interventions that only address individual behavior change may be unproductive in preventing the spread of

STIs among the population. Often, interventions are not linked and therefore may fall short of the potential benefits and increased effectiveness of the integration of behavioral and biomedical interventions together with safer sexual practices. Consequently, there are limited evaluative studies conducted to assess and compare how effective, how successful, or worthwhile and the extent of actual impact of different interventions. Evaluation limitations were mainly due to inconsistencies in types and methods of intervention, duration of implementation, differences in target populations, and the unpredictable entry and exit of people in the population (Aral, 2011). Unsuccessful implementation and failure to repeat also creates problems for evaluating the totality of interventions. Realistically, implementation of a particular intervention separately from others may not prove to be fully productive or successful in achieving the desired behavior change as a long-term outcome. Therefore, integrated approaches are strongly recommended (Kurth, Celum, Baeten, Vermund, & Wasserheit, 2011).

In the context of evidence-based STI prevention, Horowitz (2003) is reported to have applied the transtheoretical model (TTM) in health-related behavior change. This model was reportedly applied to pregnancy prevention with some degree of success. Therefore, this may arguably be the model of choice for behavior change intervention toward prevention of unwanted pregnancy. The TPB is generally considered as being more effective in predicting behavior change than the HBM and the TRA. However, none of these has been found to explain how the change in health behavior could be fostered and supported or made easy (Taylor et al., 2006). The stages of change and the related processes that are characteristic components of the TTM suggest how it can be effectively used for implementing health behavior change interventions. It is therefore found to be a useful assessment tool for behavioral change outcomes and for fostering change in health behavior and adoption of improved health behavior (Taylor et al., 2006).

Extensive research studies that directly focus on health education are necessary for substantiating evidence-based initiatives involving behavior change interventions for STI prevention. Evans and Lambert (2008) observed that implementation of the HBM requires consideration of the context of application for other prevention measures. This seems to be supported by Beh Webster and Bailey's (2013) application of qualitative methods of the behavior change model toward improvement of condom use among men. Shain et al. (2004) demonstrated the effectiveness of risk reduction interventions in decreasing sexual risk-taking behaviors and episodes of infections. These authors emphasized the importance of targeting those at high risk of gonorrhea and chlamydia infections. Their findings showed that application of theory-based behavioral risk reduction designed for a specific group facilitated achievement of reduction in chlamydia and gonorrhea infections by 38% (Shain et al., 2004) during 1 year of follow-up. Shepherd et al. (2010) also explored the impact and economic benefits of behavioral interventions designed to target an identified subgroup of young people toward prevention of STIs.

However, evidence-based practices to implement behavior change interventions of education and support may have to be further enhanced. Lazarus, Sihvonen-Riemenschneider, Laukamm-Josten, Wong, & Liljestrand, (2010) study revealed that while peer-led interventions proves to be better accepted and more effective in improving sexual knowledge, actual behavior change may not necessarily happen. Perhaps more extensive systematic reviews and critical examination of peer education and support should be given more consideration within the wider context of sexual health practice. This could certainly be implemented in the context of behavior change interventions. Carey, Senn, Vanable, Courey-Doniger, & Urban, (2010) explored brief and intensive behavior change interventions toward reducing sexual risk-taking behaviors, and there is no doubt that the delivery, content, and scope of the intervention are crucial influencing factors.

Biomedical Interventions Applied in STI and HIV Prevention

Biomedical interventions continue to gain increasing interest in STI and HIV prevention to achieve effective control. The concept encompasses implementation of multiple medical and public health principles in a composite or integrated approach to limiting the transmission and spread of STIs and HIV infection. Biomedical interventions are applied as preventive endeavors not only at population level but also to target communities, high-risk groups, and individual levels. The aim is to achieve control and prevention of HIV and STI epidemics while fostering individual self-protection.

Low (2012) explains population-level biomedical interventions as systems and procedures that incorporate treatment or prophylaxis against STIs with antibiotics and antiviral medications. Additional components include barrier methods (male and female condoms and diaphragms) with the use of microbicides. Different interventions for STIs implemented at population level may also be incorporated, as Gregson et al. (2007) demonstrated. Various biological and genetic related factors have been identified as influencing HIV transmission, which should be considered in prevention endeavors. In essence, biomedical interventions focus on curbing transmission and spread while weakening the virulence of the infective organisms and decreasing people's susceptibility, particularly among high-risk groups in the general population.

Essential Elements in Biomedical Interventions

Bacterial and viral STIs increase the risk of spread and an individual's predisposition to HIV acquisition (Low, 2012). This view led to the assumption that treating STIs and controlling the prevalence should bring about reduction in the rate of HIV transmission. However, this view has not been substantiated and firmly confirmed, as Ng, Butler, Horvath, and Rutherford (2011) also argued. Various claims about associations between different STIs and HIV have proved to be conflicting or inadequately substantiated. Malkin's (2004) claim about an association between HSV and HIV remains conflicting since other studies found no evidence to support the claim that suppression of HSV actually reduces the risk of HIV infection (Celum et al., 2010; Watson-Jones et al., 2008).

Various researchers have noted that STI treatment, control, and prevention interventions may not necessarily represent an effective strategy for achieving prevention of HIV transmission and acquisition or guarantee actual reduction in the rate of HIV infection (Gregson et al., 2007; Ng et al., 2011). Nevertheless, although transmission of HIV through sexual intercourse is found to be less efficient than other routes, the claims about association between STIs and HIV persist. Arguably, various sexual practices, including anal intercourse, increase individuals' susceptibility and risk to contracting HIV infection. Certain biological factors have also been identified as enhancing HIV infectivity and individuals' predisposition to contracting the infection. Wawer et al. (2005) maintain that individuals with raised HIV plasma viremia or advanced stage of the condition would most likely transmit the virus to their sexual partners and sexual contacts.

Other factors include concurrent or coexisting infection with localized inflammation or even vaccines that may increase the viral load. Pregnancy and the postpartum period are also considered as potential risk in terms of incident HIV acquisition and mother-to-child transmission (Chan & Ray, 2007; Drake, Wagner, Richardson, & John-Stewart, 2014; Gray et al., 2005; Modjarrad, Chamot, & Vermund, 2008). It is suggested that in relation to this, the role of antiretroviral therapy should be thoroughly explored (Bunnell et al., 2006; Chan & Ray, 2007). The strong view, however, is that the measures employed toward HIV prevention also apply to STI prevention and therefore should not be considered separately.

The rationale for STI control forms a crucial component of biomedical interventions toward HIV prevention. Key strategies include early diagnosis and treatment of STIs and effective use of microbicides together with HIV testing and counseling. It must be remembered however, that studies to assess the efficacy of the direct impact of improved STI management as a strategy for HIV prevention have revealed varied findings.

A possible explanation is that the inconsistencies seem to depend on the stage of an epidemic at which efficacy studies are conducted (Mayer et al., 2012). The effectiveness of the endeavors to deal with the complex range of viral and bacterial STIs also needs to be carefully considered for thorough evaluation. Moreover, the standard and quality of available treatments, provision of sustainable resources, and adequate staff, training, facilities, and support also present important challenges for careful consideration (Mayer et al., 2012).

Antiretroviral Therapy and Highly Active Antiretroviral Treatment as Biomedical Interventions Toward Prevention of HIV Acquisition and Transmission

The role of antiretroviral therapy (ART) and highly active antiretroviral treatment (HAART) is widely recognized throughout the world. Antiretroviral treatments cause reduction in the viral concentration of HIV in infected individuals or provide prophylaxis. Postexposure prophylaxis (PEP) may be administered to individuals who have not acquired HIV but have been exposed to possible transmission from an infected person. Apart from the nonoccupation related PEP, healthcare workers who sustain needle-prick injuries, sexual partners, and sexual contacts may receive PEP. However, in view of nonadherence problems and poor rates of PEP treatment completion due to apparent side effects, some experts suggest that this should be reconsidered. Rather, a regimen of two drugs or a simpler regimen might be better tolerated (Bassett, Freedberg, & Walensky, 2004; Liu et al., 2008). There is no doubt the identified problems may have created difficulties for conducting proper assessment of efficacy.

The use of pre-exposure prophylaxis (PrEP) is also recognized and examined. While pre-exposure chemo prophylaxis with daily doses of oral tenofovir has not been associated with significant unfavorable reactions, more extensive studies are required to test for the efficacy (Peterson et al., 2007). This prophylaxis is considered for prevention of mother-to-child transmission (MTCT) in pregnancy and postpartum together with appropriate infant feeding support for mothers living with HIV. Moreover, contraception to prevent unplanned pregnancies among HIV-positive women is an additional biomedical intervention strategy.

Some experts consider it more feasible to provide antiretroviral therapy to symptomatic individuals based on the argument that this strategy would radically reduce the rate of newly acquired HIV infections (Blower & Farmer, 2003; Wilson & Blower, 2005). Others also emphasize the importance of making ART more accessible within the context of HIV prevention and biomedical intervention (Granich, Gilks, Dye, De Cock, & Williams, 2009; Granich, Crowley, Vitoria, Lo, et al., 2010; Granich, Crowley, Vitoria, Smyth, et al., 2010). Other experts also recognize and share the view that treatment's success (in terms of effective treatment, prevention, and control) depends on appropriate measures, such as thorough treatment of STIs with genital tract inflammation, treatment adherence, safer sexual practices, and avoidance of risk-taking behaviors implemented concurrently with ART. Readers are encouraged to explore more extensive studies on the different regimens of antiretroviral therapy, such as Wilson, Coplan, Wainberg, and Blower (2008). The ensuing section examines the role of barrier methods in biomedical interventions.

Barrier Methods (Male Condoms, Female Condoms, and Diaphgrams) in Biomedical Interventions

The role of male condoms as a primary preventative measure has already been examined. However, the relevance to biomedical interventions is briefly considered here. The male condom has been a lasting device in biomedical intervention toward HIV and STI prevention. The male condom was reported earlier as highly effective in reducing the incidence of HIV by up to 95% with consistent and correct usage (Anderson, 2003). However, Foss, Watts, Vickerman, and Heise (2004) pointed out that effectiveness falls to about 70% with inconsistent and incorrect use. Therefore, they recommend that other interventional methods should be implemented. Potts et al. (2008) observed that there is lack of substantial evidence of the effectiveness of condoms in the prevention of HIV epidemics for various reasons. The Ugandan government's commitment to a comprehensive national strategy, the ABC campaign (Abstinence + Be faithful + use Condoms) (Singh, Darroch, & Bankole, 2003) revealed certain limitations despite the apparent reduction in infection rates. As Dworkin and Ehrhardt (2007) observed, the ABC project did not take account of gender relations, social inequity, injustices, and financial circumstances. These factors were linked to situations in which women may not be able to exercise personal control for ensuring safer sexual practices or the use of condoms for sexual intercourse (Minnis & Padian, 2005). Therefore, experts emphasize that female-controlled biomedical prevention methods are needed for effective protection against STIs, HIV infection, and unwanted pregnancy.

Female condoms use also has evidence to support its efficacy (Vijiyakumar, Mabude, Smit, Beksinska, & Lurie, 2006). However, while various efficacy trials for STIs seem to be available, it is unclear how extensively these have been conducted to directly assess or measure efficacy for HIV prevention Gallo, Kilbourne-Brook, & Coffey, 2012; Padian, Buve, Balks, Serwadda, & Cates, 2008; Padian et al., 2007). Associated problems are that consistent use of female condoms seems rather low because women are not able to completely conceal its application from their male sexual partners (Gallo, Kilbourne-Brook, et al., 2012; Mantell et al., 2006).

Diaphragms have been used for several years as contraception and are also used for STI and HIV prevention (Mantell et al., 2006). However, as compared to male condom use adherence, cervical diaphragms use adherence is found to be relatively low. Moreover, the efficacy against HIV prevention seems doubtful, although found to be useful with microbicides and topical antiretroviral agents (Padian et al., 2007).

Topical Microbicides: Significance in Biomedical Interventions

Topical microbicides comprise gels, sponges, foams, films, and spermicidal creams. These are applied to the vaginal or rectal mucosa and have proved to significantly reduce or prevent the risk of acquisition of STIs and HIV infection. However, the degree of effectiveness is reported to vary with the different products. The different functions include maintaining the acidity of the vaginal pH against microorganisms, causing disruption of the microbial membranes, and acting as inhibitors of viral entry and fusion, thus preventing the entering and binding processes. Others are reported to cause inhibition of viral replication (Abdool-Karim et al., 2010). As Wilson et al. (2008) reasoned, an important requirement with the use of the topical antiretroviral products is adherence. This necessitates self-discipline in making consistent use of barrier methods an essential practice in usual sexual intercourse to enhance effectiveness (Wilson et al., 2008). While specific products target inactivation and destruction of specific organisms, their spermicidal action provides the additional function of contraception in terms of sperm destruction (Abdool-Karim et al., 2010).

Male Circumcision in Biomedical Interventions

Circumcision is considered as a major preventive measure (Bailey et al., 2007; Gray et al., 2007) for the following reasons. The inner mucosal layer of the male foreskin is only minimally keratinized as opposed to the outer highly keratinized layer of skin. Consequently, the mucosal layer increases vulnerability and susceptibility to infective organisms because it contains many cells that can bind HIV and are also prone to ulceration. Thus, the role of circumcision is to remove the foreskin and the tissues that are vulnerable to HIV infection (Bailey et al., 2007; Gray et al., 2007). Nevertheless, research evidence reveals that circumcision of HIV-infected men does not directly reduce HIV transmission from males to females (Wawer et al., 2009). Moreover, various findings indicate that there could be possible increase in the risk of transmission to women if sexual intercourse is resumed while the wound is not completely healed (Wawer et al., 2009).

While circumcision could diminish the HIV epidemic by reducing male infection acquisition, another potential benefit is secondary protection of women. While life-long protection is uncertain, the cost effectiveness of circumcision could prove to be positive. Implications for public health national programs may depend on governmental support, and change of or establishment of appropriate policy regulations and guidelines, which could prove to be difficult to achieve. Health education with health promotion is important to ensure that increased sexual risk-taking behaviors do not happen among the men who are circumcised (Mayer et al., 2012; Wawer et al., 2009).

Supportive Biomedical Interventions to Curb Alcohol Abuse

Evidence from various studies has consistently indicated that heavy alcohol consumption is associated with poor judgement and neglect of self-protection with frequent unprotected sexual intercourse (Bryant, 2006; Samet, Walley, & Bridden, 2007; Silva et al., 2009). However, others argue that inconsistencies in the methodologies of the different studies make those findings rather contentious. In particular, there seemed to be lack of clarity in the implication and the link between the timing of risky sexual behavior and the alcohol consumption episode (Drumright & Colfax, 2009). Nonetheless, based on the views about the apparent association, other experts have

proposed certain supportive suggestions (Silva et al., 2009). Social needs assessment should be carried out, as supplementary to providing appropriate guidance to treatment adherence. Establishment of self-help adherence groups is reported to inspire and persuade individuals regarding the advantages of the treatment. The benefits of counseling and/or psychotherapy support should also be explained to encourage patients, partners, and relevant family members about these additional support systems available to them (Silva et al., 2009).

Supportive Biomedical Interventions to Curb Substance Abuse, Drug Dependence, and Drug Addiction

Substance abuse, drug dependence, and drug addiction; are terms used interchangeably. However, professional practitioners are cautioned to note overlaps that could cause confusion in diagnostic description of the actual problem presented by a particular patient. The seriousness of the impact on the individual's life, the family, and the wider society is recognized and the urgency for effective treatment and management strongly underscored (National Institute for Health and Care Excellence [NICE], 2007; Schifano et al., 2012). Consistently, evidence-based findings reaffirm that treatment and good management of drug dependence can achieve long-term personal health, social, and economic benefits (Schifano et al., 2012). These include abstinence from use and reduction in the rate of bloodborne virus transmission and spread of related infections. The persistent high rate of new HIV cases is attributed to increased drug use and shared injecting equipment. Therefore, in response to these issues various guidelines have been published (NICE, 2010) which emphasize staff training and supervision, collaboration between the primary and secondary sectors, standardized national guidelines and regulations, local protocols, a multidisciplinary approach, and involvement of the patient, the partner, and relevant family members (NICE, 2007).

A thorough assessment should be carried out by a multidisciplinary team and screening offered for bloodborne viral infections, including hepatitis A, B, C, and HIV, to provide appropriate treatment to those with positive results. Concurrent alcohol misuse should be recognized and treated.

As Fuller, Ford, and Rudolph (2009) maintain, effective treatment and support are essential for accomplishing effective HIV prevention.

Abstinence from Sexual Intercourse: A Supplementary Biomedical Intervention

Abstinence from all sexual activities—including vaginal, anal, and oral practices—is considered to be a most effective way of avoiding acquisition and STI transmission (Chin et al., 2012; Jemmott, Jemmott, & Fong, This is particularly vital when one or the other of sex partners or a spouse has developed an STI/RTIs or HIV and is undergoing a course of prescribed treatment. Counseling of the married couple where applicable, the sex partners, or the individual patient/client is crucial to encourage abstinence from intercourse until the treatment has been completed. Subsequent test results indicating that the individual is completely cured of the infection is reassuring for all concerned. This ensures reduction of recurrence risk and further infection transmission. It also enables young people to effectively avoid and/or reduce the problems associated with multiple and concurrent sexual partners. Moreover, this helps to reduce the risk of unplanned pregnancy and the associated potential complications of RTIs.

The Broader Implications of Biomedical Interventions

Although varying degrees of success have been reported in various applications of biomedical interventions (Hosek et al., 2013), challenges arise in applying biomedical interventions in the wider context. While it is recognized by the WHO (2013), no stipulated standardized principles exists to guide application of biomedical interventions. Social, behavioral, and economic ramifications as well as differences in human behavior, cultural values, the health service organizations, and political influences must all be considered. A particularly difficult challenge involves careful interpretation and translation of the principles into the practical context. Since biomedical interventions largely involve human behaviors this means that without recognition of appropriate social adjustments, application of the approach may not succeed on a long-term basis.

A recommended reading is Ng et al.'s (2011) study, which explored population-based STI control using biomedical interventions for reducing HIV infection. However, practitioners are also encouraged to read Low's (2012) commentary on this work, published by the WHO's Reproductive Health Library.

While many biomedical interventions are claimed to have adequate efficacy for HIV and STI protective benefits, others may not provide significant levels of efficacy. The most pragmatic strategy therefore, is to implement a mixed or composite set of biomedical interventions. The ensuing sections examine the initiatives in place and interventions employed to curb the high prevalence of STIs and unintended/unwanted pregnancies among adolescents.

Perpetually High Prevalence of STIs, Pregnancies, and Abortions Among Adolescents and Young People

While decline in the rate of teenage pregnancy rate has been reported, national and international figures reveal the relatively high teenage pregnancy and abortion rates in the United Kingdom are now comparable to other countries in Western Europe. Teenage pregnancy rate is defined as the rate of conceptions under 18 years of age. The recorded rate of births among the U.K. teenage population group was found to be seven times the rate in the Netherlands, more than twice the rate in Germany, and double the rate in France (Armstrong & Donaldson, 2005). The associated economic and social implications may amount to

tens of millions of pounds across the country in any single year, mainly attributable to abortions. Unsurprisingly, the overall implications are consistently reported as creating additional demands on specific aspects of social care and education. Similar to other countries, deprivation features as a significant associated factor (Armstrong & Donaldson, 2005; Teenage Pregnancy Associates [TPA], 2011).

Economic and Social Implications

The economic and social implications of the high rate of pregnancies under 18 years of age are recognized and rationalized in relation to the significance of the long-term outcomes for the mothers and their children. The incidence of preterm births and low-birth-weight babies is comparatively high in teenage pregnancies with relatively higher neonatal and infant morbidity and mortality. A difference of more than 60% neonatal and infant morbidity and mortality is reported in teenage pregnancies as compared to pregnancies outcomes among 20- to 39-year-old mothers (TPA, 2011). Problems associated with teenage motherhood include susceptibility to poor mental health and postnatal depression. Early interruption of education may result in long-term problems of unemployment and lack of regular income, leading to poverty and deprivation. Other social and economic implications include the costs due to the high rate of abortion and the total cost of maternity care and services. These may be followed by long-term social benefits and income support that links to significant low social and economic status (TPA, 2011).

Initiatives to Reduce the High Teenage Pregnancy Rate

Three key initiatives launched in the United Kingdom and other countries have yielded positive outcomes in the efforts to reduce the high rate of teenage pregnancy. The concept of sex and relationships education (SRE) (Blake, Emmerson, & Hayman, 2014; Emmerson, 2010, 2013; Kirby, 2007; Origanje et al., 2009) involves provision of appropriate information and the skills to enable individuals to make certain crucial personal decisions and choices. The information provided should be supported by sound evidence and delivered at a suitable level. This is crucial to empowering teenagers to make informed decisions and choices. Reasoned explanations about the importance of establishing stable relationships should be provided and safe sex practices should be clarified and emphasized. Good understanding of contraception and the importance of informed decisions about appropriate choice of methods and correct application is vital. Moreover, provision of encouragement, support and pertinent knowledge and skills about protection against STIs is also important (TPA, 2011).

Accessible Contraceptive Services for Teenagers

Provision and ease of access to contraceptive services, at carefully considered, convenient times encourages teenagers' attendance at contraceptive clinics. Generally, teenagers who attend contraceptive clinics do so to seek professional advice, evidence-based explanations, clarifications, and counseling support. Therefore, an atmosphere of genuine trust and support provided by approachable staff with nonjudgmental acceptance should be established. Recognition of individual rights and safeguarding of privacy is important. Santelli, Lindberg, Finer, and Signh's 2007 paper emphasized positive outcomes and improved use of contraception obtained by accessing contraceptive facilities set up for the teenage population subgroup. The teenage contraceptive clinics are purposefully designed, equipped, and set up to provide a range of care and services. Instructions on specific contraceptive products and supervised practice may be incorporated into ongoing health promotion and education provision. Of crucial importance is appropriate level of motivation and correct use of the particular contraceptive methods. Therefore, required training and skills development should form essential components of the contraception clinic interventions (Blake et al., 2014; Emmerson, 2010).

Timeliness of Interventions

Careful assessment of the risk factors that contribute to teenage pregnancy are important in order to design and implement appropriate prevention actions. Findings from various qualitative research studies that have explored the reasons for teenage pregnancies identified various factors and life circumstances. Multiple risk factors include low aspiration, having no particular ambition, and no specific goal or direction to pursue for the future and thus little self-worth (Harden, Brunton, Fletcher, & Oakley, 2009; TPA, 2011). Other risk factors include poor educational capability with poor achievement, lack of motivation to attend school and abandonment of school, and leaving residential care. Harden et al. (2009) identified certain key themes in connection with early motherhood and described these as dislike of school, disadvantaged childhood and poor circumstances, and low self-esteem with apathetic and unaspiring expectations of the future. These researchers reported a reduction in the teenage pregnancy rate by 39% among the participants who received early interventions as compared to those who were provided the usual standard of practice (Harden et al., 2009). They noted that early childhood interventions with youth development programs contributed to reduction in teenage pregnancies. The use of motivational interviewing in pregnancy and STI prevention counseling reported by Petersen, Albright, Garett, and Curtis (2007) failed to show any effect suggesting a need for more extensive research on the use of this method.

Other evidence indicates that a great deal of money could be saved by the health service organization through further enhancement of contraceptive services. Additionally, further improvement of accessibility for teenagers could also prove to be economically beneficial (Barham, Lewis, & Latimer, 2007; Brook & FPA, 2013; Department of Health [DH], 2013a; NICE, 2007). Arrangements to ensure easier access to sexual health services for those high-risk population groups should be considered as a national priority (DH, 2013a; Land, Van Bergen, Morré, & Postma, 2010).

SRE and Sexuality Education: Combined Interventions

SRE addresses a combination of the physical process of growth and development, the emotional aspects of human sexuality, sex, relationships and sexual health, and personal social circumstances. While no specific methods or stages have been stipulated as credible evidence-based guidelines intended for standardization, there is, nonetheless, a consensus view of what SRE should encompass (Blake & Muttock, 2012; Sex Education Forum, 2005). The general view is that SRE involves provision of pertinent information supported by the skills to enable the young person to make certain crucial personal decisions and choices. The concept is advocated throughout the United Kingdom and is recognized as a useful measure to curb the rate of STIs and reduce the incidence of teenage pregnancies. Other countries, such as the United States and Australia, also implement SRE, and various guidelines and recommendations have been published.

SRE: The Concept, Underpinning Principles, and Rationales Examined

To provide a clearer understanding of sex and relationships education, the National Children's Bureau of the Sex Education Forum (2005) describes "good" sex and relationships education as encouraging immediate reporting of sexual abuse to help to curb potential situations sexual abuse situations. It should effectively help to reduce incidence of unconsented sexual intercourse with sexual assault and abuse, reduce the rate of teenage and unplanned pregnancies, and reduce related maternal and infant mortalities. Moreover, it is envisaged that effective SRE helps to bring about change in attitude and avoidance of sexual risk-taking behaviors. It should also help to discourage unprotected sexual intercourse and STIs while helping to achieve early diagnosis and treatment. Ultimately SRE should help to reduce the gap of inequality in sexual health (Emmerson, 2010, 2016).

Various researchers have explored different aspects of SRE in an attempt to gain more insight into what young people actually need and what benefits they gain or expect to gain from this approach. Findings from various research studies suggest that effective SRE may be associated with empowering adolescents to make informed decisions and choices. Indeed, Kirby (2007) noted that while negative outcomes (such as increased earlier onset or increased frequency of sexual intercourse) were not associated with the SRE programs, positive outcomes were observed. These include delaying to start having sexual intercourse (Kirby, 2007; NICE, 2010; UNESCO, 2009) and reducing the number of sexual partners and frequency of sexual intercourse. Additionally, an increase in the use of condoms or other preferred contraceptive methods was reported in Kirby's (2007) findings. The scenario of abstinence without adequate information about contraception or without appropriate support has consistently been found to be ineffective. However, provision of relevant information, skills teaching, and appropriate contraception support are found to be associated with positive behavior changes including more disciplined use of contraceptive methods such as condoms (Kirby, 2008).

Undoubtedly, there is a shared view about the potential impact of SRE in helping to reduce the rates of STIs and teenage and unplanned pregnancies. Nevertheless, studies have shown that implementation of SRE varies in different countries in different schools and contexts and for different youth groups (Apter, 2009; Boonstra, 2010; Westwood & Mullan, 2007).

The United Nations guidance on sexuality education (UNESCO, 2009) outlines recommendations for program content, principles, and methods of implementation of the sexuality or sex and relationships education. These are applicable in all countries to be implemented for children between the ages of 5–18 despite their gender, culture, religion, ethnicity, sexual orientation or other circumstances. UNESCO urges for children in the identified age groups to be progressively guided as part of their educational curriculum to learn about human sexuality, relationships, contraception, and HIV. The importance of support in their physical and emotional development is emphasized and the main principles recommended comprise the following.

Various researchers of different studies have emphasized the importance of the quality of SRE programs, appropriate timing and methods of delivery, and well-trained educators (Gabhainn, O'Higgins, & Barry, 2010; Lockanc-Diluzio, Cobb, Harrison, & Nelson, 2007). Others have also described variations in the models of implementation and their effectiveness (Formby et al., 2011) and the need for comprehensive programs with adequate support continue to emerge. Furthermore, various surveys have revealed different forms of inadequacies in the ways in which sexuality education and SRE are implemented. From the perspective of the educators—the teachers, parents, or caretakers—the shortcomings may be due to either lack of a clear understanding of the concept, the required knowledge and skills, and/or lack of confidence. Appropriate training of the educators of sexuality education and SRE is important to young people who see their teachers as reliable and dependable resource for relevant information. Therefore, they expect the teachers to be well informed and confident in their delivery of SRE (Emmerson, 2010; Smith, Aigus, Barrett, Mitchell, & Pitts, 2009). **Box 9-1** presents the key principles of SRE. From the perspectives of the institutions and schools, the failings may be due to inadequate programming, limited content, lack of substantive detail, and unfocused sexuality education or SRE (Blake, 2010). Moreover, inadequate resources and shortfalls in the provision of required support for those who deliver the program and those at the receiving end have also been revealed. Consequently, the experiences and outcomes have been described as ineffective, disappointing, and not beneficial (Office for Standards in Education, Children's Services and Skills [Ofsted], 2007, 2010; Sex Education Forum, 2008a, 2008b). Clearly, therefore, a detailed systematic evaluation of each sexuality education program or SRE is crucial.

The timing of exposure to sexuality education or SRE is crucial, and different surveys have revealed strong views about this. The opinion among young people, relevant experts, and researchers is that these should begin before children, adolescents, and young people experience their first sexual intercourse and before they become sexually active (Emmerson, 2010; Emmerson & Lees, 2013; Martinez, Cooper, & Lees, 2013; Martinez & Emmerson, 2008). The programs should be designed to empower young people to take responsibility for their sexual relationships and provide support for safeguarding their own sexual health (Emmerson, 2010). Surveys reveal that young people would like account to be taken of their adolescent emotions, values, and ideals and norms, and for programs to reflect their social world and experiences

---

BOX 9-1 Supporting the Emotional and Physical Development of Young People: The Contexts and Related Principles

- Provision of sexuality education and SRE within the contexts of home and school.
- Training support for the providers of sexuality education and sex and relationships education.
- Incorporating wide-ranging themes with relevant issues to learn and talk about, such as contraception.
- Providing opportunities for, encouraging, and supporting the young people to examine the social standards, moral principles, and psychological influences, including their perceptions of self-worth.
- SRE should foster mutual respect, affection, devotion, and contentment in their sexual relationships to eliminate gender inequality in their interactions with full awareness of their personal human rights.
- Commencing the sexuality education and/or SRE before young adolescents begin to engage in sexual intercourse for the first time.
- Implementing interactive exercises, effective communication, and active participation.
- Organizing activities for small groups to encourage involvement by each member.

Data from Kirby, D. B. (2007). *Emerging answers: 2007 Research findings on programs to reduce teen pregnancy and sexually transmitted diseases.* Washington, DC: National Campaign to Prevent Teen and Unplanned Pregnancy; Kirby, D. B. (2008). The impact of abstinence and comprehensive sex and STD/HIV sex education programmes on adolescent sexual behaviour. *Sexuality Research and Social Policy, 5(3),* 18–27; Trivedi, D., Bunn, F., Graham, M., & Wentz, R. (2007). Preventing teenage pregnancy: Evidence from systematic reviews. In P. Baker, K. Guthrie, C. Hutchinson, R. Kane, & Wellings K. (Eds.), *Teenage pregnancy and reproductive health* (pp. 275–291). London, United Kingdom: RCOG Press.

(Blake, 2010; Gabhainn et al., 2010; Martinez & Emmerson, 2008). The consistent view among experts and the relevant researchers in their recommendations is for sexuality education and SRE programs to be clearly focused and more comprehensive, with careful consideration of subject matter, topic contents, methods of delivery with involvement of the young people, acceptability, usefulness, consistent standards, and related principles. Effectiveness and success of the programs depend on these and they should be seen as supportive and economically viable.

STI Screening Considerations in Pregnancy: Selective Versus Comprehensive

In examining the significance of prevention of specific STIs during pregnancy, account is taken of the potential adverse consequences of perinatal morbidity and mortality associated with undetected and untreated infections for mother and child. Acquisition and transmission of STIs during pregnancy can have devastating and long-term consequences for the parents and their unborn child. The severity of specific infections and the potential long-term consequences in terms of maternal and perinatal morbidity and mortality are the main concerns (Mullick, Watson-Jones, Beksinska, & Mabey, 2005). While some infections can spread from the vagina through the cervix to the uterine cavity, causing chorioamnionitis, others can cross the placental barrier directly to the fetus (Srinivas et al., 2006). In both cases, intrauterine infection and fetal illness can result, or the baby may be infected during delivery or during the neonatal period. Chorioamnionitis can result in premature rupture of the membranes, preterm birth, and a low-birth-weight baby (Mullick et al., 2005). Johnson, Ghanem, Zenilman, and Erbelding (2011) examined the adverse effects of STIs on pregnancy outcomes and suggested that early intervention should always be aimed for. They maintain that infections occurring earlier in the pregnancy are associated with higher risk of complications. Examples include puerperal infections in the women who deliver vaginally and neonatal conjunctivitis and pneumonitis. These justify rationales for screening, whether selective or routine comprehensive depending on prevalence, early detection, and appropriate treatment to reduce the potential consequences of STIs on the pregnancy outcome (CDC, 2015; Wilson, 2011).

Recognition of the increase in STIs in the United Kingdom through the recent decade does call for vigilance and necessary testing to safeguard the health of both mother and baby during pregnancy and afterward. Allstaff and Wilson (2012) share the view with other experts that a woman who presents with one STI should be considered at high risk of another STI. Such women should be offered all-inclusive STI testing together with repeat HIV testing. While some countries, such as the United States, operate a policy of routine STI and HIV screening during pregnancy, others recommend selective screening based on evidence from high-risk population groups and specific risk factors (Allstaff & Wilson, 2012).

All components of appropriate public health interventions with partner notification, health promotion/education, required counseling support and advice should be provided together with safer sexual practices and abstinence during treatment (Allstaff & Wilson, 2012). The benefit of partner notification should be emphasized and abstinence from sexual intercourse advised until the recommended period following completion of the specific prescribed medication. This is to protect individuals from being reinfected. A test of cure is also recommended because the efficacy of certain antimicrobials to eradicate particular infections could be low.

Consideration of *Chlamydia trachomatis* Screening in Pregnancy

The question arises as to whether chlamydia screening should form part of the routine antenatal screening tests instead of the existing national screening program. The trend of increase shows that women under 25 years of age are at higher risk of contracting chlamydia infection. Figures show that younger age group, frequent changes of sexual partners, and multiple sexual partners are particular risk factors among pregnant women, with 70% of infected women being asymptomatic (Chen et al., 2009). The evidence of association between chlamydia and preterm birth, low birth weight together with perinatal and infant morbidity and mortality has been contradictory. Rours et al. (2011) found that while there is an association between maternal *Chlamydia trachomatis* and preterm delivery they did not find strong association with low birth weight. Also although some earlier studies had reported an association between *Chlamydia trachomatis* infection and preterm rupture of the membranes, the evidence reported by Chow, Kang, Samuel, and Bolan (2009) revealed only a weak association. The laboratory techniques of culturing that was applied in the earlier studies reputedly had relatively low sensitivity of 60–70% (Allstaff & Wilson, 2012). These require high load of organisms and for that reason it is possible that some cases might have been missed.

Benefits and Practicality of Screening for Chlamydia trachomatis *Infection in Pregnancy*

The U.K. National Screening Committee (NSC) (National Health Service, 2011) maintains that while chlamydia screening in late pregnancy might be presumed to reduce neonatal morbidities of conjunctivitis, pneumonitis, and otitis media this should not be routinely offered to pregnant women. Nonetheless, the NSC noted the counsel by NICE (2008) that while the current level of evidence does not provide strong enough justification for recommending routine screening there should be other considerations. The possibility that treatment might reduce the incidence of prematurity, low birth weight, and related neonatal complications should be taken into consideration for research investigations. This also applies to the assumption that chlamydia screening in early pregnancy might reduce potential detrimental outcomes such as risk of preterm labor (National Health Service, 2011). Moreover, the NSC maintains its aim to reduce sexually transmitted chlamydia infection and the related reproductive complications. Where necessary, women under 25 years should be encouraged to attend their national chlamydia screening services in their local areas, and this is not necessarily linked to screening in pregnancy (National Health Service, 2011). However, the National Institute for Health and Care Excellence (NICE) emphasizes the need for in-depth research to explore the effectiveness, practicality, and acceptability of antenatal screening for *Chlamydia trachomatis* infection (NICE, 2008).

Treatment Regimens for Chlamydia trachomatis Infection in Pregnancy

The recommended antibiotics for chlamydia treatment in pregnancy comprise azithromycin, erythromycin, and amoxycillin. Pitsouni, Iavazzo, Athanasiou, and Falagas's (2007) meta-analysis of randomized controlled trials revealed that the efficacy of the three antibiotics is comparable with 90% rate of cure (Brocklehurst & Rooney, 2000; Pitsouni et al., 2007). The risk of latent infection has been reported following treatment with amoxicillin and negative test result may not be indicative of cure, so that mother-to-child transmission during birth can still happen (Brocklehurst & Rooney, 2000). Lazaro (2013) cautions that doxycycline is contraindicated in pregnancy.

Rationale for Follow-Up and Test of Cure During Pregnancy

A follow-up interview may be conducted within 2 to 4 weeks of treatment for *Chlamydia trachomatis* infection, during which tolerance and adherence to the prescribed treatment is discussed together with exposure and risk of reinfection. It is also recommended that a test of cure be carried out during pregnancy to rule out the risk of failed treatment or recurrence of infection (Allstaff & Wilson, 2012). Due to the high rate of positive tests after treatment in pregnancy possibly due to reduced treatment efficacy from poor tolerance and noncompliance and the risk of reinfection routine test of cure is recommended (BASHH, 2015). The suggestion is that all pregnant women should have test of cure 5 weeks after treatment completion. In relation to azithromycin the suggested timing for test of cure is 6 weeks after completion of treatment (Allstaff & Wilson, 2012). While there is no optimal timing for carrying out test of cure, it is recognized that NAATs can detect residual DNA/RNA 4 to 6 weeks after successful treatment. Thus, practitioners are encouraged to explore more information on the contraindications and side effects of these medications with particular attention to pregnancy and lactation.

In countries with high prevalence of *Chlamydia trachomatis* infection, prenatal screening and treatment of infected pregnant women has been reported as effective in preventing chlamydial infection in newborn babies. Nonetheless, acquisition of the infection can occur during birth through exposure to the infected cervix of the mother. The sites of infection in the baby include the mucous membranes of the eyes, oro-pharynx, urogenital tract, and rectum and in these sites the baby may remain asymptomatic. Obvious manifestations may be conjunctivitis developing 5–12 days after birth (Zar, 2005). Moreover, during the first 3 months of age the baby could develop sub-acute afebrile pneumonia (Pellowe & Pratt, 2006; Zar, 2005). *Chlamydia trachomatis* is reported to be the most common recognizable infectious cause of ophthalmia neonatorum.

Vulnerability of the Newborn Baby Exposed to Maternal Chlamydia trachomatis

Infrequent perinatal chlamydial infections, particularly ophthalmia neonatorum and neonatal pneumonia, have been attributed to intensive prenatal screening and treatment of expectant mothers. This includes the recommendation that expectant mothers who are diagnosed with *Chlamydia trachomatis* infection during the first trimester should be retested to verify chlamydial eradication. The experts maintain that babies who develop conjunctivitis at less than 30 days of age should be considered as having probably acquired *Chlamydia trachomatis*, particularly if the mother is found to have untreated chlamydial infection. Conjunctival swabs obtained from the everted eyelid are sent to the laboratory for culture and nonculture tests. It is crucial that the correct swab designed for this specific purpose is used in order to obtain accurate diagnostic test results.

Confirmation of the *Chlamydia trachomatis* infection should be followed by treatment of not only the baby but also the mother. It is also recommended that the specimen obtained from the chlamydial infected eye should be tested for *Neisseria gonorrhoeae* (CDC, 2015; Scottish Intercollegiate Guidelines Network [SIGN], 2009). The incidence of perinatal transmission is reported to be considerable and estimated at 50–70% (Pellowe & Pratt, 2006) in undiagnosed and untreated mothers with chlamydial infection (Zar, 2005). In addition to the above, other reported perinatal manifestations include oro-pharyngeal infection with otitis media, and vaginal infection in female babies. These conditions are recorded as chlamydial related morbidity in the infants of mothers infected with *Chlamydia trachomatis* (Wilson, 2011; Zar, 2005). In the United States, the recommendation is that women who are diagnosed and treated in the first trimester should be retested 3 months after treatment (CDC, 2015). See also the 2015 CDC guidelines for the management of STIs.

Consideration of Gonorrhea Screening in Pregnancy

Johnson et al. (2011) noted that complications are increased the earlier the acquisition of gonorrhea during pregnancy. These authors identified associated complications including spontaneous abortion, early rupture of the membranes, premature labor, preterm birth, low birth weight and postpartum infection (Johnson et al., 2011). Gonococcal conjunctivitis in up to 50% of babies exposed through vertical transmission during birth has also been identified (Allstaff & Wilson, 2012; Wilson, 2011).

There is a recommendation to perform gonorrhea testing on childbearing with characteristic lower genital tract symptoms and those who develop fever during labor and postpartum. This also applies to mothers whose babies develop gonococcal conjunctivitis (Allstaff & Wilson, 2012). Specimens are obtained from the endocervix, pharynx, urethra, and rectum (Bignell, 2009; Bachmann, et al., 2010).

Recommended Antimicrobial/Antibiotic Treatments for Gonorrheal Infection in Pregnancy

The national guideline provided for the management of gonorrhea in adults (Bignell & Fitzgerald, 2011) recommends ceftriaxone, spectinomycin, and cefixime for treatment of gonorrhea in pregnant women. All three antimicrobials have comparable efficacy. Ceftriaxone and azithromycin together are recommended for genital and extragenital gonococcal infection (Allstaff & Wilson, 2012). Spectinomycin, however, is found to have relatively weaker efficacy for treatment of pharyngeal gonococcal infection (Bignell & Fitzgerald, 2011; Tapsall et al., 2009).

While there has been some uncertainty about the safety of azithromycin in pregnancy, there is no strong evidence substantiating this. Moreover, the experts maintain that the efficacy of azithromycin is not weakened by pregnancy (Bignell & Fitzgerald, 2011). Generally, it is found to be safe in clinical practice but it is recommendation to be used under medical supervision (Bignell & Unemo, 2013). The advantage for prescribing azithromycin together with the recommended antimicrobials is addressed with the high incidence of coinfection with *Chlamydia trachomatis* infection (Allstaff & Wilson, 2012; Wilson, 2011). It must be noted, however, that azithromycin has been found to pass into breastmilk and therefore it is not recommended for breastfeeding mothers (Bignell & Unemo, 2013). Two other antimicrobials that are contraindicated for pregnant and breastfeeding mothers are tetracycline and fluoroquinolone (Bignell & Unemo, 2013).

In relation to concerns about antimicrobial resistance with decreased susceptibility to third-generation cephalosporins, including cefixime (Ison et al., 2013), BASHH (2011) recommends that a test of cure should be performed following treatment. The suggested timing for test of cure is 3 weeks following completion of treatment and this applies to all cases and irrespective of infection site. Practitioners should encourage partner notification and emphasize abstinence from sexual intercourse until treatment completion and the period stipulated for specific treatment regimens.

Gonorrheal Infection in the Baby

Perinatal transmission is estimated as 40% (Wilson, 2011) from mothers who have not received treatment for the gonorrheal infection. Neonatal infection is characterized by conjunctivitis with profuse, purulent discharge from the affected eye(s) together with edema of the eyelids 2 to 5 days after birth. Untreated cases can be complicated by corneal ulceration, perforation and blindness. Gram stain

and culture may be performed on a specimen obtained from the conjunctiva. Female babies may also develop vaginal infection (Wilson, 2011).

The recommended treatment:

- Ceftriaxone 25–50 mg/kg body weight administered intravenously or intramuscularly as a single dose. It is cautioned that this dosage should not exceed 125 mg.
- Cefotaxime 100 mg/kg body weight administered intramuscularly as a single dose

It is recommended that the baby's eyes should be frequently irrigated with saline (Bignell, 2009; Bignell & Unemo, 2013).

Gonorrhea Screening in Pregnancy

Comprehensive screening for gonorrhea still seems unclear in some countries while it is firmly established in others. The main indications include suspicious signs and symptoms of gonorrhea, previous gonorrheal infection, and multiple sexual partners, including new sexual partners. In the United States, the recommendation is to offer expectant women who are diagnosed with gonorrheal infection in the first trimester a repeat testing within 3 to 6 months, if possible, during the third trimester. Practitioners are encouraged to explore the current U.K. guidelines, as well as the CDC (2015) STD guidelines for more detailed information.

Consideration of Syphilis in Pregnancy

Syphilis is associated with high neonatal morbidity and mortality. Newman et al.'s (2013) finding from the multinational surveillance data revealed that the prevalence of this STI remains high in certain countries and among certain population groups. This section explores syphilis the context of STI screening in pregnancy. The consequences of syphilis in pregnancy include trans-placental transmission in the first, second, and third trimesters and can lead to abortion/miscarriage, preterm labor, still birth, and congenital syphilis (Gomez et al., 2013). Transmission risk is found to be higher during the first 2 years of the infection but has also been reported after 4 years of infection. During pregnancy, the transmission risk from mother to baby is high in the early stages of infection. Therefore, in consideration of the morbidity and mortality on newborn babies, routine prenatal screening is highly recommended for all pregnant women in all countries (Gomez et al., 2013; Hawkes, Martin, Broutet, & Low, 2011; Newman et al., 2013).

Benefits of Prenatal Screening: Overview of Syphilis Screening in the United Kingdom

The benefit of prenatal screening for syphilis is that early detection of maternal syphilis infection and appropriate treatment in early pregnancy can effectively prevent congenital syphilis (WHO, 2015). It is recommended that in addition to syphilis, other STIs should also be screened for. Currently in the United Kingdom, women are offered antenatal screening for syphilis early in pregnancy as part of the blood tests at the booking visit for screening infectious diseases in pregnancy program. The uptake, over 95% (UK-NSC, 2016) indicates women's acceptance of this routine screening test (Giraudon, Forde, Maguire, Arnold, and Permalloo, 2009). Evidence from various investigations on the effectiveness of early detection through screening with early treatment to achieve better outcomes for both mother and baby support the claims of reduced adverse effects (Carles et al., 2008; Hawkes et al., 2011; Shahrook, Mori, Ochirbat, & Gomi, 2014; Zhu et al., 2010).

The use of highly sensitive and specific testing is strongly advocated to avoid false positive results, which can cause needless maternal worry and anxiety, unnecessary antibiotic treatment, and excess demands on available resources (UK-NCSP, 2016). Referrals to appropriate professional experts for counseling and provision of required support are found to benefit women with positive screening test results (UK-NCSP, 2016). The recommended screening test for syphilis in the United Kingdom is the enzyme immunoassay (EIA), which is reputed to be highly sensitive in detecting treponemal antibodies (UK-NCSP, 2016). The other recommended tests, *Treponema pallidum* particle agglutination (TPPA) or *Treponema pallidum* hemagglutination (TPHA), are reputed to be highly sensitive, specific confirmatory tests (UK-NCSP, 2016, HPA, 2011b). Linking the EIA plate readings to the computer system is found to enhance objectivity of the results and the high sensitivity and specificity is reported to range between 85–99.5% and 98.3–100% (Seña, White, & Sparling, 2010).

Recommended Treatment for Syphilis in Pregnancy

The recommended management is that women who test positive should be tested for other STIs and HIV. Meticulous assessment is important to determine the stage of the syphilis infection in order to administer the correct treatment immediately to inhibit or curtail fetal exposure. Joint management may involve obstetric, GUM, and neonatal specialists.

The recommended treatment for primary, secondary, and early latent syphilis (early syphilis) in the first and second trimesters comprises the following:

- Benzathine penicillin 2.4 MU administered intramuscularly as a single dose (CDC, 2015; UK-NCSP, 2016; Kingston et al., 2016).

This is reputed to be effective in most cases. Nonetheless, treatment failures have been reported in mothers with higher RPR/VDRL, early stage of maternal infection and treatment in the last trimester (Kingston et al., 2016; UK-NCSP, 2016). The recommended treatment of early syphilis in the third trimester should be followed by a second dose of the following:

- Benzathine penicillin 2.4 MU intramuscularly 1 week after the first dose with careful assessment. This is to

counter lower serum levels of the drug and potential risk of treatment failure (Kingston et al., 2016).

- Recommended alternative treatment regimen includes the following:
    - Procaine penicillin G 600,000 unit IM daily for 10 days, **or**
    - Amoxycillin 500 mg orally four times daily for 14 days **in combination with**
        - Probenecid 500 mg orally four times daily for 14 days, **or**
    - Ceftriaxone 500 mg IM once daily for 10 days, **or**
    - Erythromycin 500 mg orally four times daily for 14 days, **or**
    - Azithromycin 500 mg orally once daily for 10 days

It must be noted, however, that reports about azithromycin resistance to treatment of syphilis conflicts with its use as an alternative treatment and expert advice should be sought and possibly avoid using it for this purpose.

Treatment of late syphilis in pregnancy is the same as for nonpregnant women, but doxycycline is not recommended. Some organizations consider it necessary to implement desensitization for patients who report penicillin allergy (CDC, 2015; Magpantay, Cardile, Madar, Hsue, & Belnap, 2011; Solensky, 2004). The related partner notification and follow-up programs are the same as those considered for nonpregnant patients.

Congenital Syphilis

Congenital syphilis is diagnosed by detection of *Treponema pallidum* in exudates from the infants' syphilitic lesions, such as nasal discharge or other body fluids, placental, and autopsy material. Direct or positive detection of *Treponema pallidum* by dark ground microscopy and PCR confirms the diagnosis (Rawstron, Mehta, & Bromberg, 2004). Serological tests are performed on the neonate's blood (not umbilical cord blood). If the serum screening test is positive, treponemal IgM EIA serological tests, quantitative VDRL/RPR and quantitative TPPA tests should be performed on specimens from mother and baby (Kingston et al., 2008). Positive IgM EIA test (Rawstron et al., 2004). Sustained fourfold or more increases in the VDRL/RPR or TPPA titers above the maternal serum titers that have been confirmed on a second specimen, indicate congenital syphilis. In that case, additional investigations should include full blood count, electrolytes and liver function test, CSF for cells, protein and serological tests, x-rays of the long bones, and ophthalmic examination (Kingston et al., 2016).

Detection of positive IgG serological test on the infant's specimens could be maternal antibodies that had been passively transferred to the baby who may or may not be infected. Negative IgG as well as reactive results with titers below fourfold increases in the baby's serum titers and not in the maternal serum when taken together should indicate repeat testing. Additionally, absence of congenital syphilis signs justifies repeat reactive tests at 3, 6, and 12 months of age or until negative results become evident in the tests. It is also recommended that IgM test should be repeated at 3 months of age in case of delayed response. Negative serum screening result for the infant with no signs of congenital infection indicates that no further tests are required (CDC, 2015; Kingston et al., 2016).

Clinical Manifestations of Congenital Syphilis

While congenital syphilis presents as asymptomatic in many infants, common reported signs include maculopapular and desquamation rash, hepatosplenomegaly, syphilitic snuffles, and periostitis. Manifestation of late syphilis in an infant is characterized by intestinal keratitis, Hutchinson's incisors, frontal bossing with saddle nose deformity, and deafness (Simms & Broutet, 2008; Wilson, 2011).

The recommended treatment regimen for congenital syphilis includes:

- Benzyl penicillin sodium 60–90 mg/kg daily. This is administered in divided doses of 30 mg/kg 12 hourly IV in the first 7 days of life then 8 hourly for 10 days
- Alternative treatment regimen includes
  - Procaine penicillin 50,000 µ/kg body weight administered intramuscularly daily for 10 days

It is proposed that IV treatment may be opted for children to avoid the pain of intramuscular injections (CDC, 2015; Kingston et al., 2016).

The CDC (2015) recommends that in places where optimal prenatal care is unavailable, rapid plasma reagin (RPR) card test could be carried out at the first clinic visit when the pregnancy is confirmed. Treatment is then provided if the test result is reactive. Expectant mothers who live in high syphilis-prevalent areas or who have not had previous screening should be tested early in the third trimester and at delivery. Furthermore, it is recommended that every woman who delivers a stillborn baby be screened for syphilis (CDC, 2015).

Consideration of Genital Herpes Infection in Pregnancy: HSV-1 and HSV-2 Infections

The main obstetric considerations are that maternal-child transmission can occur depending on the timing of episode, whether first episode or frequency of recurrent infections. Type-specific HSV serology examination may be used to determine the difference. Transmission rate is found to increase in pregnancy and first-episode genital herpes in the first trimester has been implicated for spontaneous abortion due to the associated viremia. Moreover, the potential risk of congenital defects continues to be investigated (Li, 2011; Pasternak & Hviid, 2010). Transmission risk to the neonate is reported to be high, 30–50%, among mothers who acquire HSV infection in late pregnancy near the time of delivery. Women who acquire primary genital HSV and are shedding HSV at the time of delivery are up to 30 times more at risk to transmit the virus to their newborn babies ((James & Kimberlin, 2015; Kimberlin & Baley, 2013; Pinninti & Kimberlin 2014b). However, among those mothers who acquire genital HSV during the first half of the pregnancy, the risk of transmission to the baby is reported to be less than 1% (CDC, 2015). A brief summary of the recommended treatment is presented here.

Three antiviral drugs that have been reported to produce positive effects for patients with genital herpes simplex infection are acyclovir, valaciclovir, and famciclovir. The recommendation is that these can be prescribed for first-episode genital HSV or recurrent infections (CDC, 2015). The main benefits reported are decrease in the duration of the HSV infection. The severity of symptoms subsides, together with diminished duration of viral shedding (CDC, 2015; Foley et al., 2014).

First and Second Trimesters

Depending on the clinical manifestation, management may involve oral or IV administration of antiviral treatment such as acyclovir. This is the preferred treatment based on evidence of its safety and effectiveness (Lazaro, 2013).

The prescribed treatment regimen may be the following:

- Acyclovir 400 mg orally three times a day usually for 5 days (Foley et al., 2014), although the CDC (2015) also recommends that a course of 7–10 days may be extended as required if not completely healed after the 10 days course of treatment.

Third Trimester

The recommendation is to aim for vaginal delivery. Therefore, antiviral suppressive therapy is commenced with acyclovir 400 mg three times daily until delivery (CDC, 2015; Foley et al., 2014; Hollier & Wendell, 2008). This is reputed to reduce HSV shedding and lesions at term. Cesarean section may be considered for women who develop first episode HSV at term, at the time of delivery or within 6 weeks of the expected delivery date (Gardella & Brown, 2011). However, continuous antiviral treatment with acyclovir throughout the last 4 weeks of pregnancy may reduce the possibility of clinical recurrence at term and delivery by cesarean section (Hollier & Wendel, 2008).

For inevitable vaginal delivery or in maternal preference for vaginal delivery, it is important that prolonged rupture of membranes and invasive procedures are avoided or kept to a minimum. Intravenous administration of acyclovir is prescribed for the woman, and the baby may also receive neonatal IV acyclovir at birth (Gardella & Brown, 2011). The obstetric team and the neonatal pediatric team should be made aware of the maternal HSV infection.

Recurrent HSV Infections in Pregnancy

The effect of recurrent HSV infections on the pregnancy has been examined through research studies. Women with recurrent HSV infection who are shedding HSV virus at delivery are less likely to transmit the virus to their newborn babies (Kimberlin & Baley, 2013). Evidence suggests that the risk of maternal HSV transmission is estimated at less than 1% among women with recurrent infection (Brown et al., 2003; Kimberlin & Baley, 2013). It is recommended that all pregnant women should be asked about previous history of genital herpes and where possible they should be asked if they have symptoms of genital herpes when admitted in labor. Women who present with symptoms should be carefully examined for herpes lesions and they may be considered for cesarean section. Fetal monitoring by scalp electrode is considered inadvisable because of inoculation and increased risk of transmission through the electrode application (Brown et al., 2003).

Recurrent episodes in the third trimester are found to be transitory without appearance of any lesions. Therefore, vaginal delivery is considered to be appropriate under those circumstances and cesarean section is not necessary to prevent the baby being infected. The benefit of acyclovir as a suppressive HSV treatment from 36 weeks' gestation is substantiated by evidence from systematic review of randomized controlled trials indicating effective reduction in clinical HSV recurrence. The suppressive antiviral therapy for recurrent HSV recommended by the CDC (2015) is acyclovir 400 mg orally three times daily or valacyclovir 500 mg orally twice a daily. Nonetheless, as Pinninti et al. (2012) noted, antenatal antiviral suppressive HSV treatment does not necessarily prevent neonatal HSV infection. Cesarean section is recommended for women with recurrent HSV lesions at onset of labor (Foley et al., 2014).

It is recommended that women who do not have genital herpes avoid sexual intercourse during the third trimester with sexual partners who have been diagnosed or are suspected to have genital herpes. Furthermore, women who have not been diagnosed with orolabial herpes should be advised to avoid receptive oral sex during the third trimester with sexual partners who are known or suspected to have orolabial herpes (CDC, 2015; Foley et al., 2014).

Counseling for Self-Protection, Recurrence, and Prevention of Transmission

The risk factors associated with transmission of HSV infection to the baby should be explained to all childbearing women, expectant mothers, and their sexual partners. Avoidance of all sexual activities with infected husband or sexual partner should be encouraged for uninfected women to reduce the risk of transmission to the baby during birth. The importance of informing the obstetric team about the HSV infection should be tactfully emphasized to the expectant mother diagnosed with HSV infection.

Despite the evidence that indicates the prevalence of asymptomatic HSV infections among women who are unaware of the infection, there is currently no vaccination program. An additional recommended reading is Schulte et al.'s (2014) study on HSV-1 and HSV-2 seroprevalence in the United States among women (Herpevac

Trial for women). Other experimental studies are still being carried out.

Neonatal HSV Infection

Both HSV-1 and HSV-2 are reported to cause neonatal herpes, with an incidence of about 1 in 60,000 live births within the United Kingdom or approximately 2/100,000 deliveries ((Royal College of Obstetricians and Gynaecologists [RCOG], 2014). This is found to be comparably lower than the incidence in some countries in Europe and the United States. While most cases are attributed to direct contact with infected maternal genital secretions during birth (James & Kimberlin, 2015), healthcare-associated sources of infection have also been reported. Most infant infections occur in asymptomatic mothers who newly acquire the HSV infections in the third trimester of pregnancy with subclinical viral shedding (Corey & Wald, 2009; Lazaro, 2013). Evidence from systematic reviews of research reveal higher incidence of this among pregnant women with primary genital herpes infection or recurrences.

Common neonatal HSV infection manifestation tends to be the skin, mouth, and eyes. Rare devastating complications of dissemination with meningoencephalitis, hepatosplenomegaly, and jaundice have been reported. These may manifest between 2 to 28 days of birth and are associated with high incidence of neonatal morbidity and mortality (Kimberlin & Baley, 2013; Kimberlin et al., 2015; Lazaro, 2013). Care and follow-up with neonatal pediatric specialists is recommended. Immediate neonatal evaluation is required if the mother acquired HSV infection near term due to the increased risk of HSV transmission to the child. Systemic treatment with acyclovir may be considered (James & Kimberlin, 2015; Pinninti & Kimberlin, 2014a). However, the treatment regimen depends on whether the infection is disseminated and involves the central nervous system and/or other sites such as the skin or mucous membranes (Pinninti & Kimberlin, 2014a). Neonatal HSV infection tends to be severe and could prove to be fatal (James & Kimberlin, 2015; Kimberlin et al., 2015). Diagnosis involves electron microscopic examination of vesicular fluid and HSV polymerase chain reaction (PCR) test (Foley et al., 2014; Kimberlin & Baley, 2013; Kimberlin et al., 2015). However, routine screening is not a recommendation.

Consideration of Anogenital Warts in Pregnancy

Although genital warts are considered to pose no adverse effects on the pregnancy and labor, the lesions are reported to undergo rapid proliferation and become friable, particularly during the last trimester (Allstaff & Wilson, 2012; Wilson, 2011). Pregnancy is reported to trigger higher levels of HPV DNA than the detectable levels that occur in nonpregnant women (Allstaff & Wilson, 2012). Treatment may involve cryotherapy, trichloroacetic acid, or surgical excision (Watts, 2008; Wilson, 2011). However, achieving total eradication or complete suppression is generally not possible. Complete resolution tends to be poor until after the pregnancy. Cesarean section is considered if extensive warts occlude the genital tract or if there would be risk of excessive hemorrhage during vaginal delivery (Allstaff & Wilson, 2012; Wilson, 2011).

Neonatal infections are rare, although laryngeal papillomatosis and genital warts are found to occur after birth during infanthood and childhood, attributable to HPV type 6 and HPV type 11 (Wilson, 2011). Goon and Sonnex (2008) reported that vertical transmission occurs in approximately 1 in 80 pregnant women with genital warts. However, the actual mode of transmission is uncertain and no substantiated evidence has been found to establish whether transmission occurs via the placenta or other routes and whether transmission occurs in relation to specific factors occurring during the perinatal or postnatal periods (Wilson, 2011). Therefore, the main concern is to significantly reduce the infant's exposure risk during and after delivery. It is also recommended that women with ano-genital warts should be provided explanation and supportive counseling regarding a small risk of warts developing on the child's larynx. This can cause recurrent respiratory papillomatosis during infancy and childhood (Watts, 2008; Wilson, 2011).

Consideration of Trichomoniasis in Pregnancy

Trichomoniasis is reported as the most common nonviral STI across the world. Prevalence is relatively low in the United Kingdom, with only 5,400 diagnoses reported in 2008 (HPA, 2011b). Potential detrimental effects associated with trichomoniasis in pregnancy include premature rupture of membranes, preterm labor, and delivery of a low-birth-weight baby (Mann et al., 2009). Prenatal testing for *Trichomonas vaginalis* is indicated if the characteristic symptoms manifest, as there is growing evidence that *Trichomonas vaginalis* may enhance HIV transmission (McLelland et al., 2007; Tanton et al., 2011) and that HIV-positive persons may be at high risk for contracting the infection (Mavedzenge et al., 2010). Nevertheless, while screening for *Trichomonas vaginalis* is not currently recommended in asymptomatic women, this may exclude with *Chlamydia trachomatis* and gonorrhea infections (Sherrard et al., 2014). Treatment of *Trichomonas vaginalis* in pregnancy is found to potentially alleviate the characteristic vaginal discharge and could prevent perinatal morbidity such as respiratory and genital infections in the newborn and may also reduce persistent transmission. The recommended treatment options include metronidazole and tinidazole regimens.

- Metronidazole 2 g orally as a single dose, **or**
- Metronidazole 400–500 mg orally twice daily for 5–7 days
- Alternative treatment includes: Tinidazole 2 g orally as a single dose (Sherrard et al., 2014)

Non-compliance and treatment failure should be carefully monitored and repeat treatment regimen prescribed as per national guidelines. Gulmezoglu and Azhar's (2011) systematic review and other related meta-analyses revealed no evidence of teratogenic effect from administration of metronidazole during the first trimester of pregnancy. Nonetheless, other studies have reported adverse effect of the treatment on the pregnancy (Kigozi, Brahmbhatt, & Wabwire-Mangen, 2003), although others also claim to have found no association with preterm delivery or low birth weight (Stringer et al., 2010).

It is recommended to explain to pregnant women with asymptomatic trichomoniasis the potential benefits and risks of treatment and be given the option to postpone treatment until 37 weeks' gestation (Wilson, 2011). However, those who present with symptoms should be provided the recommended treatment together with advice, encouragement and support regarding consistent use of condoms. The persistent risk of sexual transmission despite treatment interventions should be clearly explained to all infected pregnant women. For that reason, it is important to encourage patients to abstain from sexual intercourse until the prescribed course of treatment is completed and the recommended period has passed (Wilson, 2011). Following delivery, trichomoniasis-infected mothers receiving treatment should be advised to withhold breastfeeding during and up to the end of the recommended period following completion of the treatment regimen. The stipulated period would depend on the specific medication prescribed and administered. Sherrard et al. (2014) cite the manufacturer's recommendation that high dosages of metronidazole should be avoided for breastfeeding mothers or allow 12–24 hours following administration of a single dose before breastfeeding the baby. This ensures that the newborn babies are not exposed to the maternal medications. Partner notification is also encouraged to avoid reinfection (Wilson, 2011).

Consideration of Bacterial Vaginosis in Pregnancy

Bacterial vaginosis (BV) is reported to be the most common cause of abnormal vaginal discharge among women of child-bearing age. Regarding BV, Hay, Patel, and Daniels (2012) cited an incidence of 15% reported among pregnant women attending antenatal clinic in the United Kingdom, a considerable proportion of which were asymptomatic. Prenatal screening for asymptomatic infection has not proven to have particular benefits for pregnancy outcomes (Hay et al., 2012). Nevertheless, BV has been associated with certain unfavorable obstetric consequences, including intra-amniotic infection, late abortion, premature rupture of membranes, preterm labor, preterm birth (Brocklehurst, Gordon, Heatley, & Milan, 2013), and postpartum endometritis (Leitich et al., 2003).

Evidence from trials on the treatment of BV during pregnancy reveals that metronidazole proves to be effective therapy during pregnancy (Schwebke & Desmond, 2007a; Schwebke, Marrazzo, Beelen, & Sobel, 2015). Alternative treatment involves the use of clindamycin (Wilson, 2011). Hay et al. (2012) cited various systematic reviews and meta-analyses that revealed no evidence of teratogenic effect of metronidazole use in treating bacterial vaginosis in the first trimester of pregnancy. However, emerging evidence indicates that treatment of BV before 20 weeks' gestation may prove effective in reducing the risk of preterm birth (McDonald, Brocklehurst, & Gordon, 2007). The recommended treatment regimens include the following:

- Metronidazole 400 mg orally twice daily for 5–7 days, **or**
- Metronidazole 2 g orally as a single dose, **or**
- Alternative regimen:
  - Tinidazole 2 g orally as a single dose, **or**
  - Clindamycin 300 mg orally twice daily for 7 days (Hay et al., 2012)

Various trials have also explored the safety and efficacy of metronidazole vaginal gel (Chavoustie et al., 2015; Schwebke et al., 2015). Because no significant difference in the cure or prevention of adverse effects on pregnancy has been reported between oral and topical treatment regimens of symptomatic BV, it is recommended that symptomatic pregnant women be treated with similar oral and vaginal regimens as for nonpregnant women (CDC, 2015). Evidence from systematic reviews on the benefits of screening and treatment of asymptomatic pregnant women to prevent preterm birth have been limited and not strongly substantiated (Hay et al., 2012).

Consideration of Granuloma Inguinale (Donovanosis) in Pregnancy

This infection is caused by an intracellular gram-negative bacterium, *Klebsiella granulomatis*, and is classified as a genital ulcerative disease. The epidemiology, symptoms, diagnosis, and treatment have been examined in a previous chapter. In this section, the special considerations for pregnant women and lactating mothers in relation to the treatment regimens for granuloma inguinale as cited by BASHH (2011) are outlined; see also CDC (2015) STD guidelines.

- Erythromycin 500 mg orally four times daily for at least 3 weeks or until complete healing of the lesions (CDC, 2015)

The safety of erythromycin is also questioned by some, and practitioners may find it useful to explore this in more detail (see Kallen, Otterbald, & Danielsson, 2005). Although azithromycin is considered to be effective for treating granuloma inguinale in pregnancy, substantive evidence on this is found to be limited. However, if used, the prescribed dosage may be the following:

- Azithromycin 1 g orally weekly or 500 mg orally once daily for at least 3 weeks or until the lesions have healed (CDC, 2015)

In the treatment regimens for nonpregnant patients, it is suggested that consideration be given to the additional use of parenteral aminoglycoside, such as intravenous gentamycin 1 mg/kg every 8 hours. This is considered if symptoms persist with no improvement within a few days of treatment. However, experts caution that certain antibiotics are contraindicated in pregnancy, including gentamycin, doxycycline, ciprofloxacin, and co-trimoxazole (BASHH, 2011; CDC, 2015). The risk of infection in babies born to mothers with genital lesions of untreated granuloma inguinale is recognized and the recommendation is to consider prophylactic antibiotic treatment.

The consideration for sexual partners is that contacts within 40 days before onset of the symptoms should be examined and offered treatment as necessary. Similarly, sexual contacts who have had unprotected sexual intercourse with an index patient who has active donovanosis should be examined and offered treatment. Follow-up is recommended until the clinical signs and symptoms resolve completely (BASHH, 2011). Some centers consider a look-back period of 60 days. The benefit of screening and empirical treatment in the absence of clinical signs and symptoms has not been substantiated (BASHH, 2011).

Consideration of Screening and Monitoring of HIV Infection in Pregnancy

Screening for HIV is recommended for all pregnant women. In the United Kingdom, detection of HIV among pregnant women is currently reported as significantly high and an estimated 90% of cases are diagnosed before delivery of the baby (Wilson, 2011). This is noteworthy considering that most transmissions occur during delivery. However, transmission of HIV from mother to the child can occur in utero, at delivery, and after delivery through breastfeeding. Across the United Kingdom, monitoring of HIV incidence in pregnancy has been performed through unidentifiable survey based on dried blood spots from neonates. This information is obtained from women who give birth and is unrelated to their HIV diagnosis status. The 2009 survey covering over 400,000 women who gave birth showed a prevalence of 2.2 per 1,000 (Taylor et al., 2012). Evidence suggests that high viral load in the HIV-infected mother increases the risk of transmission to the child. Nevertheless, transmission has been found to reduce to less than 2% with highly active antiretroviral therapy (HAART) and delivery by cesarean section (Wilson, 2011). Townsend et al. (2008) reported that between 2000 and 2006 the overall transmission rate from mother to child was 1.2% among the mothers who had been diagnosed. The prevalence was reported to be less than 1% among those who had received ART for at least 14 days (Townsend et al., 2008). By 2010, more than 98% of all pregnant women diagnosed with HIV had been receiving some form of ART (Taylor et al., 2012). No substantive evidence has been reported of fetal malformations relating to maternal HAART exposure, even in the first trimester (Wilson, 2011).

Related Key Issues on HIV Screening in Pregnancy

The U.K. recommendations regarding HIV screening state that pregnant women who are newly diagnosed with HIV should receive sexual health screening. Similarly, sexual health screening is advocated for HIV-positive women who become pregnant while undergoing HIV care and related interventions. It is also recommended that treatment of genital tract infections should be based on the guidelines outlined by the clinical effectiveness group of the British Association for Sexual Health and HIV (Taylor et al., 2012).

Although there are recognized benefits to effective treatment of genital tract infection for the woman and her sexual partner, as well as the unborn child, women who are not HIV infected and are asymptomatic do not undergo screening for genital tract infections. The potential risk to the fetus in terms of mother-to-child transmission of HIV-1 should be carefully addressed (Branson et al., 2006). The risk is associated with high viral load of HIV-1 in the genital tract and/or intrauterine infection with chorioamnionitis. An additional risk of preterm labor is reported to be higher among HIV-positive women than among those who are HIV-negative (Branson et al., 2006).

It is recommended that HIV-infected women not already receiving HAART be commenced on the standard regimen during the second trimester (Wilson, 2011). The rationale is to reduce the viral load to undetectable level by 36 weeks' gestation, thus allowing for consideration of vaginal delivery. However, some women who achieve undetectable viral load still opt for elective cesarean section, and those who had not received HAART or did not achieve undetectable viral load are also recommended for elective cesarean section. It is also recommended that neonates receive postexposure prophylaxis of antiretroviral therapy during the first month of life together with total avoidance of breastfeeding and strict formula-feeding only (Wilson, 2011). Recommended tests on the baby include HIV DNA PCR on the peripheral blood lymphocytes at 1 day, 6 weeks, and 12 weeks of age (Wilson, 2011). Negative results in a baby who is not being breastfed can be reported to the parents explaining that the results of the baby's blood tests have shown HIV negative. Confirmatory tests should be performed at 18 months to establish absence of maternal HIV antibodies (Wilson, 2011).

In the United States, pregnant women who decline the HIV screening test because of previous negative result are expected to be informed of the importance of retesting in each subsequent pregnancy. The benefits of screening and treating those who have acquired infections justify the importance of aiming to reduce perinatal transmission with recommended antiretroviral therapy, together with carefully planned obstetric interventions. Thus, repeat testing is recommended in the third trimester—around 36 weeks' gestation—for those women considered to be at high risk of HIV infection (CDC, 2015), such as illicit drug users, those who have multiple sexual partners, and those who may have acquired STIs in the current pregnancy, as well as women who live in areas of high prevalence of HIV and may have an HIV-positive sexual partner(s) (CDC, 2015).

Recommendations and Rationales for Follow-up Programs and Test of Cure

Follow-up programs and test of cure are complementary services to confirm that treatment has achieved expected patient outcomes of symptom resolution with complete cure. Crucially, the rationale is to detect therapeutic failure in spite of the prescribed antibiotic treatment. Therefore, compliance and adverse reactions can be explored in addition to monitoring of possible relapse or reinfection. Furthermore, these interventions help to ensure that appropriate partner notification procedures and referrals are implemented as necessary (CDC, 2015).

Follow-up Program for *Chlamydia trachomatis* Infections

Follow-up and test of cure to detect therapeutic failure is not considered necessary for patients treated with the recommended or alternative regimen. However, if the patient fails to adhere to the regimen, symptoms persist, or reinfection occurs, repeat testing is recommended 3 to 4 weeks after treatment completion. Continued presence of nonviable chlamydial DNA may be detectable in chlamydial NAATs if tested less than 3 weeks after treatment completio (Papp, Schachter, Gaydo, & Van Der Pol, 2014; Renault et al., 2011). The U.K. BASHH 2015 guideline for management of infection with *Chlamydia trachomatis* also makes similar recommendation indicating 3 to 5 weeks to avoid false-positive results (Dukers-Muijrers et al., 2012). Moreover, women who have been treated for chlamydial infection should have a test of cure carried out but not earlier than three weeks after treatment completion of the recommended treatment regimen (CDC, 2015).

Treatment follow-up helps to identify individuals who fail to comply or who may have been reexposed to *Chlamydia trachomatis* infection to be recalled for reevaluation and retreatment. In such cases test-of-cure may be required about 5 weeks after the prescribed treatment regimen. Test of cure is also recommended for pregnant women 6 weeks after treatment with azithromycin (BASHH, 2015). It is reported that most posttreatment infections do not result from treatment failure but from reinfection due to sexual partners not being treated or due to sexual intercourse with a new infected partner. Reinfection is reported to be more common (Heijne et al., 2011, 2013; Hosenfeld et al., 2009). Evidence reveals that reinfections increase the woman's risk of developing PID.

It is recommended that all patients treated for *Chlamydia trachomatis* infection should be retested 3 months following completion of the treatment, irrespective of whether they believe their sexual partners had received treatment. The period of testing can be extended to 12 months following the initial treatment. The U.K. BASHH 2015 recommendation is for repeat testing to be done 3–6 months after treatment in individuals under 25 years of age who are diagnosed with *Chlamydia trachomatis* infection. The CDC's (2015) recommendation is for test of cure to be performed preferably by NAATs, 3 to 4 weeks following completion of treatment. This is to confirm eradication of *Chlamydia trachomatis* to avoid more serious consequences in mothers and their babies due to lingering infection. Moreover, the CDC (2015) recommends that all pregnant women diagnosed with chlamydial infection should be retested 3 months after treatment. Pregnant women under 25 years of age who have sexual partners with current STIs or have intercourse with new or multiple partners or partners with other current sexual contacts should be rescreened in the third trimester. This precautionary measure allows for treating and eradicating the infection as necessary to avoid postnatal complications and neonatal chlamydial infection.

Regarding ophthalmia neonatorum caused by *Chlamydia trachomatis*, the reported 80% efficacy of erythromycin is considered as justification for repeat course of treatment. Babies treated with azithromycin for ophthalmia neonatorum are recommended for follow-up to ascertain effectiveness of the initial treatment. The same applies to chlamydial trachomatis pneumonia, which may manifest as a concomitant infection and the follow-up after azithromycin treatment is to ascertain that the pneumonia has resolved. Further monitoring may reveal abnormal pulmonary function tests later in childhood (CDC, 2015).

Acquisition of chlamydial infection among infants should take account of the vulnerability to sexual abuse and perinatal transmission through the nasopharynx, urogenital tract, and the rectum, which could linger for 2 to 3 years. The recommended follow-up should include repeat testing by culture for test-of-cure approximately 2 weeks after completion of the treatment (CDC, 2015).

Follow-up Program for *Neisseria gonorrhoeae* Infections

In cases of gonorrheal infections various experts maintain that follow-up assessment may be advantageous after completion of the treatment to confirm the patient complied with treatment with no adverse events, to ascertain symptom resolution, and to examine current sexual history for possible reinfection risk. At the same time, partner notification, health promotion/education, and support can be provided (Bignell & Fitzgerald, 2011; Whiley et al., 2012). Test of cure may not be required following the recommended or alternative treatment regimens for uncomplicated urogenital or rectal gonococcal infections. However, for selective test of cure, priority should go to patients with persistent symptoms and signs, and patients with pharyngeal gonorrheal infection. The recommendation for patients who receive the alternative treatment regimen for pharyngeal gonorrhea is a return visit 14 days after completion of the treatment for a test-of-cure to be performed using either culture or NAATs. If the NAATs results are positive, culture should be performed for confirmation before treatment. The ongoing emergence of antimicrobial-resistant *Neisseria gonorrhoeae* justifies the recommendation that all positive cultures for test-of-cure should have antimicrobial susceptibility testing performed before further treatment is administered (CDC, 2015; Unemo, 2015; Unemo & Shafer, 2014; Whiley et al., 2012).

Patients with lingering signs and symptoms are recommended to have culture performed with or without NAATs and followed by antimicrobial susceptibility testing of the isolated gonococci (Whiley et al., 2012). However, it is important to bear in mind that persistent urethritis, proctitis, or cervicitis may be caused by other organisms (CDC, 2015).

Most posttreatment infections are not due to treatment failure but reinfection, acquired from sexual partners who have not received treatment or from sexual intercourse with a new partner who is infected. Therefore, these scenarios justify the need for ongoing patient education and their sexual partners (CDC, 2015).

It is also recommended that all patients who have been treated for gonorrhea should be retested 3 months following completion of the treatment regardless of whether they believe their sexual partners had received treatment. This period of testing can be extended to 12 months following the initial treatment (CDC, 2015).

Follow-Up Program and Test of Cure for Syphilis Infections

The follow-up program for syphilis is rather more intensive than the recommended follow-up programs for other STIs. The purpose of the repeat assessments is to make certain that cure has been achieved and to closely monitor possible relapses or reinfection. Therefore, the subsequent line of management is based on the clinical findings and the laboratory serological test results following treatment (Janier et al., 2014). The key elements outlined below draw on Kingston et al.'s (2016) U.K. national guidelines; Janier et al.'s 2014 European guideline on the management of syphilis; and the CDC's 2015 STDs treatment guidelines.

Early Syphilis

The minimum follow-up for clinical reassessments and serological monitoring involves return visits at 3, 6, and 12 months, then at intervals of every 6 months until VDRL/RPR results remain sustained as negative or serofast (Janier et al., 2014; Kingston et al., 2016). The CDC 2015 recommends more frequent review if there is concern that the patient might contract repeat infection and also points out that definite criteria for cure and treatment failure are still lacking in clarity.

Late Syphilis

The minimum follow-up for serological monitoring is return visits every 3 months until the laboratory tests show serofast results.

An increase in the VDRL or RPR titers fourfold or higher indicates reinfection or failed response to treatment. Confirmation of the latter is based on certain key findings—four times or higher nontreponemal test titers, recurrent signs/symptoms, and reinfection being ruled out (Janier et al., 2014; Kingston et al., 2016).

Cerebrospinal fluid (CSF) test, together with repeat treatment, should be considered for patients in whom the expected fourfold decrease in nontreponemal test titers fails to be achieved within 12 months of treatment. The CDC's recommendation notes that failure to achieve the expected decline 6–12 months after treatment of primary or secondary syphilis could indicate failed response to treatment. In such cases, if the CSF is found to be normal, benzathine penicillin G may be prescribed. Three doses of 2.4 MU each would be administered intramuscularly at 1-week intervals (Seña et al., 2013; Workowski & Berman, 2010). However, as Seña et al. (2013) argue, the serologic nontreponemal test titer (NTT) might not necessarily fall despite negative CSF results and the repeat treatment regimen.

Specific treponemal tests may show persistently positive results despite treatment effectiveness, which should be carefully recorded to avoid needless retreatment. Patients who develop reinfection or relapse should be retreated and supervised to help with compliance; sexual partners should also be screened and treated. Patients who remain asymptomatic with VDRL/RPR-negative or serofast at 1-year reassessment may be discharged. Experts maintain that persistent or recurrent clinical manifestations and individuals presenting at least fourfold in NTT for more than 2 weeks undoubtedly have failed response to treatment or reinfection (CDC, 2015).

The recommendation is that such patients should receive repeat treatment guided by CSF analysis results and retested for HIV infection (CDC, 2015). Patients with coexisting HIV infection should undergo the initial follow-up as previously outlined, then a program of at least yearly monitoring of syphilis serology for life. In situations of outbreaks, more frequent follow-up is scheduled at 6-month intervals and this is arranged to coincide with the HIV follow-up visits (Kingston et al., 2016). Patients are encouraged to abstain from sexual intercourse and all sexual activities until complete healing of all syphilitic lesions and until serology test results have been carefully examined in detail.

Follow-Up Program for Pelvic Inflammatory Disease (PID)

The recommendation is that outpatients should be reviewed after 72 hours of commencing treatment. Any woman who presents with fever should be reviewed within 24 hours of commencing treatment. Significant clinical improvement is characterized by resolution of fever, and subsiding of lower abdominal pain, and uterine and cervical motion tenderness within 3 days of commencing treatment. Symptom improvement is expected to occur within 3 days of treatment. However, if that fails to happen, other conditions should be considered and the diagnostic procedures reviewed. Hospitalization

may be indicated and further diagnostic tests and possible surgical intervention should be considered, with appropriate referral for specialist care, as necessary (CDC, 2015; NICE, 2015; Ross, Judlin, & Jensen, 2014). Furthermore, it is recommended that retesting be performed on all women who have been diagnosed with chlamydial or gonococcal PID, 3 months after treatment irrespective of their sexual partners having undergone treatment (Hosenfeld et al., 2009).

A follow-up after 4 weeks helps to ensure that the treatment regimen has been completed, assess that full recovery has been achieved, and where applicable, that treatment and the required management of partner(s) has been implemented. It is recommended that partners of patients with PID should receive treatment for gonorrhea and chlamydia (NICE, 2015; Ross et al., 2014).

Follow-Up Granuloma Inguinale (Donovanosis) Infection

The follow-up recommendation suggests regular reviews until the symptoms and signs have subsided and healing achieved. Treatment is found to stop the ulcer progression, with healing observed to occur from the ulcer edges inward. Prolonged therapy should be expected for granulation to occur and for epithelial regrowth. Cases of recurrence with relapse have been reported 6–18 months after the treatment has evidently achieved healing.

Management of sex partners is recommended, although the benefit of empirical treatment of asymptomatic individuals has not been established by substantive research evidence. It is recommended that sex partners who have had sexual contact with the patient with donovanosis within 60 days prior to the onset of the patient's symptoms should be examined and offered treatment (CDC, 2015). The circumstances for special consideration include cases where evidence of improvement is not observed within a few days of the prescribed treatment regimen and patients with concurrent infections of granuloma inguinale and HIV.

Vaccination and Immunization Programs and Consideration in Pregnancy: A Global Initiative Against Preventable STIs

Where it is a feasible option, pre-exposure vaccination is considered to be a most effective mode of preventing STIs. It also provides a system of controlling and reducing transmission and spread of STIs among members of a community or specific population groups. Authorized national policy and recommendations stipulate that all patients/clients who present at STI clinics should undergo thorough investigation for STIs. Individuals who fall into identified high-risk categories and who have never been vaccinated against specific vaccine-preventable infections should be offered pre-exposure vaccinations as necessary and where applicable. Internationally, different countries, including the United Kingdom, United States, Australia, some provinces in Canada, and New Zealand advocate pre-exposure vaccination against specific vaccine-preventable STIs.

Human Papillomavirus (HPV) Vaccination Program

Various research studies indicate identification of over 100 different types of HPV and two main categories have been isolated (Schiffman et al., Castle, Jeromino, Rodriguez, & Wacholder, 2007). Oncogenic or high-risk HPV, specifically HPV-16 and HPV-18, have been identified as responsible for about 70% of cervical cancers, mainly squamous cell cancer and cervical adenocarcinoma (Schiffman et al., 2007). These are also linked to anogenital cancers in both genders, affecting the anal canal, the penis, the vulva, and vagina as well as rare types of oral and pharyngeal cancers (Cogliano et al., 2005; Jayaprakash et al., 2011; McCance, 2009). The other category of HPV, specifically HPV-6 and HPV-11, is responsible for 90% of genital warts (Garland et al., 2007; Lacey, Lowndes, & Shah, 2006) and is also associated with respiratory papillomatosis (CDC, 2015; Jayaprakash et al., 2011). A particular challenge in clinical practice is that while persistent oncogenic HPV is found to increase susceptibility to development of pre-cancers and cancers, most HPV infections are unrecognized as they remain asymptomatic and subclinical (CDC, 2015; Lacey et al., 2006; McCance, 2009). Thus, national screening programs and vaccination against these (Garland et al., 2007) have become vital components of STIs/RTIs prevention.

The CDC Policy and Recommendations for HPV Vaccination

In the United States, the Advisory Committee on Immunization Practices (ACIP) recommends HPV vaccination. The recommended vaccine 9vHPV is approved for use in females from age 9 through 26 years of age and males age 9 through 15 years of age, and is administered in a two-dose schedule. Dosage is 0.5 mL, administered intramuscularly.

Special population groups: HPV vaccination is recommended for MSM through age 26 years and for immunocompromised persons (including HIV infection) who have not had previous vaccination or did not complete the two-dose series.

The precautions and contraindications stipulate the following:

- HPV vaccines are contraindicated for persons with a history of immediate hypersensitivity to any vaccine component.
- 4vHPV and 9vHPV are contraindicated for persons with a history of immediate hypersensitivity to yeast.
- 2vHPV should not be used in persons with anaphylactic latex allergy.

HPV vaccines are not recommended for use in pregnant women. If pregnancy is diagnosed after initiating the vaccination series the remainder of the series should be delayed until completion of pregnancy. Patients and healthcare providers can report an exposure to HPV vaccine during pregnancy to the Vaccine Adverse Event Reporting System (VAERS).

Cervical cancer screening is recommended beginning at age 21 years and continuing through age 65 years for both vaccinated and unvaccinated women (Moyer, 2012).

HPV vaccination should not be delayed pending availability of 9vHPV or availability of data from future clinical trial.

The U.K. Policy and Recommendations for HPV Vaccination

Within the United Kingdom, health service organizations slight variations in implementing the national policy. Two vaccines have so far been licensed for use in the United Kingdom, (Jit, Chapman, Highes, & Choi, 2011). The government's perspective on these is that both of the vaccines provide adequate protection against the specific types of HPV infections. The bivalent (2vHPV) vaccine, sold under the trade name Cervarix®, provides protection against two specific types of HPV, namely HPV-16 and HPV-18. The second licensed vaccine, Gardasil, which provides protection against HPV-16 and HPV-18, provides additional protection against two other HPV strains, namely, HPV-6 and HPV-11 (Jit et al., 2011). Thus, this product is appropriately described as a quadrivalent vaccine (4vHPV; Jit et al., 2011).

The U.K. HPV Vaccination Regimen

To achieve maximum effectiveness, the vaccine should be administered in two doses within 2 years. Optimal protection is achieved if vaccination takes place before the young girl becomes sexually active. The vaccination program comprises two injections administered to girls of 12–13 years of age over a period of 6 to 24 months, with a catch-up campaign for young adult females over 18 years of age. Following the first injection, the second dose is administered at least 6 months later, but not more than 2 years apart (National Health Service [NHS], 2014). Box 9-2 outlines the recommended schedules for HPV vaccination. Practitioners are encouraged to explore current updated recommendations, policy regulations, and guidelines

---

BOX 9-2 Schedules for Bivalent (Cervarix) and Quadrivalent (Gardasil) Human Papillomavirus Vaccine (NHS September 2014)

HPV Types 16, 18 (Cervarix)

1st Dose	0.5 mL intramuscular	
2nd Dose	0.5 mL intramuscular, 6 to 24 months after the 1st dose	

HPV Types 6, 11, 16, 18 (Gardasil)

1st Dose	0.5 mL intramuscular	
2nd Dose	0.5 mL intramuscular, 6 to 24 months after the 1st dose	

Data from UK Department of Health. (2006). Human papillomavirus (HPV). In Salisbury, D., Ramsay, M., Noakes, K. (Eds.), *The Green Book: Immunisation against infectious disease*. Norwich: The Stationary Office. Retrieved from webarchive.nationalarchives.gov.uk/20130104162126/http:// immunisation.dh.gov.uk/gb-complete-current-edition/

stipulated by the particular health service organization. For example, explore the updated 2017 recommended schedule. This evidence-based policy was substantiated by findings from published studies as well as peer review of economic modeling of cost effectiveness conducted by the Health Protection Agency (Jit, Choi, & Edmunds, 2008).

General Concerns, Knowledge, Attitudes, and Acceptability of HPV Vaccination

Some parents are uneasy about possible long-term adverse effects and the overall safety of the HPV vaccines (Marlow, 2011; Siegrist, Lewis, Eskola, Evans, & Black, 2007). A small percentage of parents had ethical reservations related to personal values and principles (Brabin, Roberts, Farzaneh, & Kitchener, 2006; Marlow, 2011; Stretch et al., 2008). They believed that consenting to the vaccination would mean conceding early commencement of sexual activity even among preteenage girls and encouraging unrestrained and promiscuous sexual behaviors and sexual risk-taking practices including unprotected sex. Nevertheless, the U.K. policy recommends that girls 16 years and older who understand what the HPV vaccination involves can give their personal consent, although ideally parental support should be encouraged (NHS, 2014). For more information regarding knowledge about HPV, the related testing, the vaccines, and vaccination programs, practitioners are urged to explore relevant recent studies, including Marlow (2011); Marlow, Zimet, McCaffery, Ostini, & Waller (2013); and Dodd et al. (2014).

Projected Impact of the Vaccination Program

There is speculation in the United Kingdom that high vaccination coverage would result in fewer abnormal cervical screening results and ultimately reduce the incidence of cervical cancer. The vaccines are considered to be very successful in preventing the specific types of HPV infection against which they were developed in women who have high risk of susceptibility. Findings from various clinical trials (Harper et al., 2006; Lu, Kumar, Castellsagué, & Guiliano, 2011) reported these as being safe and very successful in preventing long-term HPV infections and related cervical diseases. The findings from the related evaluative studies (Harper et al., 2006; Lu et al., 2011) may dispel some of the concerns and reservations among the population of adolescent girls and their parents.

The outcome of the current HPV vaccination campaign could not be realistically measured until 2015, when those who were vaccinated at 18 years of age in 2008 became eligible for cervical cancer screening. Government monitoring of vaccine coverage, safety, and the overall impact of vaccination on HPV infections may contribute toward more knowledge and understanding of HPV vaccination.

Surveillance data indicates successful reduction in the prevalence of HPV-16 and HPV-18 infection, and the evidence suggests very high vaccine effectiveness among those vaccinated. It is now obligatory that vaccination status be recorded in the local child health information system and general practitioner clinical records. This would help ensure that girls who are not up to date can be vaccinated before they reach 18 years of age.

The Department of Health and other advocates urge that women should continue to receive cervical cancer screening regardless of their vaccination status. This is sound and plausible advice, since an estimated one-third of the cancers are alleged to be attributable to HPV types that are not affected by the current vaccines (NHS, 2014). There are speculations that the quadrivalent HPV vaccine may provide some cross protection against other closely related types of human papilloma viruses; however, this has not been confirmed by empirical clinical trials. Similar to the HPV vaccines, other STIs can be prevented by pre-exposure protection with specific vaccines. The ensuing sections present overviews of the recommendations regarding hepatitis B virus (HBV).

Hepatitis Type B Virus Vaccination Program

Global estimates suggest that about 2 billion people across the world are infected with HBV (Hepatitis B Foundation, 2014), with approximately 240 million having developed the associated chronic liver disease (CDC, 2015; Heymann, 2004; Shepard, Simard, Finelli, Fiore, & Bell, 2006). The estimated mortality figures indicate that 600,000 deaths occur annually due to both acute and chronic HBV disease (Heymann, 2004; Shepard et al., 2006). Hepatitis B is a serious infection in terms of being 50 to 100 times more contagious than HIV (CDC, 2015). The incubation period is 6 weeks to 6 months, with an average of 90 days, being detectable 30–60 days after infection and persisting for varying periods of time (CDC, 2015; Chang, 2007; Heymann, 2004). HBV is distinguished by specific characteristic viral proteins: hepatitis B surface antigen (HBsAg), hepatitis B core antigen (HBcAg), and others (Dienstag, 2008). High-prevalence regions include Asia, Africa, Latin America, and Southern Europe. In Northern Europe, the United Kingdom has a low prevalence of HBV, as do North American countries, where the infection occurs mainly in adolescents and young adults (Chang, 2007). Distribution within the United Kingdom shows higher HBsAg among those who were born in high-endemic countries.

Main Clinical Manifestations

The main clinical manifestations may vary from mild to severe and include general malaise with flu-like symptoms, fever, loss of appetite, nausea, vomiting, and upper right quadrant abdominal pain. However, symptoms these may be subtle and misleading (Chang, 2007; Servoss & Friendman, 2006; Shepard et al., 2006). Laboratory results of abnormal liver function tests and the serological indicators of the hepatitis B viral proteins such as HBsAg provide confirmation of infection (Chang, 2007; Shepard et al., 2006). Thus, higher concentrations of the virus occur in the blood, with lesser concentrations in other body fluids such as semen, vaginal secretions, saliva, and wounds or ulcers (Dienstag, 2008; Shepard et al., 2006). Chronic hepatitis B infection is diagnosed when a patient has had persistent HBsAg for longer than 6 months. In this case, the patient develops fatigue, nausea, loss of appetite, and symptoms characteristic of chronic liver dysfunction with dark urine and pale stools. The risk for hepatocellular carcinoma and cirrhosis is higher in such cases (Pan & Zhang, 2005; Villeneuve, 2005).

Modes of Transmission and Significance of Vaccination

Risk of hepatitis B is a significant occupational hazard for healthcare practitioners and other health service employees (Heymann, 2004; Shepard et al., 2006). The organism can survive for at least 7 days outside the body, and during that time, direct contact with the virus can give rise to infection if the individual is not vaccinated or otherwise protected (CDC, 2015). Generally, the main modes of infection are transmission through the percutaneous tissues or through the mucous membranes as a result of direct contacts, with blood or other body fluids that contain blood (Dienstag, 2008; Heymann, 2004; Shepard et al., 2006). In Western Europe and North America, the main modes of transmission are sexual activity and injectable drug usage. However, in developing countries, transmission modes are perinatal maternal–child transmission, direct contacts with contaminated items in the house, unsafe blood transfusion, and unprotected sexual activities (Heymann, 2004; Shepard et al., 2006; WHO, 2012).

Main Risk Factors

The main risk factor pertaining for developing chronic HBV infection is age. An estimated 90% of infants who become infected in their first year of life manifest the chronic disease (Chang, 2007; Villeneuve, 2005). This figure drops to 30–50% between 1–4 years of age (DH, 2013b). An estimated 25% of adults who die from hepatitis B-associated cirrhosis of the liver or cancer of the liver had been victims of chronic hepatitis B viral infection during their childhood (Chang, 2007; DH, 2013b; Servoss & Friedman, 2006). Nevertheless, 90% of people who develop hepatitis B viral infection in adulthood recover fully within 6 months (WHO, 2012). Other particular risk factors include injection drug use and frequent changes of sexual partners, as happens among MSM and commercial sex workers.

Universal childhood HBV vaccination has received increasing positive response from several countries across the world since the World Health Assembly emphasized the importance of eradicating this health threat and economic burden. The question of introducing universal childhood vaccination against hepatitis B throughout the European Union, including the United Kingdom, is still under debate. The United Kingdom still operates a selective hepatitis B vaccination policy, and various studies have sought to argue the potential long-term health and economic benefits of introducing universal hepatitis B vaccination (English, 2006).

The U.K. Vaccination Policy for HBV

Vaccination against HBV is recommended for individuals or specific population groups considered to be at high risk of contracting the virus. Guidelines are in place for pre- and postexposure vaccination regimens. In situations requiring testing for current or previous infection status the recommendation is to administer the first dose of the vaccine while the laboratory test results are being awaited (DH, 2013b).

HBV Pre- and Postexposure Vaccination

Pre-exposure vaccination is recommended for individuals who practice frequent changes of sexual partners, including MSM and commercial sex workers. IDUs are also a particular high-risk group, whether they are current, intermittent, or potential IDUs. Non-injecting sexual partners and children of IDUs are also recommended for pre-exposure vaccination. Close family contacts of individuals with chronic HBV infection and adoptive and foster parents of children from high-prevalence countries should be offered pre-exposure HBV vaccination. Similarly, regular recipients of blood or blood products as well as patients with chronic liver disease or chronic renal failure who undergo renal dialysis are considered for pre-exposure vaccination. It is also recommended for people emigrating or travelling to countries with high HBV prevalence and those whose occupation puts them at high risk, such as healthcare practitioners and laboratory staff (DH, 2013b).

Postexposure vaccination is recommended for babies born to mothers who have acquired HBV infection as well as sexual partners of individuals with acute HBV infection. Individuals who are inadvertently inoculated through needle-prick injury or contaminated through their eyes or mouths by blood from an HBsAg-positive patient are also candidates for postexposure vaccination (DH, 2013b). The different vaccines available against HBV prevention are outlined in **Box 9-3**.

For more details of the vaccine products and dosages, practitioners are strongly urged to consult and comply with their national policy guidelines for the countries where they work. It is vital that practitioners familiarize themselves with the related contraindications, precautions, and special considerations for certain identified patients.

The U.S. recommended schedules (CDC, 2011) are presented in **Table 9-1** and **Table 9-2**.

HIV Vaccination Initiatives: Ongoing Scientific Investigations

So far, research investigations to produce an effective antibody/antigen mechanism for HIV vaccination/immunization have not been entirely achieved. Innovative attempts to generate antibodies to provide lasting protection against HIV have not proved to be confidently successful.

The UNAIDS/WHO's Joint Advocacy for HIV Vaccines Initiative

The general measures for prevention and control of HIV are not entirely different from those that are applicable to the prevention and control of STIs, and for that reason no distinction is made. Therefore, rather than duplicating the

BOX 9-3 Vaccination Schedule Against HBV Infection

Engerix B	0–15 years of age	10 µg	0.5 mL
Engerix B	16 years and over	20 µg	1.0 mL
Fendrix	Renal patients of 15 years and over	20 µg	0.5 mL
HBvaxPRO Pediatric	0–15 years	5 µg	0.5 mL
HBvaxPRO	16 years and over	10 µg	1.0 mL
HBvaxPRO40	Adult dialysis & pre-dialysis patients	40 µg	1.0 mL

Twinrix is a combined vaccine product against Hepatitis A and B.

Twinrix Paediatric (Hepatitis A/B)
3 doses at 0, 1, 6 months.
HAV dose 360 ELIZA units
HBV dose 10µg
0.5ml for age group 1-15 years of age.

Twinrix Adult (Hepatitis A/B)
3 doses at 0, 1, 6 months
HAV dose 720 ELISA units
HBV dose 20µg
1.0ml for age group 16 years or over.

Data from UK Department of Health. (2006). Hepatitis B. In Salisbury, D., Ramsay, M., Noakes, K. (Eds.), *The Green Book: Immunisation against infectious disease.* Norwich: The Stationary Office. Retrieved from webarchive.nationalarchives.gov.uk/20130104162126/http://immunisation.dh.gov.uk/gb-complete-current-edition/

Table 9-1   U.S. Vaccination Schedule Against HBV Infection

Vaccine	Age Group	Dose	Volume	Intervals
Engerix-B	0–19 years	10 µg	0.5 mL	Birth, 1–4, 6–18 months (Older child) 0, 1–2, 4 months
	20 years & over	20 µg	1.0 mL	0, 1, 6 months
Recombivax HB	0–19 years	5 µg	0.5 mL	Birth, 1–4, 6–18 months Older child, 0, 1–2, 4 months
	11–15 years	10 µg	1.0 mL	0, 4–6 months
	20 years & over	10 µg	1.0 mL	0, 1, 6 months

Data from CDC. (2016). Hepatitis B FAQs for health professionals. Retrieved from https://www.cdc.gov/hepatitis/hbv/hbvfaq.htm

Table 9-2   U.S. Schedule of Combination Hepatitis A and Hepatitis B Vaccines

Vaccine	Age Group	Volume	Intervals
Comvax	6 weeks—4 years	0.5 mL	2, 4, 12–15 months
Pediarix	6 weeks—6 years	0.5 mL	2, 4, 6 months
Twinrix	18 years & over	1.0 mL	0, 1, 6 months
HepA + HepB	18 years & over	1.0 mL	0, 7, 21–30 days, 12 months

Data from CDC. (2016). Hepatitis B FAQs for health professionals. Retrieved from https://www.cdc.gov/hepatitis/hbv/hbvfaq.htm

issues that have already been addressed, an attempt is made here to present a broad global overview of the ongoing research on an HIV vaccine (WHO, 2012).

There is a global initiative to sponsor and advocate the development of a preventive vaccine for HIV, while expediting and evaluating the prospective availability of such a vaccine. The mutual global concern is evidenced by statistics showing that from the initial HIV epidemic, 60 million people of all ages and gender have been infected by the virus (WHO, 2012). Of that, an estimated 20 million deaths have occurred due to direct consequences of the infection. Despite the fervent international response to the worldwide HIV/AIDS pandemic, transmission and spread of this infection continues. In fact, more than 14,000 newly infected people are projected each day, mostly in developing countries (WHO, 2012). Indeed, HIV/AIDS is reported as the leading cause of death in Africa and the fourth worldwide. Rehle et al. (2015) reported from their 2012 estimates that the largest number of new diagnoses of HIV infections occurs in South Africa. An estimated 1,000 new HIV infections were diagnosed each day among adults in the age range of 15–49 years during 2012. More recent statistical figures reveal that in 2014, an estimated 50,000 infected people in the United States and 2 million worldwide were diagnosed with HIV (National Institute of Allergy and Infectious Diseases [NIAID], 2016). Therefore, the need for a safe, effective, and accessible vaccine is imperative. This would help to balance and enhance the current established preventive policies and procedures in an endeavor to control the worldwide pandemic. The importance and perseverance for this initiative impelled the UNAIDS and the WHO to collaborate in establishing the new HIV Vaccine Initiative (HVI).

Each of these two organizations contributes from the wealth of its expertise in different subject areas. Thus, the UNAIDS contributes its expertise of research in social and behavioral sciences, expertise in addressing moral and ethical matters, ingenuity in political lobbying, and its pervasive association with communities. The WHO contributes through its expertise in vaccine experimentation, vaccination schemes, policies, and programs. The organization makes additional contribution through its partnerships with relevant agencies in the public and private sectors. These agencies specialize in the marketing and distribution of vaccines for public health prevention programs (WHO, 2012).

Other undertakings include enhancing the standards, while expediting the conduct of vaccine trials in developing countries through appropriate training ventures and capacity building. The HIV Vaccine Initiative is guided by the WHO/UNAIDS Vaccine Advisory Committee (VAC). This operation enables scientists, different agencies, and specialist disciplines to engage in dialogue, exchange information, and identify mutual arrangements for collaboration (WHO, 2012). Another collaborative effort involves the HIV vaccine trials network (HVTN) 100. The project involves international collaboration of scientists working on experimental investigations on HIV vaccines. A current ongoing project is the National Institute of Allergy and Infectious Diseases (NIAID)-sponsored clinical trial in South Africa that is conducting experimental tests on HIV vaccine regimens.

Conclusion

Differences in STI prevalence in different countries indicate that particular populations and subgroups are at greater risk of contracting certain STIs, and variations in the course

and associated complications also occur. The associated economic burden imposed by adverse consequences and morbidity and mortality are documented. The identified issues require special consideration in care and treatment interventions.

Specific initiatives and mechanisms are proposed for prevention and control of STIs and HIV infections. Ongoing initiatives at national and international levels have received worldwide recognition as public health concerns. To that end, systems in place for surveillance, monitoring, and control at national level have been thoroughly examined.

In essence, STI surveillance facilitates computing and determining actual incidence and estimating the prevalence of symptomatic and asymptomatic STIs. Case reporting methods include etiologic confirmatory tests for laboratory diagnosis and syndromic descriptions for making clinical diagnosis. Stipulated standard case definitions must be applied to determine recent occurrence trends of specific STIs. Surveillance data elements can be utilized to guide the planning and implementation of preventive and control interventions, as well as clinical audits and evaluative studies. Advanced or enhanced surveillance involves more detained data collection based on stipulated case definitions and more extensive analysis. Special high-level investigations such as antimicrobial resistance studies and specific prevalence studies are conducted at this level. Therefore, participating laboratories must be appropriately resourced with the required equipment and specialist knowledge and expertise. Sexual healthcare practitioners at various levels may benefit from exploring more comprehensive texts for more detailed information and clearer insight about evaluation of STI surveillance and monitoring systems.

Special laboratory tests allow for isolation of the causal organisms for particular STIs while making it possible to determine the degree of specificity and sensitivity. Additionally, better insight on the behavior of specific organisms and ensures that appropriate antibiotics and antimicrobials are prescribed for the treatment of particular infections.

Pregnancy presents the additional concern of maternal-child transmission with perinatal consequences of congenital infection and possible abnormalities. Therefore, sexual health practitioners should have adequate knowledge and insight about the significance of STIs/RTIs and HIV infection in pregnancy. The adverse consequences of specific STIs for the mother and child should be addressed in care and treatment interventions throughout pregnancy, during labor, postnatally, and the neonatal periods.

Recommended screening for STIs is an important part of routine early pregnancy assessments, where applicable. Other preventive initiatives include pertinent evidence-based patient information, education, and counseling. Screening and vaccination programs, whether general or selective, should be carefully coordinated, evaluated, and audited and the related policy regulations should be clearly defined for correct implementation. Ongoing HIV vaccine trials and other experimental studies and trials to develop HSV vaccine continue to be advocated and sponsored at national and international levels.

Specific elements in this chapter provide the bases for research in sexual and reproductive health care, including topics relating to aspects of detailed sexual history-taking. Evaluative studies could be conducted on specific issues inherent in the organizational or internal policy guidelines and recommendations. The extent to which standardization influences the effectiveness of the process of sexual history-taking could also be considered for clinical audit projects, qualitative studies, or extensive systematic review.

● ● ● **REFERENCES**

Abdool-Karim, Q., Abdool Karim, S. S., Frohlich, J. A., Grobler, A. C., Baxter, C., Mansoor, L. E., . . . CAPRISA 004 Trial Group. (2010). Effectiveness and safety of tenofovir gel, an antiretroviral microbicide, for the prevention of HIV infection in women. *Science, 329*(5996), 1168–1174.

Ahmed, N., & French, P. (2013). Interpretation of syphilis serology. *British Journal of Hospital Medicine, 74*(7), C104–C107.

Ajzen, I. (1988). *Attitudes, personality and behaviour.* Maidenhead, United Kingdom: Open University Press.

Ajzen, I., & Fishbein, M. (1980). *Understanding attitudes and predicting social behaviour.* Englewood Cliffs, NJ: Prentice Hall.

Allstaff, S., & Wilson, J. (2012). The management of sexually transmitted infections in pregnancy. *Obstetrics and Gynaecology, 14*(1), 25–32.

Anderson, J. E. (2003). Condom use and HIV risk among US adults. *American Journal of Public Health, 93*(6), 912–914.

Apter, D. (2009). Sexuality education programmes and sexual health services: Links for better sexual and reproductive health (SRH). *Entre Nous: European Magazine of Sexual & Reproductive Health,. 69*, 12–14.

American Academy of Pediatrics. (2015). Herpes Simplex. In Kimberlin, D.W. (Ed.), *Red Book: 2015 Report of the Committee on Infectious Diseases, (30th ed.)* (432). Elk Grove Village, IL: author.

Aral, S. O. (2011). Utility and delivery of behavioural interventions to prevent sexually transmitted infections. *Sexually Transmitted Infections, 87*(2), 31–33.

Aral, S. O., & Blanchard, J. F. (2011, July). *Key population and their role in STD/HIV transmission dynamics.* Presented at International Society for Sexually Transmitted Disease Research (ISSTDR), Quebec, Canada.

Aral, S. O., & Blanchard, J. F. (2012). The program science initiative: Improving the planning, implementation and evaluation of HIV/STI prevention programs. *Sexually Transmitted Infections, 88*(3), 157–159.

Aral, S. O., & Leichliter, J. S. (2010). Non-monogamy: Risk factor for STI transmission and acquisition and determinant of STI spread in populations. *Sexually Transmitted Infections 86*(3), 29–36.

Armstrong, N., & Donaldson, C. (2005). *The economics of sexual health.* London, United Kingdom: UK Family Planning Association (FPA).

Bachmann, L. H., Johnson, R. E., Cheng, H., Markowitz, L., Papp, J. R., Palella, F. J. Jr., & Hook, E. W. (3rd). (2010). Nucleic acid amplification tests for diagnosis of *Neisseria gonorrhoeae* and *Chlamydia trachomatis* rectal infections. *Journal of Clinical Microbiology, 48*(5), 1827–1832.

Bailey, R. C., Moses, S., Parker, C. B., Agot, K., Maclean, I., Krieger, J. N., . . . Ndinya-Achola, J. O. (2007). Male circumcision for HIV prevention in young men in Kisumu, Kenya: A randomised controlled trial. *The Lancet, 369*(9562), 643–656.

Barham, L., Lewis, D., & Latimer, N. (2007). One to one interventions to reduce sexually transmitted infections and under the age of 18 conceptions: A systematic review of the economic evaluations. *Sexually Transmitted Infections, 83*(6), 441–446.

Barry, P. M., Kent, C. K., Philips, C. C., & Klausner, J. D. (2010). Results of a program to test women for rectal chlamydia and gonorrhoea. *Obstetrics and Gynaecology, 115*(4), 753–759.

Barry, P. M., & Klausner, J. D. (2009). The use of cephalosporins for gonorrhoea: The impending problem of resistance. *Expert Opinions in Pharmacological Therapies, 10*(4), 555–577.

Bassett, I. V., Freedberg, K. A., & Walensky, R. P. (2004). Two drugs or three? Balancing efficacy, toxicity and resistance in postexposure prophylaxis for occupational exposure to HIV. *Clinical Infectious Diseases, 39*(3), 395–401.

Beh Webster, R., & Bailey, J. V. (2013). Development of a theory-based interactive digital intervention to improve condom use in men in sexual health clinics: And application of qualitative methods using the behaviour change wheel. *The Lancet, 382*(3), 102.

Bernstein, E. R., Bellamy, A. R., Hook, E. W.3rd, Levin, M. J., Wald, A., Ewell, M. G., . . . Belshe, R. B. (2013). Epidemiology, clinical presentation, and antibody response to primary infection with herpes simplex virus type 1 and type 2 in young women. *Clinical Infectious Diseases, 56*(3), 344–351.

Bignell, C. (2009). 2009 (UISTI/WHO) guideline on the diagnosis and treatment of gonorrhoea in adults. *International Journal of Sexually Transmitted Diseases & AIDS, 20*(7), 453–457.

Bignell, C., & Fitzgerald, M. (2011). UK National guideline for the management of gonorrhoea in adults. *International Journal of Sexually Transmitted Diseases and AIDS, 22*(10), 541–547.

Bignell, C., & Garley, J. (2010). Azithromycin in the treatment of infection with *Neisseria gonorrhoeae. Sexually Transmitted Infections, 86*(6), 422–426.

Bignell, C., & Unemo, M. (2013). 2012 European guideline on the diagnosis and management of gonorrhoea in adults. *International Journal of Sexually Transmitted Diseases and AIDS, 24*(2), 85–92.

Blake, S. (2010). *Brook responds to sexually transmitted infections.* Retrieved from https://www.sexeducationforum.org.uk/media/17706sreadvice.pdf

Blake, S., Emmerson, L., & Hayman, J. (2014). Sex and relationships education (SRE) for the 21ST century. Supplementary advice for the sex and relationship education guidance DfEE (0116/2000). Brook, London, United Kingdom: National Children's Bureau.

Blake, S., & Muttock, S. (2012). *Assessment, evaluation and sex & relationships education: A practical toolkit for education, health and community settings* (2nd ed.). London, United Kingdom: National Children's Bureau.

Blower, S. A., & Farmer, P. (2003). Predicting the public health impact of antiretrovirals: Preventing HIV in developing countries. *AIDScience, 3*(11), 2003.

Boonstra, H. D. (2010). Winning campaign: California's concerted effort to reduce its teen pregnancy rate. *Guttmacher Policy Reviews, 13*(2), 18–24.

Brabin, L., Roberts, S. A., Farzaneh, F., & Kitchener, H. C. (2006). Future acceptance of adolescent human papillomavirus vaccination: a survey of parental attitudes. *Vaccine, 24*(16), 3087–3094.

Branson, B. M., Handsfield, H. H., Lampe, M. A., Janssen, R. S., Taylor, A. W., Lyss, S. B., Clark, J E. (2006). Revised recommendations for HIV testing of adults, adolescents, and pregnant women in health-care settings. *MMWR Recommendations and Reports, 55*(14); 1–17.

Bremer, V., Marcus, U., & Hamouda, O. (2012). Syphilis on the rise again in Germany—Results from surveillance data for 2011. *European Surveillance, 17*(29), pii=20222.

British Association for Sexual Health and HIV (BASHH). (2010). *Standards for the management of sexually transmitted infections (STIs).* Published: London, United Kingdom: MEDFASH.

British Association for Sexual Health and HIV (BASHH). (2011). *United Kingdom national guideline for the management of Donovanosis (Granuloma inguinale) 2011.* London, United Kingdom: Richens University College.

British Association for Sexual Health and HIV (BASHH). (2014). *Standards for the management of sexually transmitted infections (STIs).* London, United Kingdom: MEDFASH.

British Association for Sexual Health and HIV (BASHH). (2015). *U.K. National Guideline for the management of infection with Chlamydia Trachomatis.* Retrieved from https://www.bashhguidelines.org/current-guidelines/urethritis-and-cervicitis/chlamydia-2015/

Brocklehurst, P., Gordon, A., Heatley, E., & Milan, S. J. (2013). Antibiotics for treating bacterial vaginosis in pregnancy. *Cochrane Database Systematic Reviews, (1),* CD000262.

Brocklehurst, P., & Rooney, G. (2000). Interventions for treating genital *Chlamydia trachomatis* infection in pregnancy. *Cochrane Database Systematic Reviews, (2),* CD000054.

Brook, G., Bacon, L., Evans, C., McLean, H., Roberts, C., Tipple, C., Winter, A. J., Sullivan, A. 2013 UK national guideline for consultations requiring sexual history taking. *International Journal of STD & AIDS* 0(0): 1–14.

Brook & Family Planning Association (FPA). (2013). *Unprotected nation: The financial and economic impacts of restricted contraception and sexual health services.* London, United Kingdom: Brook and FPA.

Brown, Z. A., Wald, A., Ashley, M. R., Selke, S., Zeh, J., & Corey L. (2003). Effect of serologic status and Caesarean delivery on transmission rates of herpes simplex virus from mother to child. *Journal of the American Medical Association, 289*(2), 203–209.

Bryant, K. J. (2006). Expanding research on the role of alcohol consumption and related risks in the prevention and treatment of HIV/AIDS. *Substance Use and Misuse, 41*(10–12), 1465–1507.

Bunnell, R., Ekwaru, J. P., Solberg, P., Wamai, N., Bikaako-Kajura, W., Were W., . . . Mermin, J. (2006). Changes in sexual behaviour and risk of HIV transmission after antiretroviral therapy and prevention interventions in rural Uganda. *AIDS, 20*(1), 85–92.

Burke, M., Harris, S., & Swinson, T. (2006). *National STD surveillance data dissemination: Who wants to know what?* Washington, DC: RTI International Project Number 08235 038.

California Department of Public Health. (2011). *Best practices for the prevention and early detection of repeat chlamydial and gonorrhoeal infections: Effective partner treatment and patient retesting strategies for implementation in California health care settings.* Sacramento, CA: California Department of Public Health.

Carey, M. P., Senn, T. E., Vanable, P. A., Courey-Doniger, P., & Urban, M. A. (2010). Brief and intensive behavioural interventions to promote sexual risk reduction among STD clinic patients: Results from a randomised controlled trial. *AIDS and Behavior, 14*(3), 504–517.

Carles, G., Lochet, S., Youssef, M., Guindi, W., Helou, G., Alassas, N., & Lambert, V. (2008). Syphilis and pregnancy. *Journal de gynécologie, obstétrique et biologie de la reproduction* (Paris), 37(4),353–357.

Celum, C., Wald, A., Lingappa, J. R., Magaret, A. S., Wang, R. S., Mugo, N., . . . Corey, L. (2010). Acyclovir and transmission of HIV-1 from persons infected with HIV-1 and HSV-2. *New England Journal of Medicine, 362*(5), 427–439.

Centers for Disease Control and Prevention (CDC). (2011). *Sexually transmitted disease surveillance 2010.* Atlanta, GA: US Department of Health and Human Services.

Centers for Disease Control and Prevention. (2013c). Overview of Evaluating Surveillance Systems. Atlanta, GA: Author. Retrieved from https://www.cdc.gov/globalhealth/healthprotection/fetp/training-modules/12/eval-surv-sys_fieldg_final_09262013.pdf

Centers for Disease Control and Prevention (CDC). (2015). *Sexually transmitted disease surveillance 2014.* Atlanta, GA: U.S. Department of Health and Human Services.

Centers for Disease Control and Prevention (CDC). (2017). *Fact sheet: HIV in the United States: at a Glance.* Retrieved from https://www.cdc.gov/hiv/statistics/overview/ataglance.html

Chan, D. J., & Ray, J. E. (2007). Quantification of antiretroviral drugs for HIV-1 in the male genital tract: Current data, limitations and implications for laboratory analysis. *Journal of Pharmacy and Pharmacology, 59*(11), 1451–1462.

Chang, M. H. (2007). Hepatitis B virus infection. *Seminars in Fetal and Neonatal Medicine, 12*(3), 160–167.

Chau, C., Brown, A., & Delpech, V. (2014). *HARS: The HIV and AIDS reporting system.* London, United Kingdom: Colindale.

Chavoustie, S. E., Jacobs, M., Reisman, H. A., Waldbaum, A. S., Levy, S. F., Hillier, S. L., & Nyirjesy, P. (2015). Metronidazole vaginal gel 1.3% in the treatment of bacterial vaginosis: A dose ranging-study. *Journal of Lower Genital Tract Diseases, 19*(2), 129–134.

Chen, M. Y., Fairley, C. K., De Guingand, D., Hocking, J. Tabrizi, S., Wallace, E. M., . . . Garland, S. (2009). Screening pregnant women for chlamydia: What are the predictors of infection? *Sexually Transmitted Infections, 85*(1), 31–35.

Chin, H. B., Sipe, T. A., Elder, R., Mercer, S. L., Chattopadhyay, S. K., Jacob, V., . . . Community Preventive Services Task Force. (2012). The effectiveness of group-based comprehensive risk reduction and abstinence education interventions to prevent or reduce the risk of adolescent pregnancy, human immunodeficiency virus, and sexually transmitted infections: Two systematic reviews for the guide to community preventive services. *American Journal of Preventive Medicine, 42*(3), 272–294.

Chow, J. M., Kang, M-S., Samuel, M. C., & Bolan, G. (2009). Assessment of the association of *Chlamydia trachomatis* infection and adverse perinatal outcomes with the use of population-based chlamydia case report registers and birth records. *Public Health Reports, 124*(2), 24–30.

Clutterbuck, D. (2004). *Sexually transmitted infections in the sexual health consultation. Specialist training in sexually transmitted infections and HIV.* London, United Kingdom: Mosby.

Clutterbuck, D. J., Flowers, P., Barber, T., Wilson, H., Nelson, M., Hedge, B., . . . Sullivan, A. K. (2012). UK national guidelines on safer sex advice. *International Journal of Sexually Transmitted Diseases and AIDS, 23*(6), 381–388.

Coates, T. J., Ritchter, L., & Carceres, C. (2009). HIV prevention 3. Behavioural strategies to reduce HIV transmission: How to make them work better. *The Lancet, 372*(9639), 669–684.

Cogliano, V., Baan, R., Straif, K., Grosse, Y., Secretan, B., El Ghissassi, F., & WHO International Agency for Research on Cancer. (2005). Carcinogenicity of human papillomaviruses. *Lancet Oncology, 6*(4), 204.

Cole, M. J., Unemo, M., Hoffman, S., Chisholm, S. A., Ison, C. A., & Van de Laar, M. J. (2011). The European gonococcal antimicrobial surveillance programme, 2009. *European Surveillance, 16*(42), pii 19995.

Conner, M., & Norman, P. (2005). Protection motivation theory. In M. Conner & P. Norman (Eds.), *Predicting health behaviour: Research and practice with social cognition models.* 2nd edn. (pp. 81–126) Buckingham, United Kingdom: Open University Press.

Corey, L., & Wald, A. (2009). Maternal and neonatal herpes simplex virus infections. *New England Journal of Medicine, 361*(14), 1376–1385.

Corey, L., Wald, A., Celum, C. L., & Quinn, T. C. (2004). The effects of herpes simplex virus-2 on HIV-1 acquisition and transmission: A review of two overlapping epidemics. *Journal of Acquired Immune Deficiency Syndrome, 35*(5), 435–445.

Crepaz, N., Marks, G., Liau, A., Mullins, M. M., Aupont, L. W., Marshall, K. J., . . . Wolitski, R. J. (2009). Prevalence of unprotected anal intercourse among HIV-diagnosed MSM in the United States: A meta-analysis. *AIDS, 23*(13), 1617–1629.

Crosby, R., Yarber, W., Sanders, S., Graham, C., McBride, K., Milhausen, R. R., & Arno, J. N. (2007). Men with broken condoms: Who and why? *Sexually Transmitted Infections, 83*(1), 71–75.

Delpech, V., Martin, I. M. C., Hughes, G., Nichols, T., James, L., & Ison, C. A. (2009). Epidemiology and clinical presentation of gonorrhoea in England and Wales: Findings from the Gonococcal Resistance to Antimicrobials Surveillance Programme 2001–2006. *Sexually Transmitted Infections, 85*(5), 317–321.

Department of Health. (2013a) (DH). *Framework for sexual health improvement in England.* London, United Kingdom: Author.

Department of Health (DH). (2013b). Hepatitis B: The Green Book, Chapter 18. Retrieved from https://www.gov.uk/government/publications/hepatitis-b-the-green-book-chapter-18

Department of Health Social Services and Public Safety (DHSSPS). (2011). *HIV and STI surveillance in Northern Ireland 2011: An analysis of data for the calendar year 2010.* Belfast, Northern Ireland: HSC Public Health Agency.

Dienstag, J. L. (2008). Hepatitis B virus infection. *New England Journal of Medicine, 359*(14), 1486–1500.

Dodd, R. H., McCaffery, K. J., Marlow, L. A., Ostini, R., Zimet, G. D., & Waller J. (2014). Knowledge of human papillomavirus (HPV) testing in the USA, the UK and Australia: An international survey. *Journal of Sexually Transmitted Infections, 90*(3), 201–207.

Doherty, I. A., Padian, N. S., Marlow, C., & Aral, S. O. (2005). Determinants and consequences of social networks as they affect the spread of sexually transmitted infections. *Journal of Infectious Diseases, 191*(1), S42–S54.

Drake, A. L., Wagner, A., Richardson, B., & John-Stewart, G. (2014). Incident HIV during pregnancy and postpartum and risk of mother-to-child HIV transmission: A systematic review and meta-analysis. *PLoS Medicine, 11*(2), e1001608. doi:1371/journal.pmed.1001608

Drumright, L. N., & Colfax, G. N. (2009). HIV risk and prevention for non-injection substance users. In K. Mayer & H. F. Pizer (Eds.), *HIV prevention: A comprehensive approach* (pp. 340–975). London, United Kingdom: Elsevier.

Dukers-Muijrers, N.H., Morré, S. A., Speksnijder, A., van der Sande, M. A., & Hoebe, C. J. (2012). *Chlamydia trachomatis* test-of-cure cannot be based on a single highly sensitive laboratory test taken at 3 weeks after treatment. *PLoS ONE, 7*(3), e34108.

Dworkin, S. L., & Ehrhardt, A. A. (2007). Going beyond 'ABC' to include 'GEM': Critical reflections on progress in the HIV/AIDS epidemic. *American Journal of Public Health, 97*(1), 13–18.

Emmerson, L. (2010). *Does sex and relationships education work? A Sex Education Forum evidence briefing.* London, United Kingdom: National Children's Bureau.

Emmerson, L. (2016). Overcoming the ignorance of basic sex education. *Nursing Children and Young People, 28*(8), 13.

Emmerson, L., & Lees, J. (2013). Let's get it right: A toolkit for involving primary school children in sex and relationships education. London, United Kingdom: NCB.

English, P. (2006). Should universal hepatitis B immunisation be introduced be introduced in the UK? *Archives of Diseases of Children, 94*(4), 286–289.

European Centre for Disease Prevention and Control (ECDC). (2013). *Sexually transmitted infections in Europe 2011.* Stockholm, Sweden: ECDC.

Evans, C., & Lambert, H. (2008). The limits of behaviour change theory: Condom use and contexts of HIV risk in the Kolkata sex industry. *Culture, Health and Sexuality, 10*(1), 27–42.

Ferreira, V. H., Nazli, A., Khan, G., Mian, M. F., Ashkar, A. A., Gray-Owen, S., . . . Kaushic, C. (2011). Endometrial epithelial cell responses to coinfecting viral and bacterial pathogens in the genital tract can activate HIV-1 LTR in NFκB- and AP-1–dependent manner. *Journal of Infectious Diseases, 204*(2), 229–308.

Field, E., Heel, K., Palmer, C., Vally, H., Beard, F., & McCall, B. (2010). Evaluation of clinical management of gonorrhoea using enhanced surveillance in South East Queensland. *Sexual Health, 7*(4), 448–452.

Fishbein, M., & Ajzen, I. (2005). Theory-based behaviour change interventions: Comments on Hobbis & Sutton. *Journal of Health Psychology, 10*(1), 27–31.

Foley, E., Clarke, E., Beckett, V. A., Harrison, S., Pillai, A., FitzGerald, M., . . . Patel, R. (2014). *Management of genital herpes in pregnancy.* London, United Kingdom: BASHH & Royal College of Obstetricians and Gynaecologists.

Formby, E., Coldwell, M., Stiell, B., Demack, S., Stevens, A., Shipton, L., . . . Willis, B. (2011). *Personal, social, health and economic (PSHE) Education: A mapping study of the prevalent models of delivery and their effectiveness for the Department for Education.* Sheffield, United Kingdom: Centre for Education and Inclusion Research, Sheffield Hallam University.

Foss, A. M., Watts, C. F., Vickerman, P., & Heise, L. (2004). Condoms and prevention of HIV are essential and effective, but additional methods are also needed. *BMJ, 2004; 329*(7459), 185–186.

French, P. (2011). Syphilis: Clinical features, diagnosis and management. In K. E. Rogstad (Ed.), *ABC of sexually transmitted infections* (6th ed., pp. 70–77). Chichester, United Kingdom: Wiley-Blackwell.

Frost, S. D. (2007). Using sexual affiliation networks to describe the sexual structure of a population. *Sexually Transmitted Infections, 83*(1), 37–42.

Fuller, C. M., Ford, C., & Rudolph, A. (2009). Injection drug use and HIV: Past and future considerations for HIV prevention and interventions. In K. Mayer & H. F. Pizer (Eds.), *HIV prevention: A comprehensive approach* (pp. 305–339). London, United Kingdom: Elsevier.

Gabhainn, S. N., O'Higgins, S., & Barry, M. (2010). The implementation of social, personal and health education in Irish schools. *Health Education, 110*(6), 452–470.

Gallo, M. F., Grimes, D. A., Lopez, L. M., & Schulz, K. F. (2006). Non-latex versus latex male condoms for contraception. *Cochrane Database Systematic Reviews, (1),* CD003550.

Gallo, M. F., Kilbourne-Brook, M., & Coffey, P. S. (2012). A review of the effectiveness and acceptability of the female condom for dual protection. *Sexual Health, 9*(1), 18–26.

Gallo, M. F., Macaluso, M., Warner, L., Fleenor, M. E., Hook, E. W. 3rd, Brill I., & Weaver, M. A. (2012). Bacterial vaginosis, gonorrhoea and chlamydial infection among women attending a sexually transmitted disease clinic: A longitudinal analysis of possible causal links. *Annals of Epidemiology, 22*(3), 213–220.

Galvin, S. R., & Cohen, M. S. (2004). The role of sexually transmitted diseases in HIV transmission. *Nature Reviews of Microbiology, 2*(1), 33–42.

Gardella, C., & Brown, Z. (2011). Prevention of neonatal herpes. *British Journal of Obstetrics and Gynaecology, 118*(2), 187–192.

Garland, S. M., Hernandez-Avila, M., Wheeler, C. M., Perez, G., Harper, D. M., Leodolter, S., . . . Koutsky, L. A. (2007). Quadrivalent vaccine against human papillomavirus to prevent anogenital diseases. *New England Journal of Medicine, 356*(19), 1928–1943.

Giraudon, I., Forde, J., Maguire, H., Arnold, J., & Permalloo, N. (2009). Antenatal screening and prevalence of SYPHILIS infection: surveillance in London, 2000–2007. *European Surveillance, 14*(9): 8–12.

Golparian, D., Hellmark, B., Fredlund, H., & Unemo, M. (2010). Emergence, spread and characteristics of *Neisseria gonorrhoeae* isolates with in vitro decreased susceptibility and resistance to extended-spectrum cephalosporins in Sweden. *Sexually Transmitted Infections, 86*(6), 454–460.

Gomez, G. B., Lamb, M. L., Newman, L. M., Mark, J., Boutet, N., & Hawkes, S. (2013). Untreated maternal syphilis and adverse outcomes of pregnancy: A systematic review and meta-analysis. *Bulletin of the World Health Organization, 91*(3), 217–226.

Goon, P., & Sonnex, C. (2008). Frequently asked questions about genital warts in the genitourinary medicine clinic: An update and review of recent literature. *Sexually Transmitted Infections, 84*(1), 3–7.

Granich, R., Crowley, S., Vitoria, M., Lo Y-R., Souteyrand, Y., Dye, C., . . . Williams, B. (2010). Highly active antiretroviral treatment for the prevention of HIV transmission. *Journal of the International AIDS Society, 13*, 1.

Granich, R., Crowley, S., Vitoria, M., Smyth, C., Khan, J. G., Bennett, R., . . . Williams, B. (2010). Highly active antiretroviral treatment for the prevention of HIV transmission: Review of scientific evidence and update. *Current Opinion in HIV and AIDS, 5*(4), 298–304.

Granich, R. M., Gilks, C. F., Dye, C., De Cock, K. M., & Williams, B. G. (2009). Universal voluntary HIV testing with immediate antiretroviral therapy as a strategy for elimination of HIV transmission: A mathematical model. *The Lancet, 373*(9657), 48–57.

Gray, R. H., Kigozi, G., Serwadda, D., Makumbi, F., Watya, S., Nalugoda, F., . . . Wawer, M. J. (2007). Male circumcision for HIV prevention in men in Rakai, Uganda: A randomised trial. *The Lancet, 369*(9562), 657–666.

Gray, R. H., Li X., Kigozi, G., Serwadda, D., Brahmbhatt, H., Wabwire-Mangen, F., Nalugoda, F., . . . Wawer, M. J. (2005). Increased risk of incident HIV during pregnancy in Rakai, Uganda: A prospective study. *The Lancet, 366*(9492),1182–1188.

Gregson, S., Adamson, S., Papaya, S., Mundondo, J., Nyamukapa, C. A., Mason, P. R., . . . Anderson, R. M. (2007). Impact and process evaluation of integrated community and clinic-based HIV-1 control: A cluster randomised trial in eastern Zimbabwe. *PLoS Medicine, 4*(3), 545–555.

Grimely, D. M., Annang, L., Houser, S., & Chen, H. (2005). Prevalence of condom use errors among STD clinic patients. *American Journal of Health Behavior, 29*(4), 324–330.

Groseclose, S. L., Samuel, M. C., Chow, J. M., & Weinstock, H. (2013). Surveillance for sexually transmitted diseases. In N. M. M'ikanatha, R. Lynfield, C. A. Van Beneden, & H. de Valk (Eds.), *Infectious disease surveillance* (pp. 343–361). Chichester, United Kingdom: John Wiley Ltd.

Gulmezoglu, A. M., & Azhar, M. (2011). Interventions for trichomoniasis in pregnancy. *Cochrane Database Systematic Reviews, (5),* CD000220.

Haggart, M. (2000). Promoting the health of communities. In J. Kerr (Ed.), *Community health promotion: challenges for practice* (pp. 3–25). Edinburgh, United Kingdom: Baillière Tindall.

Hall, H. I., Song, R., Rhodes, P., Prejean, J., An, Q., Lee, L. M., . . . HIV Incidence Surveillance Group (2008). Estimation of HIV incidence in the United States. *Journal of the American Medical Association, 300*(5), 520–529.

Harden, A., Brunton, G., Fletcher, A., & Oakley, A. (2009). Teenage pregnancy and social disadvantage: Systematic review integrating controlled trials and qualitative studies. *British Medical Journal, 339*, b4254.

Hargreaves, S. C., Jones, L., Madden, H. C. E., Daffin, J., Phillips-Howard, P. A., Syed, Q., . . . Cook, P. A. (2010). *HIV and AIDS in the North West of England August 2009; Liverpool John Moores University, Centre for Public Health.* Liverpool, United Kingdom: North West HIV/AIDS Monitoring Unit.

Harper, D. M., Franco, E. L., Wheeler, C. M., Moscicki, A. B., Romanowski, B., Roteli-Martins, C. M., . . . Dubin, G. (2006). Sustained efficacy up to 4.5 years of a bivalent L1 virus-like particle vaccine against human papillomavirus types 16 and 18: Follow-up from a randomised controlled trial. *The Lancet, 367*(9518), 1247–1255.

Hawkes, S., Martin, N., Broutet, N., & Low, N. (2011). Effectiveness of interventions to improve screening for syphilis in pregnancy: A systematic review and meta-analysis. *The Lancet Infectious Diseases, 11*(9), 684–691.

Hay, P., Patel, S., & Daniels, D. (2012). *UK national guideline for the management of bacterial vaginosis 2012.* https://www.guidelinecentral.com/summaries/uk-national-guideline-for-the-management-of-bacterial-vaginosis-2012/#section-society

Health Protection Agency (2010a). *Guidance for gonorrhoea testing in England and Wales.* London United Kingdom: Author.

Health Protection Agency. (2010b). Infection reports: HIV/STIs—Rise in new diagnoses of sexually transmitted infections (UK 2009). Health Protection Report, 4(34), Retrieved from http://webarchive.nationalarchives.gov.uk/20140714095645/http://www.hpa.org.uk/hpr/archives/2010/hpr3410.pdf

Health protection Agency. (2013). *HIV in the United Kingdom: Reports by PHE about HIV in the UK.* Part of HIV Surveillance, data and monitoring. Retrieved from https://www.gov.uk/government/publications/hiv-in-the-united-kingdom

Heijne, J. C., Althaus, C. L., Herzog, S. A., Kretzschmar, M., & Low, N. (2011). The role of reinfection and partner notification in the efficacy of chlamydia screening programs. *Journal of Infectious Diseases, 203*(3), 372–377.

Heijne, J. C., Herzog, S. A., Althaus, C. L., Tao, G., Kent, C. K., & Low, N. (2013). Insights into the timing of repeated testing after treatment for *Chlamydia trachomatis*: Data and modelling study. *Sexually Transmitted Infections, 89*(1), 57–62.

Hepatitis B Foundation. (2017). *What is Hepatitis B?* Doyles Town, PA: Hepatitis B Foundation. Retrieved from http://www.hepb.org/what-is-hepatitis-b/what-is-hepb/

Heymann, D. L. (2004). An official report of the American Public Health Association. In D. L. Heymann (Ed.), *Control of communicable diseases manual* (18th ed, pp. 35–37). Washington, DC: American Public Health Association.

Hollier, L. M., & Wendell G. D. (2008). Third trimester antiviral prophylaxis for preventing maternal genital herpes simplex virus (HSV) recurrences and neonatal infection. *Cochrane Database Systematic Reviews, (1),* CD004946.

Holmes, K. K., Levine, R., & Weaver, M. (2004). Effectiveness of condoms in preventing sexually transmitted infections. *Bulletin of the World Health Organization, 82*(6), 454–461.

Holmes, K. K., Sparling, P. F., Stamm, W. E., Piot, P., Wasserheit, J. N., & Corey, L. (2008). *Sexually transmitted diseases* (4th ed.). London, United Kingdom: McGraw-Hill Medical.

Horowitz, S. M. (2003). Applying the transtheoretical model to pregnancy and STD prevention: a review of the literature. *American Journal of Health Promotion, 17*(5), 304–328.

Hosek, S. G., Green, K. R., Siberry, G., Lally, M., Balthazar, C., Serrano, P. A., . . . The Adolescent Medicine Trials Network for HIV/AIDS Interventions. (2013). Integrating HIV behavioural interventions into biomedical prevention trials with youth: Lessons from Chicago's project PrEPare. *Journal of HIV AIDS and Social Services, 12*(3–4), doi: 10.1080/15381501.2013.773575

Hosenfeld, C. B., Workowski, K. A., Berman, S., Zaidi, A., Dyson, J., Mosure, D., . . . Bauer, H. M. (2009). Repeat infection with chlamydia and gonorrhoea among females: A systematic review of the literature. *Sexually Transmitted Diseases, 36*(8), 478–489.

Hughes, G., Nichols, T., & Ison, C. A. (2011). Estimating the prevalence of gonococcal resistance to antimicrobials in England and Wales. *Sexually Transmitted Infections, 87*(6), 526–531.

Hunte, T., Alcaide, M., & Castro, J. (2010). Rectal infections with chlamydia and gonorrhoea in women attending a multi ethnic sexually transmitted diseases urban clinic. *International Journal of Sexually Transmitted Diseases and AIDS, 21*(12), 819–822.

Ison, C. A., & Alexander, S. (2011). Antimicrobial resistance in Neisseria gonorrhoeae in the UK: surveillance and management. *Expert Reviews of Anti-Infective Therapies, 9*(10), 867–876.

Ison, C. A., Hussey, J., Sankar, K. N., Evans, J., & Alexander, S. (2011). Gonorrhoea treatment failures to cefixime and azithromycin in England 2010. *European Surveillance, 16*(14), pii 19833.

Ison, C. A., Town, K., Obi, C., Chisholm, S., Hughes, G., Livermore, D. M., & Lowndes, C. M. (2013). Decreased susceptibility to cephalosporins among gonococci: Data from the Gonococcal Resistance to Antimicrobials Surveillance Programme (GRASP) in England and Wales, 2007–2011. *The Lancet Infectious Diseases, 13*(9): 762–768.

Janier, M., Hegyi, V., Dupin, N., Unemo, M., Tiplica, G. S., Potocnik, M., . . . Patel, R. (2014). European guideline on the management of syphilis. *Journal of European Academy of Dermatology and Venereology, 28*(12), 1581–1593.

Janz, N. K. & Becker, M. H. (1984). The Health Belief Model: a decade later. *Health Educ Q, 11*(1): 1–49.

Javanbakth, M., Gorbach, P., Stirland, A., Chien, M., Kerndt, P., & Guerry, S. (2012). Prevalence and correlates of rectal chlamydia and gonorrhoea among female clients at sexually transmitted disease clinics. *Sexually Transmitted Diseases, 39*(12), 917–922.

Jayaprakash, V., Reid, M., Hatton, E., Merzianu, M., Riqual, N., Marshall, J., . . . Sullivan, M. (2011). Human papillomavirus types 16 and 18 in epithelial dysplasia of oral cavity and oropharynx: A meta-analysis, 1985–2010. *Oral Oncology, 47*(11), 1048–1054.

Jit, M., Choi, Y. H., & Edmunds, W. J. (2008). Economic evaluation of human papillomavirus vaccination in the United Kingdom. *British Medical Journal, 337,* a769.

Jemmott, J., Jemmott, L., & Fong, G. (2010). Efficacy of a theory-based abstinence-only intervention over 24 months: A randomised controlled trial with young adolescents. *Archives of Pediatric and Adolescent Medicine, 164*(2), 152–159.

Jit, M., Chapman, R., Hughes, O., & Choi, Y. H. (2011). Comparing bivalent and quadrivalent human papillomavirus vaccines: Economic evaluation based on transmission model. *British Medical Journal, 343,* d5775.

Johnson, H. L., Ghanem, K. G., Zenilman, J. M., & Erbelding, E. J. (2011). Sexually transmitted infections and adverse pregnancy outcomes among women attending inner city public sexually transmitted diseases clinics. *Sexually Transmitted Diseases, 38*(3), 167–171.

Kallen, B. A., Otterbald, O. P., & Danielsson, B. R. (2005). Is erythromycin therapy teratogenic in humans? *Reproductive Toxicology, 20*(2), 209–214.

Kent, C. (2007). STD surveillance: Critical and costly but do we know if it works? *Sexually Transmitted Diseases, 34*(2), 81–82.

Kenyon, C., Buyze, J., & Colebunders, R. (2014). Classification of incidence and prevalence of certain sexually transmitted infections by world regions. *International Journal of Infectious Diseases, 18*, 73–80.

Kerrigan, D., Moreno, L., Rosario, S., Gomez, B., Jerez, H., Barrington, C., Weiss, E., & Sweat, M. (2006). Environmental-structural interventions to reduce HIV/STI risk among female sex workers in the Dominican Republic. *American Journal of Public Health, 96*(1), 120–125.

Kigozi, G. G., Brahmbhatt, H., & Wabwire-Mangen, F. (2003). Treatment of trichomonas in pregnancy and adverse outcomes of pregnancy: A sub analysis of a randomized trial in Rakai, Uganda. *American Journal of Obstetrics and Gynecology, 189*(5), 1398–1400.

Kimberlin, D. W., & Baley, J., (2013). Guidance on management of asymptomatic neonates born to women with active genital herpes lesions. *Pediatrics, 131* (2): e635–e645.

Kingsberg, S. A. (2006). Taking sexual history. *Obstetric and Gynecology Clinics of North America, 33*(4), 535–547.

Kingsberg, S. A., & Janata J. W. (2007). Female sexual disorders: Assessment, diagnosis and treatment. *Urology Clinics of North America, 34*(4), 497–506.

Kingston, M., French, P., Goh, B., Goold, P., Higgins, S., Sukthankar, A., . . . Young, H. (2008). UK national guidelines on the management of syphilis 2008. *International Journal of Sexually Transmitted Diseases and AIDS, 19*(11), 729–740.

Kingston, M., French, P., Higgins, S., McQuillan, O., Sukthankar, A., Scott, C., . . . Sullivan, A. (2016). UK National guidelines on the management of syphilis 2015. *International Journal of Sexually Transmitted Diseases and AIDS, 27*(6), 421–446.

Kirby, D. B. (2007). *Emerging answers: 2007 Research findings on programs to reduce teen pregnancy and sexually transmitted diseases.* Washington, DC: National Campaign to Prevent Teen and Unplanned Pregnancy.

Kirby, D. B. (2008). The impact of abstinence and comprehensive sex and STD/HIV sex education programmes on adolescent sexual behaviour. *Sexuality Research and Social Policy, 5*(3), 18–27.

Kirkcaldy, R. D., Kidd, S., Weinstock, H. S., Papp, J. R., & Bolan, G. A. (2013). Trends in antimicrobial resistance in Neisseria gonorrhoeae in the USA: The Gonococcal Isolate Surveillance Project (GISP), January 2006-June 2012. *Sexually Transmitted Infections, 89*(4), iv5–iv10.

Koedijk, F. D. H., van Bergen, J. E. A. M., Dukers-Muijrers, N. H. T. M., van Leeuwen, A. P., Hoebe, C. J. P. A., & van der Sande, M. A. B. (2012). The value of testing multiple anatomic sites for gonorrhoea and chlamydia in sexually transmitted infection centres in the Netherlands, 2006–2010. *International Journal of Sexually Transmitted Diseases and AIDS, 23*(9), 626–631.

Koedijk, F. D. H., van Veen, M. G., de Neeling, A. J., Linde, G. B., & van der Sande, M. A. B. (2010). Increasing trend in gonococcal resistance to ciprofloxacin in the Netherlands 2006-8. *Sexually Transmitted Infections, 86*(1), 41–45.

Koss, C. A., Dunne, E. F., & Warner, L. (2009). A systematic review of epidemiologic studies assessing condom use and risk of syphilis. *Sexually Transmitted Diseases, 36*(7), 401–405.

Kurth, A. E., Celum, C., Baeten, J. M., Vermund, S. H., & Wasserheit, J. N. (2011). Combination HIV prevention: Significance, challenged, and opportunities. *Current HIV/AIDS Report, 8*(1), 62–72.

Lacey, C. J., Lowndes., C. M., & Shah, K. V. (2006). Burden and management of non-cancerous HPV-related conditions HPV6/11 disease. *Vaccine, 24*(3), 35–41.

Land, J. A., Van Bergen, J. E., Morré, S. A., & Postma, M. J. (2010). Epidemiology of *Chlamydia trachomatis* infection in women and the cost-effectiveness of screening. *Human Reproductive Update, 16*(2), 189–204.

Lazaro, N. (2013). *Sexually Transmitted Infections in Primary Care* (2d ed.). Lancashire, UK: RCGP/BASHH. Retrieved from www.rcpg.org and www.bashh.org/guidelines

Lazarus, J. V., Sihvonen-Riemenschneider, H., Laukamm-Josten, U., Wong, F., & Liljestrand, J. (2010). Systematic review of interventions to reduce spread of sexually transmitted infections, including HIV, among young people in Europe. *Croatian Medical Journal, 51*(1), 74–84.

Leitich, H., Bodner-Alder, B., Brunbauer, M., Kaider, A., Egarter, C., & Husslein, P. (2003). Bacterial vaginosis as a risk factor for preterm delivery: A meta-analysis. *American Journal of Obstetrics and Gynecology, 189*(1), 139–147.

Lewis, D. A. (2003). Chancroid: Clinical manifestations, diagnosis and management. *Sexually Transmitted Infections, 79*(1), 68–71.

Lewis, D. A. (2010). The gonococcus fights back: Is this time a knock out? *Sexually Transmitted Infections, 86*(6), 415–421.

Li, D. K. (2011). Does antiviral medication for treating herpes simplex during pregnancy increase the risk of birth defects in offspring? *Evidence Based Medicine, 16*(1), 30.

Lockanc-Diluzio, W., Cobb, H., Harrison, R., & Nelson, A. (2007). Building capacity to talk, teach and tackle sexual health. *Canadian Journal of Human Sexuality, 16*(3–4), 135–143.

Looker, K. J., Garnett, G. P., & Schmid, G. P. (2008). An estimate of the global prevalence and incidence of herpes simplex virus type 2 infection. *Bulletin of the World Health Organization, 86*(10), 805–812.

Low, N. (2012). Population-based biomedical sexually transmitted infection control interventions for reducing HIV infection: RHL commentary. Geneva, Switzerland: World Health Organization.

Low, N., Broutet, N., Adu-Sarkodie, Y., Barton, P., Hossain, M., & Hawkes, S. (2006). Global control of sexually transmitted infections. *The Lancet, 368*(9551), 2001–2016.

Lowndes, C. M. & Fenton, K. A. (2004). Surveillance systems for sexually transmitted infections in the European Union. *Sexually Transmitted Infections, 80*(4), 264–271.

Lu, B., Kumar, A., Castellsagué, X., & Guiliano, A. R. (2011). Efficacy and safety of prophylactic vaccines against cervical HPV infection and diseases among women: A systematic review and meta-analysis. *BMC Infectious Diseases, 11*, 13.

Magpantay, G., Cardile, A. P., Madar, C. S., Hsue, G., & Belnap, C. (2011). Antibiotic desensitization therapy in secondary syphilis and listeria infection: Case reports and review of desensitization therapy. *Hawaii Medicine Journal, 70*(12), 266–268.

Malkin, J. E. (2004). Epidemiology of genital herpes simplex virus infection in developed countries. *Herpes 11*(1), 2A–23A.

Manhart, L. E., & Holmes, K. K. (2005). Randomised controlled trials of individual-level, population level, and multilevel interventions for preventing sexually transmitted infections: What has worked? *Journal of Infectious Diseases, 191*(1), 7–24.

Mann, J. R., McDermott, S., Barnes, T. L., Harding, J., Bao, H., & Zhou, L. (2009). Trichomoniasis in pregnancy and mental retardation in children. *Annals of Epidemiology, 19*(12), 891–899.

Mantell, J. E., Dworkin, S. L., Exner, T. M., Hoffman, S., Smit, J. A., & Susser, I. (2006). The promise and limitations of female-initiated methods of HIV/STI protection 1998–2009. *Social Science and Medicine, 63*(8), 1998–2009.

Marks, G., Gardner, L. I., Craw, J., & Crepaz, N. (2010). Entry and retention in medical care among HIV-diagnosed persons: A meta-analysis. *AIDS, 24*(17), 2665–2678.

Marlow, L. A. V. (2011). HPV vaccination among ethnic minorities in the UK: Knowledge, acceptability and attitudes. *British Journal of Cancer, 105*(4), 486–492.

Marlow, L. A., Zimet, G. D., McCaffery, K. J., Ostini, R., & Waller, J. (2013). Knowledge of human papillomavirus (HPV) and HPV vaccination: an international comparison. *Vaccine, 31*(5), 763–769.

Martinez, A., Cooper, V., & Lees, J. (2013). *Laying the foundations: A guide to sex and relationships education in primary schools.* (2nd ed.). London, United Kingdom: National Children's Bureau.

Martinez, A., & Emmerson, L. (2008). *Key findings: Young people's survey on sex and relationships education: Sex Education Forum Briefing Paper.* London, United Kingdom: National Children's Bureau.

Mavedzenge, S. N., Pol, B. V., Cheng, H., Montgomery, E. T., Blanchart, K., de Bruyn, G., . . . Straten, A. V. (2010). Epidemiological synergy of *Trichomonas vaginalis* and HIV in Zimbabwean and South African women. *Sexually Transmitted Diseases, 37*(7), 460–466.

Mayer, K. H., Bush, T., Henry, K., Overton, E. T., Hammer, J., Richardson, J., . . . SUN Investigators. (2012). Ongoing sexually transmitted disease acquisition and risk-taking behaviour among US HIV-infected patients in primary care: Implications for prevention interventions. *Sexually Transmitted Diseases, 39*(1), 1–7.

McCance, D. J. (2009). Papillomaviruses. In A. J. Zuchermak, J. E. Banatvala, J. R. Pattison, P. Griffiths, & B. Schoub (Eds.) *Principles and practice of clinical virology.* (6th ed., pp.807–822). Oxford: John Wiley & Sons Ltd.

McDonald, H. M., Brocklehurst, P., & Gordon, A. (2007). Antibiotics for treating bacterial vaginosis in pregnancy. *Cochrane Database of Systematic Reviews,* (1), CD000262.

McLean, H., Radcliffe, K., Sullivan, A., & Ahmed-Jushuf, I. (2013). BASHH Statement on partner notification for sexually transmissible infections. *International Journal of Sexually Transmitted Diseases and AIDS, 24*(4), 253–261.

McLelland, R. S., Sangare, L., Hassan, W. M., Lavreys, L., Mandaliya, K., Kiarie, J., . . . Baeten, J. M. (2007). Infection with *Trichomonas vaginalis* increases the risk of HIV-1 acquisition. *Journal of Infectious Diseases, 195*(5), 698–702.

M'ikanatha, N. M., Lynfield, R., Van Beneden, C. A., & de Valk, H. (2013). *Infectious disease surveillance* (2nd ed.). Hoboken, NJ: Wiley-Blackwell.

Minnis, A. S., & Padian, N. S. (2005). Effectiveness of female controlled barrier methods in preventing sexually transmitted infections and HIV: Current evidence and future research directions. *Journal of Sexually Transmitted Infections, 81*(3), 193–200.

Modjarrad, K., Chamot, E., & Vermund, S. H. (2008). Impact of small reductions in plasma HIV RNA levels on the risk of heterosexual transmission and disease progression. *AIDS, 22*(16), 2179–2185.

Moyer, V. A. (2012). Screening for cervical cancer: US Preventive Services Task Force recommendation statement. *Annals of Internal Medicine, 156*(12), 880–891, W312.

Mullick, S., Watson-Jones, D., Beksinska, M., & Mabey, D. (2005). Sexually transmitted infections in pregnancy: Prevalence, impact on pregnancy outcomes, and approach to treatment in developing countries. *Sexually Transmitted Infections, 81*(4), 294–302.

Naidoo, J. & Wills, J. (2000). *Health promotion: Foundations for practice* (2nd ed.). Edinburgh, United Kingdom: Baillière Tindall.

National Health Service (NHS). (2014). *HPV vaccine.* Retrieved from http://www.nhs.uk/conditions/vaccinations/pages/hpv-human-papillomavirus-vaccine.aspx

National Health Service (NHS). (2011). *The UK NSC recommendation on Chlamydia screening in pregnancy.* Retrieved from https://legacyscreening.phe.org.uk/chlamydia-pregnancy (accessed September 13, 2017).

National Institute of Allergy and Infectious Diseases. (2016). *Large-Scale HIV Vaccine Trial to Launch in South Africa.* Retrieved from https://www.niaid.nih.gov/news-events/large-scale-hiv-vaccine-trial-launch-south-africa

National Institute for Health and Care Excellence (NICE). (2007). *One to one interventions to reduce the transmission of sexually transmitted infections (STIs) including HIV, and to reduce the rate of under 18 conceptions especially among vulnerable and at risk groups.* London, United Kingdom: Author.

National Institute for Health and Care Excellence. (2008). *Antenatal care for uncomplicated pregnancies* (Rev. ed 2017). London, U.K.: author.

National Institute for Health and Care Excellence (NICE). (2010). *Public health draft guidance: School, college and community-based personal, social, health and economic education focusing on sex and relationships and alcohol education.* Retrieved from https://www.nice.org.uk/guidance/development/gid-phg0/documents

National Institute for Health and Care Excellence (NICE). (2015). *Pelvic inflammatory disease.* London, United Kingdom: Author.

Newman, L., Kamb, Hawkes, S., Gomez, G., Say, L., Seuc, A., & Broutet, N. (2013). Global estimates of syphilis in pregnancy and associated adverse outcomes: Analysis of multinational antenatal surveillance data. *PLoS Medicine, 10*(2),e1001396.

Niccolai, L. M., Rowhani-Rahbar, A., Jenkins, H., Green, S., & Dunne, D. W. (2005). Condom effectiveness for prevention of *Chlamydia trachomatis* infection. *Sexually Transmitted Infections, 81*(4), 323–325.

Ng, B. E., Butler, L. M., Horvath, T., & Rutherford, G. W. (2011). Population-based biomedical sexually transmitted infection control interventions for reducing HIV infection. *Cochrane Database Systematic Reviews,* (3), CD001220.

Noar, S. M., Cole, C., & Carlyle, K. (2006). Condom use measurement in 56 studies of sexual risk behaviour: Review and recommendations. *Archives of Sexual Behavior, 35*(3), 327–345.

Office for Standards in Education, Children's Services and Skills. (2007). *Time for change? Personal, social and health education.* London, United Kingdom: Ofsted.

Office for Standards in Education, Children's Services and Skills. (2010). *Personal, social and health and economic education in schools.* London, United Kingdom: Ofsted.

Origanje, C., Meremikwu, M. M., Eko, H., Esu, E., Meremikwu A., & Ehiri, J. E. (2009). Interventions for preventing unintended pregnancies among adolescents. *Cochrane Database Systematic Reviews, (4),* CD005215.

Padian, N. S., Buve, A., Balks, J., Serwadda, D., & Cates, W. Jr. (2008). Biomedical interventions to prevent HIV infection: Evidence, challenges, and the way forward. *The Lancet, 372*(9638), 585–599.

Padian, N. S., Van Der Straten, A., Ramjee, G., Chipato, T., de Bruyn, G., Blanchard, K., . . . McIntyre, J. (2007). Diaphragm and lubricant gel for prevention of HIV acquisition in Southern African women: A randomised controlled trial. *The Lancet, 370*(9583), 251–261.

Pan, C. Q., & Zhang, J. X. (2005). Natural history and clinical consequences of hepatitis B virus infection. *International Journal of Medicine and Science, 2*(1), 36–40.

Papp, J. R., Schachter, J., Gaydos, C. A., & Van Der Pol, B. (2014). Recommendations for the laboratory-based detection of *Chlamydia trachomatis* and *Neisseria gonorrhoeae. Morbidity and Mortality Weekly Reports: Recommendations and Reports, 63*(RR02), 1–19.

Pasternak, B., & Hviid, A. (2010). Use of acyclovir, valacyclovir and famciclovir in the first trimester of pregnancy and the risk of birth defects. *Journal of the American Medical Association, 304*(8), 859–866.

Peeling, R. W. (2009). Utilisation of rapid tests for sexually transmitted infections: Promises and challenges. *Open Infectious Diseases Journal, 3*(1), 156–163.

Peeling, R. W. (2011). Applying new technologies for diagnosing sexually transmitted infections in resource-poor settings. *Sexually Transmitted Infections, 87*(2), ii28–ii30

Peeling, R. W., & Ye, H. (2004). Diagnostic tools for preventing and managing maternal and congenital syphilis: An overview. *Bulletin of the World Health Organization, 82*(6), 439–446.

Pellowe, C., & Pratt, R. J. (2006). Neonatal conjunctivitis and pneumonia due to chlamydia infection. *Infant, 2*(1), 16–17.

Peterson, L., Taylor, D., Roddy, R., Belai, G., Philips, P., Nanda, K., . . . Cates W. (2007). Tenofovir disoproxil fumerate for prevention of HIV infection in women: A phase 2, double-blind, randomised placebo-controlled trial. *PLoS Clinical Trials, 2*(5), e27.

Petersen, R., Albright, J., Garett, J. M., & Curtis, K. M. (2007). Pregnancy and STD prevention counselling using an adaptation of motivational interviewing: A randomised controlled trial. *Perspectives in Sexual and Reproductive Health, 39*(1), 21–28.

Pinninti, S. G., Angara, R., Feja, K. N., Kimberlin, D. W., Leach, C. T., Conrad, D. A., . . . Tolan R. W. Jr. (2012). Neonatal herpes disease following maternal antenatal antiviral suppressive therapy: a multicentre case series. *Journal of Pediatrics, 161*(1), 134–138.

Pinninti, S. G., & Kimberlin, D. W. (2014a). Management of neonatal herpes simplex virus infection and exposure. *Archives*

of Diseases in Childhood Fetal and Neonatal Edition. 99(3), F240–F244.

Pitsouni, E., Iavazzo, C., Athanasiou, S., & Falagas, M. E. (2007). Single-dose Azithromycin versus Erythromycin or Amoxicillin for *Chlamydia trachomatis* infection during pregnancy: a meta-analysis of randomised controlled trials. *International Journal of Antimicrobial Agents, 30*(3), 213–221.

Potts, M., Halperin, D., Kirby, T., Swidler, A., Marseille, E., Klausner, J. D., . . . Walsh, J. (2008). Reassessing HIV prevention. *Science, 320*(5877), 749–750.

Public Health England. (2013). *The Green Book: Immunisation against infectious disease.* Retrieved from https://www.gov.uk /government/collections/immunisation-against-infectious-disease -the-green-book

Public Health England. (2014). *Sexually Transmitted Infections (STIs): surveillance, data, screening and management.* Retrieved from https://www.gov.uk/government/collections/sexually-trans-mitted-infections-stis-surveillance-data-screening-and-management

Public Health England. (2016). U.K. National chlamydia screening programme standards. (7th ed.). Retrieved from https://www .gov.uk/government/publications/ncsp-standards

Rawstron, S. A., Mehta, S., & Bromberg, K. (2004). Evaluation of the treponema pallidum-specific IgM enzyme immunoassay and treponema pallidum Western blot antibody detection in the diagnosis of maternal and congenital syphilis. *Sexually Transmitted Diseases, 31*(2), 123–126.

Rehle, T. M., Hallett, T. B., Shisana, O., Pillay-van-Wyk, V., Zuma, K., Carrara, H., & Jooste, S. (2010). A decline in new HIV infections in South Africa: estimating HIV incidence from three national HIV surveys in 2002, 2005 and 2008. *PLoS ONE, 5*(6), e11094.

Rehle, T., Johnson, L., Hallett, T., Mahy, M., Kim, A., Odido, H., . . . Stover, J. (2015). A comparison of South African National HIV Estimates: A critical appraisal of different methods. *PLoS ONE, 10*(7), e0133255.

Renault, C. A., Israelski, D. M., Levy, V., Fujikawa, B. J., Kellogg, T. A., & Klausner, J. D. (2011). Time to clearance of *Chlamydia trachomatis* ribosomal RNA in women treated for chlamydial infection. *Sexual Health, 8*(1),69–73.

Richens, J. (2011). Main presentations of sexually transmitted infections in male patients. In K. E. Rogstad (Ed.), *ABC of sexually transmitted infections* (6th ed., pp. 29–34). Chichester, United Kingdom: Wiley-Blackwell.

Rietmeijer, C. A., Donnelly, J., Bernstein, K. T., Bissett, J. M., Martins, S., Pathela, P., . . . Newman, L. M. (2009). Here comes the SSuN: Early experiences with the STD surveillance network. *Public Health Reports, 124*(2), 72–77.

Roett, M. A., Mayor, M. T., & Uduhiri, K. A. (2012). Diagnosis and management of genital ulcers. *American Family Physician, 85*(3), 254–262.

Ross, J., Judlin, P., & Jensen, J. (2014). 2012 European guideline for the Management of Pelvic Inflammatory Disease. *International Journal of Sexually Transmitted Diseases and AIDS, 25*(1), 1–7.

Rours, G. I. J. G., Duijts, L., Moll, H. A., Arends, L. R., de Groot, R., Jaddoe, V. W., . . . Verburgh, H. A. (2011). Chamydia trachomatis infection during pregnancy associated with preterm delivery: A population-based prospective cohort study. *European Journal of Epidemiology, 26*(6), 493–502.

Royal College of Obstetricians & Gynecologicals. (2014). *Joint RCOG/BASHH Release: Managing genital herpes in pregnancy – new information published*. London, U.K.: RCOG. Retrieved from https://www.rcog.org.uk/en/news/joint-rcogbashh-release-managing-genital-herpes-in-pregnancy--new-information-published/

Samet, J. H., Walley, A. Y., & Bridden, C. (2007). Illicit drugs, alcohol and addiction in human immunodeficiency virus. *Panminerva Medicine, 49*(2), 67–77.

Santelli, J. S., Lindberg, L. D., Finer, L. B., & Singh, S. (2007). Explaining recent declines in adolescent pregnancy in the United States: the contribution of abstinence and improved contraceptive use. *American Journal of Public Health, 97*(1), 150–156.

Savage, E. J., Marsh, K., Duffell, S., Ison, C. A., Zaman, A., & Hughes, G. (2012). Rapid increase in gonorrhoea and syphilis diagnoses in England. *European Surveillance, 17*(29), pii=20224. Available online: http://www.eurosurveillance.org/ViewArticle.aspx?Articled=20224

Schifano, F., Martinotti, G., Cunniff, A., Reissner, V., Scherbaum, N., & Ghodse, H. (2012). Impact of an 18-month, NHS-based, treatment exposure for heroin dependence: Results from the London Area Treat 2000 Study. *American Journal of Addiction, 21*(3), 268–273.

Schiffman, M., Castle, P. E., Jeromino, J., Rodriguez, A. C., & Wacholder, S. (2007). Human papillomavirus and cervical cancer. *The Lancet, 370*(9590), 890–907.

Schulte, J. M., Bellamy, A. R., Hook, E. W. 3rd, Bernstein, D. I., Levin, M. J., Leon, P. A., . . . Belshe, R. B. (2014). HSV-1 and HSV-2 Seroprevalence in the United States among asymptomatic women unaware of any herpes simplex virus infection (Herpevac Trial for women). *Southern Medicine Journal, 107*(2), 79–84.

Schwebke, J. R., & Desmond, R. K. (2007b). A randomised trial of metronidazole in asymptomatic bacterial vaginosis to prevent the acquisition of sexually transmitted diseases. *American Journal of Obstetrics and Gynecology, 196*(6), 517e1–e6.

Schwebke, J. R., Marrazzo, J., Beelen, A. P., & Sobel, J. D. (2015). A phase 3, multicentre, randomised, double-blind, vehicle-controlled study evaluating the safety and efficacy of Metronidazole Vaginal Gel 1.3% in the treatment of bacterial vaginosis. *Sexually Transmitted Diseases, 42*(7), 376–381.

Scottish Intercollegiate Guidelines Network (SIGN). (2009). Management of genital *Chlamydia trachomatis* infection: A national clinical guideline. Edinburgh, United Kingdom: Scottish Intercollegiate Guidance Network.

Seña, A. C., White, B. L., & Sparling, P. F. (2010). Novel treponema pallidum serologic tests: A paradigm shift in syphilis screening for the 21st century. *Clinical Infectious Diseases, 51*(6), 700–708.

Seña, A. C., Wolff, M., Behets, F., Van Damme, K., Martin, D. H., Leone, P., . . . Hook, E. W. (2013). Response to therapy following retreatment of serofast early syphilis patients with Benzathine Penicillin. *Clinical Infectious Diseases, 56*(3), 420–422.

Servoss, J. C., & Friedman, L. S. (2006). Serologic and molecular diagnosis of hepatitis B virus. *Infectious Disease Clinics of North America, 20*(1), 47–61.

Sex Education Forum. (2005). *Sex and relationships education framework*. London, United Kingdom: NCB.

Sex Education Forum. (2008b). *Key findings: Young people's survey on sex and relationships education*. London, United Kingdom: NCB.

Sex Education Forum. (2008a). *National mapping survey of on-site sexual health services in education settings: Provision in further education and sixth form colleges*. London, United Kingdom: NCB.

Shahrook, S., Mori, R., Ochirbat, T., & Gomi, H. (2014). Strategies of testing for syphilis in pregnancy. *Cochrane Database Systematic Reviews, 10*, CD010385.

Shain, R. N., Piper, J. M., Holden, A. E., Champion, J. D., Perdue, S. T., Korte, J. E., & Guerra, F. A. (2004). Prevention of gonorrhoea and chlamydia through behavioural intervention: Results of a two-year controlled randomised trial in minority women. *Sexually Transmitted Diseases, 31*(7), 401–408.

Shepard, C. W., Simard, E. P., Finelli, L., Fiore, A. E., & Bell, B. P. (2006). Hepatitis B virus infection: Epidemiology and vaccination. *Epidemiologic Reviews, 28*(1), 112–125.

Shepherd, J., Kavanagh, J., Picot, J., Cooper, K., Harden, A., Bardett-Page, E., . . . Price, A. (2010). The effectiveness and cost effectiveness of behavioural interventions for the prevention of sexually transmitted infections in young people aged 13–19: A systematic review and economic evaluation. *Health Technology Assessment, 14*(7), 1–206.

Sherrard, J., Ison, C., Moody, J., Wainwright, E., Wilson, J., & Sullivan, A. (2014). *United Kingdom national guideline on the management of* Trichomonas vaginalis *2014*. London, United Kingdom: BASHH.

Shisana, O., Rehle, T., Simbayi, L. C., Zuma, K., Jooste, S., Pillay-van-wyk, V., . . . The SABSSM III Implementation Team. (2009). *South African National HIV prevalence, incidence, behaviour and communication survey 2008: A turning tide among teenagers?* Cape Town, South Africa: HSRC Press.

Siegrist, C-A., Lewis, E. M., Eskola, J., Evans, S. J. W., & Black, S. B. (2007). Human papillomavirus immunization in adolescent and young adults: A cohort study to illustrate what events might be mistaken for adverse reactions. *Pediatric Infectious Disease Journal, 26*(11), 979–984.

Silva, M. C., Ximenes, R. A., Miranda, Filho, D. B., Arraes, L. W., Mendes, M., Melo, A. C., & Fernandes, P. R. (2009). Risk factors for non-adherence to antiretroviral therapy. *Revista do Instituto de Medicina Tropical de São Paulo, 51*(3), 135–139.

Simms, I., & Broutet, N. (2008). Congenital syphilis re-emerging. *ournal der Deutschen Dermatologischen Gesellschaft, 6*(4), 269–272.

Simms, I., McDonald, N., Ison, C., Alexander, S., Lowndes, C. M., & Fenton, K. A. (2004). Enhanced surveillance of lymphogranuloma venereum (LGV) begins in England. *European Surveillance, 8*(41), pii. 2565.

Singh, S., Darroch, J. E., & Bankole, A. (2003). A, B and C in Uganda: The roles of abstinence, monogamy and condom use in HIV decline. *Reproductive Health Matters, 12*(23), 129131.

Slater, W., Sadler, K., Cassell, J. A., Horner, P., & Low, N. (2007). What can be gained from comprehensive disaggregate surveillance? The Avon surveillance system for sexually transmitted infections. *Sexually Transmitted Infections, 83*(5), 411–415.

Slutkin, G., Okware, S., Naamara, W., Sutherland, D., Flanagan, D., Carael, M., . . . Tarantola, D. (2006). How Uganda reversed its HIV epidemic. *AIDS and Behavior, 10*(4), 351–360.

Smith, A., Aigus, P., Barrett, A., Mitchell, C., & Pitts, M. (2009). *Results of the 4th national survey of Australian Secondary School Students, HIV/AIDS and sexual health*. Melbourne, Australia: Australia Research Centre in Sex, Health & Society.

Solensky, R. (2004). Drug desensitization. *Immunology and Allergy Clinics of North America, 24*(3), 425.

Srinivas, S. K., Ma, Y., Sammel, M. D., Chou, D., McGrath, C., Parry, S., & Elovitz, M. A. (2006). Placental inflammation and viral infection are implicated in second trimester pregnancy loss. *American Journal of Obstetrics and Gynecology, 195*(3), 797–802.

Steen, R., Wi, T. E., Kamali, A., & Ndowa, F. (2009). Control of sexually transmitted infections and prevention of HIV Transmission: mending a fractured paradigm. *Bulletin of the World Health Organization, 87*(11), 805–884.

Stoneburner, R. L., & Low-Beer, D. (2004). Population-level HIV declines and behavioural risk avoidance in Uganda. *Science, 304*(5671), 714–718. (Erratum in *Science, 306*(5701), 1477).

Stretch, R., Roberts, S. A., McCann, R., Baxter D., Chambers, G., Kitchener, H., & Brabin, L. (2008). Parental attitudes and information needs in an adolescent HPV vaccination programme. *British Journal of Cancer, 99*(11), 1908–1911.

Stringer, E., Read, J. S., Hoffman, I., Valentine, M., Aboud, S., & Goldenberg, R. L. (2010). Treatment of trichomonas in pregnancy in Sub-Saharan Africa does not appear to be associated with low birth weight or preterm birth. *South African Medical Journal, 100*(1), 58–64.

Tanton, C., Weiss, H. A., Le Goff, J., Changalucha, J., Rosizoka, M., Baisley K., . . . Watson-Jones D. (2011). Correlates of HIV-1 genital shedding in Tanzanian women. *PLoS ONE, 6*(3), e17480.

Tapsall, J. W., Ndowa, F., Lewis, D.A., & Unemo, M. (2009). Meeting the public health challenge of multidrug- and extensively drug-resistant *Neisseria gonorrhoeae*. *Expert Review of Anti-Infective Therapy 7*(7), 821–834.

Taylor, D., Bury, M., Campling, N., Carter, S., Garfield, S., Newbould, J., & Rennie, T. (2006). *A review of the use of the health belief model (HBM), the theory of reasoned action (TRA), the theory of planned behaviour (TPB) and the trans theoretical model (TTM) to study and predict health related behaviour change*. London, United Kingdom: NICE.

Taylor, G. P., Clayden, P., Dhar, J., Ghandi, K., Gileece, Y., Harding, K., . . . de Ruiter, A. (2012). British HIV Association guidelines for the management of HIV infection in pregnant women 2012. *HIV Medicine, 13*(2), 87–157.

Teenage Pregnancy Associates (TPA). (2011). *Teenage pregnancy: The evidence*. London, United Kingdom: Teenage Pregnancy Associates.

Townsend, C. L., Cortina-Borja, M., Peckham, C. S., de Ruiter, A., Lyall, H., & Tookey, P. A. (2008). Low rates of mother-to-child transmission of HIV following effective pregnancy interventions in the United Kingdom and Ireland, 2000–2006. *AIDS, 22*(8), 973–981.

Trivedi, D., Bunn, F., Graham, M., & Wentz, R. (2007). Preventing teenage pregnancy: Evidence from systematic reviews. In P. Baker, K. Guthrie, C. Hutchinson, R. Kane, & Wellings K. (Eds.), *Teenage pregnancy and reproductive health* (pp. 275–291). London, United Kingdom: RCOG Press.

UNAIDS/WHO Working Group on Global HIV/AIDS and STI Surveillance. (2012). *Strategies and laboratory methods for strengthening surveillance of sexually transmitted infection*. Geneva: WHO.

UNAIDS Global Report. (2010). *UNAIDS report on the global AIDS epidemic 2010*. Retrieved from http://www.unaids.org/globalreport/Global_report.htm

Unemo, M. (2015). Current and future antimicrobial treatment of gonorrhoea: The rapidly evolving Neisseria gonorrhoeae continues to challenge. *BMC Infectious Diseases, 15*, 364.

Unemo, M., Golparian, D., Syversen, G., Vestrheim, D. F., & Moi, H. (2010). Two cases of verified clinical failures using internationally recommended first-line cefixime for gonorrhoea treatment, Norway, 2010. *European Surveillance, 15*(47), pii 19721.

Unemo, M., & Nicholas, R. A. (2012). Emergence of multi-drug resistance and untreatable gonorrhoea. *Future Microbiology, 7*(12), 1401–1422.

Unemo, M., & Shafer, W. M. (2014). Antimicrobial resistance in *Neisseria gonorrhoeae* in the 21st century: Past, evolution, and future. *Clinical Microbiology Reviews, 27*(3), 587–613.

UNESCO. (2009). *International guidelines on sexuality education: An evidence informed approach to effective sex, relationships and HIV/STI education*. Paris, France: UNESCO.

Villeneuve, J. P. (2005). The natural history of chronic hepatitis B virus infection. *Journal of Clinical Virology, 34*(1), S139–S142.

Vijiyakumar, G., Mabude, Z., Smit, J., Beksinska, M., & Lurie, M. (2006). A review of female condom effectiveness: Patterns of use and impact on protected sex acts and STI incidence. *International Journal of Sexually Transmitted Diseases and AIDS, 17*(10), 652–659.

Ward, H., & Rönn, M. (2010). Contribution of sexually transmitted infections to the sexual transmission of HIV. *Current Opinion in HIV and AIDS, 5*(4), 305–310.

Warner, L., Newman, D. R., Austin, H. D., Kamb, M., Douglas, J. M. Jr., Malotte, C. K., . . . Project RESPECT Study Group. (2004). Condom effectiveness for reducing transmission of gonorrhoea and chlamydia: the importance of assessing partner infection status. *American Journal of Epidemiology, 159*(3), 242–251.

Warner, L., Newman, D. L., Kamb, M. L., Fishbein, M., Douglas, J. M. Jr., Zenilman, J., . . . Project RESPECT Study Group. (2008). Problems with condom use among patients attending sexually transmitted disease clinics: Prevalence, predictors, and relation to incident gonorrhea and chlamydia. *American Journal of Epidemiology, 167*(3), 341–349.

Warner, L., Stone, K. M., Macaluso, M., Buehler, J. W., & Austin, H. D. (2006). Condom use and risk of gonorrhoea and chlamydia: A systematic review of design and measurement factors assessed in epidemiologic studies. *Sexually Transmitted Diseases, 33*(1), 36–51.

Watson-Jones, D., Weiss, H. A., Rusizoka, M., Changalucha, J., Baisley, K., Mugeye, K., . . . HSV trial team; Steering and Data Monitoring Committees. (2008). Effect of herpes simplex suppression on incidence of HIV among women in Tanzania. *New England Journal of Medicine, 358*(15), 1560–1571.

Watts, D. H. (2008). Pregnancy and viral sexually transmitted infections. In K. K. Holmes, P. F. Sparling, W. E. Stamm, P. Piot, J. N. Wasserheit, L. Corey, & M. S. Cohen (Eds.) *Sexually transmitted diseases* (4th ed., pp. 1563–1576). New York, NY: McGraw-Hill Medical.

Wawer, M. J., Gray, R. H., Sewankambo, N. K., Serwadda, D., Xianbin, L., Laeyendecker, O., . . . Quinn, T. C. (2005). Rates of HIV-1 transmission per coital act, by stage of HIV-1 infection, in Rakai, Uganda. *Journal of Infectious Diseases, 191*(9), 1403–1409.

Wawer, M. J., Makumbi, F., Kigozi, G., Serwadda, D., Watya, S., Nalugoda, F., . . . Gray, R. H. (2009). Circumcision in HIV infected men and its effect on HIV transmission to female partners in Rakai, Uganda: A randomised controlled trial. *The Lancet, 374*(9685), 229–237.

Weinstock, H., Berman, S., & Cates, W., Jr. (2004). Sexually transmitted diseases among American youth: Incidence and prevalence estimates 2000. *Perspectives in Sexual and Reproductive Health, 36*(1), 6–10.

Weller, S. C., & Davis-Beaty, K. (2007). Condom effectiveness in reducing heterosexual HIV transmission. *Cochrane Database of Systematic Reviews, (4)*, CD003255.

Westwood, J., & Mullan, B. (2007). Knowledge and attitudes of secondary school teachers regarding sexual health education in England. *Sex Education, 7*(2),143–159.

Wetmore, C. M., Manhart, L. E., & Wasserheit, J. N. (2010). Randomised controlled trials of interventions to prevent sexually transmitted infections: Learning from the past to plan for the future. *Epidemiology Reviews, 32*(1), 212–136.

Whiley, D. M., Goire, N., Lahara, M. M., Donovan, B., Limnios, A. E., Nissen, M. D., & Sloots, T. P. (2012). The ticking time bomb: escalating antibiotic resistance in Neisseria gonorrhoeae is a public health disaster in waiting. *Journal of Antimicrobial Chemotherapy, 67*(9), 2059–2061.

Wilson, D. P., & Blower, S. M. (2005). Allocating antiretrovirals in South Africa: Using modeling to determine treatment equity. *PLoS Medicine, 2*(6), e155.

Wilson, D. P., Coplan, P. M., Wainberg, M. A., & Blower, S. M. (2008). The paradoxical effects of using antiretroviral-based microbicides to control HIV epidemics. *Proceedings of the National Academies of Sciences, USA, 105*(28), 9835–9840.

Wilson, J. (2011). Sexually transmitted infections and HIV in pregnancy. In K.E. Rogstad (Ed.)., *ABC of sexually transmitted infections* (6th ed., pp. 59–63). Chichester, United Kingdom: Wiley-Blackwell.

World Health Organization (WHO). (2005a). *The global elimination of congenital syphilis: Rationale and strategy for action.* Geneva, Switzerland: WHO Department of Reproductive Health and Research.

World Health Organization (WHO). (2005b) *Sexually transmitted and other reproductive tract infections: A guide to essential practice.* Geneva, Switzerland: Author.

World Health Organization (WHO). (2007). *Global strategy for the prevention and control of sexually transmitted infections 2005-2015.* Geneva, Switzerland: Author.

World Health Organization (WHO). (2008). *Consultation on STI interventions for preventing HIV: Appraisal of the evidence.* Geneva, Switzerland: World Health Organization/Joint United Nations Programme on HIV/AIDS.

World Health Organization (WHO). (2012). *Global incidence and prevalence of selected curable sexually transmitted infections—2008.* Geneva: World Health Organization.

World Health Organization (WHO). (2013). *Sexually transmitted infections.* Geneva: World Health Organization.

World Health Organization (WHO). (2015). *Sexually transmitted infections. Fact Sheet No. 110.* Geneva, Switzerland: World Health Organization.

World Health Organization/United Nations Working Group on Global HIV/AIDS and STI Surveillance. (2013). *Evaluating a national surveillance system.* Geneva, Switzerland: World Health Organization.

Workowski, K. A., & Berman, S. (2010). Centers for Disease Control and Prevention sexually transmitted disease treatment guidelines 2010. *Morbidity and Mortality Weekly Report: Recommendations and Reports, 59*(RR-12), 1–110.

Workowski, K. A., & Bolan, G A. (2015). Centers for Disease Control and Prevention sexually transmitted diseases treatment guidelines, 2015. *Morbidity and Mortality Weekly Report: Recommendations and Reports, 64*, 1–137.

Youm, Y. (2010). A sociological interpretation of emerging properties in STI transmission dynamics: Walk-betweeness of sexual networks. *Sexually Transmitted Infections, 86*(3), iii24–iii28.

Zar, H. J. (2005). Neonatal chlamydial infections. *Pediatric Drugs, 7*(2), 103–110.

Zhu, L., Qin, M., Du, L., Xie, R. H., Wong, T., & Wen, S. W. (2010). Maternal and congenital syphilis in Shanghai, China, 2002–2006. *International Journal of Infectious Diseases, 14*(3), e45–e48.

• • • SUGGESTED FURTHER READING

Ajzen, I. (1988). *Attitudes, personality and behaviour.* Maidenhead, United Kingdom: Open University Press.

Beh, Taylor, D., Bury, M., Campling, N., Carter, S., Garfield, S., Newbould, J., & Rennie, T. (2006). *A review of the use of the health belief model (HBM), the theory of reasoned action (TRA), the theory of planned behaviour (TPB) and the trans theoretical model (TTM) to study and predict health related behaviour change.* London, United Kingdom: NICE.

Brown, Z. A., Gardella, C., Wald, R. A., Marrow, A., & Corey, L. (2005). Genital herpes complicating pregnancy. *Obstetrics and Gynaecology, 106*(4),845–856.

Buchbinder, S. P., Mehrotra, D. V., Duerr, A., Fitzgerald, D. W., Mogg, R., Li D., . . . Step Study Protocol Team. (2008). Efficacy assessment of a cell mediated immunity HIV-1 vaccine (the Step Study): A double blind randomised, placebo-controlled, test-of-concept trial. *The Lancet, 372*(9653), 1881–1893.

Centers for Disease Control and Prevention (CDC). (2013a). *Diagnoses of HIV infection in the United States and dependent areas, 2011: HIV Surveillance Report, Vol. 23.* Retrieved from https://www.cdc.gov/hiv/pdf/statistics_2011_HIV_Surveillance_Report_vol_23.pdf

Centers for Disease Control and Prevention (2013b). Testing for HCV infection: An update of guidance for clinicians and laboratorians. *Morbidity and Mortality Weekly Report, 62*(18), 362–365.

Christophers, H., Mann, S., & Lowbury, R. (2008). *Progress and priorities—Working together for high quality sexual health. Review of the national strategy for sexual health and HIV.* London, United Kingdom: Medical Foundations for AIDS and Sexual

Health (MedFASH). Retrieved from http://www.medfash.org.uk/uploads/files/p17abl1iai1e961d438j2pjl1rp7p.pdf

Da Costa, N. (2011). *Relationships and sex education: Exploring the process of quality assuring the content, delivery and training.* Bristol, United Kingdom: Brook Bristol.

Department of Education for Northern Ireland. (2012). *Guidance on relationships and sexuality education.* Circular No. 2010/01. Belfast, Northern Ireland: FPA.

Emmerson, L. (2014). The issue of consent. *Sex Educational Supplement, 1*(2), Pages 1–24.

European Centre for Disease Prevention and Control (ECDC). (2013). *Technical report—A comprehensive approach to HIV/STI prevention in the context of sexual health in the European Union/European Economic Area (EU/EEA).* Stockholm, Sweden: European Centre for Disease Prevention and Control.

Evans, C. (2013). Teenage pregnancy and sexual health. *Nursing Times, 109*(46), 22–27.

Food and Drug Administration (FDA). (2014). *Highlights of prescribing information: Gardasil 9 (human papillomavirus 9-valent vaccine, recombinant).* Silver Spring, MD: Author. Retrieved from http://www.fda.gov/downloads/BiologicBloodVaccines/Vaccines/ApprovedProducts/UCM426457.pdf

Flynn, N., Forthal, E. N., Harro, C. D., Judson, F. N., Mayer, K. H., Para, M. F.; The rgp120 HIV Vaccine Study Group. (2005). Placebo-controlled phase 3 trial of a recombinant glycoprotein 120 vaccine to prevent HIV-1 infection. *Journal of Infectious Diseases, 191*(5), 654–665.

Health Protection Agency. (2011a). Gonococcal resistance to antimicrobials surveillance programme in England and Wales (GRASP), 2010 report. *Health Protection Report, 4*(34).

Health Protection Agency (2011b). Annual Data: Sexually transmitted infections in England 2008–2010. *Health Protection Report, 5*(24). Retrieved from http://webarchive.nationalarchives.gov.uk/20140714093213/http://www.hpa.org.uk/hpr/archives/2011/hpr2411.pdf

Ihekweazu, C., Maxwell, N., Organ, S., & Oliver, I. (2007). Is STI surveillance in England meeting the requirements of the 21st century? An evaluation of data from the South West Region. *European Surveillance, 12*(5), pii=708.

International Group on Analysis of Trends in HIV prevalence and behaviours in young people in countries most affected by HIV. (2010). Trends in HIV prevalence and sexual behaviour among young people aged 15–24 years in countries most affected by HIV. *Sexually Transmitted Infections, 86* (Suppl. 2), ii72–ii83. Erratum in: *Sexually Transmitted Infections, 87*(1), 8.

James, S. H., & Kimberlin, D. W. (2015). Neonatal herpes simplex virus infection: Epidemiology and treatment. *Clinical Perinatology, 42*(1), 47–59.

Kimberlin, D. W. (2004). Neonatal herpes simplex infection. *Clinical Microbiology Reviews, 17*(1), 1–13.

Kimberlin, D. W., & Gutierrez, K. M. (2016). Herpes simplex virus infections. In C. B. Wilson, V. Nizet, Y. Maldonaldo, J. S. Remington, & J. O. Klein (2015). (Eds.), *Remington and Klein's infectious diseases of the fetus and newborn infant* (8th ed., pp. 843–865). Philadelphia: Elsevier Saunders.

Lanjouw, E., Ouburg, S., de Vries, H. J., Stary, A., Radcliffe, K., & Unemo, M. (2015). European guideline on the management of *Chlamydia trachomatis* infections. *International Journal of Sexually Transmitted Disease and AIDS, 27*(5), 333–348.

Liu, A. Y., Kittredge, P. V., Vittinghoff, E., Raymond, H. E., Ahrensk, K., Matheson, T., . . . Buchbinder, S. P. (2008). Limited knowledge and use of HIV post- and pre-exposure prophylaxis among gay and bisexual men. *Journal of Acquired Immune Deficiency Syndrome, 47*(2), 241–247.

Lumbiganon, P. (2004). Management of gonorrhoea and *Chlamydia trachomatis* infection in pregnancy: RHL Practical aspects. Geneva, Switzerland: The World Health Organization.

Martin, A., & Lemon, S. M. (2006). Hepatitis A virus: From discovery to vaccines. *Hepatology, 43*(2 Suppl. 1), S164–S172.

Mayer, K. H., Maslankowski, L. A., Gai, F., El-Sadr, W. M., Justman, J., Kwiecien, A., . . . Soto-Torres, L. 2006). Safety and tolerability of tenofovir vaginal gel in abstinent and sexually active HIV-infected and uninfected women. *AIDS, 20*(4), 543–551.

Medical Foundation for AIDS & Sexual Health (MEDFASH). (2010). *Standards for the management of sexually transmitted infections (STIs).* Retrieved from http://www.medfash.org.uk/uploads/files/p17abl5efr149kqsu10811h21i3tt.pdf

M'ikanatha, N. M., & Iskander, J. (2014). *Concepts and methods in infectious disease surveillance.* Hoboken, NJ: Wiley-Blackwell.

Moyer, V. A. (2013). Screening for hepatitis C virus infection in adults: U.S. Preventive Services Task Force recommendation statement. *Annals of Internal Medicine, 159*(5), 349–357.

Nainan, O. V., Xia, G., Vaughan, G., & Margolis, H. S. (2006). Diagnosis of hepatitis A virus infection: A molecular approach. *Clinical Microbiol Reviews, 19*(1), 63–79.

National AIDS Trust (NAT) (2014). *HIV patient information and NHS confidentiality.* London, United Kingdom: Author. Retrieved from http://www.nat.org.uk/sites/default/files/publicatins/Jan-2014-HIV-Patient-Confidentiality-NHS.pdf

National AIDS Trust. (2014). *HIV patient information and NHS confidentiality.* London, United Kingdom: National Aids Trust. https://www.nat.org.uk/sites/default/files/publications/Jan-2014-HIV-Patient-Confidentiality-NHS.pdf

National Center for Health Statistics. Health United States 2009: With Special Features on Medical Technology. Hyattsville, Maryland. http://www.cdc.gov/hiv/topics/surveillance.

Padian, N. S., McCoy, S. I., Balkus, J. E., & Wasserheit, J. N. (2010). Weighing the gold in the gold standard: Challenges in HIV prevention research. *AIDS, 24*(5), 621–635.

Petrosky, E., Bocchini, J. A., Hariri, S., Chesson, H., Curtis, C. R., Saraiya, M., . . . Markowitz, L. E. (2015). Use of 9-Valent Human Papillomavirus (HPV) vaccine: Updated HPV vaccination recommendations of the Advisory Committee on Immunization Practices. *Morbidity and Mortality Weekly Report, 64*(11), 300–304.

Pinninti, S. G., & Kimberlin, D. W. (2014b). Preventing herpes simplex virus in the newborn. *Clinical Perinatology, 41*(4), 945–955.

Poulton, M. (2013). Patient confidentiality in sexual health services and electronic patient records. *Sexually Transmitted Infections, 89*(2), 90.

Public Health England. (2015a). Human papillomavirus (HPV) immunisation programme review: 2008-2014. Retrieved from https:

//www.gov.uk/government/publications/human-papillomavirus-hpv-immunisation-programme-review-2008-to-2014

Public Health England. (2015b). Vaccine uptake guidance and the latest coverage data. *PHE Publications Gateway*, 2014797.

Ray, K., Muralidhar, S., Bala, M., Kumari, M., Salhan, S., Gupta, S. M., & Bhattacharya, M. (2010). Comparative study of syndromic and etiologic diagnosis of reproductive tract infections/sexually transmitted infections in women in Delhi. *International Journal of Infectious Diseases, 13*(6), e352–e359.

Rerks-Ngarm, S., Pitisuttithum, P., Nitayaphan, S., Kwaekungwal, J., Chiu, J., Paris, R., . . . MOPH TAVEG Investigators. (2009). Vaccination with ALVAC and AIDSVAX to prevent HIV-1 infection in Thailand. *New England Journal of Medicine, 361*(23), 2209–2220.

Risley, C. L., Ward, H., Choudhury, B., Bishop, C. J., Fenton, K. A., Spratt, B. G., . . . Ghani, A. C. (2009). Geographical and demographic clustering of gonorrhoea in London. *Sexually Transmitted Infections, 83*(6), 481–187.

Ross, J., & McCarthy, G. (2011). UK National guideline for the management of Pelvic Inflammatory Disease 2011. London, United Kingdom: BASHH. Retrieved from https://www.bashh.org/documents/3572.pdf

Royal College of Obstetricians and Gynecologists. (2014). *Management of genital herpes in pregnancy*. Retrieved from https://www.rcog.org.uk/globalassets/documents/guidelines/management-genital-herpes.pdf

Ryder, N., & McNulty, A. M. (2009). Confidentiality and access to sexual health services. *Sexual Health, 6*(2), 153–155.

Savage, E. J., Mohammed, H., Leong, G., Duffell, S., & Hughes, G. (2014). Improving surveillance of sexually transmitted infections using mandatory electronic clinical reporting: The genitourinary medicine clinic activity dataset, England, 2009–2013. *European Surveillance, 19*(48), 20981.

Savage, E. J., Marsh, K., Duffell, S., Ison, C. A., Zaman, A., & Hughes, G. (2012). Rapid increase in gonorrhoea and syphilis diagnoses in England. *European Surveillance, 17*(29), pii=20224.

Schwebke, J. R., & Desmond, R. K. (2007a). A randomised trial of the duration of therapy with metronidaxole plus or minus azithromycin for treatment of symptomatic bacterial vaginosis. *Clinical Infectious Diseases, 44*(2), 213–219.

Schwebke, J. R., & Desmond, R. K. (2011). Tinidazole vs metronidazole for the treatment of bacterial vaginosis. *American Journal of Obstetrics and Gynecology, 204*(3), 211–216.

Shahrook, S., Mori, R., Ochirbat, T., & Gomi, H. (2014). Strategies of testing for syphilis in pregnancy. *Cochrane Database Systematic Reviews, 10*, CD010385.

Sherrard, J., Donders, G., White, D., Jensen, J. S. & European IUSTI. (2011). European IUSTI/WHO guideline on the management of vaginal discharge, 2011. *International Journal of Sexually Transmitted Diseases and AIDS, 22*(8), 421–429.

Taylor, B. D., & Haggerty, C. L. (2011). Management of *Chlamydia trachomatis* genital tract infection: Screening and treatment challenges. *Infection and Drug Resistance, 2011*(4), 19–29.

Terrault, N. A., Dodge, J. L., Murphy, E. L., Tavis, J. E., Kiss, A., Levin, T. R., . . . Alter, M. J. (2013). Sexual transmission of hepatitis C virus among monogamous heterosexual couples: The HCV partners study. *Hepatology, 57*(3), 881–889.

United Nations Educational, Scientific, and Cultural Organization (UNESCO). (2011). *Cost and cost-effectiveness of school-based sexuality education programmes in six countries*. Paris, France: Author. Retrieved from http://unesdoc.unesco.org/images/0021/002116/211604e.pdf

United Nations Programme on HIV/AIDS. *Report on the global AIDS epidemic: 2010*. Geneva, Switzerland: UNAIDS.

Usher, E. L., & Pajares, F. (2008). Self-efficacy for self-regulated learning: A validation study. *Educational and Psychological Measurement, 68*(3), 443–463.

Wasley, A., Fiore, A., & Bell, B. P. (2006). Hepatitis A in the era of vaccination. *Epidemiology Reviews, 28*(1), 101–111.

World Health Organization (WHO). (2007). *Global strategy for the prevention and control of sexually transmitted infections 2005–2015*. Geneva-and-proge, Switzerland: Author.

World Health Organization (WHO). (2010). *Human papillomavirus (HPV)*. Geneva, Switzerland: Author. Retrieved from www.who.int/immunization/topics/**hpv**/en/

World Health Organization (WHO). (2010). *Standards for Sexuality Education in Europe: A framework for policy makers, educational and health authorities and specialists*. Cologne, Germany: Federal Centre for Health Education (BZgA) and World Health Organization Regional Office for Europe.

World Health Organization (WHO). (2011). *Rio political declaration on social determinants of health*. Geneva, Switzerland: Author.

WHO/UNAIDS. (1999). *Sexually transmitted diseases: Policies and principles for prevention and care*. Retrieved from http://data.unaids.org/publications/IRC-pub04/una97–6_en.pdf

The WHO/UNAIDS is comprised of six international organizations, including the United Nations International Children's Fund (UNICEF); United Nations Development Programme (UNDP); United Nations Fund for Population Activities (UNFPA); United Nations Educational, Scientific and Cultural Organisation (UNESCO); World Health Organization (WHO); and the World Bank.

10

Subfertility and Its Impact

JILL STEWART-MOORE

CHAPTER OBJECTIVES

The main objectives of this chapter are to:

- Provide an overview of pre-existing diseases or conditions, such as epilepsy, diabetes, congenital or known acquired cardiac disease, autoimmune disorders, and severe mental illness, that affect women
- Explore the psychological effects of subfertility
- Explain the feminist perspective

Introduction

This chapter aims to provide the practitioner with holistic information to be shared with patients to enhance the probability of conception. The health professional may be informed that a couple has been trying to conceive for some time, yet finds that the couple is reluctant to be referred to specialist infertility services. The opportunity to provide a couple with advice commonly arises after a negative pregnancy test result is confirmed. This chapter will address fundamental aspects of health that may impact subfertility.

Subfertility Issues

It is estimated that one in six couples will experience difficulties in achieving a pregnancy. A common question, especially after discontinuation of contraception is: How long will it take to conceive? Specialist examination may reveal common female causes of subfertility: polycystic ovaries, hyperprolactinemia, thyroid dysfunction, endometriosis, uterine fibroids, and tubal abnormalities (Senie, 2014). Male causes may include urogenital abnormalities, malignancies, infections, increased scrotal temperature, and genetic and immunological causes (Jungwirth et al., 2015). *Unexplained subfertility* is diagnosed when results of standard investigations (tests for ovulation, tubal patency, and semen analysis) are all normal. Between 30% and 40% of subfertile couples fall into this category (Nandi & Homburg, 2016). Experts vary in their opinion on how long to wait before intervention; a wait of up to 1 year is advised by the American Society for Reproductive Medicine Practice Committee (2013). Nandi & Homburg (2016) summarize the investigations and treatments available to these couples but acknowledge that without clear evidence for treatment, some couples may be advised to try to conceive naturally for 2 years before they are offered treatment.

Frequency of intercourse deserves exploring, as some couples are only able to engage in sexual intercourse on weekends, as the week is too busy. The timing of female ovulation is not always predictable, even in a 28-day cycle, with the ovum viable a maximum of 48 hours. Conception is only possible from about 5 days before and up to several hours after ovulation. Manders et al. (2015) reviewed the evidence of ovulation prediction methods for the timing of intercourse in couples trying to conceive. Methods such as urinary fertility monitoring, calendar charting, observation of cervical mucus and basal body temperature changes, and follicular maturation on ultrasonic scanning were compared. The authors concluded that imprecise evidence and poor reporting resulted in a recommendation to exercise caution in recommending any of these methods. Intercourse needs to take place every 2 to 3 days to optimize the chance of conception. Practitioners need to inquire about the satisfaction of intercourse, as problems such as erectile dysfunction or dyspareunia will reduce the chance of conception (Jungwirth et al., 2015).

Case Scenario

Hilary, a 36-year-old nulliparous woman, presents with an early morning urine specimen for a pregnancy test. She has attended three times already this year for the same reason. Her demeanour is somewhat agitated, and on preliminary questioning, you learn that this is a wanted pregnancy. On receipt of her negative result, she is upset and frustrated at not conceiving. What is your response?

According to the Six Category Intervention Analysis (Heron, 2001), there are six categories of intervention a health professional could use with a patient. Within an overall setting of concern for the patient's best interests, the interventions fall into one or more of these six categories:

1. *Prescriptive*: Giving advice or instructions, being critical or directive. Advice may include frequency of intercourse, referral to physician about a pre-existing disorder, or attention to lifestyle.

2. *Informative*: Imparting new knowledge, instructing, or interpreting. Information may be offered about support services such as anti-obesity clinics, folic acid supplementation, or the impact of previous contraception—such as use of the injectable contraception—that may delay ovulation for a year or longer after discontinuation (Spevack, 2013).

3. *Confronting*: Challenging a restrictive attitude or behavior, giving direct feedback within a caring context. For example, confronting habits such as smoking, excessive alcohol intake, or use of illicit drugs, all of which are teratogens that interrupt normal fetal growth, depending on the timing and amount of consumption.

4. *Cathartic*: Seeking to release emotion in the form of weeping, laughter, or anger. This may be the first time the patient has talked about this very private matter.

5. *Catalytic*: Encouraging the patient to discover and explore his/her own latent thoughts and feelings. There may be relationship issues that are interfering with successful sexual function.

6. *Supportive*: Offering comfort and approval, affirming the patient's intrinsic value. Patients may be embarrassed to discuss this issue and need positive affirmation to address it.

Addressing Lifestyle Factors Affecting Fertility

Alcohol

In 2005, the U.S. Surgeon General advised that pregnant women and women of childbearing age who are considering becoming pregnant should not drink alcohol. The risk of having a child with a fetal alcohol spectrum disorder (FASD), such as fetal alcohol syndrome, alcohol-related neurodevelopmental disorder, or alcohol-related birth defects, is increased in women who are more than 30 years of age, which is often the age group of women seeking help with subfertility. Fetal alcohol syndrome, characterized by facial anomalies, retarded growth, and neurological abnormalities, is a well-recognized sequelae of alcohol overuse (Senie, 2014). Excessive alcohol consumption over 5 drinks a week can adversely affect sperm quality in men and decrease implantation rates in women (Nandi & Homburg, 2016; **Figure 10-1**). Alcohol consumption can also adversely affect male ejaculation (Jungwirth et al., 2015). High levels

of alcohol consumption during pregnancy can result in any one of the FASD. More information can be obtained from the National Organization on Fetal Alcohol Syndrome (NOFAS) at http://www.nofas.org or through the Centers for Disease Control and Prevention (CDC). Features of FASD include fetal growth retarding, intellectual disability, facial anomalies, poor coordination, low body weight, speech and language delays, and difficulty with attention. Attendance at alcohol abuse prevention programs is to be encouraged in individuals or couples who consume alcohol to excess or who express concern about abstaining from alcohol during pregnancy. Local Alcoholics Anonymous organizations are identified at http://www.aa.org (Schub and Pravikoff, 2016).

Smoking

Similarly, women should be informed that active and passive smoking is likely to reduce their fertility, and men should be informed there is an association between smoking and semen quality (Nandi & Homburg, 2016). Regarding caffeinated beverages, there is no consistent evidence of an association between caffeine consumption and fertility problems (Nandi & Homburg, 2016). Nonetheless, heavy caffeine users should restrict consumption to no more than 5 caffeinated drinks per day.

Obesity and Overweight

The dangers of obesity and pregnancy are too complex for detailed discussion, but a brief review is relevant. Women who have a body mass index of greater than 29 should be informed that they are likely to take longer to conceive. Both men and women should achieve a normal weight for their height. Obesity in men can cause DNA damage to sperm, decreased libido, and erectile dysfunction (Nandi & Homburg, 2016). Regular cardiovascular exercise of at least 20 to 30 minutes per day will help. More seriously, in the U.K. *Saving Lives, Improving Mothers' Care Report,*

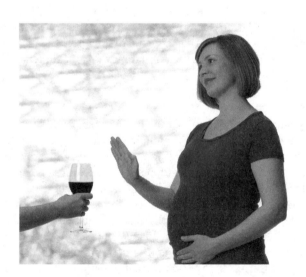

Courtesy of CDC

Figure 10-1 Excessive alcohol consumption before pregnancy in either parent can adversely affect pregnancy prospects

Knight et al. (2015) have identified that 30% of the women who died during pregnancy or postpartum were obese. In this report, the reasons why women die in pregnancy and in the postnatal period in the United Kingdom are quantified and confirmed. This edition specifically examined surveillance information for 575 women who died during or up to 1 year after the end of pregnancy between 2011 and 2013. Medical comorbidities such as obesity were significantly associated with higher odds of dying from specific pregnancy complications such as thromboembolism. Where possible, obese women should be helped to lose weight prior to conception or receipt of any form of assisted reproductive technologies. Health education for couples trying to conceive regarding folic acid supplementation and reduction in obesity and smoking will enhance the general health of the individuals, but the current evidence is limited to support assurance that the couple will conceive as a consequence.

Nutrition and Diet

Advice should include attention to lifestyle and dietary factors. Folate is a water-soluble B vitamin that occurs naturally in food. Folic acid is the synthetic form of folate found in supplements and added to fortified foods, such as bread and cereal in the United States and United Kingdom Folate helps produce and maintain new cells, which is especially important during periods of rapid cell division and growth, such as in pregnancy. Importantly, folic acid supplementation not only decreases the likelihood of fetal abnormalities such as the neural tube defect spina bifida, it also enhances the absorption of folate, important for oocyte quality, maturation, and implantation. A balance of folate and zinc is required in the body for effective reproduction. Dietary supplementation with folic acid before conception and up to 12 weeks' gestation is recommended. For women who have previously had an infant affected by a neural tube defect or who are taking anti-epileptic medication, a higher dose is recommended (Wilson et al., 2015). Vitamin supplements other than folic acid are of doubtful benefit in natural conception for either sex. Additionally, there is no evidence to support magnesium supplementation (Jungwirth et al., 2015).

Infectious Diseases Affecting Fertility

Early detection and treatment of chlamydia is a fundamental principle of subfertility care. *Chlamydia trachomatis* infection of the genital tract is commonly asymptomatic, which promotes bacterial progression to the upper genital tract, causing complications, namely, pelvic inflammatory disease, ectopic pregnancy, and infertility in women (Keltz et al., 2016; **Figure 10-2**). Noninvasive self-swabbing of the vagina, collection of first-void urine, an endocervical swab at the time of cervical smear, or pharyngeal specimen should be offered to detect and treat early-stage infection. This investigation is important before undergoing uterine instrumentation as part of fertility treatment. Untreated, the antibody response to chlamydia may be sensitized and

contribute to chronic, persistent, or repeated infection in susceptible individuals. Even mild forms of gonorrhea or chlamydia infection can cause tubal function defects without causing overt occlusion (Nandi & Homburg, 2016). Evidence from a prospective observational study was performed at Columbia University, New York (Keltz et al., 2013) confirms that clinical pregnancy without in vitro fertilization (IVF) was significantly lower among chlamydia-positive patients. New infertility patients (1,279) seen at the center underwent chlamydia screening. Charts were later reviewed for evidence of subsequent spontaneous intrauterine pregnancies and identified tubal block and tubal damage. Comparing results between chlamydia-positive and chlamydia-negative patients at initial assessment, the conclusion was reached that a positive chlamydia serology result is predictive of both tubal damage and a reduced cumulative pregnancy rate when excluding treatment with IVF (Keltz et al., 2013).

Another fundamental aspect of preconception care is attention to whether the woman has been vaccinated against rubella (German measles) infection. If a new mother contracts rubella in the first trimester of pregnancy, the infant has a very high risk of being born blind, deaf, and mentally disabled. Today, parents of children in the United States and United Kingdom are offered one or two vaccinations to protect children who are 12 months through to 12 years old against measles, mumps, rubella, and varicella (chickenpox). Older women and women born outside of the United States and United Kingdom, as well as women who are doubtful if they were vaccinated, should be tested for immunity status and vaccinated as indicated (Centers for Disease Control and Prevention [CDC], 2010, National Collaborating Centre for Women's and Children's Health, 2013).

Women should be advised to be up to date with cervical cytology before embarking on a pregnancy. Cervical screening is offered in the United Kingdom to women age 25 to 60 years at 3- to 5-year intervals (Public Health England [PHE], 2015;

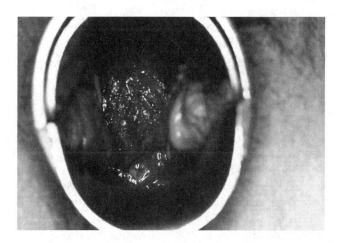

Figure 10-2 This woman's cervix has manifested signs of an erosion and erythema due to chlamydial infection
Courtesy of CDC/Dr. Lourdes Fraw, Jim Pledger.

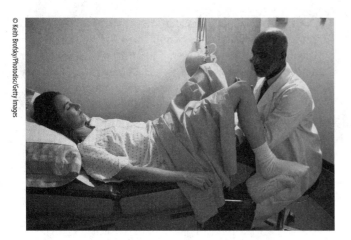

© Keith Brofsky/Photodisc/Getty Images

Figure 10-3 Regular cervical screening is advised

Figure 10-3). In the United States cervical screening is recommended for women aged 21–65 years every 3 years (CDC, 2016). Human papillomavirus (HPV) infection is believed to be a primary cause of cervical cancer, with an estimated prevalence of over 99% of all cervical cancers. Two subtypes of the virus HPV (16 and 18) are present in over 80% of invasive cervical cancers. In uninfected females, the recently available vaccine effectively prevents HPV 16 and 18 associated with cervical cancer. This HPV vaccine is currently offered to girls aged 12 to 13 (CDC, 2015; PHE, 2015), which will not be of benefit to women presenting today with subfertility. The exact cause of cervical cancer is multifactorial, thus prevention is the main reason for cervical screening programs.

Women with Pre-existing Diseases or Conditions

Couples preparing for pregnancy need to be aware of the risks imposed on a mother's health if pre-existing medical conditions exist. Several chronic diseases and the medication required for treatment have implications for fetal health. In addition, pregnancy and labor may worsen pre-existing maternal diseases. Mhyre, Bateman, and Leffert (2011) studied data from the U.S. Nationwide Inpatient Sample and concluded that complications of pre-existing medical conditions appear to be the fastest rising category of U.S. maternal death. The U.K. *Saving Lives, Improving Mothers' Care* report (Knight et al., 2015) has identified that many of the women who died from thrombosis and thromboembolism would have benefited from a risk assessment prepregnancy or in early pregnancy. Women with pre-existing medical conditions should have prepregnancy counseling by physicians with experience of managing the specific disorder in pregnancy. Women with major risk factors for maternal death who received treatment for infertility have been notable in the U.K. report and previous reports. The authors recommend that a full assessment of coexisting medical conditions and obstetric history must be undertaken before any form of infertility treatment, including ovulation induction and particularly IVF, is offered. Referral for psychological counseling is advised where a woman's health history suggests that infertility treatment is contraindicated. Before IVF is started, a woman's previous medical and obstetric history must be taken into account when determining the safest embryo transfer strategy. The more common conditions that require prepregnancy counseling and advice are epilepsy, diabetes, congenital or known acquired cardiac disease, autoimmune disorders, and severe pre-existing or past mental illness (Lewis, 2007; Mhyre et al., 2011).

Epilepsy

Women who have epilepsy and are preparing for pregnancy will need careful physician and contraceptive support while changing anti-epileptic medication to drugs that are not harmful to the fetus. Epilepsy may be more difficult to control in pregnancy, thus increasing the risk of sudden unexpected deaths in female epileptic patients (Knight et al., 2015). Pregnant women with type 1 or type 2 diabetes are at a greater risk of adverse outcomes in pregnancy, such as high blood pressure (gestational hypertension) and preterm births. Pregnancy can also accelerate the development of diabetic complications such as retinopathy, nephropathy, neuropathy, ischemic heart disease, cerebrovascular disease, and peripheral vascular disease. The number of women in the United Kingdom and United States dying in childbirth from heart disease, both congenital and acquired, is of concern (Mhyre et al., 2011).

Cardiac Disease and Mortality

Cardiac disease is the leading cause of indirect maternal deaths in the United Kingdom (Knight et al., 2016); this risk is higher in older women. Women who present for subfertility advice are more likely to be older women, some of whom may have followed the U.K. trend for delayed childbearing. Women who died of cardiac disease had identifiable risk factors, including:

- Obesity
- Older age and higher parity
- Smoking
- Diabetes
- Pre-existing hypertension
- Family history

Pregnancy can impose strain on congenitally abnormal heart conditions, such as in women with repaired Fallot's tetralogy. In some cases, this has led to maternal death. Although extremely rare in the United States and United Kingdom rheumatic heart disease is still common in less-developed countries, and mitral valve stenosis often complicates pregnancy. Immigrants may have relatively poor overall general health and are at risk from illnesses, such as tuberculosis, that have largely disappeared from the United States and United Kingdom Some are also more likely to be at risk of HIV infection. Newly arrived women from developing countries, who may well have come to the United Kingdom for subfertility treatment they cannot receive in their home country, therefore require a full physical examination when they present. In the United States, Niemczyk (2015) observes that non-Hispanic black women are disproportionately represented among patients with near-miss maternal morbidity and mortality. They were more likely to have late entry to prenatal care, were younger, and had less education. It is suggested that they may enter pregnancy with pre-existing chronic medical conditions that might particularly benefit from preconception care. These very pre-existing medical conditions may contribute to subfertility.

The growing incidence of acquired heart disease in women is related to less healthy diets, smoking, alcohol use, and the growing obesity epidemic (Knight et al., 2016). In the United States it is observed that the rise in maternal mortality, particularly cardiovascular disease-related deaths, can be attributed to advances in cardiac care (Castellucci 2015). That is, women who had a congenital, heart defect or a cardiac condition when they were younger and had reparative surgery are now living longer and are consequently trying to conceive. All of these women may present with subfertility.

Mental Illness

Assessment of medication for women with severe pre-existing or past mental illness such as bipolar disorder or schizophrenia requires review and adjustment to minimize fetal risks. According to the severity of the illness, a full review by a psychiatrist may be necessary.

There is a need for practical national guidance for the management of women with multiple morbidities and social factors prior to, during, and after pregnancy (Knight et al., 2016). Women with serious pre-existing medical conditions should have prepregnancy counseling at every opportunity, even if they are not immediately seeking to achieve pregnancy. This is especially the case if they seek assisted reproduction. A careful selection and adjustment of medication may be required prior to pregnancy.

Psychological Effects of Subfertility

Being unable to conceive can be a distressing experience. This psychological distress may lead to a reduction in libido and thus the frequency of intercourse, which can further compound the problem. Some couples may find it helpful to contact a fertility support group such as www.fertilityfriends.co.uk, a worldwide organization with forums to support members (**Figure 10-4**). Distress can manifest as depression, anxiety, sexual difficulty, and relationship problems with the partner, family, or friends, any or all of which can lead to an increased sense of self-blame and guilt.

Women may become more prone to psychological distress if they go on to receive assisted reproductive treatment. Women often undergo numerous invasive procedures, as well. The drugs and hormones used to treat infertility may have various psychological side effects. Times of high stress for couples can be during egg retrieval, embryo transfer, and pregnancy tests that follow the in vitro fertilization procedure. A systematic review from Weill Cornell Medical College (Stellar, 2016) identified that subfertility may be a risk factor for intimate partner violence (IPV). IPV can include emotional, psychological, and economic elements in addition to physical and sexual components. The study built on previous knowledge that infertility has been linked to high levels of marital discord, separation, divorce, and multiple sexual partners. The review was based on 21 studies from 11 countries, representing 1 high income country and 10 low- and middle-income countries as defined by the World Bank. Findings included that infertile men and women are commonly stigmatized, are not allowed to participate in community activities, and experience higher rates of divorce, remarriage, and polygamy relative to their fertile counterparts. They can experience feelings of alienation and high levels of distress, depression, and low self-esteem.

Infertile women could also find themselves at higher risk for exposure to sexually transmitted infections and/or HIV due to willingness to engage in unprotected sex with multiple partners in the hope of achieving a pregnancy. Regardless of diverse populations and culture, the effects of infertility on couples are not population specific or culturally bound (Luk & Loke, 2015). Couples considering, fertility technologies should be offered counseling from someone independent of the treatment unit, regarding all the physical and psychological implications of treatment (National Collaborating Centre for Womens' and Childrens' Health, 2013). In addition, certain physical conditions may impact fertility. Women with polycystic ovarian syndrome (PCOS), one of the commonly diagnosed causes of subfertility,

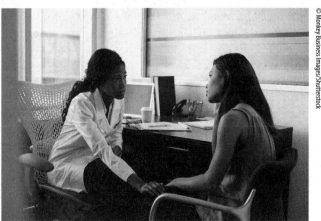

© Monkey Business Images/Shutterstock

Figure 10-4 Women who are having difficulty conceiving may need psychological support

are more likely to experience a negative impact on their sexuality because of excessive hair growth and increased weight associated with the condition. This has been demonstrated in lower levels of health-related quality-of-life measurement in women with PCOS (Sanchez, 2015).

A Feminist Perspective

It is useful to balance the scientific approach to subfertility treatment with the more circumspect view within the feminist paradigm. Over 30 years ago, Klein (1986) drew attention to the commercialization of infertility treatments globally and the abuses therein. Some clinics offered artificial reproductive technologies, yet unbeknownst to the clients, had not one successful outcome. Padamsee (2011) analyzed a pharmaceutical company's journal content over a 13-year period, which was targeted at the medical profession. She argues that the company invested substantial resources to influence doctors' disposition and prescribing behaviors to develop the medicalization of fertility and infertility. Female patients were portrayed as passive, disempowered objects of medical practice. The high failure rates and negative experiences that patients undergoing infertility treatments endured were missing from the company's journal. Padamsee (2011) explains that the perceived epidemic of infertility and availability of artificial reproductive technologies has changed the dynamics of the social construction of reproduction and infertility. Within the medical profession, there have been reservations about the "overtreatment" of subfertility. Concern at the rising incidence of the fatal ovarian hyperstimulation syndrome and multiple births has shifted drug regimens to aim for mild ovarian stimulation and single-embryo transfer (Romundstad, Opdahl, & Pinburg, 2015). In a study from the Netherlands, couples with unexplained subfertility and an intermediate prognosis of natural conception were randomly allocated to a 6-month expectant management group and an immediate start group with intrauterine insemination and controlled ovarian stimulation (Custers et al., 2012). Time to ongoing pregnancy did not differ between the groups. The expectant management group saved half the cost of treatment in the intervention group. This evidence-based knowledge supports professionals advising expectant management, especially if after initial investigations the couple have unexplained infertility. The chances of spontaneous conception remain high in couples with unexplained subfertility (Nandi & Homburg, 2016).

In the author's professional practice in England and Northern Ireland, couples sometimes wait 5 to 10 years to successfully conceive—whether for religious reasons, fear of reproductive technologies, or concern about the costs involved. Even where health services are provided free, time out from work and travel costs may not affordable. Views on subfertility and its social construction vary from being a nuisance, to bad luck but acceptable, to a body dysfunction or a disease.

Against the background of global economic austerity and a supportive business entrepreneur ethic, couples may be attracted to seek increasingly available private fertility care. An appropriate and cautious approach is advised.

Conclusion

In conclusion, before referral to specialist services, health professionals can guide the couple trying for a pregnancy to improve their success at conception. Simple lifestyle changes, with attention to stable control of pre-existing illnesses and avoiding teratogenic medication, will improve the chances of success. As a group, women with subfertility are likely to be older. Those affected by a pre-existing illness may find the illness is exacerbated during pregnancy. In giving couples the correct information about preparing for pregnancy, health professionals may not only help them succeed in a pregnancy, but also avoid increased maternal morbidity or mortality.

● ● ● REFERENCES

American Society for Reproductive Medicine Practice Committee. (2013). Definitions of infertility and recurrent pregnancy loss: A committee opinion. *Fertility and Sterility, 99*, 63.

Castellucci, M. (2015). Pre-existing conditions contribute to rising U.S. maternal mortality rates. *Modern Healthcare, 45*(50), 14. Retrieved from http://www.modernhealthcare.com/article/20151212/MAGAZINE/312129961

Centers for Disease Control and Prevention (CDC). (2016). National breast and cervical cancer early detection program. Retrieved from http://www.cdc.gov/cancer/nbccedp/about.htm.

Centers for Disease Control and Prevention (CDC). (2010). Measles, mumps, and rubella (MMR) vaccination: What everyone should know. Retrieved from http://www.cdc.gov/vaccines/vpd-vac/combo-vaccines/mmrv/vacopt.htm.

Centers for Disease Control and Prevention (CDC). (2015). *HPV vaccine for preteens and teens.* Retrieved from http://www.cdc.gov/vaccines/parents/diseases/teen/hpv.html.

Custers, I., Van Rumste, M., Van Der, Steeg J., Van Wely, M., Hompes, P., Bossuyt, P., . . . CECERM. (2012). Long-term outcome in couples with unexplained subfertility and an intermediate prognosis initially randomized between expectant management and immediate treatment. *Human Reproduction, 27*, 444–450.

Heron, J. (2001). *Helping the client: A creative practical guide* (5th ed). London, United Kingdom: Sage.

Jungwirth, A., Diemer, T., Dohle, G., Giwercman, A., Kopa, Z., Krausz, C., & Tournaye, H. (2015). European Association of Urology Guidelines on Male Infertility. *European Urology.* 62(2), 324–332.

Keltz, M., Sauerbrun-Cutler, M., Durante, M., Moshier, E., Stein, D., & Gonzales, E. (2013). Positive *Chlamydia trachomatis* serology result in women seeking care for infertility is a negative prognosticator for intrauterine pregnancy. *Sexually Transmitted Diseases, 40*(11), 842–845.

Klein, R. (1986). *Infertility: Women speak out about their experiences of reproductive medicine.* London, United Kingdom: Pandora Press.

Knight, M., Nair, M., Tuffnell, D., Kenyon, S., Shakespeare, J., Brocklehurst, P., & Kurinczuk, J. J. (Eds.). (2016). *Saving lives, Improving mothers' care: Surveillance of maternal deaths in the UK 2012-14 and lessons learned to inform maternity care from the UK and Ireland Confidential Enquiries into Maternal Deaths and Morbidity 2009-14.* Oxford, United Kingdom: National Perinatal Epidemiology Unit, University of Oxford.

Knight, M., Tuffnell, D., Kenyon, S., Shakespeare, J., Gray, R., & Kurinczuk, J. J. (Eds.). (2015). *Saving lives, Improving mothers' care: Surveillance of maternal deaths in the UK 2011-13 and lessons learned to inform maternity care from the UK and Ireland Confidential Enquiries into Maternal Deaths and Morbidity 2009-13.* Oxford, United Kingdom: National Perinatal Epidemiology Unit, University of Oxford.

Lewis, G. (2007). *Saving mothers' lives: Reviewing maternal deaths to make motherhood safer, 2003-2005.* London, United Kingdom: Confidential Enquiry into Maternal and Child Health.

Luk, B., & Loke, A. (2015). The impact of infertility on the psychological well-being, marital relationships, sexual relationships, and quality of life of couples: a systematic review. *Journal of Sex & Marital Therapy, 41*(6), 610–625.

Manders, M., McLindon, L., Schulze, B., Beckmann, M. M., Kremer, J. A. M., & Farquhar, C. (2015). Timed intercourse for couples trying to conceive. *Cochrane Database of Systematic Review, (3)*, CD0011345.

Mhyre, J., Bateman, B., & Leffert, L. (2011). Influence of patient comorbidities on the risk of near-miss maternal morbidity or mortality. *Anesthesiology, 115,* 963–972.

Nandi, A., & Homburg, R. (2016). Unexplained subfertility: Diagnosis and management. *Obstetrics & Gynecology, 18,* 107–115.

National Collaborating Centre for Women's and Children's Health. (2013). *Fertility: Assessment and treatment for people with fertility problems (full NICE guideline 156).* Retrieved from https://www.nice.org.uk/guidance/cg156/.

Niemczyk, N. (2015). Causes of pregnancy-related mortality change, but racial disparities remain. *Journal of Midwifery & Women's Health, 60,* 623–624.

Padamsee, T. J. (2011). The pharmaceutical corporation and the 'good work' of managing women's bodies. *Social Science & Medicine, 72*(8), 1342–1350.

Public Health England (PHE). (2015). *Cervical screening: Programme overview.* Retrieved from https://www.gov.uk guidance/cervical screeningprogramme.

Romundstad, L., Opdahl, S., & Pinburg, A. (2015). Which treatment option for couples with unexplained or mild male subfertility? *BMJ, 350,* g7843.

Sanchez, N. (2015). *Polycystic ovary syndrome, absent from national surveillance and present online: Implications for mental and behavioral health* (Unpublished doctoral dissertation). University of Michigan.

Schub, T., & Pravikoff, D. (2016 Apr 8). Fetal alcohol syndrome. Cinahl Information Systems. Glendale, CA: CINAHL Nursing Guide.

Senie, R. (2014). *Epidemiology of women's health.* Burlington, MA: Jones & Bartlett.

Spevack, E. (2013). The long-term health implications of Depo-Provera. *Integrative Medicine, 12*(10), 27–34.

Stellar, C. (2016). A systematic review and narrative report of the relationship between infertility, subfertility, and intimate partner violence. *International Journal of Gynecology & Obstetrics, 133*(1), 3–8.

Wilson, R., Audibert, F., Brock, J., Carroll, J., Cartier, L., Gagnon, A., . . . Van den Hof, M. (2015). Pre-conception folic acid and multivitamin supplementation for the primary and secondary prevention of neural tube defects and other folic acid-sensitive congenital anomalies. *Journal of Obstetrics and Gynaecology Canada, 37*(6), 534–552.

Identifying Special Client Groups with Recommended Screening Services and Referral Systems

JILL STEWART-MOORE

CHAPTER OBJECTIVES

The main objectives of this chapter are to:

- Explore young people's sexual health issues
- Examine good practices for people with learning disability and clients with mental health issues
- Recognize sexual health problems among clients in prison and commercial sex workers
- Identify the challenges of sexual health care for clients with specific medical conditions
- Describe elderly clients and "hidden" sexual health problems

Introduction

This chapter addresses specific health issues on account of age, disability, or discrimination that the sexual health practitioner may encounter. Each section is intended to give the reader an overview of the current knowledge and factors to consider. Good practice examples are highlighted and resources to support developmental work are indicated.

Young Peoples' Sexual Health Issues

Debates about young people's sexuality and their sexual health challenge the health professional to be nonjudgmental in care giving. A knowledge of good working practice in adolescent sexual healthcare enables the practitioner to help young people make the right choices in contraception and disease prevention. Background trends, a user-friendly service, legal issues including consent, sexual behavior, and contraceptive choices will be addressed. The objective is to enable the practitioner to assess the young person's needs and guide them to safe health-promoting behavior.

Background Trends

Compared to other European countries, teenage pregnancy rates and numbers of young people affected by sexually transmitted infections (STIs) in the United Kingdom were higher than elsewhere. Implementation of a 10-year Teenage Pregnancy Strategy for England (1999–2010) has achieved impressive results. The lessons learned from this experience are applicable elsewhere (Hadley, Chandra-Mouli, & Ingham, 2016). There are certain groups who are more likely to become teenage parents. These groups include those who are in care or leaving care; the homeless; those underachieving at school; children of teenage parents; members of specific ethnic groups such as Caribbean, Pakistani, and Bangladeshi; and those involved in crime or living in areas with higher social deprivation (Cook & Cameron, 2015). Similarly, teenage birth rates in the United States have declined to the lowest rates seen in 70 years, yet still rank highest among developed countries. It is a goal of the U.S. Healthy People 2020 initiative to eliminate disparities and improve health in all social groups. However, birth rates to Hispanic and non-Hispanic black teenagers are twice as high compared to non-Hispanic teenagers, and Hispanic teen birth rates were still more than twice as high as for non-Hispanic white teens. Teenage birth rates to American Indian/Alaska natives remain more than 1.5 times higher than the non-Hispanic white teen birth rates. The Centers for Disease Control and Prevention (CDC) is supporting specific organizations from 2015–2020 to enhance youth-friendly sexual and reproductive health services in publicly funded health centers and increase the number of young people accessing the services (CDC, 2016a).

During the initial interview, the health professional needs to be alert to such high-risk factors in assessing the young person's vulnerability. Expert communication skills are required to inspire the trust necessary for such information sharing. Often, young clients can be frightened and reluctant to divulge personal details for fear of a break in confidentiality. Early in the interview, the health professional should explain their rights and the limits of confidentiality.

A User-Friendly Service

A user-friendly service means that not only the staff should be friendly but the decor, signposting, and atmosphere of the clinic needs to be youth friendly. See **Figure 11-1** depicting individuals to attract to the service. The experience of Brook Advisory Centres (Institute of Child Care Research, 2011) in the United Kingdom has produced a successful model of youth-friendly clinics that has resulted in increasing numbers of clients accessing the service. Signposting includes online resources that direct young people to their nearest clinic, along with information sharing about sexual health. Brook also offers a confidential helpline and a text messaging service, with links to social networking sites. The CDC (2013) recommends a minimally invasive approach. The advice to providers is to inform young people that they can get birth control without a Pap smear or pelvic examination. They should also be informed that they can receive STI/HIV counseling, testing, and treatment without having an examination. Selkie, Benson, and Moreno (2011) undertook qualitative research with 29 adolescents in 5 focus groups in Wisconsin. The authors suggest that adolescents choose sexual health resources that offer information in a nonthreatening way and this explains the success of text messaging and social networking sites.

Brook services provide integrated counseling and care alongside a mixture of medical and nurse-led clinical services. Staff respond flexibly to young people's needs, making the connections between sexual and emotional health and the impact of alcohol, drugs, and peer pressure on behavior. Young people are involved in making decisions about everything from the color of the walls to the service's locations and opening times. To make young people believe their sexual health matters, attention to a youth-friendly environment is necessary. Inconvenient clinic hours or location, a lack of transportation, and fear of a lack of confidentiality are obstacles to accessing services (Brittain Williams, Zapata, Pazol, & Romero, 2015). In a study comparing Brook services and the statutory sector (Institute of Child Health, 2011), the environment, privacy, and ease of access were better rated at Brook than the statutory clinic. "Drop-in" clinics appear to be preferred by young people rather than advance arranged appointments. Visits are encouraged from youth groups so that young people become familiar with the center. Staff engage in an advocacy role, contributing to sexual health policy making and discussions in the media about sexual health. Successful service provision depends on working with service users, the community, and staff in partnership. The Department of Health (2011) has developed a self-review tool for young people-friendly health services. The "You're Welcome" quality criteria cover eight themes:

- Accessibility
- Publicity
- Confidentiality and consent
- Environment
- Staff training, skills, attitudes, and values
- Joined-up working
- Young people's involvement in monitoring and evaluation of patient experience
- Health issues for young people

Service providers will have to demonstrate that they are fulfilling these criteria to be assured of continued funding. A systematic review (Brittain et al., 2015) examined the evidence for youth-friendly services and identified similar service characteristics that should be considered when setting up youth-friendly family planning interventions.

Legal Issues

Both staff and young people express concern about their legal rights and duties in sexual health care. Young people want confidential advice, yet staff may be unsure about the boundaries of that confidentiality. Article 8 of the European Convention on Human Rights emphasizes the right to privacy and strengthens the legal basis of confidentiality. In the United Kingdom contraceptive advice may be provided to a competent young person under the following circumstances:

- The young person understands the advice and has sufficient maturity to understand what is involved.

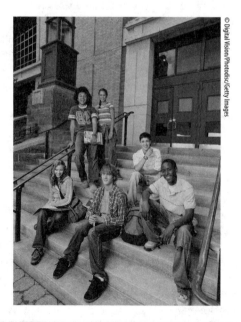

Figure 11-1 A Service that Welcomes Young People is Required

- The doctor could not persuade the young person to inform their parents, nor to allow the doctor to inform them.
- The young person would be very likely to begin or continue having sexual intercourse with or without contraceptive treatment.
- Without contraceptive advice or treatment, the young person's physical or mental health would suffer.
- It would be in the young person's best interest to give such advice or treatment without parental consent.

The use of standardized proforma with these criteria is useful for completion at each visit of an under-16-year-old. Regular reassessment is necessary, as young people's home situation can change quickly.

In the United States efforts to provide clinical care to young people may be complicated by a lack of clarity regarding parental consent requirements with respect to medical services. Several competing interests are involved. They include parental rights to make medical decisions for their children, confidentiality between physician and patient, and privacy rights of young people with respect to sexual health care. Currently, 20 states restrict some minors' ability to consent to contraceptive services; young people may not avail themselves of the services if they are forced to inform their parents (Guttmacher Institute, 2016b).

In addition, in the United Kingdom the health professional also has a legal duty to protect the under 16-year-old from harm and assess their vulnerability to abuse. This duty has become more prominent as incidences of historic covert sexual abuse have been uncovered. The National Institute of Clinical Excellence (NICE, 2009) suggests that abuse should be considered when a young woman aged 16 or 17 years is diagnosed with a sexually transmitted infection (STI) and there is "no clear evidence of blood contamination or that the STI was acquired from consensual sexual activity and a clear difference in power or mental capacity between the young person and their sexual partner (in particular when the relationship is incestuous or with a person in a position of trust) or concern that the young person is being exploited" (NICE, 2009).

It is essential to ask the age of the partner, as in the United Kingdom and the United States a person of any age who engages in sexual activity with a person under the legal age of consent—which varies by state but is generally 16–18 years of age—is committing a criminal offense, regardless of whether the underage person participates willingly. In the United Kingdom the health professional must mandatorily refer cases to social work services and authorities where the partner engaging in sexual activity with an underage person is over 18. The Family Planning Association (FPA, 2011) argues that the law is not intended to prosecute mutually agreed-upon teenage sexual activity between young people of a similar age, unless it involves abuse or exploitation. In the United States the law varies. In some states, no one under 16 is capable of consent and any sex between a minor and a person over 17 is statutory

rape. In others, statutory rape is considered only if the partners are more than 2 years apart in age. When a child is under the legal age reports engaging in sexual activity, the law requires mandatory social work and police referral. Health professionals are advised to adhere to the latest professional guidance in their workplace and discuss cases with their team leader. Young people engaged in same-sex relationships are subject to the same child protection laws, which are gender neutral.

Sexual Behavior

Central to providing a service for young people is an understanding of the pressures and environment young people encounter. The cases described in another chapter illustrate these pressures. Getting young people to discuss their needs can be difficult. For example, asking clients to put down the mobile phone so that they can focus on the discussion may be required! Mobile phones, web cams, social websites, and internet pornography are all part of the cyberspace revolution that poses opportunities and risks in social contacts (Ketting & Winkelmann, 2011; **Figure 11-2**). While knowledge of sexual health can be easily accessed on the internet, exposure to scenes of sexual abuse and violence can also be viewed. Inappropriate social contacts may be arranged with dangerous consequences. In this section, these consequences and the "sex as a risk" paradigm will be examined, followed by the conditions for positive sexual experiences and the resultant effects on contraceptive choices.

Surveys suggest that one in three young people in the United Kingdom and United States have had sexual intercourse by the age of 16 (Cook & Cameron, 2015; Finer & Philbin, 2013). The risks of sexual behavior include regret at first intercourse, unplanned pregnancy, and sexually transmitted infections. Regret has been associated with less control, such as feeling pressured, being drunk or under the influence of drugs, and less intimacy, involving sex with a casual partner (Wight et al., 2008). In a series of extended discussion groups, the Family Planning Association (2007) concluded that many young people have

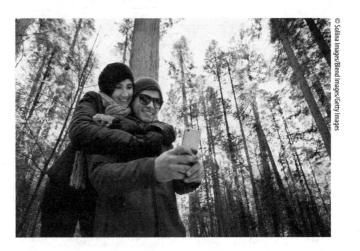

Figure 11-2 Mobile Phones are Part of Today's Cyberspace Revolution

problems communicating with the opposite gender about sexual relationships. Young people aged 16 to 24 are more likely to report at least one new sexual partner in the last year. People in this group continue to experience the highest rates of sexually transmitted infections (Public Health England [PHE], 2015).

Another emerging concern is around infections acquired through noncoital sex. There is a greater perceived safety of noncoital sexual activity compared with vaginal sex; however, noncoital sex is not necessarily safe sex. In a study of African American and Mexican American women aged 14 to 18, Champion and Roye (2014) examined the practice of anal sex in relationships. The study was prompted by the knowledge that unprotected anal sex is riskier in HIV acquisition than vaginal sex. If anal sex is receptive, there is a higher risk of exposure to infection. The study identified that there was an increased prevalence of anal sex in bisexual young women. The authors suggest that education programs that previously have not attached much attention to this practice should now include the risks of unprotected anal sex. Oral sex has also been perceived as less risky. Saliva has some components that inactivate some viruses, although transmission of viral infections such as non-gonococcal urethritis, adenoviruses, herpes simplex virus 1, and hepatitis have been associated with unprotected oral sex. In addition, bacterial infections can also be transmitted by oral-genital contact, including gonorrhea, syphilis, chlamydia, and chancroid (Edwards & Carne, 1998). In assessing risk, practitioners should consider whether the client has engaged in oral sex or anal sex and the gender and number of sexual partners. Multiple sexual partnerships increase the risk of exposure to infection; correct and consistent use of a condom or oral shield should be encouraged.

The sex-as-a-risk paradigm has been presented. However, risk-taking is part of the transition to adulthood. Focusing on the either/or activity negates the continuum that we pass through to achieve positive sexual enjoyment. Schalet (2011) argues that it pays little attention to the skills acquisition required to discern and communicate sexual wishes and boundaries in relationships. An alternative model is presented for creating the conditions for more positive sexual experiences (Schalet, 2011). The model uses the acronym "ABCD" (Figure 11-3); A is for Autonomy of the sexual self, in which gaining that autonomy involves learning about sexual desire and comfort levels at their own pace, giving a greater sense of control. B is for Building good romantic relationships by getting to know another person, building trust over time, dealing with conflict, and having fun (Figure 11-4). C is for Connectedness with parents and other care givers to discuss sexuality in a positive, comfortable manner. D is for recognizing Diversities and removing Disparities in accessing resources. Working toward equality of access to resources is vital to adolescent sexual health. This model proposes the positive components of adolescents' sexuality, pleasure, intimacy, and discovery

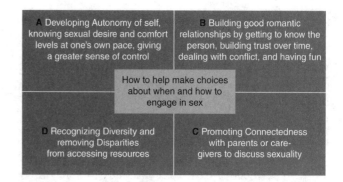

Figure 11-3 Creating Conditions for Positive Transition to Sexual Experiences and Adulthood
Concepts from Schalet (2011).

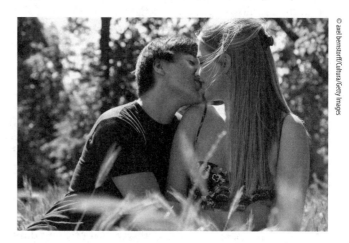

Figure 11-4 Enjoying a Romantic Relationship

to equip young people to make intentional and respectful choices about when and how to engage in sex. Concerns have been raised in the United Kingdom (Family Planning Association, 2013) that sex and relationships education has not been made compulsory in schools. Education needs to explore sex in the wider context of emotions and relationships, the positive side of sex, and the implications of being in a relationship. Discussing this positive side can be part of clinical professional practice. Without this education, the potential outcome is sexual ill health, including dysfunctional relationships. In the United States between 2006 and 2013, there were significant declines in teenage girls' reports of receiving formal instruction about birth control, saying no to sex, and formal instruction about STI's, particularly in rural areas (Lindberg, Maddow-Zimet, & Boonstra, 2016).

Part of acknowledging the autonomy of young people to develop their experiences is to provide access to contraceptive services. That respect for their autonomy also recognizes the occasional nature of sexual engagement.

Contraceptive Choices

As adolescence is a time of experimentation, requests for emergency contraception are common. One of the advantages for young people coming to discuss emergency contraception is that it creates an opportunity to discuss regular contraception. Some young people have no intention of taking further contraception, as they regret the initiating event. Others are happy to discuss their contraceptive options. In England, the contraceptive pill remains the most commonly used method in use, being the main method for 45% of women (NHS Digital, 2016). In the United States the majority of young people rely on the pill; a significant proportion rely on other hormonal methods, including the implant, injectable, patch and ring; and a small minority rely on an intrauterine device (IUD) (Guttmacher Institute, 2016a). Requests to start oral contraception are frequent and assessment includes taking a personal and first-degree relative family health history, taking particular note of thromboembolic disorders, cancer, and liver disorders. Height, weight, and blood pressure measurement are performed. An explanation of the two main groups of oral contraception, the combined hormonal contraception and progestogen-only pill are given. Patients are offered a choice of contraception. Obesity or focal migraine are frequent contraindications in young people to starting combined hormonal contraception, so the progestogen-only pill is recommended in those situations (Faculty of Sexual & Reproductive Healthcare [FSRH], 2016). A 3-month supply may be prescribed to start and then if the method suits, further supplies may be given. Clients are encouraged to return earlier if they experience side effects such as persistent nausea, breast tenderness, or breakthrough bleeding in the first three months. Another estrogen-progestogen combination may be indicated. Discontinuation or intermittent use of the method is not uncommon, as relationships may be short lived or the method unsatisfactory. A sympathetic but methodical approach is called for by the practitioner to achieve a more suitable method. The same regimen is available in patch or vaginal ring form, both providing a steady release of combined estrogen and progesterone hormones. These new methods may appeal particularly to young people.

Dual protection with a male or female condom is advised. The diaphragm or cervical cap can be offered but are rarely chosen by young people in the United Kingdom because of their unacceptable invasiveness. Condoms and the contraceptive pill are called the "double Dutch" or "belt and braces" method, giving give dual protection from pregnancy and infection. If the condom alone is chosen, full details of emergency contraception methods are given as back up in cases of method failure. Over-the-counter access to emergency contraception has been a complicated religious and political battle in many countries. Worldwide efforts to expand access have resulted in access to contraception via the internet. Young women are users of both mobile devices and oral contraception. However, costs have not reduced, which limits access for many (Gawron & Turok, 2015).

Oral contraception may be a bridging method while the young person considers a long-term method of contraception. Use of long-acting reversible contraceptives (LARCs) now accounts for 30% of primary methods of contraception among women who attended National Health Service (NHS) community contraceptive clinics in the United Kingdom (NHS Contraceptive Services, England, 2014). The implant and injection were the most commonly used methods. There is increasing popularity with young people in the use of the contraceptive implant that lasts for 3 years. Depot injections are reliable and provide a contraceptive effect for 8–12 weeks. Martinez and Abma (2015) noted that compared with 2006–2010, in 2011–2013 a smaller percentage of U.S. female teenagers ever used depot medroxyprogesterone acetate (DMPA; trade name DepoProvera), dropping from 20% to 15%. The availability of the 1-month injection Lunelle may account for some of this drop in use. However, there are concerns about the loss of bone mineral density that usually recovers after discontinuation of the method. Young people should also be informed that there can be a delay of up to a year in the return of fertility after discontinuing this injection (FSRH, 2010).

A cautious approach to the appropriateness of IUDs for adolescents is suggested. Deans and Grimes (2009) conducted a systematic review of the literature concerning IUD use in adolescents. They examined six cohort studies and seven case-series reports and concluded that the results were reassuring, but that further research needs to be done. There is a small increase in risk of pelvic infection in the 20 days after IUD insertion, but there is no increased risk after the first 20 days.

Table 11-1 describes the UK Medical Eligibility Criteria for Contraceptive Use (UKMEC) categories based on age. All methods for use from menarche are UKMEC category 1 or 2. Category 1 is when there is no restriction for the use of the contraceptive method. Category 2 is when the advantages of using the method generally outweigh the theoretical or proven risks. Age alone should not limit contraceptive choices, including intrauterine methods (FSRH, 2010).

Say and Mansour (2009) in a qualitative study of 127 young people in Newcastle, United Kingdom, found that interest in the patch, vaginal ring, or implant was low. Young people wanted to know about convenience, effectiveness, and safety along with side effects, invasiveness, and discretion of the methods. The authors suggest that practitioners should educate young people about these issues in particular. With the increased availability of emergency contraception young people are presenting at clinics describing recent unprotected vaginal intercourse, requesting emergency contraception. This suggests a considerably sexually active population who are not safeguarding their sexual health. The Public Health England (2014) suggests embedding chlamydia screening within primary care and sexual health services to ensure that young adults are offered screening as part of a routine consultation. Around 75% of young adults visit their family doctor every year, providing opportunities to offer an annual chlamydia screen. However, in financially stringent health services, money to fund this screening

Table 11-1	U.K. Medical Eligibility Criteria for Contraceptive Use (UKMEC), Categories Based on Age	
Method	**Age**	**UKMEC Category**
Combined hormonal contraception (combined oral contraception, vaginal ring, patch)	Menarche to <40 years	1
	≥40 years	2
Progestogen-only pill	Menarche onward	1
Progestogen-only implant	Menarche onward	1
Progestogen-only injectable (DMPA or NET-EN)	Menarche to <18 years	2
	18–45 years	1
	>45	2
Barrier methods (condoms, diaphragms, cervical caps)	Menarche onward	1
Copper-bearing intrauterine device	Menarche to <20 years	2
	≥20 years	1
Levonorgestrel-releasing intrauterine system	Menarche to <20 years	2
	≥20 years	1

DMPA, depot medroxyprogesterone acetate; NET-EN, norethisterone enantate.

Reproduced from Faculty of Sexual health and Reproductive Healthcare. (2010b). Contraceptive Choices for Young People Clinical Guidance. Reproduced from http://www.fsrh.org

has yet to be fully available. In the United States a lack of insurance coverage, particularly young people who want to keep their sexual health confidential and not shared to their parents whose insurance may cover access, continues to be a barrier to diagnosis and treatment.

A group of young people of particular concern are those who go on to have repeat pregnancies in the teenage years, both in the United Kingdom and globally. Among young women younger than 20 years old in England and Wales, there has been a significant increase in the proportion of abortions that are subsequent to a previous birth and an increase in the number of abortions subsequent to a previous abortion (Collier, 2009; Collier, 2014). Globally, the World Health Organization (WHO) (Ganchimeg et al., 2014) reports that there is radical increase in the proportion of abortions that are subsequent to a previous abortion. From personal observation in the United Kingdom some abortion providers are setting staff targets to engage with clients who are medically eligible to consent to the administration of long-acting reversible contraceptives (LARC) on the same day, following the abortion. Teen pregnancy is a marker for future sexual risk behavior. Service providers are urged to consider this group a priority for sexual health interventions.

Unintended pregnancy in young women can have several adverse outcomes such as an inability to complete school education, which may limit future social and economic opportunities; abandonment by their partners; and an increase in complications of childbirth and for the infant (Oringanje et al., 2010). Practitioners are challenged to provide a youth-friendly service that young people will avail of and return to throughout their transition to adulthood.

Male Sexual and Reproductive Health

Women have a limited reproductive phase in their life, from puberty to menopause, yet men remain fertile from puberty to the end of their life. Female fertility is easier to control and influence, as only one egg a month is normally released. At each ejaculation men release millions of sperm with the potential to fertilize the female egg. Complete control over male fertility, as a consequence, is more difficult to achieve. In this section, progress on the development of male contraception will be discussed. Advances in gender issues and, in particular, problems faced by transgender persons will be explored.

The pace of progress in research into male contraception has been slow. Both hormonal and nonhormonal methods disrupt male fertility by one or more mechanisms. Methods comprise suppression of sperm production, disruption of sperm maturation, or the disruption of sperm transport or motility. Although records indicate 80 years of research, available options for male contraception are restricted to condoms, vasectomy, withdrawal, and abstinence (Dorman & Bishai, 2012).

Nonhormonal Male Contraception

Nonhormonal methods aim to disrupt the production, function, or motility of sperm. Blockage of the flow of sperm has been studied. One method in China under development is a temporary and reversible vasectomy. The intravas device consists of tiny implants that block the flow of sperm through the vas deferens. Alternatively, a chemical injection of gel into the vas that inactivates sperm has been developed. Both involve interventions that demand medical expertise and acceptability. Oral drugs known to stop ejaculation during orgasm need further work to improve the adverse effects on blood pressure and mood. Preliminary work in the United States reviewed by Dorman and Bishai (2012), has been the development of immunology using antigens and antibodies to induce infertility. The safety of these nonhormonal methods has yet to be demonstrated. Condom use and vasectomy are covered in other chapters.

Hormonal Contraception

In a review of chemical trials performed over the previous 15 years, Liu, Swerdloff, and Wang (2010) examined studies of hormonal male contraception aimed at reducing sperm output and thereby regulating male fertility. Modern androgen and androgen-progestin combinations were found to suppress sperm production in 80–95% of men. Universal suppression of sperm in all men was seen to be unrealistic and work has focused on predicting which men would be suitable for male hormonal contraception. For example, ethnicity was identified as a possible factor. Confusion has arisen because Caucasian men suppressed sperm output faster initially but to a lesser extent than Asian men (Mahmoud & T'Sjoen, 2012).

In evaluating the success of male hormonal contraception, adverse effects are closely monitored. Short-term adverse effects included acne, fatigue, night sweats, increased weight, aggression, altered mood, disturbed sleep, libido change, and reduced testes size. These adverse effects create a high commercial and litigation risk for the pharmaceutical industry, especially in the United States. Long-term adverse effects have yet to be assessed, until male hormonal contraception is more widely available. Despite these effects multiple global studies (Liu, Swerdloff, & Wang, 2010) indicate that male hormonal contraception was acceptable to couples. Full recovery of spermatogenesis was seen to be realistic after hormonal contraception regimens, with an average of 4 to 5 months required for full recovery of normal sperm concentration. A 2- to 3-month delay in action of male hormonal contraception compared favorably to vasectomy. This delay in suppression and recovery of spermatogenesis is partly explained by the time taken to produce spermatozoa, which is 64 days on average (Mahmoud & T'Sjoen, 2012).

The method of hormonal administration has been varied. Ilani et al. (2012) reported results of a randomized trial of a combination testosterone and progestin gel demonstrating successful suppression of sperm concentration in nearly 90% of men. This combination of hormones in a gel is seen as the most promising regimen so far (Mahmoud & T'Sjoen, 2012).

The tolerability, though, of testosterone in either parenteral or subdermal delivery is called into question (Dorman & Bishai, 2012). The authors report discomfort at the injection site and injection schedules such as weekly injection being unacceptable. With transdermal gels, the need for daily application of the gel and the potential of transfer to female partners or children as a concern was explained by Chao et al. (2014). Long-acting testosterone preparations such as implants are being studied. In a multicenter study in Germany, Chile, and the Dominican Republic, work is continuing to develop implants that release high levels of hormone over a sustained period, such as a year (Nieschlag, Kumar, & Sitruk-Ware, 2013).

However, the challenge remains to develop methods that render males infertile and are fully reversible and safe for long-term use, as men may practice the method over many years. Advantages of hormonal male contraception comprise easy reversibility and a lack of interference with sexual pleasure. Many of the methods developed have had adverse effects or poor acceptability. There is still no commercially viable option for male contraception. Dorman and Bishai (2012) suggest that if methods could be developed that have an additional benefit to men's health, similar to oral contraception in women where the risk of endometrial and ovarian cancer has been reduced, further investment may be attracted from the pharmaceutical companies. To progress with research into male contraception, further multicultural and long-term studies are needed to measure the side effects, efficacy of birth control, and reliable reversibility of the methods. Funding for these studies will depend on government bodies or agencies such as the World Health Organization (WHO).

Gender Identity Issues and Advances in Transgender Knowledge

Increasingly, gender issues have come more to the fore in the media and public domain. In the United Kingdom three specialist units provide services of genital and gonadal male-to-female reassignment procedures for 480 patients annually (Suchak et al., 2015). Transgender is an umbrella term for individuals whose gender presentation is different to the sex assigned to them at birth. It includes intersex people who are born with both female and male sex characteristics. They often will have undergone surgery to construct genitals that are definitely male or female. Their internal organs, however, remain different to their external presentation. It also includes transmen, transwomen, butch women, and crossdressers (Levitt & Ippolito, 2014). Transgender can be differentiated between male-to-female transgender women who were assigned a male identity at birth but identify as female and female-to-male transgender men who were assigned a female identity at birth but identify as male (Reisner, White, Mayer, & Mimiaga, 2014).

Researchers in the United States (Levitt & Ippolito, 2014) reported that some patients suffer extreme mental turmoil as they hide their true self from family and friends.

Some turn to drug or alcohol addiction to escape. They are a vulnerable and at-risk group. Some suffer social isolation and stares by the public and search for affirming communities to provide safety and support. They may find a safe place to experiment in their identity-development process, away from their homes, frequently in cities. A U.K. transgender person who has lived exclusively in their new gender for at least 2 years can apply for a gender recognition certificate. Once they have this certificate, they can obtain a new birth certificate (Suchak et al., 2015).

Evidence from Guatemala suggests that transgender persons, in common with other sexual minorities, are disproportionately affected by HIV, AIDS, and STIs, notably syphilis. The epidemic of HIV is concentrated in Guatemala City. Alcohol and drug use was reported as a leading cause of unprotected sex. Some of the study participants reported the need for housing options, as they found themselves homeless after parents and families ejected them from the home. The families did not accept their gender change. Some transgender persons sold sex to survive in the city (Rhodes et al., 2014).

Evidence from Boston, Massachusetts examined HIV and STI sexual risk behavior in female-to-male transgender men. The authors (Reisner et al., 2014) report that there can be a synergistic effect in the lives of transgender individuals. Under conditions of social marginalization, mental health and psychosocial problems such as depression, anxiety, psychological stress, and violence are frequently reported in transgender persons. They are vulnerable to HIV-risk behaviors. In a study of 23 transgender men, use of hormones such as testosterone was frequently reported. Some had had top surgery (mastectomy and chest reconstruction) and/or abdominal surgery, hysterectomy, or oophorectomy. Over half of the transgender men studied identified as bisexual and had diverse sexual identities. Changes in sexual attractions, identities, and behaviors throughout the gender transition are described. Some transgender men engage in both receptive anal and frontal vaginal sex. Clinicians need to be aware of this diversity and be specific in history taking about sexual behaviors, to identify risk (Reisner et al., 2014).

Testosterone treatment and chest reconstruction can positively affect the mental health and sexuality of female-to-male transgender men. In a study of 210 transgender men, participants in San Francisco who were receiving testosterone endorsed fewer symptoms of anxiety and depression as well as less anger than the untreated group (Davis & Meier, 2014). Participants who had chest reconstruction surgery as well as testosterone treatment reported less body dissatisfaction than the control group. Some transgender persons in the United States report unfavorable experiences of medical care and health insurance providers (Roller, Sedlak, & Draucker, 2015). Many experienced uncertainty and ambivalence when engaging with healthcare professionals and systems not prepared to meet their primary care and transition-related health needs. Indeed, in a study of 433 transgender persons in Ontario,

Canada, the negative experiences with providers, along with limited financial resources and a lack of access to transition-related services, led to nonprescribed hormone use and self-performed surgery. Participants had obtained hormones from nonmedical sources and others reported having performed or attempted surgical procedures on themselves such as orchiectomy or mastectomy (Rotondi et al., 2013). Work in the United States has been done to identify (Khalili, Leung, Diamant, 2015) health professionals who are LGBT competent. Where professional training was available, the professionals were more willing to develop policies and procedures for caring for this minority group. There are several issues to consider. For example, data on computer programs normally requires a definitive male or female classification. Individuals may vary in their gender identity as they go through the transition process. Policies need to be developed that all staff agree to stay with the client's original identity or the changed identity. Alternatively, the data needs a facility for altering gender according to the one expressed that day by the client. An e-learning course for general practitioners open to all healthcare professionals can be accessed at http://elearning.rcgp.org.uk/gendervariance.

While more transgender persons emerge from secrecy, healthcare services will be challenged to provide the mental health support, STI screening, and hormonal and surgical treatment for the gender change process. As we develop a better understanding of individual gender transition processes, we can plan and secure funding for the care of this minority group.

People with Learning Disability

In the United Kingdom, the primary healthcare team can have a small caseload of people with learning disability (PLD) and work with the community disability teams to meet those needs. Many healthcare professionals have little or no training in this role and have been open to criticism (McCarthy, 2010). In the United States, Quint (2016) explains the clinical challenges that may be experienced in caring for teenagers with special needs. Parents may seek anticipatory guidance from health professionals in identifying their options. Menstrual avoidance can be a priority if hygiene is problematic already. Some teenagers are unable to tolerate dysmenorrhea or the mood fluctuations associated with the menstrual cycle.

A recent inquiry (Hollins & Tuffrey-Wijne, 2013) highlights failings in the delivery of care to people with learning disabilities. Deaths in the United Kingdom were reviewed and it was found that men with severe learning disabilities died on average 13 years earlier than men in the general population, and that this figure was 20 years for women. Intellectual disability mortality reviews established in 15 U.S. states have been shown to be effective. Suggestions were made that families should be included as care partners, and their care should be adjusted to take account of particular vulnerabilities, which would include unwanted pregnancy and STIs.

Learning disability has a spectrum from mild and moderate to severe and profound, with an increase in autistic spectrum disorders and attention deficit hyperactivity disorders (Quint, 2016). Article 5 of the International Planned Parenthood Federation Declaration (2008) on sexual rights states that everyone has the right to sexual freedom, which encompasses the opportunity for individuals to have control and decide freely on matters related to sexuality, and to choose their sexual partners. As teenagers with special needs approach adolescence, they may experience challenges that affect them and their caregivers.

It is the assessment of capacity to consent to a plan of care that challenges the health professional. Communication problems during the consultation, along with a lack of time to conduct an adequate consultation, difficulties in obtaining a health history, and patient inhibitions make for barriers for PLD seeking healthcare (McCarthy, 2010). In England changes in the law with the implementation of the Mental Capacity Act (Office of the Public Guardian, 2007) mean that a client must be presumed competent unless demonstrated otherwise. Serious decisions such as sterilization or abortion are dealt with by the Court of Protection. Mental capacity is defined as the ability to make decisions or take actions oneself. A person is unable to make a decision if they cannot do one of the following:

- Understand the information given to them
- Retain the information long enough to make the decision
- Use or weigh up the information as part of the decision-making process
- Communicate their decision (Rowlands, 2011)

Information needs to be presented to these patients in simplified language or by use of visual aids such as pictures, objects, or electronic media. Professionals must consider also the views of anyone engaged in caring for the person or who is interested in their welfare (Rowlands, 2011). The health professional also has to balance the rights of the carer to support and the rights of the PLD to privacy and confidentiality. In a project where women with learning disability were interviewed about their experience gaining contraception, McCarthy (2010) found that women appreciated a companion being present and the majority of physicians interviewed also found it helpful. However, a lack of autonomy in decision-making about contraceptive use was reported by women in the study. While the Mental Capacity Act (Department of Health, 2005) requires that people be supported in making their decisions, the others involved may take over. The sexual partner of the client or the client's parents may seek to impose their views. The health professional is required to make a formal assessment of capacity to consent. If the PLD is incompetent, the Mental Capacity Act Code of Practice (Office of the Public Guardian, 2007) needs to be followed.

Records need to include the following:

- How the decision about the person's best interest was reached
- What the reasons for reaching the decision were
- Who was consulted to help work out the best interests
- What particular factors were taken into account

Conflicts have arisen for professionals between the protection of the client from pregnancy and empowerment of the client. There has been a disproportionate use of DMPA, IUDs, and sterilization for women with disability. These methods require no active participation (McCarthy, 2010; Rowlands, 2011). A balance is needed between protection and empowerment. Many women with learning disabilities often live isolated lives, making them vulnerable to sexual abuse. Health professionals are expected to be aware of the signs and symptoms of abuse. Educational initiatives have been developed to empower PLD (http://www.fpa.org.uk). Training is provided by the Family Planning Association for health professionals on legal issues and working effectively with PLD. The Open University (Bodley-Tickell et al., 2015) has useful guidance on talking about sex, sexuality, and relationships for those working with young people with life-limiting or life-threatening conditions.

Appropriate sex education and use of emergency contraception are the way forward to counter real concerns of unwanted pregnancy in teenagers who are mildly intellectually disabled. O'Connor (2011) details the challenges experienced by mothers with learning disability, such as poverty, anxiety, social isolation, and poor support for such crisis pregnancies. In the United States a study using longitudinal data collected in Massachusetts identified an increase in negative birth outcomes in women with intellectual and developmental disabilities. The study found a low rate of paternity establishment, which resulted in a lack of paternal involvement in parenthood (Mitra, Parish, Clements, Cui, & Diop, 2015). The Mental Capacity Act (Department of Health, 2005) has clarified the referral path for the disability team to take in seeking the judgment of the Court of Protection in cases where the client lacks the capacity to make health-related decisions. Effective contraception may be one of those decisions. As sterilization laws vary from state to state in the United States, the American Congress of Obstetricians and Gynecologists recommends that hysterectomy solely for the purpose of sterilization should not usually be performed (Quint, 2016).

Clients with Mental Health Issues

Clients with established mental health issues may be undergoing prescribed treatment regimens that could interact with hormonal contraceptives. The Faculty of Sexual and Reproductive Health (2017) have produced comprehensive guidance about drug interactions and hormonal contraceptive methods. Women should be asked about their current and previous drug use, including prescription, over-the-counter, herbal, and recreational drugs and dietary supplements. For example, St. John's Wort, an herbal remedy taken to relieve depression, is an enzyme-inducing drug that may interfere with the absorption of estrogen and progesterone.

Wirehn, Foldemo, Josefsson, and Lindberg (2010) investigated the link between hormonal contraceptives and antidepressant therapy in Sweden. They found that antidepressant therapy use was higher in users of progesterone-only therapy including, injections, implants, and patches, in every age group, but particularly among women 16 to 19 years old. This study used a population register and it was not possible to investigate variables such as life events that may cause depression. The use of antidepressants was higher in the progesterone-only users compared to the combined hormonal methods. The authors suggest progesterone-only contraceptives are a precipitating or perpetuating factor in mood disorders in vulnerable women and this should be taken into account in giving contraceptive advice. As well as the burden of depression, the risk of suicide is increased.

Attention is drawn to the link between depression and adverse reproductive health. Women are more likely to self-harm and attempt suicide if they have experienced childhood abuse or sexual or domestic violence. The World Health Organization (2009), in a global review of the literature, calls on family planning programs to be aware of how psychological issues related to sexuality can affect health. The authors argue that the relationship between broader situational and interpersonal determinants of contraceptive use, decision-making and the development of emotional distress, depression and other psychological disorders in women has not been adequately investigated. Women may not comply with use or be consistent in the use of contraceptives if they lack autonomy at home.

Often, the practitioner will signpost clients to further help for STIs, including HIV/AIDS, reproductive tract surgery, sterilization, premarital pregnancy, menopause, and infertility. Listening to clients and knowing local services is part of sexual health work.

Sexual Health Problems Among Clients in Prison

There has been increasing awareness over the last decade of how disadvantaged women in the prison system can be helped by access to sexual and reproductive services. Because of their short time in prison, it may be thought not worthwhile to provide such access, particularly if the prisoner has to be transported to specialist services outside of prison. In the United States, Sufrin, Kolbi-Molinas, and Roth (2015) report that the majority of incarcerated women are not allowed to continue birth control methods that they were already using, and very few facilities provide on-site access to contraceptives in preparation for their release. This lapse in use of effective contraceptives puts women at risk of unintended pregnancies when they are released.

In a cross-sectional study of newly arrested women in a busy urban jail in San Francisco, Sufrin, Tulsky, Goldenson, Winter, and Cohanet (2010) examined the proportion and characteristics of women who would be eligible and willing to take emergency contraception upon incarceration. Subjects (n = 290) completed a 20-minute audio computer-assisted interview survey. Nearly one-third of these newly arrested women had had unprotected sex within 5 days of coming to jail, and half of them would take emergency contraception if offered to them. The cohort was representative of incarcerated women in the United States who are likely to be of reproductive age, poorly educated, and from ethnic minority groups.

Subsequently, the Sufrin et al. (2015) studied the feasibility of providing long-acting reversible contraception at the initial women's health exam at entry to prison. Of those who accepted either an implant or intrauterine device, the median duration of known use was 11–13 months.

During imprisonment in the United States, Pardue, Bruce, and Murphy (2011) describe a spectrum of sexual behaviors reported in prisons involving extensive sexual victimization, exploitation, and sexual violence perpetrated by other prisoners. They report that incarcerated women have significantly higher rates of STIs compared to the general population.

Certain groups, such as lesbian, gay, bisexual, and transgender (LGBT) persons, are at increased risk of HIV infection and are vulnerable to increased stigma and discrimination inside and outside prison (Torriente, Tadion, & Hsu, 2016). There is a higher incidence of HIV and hepatitis in prisoners. Williams, Axten, Makia, Teague, and Fox (2011) report that 15% to 20% of prisoners in HM Prison Brixton in the United Kingdom are HIV positive. In the United States, the rate of HIV infection in prison was estimated to be nearly 13 times as high as the general population (Fogul et al., 2015). HIV and hepatitis C screening is not offered universally to all prisoners. While imprisoned, some prisoners are more likely to adopt riskier lifestyles, such as sharing needles (**Figure 11-5**).

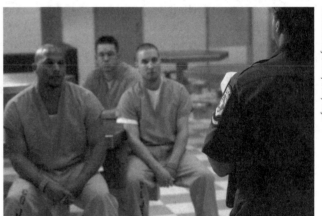

Figure 11-5 Sexual Health in Jail

A Hepatitis B vaccination programme for prisoners has the potential to significantly decrease the incidence of the disease in all injecting drug users countrywide. For that reason, it is now policy that hepatitis B immunization is recommended for all sentenced prisoners and all new inmates entering prison in the United Kingdom (Public Health England, 2016). There has also been an increase in the uptake of screening for chlamydia in prisons, which is encouraging further its infectious disease prevention work in prisons. A national survey of sexual health services in U.K. prisons (Tang, Maw, & Kell, 2010) revealed a wide variation in the quality of services provided. Tang (2011) has outlined a framework for further involvement of genitourinary services in prison and urges sexual health professionals to respond positively to the commissioning of services being located in prisons, rather than prisoners coming to hospital service in shackles. In the same year, the British Association for Sexual Health and HIV (BASHH, 2011) issued guidance for commissioning sexual health services in prisons. One of the key performance indicators was to have access to a voluntary genitourinary service on-site, in prison. There is a potential for women to feel coerced into contraceptive methods, such as sterilization, in some cases. There are reports that over 100 women in California's prison system were unlawfully sterilized from 2006–2010 (Sufrin et al., 2015).

Positive interventions point the way for future service development. In the United States Fogul et al. (2015) conducted a randomized controlled trial with 52 incarcerated women aged 18 to 60 years in correctional facilities in North Carolina. The authors used an adapted existing HIV/STI intervention program. Over an average of 5.8 sessions, the intervention group engaged in discussions about risk reduction both in prison and after release. At 6 months after release from prison, the intervention group reported less risky behavior, such as having unprotected sex with a non-main partner, and increased condom use with their main partner.

Sufrin et al. (2010) argue that by addressing the reproductive health needs of this marginalized high-risk population, the provision of contraceptives and treatment of infections would contribute to the larger goals of reducing health disparities in the United States.

Commercial Sex Workers

Sex workers are defined as female, male, and transgender adults and young people who receive money or goods in exchange for sexual services, either regularly or occasionally, who may or may not consciously define their activities as income generating (UNAIDS, 2002). Sex workers may not disclose their occupation voluntarily, particularly if they are underage or a victim of trafficking. Women selling sex experience a disproportionate burden of sexually transmitted diseases including HIV (Robertson et al., 2014). Multiagency outreach projects have proved successful. The evidence differentiates between street sex workers and indoor sex workers. Indoor sex work refers to the exchange of sex for money in settings where the negotiation of the exchange does not occur in a street-based setting. Common indoor settings include massage parlors, escort agencies, bars, hotels, and apartments. In a Canadian study examining the sexual health and safety practices of massage-parlor-based sex workers and clients, Kolar, Atchison, and Bungay (2014) reported high rates of condom use for vaginal/anal intercourse. Both groups, sex workers and their clients, reported lower rates of condom use for oral sex during sex transactions. Condom use with non-commercial sex partners was reported to be less consistent by both groups. STI testing was higher among sex workers than clients. Initiatives targeting clients of massage-parlor-based sex workers for STI education and testing are needed.

These results support previous research suggesting that education and outreach initiatives in Vancouver may be positively impacting condom use and STI and HIV testing among these populations. Parlor-based sex workers tended to be younger, single, have lower levels of education, and more often identified as immigrants and from minority groups than clients.

Pursuing the link between sex work and drugs, Robertson et al. (2014) studied street-based female sex workers on the northern Mexican border. Drug use, including injecting drug use, is common and compromises the female sex workers' ability to negotiate safe sex. In these cities along the Mexican border, female sex workers' HIV positivity was associated with smoking, snorting, inhaling, and injecting drugs. The authors examined the behaviors of female sex workers with their non-commercial male partners, with whom they were less likely to have protected sex. Nearly 1 in 10 of non-commercial partners tested positive for HIV/AIDS. In common with Kolar et al. (2014), they too recommended more intervention programs aimed at the regular male partners.

Another initiative is hepatitis B vaccination. Hepatitis B virus (HBV) is a blood-borne virus that causes hepatitis and can cause long-term liver damage. It can be transmitted by sexual contact. Outreach health professionals from specialist sexual health services are involved in massage parlors and other gay venues, offering testing and vaccination.

Caution is urged in studying sex workers. They are a clandestine and mobile group, which makes follow up difficult. Other negative ramifications of targeting sex workers for sexual health promotion are stigma and violence that could drive sex workers further underground (Shahmanesh, Patel, Mabey, & Cowan, 2008).

Challenges of Sexual Health Care for Clients with Specific Medical Conditions

With advances in modern medicine, increasing numbers of women with severe health complications are living longer and are considering planning a family. For some, the toll of a pregnancy on their physical well-being necessitates them being closely monitored under consultant care in the pregnancy, with periods of hospitalization. This can cause stress in the family network, especially if there are other children needing care. After childbirth, the mother and baby may take some time to recover and another pregnancy is not planned for a long time. Effective contraception for this group is particularly important and may be life preserving. There is some evidence that, as a group, they are less likely to plan a pregnancy. Chor, Rankin, Harwood, and Handler (2011) followed up new mothers with chronic medical disease in Florida and compared their pregnancy plans—intended pregnancy—with a control group. More women in the group with chronic medical disease were likely not to have planned their pregnancy. The authors recommended that more contraceptive advice needs to be given to this group to help avoid unintended pregnancy and reduce potential morbidity and mortality.

Moreover, there is a misperception of the risks of hormonal contraception. Nelson and Rezvan (2011) studied women's knowledge of the health risks of pregnancy and how their assessment of pregnancy risks compared to estimates of oral contraception risks. Of 248 women surveyed on a research institute campus in California, over one-quarter of women could not correctly name any health risk associated with pregnancy. Over 75% of respondents rated birth control pills more hazardous to a woman's health than pregnancy. For women with chronic medical conditions, the risks of pregnancy are even higher. These women have more disjointed health care with many health professionals and are already taking many medications. Some health professionals may be reluctant to advise due to the complexity of the case and lack of familiarity with different contraceptive methods (Chor et al., 2011). A major advance has been taken by the WHO (2015) publishing the *Medical Eligibility Criteria for Contraceptive Use*. This provides evidence-based recommendations on whether an individual can safely take a contraceptive method. The Faculty of Reproductive and Sexual Health (2016) has published summary sheets for use in the United Kingdom differentiating between the criteria for initiating a method or the client developing a condition that may restrict her from continuing with the method. These simple tables have made it much easier to make clinical judgments about the suitability of the method. Furthermore, the Faculty of Reproductive and Sexual Health Care Clinical Effectiveness Unit (2017) has guidance which tabulates the effects of drugs on the absorption of hormonal contraception, particularly liver enzyme-inducing drugs that interfere with hormonal absorption. The methods of absorption and metabolism of different groups of drugs are explained. Potential drug interactions between medications and hormonal contraceptives can be checked using an online drug interaction checker such as

http://reference.medscape.com/drug-interactionchecker. In the United States, the CDC (2016b) has published similar guidelines for practitioners.

Epilepsy

Epileptic women controlled on certain anti-epileptic drugs may find their contraceptive choices restricted. Some drugs induce liver enzymes that reduce the efficacy of combined hormonal contraception and progesterone-only contraception. In particular, combined hormonal contraception may increase the clearance of lamotrigine monotherapy and the clearance of sodium valproate if taken as monotherapy (FSRH, 2017); seizure frequency may increase. Some levels of progesterone may be reduced by lamotrigine, but data have yet to be finalized. Caution is required in using hormonal methods with anti-epileptic drugs and the latest guidance followed. Currently, the Faculty of Sexual and Reproductive Health Care (2017) do not consider the efficacy of the progestogen-only injectable or intrauterine methods to be affected by these enzyme-inducing drugs.

Epileptic women who require emergency contraception while using liver enzyme-inducing drugs are advised that an intrauterine device is the preferred option. As well as a careful choice of contraceptive methods, some anti-epileptic drugs that give good seizure control are teratogenic. Epileptic women preparing for pregnancy will need careful contraceptive support while changing anti-epileptic medication to nonharmful drugs. Their lifestyles may be disrupted by increased seizures. It is suggested that partners are taught resuscitation skills. There are case reports of sudden unexpected death in childbearing women with epilepsy who discontinued their anti-epileptic medication without seeking medical advice (Knight et al., 2015), believing that they were seizure free. Sudden unexpected death in childbearing women with epilepsy occurred when alone with their baby. Decisions are taken on an individual basis, weighing up the risks of the contraceptive against the risks of an unwanted pregnancy.

Obesity

Another common example is obesity. Overweight and obesity are determined with the body mass index (BMI) based on a weight to height ratio. Frequently used BMI categories are 25–29.9 (kg/m2) for overweight and 30 or higher for obesity (Lopez, Grimes, Gallo, & Schulz, 2010). In a Cochrane review, Lopez et al. (2010) examined the evidence that metabolic changes and greater body mass may lead to reduced effectiveness of hormonal contraception. Two studies of the implant and one of the injectable contraceptive suggested that the methods may be unaffected by body mass. One trial examined hormonal contraception and found a higher pregnancy risk for overweight women. The authors concluded that the evidence on effectiveness due to obesity is limited for specific contraceptive methods. When women develop a BMI over 35 kg/m2, the risks, namely venous thromboembolism, of continuing on the combined hormonal methods outweigh the advantages. A progesterone-only method is advised.

Having established that obese women have limited contraceptive choices, unplanned pregnancy could be dangerous for this group. Obesity is a risk factor in maternal death in childbirth (The Centre for Maternal and Child Enquiries [CMACE] & the Royal College of Obstetricians and Gynaecologists [RCOG], 2010). Serious adverse outcomes that are more prevalent are miscarriage, fetal congenital anomaly, thromboembolism, gestational diabetes, pre-eclampsia, dysfunctional labor, postpartum hemorrhage, wound infections, stillbirth, and neonatal death. Inter-pregnancy weight reduction among women with obesity has been shown to significantly reduce the risk of developing gestational diabetes. CMACE and RCOG (2010) advise that all women of reproductive age should be urged to optimize their weight before pregnancy. Advice on weight, particularly for women with a BMI of 30 kg/m2 or more, should be included in contraceptive consultations and weight and body mass index should be regularly monitored.

The importance of pre-conception care is outlined further by the authors of the *Saving Mothers' Lives Report* in the United Kingdom (Knight et al., 2014). Women with pre-existing serious medical or mental health conditions that may be aggravated by pregnancy should be counseled and supported to prepare for pregnancy. As well as obese women and epileptics, women with diabetes, those with auto-immune disorders, severe pre-existing or past mental illness, and cardiac disease should be identified for pre-conception care, which may require referral to a specialist physician. The health of women with medical conditions, especially rare disorders and multiple morbidities should be reviewed prior to conception to identify any potential pregnancy-related risks. All women should undergo a documented assessment of risk factors for venous thromboembolism in pre-pregnancy (Knight et al., 2015). Poor maternal preconception health in the United States is identified as contributing to infant mortality (Senie, 2014).

Chronically ill physically disabled women who are immobile will find contraceptive choices restricted due to risk of venous thromboembolism. Similarly, if women have multiple risks factors for cardiovascular disease, they are less likely to be prescribed combined hormonal methods. The proven risks of using combined hormonal contraception outweigh the advantages of use for this group (FSRH, 2016). However, other methods such as progesterone-only contraception or the intrauterine device are considered suitable while preparing for optimum health before a pregnancy, or at least avoiding an unplanned pregnancy.

Guiding the client with medical health complications to an effective contraceptive choice may be problematic, yet the alternative of an unplanned pregnancy may have further adverse health and social consequences.

Elderly Clients and "Hidden" Sexual Health Problems

Sexuality in the older person can be the subject of triviality and mirth with others either ignoring or deriding the sexual health needs of the elderly (Kessel, 2001). From a public health perspective the rise in people over 45 attending genitourinary medicine clinics, with those age 55 to 59 years of age being significantly more likely to be infected, gives cause for concern (Bodley-Ticknall et al., 2011). The CDC (2015) report that in the United States people aged 55 and older accounted for one-quarter of all Americans living with HIV in 2012 and that older Americans are more likely to be diagnosed with HIV infection later in the course of their disease. They recommend routine HIV/AIDS testing to those under 65 years and assessing risk factors for those over 65 with counseling for HIV/AIDS testing where indicated (**Figure 11-6**).

Studies of the sexual health of the elderly are few and have their limitations, due to the sensitivity and complexity of the subject. The reader will note the varying age ranges given for defining the "older person," as well as the real difficulties of recruiting subjects willing to participate in research.

Evidence-based knowledge that has emerged is that a lack of partner and a lack of privacy affects the ability to enjoy sex. Elderly living in institutions find a lack of privacy particularly difficult. Some older people were embarrassed to attempt intercourse if caught by their children.

According to an Australian study, male health problems seemed to be the primary reason for ceasing sexual activity (Hyde et al., 2010). Medical factors such as osteoporosis, prostate cancer, diabetes, and partner's physical limitations were associated with reduced sexual activity. Medication use affects sexual performance. Use of antidepressants affects

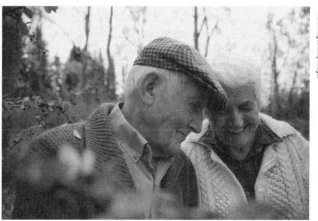

Figure 11-6 Sexual Health in Older People

sex, particularly selective serotonin reuptake inhibitors, which are associated with sexual difficulties. In an Australian population-based cohort study, those elderly men taking beta-blockers were more likely to be sexually inactive (Hyde et al., 2010). Advances in the treatment of erectile dysfunction have varying success. Male-centered sexual fulfilment is culturally conceptualized as being focused on penile penetration. Gledhill and Schweitzer (2014) found in an Australian qualitative study that pharmaceuticals for sexual enhancement can have disappointing results, yet sexual desire can persist regardless of age, health, or sexual function. However, a careful history and examination will elicit risk factors such as cardiovascular disease, relationship problems, or previous sexual abuse. Enquiries about early morning erections and successful masturbation are made. A measure of morning testosterone levels is suggested, as hypogonadism may be the cause. In the United Kingdom in 75% of patients at low risk of cardiovascular disease, treatment with oral phosphodiesterase inhibitors is successful (Edwards & Bunker, 2011). Addressing risk factors such as depression, diabetes, and medication use may improve sexual activity for some (Hyde et al., 2010). Films, literature, and devices designed to increase sexual pleasure can help men overcome difficulties with achieving or maintaining an erection. Penile rings have been found to help men maintain an erection in an Australia and U.K. review, and a penile pump can help with achieving an erection (Buttaro, Koeniger-Donohue, & Hawkins, 2014). Increased physical activity has been suggested to help erectile dysfunction for obese men (Wylie, Wood, & Abbasi, 2011).

Inappropriate sexual behavior is seen in older persons with dementia, particularly men (Ni Lochlainn & Kenny, 2013). This can cause a conflict between respecting the patient's autonomy and preventing emotional and physical trauma for the patient and others. Behavioral therapy and pharmacological therapy are indicated, but as yet there is no clear evidence on the treatments.

For women, the most common problems are lack of estrogen, frequent lower urinary tract infections, problems with arousal and achieving orgasm, lack of libido, pain with intercourse, and negative body image. The use of lubricants, vaginal estrogen tablets, rings, or creams, when appropriate, help significantly in treating the dyspareunia associated with menopause. These may also help vaginal dryness associated with chronic atrophic vaginitis (Buttaro et al., 2014). Use of vibrators may help with stimulation. There is also an association between obesity and lower satisfaction in women's sexual life. Illnesses such as cardiovascular disorders and joint or muscle problems can be disabling and have a negative effect on well-being and self-esteem.

Some accept a lack of sexual interest as part of aging. Gledhill and Schweitzer (2014) argue that acknowledgement of the older person as a sexual being is slow to develop in Western society. A knowledge of sexual aids is advised. Concerns about comorbidities and polypharmacy in older adults limit the biomedical approach (Buttaro et al., 2014).

Conclusion

In conclusion, when clients are identified as being in a special client group, practitioners need to be aware of the latest national medical eligibility criteria for contraceptive methods, such as Medical Eligibility Criteria for Contraceptive Use (World Health Organization, 2015), the U.S. Centers for Disease Control (2016b), and U.K. Faculty of Sexual and Reproductive Healthcare (2016). In clients with complicated medical histories, specialist medical help should be sought to recommend the most effective contraceptive and sexual health advice available. Knowledge of local and web-based specialist referral agencies will help.

● ● ● REFERENCES

Bodley-Tickell, A. T., Olowokure, B., Bhaduri, S., White, D. J., Ward, D., & Ross, J. D. C. (2011). Trends in sexually transmitted infections (other than HIV) in older people: Analysis of data from an enhanced surveillance system. *Sexually Transmitted Infections, 84*(4): 312–317.

British Association for Sexual Health and HIV (BASHH). (2011). *National guidance on commissioning sexual health and blood borne virus services in prisons*. Retrieved from http://www.bashh.org/documents/3829.pdf

Brittain, A., Williams, J., Zapata, L., Pazol, K., & Romero, L. (2015). Youth-friendly family planning services for young people: A systematic review. *American Journal of Preventive Medicine, 49*(2S1):S73–S84.

Buttaro, T., Koeniger-Donohue, R., & Hawkins, J. (2014). Sexuality and quality of life in aging: Implications for practice. *Journal for Nurse Practitioners, 10*(7): 480–485.

Centers for Disease Control and Prevention (CDC). (2013). *Teens visiting a health clinic*. Retrieved from http://www.cdc.gov/teenpregnancy/health-care-providers/teen-friendly-health-visit.htm

Centers for Disease Control and Prevention (CDC). (2015). HIV among older Americans. Retrieved from http://www.cdc.gov/hiv/risk/age/olderamericans/index.html. (Updated October 7, 2015; accessed September 9, 2017).

Centers for Disease Control and Prevention (CDC). (2016a). *Social determinants and eliminating disparities in teen pregnancy*. Retrieved from https://www.cdc.gov/teenpregnancy/about/social-determinants-disparities-teen-pregnancy.htm

Centers for Disease Control and Prevention (CDC). (2016b). *US medical eligibility criteria (US MEC) for contraceptive use* (5th ed.). Retrieved from https://www.cdc.gov/reproductivehealth/contraception/mmwr/mec/intro.html

Centre for Maternal and Child Enquiries (CMACE) and the Royal College of Obstetricians and Gynaecologists (RCOG). (2010). *Management of women with obesity in pregnancy*. Retrieved from https://www.rcog.org.uk/en/guidelines-research-services/guidelines/management-of-women-with-obesity-in-pregnancy/

Champion, J., & Roye, C. (2014). Toward an understanding of the context of anal sex behavior in ethnic minority adolescent women. *Issues in Mental Health Nursing, 35*, 509–516.

Chao, J., Page, S., & Anderson, R. (2014). Male contraception. *Best Practice & Research: Clinical Obstetrics & Gynacology, 28*, 845–857.

Chor, J., Rankin, K., Harwood, B., & Handler, A. (2011). Unintended pregnancy and postpartum contraceptive use in women with and without chronic medical disease who experienced a live birth. *Contraception, 84*(1), 57–63.

Collier, J. (2009). The rising proportion of repeat teenage pregnancies in young women presenting for termination of pregnancy from 1991 to 2007. *Contraception, 79*(5), 393–396.

Collier, J. (2014). The rising proportion of repeat teenage pregnancies in young women presenting for termination of pregnancy from 1991 to 2007. *Contraception, 89*(5), 475–477.

Cook, S., & Cameron, C. (2015). Social issues of teenage pregnancy. *Obstetrics, Gynaecology, and Reproductive Medicine, 25*(9), 243–248.

Davis, S., & Meier, S. (2014). Effects of testosterone treatment and chest reconstruction surgery on mental health and sexuality in female-to-male transgender people. *International Journal of Sexual Health, 26*, 113–128.

Deans, E., & Grimes, D. A. (2009). Intrauterine devices for adolescents: a systematic review. *Contraception, 79*(6), 418–423.

Department of Health. (2011). *"You're Welcome" Self review tool for quality criteria for young people friendly services.* Retrieved from https://www.gov.uk/government/publications/self-review -tool-for-quality-criteria-for-young-people-friendly-health-services

Department of Health. (2005). *Mental Capacity Act. London, HMSO.* Retrieved from http://www.legislation.gov.uk/ukpga/2005 /9/contents/enacted

Dorman, E., & Bishai, D. (2012). Demand for male contraception. *Expert Review of Pharmacoeconomics & Outcomes Research, 12*(5), 605–613.

Edwards, S., & Bunker, C. (2011). Other conditions affecting the male genitalia. In K. E. Rogstad (Ed.), *ABC of Sexually Transmitted Infections* (6th ed., pp. 35–41). Chichester, United Kingdom: Wiley-Blackwell/BMJ Books.

Edwards, S., & Carne, C. (1998). Oral sex and the transmission of non-viral STIs. *Sexually Transmitted Infections, 74*(2): 95–100.

Faculty of Sexual Health and Reproductive Healthcare (FSRH). (2010). *Contraceptive choices for young people: Clinical guidance.* Retrieved from https://www.fsrh.org/standards-and-guidance /documents/cec-ceu-guidance-young-people-mar-2010/

Faculty of Sexual Health and Reproductive Healthcare (FSRH). (2016). *UK medical eligibility criteria for contraceptive use (UK-MEC).* Retrieved from https://www.fsrh.org/standards-and-guidance /uk-medical-eligibility-criteria-for-contraceptive-use-ukmec/

Faculty of Sexual and Reproductive Healthcare (FSRH). (2017). *Clinical guidance: drug interactions with hormonal contraception.* Retrieved from https://www.fsrh.org/news/updated-clinical-guideline -published-drug-interaction-with/

Family Planning Association (FPA). (2007). *Are you ready? Young people's views of sex and relationships.* London, United Kingdom: Family Planning Association.

Family Planning Association (FPA). (2011).*The law on sex. Members area fact sheet January 2011.* London, United Kingdom: Family Planning Association.

Family Planning Association (FPA). (2013). *FPA responds to ministerial statement on PSHE education 21st March.* London, United Kingdom: Family Planning Association. Retrieved from www.fpa.org.uk/news /fpa-responds-ministerial-statement-pshe-education

Finer, L., & Philbin, J. (2013). Sexual initiation, contraceptive use, and pregnancy among young adolescents. *Pediatrics, 131*(5), 886–891.

Fogul, C., Crandell, J., Neevel, B., Parker, S., Carry, M., White, B., ... Gelaude, D. J. (2015). Efficacy of an adapted HIV and sexually transmitted infection prevention intervention for incarcerated women: A randomized controlled trial. *American Journal of Public Health, 105*, 802–809.

Ganchimeg, T., Ota, E., Morisaki, N., Laopaiboon, M., Lumbiganon, P., Zhang, J., ... Mori, R. (2014). Pregnancy and childbirth outcomes among adolescent mothers: A World Health Organization multicountry study. *BJOG, 121*(Suppl 1), 40–48.

Gawron, L., & Turok, D. (2015). Pills on the World Wide Web: Reducing barriers through technology. *American Journal of Obstetrics and Gynecology, 213*(4), 500.e1–500.e4.

Gledhill, S., & Schweitzer, R. (2014). Sexual desire, erectile dysfunction and the biomedicalization of sex in older heterosexual men. *Journal of Advanced Nursing, 70*(4), 894–903.

Guttmacher Institute. (2016a). *Contraceptive use in the United States.* New York, NY: Author. Retrieved from https://www .guttmacher.org/fact-sheet/contraceptive-use-united-states

Guttmacher Institute. (2016b). *An overview of minors' consent law: state policies in brief.* New York, NY: Author. Retrieved from http://www.guttmacher.org/statecenter/spibs /spib_OMCL.pdf

Hadley, A., Chandra-Mouli, V., & Ingham, R. (2016). Implementing the United Kingdom Government's 10-year teenage pregnancy strategy for England (1999e2010): Applicable lessons for other countries. *Journal of Adolescent Health, 59*, 68–74.

Hollins, S, & Tuffrey-Wijne, I. (2013). Meeting the needs of patients with learning disabilities, *BMJ. 346*, f3421. doi: https:// doi.org/10.1136/bmj.f3421

Hyde, Z., Flicker, L., Hankey, G. J., Almeida, O. P., McCaul, K. A., Chubb, S. A., & Yeap, B. B. (2010). Prevalence of sexual activity and associated factors in men aged 75 to 95 years: A cohort study. *Annals of Internal Medicine, 153*(11), 693–702.

Ilani, N., Roth, M., Amory, J., Swerdloff, R., Dart, C., & Page, S. (2012, June). A combination of testosterone and Nesterone transdermal gels for male hormonal contraception. Presented June at Endocrine Society 94th Annual Meeting, Houston, TX.

Institute of Child Care Research. (2011). *Evaluation of the Brook Sexual Health Clinic: Coleraine & Outreach Service Belfast.* Retrieved from http://www.effectiveservices.org/downloads /evaluation_of_the_brook_sexual_health_clinic.pdf

International Planned Parenthood Federation. (2008). *Sexual rights: An IPPF declaration.* London, United Kingdom: Author. Retrieved from http://www.ippf.org/resource /sexual-rights-ippf-declaration (accessed September 9, 2017).

Kessel, B. (2001). Sexuality in the older person. *Age and Ageing, 30,* 121–124.

Ketting, E., & Winkelmann, C. (2011). Sexual health of young people in the European Region. *Entre Nous, 72,* 12–13.

Khalili, J., Leung, L., & Diamant, A. (2015). Finding the perfect doctor: Identifying lesbian, gay, bisexual, and transgender-competent physicians. *American Journal of Public Health, 105*(6), 1114–1119.

Knight, M., Kenyon, S., Brocklehurst, P., Neilson, J., Shakespeare, J., Gray, R., & Kurinczuk, J. (Eds.). (2014). *Saving lives, Improving mothers' care.* Oxford, United Kingdom: National Perinatal Epidemiology Unit, University of Oxford.

Knight, M., Tuffnell, D., Kenyon, S., Shakespeare, J., Gray R., & Kurinczuk, J. J. (Eds.). (2015). *Saving lives, Improving mothers' care.* Oxford, United Kingdom: National Perinatal Epidemiology Unit, University of Oxford.

Kolar, K., Atchison, C., & Bungay, V. (2014). Sexual safety practices of massage parlor-based sex workers and their clients. *AIDS Care, 26*(9), 1100–1104.

Levitt, H., & Ippolito, M. (2014). Being transgender: The experience of transgender identity development. *Journal of Homosexuality, 61*(12), 1727–1758.

Lindberg, L., Maddow-Zimet, I., & Boonstra, H. (2016). Changes in adolescents' receipt of sex education, 2006–2013. *Journal of Adolescent Health, 58*(6), 621–627.

Liu, P., Swerdloff, R., & Wang, C. (2010). Recent methodological advances in male hormonal contraception. *Contraception, 82*(5), 471–475.

Lopez, L., Grimes, D., Gallo, M., & Schulz, K. (2010). Skin patch and vaginal ring versus combined oral contraceptives for contraception. Chichester, United Kingdom: John Wiley & Sons.

Mahmoud, A., & T'Sjoen, G. (2012). Male hormonal contraception: Where do we stand? *European Journal of Contraception & Reproductive Health, 17*(3), 179–186.

McCarthy, M. (2010). Exercising choice and control-women with learning disabilities and contraception. *British Journal of Learning Disabilities, 38*(4), 293–302.

Martinez, G., & Abma, J. (2015). *Sexual activity, contraceptive use, and childbearing of teenagers.* NCHS Data Brief No. 209. Retrieved from http://www.cdc.gov/nchs/products/databriefs/db209.htm

Mitra, M., Parish, S., Clements, K., Cui, X., & Diop, H. (2015). Pregnancy outcomes among women with intellectual and developmental disabilities. *American Journal of Preventive Medicine, 48*(3), 300–308.

National Institute of Clinical Excellence (NICE). (2009). *When to suspect child maltreatment: NICE guideline CG89.* London, United Kingdom: Author.

Nelson, A., & Rezvan, A. (2011). A pilot study of women's knowledge of pregnancy health risks: Implications for contraception. *Contraception, 85*(1), 78–82.

NHS Contraceptive Services, England. (2014). *Community contraceptive clinics 2013–14.* Retrieved from www.hscic.gov.uk/catalogue/PUB15746

NHS Digital. (2016). *Sexual and Reproductive Health Services, England - 2015-16.* Retrieved from http://digital.nhs.uk/catalogue/PUB21969

Ni Lochlainn, M., & Kenny, R. (2013). Sexual activity and aging. *Journal of the American Medical Directors Association, 14*(8), 565–572.

Nieschlag, E., Kumar, N., & Sitruk-Ware, R. (2013). 7a-Methyl-19-nortsosterone (MENT): The Population Council's contribution to research on male contraception and treatment of hypogonadism. *Contraception, 87,* 288–295.

O'Connor, J. (2011). *Literature review on provision of appropriate and accessible support to people with an intellectual disability who are experiencing crisis pregnancy.* Retrieved from http://crisispregnancy.ie/wp-content/uploads/2012/05/Literature-Review-on-Provision-of-Appropriate-and-AccessibleSupport-to-People-with-an-Intellectual-Disability-who-areExperiencing-Crisis-Pregnancy.pdf

Department of Health. (2005). *Mental Capacity Act. London, HMSO.* Retrieved from http://www.legislation.gov.uk/ukpga/2005/9/contents/enacted

Oringanje, C., Meremikwu, M., Eko, H., Esu, E., Meremikwu, A., & Ehiri, J. (2010). Interventions for preventing unintended pregnancies among adolescents. *Cochrane Database of Systematic Reviews, 2,* CD005215. doi: 10.1002/14651858.CD005215.pub3

Pardue, A., Bruce, A., & Murphy, D. (2011). Sex and sexuality in women's prisons: A preliminary typological investigation. *Prison Journal, 91*(3), 279–304.

Public Health England. (2014). *Developing integrated chlamydia screening provision locally.* Retrieved from https://www.gov.uk/government/uploads/system/uploads/attachment_data/file/373133/Developing_NCSP_services_locally.pdf

Public Health England (PHE). (2015). Sexually transmitted infections and chlamydia screening in England, 2014. *Health Protection Report, 9*(22), news.

Public Health England (PHE). (2016). *Immunisation against infectious diseases and Hepatitis B guidance, data and analysis.* Green Book chapter 18 v.30. Retrieved from https://www.gov.uk/government/publications/hepatitis-b-the-green-book-chapter-18

Quint, E. (2016). *Adolescents with Special Needs: Clinical Challenges in Reproductive Health Care Journal of Pediatric and Adolescent Gynecology, 29*(1), 2–6.

Reisner, S., White, J., Mayer, K., & Mimiaga, M. (2014). Sexual risk behaviors and psychosocial health concerns of female-to-male transgender men screening for STDs at an urban community health center. *AIDS Care, 26*(7), 857–864.

Rhodes, S., Alonzo, J., Mann, L., Downs, M., Siman, F., Andrade, M., . . . Bachmann, L. H. (2014). Novel approaches to HIV prevention and sexual health promotion among Guatemalan gay and bisexual men, MSM, and transgender persons. *AIDS Education and Prevention, 26*(4), 345–361.

Robertson, A., Syvertsen, J., Ulibarri, M., Rangel, M, Martinez, G., & Strathdee, S. (2014). Prevalence and correlates of HIV and sexually transmitted infections among female sex workers and their non-commercial male partners in two Mexico-USA border cities. *Journal of Urban Health, 91*(4), 752–767

Roller, C., Sedlak, C. & Draucker, C. (2015). Navigating the system: how transgender individuals engage in health care services. *Journal of School Nursing, 47*(5), 417–424.

Rotondi, N., Bauer, G., Scanlon, K., Kaay, M., Travers, R., & Travers, A. (2013). Nonprescribed hormone use and self-performed surgeries: "Do-it-yourself" transitions in transgender communities in Ontario, Canada. *American Journal of Public Health, 103*(10), 1830–1836.

Rowlands, S. (2010). Sharing personal information: How to decide whether or not. *Journal of Family Planning and Reproductive Health Care, 36*(3), 161–165.

Rowlands, S. (2011). Learning disability and contraceptive decision-making. *Journal of Family Planning and Reproductive Health Care, 37*(3), 173–178.

Say, R., & Mansour, D. (2009). Contraceptive choice for young people. *Journal of Family Planning and Reproductive Health Care, 35*(2), 81–85.

Schalet, A. (2011). Beyond abstinence and risk: A new paradigm for adolescent sexual health *Women's Health Issues, 21*(3 Suppl), S5–S7.

Senie, R. (2014). Epidemiology of Reproductive Health In R. Senie (Ed.) *Epidemiology of Women's Health* (125–152). Burlington, MA: Jones & Bartlett Learning.

Selkie, E., Benson, M., & Moreno, M. (2011). Adolescents' views regarding uses of social networking websites and text messaging for adolescent sexual health education. *American Journal of Health Education, 42*(4), 205–212.

Shahmanesh, M., Patel, V., Mabey, D., & Cowan, F. (2008). *Tropical Medicine and International Health, 13*(5), 659–679.

Sufrin, C., Kolbi-Molinas, A., & Roth, R. (2015). Reproductive justice, health disparities and incarcerated women in the United States. *Perspectives on Sexual and Reproductive Health, 47*(4), 213–219.

Suchak, T., Hussey, J., Takhar, M., & Bellringe, J., (2015). Post-operative trans women in sexual health clinics: managing common problems after vaginoplasty. *Journal of Family Planning and Reproductive Health Care, 41*(4), 245-247.

Sufrin, C., Tulsky, J., Goldenson, J., Winter, K., & Cohanet, D. (2010). Emergency contraception for newly arrested women: Evidence for an unrecognized public health opportunity. *Journal of Urban Health, 87*(2), 244–253.

Tang, A. (2011). How to run a prison STI service. *Sexually Transmitted Infections, 87*(4), 269–271.

Tang, A., Maw, R., & Kell, P. (2010). A survey of sexual health services in UK prisons. *International Journal of STD and AIDS, 21,* 638–641.

Torriente, A., Tadion, A. & Hsu, L. (2016). Opening the door to zero new HIV infections in closed settings. *Health and Human Rights, 18*(1), 157–168.

UNAIDS. (2002). Sex work and HIV/AIDS. Geneva, Switzerland: Author. Retrieved from http://data.unaids.org/publications /irc-pub02/jc705-sexwork-tu_en.pdf

Wight, D., Parkes, A., Strange, V., Allen, E., Bonell, C., & Henderson M. (2008). The quality of young people's heterosexual relationships: a longitudinal analysis of characteristics shaping subjective experience. *Perspectives on Sexual and Reproductive Health, 40*(4), 226–237.

Williams, H., Axten, D., Makia, F., Teague, A., & Fox, J. (2011). HIV and hepatitis C prevalence in individuals leaving prison and entering drug and alcohol services in the area of highest HIV prevalence in the in the UK. *Sexually Transmitted Infections, 87,* A356–A357.

Wirehn, A., Foldemo, A., Josefsson, A., & Lindberg, M. (2010). Use of hormonal contraceptives in relation to antidepressant therapy: A nationwide population-based study. *European Journal of Contraceptive and Reproductive Health Care, 15*(1), 41–47.

World Health Organization (WHO). (2015). *Medical eligibility criteria for contraceptive use.* (5th ed.). Geneva, Switzerland: Author. Retrieved from www.who.int/reproductivehealth/publications /family_planning/MEC-5/en/

World Health Organzation (WHO). (2009). *Mental health aspects of women's reproductive health: A global review of the literature.* Geneva, Switzerland: Author.

Wylie, K., Wood, A., & Abbasi, Y. (2011). Challenges of the sexual health of the elderly in Europe. *Entre Nous, 72,* 16–17.

CHAPTER

12

Lesbian, Gay, Bisexual, Transgender, Transsexual, and Questioning Dispositions

THEODORA D. KWANSA

Introduction

Various terms are used to describe individuals who identify with a particular sexuality, gender, sexual orientation, or sexual inclination. Thus, lesbian, gay, bisexual, transgender, transsexual, and questioning (LGBTQ) dispositions are descriptive. To avoid causing offense or confusion by using the controversial connotations of homosexual and homosexuality, the terms same-sex, same-gender, gay, lesbian, and bisexual are used in this section as appropriate. Similar to other categories of population groups and subgroups, various research studies have reported certain risky lifestyle behaviors with sexual risk-taking practices. These behaviors should be carefully examined to inform development of appropriately targeted interventions toward improved sexual health.

Published studies exploring the occurrence of specific sexually transmitted infections (STIs) and HIV infection among different categories of same-sex oriented relationships appear to be varied, and studies on specific issues are apparently limited in different countries. Therefore, sexual healthcare professionals are urged to conduct more extensive studies on related issues of concern to identified groups. Findings from various studies have consistently revealed that STIs and HIV infections are particularly prevalent among the LGBTQ communities. This section examines the factors associated with the prevalence of STIs and HIV infection among same-sex oriented groups.

Same-Sex Relationships: Overview of the Prevalence of Drug Use Among LGBT Patients

The World Health Organization's (WHO's) (2006) definition of sexual health involves not only freedom from or the absence of sexual ill health, abnormal conditions, infections, and the associated diseases, but also involves the experience of normality and constancy of healthy, non-violent, and non-risky sexual practices, healthful lifestyle behavior with respect, contentment, and stable sexual relationships. Individuals should feel confident in their sexuality as an element of their fundamental human rights. The promotion of safer sex, respect, and responsibility is intended to foster these rights through sexual health promotion.

Various factors influence the way that individuals' express their sexuality. Bregman, Malik, Page, Makynen, and Lindahl (2013) examine the significance of family influences, while Savin-Williams and Cohen (2015) explore the developmental progression, self-labeling, and disclosure of LGBT. Chatterjee (2014) examines the impact of problems encountered by LGBT individuals including conflicts, rejection, bullying, prejudices, and discrimination within family, education, and employment contexts. Marginalization and isolation with inaccessibility to certain public amenities in some wider societies are also among problems that may be experienced by LGBT individuals.

Consequently, their sexual health status, behaviors, and predisposition to abuse and harm are likewise affected by multiple factors.

Damage to reproductive structures and function—and long-term disease—can be attributed mainly to STIs and HIV infection acquired through risky sexual practices. For instance, Wolitski and Fenton (2011) noted that men who have sex with men (MSM) are more susceptible to contract HIV and STIs than other men in the general population. Practitioners are encouraged to explore the current evidence-based national and international policy recommendations and guidelines upon which implementation of LGBT care and services are based (**Box 12-1**).

BOX 12-1 Useful LGBT Policy Reports, Recommendations, Evidence-Based Care, and Therapeutic Intervention Guidelines

- CDC National Center for HIV/AIDS, Viral Hepatitis, STD, and TB Prevention: Division of HIV/AIDS Prevention. HIV and Transgender Communities, CDC September 2016.

- Deutsch, M. B. (Ed.). (2016). *Guidelines for the primary and gender-affirming care of transgender and gender nonbinary people* (2nd ed.). UCSF Center of Excellence for Transgender Health. San Francisco, CA: University of California.

- National LGBT Health Education Center. (2015). *Taking routine histories of sexual health: A system-wide approach for health centers.* Retrieved from www.lgbthealtheducation.org /wp-content/uploads/COM-827-sexual-history _toolkit_2015.pdf

- Sevelius, J. (2013). *Transgender issues in HIV.* American Academy of HIV Medicine. San Francisco, CA: University of California.

- Institute of Medicine. (2011). *The health of lesbian, gay, bisexual, and transgender people: Building a foundation for better understanding.* Institute of Medicine Consensus Report. Washington, DC: National Academies Press.

- United Nations Development Programme. (2016). *Implementing comprehensive HIV prevention programmes with transgender people.* Retrieved from http://www.undp.org /content/undp/en/home/librarypage/hiv-aids /implementing-comprehensive-hiv-and-sti -programmes-with-transgend.html

- World Health Organization (WHO). (2015). *Policy brief: Transgender people and HIV.* Geneva, Switzerland: Author.

See: The Center of Excellence for Transgender Health: Learning Center: Guidelines and Reports. http://transhealth .ucsf.edu/trans?page=lib-00-02

Perspectives of the U.K. Drugs Policy Commission and the CDC

The U.K. Drug Policy Commission (UKDPC) (2010) identified that unrelated to gender or age groupings, the use of drugs among LGBT groups is higher than among heterosexual groups. The higher incidence of drug use in gay men is primarily attributed to rampant stimulant use, such as amyl nitrite. Cannabis is found to be the most commonly used drug among the lesbian group. Additional evidence reveals higher incidence of use of recreational drugs and emerging new drugs among gay men much earlier than they occur among other population groups. Gay men are also reported to be inclined to misuse other drugs such as steroids and sildenafil (Viagra), with the latter often used to offset or minimize the adverse side effects of misused stimulant drugs. Apart from the higher incidence of STIs and HIV infection, erectile dysfunction, cardiovascular conditions, and mental health problems are associated with the misuse of stimulant drugs. Other researchers concur with the association between drug use to treat erectile dysfunction in MSM and increased sexual risk behaviors that promote HIV and STI transmission (Purcell et al., 2005).

The Centers for Disease Control and Prevention (CDC, 2010) revealed from its recent HIV/AIDS surveillance that MSM comprise more than half the total number of newly diagnosed HIV individuals in the United States each year. This rate far exceeds the prevalence among men in the general population and continues to increase. Wolitski and Fenton (2011) maintain that irrespective of progressive developments in the social, political, and human rights activities and campaigns, the sexual health of gay, bisexual, and other MSM remains unimproved. Similar to findings from other studies, these authors noted that the prevalence of HIV infection and STIs among MSM has continued to increase over almost 2 decades. Similar findings have been reported in other North American countries, Western Europe, and Australia (Dougan, Evanns, & Elford, 2007;

Fenton & Imrie, 2005; Sullivan et al., 2009). Other evidence indicates similar trends of increased risk of HIV among MSM in low- and middle-income countries (Baral, Sifakis, Cleghorn, & Beyrer, 2007).

Identified Social Circumstances, Demographic Characteristics, and Lifestyle Behaviors

Factors influencing sexual risk-taking behaviors include individual circumstances, age, sexual inclination (bisexual, gay transgender, or questioning), level of education attained, marital status, employment status, and alcohol and drug misuse (Brito et al., 2015). Identified risky sexual practices include frequent changes of sexual partners and engagement with numerous sexual contacts of varied backgrounds such as casual sexual contacts, sex workers, sex clients, and tourists. Condom use may be neglected or inconsistent, the sexual identity of partners/contacts may vary in terms of same-sex or bisexual, and sexual intercourse modes may vary, including vaginal, anal, oral, or combination. Infection transmission through tissue damage due to mucosal trauma and tears has been reported. Moreover, complications arising from particular serious infections, emotional and psychological trauma, victimization, stigmatization, discrimination, violence, and physical abuse are also recognized.

Interconnected Influences: Perceptions About Diminished Intimacy Determining Condom Use and Other Factors

Golub, Starks, Payton, and Parsons (2012) noted that among gay and bisexual men who engage in risky sexual practices, individuals' perception and belief about diminution of intimacy determined their decisions about condom use. This finding was particularly common among substance-using gay and bisexual men who engage in casual sexual partnerships. Moreover, these authors noted that perception about decrease in sexual pleasure was also found to influence individuals' decisions about condom use. These findings suggest that compared to sexual and emotional intimacy and pleasure, risk reduction in terms of HIV and STI prevention seems to be a less important concern among this group. Furthermore, the HIV prevention advice and guidance provided through various interventions apparently promotes mistrust among sexual partners regarding their commitment to monogamy and disclosure of each other's HIV status. Rietmeijer (2007) cited earlier studies that explained the increase in rate of STIs among MSM as associated with multiple sex partners and the risky practice of anal sex. Everette, Schnarrs, Rosario, Garofalo, and Mutanski's (2014) finding indicated that among adolescent males, those who identified as bisexuals presented a characteristic commonality of particular risk behaviors associated with STI transmission. They maintain that disparities in sexual health become apparent in the early stages of life and the disparate sexual behaviors manifest with particular sexual identities. These findings support Everette's (2013) deduction that these factors are interconnected and associated with acquisition and spread of sexually transmitted infections.

Delays in Uptake of Preventive Interventions, Early Diagnosis, and Commencement of Therapeutic Interventions

Delayed uptake of preventive interventions, late diagnosis, and delayed commencement of the therapeutic interventions for HIV and STIs may be associated with reluctance to disclose personal HIV status due to insecurity about own sexual inclination (Nelson et al., 2010). In relation to these, Nelson et al. emphasize the importance of thorough examination of the types of patients and the circumstances that lead to late diagnosis among MSM. This would help in developing appropriate outreach programs and interventions specifically designed for prevention, early detection, appropriate treatment and care.

Furthermore, Nelson et al. (2014) maintain that the experience of many different stresses in life, either personal or contextual, very possibly result in delayed HIV diagnosis. The more vulnerable are those MSM who do not receive mental health and social support or who do not have the capacity or self-efficacy to adopt the preventive and protective interventions provided for them. Such interventions should enable them to cope with the multiple life stresses to which they are exposed. Fear of stigma and discrimination as well as anxiety about rejection or breakdown of relationships with sexual partners and sexual contacts may also be significant contributing factors.

Wall, Khosropour, and Sullivan (2010) noted that following the CDC's recommendation in 2006 for healthcare providers to offer at least annual HIV testing to MSM, coverage of regular screening has not been adequately explored. They noted that only one-third of MSM presenting to their healthcare provider confirmed that they had been offered routine HIV testing. Therefore, they propose that healthcare providers should thoroughly and realistically explore the risks associated with MSM sexual activities and provide adequate screening programs for early diagnosis and preventive interventions.

Sexual Dysfunction and Erectile Problems Among Men Who Have Sex with Men

Research evidence in both the United States and United Kingdom indicates that various forms of sexual dysfunction are commonly experienced among MSM. The problem is reported to be more common among those MSM who are living with HIV infection (Bourne, Hickson, Keogh, Reid, & Weatherburn, 2012; Wolitski & Fenton, 2011). In particular, erectile dysfunction is found to be associated with poor adherence to HIV treatment (Sullivan et al., 2009). The perception among MSM is that side effects of HIV medication include sexual dysfunction and therefore, as

Trotta et al. (2008) noted, a particularly common problem is negligence in antiretroviral medication adherence. Other experts present their deduction about complex interactions between sexual dysfunction, sexual risk taking, HIV infection, depression, and the general health state of men who actively engage in same-sex activities (Mao et al., 2009). The experts' view is that multiple factors contribute to different forms of sexual dysfunction (Asboe et al., 2007). Erectile problems are reported to be associated with performance anxiety, low desire, unfulfilled/unsatisfied pleasure, hypoactive sexual desire disorder, or pain during anal intercourse (Hirshfield et al., 2010). Drug use is also identified as a common factor associated with sexual dysfunction (Cook et al., 2010). Various studies consistently indicate that sexual dysfunction and erectile dysfunction treatment regimens (in particular methamphetamine and sildenafil [Viagra]) have been associated with risky sexual behavior (Fisher et al., 2011). Moreover, increased incidence of HIV is associated with increased rate of acquisition and diagnosis. Also evident is increased transmission of STIs among those MSM who self-report both sexual dysfunction and use of erectile dysfunction treatment medications (Cook et al., 2010; Fisher et al., 2011; Mao et al., 2009; Marks et al., 2005).

Shindel, Horberg, Smith, & Breyer (2011) maintain that it is important to thoroughly explore the prevalence, personal distress, and social encumbrance created by sexual dysfunction. Gaining better insight to and understanding of the factors associated with sexual risk-taking behaviors would help to inform and guide the development of effective intervention programs. Ultimately, the aim is to provide therapeutic interventions, health promotion/education, and necessary support for the identified group and reduce the prevalence of sexual dysfunction among MSM and HIV-infected patients.

Jena, Goldman, Kamdar, Lakdawalla, and Lu (2010) maintain that the association between erectile dysfunction medication use and rates of STI/HIV acquisition may not necessarily be related to accessibility and convenience. Instead, the authors call for attention to individual characteristics of men who use erectile dysfunction drugs to provide appropriate risk reduction counseling and related interventions. Hirshfield et al. (2010) propose that empirical studies conducted collaboratively by researchers and clinicians would help to gain better understanding and clearer insight into this problem by exploring the sociocultural aspects and physical mechanisms involved.

The Need for Responsive Services

Crucially, sexual and reproductive health care and services should be responsive in taking account of the needs of a particular community and ultimately aimed at supporting sexually healthy populations. The United Kingdom Drugs Policy Commission (UKDPC, 2010) recommends that policy makers and local commissioners should take account of the high incidence of drug use among LGBT groups to more effectively meet their needs. Wolitski and Fenton (2011)

also call for an obligatory reexamination of interventions to reduce HIV infection and STIs among this group. They propose a thorough examination of sexual behavior patterns, nature of relationships among MSM, and the impact on individuals' mental health and physical well-being.

Wolitski and Fenton (2011) maintain that a sexual health approach presents the ideal context and opportunity to understand the sexual behaviors, practices, and relationships among MSM. Moreover, the context of sexual healthcare offers the ideal milieu for HIV and STI risk-reduction interventions. As Rietmeijer (2005) pointed out, keenness to embrace safer sex practices with fewer sexual partners and more consistent condom use among MSM has led to a reduction in the prevalence of syphilis and gonorrhea. However, this is undeniably due to greater societal awareness about the risk of HIV and related complications rather than implementation of public health risk-reduction interventions. Bourne et al. (2012) emphasize the importance of continual support and enhancement of services to meet the needs of HIV-diagnosed MSM. They deduce that there is a link between these problems and the physical and emotional capacity of MSM to achieve pleasurable sexual performance. No doubt these also link to sexual dysfunction and the related problem of drug use.

The expert opinion is that healthcare professionals (practitioners, managers, and policy decision-makers) should recognize the favorable impact that sexuality can have on individuals' lives. As the UK Drugs Policy Commission (UKDPC, 2010) points out, healthcare professionals should avoid considering all of these population subgroups as homogenous and as having the same sexual identity with indistinguishable characteristics, problems, and needs. Differences in the sexual practices among the different subgroups possibly influence variations in the prevalence of specific STIs, HIV infection, and other related disease consequences.

There is a need for ongoing research. Consequently, the CDC supports a range of behavioral research to develop and test interventions aimed at reducing risk behaviors associated with HIV infection among MSM. Current technologies such as mobile phone and internet-based interventions are being utilized to target high-risk MSM—in particular, alcohol and substance-using MSM who engage in unsafe sexual practices. Various MSM monitoring projects and enhanced surveillance of specific STIs are also advocated.

Pre-Exposure Prophylaxis (PrEP)

The use of pre-exposure prophylaxis (PrEP) is reputed to be a means of reducing HIV infection. Studies in the United States and the United Kingdom reveal effectiveness rates up to of 92% and 86%, respectively. PrEP is an intervention intended to reduce the risk of HIV infection. The procedure involves identifying people who are considered to be at high risk of acquiring HIV infection, but who are HIV seronegative, to take the prescribed daily antiretroviral medication. The recommended antiretroviral

HIV medication, sold under the name Truvada®, consists of tenofovir and emtricitabine (TDF/FTC) (CDC, 2014; NICE [ESNM78], 2016; Medicines & Healthcare products Regulatory Agency [MHRA], 2017). Conventionally, this is prescribed in combination with other medications for treating HIV infection. Evidence indicates the importance of strict medication adherence to achieve high degree of effectiveness. Koening , Lyles and Smith (2013) noted that variations in efficiency reported in different PrEP studies were evidently affected by the degree of self-discipline and conscientious adherence to the daily doses. These researchers explored adherence analysis and examined the available published literature on antiretroviral therapy and suggest that more extensive scientific studies are warranted. Other researchers also emphasize the need for enhanced medication adherence counseling (Hosek et al., 2013). Thrun (2013) suggests that the consultation interaction should include asking the individual about his ongoing HIV-risk behavior by using standard or routine questions. Relevant routine screening procedures should also be implemented at each clinic visit together with provision of health promotion preventive messages and development of action plans to reduce identified risk behaviors.

Within the United Kingdom a pilot study was carried out in England to measure the effectiveness of daily doses of pre-exposure prophylaxis for gay men and other MSM. The PROUD pilot study (officially "Pre-exposure Option for Reducing HIV in the UK: An Open-Label Randomization to Immediate or Deferred Daily Truvada for HIV Negative Gay Men") involved a 2-year recruitment of HIV-negative volunteers during the period from 2012 to 2014. Study participants were prescribed daily doses of TDF/FTC, which was administered in sexual health clinics. The results from the pilot study published in early 2015 showed that a high degree of protection is achievable with the use of PrEP for HIV-negative gay men and other MSM who are at high risk of acquiring HIV infection (NICE [ESNM78], 2016; Medicines & Healthcare products Regulatory Agency [MHRA], 2017). However, as yet there is no license with approved policy guideline for the administration of this prophylactic medication in the United Kingdom and other E.U. countries. In both the United Kingdom and the United States, changes were made to the deferment period for daily TDF/FTC administration for certain study participants, and the need for additional HIV-prevention measures was also emphasized.

Women Who Have Sex with Women

Similar to the MSM community, women who have sex with women (WSW) also present disparate sexual identities such as gay, lesbian, and bisexual (Marrazzo & Gorgos, 2012). Xu, Sternberg, and Markowitz (2010) noted that comparative to heterosexual or bisexual women, self-reported same-sex behaviors have become increasingly more prevalent among younger women. The sexual practices among WSW also involve risk behaviors and unsafe sexual activities (Gorgos & Marrazzo, 2011). Consequently, the risk of tissue damage in terms of mucosal trauma and tears is inevitable and their susceptibility to STIs/HIV infection is reported to be high. Organisms such as *Chlamydia trachomatis*, *Neisseria gonorrhoeae*, HIV, human papillomavirus (HPV), syphilis (*Treponema pallidum*), herpes simplex virus (HSV), and bacterial vaginosis are sexually transmissible between women (CDC, 2015). Transmission may occur via cervical fluid or directly through the mucosa of the genital tract (Gorgos & Marrazzo, 2011; Marrazzo, Coffey, & Bingham, 2005). Thus, sexual partners and sexual contacts are at high risk of repeatedly contracting many different STIs, such as trichomoniasis (Singh, Fine, & Marrazzo, 2011), HPV, genital herpes, and HIV (Gorgos & Marrazzo, 2011). Xu et al. (2010) noted that comparatively, WSW present higher HSV-2 seroprevalence with higher incidence of HSV-2 infection than heterosexual and bisexual women. Frenkl & Potts (2008) reported that HSV-2 acquisition risk is associated with the practice of oral-genital sex. Moreover, Singh et al. (2011) reported high incidence of positive chlamydial infection among women reporting same-sex relationships.

Penetrative and Non-Penetrative Sexual Practices

Transmission of infective organisms may occur through contact with the hands and fingers as well as through items used during the sexual activities without appropriate preventive measures. Marrazzo et al. (2005) categorized sexual practices as penetrative in terms of use of vaginal or anal dilators, vibrators, and domestic items. The use of fingers, hands, or sex toys that involve sharing by the sexual partners predictably increases the risk of STI transmission. Non-penetrative practices, on the other hand, relate to oral-vaginal, oral-anal, and genital-to-genital sexual activities. Identified portals of entry include direct contact with the mucosa and/or secretions from the cervix and vagina as well as through menstrual discharge.

Recommended Risk-Reduction Measures

Regarding transmission of HPV between sexual partners of WSW, Marrazzo and Gorgos (2012) emphasize the importance of following recommended guidelines for Pap smears. These include screening for early diagnosis and early treatment of other identified STIs. Hand hygiene, use of rubber gloves, thorough cleaning of sex toys, and protective condoms and oral shield use are crucial and should be strongly encouraged among WSW. Singh et al. (2011) argue that biological susceptibility and the sexual identity should be included in future investigations. Sexual behaviors, sexual network, disclosure, and assessment and routine screening for *Chlamydia trachomatis* infection should also be given careful consideration. Fine, Thomas, Nakatsukasa-Ono, and Marrazzo (2012) noted persistent racial and ethnic disproportions in the prevalence of chlamydial infections that were not related to or influenced by social and economic circumstances, traditions, or practices. They propose that carefully considered plans and purposeful approaches are necessary for dealing with the racial/ethnic occurrences of chlamydial infection among women attending family planning clinics, and sexual and other reproductive health clinics.

Need for Distinguishing Among WSW Subgroups

Gorgos and Marrazzo (2011) emphasize that WSW represent a diverse group with differences in sexual identities, sexual behaviors, sexual practices, and risk behaviors. WSW are at risk of acquiring bacterial, viral, and protozoal STIs from their existing and former male and female sexual partners. Bacterial vaginosis (BV) is reported to be common among the general population of women and more so among women who have female sexual partners. WSW should not be assumed to be at lower risk of acquiring STIs on the basis of their sexual identity or simply because they report involvement in same-sex relationships. These factors should not dissuade or prevent service providers from offering and performing STI screening programs in fulfilment of current policy regulations. The recommendation is that programs aimed at bisexual women should emphasize the possibility of STI transmission between women and encourage personal responsibility for the care, support, and well-being of their partners and sexual contacts. Tao (2008) argued that a clear distinction should be made between the sexual practices of women who identify as lesbians and those who identify as bisexual women. The intervention programs provided should target identified sexual practices and provide guidance on appropriate protection for safer and healthier sexual practices.

The provision of sexual health services for WSW requires an all-embracing discussion that reflects honesty, evidence-based facts, and transparency. In this way professionals and patients could effectively address sexual and behavioral risks based on a holistic framework. This should represent a shared concern between care providers and the relevant communities.

Prevalence of Bacterial Vaginosis Among Lesbians and Heterosexual Women

Bacterial vaginosis is a common genital-tract infection among women of childbearing age in the United States, and some studies have reported this to be more highly prevalent among sexual partners of WSW, particularly lesbians (Gorgos & Marrazzo, 2011; Marrazzo, Thomas, & Ringwood, 2011). Transmission occurs through transfer of vaginal secretions between the sexual partners (Gorgos & Marrazzo, 2011). The challenges with this condition have been reinfection, relapses, recurrence, or resistance, as critically considered by Eschenbach (2007). Such challenges have emerged in various studies on the medication regimens used for BV (Donders, Zodzika, & Rezeberga, 2014; Schwebke & Desmond, 2007). Research evidence

reveals that in 28% of those affected, early treatment failure occurs (Marrazzo et al., 2011). These researchers observed substantial increase in the use of gloves during digital vaginal sex following BV treatment and only occasional sharing of sex toys by sexual partners. Nonetheless, they found no association between these and the persistence of BV. Thus, an individual's risk of acquiring particular species and communities of vaginal bacteria may relate to specific sexual practices such as unprotected vaginal or oral sex. Bacterial vaginosis was also reported as the commonest complaint of vaginal discharge among women in the United Kingdom (Evans, Scally, Wellard, & Wilson, 2007). These researchers noted that higher concordance and exchange of microorganisms between lesbian couples probably reinforces the assumption of common sexually transmissible risk factors linked to the acquisition of STIs among that group.

Complex Manifestations of Bacterial Vaginosis

Bacterial vaginosis (BV) is a heterogeneous syndrome caused by different clusters of vaginal bacteria mainly brought about by a change in the composition of the microorganisms. Malaguti, Bahls, Uchimura, Gimenes, and Consolaro (2015) describe BV as proliferation of multiple anaerobic microorganisms with depletion of the natural lactobacilli within the vagina. The condition is explained as replacement or imbalance of the normal vaginal bacterial flora by anaerobic bacteria of the *Gardnerella* and *Mobilunculus* species, causing multiple upper genital tract infections. Therefore, the manifestation of BV is a disproportion of complex mix of microorganisms within the vagina with clusters of these forming different subcategories of BV (Datcu, 2014). However, the actual causation of pathogenic conditions is not clearly understood. Malaguti et al. (2015) maintain that methods for diagnosing BV are evidently imperfect at this time. The general view is that detailed studies of BV characteristics in locations other than the vagina (such as the rectum and oropharynx) may help explain how specific microorganisms manifest in abundance.

Variations are reported in the multitude of vaginal bacteria identified in different women, and BV is associated with particularly numerous varieties of vaginal bacteria that are exchanged among WSW (Oakley, Fiedler, Marrazzo, & Fredricks, 2008). Examination of the distribution of bacteria within the vagina and rectum and the pattern of exchange among the sexual partners of WSW was deemed to be crucial (Marrazzo, Antonio, Agnew, & Hillier, 2009). This enabled researchers to determine the type of bacteria associated with particular sexual practices. Findings from tests to determine if specific strains of *Lactobacillus* are common to female sex partners reveal that the strain of *Lactobacillus crispatus* is more prevalent in most women. The strain of *Lactobacillus gasseri* tends to be an indication of recent sexual activity involving penetrative digital-vaginal sexual activity. Furthermore, BV is found to be associated with early treatment failure with the metronidazole single-dose regimen prescribed for treating *Trichomonas vaginalis*. Clinical researchers are urged to conduct further studies to gain better insight and understanding of this complex condition.

Ongoing Research on Bacterial Vaginosis

Other studies have revealed that co-occurrence of BV and *Trichomonas vaginalis* increases susceptibility to acquisition of HIV infection through various mechanisms. The researchers explain that inflammatory damage and breakdown of mucosal barrier function increases risk of HIV infection (Mirmonsef, Krass, Landay, & Spear, 2012). Gatski, Martine, Levindon, et al., (2011) also report a high rate of BV among HIV-positive women who have *Trichomonas vaginalis* infection. They proposed that HIV-positive women should be made aware of the high incidence of coinfection among that subgroup of women. Additionally, these researchers maintain that more extensive studies are needed to examine the effects of interaction between these concurrent conditions on the progress and treatment of HIV-positive women. Fastring et al. (2011) reported an association between the co-occurrence of trichomoniasis/BV and vaginal shedding of HIV-1 RNA. They emphasize the importance of screening in order to offer immediate treatment for these two conditions among HIV-positive women and for implementation of HIV-prevention interventions.

Muzny, Harbison et al., (2013) maintain that southern African American WSW/WSWM (women who have sex with women and men) demonstrate awareness of their sexual risk behaviors and risk of STI transmission. Bisexual women also demonstrate awareness of their increased vulnerability to exposure and acquisition of STIs from sexual activities with their male sexual partners and contacts. Therefore, these subgroups require appropriate health promotion/education together with effective evidence-based targeted information, guidance, and support regarding measures for safer sex practices. The preventive interventional programs should include accurate explanation and facts about the modes of STI transmission through heterosexual relationships as well as protection of their contacts in their female sexual partnerships.

Marrazzo (2011) considers that contemporary techniques in microbiology continue to reveal the complex nature of BV and the multiplicity of the different species. Other contemporary techniques are also being employed to study and determine what microorganisms specifically cause BV by acting with other bacteria. However, the stages of BV development still remain unclear, and the biological basis of symptoms accompanying the proliferative change in vaginal microorganisms in some women and not in other women is also not clearly understood. Marrazzo (2011) urges for more research to explain high recurrence rates. Further studies are also needed to investigate whether specific species or clusters of vaginal microorganisms are more strongly pathogenic in causing damaging disease consequences than others.

The suggestion is that future research should consider frequent prospective sampling of the vaginal microorganisms,

taking account of simultaneous sexual practices. Additionally, the preventive measures of hygiene that are employed and the inherent characteristics of the existing bacterial community should be considered. Understanding the characteristics of extra-vaginal sites for BV in terms of the rectum and oropharynx may also help to explain the modes and processes by which these bacteria establish proliferation.

Mental and Psychological Health Issues Among Lesbian, Gay, and Bisexual (LGB) Men and Women

Research evidence reveals that the incidence of mental and psychological health problems among LGB men and women is consistently higher than it is among heterosexual men and women (Warner et al., 2004; Chakraborty et al., 2011; Bostwick, 2012). Depression and anxiety are common problems reported by bisexual men and women. These problems, together with a high risk of suicide, tend to be more serious among those who conceal disclosure of their sexual identity. This is a common problem among adolescents and young adults. King et al.'s (2008) finding revealed that compared to heterosexual men, lifetime suicide attempts among gay and bisexual men were recorded four times higher. These researchers also discovered that adolescent and adult LGBs were more than twice as likely to have attempted suicide in the past year as compared to heterosexual adolescents and adults. The CDC (2014) indicated that LGBT youth demonstrate higher risk of contemplating suicide, suicidal behaviors, attempting suicide, and actually carrying out acts of suicide.

Specific Mental Health Problems Reported

Factors influencing mental health include substance misuse (McCabe, Hughes, Bostwick, West, & Boyd, 2009), alcohol abuse and a combination of these together with risky sexual practices (Chakraborty et al., 2011; King et al., 2008). Some researchers had noted that gay, lesbian, and bisexual men and women frequently report significant levels of mental disorders with planned and/or actual self-harm. A noteworthy associated factor seems to be exposure to discrimination (Warner et al., 2004). Discrimination related to sexual orientation is an apparent predictor of specific neurotic disorders. These authors uphold the idea that perception of discrimination among these subgroups creates a social stress factor that cultivates development of mental health problems. Consequently, they noted more frequent use of mental health services by these subgroups. Bostwick (2012) also noted that compared to heterosexual women and lesbians, bisexual women present higher incidence of mental health problems, particularly depression. Findings indicated this is related level of stigma to which bisexual women might be exposed. That could also operate as a stress factor associated with mental health problems.

Lea, de Wit, and Reynolds (2014) also noted that compared to their heterosexual peers, lesbian, gay, bisexual, and other same-sex attracted youngsters demonstrated higher risk of mental health problems, including depression, anxiety, suicidal tendencies, and substance abuse. The experiences reported include homophobic prejudices, stigmatization, perceived and actual physical abuse, together with psychological anguish and torment. Schneeberger, Dietl, Muenzenmaier, Huber, and Lang (2014) assert that LGBT population groups present with high incidences of stressful childhood experiences that manifest as psychiatric symptoms, physical illnesses, alcohol and drug misuse, and victimization experiences. Comparatively, heterosexual controls present at lower risk of being victims of stressful childhood experiences. It must be noted, however, that the majority of studies exploring this issue have been conducted in the United States. Therefore, the researchers urge that future studies should aim to target culturally diverse populations in other countries.

Other mental health problems identified by Chakraborty et al. (2011) include phobic and psychotic disorders as well as tendencies to commit suicide, self-harm, and high incidence of drug and alcohol misuse. Talley (2013) maintains that empirical research activities aimed at exploring, designing, and implementing cultural-specific interventions for dealing with substance use disorders (SUD) have intensified. This author urges for more extensive studies on interventions that take account of the specific circumstances, problems, and needs of lesbian, gay, and bisexual (LGB) individuals who abuse or are dependent on substances. Therefore, existing general interventions should be reexamined, modified, or adjusted to reflect the cultural characteristics of specific target groups.

Proposed Interventions and Research

Implementation of comprehensive evidence-based treatment interventions involve various approaches. The process of 12-step facilitation, cognitive behavioral therapy, contingency management, or motivational interviewing are suggested (Talley, 2013). In relation to these, practitioners would find the recent studies by Glasner-Edwards et al. (2007), Donovan et al. (2012), and Donovan, Ingalsbe, Benbow, and Daley (2013) particularly useful. Research findings emphasize that the materials, content, and communication should reflect the identified characteristics of the target group. Therefore, it is crucial that recruitment of representative participants be conducted within relevant LGB-responsive and sociable settings (Talley, 2013).

Interventions should address social, cultural, environmental, and psychological aspects relating to previous events that may be contributory factors toward substance abuse in LGB groups. The core component of the interventions should specifically address issues of special concern to the LGB population and should be directly pertinent to the problem of substance misuse and addiction. Therefore, self-acceptance of own sexual identity and disclosure, along with experiences of childhood and adult victimization should be examined. Additionally, the problem of family rejection and coping strategies in situations of peer group

substance misuse should be carefully explored (Talley, 2013). This author argues for increased clinical training in LGBT cultural sensitivity with the aim of improving the care and services provided for treating and supporting individuals who present with substance abuse.

Patterns of Substance Abuse and Implications of Treatment Outcome

Green and Feinstein's (2012) review provides an update on the patterns of substance abuse and treatment outcomes and examines the clinical implications of the findings. They emphasize the need for more advanced empirical studies on representative study samples to explore the multiple dimensions of sexual orientation in relation to substance misuse. These researchers noted that lesbians present greater risk of alcohol and drug abuse disorders and related problems, while gay and bisexual men present higher risk of illicit drug use and related problems. Identified sociocultural factors include membership in terms of belonging of the gay culture as well as HIV status, and variations in demographic characteristics. They claim that compared to the heterosexual groups, older age and female gender do not necessarily represent strong protective factors against substance abuse among LGB individuals. Bisexual identity was found to be related to increased risk of substance abuse.

In terms of treatment outcome, they noted that research evidence seems to be insufficient for substantiating LGB-specific interventions and therefore suggest that more studies are needed. They suggest that based on the clinical implications of the findings, moderation versus abstinence be explored and targets for intervention should be linked to specific treatment modalities (Green & Feinstein, 2012). The researchers argue that efforts for enhancing treatment intervention effectiveness should continually improve by tailoring them for specific population subgroups. Additionally, appropriate interventions are needed for reducing factors that prevent individuals from seeking the treatment and support that are designed for the particular groups.

Shame and Guilt Associated with Drug, Alcohol, and Substance Abuse

Hequembourg and Dearing (2013) examined associations between proneness to shame, guilt, "internalized heterosexism," and the problems of substance abuse. These researchers found alcohol and drug abuse to be positively linked to proneness to shame and negatively linked to proneness to guilt. However, they reported that compared to gay men and lesbians, bisexual people presented higher risk of substance abuse and higher prevalence of heterosexual inclination but less proneness to guilt.

These researchers propose that it is important to make a distinction between guilt and shame. They noted that these may play a role in a person's decision to seek therapeutic support and required treatment. The findings clearly indicate the need for more studies to examine these associations in order to enhance existing knowledge and insight about sexual minority stress and to guide development of preventive and therapeutic interventions for sexual minorities.

Commonly Used Drugs

Chow et al.'s (2013) findings from samples drawn from different cities in Canada during 2008–2012 corroborated other research findings. They noted that compared to their equivalents sexual minority groups are more at risk of misuse of illegal substances and the associated impairment of health. Their findings revealed that commonly used drugs include ecstasy, ketamine, marijuana, cocaine, crack, and alcohol. They found that LGB individuals are particularly more prone to have used ecstasy, ketamine, and alcohol in the recent 30 days. Gender, age, education, housing, and employment influenced variations in drug use and self-harm among the different subgroups. They urge for development and implementation of interventions aimed at reduction of drug use and harm among high-risk sexual minority drug users. Moreover, they urge for more provision of secure housing accommodations aimed at reducing drug use among these population subgroups.

Conclusion

This chapter explored the sexual health issues relating to the diverse population communities and subgroups of lesbian, gay, bisexual, transgender, and questioning. Healthcare providers and practitioners, together with providers of related supportive services, are encouraged to consider the positive aspects of sexuality and sexual identity. Nonetheless, evidence from many studies reveals various high-risk behaviors and associated problems that need careful consideration. Factors associated with risky sexual practices are mainly drugs and substance and alcohol abuse. Disregard of preventive practices including neglect and inconsistent condom use have been reported as a persistent problem among many same-sex partnerships and relationships. These are found to be associated with perceptions of reduced intimacy and reduced pleasure with indifferent attitude to commitment in the relationships.

Evidence from various studies has revealed the potential benefit of pre-exposure prophylaxis as a protective intervention for HIV-negative individuals at high risk of acquiring HIV infection. This is considered to be a way to prevent and reduce the transmission rate and spread among high-risk groups. However, routine administration requires approval and licensing at the government level to enable the relevant health service providers to consider this preventive measure.

The prevalence and persistence of BV presents a particular challenge in the care and services and support provision for same-sex partnerships among women.

The repercussions of vulnerability and acquisition of STIs and HIV, as well as sexual dysfunction and mental and psychological health problems vary among the different same-sex relationship subgroups.

Depression, anxiety, and suicidal tendencies are more commonly reported by bisexual men and women than by their heterosexual counterparts. Moreover, experiences of guilt, shame, and suicidal tendencies have been associated with fear of homophobic prejudices, discrimination, stigmatization, victimization, and rejection by family members and sexual partners. Consequently, the predilection to drugs, substance, and alcohol abuse and risky sexual practices is commonly reported and linked to stressful childhood experiences.

The importance of substantial evidence to support evidence-based interventions is emphasized by various researchers. They propose targeted prevention and treatment programs for the identified groups. This requires clear characterization of the different sexual identities and distinguishing between guilt and shame.

● ● ● REFERENCES

Asboe, D., Catalan, J., Mandalia, S., Dedes, N., Florence, E., Schrooten, W., . . . Colebunders, R. (2007). A cross-sectional study to evaluate the association of hyperbilirubinaemia on markers of cardiovascular disease, neurocognitive function, bone mineral density and renal markers in HIV-1 infected subjects on protease inhibitors. *AIDS Care, 19*(8), 955–965.

Baral, S., Sifakis, F., Cleghorn, F., & Beyrer, C. (2007). Elevated risk for HIV infection among men who have sex with men in low- and middle-income countries 2000–2006: A systematic review. *PLoS Med, 4*(12), e339.

Bostwick, W. (2012). Assessing bisexual stigma and mental health status: A brief report. *Journal of Bisexuality. 12*(2): 214–222.

Bourne, A., Hickson, F., Keogh, P., Reid, D., & Weatherburn, P. (2012). Problems with sex among gay and bisexual men with diagnosed HIV in the United Kingdom. *BMC Public Health, 12*(916), 916.

Bregman, H. R., Malik, N. M., Page, M. J., Makynen, E., & Lindahl, K. M. (2013). Identity profiles in lesbian, gay, and bisexual youth: The role of family influences. *Journal of Youth and Adolescence, 42*(3), 417–430.

Brito, M. O., Hodge, D., Donastorg, Y., Khosla, S., Lerebours, L., & Pope, Z. (2015). Risk behaviours and prevalence of sexually transmitted infections and HIV in a group of Dominican gay men, other men who have sex with men and transgender women. *BMJ Open, 5,* e007747. doi: 10. 1136/bmjopen-2015-007747

Centers for Disease Control and Prevention (CDC). (2010). *HIV/AIDS surveillance report, 2008.* Atlanta, GA: U.S. Department of Health and Human Services.

Centers for Disease Control and Prevention (CDC). (2015). *Sexually Transmitted Diseases Treatment Guidelines.* Retrieved from https://www.cdc.gov/std/tg2015/default.htm

Centers for Disease Control and Prevention (CDC). (2014). *LGBT youth.* Retrieved from https://www.cdc.gov/lgbthealth/youth.htm

Chakraborti, A., McManus, S., Brugha, T.S., Bebbibgton, P., King, M. (2011). Mental health of the non-heterosexual population of England. *Br J Psychiatry.* 2011 Feb; *198*(2): 143–148.

Chatterjee, S. (2014). Problems faced by LGBT people in the mainstream society: Some recommendations. *International Journal of Interdisciplinary and Multidisciplinary Studies, 1*(5), 317–331.

Chow, C., Vallance, K., Stockwell, T., Macdonald, S., Martin, G., Ivsins, A., Duff, C. (2013). Sexual identity and drug use harm among high-risk active substance users. *Culture, Health & Sexuality, 15*(3), 311–326.

Cook, R. L., McGinnis, K. A., Samet, J. H., Fiellin, D. A., Rodriguez-Barradas, M. C., Kraemer, K. L., . . . Justice, A. C. (2010). Erectile dysfunction drug receipt, risky sexual behaviour and sexually transmitted diseases in HIV-infected and HIV-uninfected men. *Journal of General Internal Medicine, 25*(2), 115–121.

Datcu, R. (2014). Characterisation of the vaginal microflora in health and disease. *Danish Medicine Journal, 61*(4), B 483.

Donders, G. G., Zodzika, J., & Rezeberga, D. (2014). Treatment of bacterial vaginosis: What we have and what we miss. *Expert Opinion on Pharmacotherapy, 15*(5), 645–657.

Donovan, D. M., Daley, D. C., Bringham, G. S., Hodkins, C. C., Perl, H. J., Garrett, S. B., . . . Zammarelli, L. (2012). Stimulant abuser groups to engage in 12-step (STAGE-12): A multisite trial in the National Institute on Drug Abuse Clinical Trials Network. *Journal of Substance Abuse Treatment, 44*(1), 103–114.

Donovan, D. M., Ingalsbe, M. H., Benbow, J., & Daley, D. C. (2013). 12-step interventions and mutual support programs for substance use disorders: an overview. *Social Work in Public Health, 28*(3-4), 312–332.

Dougan, S., Evans, B. G., & Elford, J. (2007). Sexually transmitted infections in Western Europe among HIV-positive men who have sex with men. *Sexually Transmitted Diseases, 24*(10), 783–790.

Eschenbach, D. A. (2007). Bacterial vaginosis: Resistance, recurrence, and/or reinfection? *Clinical Infectious Diseases, 44*(2), 220–221.

Evans, A. L., Scally, A. J., Wellard, S. J., & Wilson, J. D. (2007). Prevalence of bacterial vaginosis in lesbians and heterosexual women in a community setting. *Sexually Transmitted Infections, 83*(6), 470–475.

Everette, B. G. (2013). Sexual orientation disparities in sexually transmitted infections: Examining the intersection between sexual identity and sexual behaviour. *Archives of Sexual Behavior, 42*(2), 225–236.

Everette, B. G., Schnarrs, P. W., Rosario, M., Garofalo, R., & Mustanski, B. (2014). Sexual orientation disparities in sexually transmitted infections risk behaviours and risk determinants among sexually active adolescent males: Results from a school-based sample. *American Journal of Public Health, 104*(6), 1107–1112.

Fastring, D. R., Amedee, A., Gatski, M., Clark, R. A., Mena, L. A., Levison, J., . . . Kissinger, P. (2011). Co-occurrence of Trichomonas vaginalis and bacterial vaginosis and vaginal shedding of HIV-1 RNA. *Sexually Transmitted Diseases, 41*(3), 173–179.

Fenton, K. A., & Imrie, J. (2005). Increasing rates of sexually transmitted diseases in homosexual men in Western Europe and the United States: Why? *Infectious Disease Clinics of North America, 19*(2), 311–331.

Fine, D., Thomas, K. K., Nakatsukasa-Ono, W., & Marrazzo, J. M. (2012). Chlamydia positivity in women screened in family planning clinics: Racial/ethnic differences and trends in the Northwest U.S. 1997-2006. *Public Health Reports, 127*(1), 38–51.

Fisher, D. G., Reynolds, G. L., Ware, M. R., & Napper, L. E. (2011). Methamphetamine and Viagra use: Relationship to sexual risk behaviours. *Archives of Sexual Behavior, 40*(2), 273–279.

Frenkl, T. L., & Potts, J. (2008). Sexually transmitted infections. *Urologic Clinics of North America, 35*(1), 33–46.

Gatski, M., Martin, D. H., Levidon, J., Mena, L. A., Clark, R. A., Murphy, M., . . . Kissinger, P. (2011). The influence of bacterial vaginosis on the response to *Trichomonas vaginalis* treatment among HIV-infected women. *Sexually Transmitted Infections, 87*(3), 205–208.

Glasner-Edwards, S., Tate, S. R., McQuaid, J. R., Cummins, K., Granholm, E., & Brown, S. A. (2007). Mechanisms of action in integrated cognitive-behavioural treatment versus twelve-step facilitation for substance-dependent adults with comorbid major depression. *Journal of Studies on Alcohol and Drugs, 68*(5), 663–672.

Golub, S. A., Starks, T. J., Payton, G., & Parsons, J. T. (2012). The critical role of intimacy in the sexual risk behaviours of gay and bisexual men. *AIDS Behavior, 16*(3), 626–632.

Gorgos, L. M., & Marrazzo, J. M. (2011). Sexually transmitted infections among women who have sex with women. *Clinical Infectious Diseases, 53*(3), S84–S91.

Green, K. E., & Feinstein, B. A. (2012). Substance use in lesbian, gay and bisexual populations: An update on empirical research and implications for treatment. *Psychology of Addictive Behaviors, 26*(2), 265–278.

Hequembourg, A. L., & Dearing, R. L. (2013). Exploring shame, guilt, and risky substance use among sexual minority men and women. *Journal of Homosexuality, 60*(4), 615–638.

Hirshfield, S., Chiasson, M. A., Wagmiller, R. L., Remien, R. H., Humberstone, M., Scheinmann, R., & Grov, C. (2010). Sexual dysfunction in an internet sample of US men who have sex with men. *Journal of Sexual Medicine, 7*(9), 3104–3114.

Hosek, S., Siberry, G., Bell, M., Lally, M., Kapogiannis, B., Green, K., . . . Wilson, C. M. (2013). Project PrEPare (ATN082): The acceptability and feasibility of an HIV pre-exposure prophylaxis (PrEP) trial with young men who have sex with men (YMSM). *JAIDS, 62*(4), 447–456.

Jena, A. B., Goldman, D. P., Kamdar, A., Lakdawalla, D. N., & Lu, Y. (2010). Sexually transmitted diseases among users of erectile dysfunction drugs: analysis of claims data. *Annals of Internal Medicine, 153*(1), 1–7.

King, M., Semlyen, J., Tai S. S., Killaspy, H., Osborn, D., Popelyuk, D., & Nazareth, I. (2008). A systematic review of mental disorder, suicide, and deliberate self-harm in lesbian, gay and bisexual people. *BMC Psychiatry, 8,* 70.

Koening, L. J., Lyles, C., & Smith, D. K. (2013). Adherence to antiretroviral medications for HIV Pre-exposure prophylaxis: Lessons learned from trials and treatment studies. *American Journal of Preventive Medicine, 44*(1 Suppl. 2), S91–S98.

Lea, T., de Wit, J., & Reynolds, R. (2014). Minority stress in lesbian, gay, and bisexual young adults in Australia: Associations with psychological distress. *Archives of Sexual Behavior, 43*(8), 1571–1578.

Malaguti, N., Bahls, L. D., Uchimura, N. S., Gimenes, F., & Consolaro, M. E. L. (2015). Sensitive detection of thirteen bacterial vaginosis-associated agents using multiplex polymerase chain reaction *BioMed Research International, 2015,* 645853.

Mao, L., Newman, C. E., Kidd, M. R., Saltman, D. C., Rogers, G. D., & Kippax, S. C. (2009). Self-reported sexual difficulties and their association with depression and other factors among gay men attending high HIV-caseload general practices in Australia. *Journal of Sexual Medicine, 6*(5), 1378–1385.

Marks, G., Richardson, J. L., Milam, J., Bolan R., Stoyanoff, S., & McCutchan, A. (2005). Use of erectile function medication and unsafe sex among HIV + men who have sex with men in care. *International Journal of STDs and AIDS, 16*(3), 271–272.

Marrazzo, J. M. (2011). Interpreting the epidemiology and natural history of bacterial vaginosis: Are we still confused? *Anaerobe, 17*(4), 186–190.

Marrazzo, J. M., Antonio, M., Agnew, K., & Hillier, S. L. (2009). Distribution of genital Lactobacillus strains shared by female sex partners. *Journal of Infectious Diseases, 199*(5), 680–683.

Marrazzo, J. M., Coffey, P., Bingham, A., (2005). Sexual practices, risk perception and knowledge of sexually transmitted disease risk among lesbian and bisexual women. *Perspectives on Sexual and Reproductive Health, 37*(1), 6–12.

Marrazzo, J. M., & Gorgos, L. M. (2012). Emerging sexual health issues among women who have sex with women. *Current Infectious Disease Reports, 14*(2), 204–211.

Marrazzo, J. M., Thomas, K. K., & Ringwood, K. (2011). A behavioural intervention to reduce persistence of bacterial vaginosis among women who report sex with women: A randomised trial. *Sexually Transmitted Infections, 87*(5), 399–405.

McCabe, S. E., Hughes, T. L., Bostwick, W. B., West, B. T., & Boyd, C. J. (2009). Sexual orientation, substance use behaviours and substance dependence in the United States. *Addiction, 104*(8), 1333–1345.

Medicines & Healthcare products Regulatory Agency (MHRA). (2017). *Decentralised Procedure. Emtricitabine and tenofovir disoproxil phosphate.* Retrieved from https://www.mhra.gov.uk/home/groups/par/documents/websiteresources/con79286.pdf

Mirmonsef, P., Krass, L., Landay, A., & Spear, G. T. (2012). The role of bacterial vaginosis and Trichomonas in HIV transmission across the female genital tract. *Current HIV Research, 10*(3), 202–210.

Muzny, C. A., Austin, E. L., Harbison, H. S., & Hook, E. W. (2014). Sexual partnership characteristics of African American women who have sex with women: Impact on sexually transmitted infection risk. *Sexually Transmitted Diseases, 41*(10), 611–617

Muzny, C. A., Harbison, H. S., Pembleton, E. S., & Austin, E. L. (2013). Sexual behaviour, perception of sexually transmitted infection risk, and practice of safe sex among southern African American women who have sex with women. *Sexually Transmitted Diseases, 40*(5), 395–400.

National Institute for Health and Care Excellence (NICE). (2016). *Pre-exposure prophylaxis of HIV in adults at high risk: Truvada (emtricitabine/tenofovir disoproxil). Guidance and guidelines.* Retrieved from https://www.nice.org.uk/advice/esnm78/chapter/key-points-from-the-evicence#introduction-and-current-guidance

Nelson, K. M., Thiede, H., Hawes, S. E., Golden, M. R., Hutcheson, R., Carey, J. W., . . . Jenkins, R. A. (2010). Why the wait? Delayed HIV diagnosis among men who have sex with men. *Journal of Urban Health, 87*(4), 642–655.

Nelson, K. M., Thiede, H., Jenkins, R. A. Carey, J. W., Hutcheson, R., & Golden, M. R. (2014). Personal and contextual factors related to delayed HIV diagnosis among men who have sex with men. *AIDS Education and Prevention, 26*(2), 122–133.

Oakley, B. B., Fiedler, T. L., Marrazzo, J. M., & Fredricks, D. N. (2008). Diversity of human vaginal bacterial communities and associations with clinically defined bacterial vaginosis. *Applied Environmental Microbiology, 74*(15), 4898–4909.

Purcell, D. W., Wolitski, R. J., Hoff, C. C., Parsons, J. T., Woods, W. J., & Halkitis, P. N. (2005). Predictors of the use of Viagra, testosterone and antidepressants among HIV-seropositive gay and bisexual men. *AIDS, 19*(1), S57–S66.

Rietmeijer, C. A. (2005). Resurgence of risk behaviours among men who have sex with men: The case for HAART realism. *Sexually Transmitted Diseases, 32*(3), 176–177.

Rietmeijer, C. A. (2007). Risk reduction counselling for prevention of sexually transmitted infections: How it works and how to make it work. *Sexually Transmitted Infections, 83*(1), 2–9.

Savin-Williams, R. C., & Cohen, K. M. (2015). Developmental trajectories and milestones of lesbian, gay, and bisexual young people. *International Review of Psychiatry, 27*(5), 357–366.

Schneeberger, A. R., Dietl, M. F., Muenzenmaier, K. H., Huber, C. G., & Lang, U. E. (2014). Stressful childhood experiences and health outcomes in sexual minority populations: A systematic review. *Social Psychology and Psychiatric Epidemiology, 49*(9), 1427–1445.

Schwebke, J. R., & Desmond, R. A. (2007). A randomised trial of the duration of therapy with metronidazole plus or minus azithromycin for treatment of symptomatic bacterial vaginosis *Clinical Infections Diseases, 44*(2), 212–219.

Shindel, A. W., Horberg, M. A., Smith, J. F., & Breyer, B. N. (2011). Sexual dysfunction, HIV and AIDS in men who have sex with men. *AIDS Patient Care and STDs, 25*(6), 341–349.

Singh, D., Fine, D. N., & Marrazzo, J. M. (2011). Chlamydia trachomatis infection among women reporting sexual activity with women screened in family planning clinics in the Pacific Northwest, 1997-2005. *American Journal of Public Health, 101*(7), 1284–1290.

Sullivan, P. S., Hamouda, O., Delpech, V., Geduld, J. E., Prejean, J., Semaille, C., . . . Fenton, K. A. (2009). Reemergence of the HIV epidemic among men who have sex with men in North America, Western Europe, and Australia, 1996-2005. *Annals of Epidemiology, 19*(6), 423–431.

Talley, A. E. (2013). Recommendations for improving substance abuse treatment interventions for sexual minority substance abusers. *Drug and Alcohol Review, 32*(5), 539–540.

Thrun, M. W. (2013). Provider-initiated HIV risk-behaviour counselling: Ask, screen, intervene in the context of HIV pre-exposure prophylaxis. *American Journal of Preventive Medicine, 44* (1 Suppl. 2), S108–S111.

Trotta, M. P., Ammassari, A., Murri, R., Marconi, P., Zaccarelli, M., Cozzi-Lepri, A., . . . Antinori, A. (2008). Self-reported sexual dysfunction is frequent among HIV-infected persons and is associated with suboptimal adherence to antiretrovirals. *AIDS Patient Care and STDs, 22*(4), 291–299.

UK Drug Policy Commission (UKDPC). (2010). Drugs and diversity: Lesbian, Gay, Bisexual and Transgender (LGBT)

communities: Learning from the evidence. Retrieved from www .ukdpc.org.uk/wp-content/uploads/a-fresh-approach-to-drugs -the-final-report-of-the-uk-drug-policy-commission.pdf

Wall, K. M., Khosropour, C. M., & Sullivan, P. S. (2010). Offering of HIV screening to men who have sex with men by their health-care providers and associated factors. *Journal of the International Association of Physicians in AIDS care (Chicago), 9*(5), 284–288.

Warner, J., McKeown, E., Griffin, M., Johnson, K., Ramsay, A., Cort, C., & King, M. (2004). Rates and predictors of mental illness in gay men, lesbians and bisexual men and women. *British Journal of Psychiatry, 185*(6), 479–485.

Wolitski, R. J., & Fenton, K. A. (2011). Sexual health, HIV and sexually transmitted infections among gay, bisexual and other men who have sex with men in the United States. *AIDS Behavior, 15*(1), S9–S17.

World Health Organization (WHO). (2006). Defining sexual health: Report of a technical consultation on sexual health. Geneva, Switzerland: Author.

Xu, F., Sternberg, M. R., & Markowitz, L. E. (2010). Women who have sex with women in the United States: Prevalence, sexual behaviour and prevalence of herpes simplex virus type 2 infection - results from national health and nutrition examination survey 2001-2006. *Sexually Transmitted Diseases, 37*(7), 407–413.

● ● ● SUGGESTED FURTHER READING

American Psychological Association. (n.d.). *Understanding sexual orientation and gender identity*. Retrieved from http://www.apa.org /helpcenter/sexual-orientation.aspx

Centers for Disease Control and Prevention (CDC). (2014). *Pre-exposure prophylaxis for the prevention of HIV infection in the United States – 2014: A clinical practice guideline*. Retrieved from https://www.cdc.gov/hiv/pdf/prepguidelines2014.pdf

Egleston, B. L., Dunbrack, R. L. Jr., & Hall, M. J. (2010). Clinical trials that explicitly exclude gay and lesbian patients. *New England Journal of Medicine, 362*(11), 1054–1055.

Gatski, M., Martin, D. H., Clark, R. A., Harville, E., Schmidt, N., & Kissinger, P. (2011). Co-occurrence of *Trichomonas vaginalis* and bacterial vaginosis among HIV-positive women *Sexually Transmitted Diseases, 38*(3), 163–166.

McDermott, E. S., Hughes, E., Rawlings, V. E. (2016). *Queer Future Final Report: Understanding lesbian, gay, bisexual and trans (LGBT) adolescents' suicide, self-harm and help-seeking behaviour*. Lancaster, UK: Lancaster University, Research Directory. Retrieved from http://www.queerfutures.co.uk/wp-content /uploads/2016/06/Queer-Futures-Final-Report.pdf

Mastromarino, P., Vitali, B., & Mosca, L. (2013). Bacterial vaginosis: A review on clinical trials with probiotics. *Microbiology, 36*(3), 229–238.

Muzny, C. A., Sunesara, I. R., Austin, E. L., Mena, L. A., & Schwebke, J. R. (2013). Bacterial vaginosis among African American women who have sex with women. *Sexually Transmitted Diseases, 40*(9), 751–755.

PROUD – Medical Research Council, University College London, Public Health England. (2012–2015). *PROUD Results Key Messages and Q&A*. Retrieved from www.proud.mrc.ac.uk/97173/97177 /proud_results_key_messages_qa_v2.0_10dec2015

CHAPTER

13

Applied Psychology and Sexual Health: The Roles of Clinical and Health Psychologists

MANDY J. FORBES AND HANNAH L. DALE

CHAPTER OBJECTIVES

The main objectives of this chapter are to:

- Consider the significance of applied psychology within the context of primary, secondary, and tertiary prevention
- Examine the wider roles of applied psychology, including research, consultancy, and service development
- Demonstrate where both clinical and health psychologists may provide input to an individual case using a case example of human immunodeficiency virus (HIV)
- Illustrate the use of research, theory, and evidence in the development of a behavior change intervention for young people in foster care or group homes

Introduction

Patients attempting to achieve, or trying to maintain, positive sexual health, as well as those with a sexually transmitted infection (STI) or bloodborne virus (BBV), may require support. In the United Kingdom, greater awareness and evidence-based data on psychological therapies has resulted in the acknowledgement that psychologists can successfully address the needs of specific populations, including those struggling with positive sexual health. *Applied psychology* is defined as the use of psychological knowledge to address problems associated with human behavior (Davey, 2011).

Psychologists in the United Kingdom are registered with the Health and Care Professional Council (HCPC) and must have followed an undergraduate degree in psychology with 3 years of postgraduate training.

The purpose of this chapter is to apply the roles of clinical and health psychology to sexual health. It is not the authors' intentions to exclude the role of other health professionals and colleagues within the healthcare, social, and voluntary sector in the delivery of psychological and behavior-change support. However, it is beyond the scope of this chapter to identify the role for others providing such services.

Within the domain of sexual health, both clinical and health psychologists provide specialist psychological knowledge, enabling assessment and treatment interventions based on psychological theories and concepts such as cognitive behavioral therapy (CBT), motivational interviewing (MI), the theory of planned behavior (Ajzen, 1985), and the health action process approach (Schwartzer, 1992).

Clinical Psychology Specialization

In the United Kingdom, clinical psychology training focuses on the following core competencies (British Psychological Society, 2010):

- Psychological assessment
- Psychological formulation grounded in psychological theory and evidence
- Psychological intervention
- Audit and evaluation
- Research, including qualitative and quantitative analysis
- Communication and teaching

- Personal and professional skills
- Service delivery skills
- Transferable skills

All training courses teach at least two evidence-based models of psychological therapy, one of which must be CBT (British Psychological Society, 2010). In addition, interpersonal, societal, cultural, and biological factors are applied to psychological formulations and understanding the individual patient's needs. Clinical training is structured to encompass problems across the lifespan, with clinical placements in Child and Adolescent, Adult Mental Health, Older Adults, and Learning Disabilities, with the addition of specialist elective clinical placements, such as Physical Health, Physical Rehabilitation, Forensic, and Addictions. Clinical psychologists may work in a range of areas, including working with individuals who have psychological issues related to physical health problems. Problems may range from early cancer diagnosis or chronic pain, to HIV, diabetes, or end-of-life issues. Across the spectrum of health concerns, individuals may present with complex psychological problems that existed prior to their physical health problem, which can impact their medical condition.

Clinical psychologists implement evidence-based psychological interventions such as CBT, interpersonal therapy, person-centered therapy, and systemic and family therapy. Other therapies specific to presenting problems are also implemented; for example, eye movement desensitization and reprocessing in relation to post-traumatic stress disorder. These skills are not unique to clinical psychologists, but are skills that a range of health professionals may have as a result of training.

In relation to HIV, treatment guidelines (British Psychological Society, British HIV Association, & Medical Foundation for AIDS and Sexual Health [BOS/BHA/MFASH], 2011) encompass a stepped approach to psychological care and treatment in which clinical psychologists assess and deliver therapy to patients presenting with complex psychological problems. The guidelines highlight the complexity of the individual's needs, practitioner training, specialty training in psychological and psychiatric problems, and the competency required for providers serving patients with HIV. This ensures support and interventions are targeted over a spectrum of presenting problems and delivered by individuals competent to provide psychological support, assessments, and interventions at the individual, social, and cultural levels (**Figure 13-1**).

In the United States, the American Psychological Association currently accredits 391 programs. A large number of clinical psychology graduate programs provide PhD-level studies, which mainly concentrate on research, while programs of PsyD-level studies concentrate on practice. The American Psychological Association endorses both types of programs by accreditation. A relatively small number of clinical psychology programs offered at post-baccalaureate level allow students to graduate with a masters degree awarded over a period of 3 years. Similar to the United Kingdom Canada,

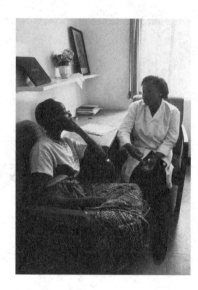

Figure 13-1 Communication and Teaching Interaction in a Non-Threatening Environment

and other countries, official licensing is required for practice in the United States. Three key prerequisites that apply in all states stipulate (1) graduation with an appropriate degree from an accredited educational institution, (2) completion of supervised internship or clinical experience, and (3) a passing grade on a written exam (with or without an oral exam).

Principal Components of Clinical Psychology Competencies

The following elements are functional and foundational competencies that must be developed and applied to clinical practice:

- Foundational competencies
- Relationships
- Individual and cultural diversity
- Ethical and legal standards/policy
- Professionalism
- Reflective practice/self-assessment/self-care
- Science, knowledge, and methods
- Interdisciplinary systems
- Evidence-based practice
- Functional competencies
- Assessment/diagnosis/conceptualization
- Intervention
- Consultation
- Research and/or evaluation
- Supervision
- Teaching
- Management/administration
- Advocacy

In the United States, the code of ethics in clinical psychology is specified by the American Psychological

Association (APA) Code of Conduct. The Code is designed to guide responsible behavior, protect clients, and uphold the rights of individuals, organizations, and society. The APA Code is underpinned by five principles:

- Beneficence and non-maleficence
- Fidelity and responsibility
- Integrity
- Justice
- Respect for people's rights and dignity

The key elements addressed include process of resolving ethical issues, human relations, privacy and confidentiality, competence, assessment and therapy, record keeping, training, research, publication, advertising, and fees.

Accessible Integrated Care in Collaboration with Clinical and Health Psychology

Broadly, integrated sexual and reproductive healthcare (SRH) aims to provide easily accessible care. An integrated SRH system should specify details for various levels of care and service provision, as well as stipulations for required professional and other quality standards. Importantly, there should be collaboration with other services, such as pregnancy termination, clinical psychology, and mental health services (Parma, 2013). Steinberg and Rubin (2014) identified areas in women's reproductive health that require psychological support, including adolescence, sexual health, puberty, sexuality, body image, sex education, menstrual cycle, contraception, unintended pregnancy and abortion, conception, childbirth, miscarriage, assisted reproductive technology, menopause, and reproductive aging. Each of these may potentially be associated with emotional, psychological, and mental health experiences, such as depressive symptoms or anxiety.

Research evidence lacks clarity in the association between hormonal contraceptives and depressive symptoms, although Steinberg & Rubin (2014) maintain association of psychological health with contraceptive use. Evidence suggests that 95% of unintended pregnancies are due to flaws in contraceptive use. Therefore, the suggestion is for more extensive studies that examine the association of psychological states on risky sexual behaviors.

While mental health problems may influence contraceptive behavior and risk of unintended pregnancy, the question arises as to how mental health influences pregnancy decision-making when unintended pregnancy occurs (Steinberg & Rubin, 2014). They maintain that there is no clear evidence to substantiate an association in the use of hormonal contraception and depression or depressive symptoms. The point is made that depression and other mental health problems should not be assumed to be the aftereffects of having an abortion; they argue that although abortion itself may not cause mental health problems, women having abortions are more likely to have had mental health problems. It is important to consider the assumption that women who have abortions who very likely have histories of mental health

problems (Steinberg & Finer, 2011; Steinberg, McCulloch, & Adler, 2014) may not have received appropriate treatment. Therefore, appropriate provision could be made for mental health screening and interventions within the abortion care setting. That would certainly ensure a shared care provision approach with clinical and health psychologists.

Joint Care with Referral to Clinical/Health Psychologists

Generally, U.S. abortion policies are not informed by psychological science. Yet, some U.S. policies and court decisions are based on the assumption that abortion does cause harmful effects to women's mental health. However, as Steinberg and Rubin (2014) point out, policies that emphasize potential mental health harm to women seeking abortions are not adequately substantiated by strong evidence. The researchers emphasize that clinical practice and related policies should be informed by psychological science. They propose that abortion clinics may be appropriate settings in which to integrate mental health services (Steinberg & Rubin, 2014). There is evidence to suggest an association between unintended pregnancies resulting in births and subsequent maternal depression. Therefore, policies that provide paid maternity leave and subsidized child care may relieve stress for many women having unintended pregnancies (Lopez, Tolley, Grimes, Chen, & Stockton, 2013).

Health Psychology Specialism

A student specializing in health psychology is trained in the following broad areas (adapted from British Psychological Society, 2010):

- Context and perspectives in health psychology, including social and cultural factors
- Epidemiology of health and illness, including inequalities and causes of mortality and morbidity
- Biological mechanisms of health and disease
- Health-related behavior, including theoretical models and behavioral risk factors
- Health-related cognitions, including efficacy and control beliefs and symptom perception
- Individual differences in health and illness
- Stress, health, and illness
- Long-term conditions/disability, including coping, pain, and interventions
- Lifespan, gender, and cross-cultural perspectives in health psychology
- Health care in professional settings
- Applications of health psychology
- Research methods
- Measurement issues
- Professional issues

Health psychologists work in a range of areas, but particularly focus on working with people who have certain physical health conditions. Their work involves assessment, formulation, treatment planning, and interventions to help patients adjust emotionally and cope with a diagnosis and living with an illness or long-term condition (e.g., diabetes, heart disease, or HIV). The aim is to improve functional and emotional well-being and self-management, in addition to health behavior change and medication adherence. Health psychologists specialize in health behavior change by drawing on psychological theories, therapies, techniques, and evidence to help people improve their health. This may be primary prevention in well populations, or secondary prevention to reduce the risk of infection transmission, or tertiary prevention to prevent further disease or infirmity in those who are already ill. Health psychologists design and deliver interventions on an individual, dyad, group, or community level. They may also work around healthcare systems and communication, examining and implementing change to assist in developing more effective systems for patients and organizations (British Psychological Society, 2011).

In relation to sexual health, a health psychologist would therefore understand the determinants of behavior, including risky sexual behavior, and have the skills to develop, deliver, and evaluate individual, dyad, group, or community-level preventative interventions. They would understand the potential impact of a diagnosis of an illness or a disease that may be a result of sexual activity (or other risk-taking behavior), the factors affecting individual reactions, and implement treatments or interventions for people who are finding it difficult to cope with or adjust to a diagnosis or live with a long-term condition. Lastly, health psychologists work around secondary prevention and medication adherence with patients, including those who have a BBV or other STI.

Practitioner Psychologists and Sexual Health

As with other healthcare professions, further specialization in addition to the core training in clinical or health psychology is required for working in the field of sexual health. Practitioners must understand the mode of transmission for illnesses from chlamydia to HIV; contraception and side effects; the symptoms, treatment and prognosis of illnesses; and local knowledge of the healthcare system surrounding each illness. Primary prevention care may require knowledge of local areas and special factors that may affect infection risk and transmission, including pockets of deprivation and local practices. For psychological intervention, knowledge of the evidence base for prevention and treatment of specific illnesses is required.

The Role of Psychology in Primary Prevention

Primary prevention is essential to reducing unwanted pregnancies and STIs. Over the years, a wealth of literature has been developed targeting specific and general populations on individual, group, and community levels. In order to develop effective interventions for prevention on any of these levels, it is important to understand the needs of the population being targeted, and a "one size fits all" approach is unlikely to suffice (de Visser, 2005). Once the characteristics and needs of the target population are known, the research literature can be further used to inform the development of interventions through applying the evidence, along with drawing on a range of behavioral theories and behavior change techniques. Tailored interventions based on a combination of theoretical, behavioral, and demographic factors are likely to be more effective than those using one factor alone (Noar, Benac, & Harris, 2007).

Evidence of success in pregnancy prevention programs requires careful analysis. For example, one review indicated promise for programs integrating skill building, education, and contraceptive promotion; however, pooled results of the interventions remained inconclusive (Oringanje et al., 2009). Another review on group-based sexual health interventions showed no positive effects on birth control or pregnancies (DiCenso, Guyatt, Willan, & Griffith, 2002). One reason for this may have been a lack of integration of theory, or targeting of wider factors impacting contraceptive use. Other studies, for example, have shown positive effects on contraceptive use and pregnancy prevention by tackling social disadvantage through youth development programs that aim to improve enjoyment of school and raise expectations and ambitions for the future (Harden, Brunton, Fletcher, & Oakley, 2009) or those grounded in theory, since these integrate how people learn, think and behave (Lopez, Tolley, Grimes, & Chen-Mok, 2009). In addition to simply increasing the uptake of contraceptives for individuals who are sexually active and wanting to avoid pregnancy, the effective use of contraceptives is essential. The addition of behavior-change techniques has been shown to reduce emergency contraceptive use and pregnancy rates (Martin, Sheeran, Slade, Wright, & Dibble, 2011). Behavior-change techniques prompt participants to make plans for any event that may put their contraceptive effectiveness at risk. Having solutions to events prior to them happening helps facilitate more effective contraceptive use.

STI prevention research often focuses on HIV, and a range of studies and reviews have been undertaken. However, some reviews have not indicated the important intervention components required to effectively reduce STI transmission, and others have not found conclusive evidence from interventions to show they are effective at STI prevention (Lyles et al., 2007; Picot et al., 2012; Sangani, Rutherford, & Wilkinson, 2004). Ellis et al. (2003) indicate that effective programs may need to include cognitive behavioral group work, and target risk reduction, sexual negotiation, and communication skills. Negotiation skill development, along with interventions based on socio-psychological models, have also been found to be effective components of cervical cancer risk reduction (Shepherd, Weston, Peersman, & Napuli, 2000). Another review looking at HIV risk reduction among men who have sex with men, found that individual, group, and community-based behavioral interventions are largely effective (Herbst et al., 2007).

It is particularly important to tailor interventions to the needs of the population and not use a one-size-fits-all approach, because primary prevention around sexual health can potentially target the majority of the population through community-level interventions. On a community or population level, theory-based informational messages could utilize theory and evidence more to assist in targeting the cognitive and behavioral determinants of behavior; however, most do not draw on these factors but may be more effective if they did so (Abraham, Krahe, Dominic, & Fritsche, 2002). Technology interventions also compare favorably to interventions delivered by human facilitators (McLellan & Dale, 2013; Noar et al., 2009). Interactive interventions using computers and mobile phones may prove more effective than leaflets on a population level (Bailey et al., 2010) and may be more acceptable to young people in particular. Some of these approaches may be appropriate to target both primary and secondary prevention; however, referring to the literature is an important step in identifying key intervention components. Therefore, utilizing the evidence-based theory and behavior change techniques is crucial in developing interventions around sexual health.

The Role of Psychology in Secondary Prevention

Secondary prevention is arguably one of the most cost-effective ways to reduce STI transmission, particularly infections without a cure. Secondary prevention can include interventions to promote testing for STIs; routine STI screenings, for example, in pregnant women; and prevention of onward transmission of STIs. The research literature indicates that a range of psychological factors are involved in people's decisions whether or not to get an STI test. Mass media campaigns are the most common method of promoting testing and treatment detailed in the research literature. Most focus on HIV and have some positive effects (Coleman & Ford, 1996; Vidanapathirana, Abramson, Forbes, & Fairley, 2005). However, the review by Vidanapathirana and colleagues (2005) suggests that campaigns don't reach those most at risk of HIV, because interventions have not increased diagnoses of HIV. Therefore, more targeted messages may be required. More recently, research examining the psychological determinants of self-testing for HIV revealed several that affect uptake, including perceived susceptibility, perceived benefits, and self-efficacy (Grispen et al., 2011). Motivational interviewing, which is described in more depth in the following sections, has been found to be an effective one-to-one intervention

---

Case Study 13-1

In Fife, a project initiated in 2008 focusing on the sexual health of a vulnerable group—young people in foster care or group homes—utilized the skills of a health psychologist to work in primary prevention. The project commenced with qualitative interviews exploring the sexual health needs of young people (Dale, Watson, Adair, Moy, & Humphris, 2011). These interviews revealed a need for additional interventions around sexual health and other lifestyle risk behaviors, including healthy eating, smoking, and alcohol use. The theory and evidence base were then consulted to further inform the development of a pilot service, which has now been established and has been running for 3 years. The intervention draws on a range of motivational and volitional behavior-change techniques and therapeutic approaches, including motivational interviewing, action and coping planning, restructuring the environment, and planning social support to help achieve goals. A feasibility evaluation showed it was well received and early behavior change data was positive (Dale, Watson, Adair, & Humphris, 2012). In addition to the core patient work, consultancy is offered to caregivers and workers, providing information and advising on effective ways of discussing risk behaviors with young people. Training around sexual health has been provided to residential care staff and foster caregivers. Population-level interventions have also been developed through working together with colleagues and involving the at-risk youth audience to develop concise literature on contraceptives and STIs. This gives a flavor for the range and scope of primary prevention sexual health work that a health psychologist could undertake.

Case Study 13-2

Research around STI screening in pregnancy has also focused on HIV. The following case study provides an example of how research can influence practice, and demonstrates the range of skills psychologists bring to a team.

An initial large-scale randomized controlled trial (RCT) found that offering an opt-in for HIV testing involving combinations of written and verbal information led to significantly greater uptake than standard care, which offered HIV testing only on request, without causing an increase in anxiety or dissatisfaction (Simpson, Johnstone, Boyd et al., 1998). Looking further at reasons for and against uptake, Simpson, Johnstone, Hart, Boyd, and Goldberg (1998) explored cognitions and behavior of pregnant women who were offered an HIV test. It suggested attitudes and beliefs toward testing were the highest predictors of uptake to HIV screening. One recommended way to achieve more positive attitudes toward the test was making the test more routine, and therefore increasing its acceptability. In a further study, providing HIV testing routinely by offering an opt-out of having the test done achieved a significantly higher rate of testing; 88% compared to 35% in their earlier study

(Simpson, Johnstone, Goldberg, Gormley, & Hart, 1999). This series of studies made a considerable contribution toward policy changes with HIV testing becoming standard and the test only not being undertaken if a woman chooses to opt out of it.

The majority of research looking at preventing people with STIs from transmitting them to other people concentrates on HIV secondary prevention. Reviews show that interventions guided by behavioral theory and that are on a one-to-one basis are most effective and may include condom use skills building, communication skills guidance and practice, and skills increasing self-efficacy for condom use (Crepaz et al., 2006). Similar interventions may be developed for other modes of transmission for HIV and hepatitis. There are therefore a range of psychological theories, techniques, and interventions that can play a role in secondary prevention and contribute toward improved outcomes.

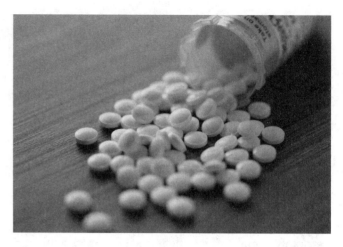

Figure 13-2 HIV-Related Neurocognitive Impairment: Problematic. Evidence-Based Psychological Interventions Crucial to Improve Medication Adherence

in increasing uptake to HIV testing (Foley et al., 2005). Because similar psychological processes will be involved in any mode of STI testing, campaigns to increase uptake may need to integrate psychology to effectively target these factors and increase their effectiveness.

The Role of Psychology in Tertiary Prevention

Medication Adherence

Medication adherence can be especially problematic people who have an illness such as HIV, which can have complex medication regimens. Although a number of factors may contribute to difficulty in medication adherence, some individuals presenting with such difficulties suffer from HIV-related neurocognitive impairment (**Figure 13-2**). Before the advent of effective antiretroviral medication, AIDS dementia complex was one of the recognized AIDS-defining illnesses (Centers for Disease Control and Prevention [CDC], 1987). As medical treatment advanced with the introduction of highly active antiretroviral therapy (HAART), AIDS dementia complex became less commonly observed (Sacktor et al., 2001). However, in 2005, a refined definition of HIV-related cognitive deficits was developed: HIV-associated neurocognitive disorders (HAND) (Anitinori et al., 2007). Rackstraw (2011), in a review of HIV-related neurocognitive impairment, reported these definitions of HAND: asymptomatic neurocognitive impairment (ANI), mild neurocognitive disorder (MND), and HIV-associated dementia (HAD). Impairments that HIV can affect are attention, information processing, language skills, sensory perception, and memory (including learning and recall) (Rackstraw, 2011). Rackstraw reports a cohort study of 1,500 patients (CNS HIV Antiretroviral Therapy Effects Research Project) carried out between 2003 and 2007, which appeared to show that over 50% of patients had a HAND diagnosis, with 25% of the cohort presenting

with cognitive impairments that interfered with activities of daily living. Rackstraw (2011) concludes in his review that although severe neurocognitive impairment is now less common, less severe impairments have become more prevalent. In addition to cognitive impairments, depression, anxiety, and associated mental health problems can also interfere with medication adherence (Harding et al., 2010).

Psychologists, therefore, have an important role in assessing and identifying the factors impacting treatment adherence and delivering interventions based on those factors. Evidence-based interventions that aim to improve medication adherence targeting multiple components may be most effective in achieving change. Interventions may include regimen-related interventions looking at scheduling of medication, or reminders such as text messages or beepers; targeting psychological factors such as self-efficacy or motivation; developing action and coping plans to help patients anticipate possible barriers and ways around them; and developing greater social support to assist in maintaining improved regimens (Fogarty et al., 2002; Reisner et al., 2009; Smith, Rublein, Marcus, Brock, & Chesney, 2003; Thrasher et al., 2006; Wise & Operario, 2008).

Cognitive Behavioral Therapy

Cognitive behavioral psychotherapies are structured, active, and time-limited psychological approaches supported by empirical data to be effective for a number of psychological problems, including depression and anxiety disorders (National Institute for Health and Clinical Excellence [NICE], 2009, 2011). Cognitive behavioral therapy (CBT) comprises both cognitive and behavioral interventions and can be delivered in individual therapy, group therapy, and more recently, computerized CBT. Interested readers may wish to read the historical perspective of the cognitive model (Beck, Rush, Shaw, & Emery, 1979), which gives an overview of the development of cognitive therapy and the contributions made by a number of writers.

As noted, psychological problems exist within the HIV population at a higher level than the general population (Clucas et al., 2011; Whetten, Reif, & Murphy-McMillan, 2008). Sherr, Clucas, Harding, Sibley, and Catalan (2011) reported that psychological interventions and those that incorporated a cognitive behavioral approach were generally effective in the treatment of depression among individuals with HIV infection. In the systematic review carried out by Clucas et al. (2011), cognitive behavioral stress management interventions were found to be useful in reducing anxiety. However, this study noted a lack of harmonized measurement of anxiety as well as a clear understanding of anxiety triggers and course of anxiety over time (Clucas et al., 2011). The authors further argue that mental health—and anxiety specifically—needs to be constantly examined and understood in the management of HIV infection. It is therefore timely that psychological standards in relation to HIV infection have been published to address such issues.

Motivational Interviewing

Motivational interviewing (MI) is "a directive, client-centered communication style for eliciting behavior change by helping clients to explore and resolve ambivalence. Compared with non-directive counseling it is more focused and goal directed. The examination and resolution of ambivalence is its central purpose, and the counselor is intentionally directive in pursuing this goal" (Rollnick & Miller, 1995). The therapeutic approach used in MI aims to work with patients to explore their own motivations for engaging or not engaging in behaviors. The approach avoids telling the patient what to do, uses empathic listening to help the patient realize some of the answers themselves, and helps empower and motivate the patient to improve their health (Rollnick, Miller, & Butler, 2008). In addition to the therapeutic approach, tools that may assist with MI include decisional balance, where the advantages and disadvantages of current behavior and behavior change are explored; two futures, where the patient is prompted to imagine their future if they continue as they are versus if they are able to make changes; motivation and confidence rulers, to help assess the patient's motivation and confidence in engaging in a behavior; and informing the patient of the consequences of behavior or suggestions for change, which would be done with their permission, and options for change provided. MI has shown promise in a range of tertiary prevention areas, including HIV management and medication adherence (Holstad, Dilorio, Kelley, Resnicow, & Sharma, 2011; Parsons, Rosof, Punzalan, & Di Maria, 2005; Thrasher et al., 2006). It is also an effective technique in primary and secondary prevention in improving health protective behaviors in sexual health (Britt, Hudson, & Blampied, 2004; Golin et al., 2012; Ruback, Sandbæk, Lauritzen, & Christensen, 2005). MI can therefore play a key role in helping motivate people around primary and secondary prevention, and around illness management where behaviors impact the patient's well-being, medication management, or symptoms.

Complementary Skills of Clinical and Health Psychologists

Because there is some overlap in the core training of clinical and health psychologists, the skills of both professions overlap at times. The diagram in **Figure 13-3** is a guide to the core areas of unique and complementary skills. This has been developed based on joint work in the National Health Service of Fife, Scotland, between clinical and health psychologists; it has since been adapted for sexual health. While this has been provided as a guide, each individual may have additional experience and skills; therefore, there may be potential for a health psychologist to work in some areas defined as primarily clinical psychology and vice versa.

Psychology and HIV

Individuals with HIV in particular may present with complex psychological needs that may have existed prior to their diagnosis, and may be exacerbated by their disease or as a consequence of treatment side effects (Sherr et al., 2011). Although medical treatment advances have increased the life expectancy of individuals with HIV, psychological problems are known to exist within this population at a higher level than the general population (Clucas et al., 2011; Whetten et al., 2008). Standards emphasize that psychological health and well-being are essential to individuals diagnosed with HIV (BPS/BHA/MFASH, 2011). Psychological difficulties are known to complicate the clinical management of HIV-positive individuals regarding reduction in quality of life, decreased rates of anti-retroviral adherence, and mortality (Sherr et al., 2011). Depression is also associated with HIV. Ciesla and Roberts (2001) carried out a meta-analysis and concluded that HIV infection was associated with a greater risk for major depression. Another recent systematic review (Catalan et al., 2011) highlighted the need for routine clinical care in relation to suicidality and self-harming behaviors among individuals diagnosed with HIV infection.

Anxiety disorders have also been identified within the HIV population at a higher level than that of the general population (Clucas et al., 2011). Various difficult emotional issues exist within this population, from the decision to go for testing, diagnosis, disclosure to others, and long-term antiretroviral treatment with a high adherence demand. Stigma of being diagnosed with HIV may lead to associated problems such as prejudice and discrimination from others in respect to the attitudes regarding HIV transmission methods (Crandall, 1991; Herek & Glunt, 1988), such as intravenous drug use or gay sex. Such experiences may trigger anxiety levels that may fluctuate as a response to the stressors associated with HIV infection and the changing nature of the disease. Therefore, screening for psychological problems over the course of HIV disease should be an important aspect of routine clinical care (BPS/BHA/MFASH, 2011; Healthcare Improvement Scotland, 2011).

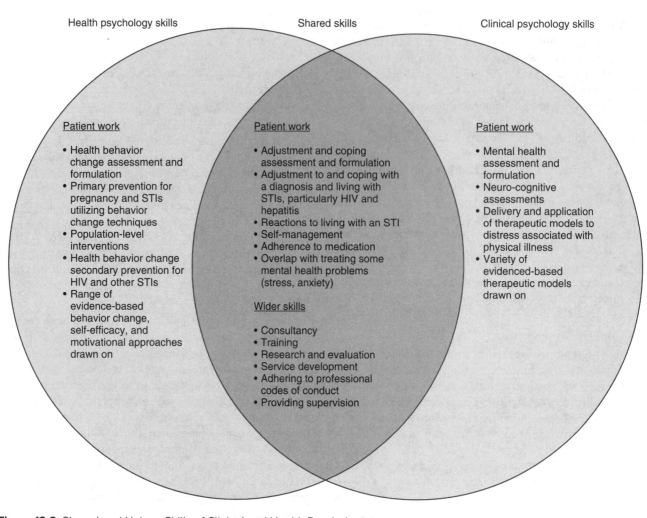

Health psychology skills   Shared skills   Clinical psychology skills

Patient work

- Health behavior change assessment and formulation
- Primary prevention for pregnancy and STIs utilizing behavior change techniques
- Population-level interventions
- Health behavior change secondary prevention for HIV and other STIs
- Range of evidence-based behavior change, self-efficacy, and motivational approaches drawn on

Patient work

- Adjustment and coping assessment and formulation
- Adjustment to and coping with a diagnosis and living with STIs, particularly HIV and hepatitis
- Reactions to living with an STI
- Self-management
- Adherence to medication
- Overlap with treating some mental health problems (stress, anxiety)

Wider skills

- Consultancy
- Training
- Research and evaluation
- Service development
- Adhering to professional codes of conduct
- Providing supervision

Patient work

- Mental health assessment and formulation
- Neuro-cognitive assessments
- Delivery and application of therapeutic models to distress associated with physical illness
- Variety of evidenced-based therapeutic models drawn on

Figure 13-3 Shared and Unique Skills of Clinical and Health Psychologists

---

Case Study 13-3

The following case example is fictional, based on an amalgamation of common presentations in psychology services of people living with HIV in the United Kingdom.

John is a student who was diagnosed with HIV 2 months ago. He contracted HIV through unprotected sex. Since his HIV diagnosis, he has admitted to feeling "down" and tearful. He has not disclosed his HIV diagnosis to family or friends due to concerns that they would disown him. He acknowledges feelings of loneliness. When reviewed at his medical appointment he did not describe any suicidal thoughts but did "not know where to turn." He had been experiencing palpitations and had started to experience episodes of "panic" when attending lectures. Over the 2 months since his HIV diagnosis, his attendance at University had declined due to feeling low in mood. He had no previous history of depression; however, described difficulty in accepting his sexuality, which affects his self-esteem. In relation to his sexual history, he described himself as passive and not feeling confident to ask others to use condoms. He had

not disclosed that he was gay to his family but had told two close friends. He met his sexual partners through internet sites. He acknowledged that he will consume alcohol prior to sexual activity to try and boost his confidence; however, this strategy was never helpful in negotiating condom use with his sexual partners, and he feels he is unlikely to use condoms. He has not engaged in any sexual activity since his HIV diagnosis. John has commenced anti-retroviral medication; however, he identified concerns in relation to how he will "hide" his tablets if staying at home with his family and is struggling to maintain the rigorous routines for medication adherence.

Clearly, John presents with issues that pre-date his HIV infection diagnosis in addition to difficulties that have developed as a result of his diagnosis.

Both clinical and health psychologists could have a role in helping John adjust to his diagnosis, including exploring his initial feelings and normalizing these within the context of a range of normal reactions.

As health beliefs are known to influence treatment outcomes, including medical adherence, it is important to explore with John his understanding of HIV, its transmission, treatment, and factors that may impact his health, such as his alcohol use.

As his mood is "down" and he is tearful, screening of his mood is essential, including any risk of suicidal and or self-harming behaviors. Although John did not admit to any previous history of depression, it is important to establish if he has experienced any other psychological problems. His past and current coping strategies (using alcohol to boost confidence) should be addressed, as well as feelings of low self-esteem around his sexuality and his anxiety symptoms. John's unease at disclosing his diagnosis and sexuality are important factors, as are his difficulties in identifying any positive emotional or practical supports.

To improve his adherence to medication, it may be beneficial for a clinical psychologist to first work with John around his mood, because mood and anxiety can impact medication adherence (Reisner et al., 2009) and other factors, including poorer health behaviors (Safren et al., 2010). Therefore, some improvements in adherence and health behaviors may be seen if anxiety and depression symptoms reduce. Conversely, some improvement in health behaviors—particularly exercise—may in fact enhance John's mood. Lower alcohol and drug use and greater coping skills contribute to improved medication adherence (Reisner et al., 2009). Additional work around these factors may be conducted by a clinical or health psychologist to further assist in adherence.

Secondary prevention is important to help John avoid passing HIV on to a sexual partner. The health psychologist could draw on behavior change techniques to assist John in protecting others from HIV. Initially, his motivation for using or not using condoms may need to be explored to assist the psychologist's understanding and acknowledge his autonomy, which is important therapeutically. Techniques may also include building his skills and confidence to negotiate condom use and use condoms effectively. Similar techniques could be utilized to help build his motivation and skills to adhere to his medication regimen.

It is first necessary to carry out an assessment with John. As has been highlighted earlier, both clinical and health psychologists would have a role in this process. Listed here are areas in relation to his assessment, formulation, and intervention.

Assessment

- Assessment of John's mood, anxiety, and any previous psychological problems.
- Assessment of any risk such as suicidal ideation or any self-harming behaviors.
- History of his panic episodes, including the symptoms he experiences and their development.
- John's psychological developmental history, including his family history. How did John function prior to his diagnosis?
- His practical knowledge in relation to HIV and his treatment regimen.
- Assessment of his self-efficacy beliefs, specifically focusing on his adherence to medications and condom use. Identify the difficulties that John is experiencing in relation to his medicine regimen.
- How do John's mood and beliefs impact on his behavior, including his medication use, condom use, and his social interactions?
- Impact of other social and environmental factors on his mood and behavior.
- Day-to-day coping with his diagnosis: acceptance/denial.
- Any impact on sleep.
- Assessment of his memory and cognitive functioning.
- Attitude toward protecting others from HIV.
- Social norms of condom use within peer group.
- Outcome expectancies of medication use, unprotected sex, and not disclosing his HIV diagnosis to his family.
- His concerns around his sexuality and, if appropriate, his sexual history.

Formulation

Johnstone and Dallos (2006) suggest that essential features of a psychological formulation should include a summary of the individual's core problems and indicate how the problems may relate to each other by drawing on psychological theories and principles. They also suggest that a psychological formulation should explain the development and maintenance of the individual's problems and indicate a plan of intervention based on the psychological processes identified. Formulations are also open to revision and reformulation.

Development and maintaining factors identified in John's presentation may include the cycle of low mood and anxiety impacting his day-to-day functioning, such as missing some of his lectures.

His adjustment and concerns surrounding his HIV diagnosis may have further impacted his self-esteem, which he had already identified as a concern in relation to his sexuality.

Environment of not disclosing sexuality and fear of doing so, along with shame of having HIV, may further impact his low self-esteem and anxiety.

Low self-efficacy, self-esteem, and confidence negotiating condom use further impacting both condom use and medication adherence.

The relationship among his thoughts, feelings, behavior, and health beliefs and how these may maintain his current core problems.

Interventions

Exploring with John how he feels about his diagnosis, how his feelings and thoughts have changed over the 2 months since being diagnosed, and identifying any thinking that may be mood or anxiety influenced. This can be achieved by asking John to keep a diary of his thoughts, feelings, and behaviors and introducing John to the CBT model of intervention.

This helps with normalizing some of these feelings as a typical reaction to a diagnosis of HIV or other life-threatening illness. This may be through psycho-education, including suggested reading or information about other HIV-related agencies that John may wish to contact for support and advice.

Exploring his daily routine, how his diagnosis has affected it, and his day-to-day coping. It again may be helpful to ask John to keep a diary to record his panic episodes and how often he is missing his lectures. Activity scheduling, asking John to record his daily routine in terms of any activities he might be enjoying, may allow John to build up a repertoire of positive activities.

Building effective coping strategies through drawing on his ways of coping with other major life events and eliciting from him what might help him, along with suggesting helpful coping strategies, such as building confidence in discussing his health and associated problems with his family. Identifying both practical and emotional support networks may also be helpful to John.

Exploring his feelings around taking medications and his expectations about their role in his treatment would be indicated, with any medical issues surrounding his medication being highlighted to his medical team for clarification and explanation.

MI would be indicated to explore his reasons for not using condoms or adhering to medication and build his motivation to discuss why these actions (condom use, medication adherence) might be beneficial. Moving on to discuss reasons against and for changing and exploring his ambivalence around this would be part of this process as well as building in his values and highlighting discrepancies between these and his current behavior.

Exploring John's issues of low self-esteem related to his sexuality may help him process his concerns and beliefs. As can be seen, identifying John's core concerns and developing a formulation and intervention plan are some of the roles carried out by both clinical and health psychologists.

Additional Roles of Psychologists Working in Applied Settings

Consultancy and Team Working

Particularly for BBV illnesses, working closely with the team of health professionals is important in managing each patient. Being fully integrated into a multi-agency team is optimal and will assist with patient management. This integration may assist in being able to provide consultancy to staff or teams who would welcome advice or training. Sharing a formulation may help other health professionals understand the psychological processes involved related to patient presentations. The types of consultancy and training provided by health and clinical psychologists may differ. For example, a clinical psychologist may provide guidance on working with individuals around psychological issues, including mental health issues. Both clinical and health psychologists may provide advice around self-management, adjusting to living with and coping with an illness, and other areas of functioning, such as quality of life. They may also recommend screening measures that may be used to assess for risk behaviors, readiness for treatment, anxiety disorders, and depression. A health psychologist may provide training in behavior change for primary and secondary prevention or medication adherence, and may develop persuasive theory-based written or technology-based information to assist people in preventing unwanted pregnancies and STIs or manage an illness more effectively.

Service Developments

Clinical and health psychologists both possess skills in developing interventions and service developments. This may include setting up or further developing a psychological service for people with HIV to assist individuals to cope with and adjust to a diagnosis, and to reduce symptoms of anxiety and depression. It may also include developing interventions for adherence to medication, primary or secondary prevention, and population-level interventions.

Research and Evaluation

Research and evaluation are core parts of all psychology training. The focus may be on research to understand the needs of a local population, or to better understand an issue not previously researched, in order to develop new services or interventions. Evaluation is crucial to understand the impact of services. Psychologists may take the lead on the design, conduction, and analysis of evaluations for both their own work and that of others. This may be to assess how a new service has been received, examine the way a service has been used, or explore the impact of a service looking at pre- and postintervention scores for psychological health or health behaviors. Research and evaluation may be quantitative or qualitative, drawing on a range of methods and analytical techniques. Psychologists may be based in applied settings, or at a university, which may provide the infrastructure for larger pieces of research. Collaborations between university and applied staff may provide an ideal partnership for research. A prime example of influential work in the sexual health field is a series of studies at the University of Edinburgh that explored HIV testing in pregnancy, as detailed in the secondary prevention section (Simpson, Johnstone, Boyd, et al., 1998; Simpson, Johnstone, Hart, et al., 1998). This work provides an example of research that can lead to important changes to improve sexual health and, specifically, reduce HIV transmission.

Conclusion

This chapter has provided an overview of the training, core competencies, and applications of health and clinical psychologists to the area of sexual health. Clinical psychologists are specialists in assessment and treatment for complex problems incorporating mental health difficulties, while health psychologists are specialists in assessment and treatment for complex behavior change within primary and secondary prevention. However, there are overlapping areas of focus for clinical and health psychologists, particularly around emotional adjustment, coping, and illness management, along with research, evaluation, service development, consultancy, and training skills. If services are able to employ both clinical and health psychologists, as appropriate, this may lead to greater benefits to patients in the areas of sexual health and BBV.

● ● ● REFERENCES

Abraham, C., Krahe, B., Dominic, R., & Fritsche, I. (2002). Do health promotion messages target cognitive and behavioural correlates of condom use? A content analysis of safer-sex promotion leaflets in two countries. *British Journal of Health Psychology, 7,* 227–246.

Ajzen, I. (1991). The theory of planned behavior. *Organizational Behavior and Human Decision Process, 50,* 179–211.

Antinori, A., Arendt, G., Becker, J. T., Brew, B. J., Byrd, D., & Wojna, V. E. (2007). Updated research nosology for HIV-associated neurocognitive disorders. *Neurology, 69,* 1789–1799.

Bailey, J. V., Rait, M. E., Mercer, C. H., Morris, R. W., Peacock, R., Cassell, J., & Nazareth, I. (2010). Interactive computer-based interventions for sexual health promotion (Review). *The Cochrane Database of Systematic Reviews, 9,* CD006483. doi: 10.1002/14651858 .CD006483.pub2

Beck, A., T, Rush, A. J., Shaw, B. E., & Emery, G. (1979). *Cognitive therapy of depression.* New York, NY: Guildford Press.

British Psychological Society. (2010). *Masters programmes in health psychology: Academic knowledge base mapping document.* Leicester, United Kingdom: British Psychological Society. Retrieved from http://www.bps.org.uk

British Psychological Society, British HIV Association, Medical Foundation for AIDS, & Sexual Health (BPS/BHA/MFASH). (2011). *Standards for psychological support for adults living with HIV: A guide for employers.* Leicester, United Kingdom: The British Psychological Society.

Britt, E., Hudson, S. M., & Blampied, N. M. (2004). Motivational interviewing in health settings: a review. *Patient Educ Couns.* 53, 147–155.

Catalan, J., Harding, R., Sibley, E., Clucas, C., Croome, N., & Sherr, L. (2011). HIV infection and mental health: Suicidal behaviour—Systematic review. *Psychology, Health & Medicine, 16(5),* 588–611.

Centers for Disease Control and Prevention (CDC). (1987). Revision of the CDC surveillance case definition for acquired immunodeficiency syndrome. *MMWR Supplements, 36(1),* 1S–15S.

Ciesla, J. A., & Roberts, J. E. (2001). Meta-analysis of the relationship between HIV infection and risk for depressive disorders. The *American Journal of Psychiatry, 158,* 725–730.

Clucas, C., Sibley, E., Harding, R., Liu, L., Catalan, J., & Sherr, L. (2011). A systematic review of Interventions for anxiety in people with HIV. *Psychology, Health & Medicine, 16(5),* 528–547.

Coleman, L. M. & Ford, N. J. (1996). An extensive literature review of the evaluation of HIV prevention programmes. *Health Education Research: Theory & Practice, 11,* 327–338.

Crandall, C. S. (1991). Multiple stigma and AIDS: Illness stigma and attitudes toward homosexuals and IV drug users in AIDS-related stigmatization. *Journal of Community & Applied Social Psychology, 1,* 165–172.

Crepaz, N., Lyles, C. M., Wolitski, R. J., Passin, W. F., Rama, S. M., Herbst, J. H., . . . HIV/AIDS Prevention Research Synthesis (PRS) Team. (2006). Do prevention interventions reduce HIV risk behaviours among people living with HIV? A meta-analytic review of controlled trials. *AIDS, 20,* 143–157.

Dale, H., Watson, L., Adair, P., & Humphris, G. (2012). Assessment of an innovative behaviour change intervention for looked after young people through applying health psychology and public health. *Lancet, 380,* 12-4906 (Poster).

Dale, H., Watson, L., Adair, P., Moy, M., & Humphris, G. (2011). The sexual health needs of looked after young people; findings from a qualitative study led through a partnership between public health and health psychology. *Journal of Public Health, 33,* 86–92.

Davey, G. (2011). *Introduction in applied psychology.* Chichester, United Kingdom: John Wiley and Sons Ltd.

de Visser, R. (2005). One size fits all? Promoting condom use for sexually transmitted infection prevention among heterosexual young adults. *Health Education Research: Theory & Practice, 20,* 557–556.

DiCenso, A., Guyatt, G., Willan, A., & Griffith, W. L. (2002). Interventions to reduce unintended pregnancies among adolescents: Systematic review of randomized controlled trials. *BMJ, 324.*

Ellis, S., Barnett-Page, E., Morgan, A., Taylor, L., Walters, R. & Goodrich, J. (2003). *HIV prevention: A review of reviews assessing the effectiveness of interventions to reduce the risk of sexual transmission.* London, United Kingdom: Health Development Agency.

Fogarty, L., Roter, D., Larson, S., Burke, J., Gillespie, J. & Levy, R. (2002). Patient adherence to HIV medication regimens: A review of published and abstract reports. *Patient Education and Counseling, 46,* 93–108.

Foley, K., Duran, B., Morris, P., Lucero, J., Jiang, Y., Baxter, B., et al. (2005). Using motivational interviewing to promote HIV testing at an American Indian substance abuse treatment facility. *Journal of Psychoactive Drugs, 37,* 321–329.

Golin, C. E., Earp, J. A., Grodensky, A., Patel, S. P., Suchindran, C., Parikh, M., . . . Groves, J. (2012). Longitudinal effects of SafeTalk, a motivational interviewing-base program to improve safer sex practices among people living with HIV/AIDS. *AIDS Behavior, 16(5),* 1182–1191. doi: 10.1007/s10461-011-0025-9

Grispen, J. E. J., Ronda, G., Dinant, G-J., de Vries, N. K., & van der Weijden, T. (2011). To test or not to test: A cross-sectional survey of the psychosocial determinants of self-testing for cholesterol, glucose, and HIV. *BMC Public Health, 11,* 112.

Harden, A., Brunton, G., Fletcher, A., & Oakley, A. (2009). Teenage pregnancy and social disadvantage: Systematic review integrating controlled trials and qualitative studies. *BMJ, 339,* b4254.

Harding, R., Lampe, F. C., Norwood, S., Date, H. L., Clucas, C., Fisher, M., & Sherr, L. (2010). Symptoms are highly prevalent among HIV outpatients and associated with poor adherence and unprotected sexual intercourse. *Sexually Transmitted Infections, 86*(7), 520–524.

Healthcare Improvement Scotland. (2011). *Human immunodeficiency virus (HIV) standards, July, 2011.* Retrieved from http://www.hivscotland.com/downloads/1311590607-20110707_FINAL_STANDARDS_FOR_HIV_SERVICES_PUBLICATION_VERSION_JULY_2011.pdf

Herbst, J. H., Beeker, C., Mathew, A., McNally, T., Passin, W. F., Kay, L. D., . . . Task Force on Community Preventive Services. (2007). The effectiveness of individual-, group-, and community-level HIV behavioural risk-reduction interventions for adult men who have sex with men. *American Journal of Preventive Medicine, 32,* S38–S67.

Herek, G., & Glunt, E. (1988). An epidemic of stigma: Public reactions to AIDS. *American Psychologist, 43*(11), 886–891.

Holstad, M. M., Dilorio, C., Kelley, M. E., Resnicow, K., & Sharma, S. (2011). Group motivational interviewing to promote adherence to antiretroviral medications and risk reduction behaviors in HIV infected women. *AIDS and Behavior, 15,* 885–896.

Johnstone, L., & Dallos, R. (2006). Introduction to formulation. In L. Johnstone & R. Dallos (Eds.), *Formulation in psychology and psychotherapy: Making sense of people's problems* (pp. 1–16). New York, NY: Routledge.

Lopez, L. M., Tolley, E. E., Grimes, D. A., & Chen-Mok, M. (2009). Theory-based interventions for contraception. *The Cochrane Database of Systematic Reviews, 1,* CD007249. doi: 10.1002/14651858.CD007249.pub2

Lopez, L. M., Tolley, E. E., Grimes, D. A., Chen, M., & Stockton, L. L. (2013). Theory-based interventions for contraception. *The Cochrane Database of Systematic Reviews, 8,* CD007249. doi: 10.1002/14651858.CD007249.pub4

Lyles, C. M., Kay, L. S., Crepaz, N., Herbst, J. H., Passin, W. F., Kim, A. S., . . . HIV/AIDS Prevention Research Synthesis Team. (2007). Best-evidence interventions: Findings from a systematic review of HIV behavioural interventions for US populations at high risk, 2000-2001. *American Journal of Public Health, 97,* 133–143.

Martin, J., Sheeran, P., Slade, P., Wright, A., & Dibble, T. (2011). Durable effects of implementation intentions: Reduced rates of confirmed pregnancy at 2 years. *Health Psychology, 30,* 368–373.

McLellan, J., & Dale, H. (2013). Can technology be effective in interventions targeting sexual health and substance use in young people; a systematic review. *Health and Technology. doi:*10.1007/s12553-013-0059-2

National Institute for Health and Clinical Excellence (NICE). (2009). *Depression in adults.* Clinical Guideline CG90. Available at http://publications.nice.org.uk/depression-in-adults-cg90

National Institute for Health and Clinical Excellence (NICE). (2011). *Generalised anxiety disorder and panic disorder in adults: Management.*Clinical Guideline CG113. Retrieved from http://guidance.nice.org.uk/CG113

Noar, S. M., Benac, C. N., & Harris, M. S. (2007). Does tailoring matter? Meta-analytic review of tailored print health behaviour change interventions. *Psychological Bulletin, 133,* 673–693.

Oringanje, C., Meremikwu, M. M., Eko, H., Esu, E., Meremikuwu, A., & Ehiri, J. E. (2009). Interventions for preventing unintended pregnancies among adolescents. *The Cochrane Database Systematic Reviews, 4,* CD005215. doi: 10.1002/14651858.CD005215.pub2

Parma, S. (2013). Integrated sexual health services: National service specification. London, United Kingdom: Department of Health. Retrieved from https://www.gov.uk/dh

Parsons, J. T., Rosof, E., Punzalan, J. C., & Di, Maria L. (2005). Integration of motivational interviewing and cognitive behavioural therapy to improve HIV medication adherence and reduce substance use among HIV-positive men and women: Results of a pilot project. *AIDS Patient Care and STDs, 19,* 31–39.

Picot, J., Shepherd, J., Kavanagh, J., Cooper, J., Harden, A., Barnett-Page, E., . . . Frampton, G. K. (2012). Behavioural interventions for the prevention of sexually transmitted infections in young people aged 13-19 years: A systematic review. *Health Educaton Research, 27,* 495–512.

Rackstraw, S. (2011). HIV-related neurocognitive impairment—A review. *Psychology, Health & Medicine, 16*(5), 548–563.

Reisner, S. L., Mimlaga, M. J., Skeer, M., Perkovich, B., Johnson, C. V., & Safren, S. A. (2009). A review of HIV antiretroviral adherence and intervention studies among HIV-infected youth. *Adher Interv Youth.* 17, 14–25.

Rollnick, S., & Miller, W. R. (1995). What is motivational interviewing? *Behavioural and Cognitive Psychotherapy, 23,* 325–334.

Rollnick, S., Miller, W. R., & Butler, C. C. (2008). *Motivational Interviewing in Health Care.* New York, NY: The Guilford Press.

Rubak, S., Sandbæk, A., Lauritzen, T., & Christensen, B. (2005). Motivational interviewing: A systematic review and meta-analysis. *British Journal of General Practice, 55,* 305–312.

Sacktor, N., Lyles, R. H., Skolasky, R., Kleeberger, C., Selnes, O. A., Miller, E. N., & McArthur, J. C. (2001). Multicenter AIDS cohort Study, 1990–1998. *Neurology, 56,* 257–260.

Safren, A. A., Traeger, L., Skeer, M. R., O'Cleirigh, C., Meade, C. S., Covahey, C. & Mayer, K. M. (2010). Testing a social-cognitive model of HIV transmission risk behaviors in HIV-infected MSM with and without depression. *Health Psychology, 29,* 215–221.

Sangani, P., Rutherford, G., & Wilkinson, D. (2004). Population-based interventions for reducing sexually transmitted infections, including HIV infection. *The Cochrane Database of Systematic Reviews, 2,* CD001220.

Shepherd, J., Weston, R., Peersman, G., & Napuli, I. Z. (2000). Interventions for encouraging sexual lifestyles and behaviours intended to prevent cervical cancer. *Cochrane Database Syst Rev.* (2):CD001035.

Sherr, D. L., Clucas, C., Harding, R., Sibley, E., & Catalan, J. (2011). HIV and depression - a systematic review of interventions. *Psychol Health Med.* 16(5), 493–527.

Simpson, W. M., Johnstone, F. D., Boyd, F. M., Goldberg, D. J., Hart, G. J., & Prescott, R. J. (1998). Uptake and acceptability of antenatal HIV testing: Randomized controlled trial of different methods of offering the test. *BMJ, 3,* 262–267.

Simpson, W. M., Johnstone, F. D., Goldberg, D. J., Gormley, S. M., & Hart, G. J. (1999). Antenatal HIV testing: Assessment of a routine voluntary approach. *BMJ, 318,* 1660–1661.

Simpson, W. M., Johnstone, F. D., Hart, G. J., Boyd, F. M., & Goldberg, D. J. (1998). To test or not to test? What makes pregnant women decide to take an HIV test? *Psychology, Health & Medicine, 3,* 327–355.

Smith, S. R., Rublein, J. C., Marcus, C., Brock, T. P., & Chesney, M. A. (2003). A medication self-management program to improve adherence to HIV therapy regimes. *Patient Education and Counseling, 50,* 187–199.

Steinberg, J. R., & Finer, L. B. (2011). Examining the association of abortion history and current mental health: A reanalysis of the National Comorbidity Survey using a common-risk-factors model. *Social Science & Medicine, 72*(1): 72–82.

Steinberg, J. R., McCulloch, C. E., & Adler, N. E. (2014). Abortion and mental health: Findings from the National comorbidity Survey-Replication. *Obstetrics & Gynecology, 123*(2, Pt.1): 263–270.

Steinberg, J. R., & Rubin, L. R. (2014). Psychological aspects of contraception, unintended pregnancy and abortion.

Policy Insights from the Behavioral and Brain Sciences, 1(1): 239–247.

Thrasher, A. D., Golin, C. E., Earp, J. A., Tien, H., Porter, C., & Howie, L. (2006). Motivational interviewing to support antiretroviral therapy adherence: The role of quality counseling. *Patient Education and Counseling, 62,* 64–71.

Vidanapathirana, J., Abramson, M. J., Forbes, A., & Fairley, C. (2005). Mass media interventions for promoting HIV testing. *The Cochrane Database of Systematic Reviews, 3,* CD004775.

Whetten, K., Reif S., & Murphy-McMillan, L. K. (2008). Trauma, mental health, distrust and stigma among HIV-positive persons: Implications for effective care. *Psychosomatic Medicine, 70*(5), 531–538.

Wise, J., & Operario, D. (2008). Use of electronic reminder devices to improve adherence to antiretroviral therapy: A systematic review. *AIDS Patient Care and STDs, 22,* 495–504.

CHAPTER

14

Counseling and Psychotherapeutic Interventions in Sexual Health Care

TINA CAMPBELL

Introduction

Advances in medical practice and insight gained from times of difficulty have enabled a deeper appreciation of the impact of physical health upon emotional well-being and vice versa. The same applies therefore to the links between sexual and emotional or psychological health. The social model of health appropriately captures the complex interactions among cultural, environmental, economic, and political factors; personal characteristics, lifestyle, individuals' risk-taking behaviors, and personal health decisions. Thus, the Sandyford sexual and reproductive healthcare center in Glasgow, Scotland, has grown to encompass several programs addressing different facets of sexual health care. Broadly, Sandyford sexual health care involves multi-agency, integrated care and service provision, including the following:

- Contraception and sexual health clinics
- Sexually transmitted infection (STI) testing and treatment
- Community pharmacies
- Sexual and reproductive health information
- Relationships and sexual problems support
- Support for survivors of sexual abuse/sexual assault
- HIV and AIDS care and support
- Lesbian, gay, bisexual, transgender (LGBT) support
- Support for parents and caregivers
- Services for young people

This chapter offers a practitioner and managerial perspective on counseling and psychotherapeutic interventions in sexual health care by describing the Sandyford Model and exploring a variety of therapeutic modalities. It will argue the case for an integrated service, which can offer a more holistic treatment and care plan for patients. The chapter will also explore the impact of historical sexual abuse, the role of attachment theory, how depression can affect sexual health, and the range of therapeutic interventions that can assist a client in their journey toward sustaining a healthy, fully integrated sense of what it means to be human.

The experience of the Sandyford Model is be illustrated in Case Study 14-1.

Case Study 14-1

Liz is 48 and in her third long-term relationship. She attends the sexual health service for a routine cervical smear test. During her consultation, she becomes distressed and admits that she is emotionally exhausted due to a series of abusive relationships. She has four children who are teenagers and feels out of her depth with her older son because of his challenging behaviors. Liz feels unable to cope. Her distress is so significant that she feels unable to remain in the clinic. The nurse encourages her to have some time out within the counseling service, and Liz is able to find some space and the opportunity to talk to the Listening Ear support worker.

Integrating Psychological Well-Being into Sexual Health: The Sandyford Model

McCormack et al. (2008) noted the observation that clients present for counseling with a range of issues including serious physical illness or long-term mental health problems. Counseling may address developmental issues, particular personal problems, decision-making, dealing with crisis, feelings of inner conflict, perceptiveness, comprehension, and relationships with others. The counselor maintains a facilitative role while respecting the individual's values, resources, and self-determining capability.

Historically, counseling has been a dimension of some sexual and reproductive health services, providing, for example, pre- and post-termination counseling, addressing psychosexual issues, and perhaps almost coincidentally working with emotional issues that might have emerged from a patient consultation. The formation of Sandyford evidenced a very clear strategic decision to fully integrate counseling and psychotherapy within the context of sexual health. The Sandyford Model thereby has been able to capture the very essence of how an integrated service can enhance the sexual health, reproductive care, and emotional well-being of everyone.

Sandyford Counseling and Support Service (SCASS) is an important dimension of patient care at Sandyford. SCASS has a major role in ensuring that emotional and mental health are key factors in positive sexual and reproductive health. Not only placing but also developing and sustaining such an extensive and therapeutically robust counseling service within the context of sexual health remains unique in the United Kingdom.

Historical Development

Historically, the counseling service began as the Center for Women's Health in 1998, and was innovative in offering open-ended/long-term counseling and therapeutic support to women within Greater Glasgow and beyond. Initially, the Center for Women's Health had provided a safe space for women to come and talk. As it became evident that some women were looking for therapy, volunteer counselors began to offer volunteer hours in this women-only space. The Social Model of Health helped gain National Health Service (NHS) support for open access to counseling for women who presented with a range of issues. It was also regarded as a positive step on a political and socioeconomic level toward the reduction of mental health problems caused by social deprivation, all forms of abuse, sexual assault, rape, and gender-based violence. The Glasgow City Council began to fund the program, and in 2005, additional funding from the Scottish Government's "Survivor Scotland" initiative was secured and assisted in the development of counseling for male survivors of historical childhood sexual abuse (CSA).

In 2003, the majority of women attending were in long-term counseling (in excess of 2–3 years). The Service was staffed primarily by contracted counselors, working a range of hours, but the majority only working 4 hours per week. There were a number of volunteer counselors (already qualified) and a few trainees (currently in training). However, the waiting list became unmanageable with increasing demand for long-term counseling. A number of groups for women were offered, including Self-Esteem and Writing Groups, following disclosure of CSA. The social benefits of group work proved to be as valuable as the therapeutic input for some women.

Integration and Service Redesign, 2006

It is evident that a counseling service should parallel the process of a therapeutic relationship of psychological growth in that it will be open to both challenge and opportunities for change. Since 2003, the Sandyford Counseling Services Model has experienced a significant transition. Sometimes that has been in response to the challenges of the financial climate, but often it has been through systematic reviews that have tried to determine how the service might best meet the needs of our clients. It makes sense, therefore, for any psychological service, but perhaps more specifically within sexual health, to evolve and engage in the review process. Thankfully, the world of psychological therapies does not stand still, and it is imperative that service providers seek to deliver the highest standard of evidenced-based therapies to those who are seeking help. Previous reviews have resulted in a restructuring of the service to address gender inequalities, more clearly defined criteria, enhanced services, a rigorous assessment process, and the development of more specialized evidence-based therapeutic interventions.

In 2006, Sandyford Counseling Services underwent a service redesign based on client review. Changes were both clinical and operational in nature, such as expanded staff hours and adding to the range of therapeutic modalities offered. In addition, male counselors were brought on staff to offer counseling services for men, such as Thrive and the Steve Retson Project.

The Counseling Services division of Sandyford has worked to implement the Standards Framework for counselors and Counseling Services (McCormack et al., 2008). The staff has addressed areas of clinical governance, time management, supervision, and the importance of maintaining a high level of professionalism. SCASS is therefore an integral part of Sandyford, but also by informal agreement and function works in partnership with the Primary Care Mental Health Teams (PCMHTs). As such, SCASS regards itself as a similar but also specialist service in terms of the clients who are seen. It remains unique as a self-referral service to a specialist team. The function of PCMHTs is to work with clients presenting with mild to moderate mental health issues. SCASS receives professional referrals or self-referrals from clients who can present with moderate to severe and severe to enduring mental health difficulties. SCASS is recognized as a specialist service for therapeutic treatment of sexual abuse and other issues related to sexual identity and inequalities. Though we rarely turn clients away, it is important that the counselors are not expected to work beyond their capabilities, such as therapeutic work with registered sex offenders or clients who are currently engaged in the criminal justice system following charges in relation to sexual offenses, or clients who are cared for within tertiary services and who are too unstable to engage in therapy. However, clients are referred from both PCMHTs and Community Mental Health Teams (CMHTs) within NHS Greater Glasgow and Clyde Board (NHSGGC) and beyond, with approximately 19% of clients annually accessing counseling from other Health Board areas.

Current Service Delivery

In 2012, the staffing of the service was structured as shown in **Figure 14-1**.

Generic Counseling for Men and Women

The counselors at Sandyford all belong to one or more dedicated specialist teams. The "generic service" embraces those clients who might not attend specific Sandyford services such as Thrive or the Steve Retson Project. The term *generic* does not completely or adequately capture the significant number of people who present within this category with moderate to severe—and sometimes severe and enduring—psychological presentations. Some 70–80% of clients who are seen predominantly present with (historical) CSA. Many will report other abuse that might be either past and present. It is the experience of many survivors of sexual abuse that sexual harm does not stand alone and is often within the context of emotional and physical abuse or neglect. It is not unusual for men and women who have suffered abuse in the past to engage in repetitive abusive adult relationships. This is often a result of poor early attachment. Attachment theory can provide a model for understanding how attachment styles formed

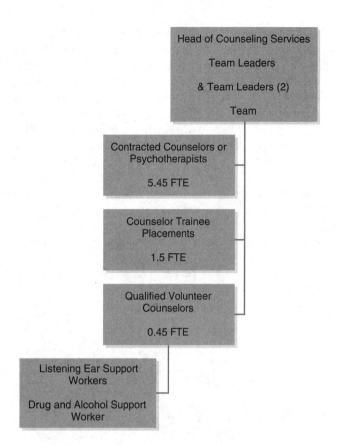

Figure 14-1 SCASS Service Delivery Structure, 2012

in infancy systematically affect subsequent psychological functions and functioning across the lifespan of individuals (Shorey & Snyder, 2006).

Attachment styles formed very early in infancy can indeed impact not only cognitive and emotional development but can also influence the ability to respond to and process trauma. Early attachments can set a template for future coping mechanisms in adulthood: "Attachment Theory proposes that interactions with a primary caregiver in childhood result in episodic memories that form secure or insecure working models of relationships in adulthood" (Shorey & Snyder, 2006, p. 7).

A clear determinant of attachment styles is the messages the infant receives from the caregiver when responding to difficult experiences. Learned behavior and generational patterns also impact outcomes. Not only do the primary caregiver and family of origin influence attachment styles, but they also model behavior and attitudes in relation to sexual values.

Shorey and Snyder (2006) argue that an understanding of attachment theory facilitates the conceptualization of a client's problems and the selection of appropriate interventions. Reassuringly, they conclude that attachment styles should be assessed as a standard part of treatment planning in psychological services. Indeed, this is evident in sexual health services where clients might act out a disruptive attachment pattern or style in therapy but also within the relationships they establish with other healthcare professionals. The very nature of engaging with sexual health services implies willingness from the patient or client to feel potentially vulnerable and to also feel safe enough to disclose sometimes intensely personal details and information. For some, this might be the first time they have been able to engage in such disclosure within a safe, boundaried professional relationship if their early attachment relationships were disorganized or avoidant. An exploration of early attachment history in therapy is indeed most important for clients as they start to engage in a therapeutic alliance. It is not uncommon, for example, for an avoidant, ambivalent attachment style to be a contributory factor in sexual risk-taking behaviors.

Emotional Support in Times of Crisis: The Listening Ear Service

---

Case Study 14-2

Ann has been to see her general practitioner (GP) at various times over the past year with some medically unexplained symptoms. She has persistent low mood. A demanding job has increased her stress levels. When her younger sister becomes pregnant, Ann becomes very distressed. Her GP refers her to the Listening Ear service where she shares her deep distress at not being in a relationship and her longing for children.

The Listening Ear (LE) service at Sandyford is an innovative post within mental health and it encapsulates the ethos of the foundation of the Counseling Services (formerly the Center for Women's Health) more than 13 years ago. The LE system was originally put in place to meet the increasing demand by women to have a safe place to speak, to address their concerns, and to address identified gaps within service provision. Many of those concerns were issues that regrettably remain current (if not further compounded) today, such as domestic abuse, gender-based violence, addictive behaviors, challenges to parenting, historical sexual abuse, rape, and sexual assault.

In more recent years, the LE service is primarily delivered by one LE support worker in collaboration with the Sandyford drug and alcohol support worker. The service is in constant demand and the waiting times are closely monitored, which is important given the high levels of risk and vulnerability among those who attend. Men, women, and young people aged 18 and over attend this service. Sometimes couples might attend, or a client might wish to have a support worker, caregiver, or family member attend with them.

Patients and clients self-refer to this service and are referred by other health professionals on a daily basis. It offers an immediate intervention to men, women, and young people, who can often drop in and are in need of emotional support. Within Sandyford, patients are regularly brought to the LE service by clinicians due to high levels of distress or following the painful disclosure of significant risks or losses that impact the emotional and mental health of the patient. Some patients attend and, having had an opportunity to explore their thoughts and feelings, reach a decision quite spontaneously about what they need to do in relation to their difficulties.

Referrals to the LE service from outside Sandyford come from GP practices, community addiction teams, crisis teams, community mental health teams, and numerous voluntary organizations that are not able to offer such a service.

Clients who attend the LE service can receive up to three sessions. Our policy is to be very clear that this is emotional support and often practical intervention rather than a counseling relationship. The service also includes advocacy work, and the LE support worker can make referrals to other agencies, find resources for clients, and explore appropriate counseling for their needs. The LE service is a vital resource not only within Sandyford, but for many professionals and service users within the Greater Glasgow and Clyde area of Scotland. As a model of service, it serves not only as an immediate and often "emergency" service, but sometimes as an informal introduction to a potential counseling relationship. Clients often present to the LE service with high levels of anxiety; many will have already been seen within the mental health system, and some will have found engagement difficult. Chaotic life styles, addictions, poor attachments, and abusive relationships commonly form part of the client story when presenting for an LE appointment. Even though this is a brief intervention, it can indeed model for patients and clients what a supportive therapeutic relationship might be like. In that sense, it can also serve to provide a pre-therapy model to establish contact with those who might find that difficult.

The Place Counseling Service for Young People (14- to 18-Year-Olds)

The Place (now more often known as the Young People's Service) is the special sexual health services for young people up to age 18. The Place is an integral part of Sandyford, and only young people can use the sexual health service during the times The Place is operational. The counseling service within The Place runs alongside but also independently within Sandyford. The Place captures an excellent model of integrated work within multidisciplinary teams. The Place has a consultant lead and a lead nurse, both of whom are very experienced in working with young people. The lead nurse in particular has a good working relationship with both The Place's cognitive behavioral therapist and the drug and alcohol support worker. The Place staff play a key role in the Sandyford Child Protection Standing Committee and also have good professional links with Social Work, the Family Protection Unit, and other statutory authorities and agencies.

The Place offers a full range of sexual health and relationships services, treatment, advice, and information. It provides regular ongoing contraception and emergency contraception, free condoms, testing and treatment for sexually transmitted infections, pregnancy testing, advice, and counseling around pregnancy choices.

Young people are encouraged to reflect upon their risk-taking behaviors in terms of their sexual health, relationships, life style patterns, and choices. This clearly includes choices around alcohol and tobacco.

There is a specific focus on the impact of excessive alcohol consumption in working with young people who attend The Place. The literature review of Kenny (2010) produced a summary of key findings on sexual risk taking and the role of alcohol among potentially high-risk groups. Some of the findings are as follows:

- Young people are more likely to take sexual risks when consuming or having just consumed excessive alcohol.
- Sexualized gender stereotypes and the significant impact of the media's portrayal of alcohol use and sexual activity among young celebrities has a negative influence on young people.
- Alcohol is the main reason given by many young people for having sex, especially early sex or sex with someone they had not known very long.
- Alcohol is a main contributing factor to first sex using no contraception.
- Alcohol consumption can result in lowered inhibitions and poor judgments regarding sexual activity and risky sexual behaviors.
- Poor mental health, including depression, has been linked to higher numbers of sexual partners and failure to use condoms.
- Young people who drink are more likely to take other risks and engage in sexually risky behaviors.

Further, Prescription for Change (Hunt & Fish, 2008), the lesbian and bisexual women's health review produced by both De Monfort University Leicester and Sigma Research, found that 90% of lesbian and bisexual women drink, and 40% drink three times a week compared to 25% of women in general.

The correlation between alcohol and risk-taking behaviors has led to the decision to screen all young people who attend The Place. The young person completes the tool in the reception area while waiting to be seen at the clinic. If help is required to complete the screening tool, a staff member or clinician is available to assist. Although completion of the tool is voluntary, staff are trained to both encourage and support young people to complete it. Data from the screening remains confidential to Sandyford but is extremely useful in terms of data capture and reviewing trends. Alcohol screening is an effective preventative intervention aimed at young people. Encouraging self-monitoring through screening increases awareness of alcohol consumption and will hopefully identify either risky or harmful drinking before it becomes too problematic. It also monitors individual patterns by screening at each visit to the clinic. By its very nature, it encourages young people to experience a holistic approach toward their sexual health. It is educational in that young people are encouraged to reflect upon the links between alcohol consumption, sexual health, and risk-taking behaviors. The same voluntary alcohol screening has been made available in adult services with an option for any patient to have a call from the alcohol and drugs worker to follow up on any concerns.

Alcohol Brief Intervention for Young People

The Sandyford website has an online program called the Alcolator, which can be used to calculate how many units someone might drink; this is followed by access to a survey to see if the young person would benefit from some tips on sensible drinking. The Alcohol Brief Intervention is essentially relaxed and helpful, not confrontational or judgmental. It is seen as a supportive conversation that aims to raise awareness to motivate and encourage a reduction in drinking. The intervention is offered by the drug and alcohol support worker. It can be either requested by a young person or referred via one of the healthcare professionals. There is additional access to Sandyford's drug and alcohol support worker for young people, who offer support if a young person is worried about their own drinking or if they are worried about someone close to them who is drinking to excess.

Alcohol is not the only significant factor in sexual risk-taking behaviors. Increased levels of poor mental health, low motivation, self-worth, and sense of purpose all have a significant impact. To address some of the more complex psychological issues, there is one part-time highly skilled cognitive behavioral therapist working in The Place who is qualified in cognitive behavioral therapy (CBT) training and relationship (couples) counseling and is also an eye movement desensitization and reprocessing (EMDR) practitioner. The majority of clients self-refer or come via the sexual health clinic at The Place. External referrals come from GPs, health visitors, and CMHTs.

The gender of clients presenting for counseling is now balanced equally and this has been an encouraging change over recent years. Initially, clients presenting for counseling within The Place were predominantly female. There has been a noticeable increase in males attending for counseling. Young people are made aware that they can have direct access to The Place Counseling Service without necessarily having to go via the sexual health clinic. Young people can also access a Listening Ear service in an emergency with any of the Sandyford counselors.

Couples Counseling

....

> ### Case Study 14-3
>
> John is in a long-term relationship, and the couple has two young children. His work often takes him away from home. He attends the sexual health service for a sexual health screen. When he is diagnosed with an STI, he has to tell his partner, who also needs to attend the sexual health clinic. During the consultation, his use of escort services comes to light. John and his partner are referred for couples counseling.

Couples counseling is a key service within sexual health. However, apart from couples who might access counseling together in the Psychosex Service, there has historically been a lack of support and therapeutic interventions for couples who attend sexual health services. The benefits of couples' therapy in Sandyford enabled clients who did not meet the criteria of requiring psychosexual therapy an opportunity to work together as a couple on relationship issues directly related to sexual health. A couple presenting for sexual health screening when one or the other has engaged in risk-taking sexual activity is not unusual, and the benefit of couples' therapy is that it enables them to work together, rather than as individuals, in resolving the issues and essentially understanding and changing behaviors.

Working with couples requires a specific and different set of therapeutic skills, and it would not therefore be appropriate for anyone to work in this area without specialist training. Although there are several voluntary agencies offering counseling—some for a fixed fee and others for a donation—it remains a gap in service provision within Sandyford. Within NHSGGC, couples counseling is only available through psychosexual services. Any couples wishing to access therapy together would be required to do so privately and pay a fee per session.

Psychosexual Therapy Working Alongside Counseling

> ### Case Study 14-4
>
> Martin and Sarah are referred by their GP to the Psychosex Team for assessment. They have been married for 3 years and were in a relationship for 18 months prior to being married. For religious reasons, they had both agreed to wait until after they were married to have sexual intercourse. Sarah finds intercourse painful and yet wants to become pregnant. Martin believes that Sarah does not really love him and that she does not want sex, but shares the desire for a child. He has stopped initiating sex because it frequently concludes with Sarah becoming very upset and in pain. They seek help, and during the sexual history-taking aspect of their assessment, Sarah discloses that she was sexually abused by an uncle when she was 8 years old.

As a medical discipline in itself, psychosexual counseling developed from the integration of family planning and psychotherapy services. Initially, a client might be seen individually or with their partner by a specialist with training in psychosexual medicine, who will explore the possibility of physical causes for the presenting sexual difficulties. If there are indeed indicators of physical problems, then there are a range of both medical and surgical possibilities. Psychosexual counseling might be considered to explore related psychological factors.

A major benefit of an integrated sexual health and counseling service is that patients can be appropriately assessed and given a package of care to help them understand the possible connections between their emotional and physical well-being. It is not unusual for patients to underestimate the impact that mental ill health can have on sexual health and thereby on reproductive functioning. The Sandyford integrated service means that the Psychosex Team works closely with the head of counseling services to deliver a personalized package of care. Referrals to the Psychosex Team usually come from GPs, but patients can self-refer and there are referrals from other health professionals within Sandyford. Patients who are referred for counseling usually have disclosed historical CSA, a history of abusive relationships, issues in terms of sexual functioning related to previous terminations or miscarriages, and more recently, a notable increase of referrals for patients who disclose the impact of sexual addiction on their sexual health.

Ultimately, it is most important that patients are not sent from one department to another, having to discuss their difficulties repeatedly and with a different person each time. A close working relationship within the teams can assist what can be a potentially complex experience for patients in disclosing highly sensitive information.

Psychosexual Issues: The Impact of the Loss of Intimacy on Sexual Health and Well-Being

In meeting a patient's psychosexual concerns, it is important to explore the patient's general emotional health. A couple may present with communication difficulties that are often described as episodes of tension, arguments, and an inability to problem solve. Probing underneath the surface of these tensions, there will be a myriad of difficulties and events, but what couples have in common is often a lack of both physical and emotional intimacy. For some, this loss can be linked to depression, but it can also be a cause of depression, which in itself can be problematic for a health practitioner. (The role of depression and the impact on sexual health is discussed later in this chapter, together with an exploration of appropriate therapeutic approaches and modalities.) The loss or diminishing of libido is often one of the first consequences of depression and one of the last factors to be resolved once a depressive phase has started to dissipate. Some of the side effects of depression, however, can be rather (distressingly) subtle, and it is perhaps understandable that health practitioners focus upon the signs such as low mood, tearfulness, and insomnia rather than asking about libido or levels of emotional intimacy.

Gilbert and Shmukler (1992) suggest that much psychological pain can be relieved if sexual issues are explored sensitively and openly by therapists. They also explore the importance of therapists being comfortable with their own sexuality in order to feel confident in working with the complexities of psychosexual issues in the therapeutic room.

It might be difficult for therapists to explore psychosexual issues, particularly if an individual or couple present with other issues. The same might apply when sexual health concerns are raised by the therapist, and it is not unusual for a client's response to be that they "cannot be bothered" or indeed to consider an active sex life to be something that was an aspect of the early years of the relationship that is not as relevant now. The therapeutic world has continued to strive to maintain a holistic approach to the needs of anyone seeking therapy. Developments have included acknowledging the spiritual needs of an individual. In the same way, there has been a strategic decision to ensure that risk assessments of clients who might present with suicidal ideation are a key element of the therapeutic relationship. It seems of equal importance that due attention is given to the sexual health needs of both individuals and couples who present for therapy.

Therapists should feel confident in exploring the impact of a loss of intimacy and how it might be related to a loss of libido, which can occur at any time during the life cycle of both men and women. Each physical and psychological developmental stage can offer its own challenges and raise personal and intimate questions for individuals in relation to their sexual self. At the point at which someone requests counseling, some of these issues have reached crisis point and there is often a correlation between the presenting issues, the crisis, and the life stage in which that individual finds themselves. It can be very easy for a therapist to overlook some of this and neglect having a holistic approach.

Other causes of low libido can be due to past sexual abuse, rape, and sexual assault or previous complex relationships. If there is an emotional void in a relationship, it can directly negatively influence the ability to engage in physical contact. If either partner in a relationship is feeling emotional instability, and their thought processes are by default negative, then erotic thoughts and fantasies are replaced with dark feelings of abandonment and isolation. In such instances, it becomes impossible for either partner to contemplate even non-genital signs of affection, let alone penetrative sex.

Consideration of appropriate therapeutic approaches for psychosexual difficulties should include CBT. This might not suit every individual or couple, but for some it can prove to be highly effective. CBT can be a useful technique in the assessment of levels of desire in a couple with psychosexual difficulties. Chambless and Ollendick (2001) support the understanding that clients will seek CBT if they have already had a positive experience of it as a therapeutic intervention. The very ethos of CBT is a problem-oriented focus where setting goals is an important dimension of the therapeutic engagement.

Exploring Beyond the Presenting Issue: Eating Disorders Counseling in Sexual Health

Interestingly, the Sandyford Model placed a specific counseling service for eating disorders within sexual health. There is a high correlation between sexual abuse (or other sexually related trauma) and development of eating disorders, where there are clear indications of early trauma and the need for the patient to take control over their own body (Anderson, 1990; Gleaves & Eberenz, 1994; Palmer, Oppenheimer, Dignon, Chaloner, & Howells, 1990; Waller, Ruddock, & Cureton, 1995) and while CSA is not necessarily a cause of eating disorders, it is an indication of how survivors manifest the trauma:

> [F]or many survivors of CSA, eating disorders are a re-enactment of their experiences of CSA, in which the survivor is forced to take something through the mouth and into the body, which he then wishes to rid himself of. (Sanderson, 2008, p. 292)

Even when dissociation might prevent or cloud the memory, the behavioral acting out remains. Food can also serve as a transitional object for patients in terms of relationship development when the risk of engagement with other human beings is perceived as too dangerous (Schwartz & Cohn, 1996).

In some clients, where there has been no CSA, an eating disorder can develop following a sexual assault. Early disclosures are regarded as beneficial for the patient and treatment can become rapidly more effective (Tice, Hall, Beresford, Quinones, & Hall, 1989).

In recognition of these factors, the eating disorders service was established in 2006 (at the point of Service Redesign and Integration), and offered a range of approaches in both early intervention and therapeutic support that was not being offered elsewhere. The service was available to both male and female clients; although statistically more women than men present with eating disorders, the number of male clients has increased in recent years among adolescents.

The eating disorder service incorporates a rigorous evaluation process, regular reporting to the Women's

Health team, "one-off" sessions for patients and caregivers, "joint work" for patients and partners, a drop-in support group, and advice and supervision sessions for other health professionals.

In the autumn of 2010, a pre-therapy group for women coping with an eating disorder was offered for the first time. It was remarkably successful, with some women not needing individual therapy and others needing far less time in therapy than they would if they had not attended the group.

Supporting Male Survivors of Childhood Sexual Abuse: Thrive

Thrive is a dedicated counseling service for non-offending male survivors of historical CSA. It began in 2005 and was initially part funded by Choose Life in recognition of working with vulnerable young males and helping to reduce the high suicide rates among young adult males, particularly in Scotland. Partial funding continues to be provided by the Scottish Government through the Survivor Scotland Network. Funding requires rigorous monitoring reports, and it is hoped that further grants will be available from the Scottish Government for the continuation of this service.

Thrive has been an innovative service within the NHS in Scotland and remains one of the few dedicated services for male survivors of CSA. The new team of therapists appointed to work in this service were able to work creatively to engage men to attend. Pre-therapy and post-therapy groups have been important to help men make the transitions both to and from individual therapy. There has also been some greater degree of flexibility to offer longer-term therapy and the opportunity to return for further support should major life adjustments result in the resurgence of symptoms such as flashbacks. Such life adjustments might include starting a new relationship, the loss of a significant other, becoming a parent, and more commonly, death of the perpetrator.

The service was evaluated in 2006, with significant consultation of service users, resulting in further service development. Therapy has helped to reduce suicidal ideation among the client group by acknowledging the impact of CSA for men. Counselors were trained to acknowledge the level of stigma for men both in seeking help and in disclosing the abuse. For some men, the disclosure is even more complex if the perpetrator was the mother or another female caregiver. The impact of historical sexual abuse is by its very nature complex, and Thrive service clients are able to regard recovery as an attainable and sustainable goal. Therefore, the importance of having an individualized service package for each client is seen as a priority.

Additional activities offered include a long-term post-therapy support group, where male clients are able to attend as part of their transition from counseling to more independence and recovery. The design and implementation of a Befriending Program was certainly an unusual step within a NHS service, and had limited uptake from clients.

However, for those who did use the service, it was helpful to reduce isolation and develop manageable goals for daily living.

The counselors now work within a time-limited framework so that clients are no longer in therapy for a minimum of 1 to 2 years. However, men who present with CSA are also attending SCASS to see non-Thrive counselors and have done so since the last service redesign in 2006.

Therapeutic Interventions Following Rape and Sexual Assault: Archway Glasgow

Archway is Scotland's first Sexual Assault Referral Center (SARC) and it is both based within and delivered by Sandyford medical, nursing, and counseling staff. It is the first Rape and Sexual Assault Referral Center in Scotland and was established in April 2007. It is a collaborative service between the NHS, Strathclyde Police, and Greater Glasgow City Council.

The main function and purpose of a SARC is to offer a holistic service to men, women, and young people from the age of 14 who have been recently raped or sexually assaulted. The service combines both medical and psychological support with an integrated forensic service.

Archway offers clients forensic services (including storage of forensic samples), immediate medical care for minor injuries, emergency contraception, STI prophylaxis, support services, follow-up STI screening, and counseling. The service is open 24 hours a day, 365 days a year, and is in significant demand. Counselors at Archway offer a robust, mixed modality of therapeutic interventions such as CBT, gestalt, integrative, psychodynamic, and person-centered therapy. Nearly all the counselors and psychotherapists are also trained in EMDR, which is recommended as treatment for posttraumatic stress disorder (PTSD) by National Institute for Clinical Excellence (NICE) Guidelines. PTSD is common indicator among Archway attendees.

Appointments are available for Archway clients on a weekly basis. Archway clients are given a longer time in therapy than generic service clients and may return or request further counseling or additional support at the time of a court case. Some clients might return when life events trigger past trauma. Presence of a male counselor has enabled clients to indicate a preference for the gender of their counselor.

The Role of the Archway Support Workers

Initially, at the time when Archway opened, emotional support was offered through some partnership working with Rape Crisis. This continued as the service became established and a full-time support worker was appointed, which expanded to two full-time workers as the number of referrals increased. Both support workers offer an individual approach, and client feedback is positive. The number of clients presenting for counseling is an indication of their skill in assessing client needs. It is important to always have two support workers available, to increase client choice, which is important in a context where choice and control have been seriously compromised following a sexual assault or rape. Enabling clients to have a choice about appropriate support and therapeutic options can enable them to regain some of the skills that they perceive as having been compromised. The Archway support workers are fully aware of the modalities offered by the Archway counselors and work in collaboration to ensure a good "therapeutic fit" for the client.

The Archway Client Journey

Although Archway clients have many common threads in terms of symptomatic presentations, emotions, and outcomes, each client is regarded as an individual. The most important focus is on client choice, which begins with whether to immediately disclose the rape/assault to police. The benefit of available forensic services is the ability to take samples, and record and store them until the client is ready to report. Client choice also includes the offer of counseling or meeting with a support worker. Some clients choose one or the other, some choose neither, and some engage with both service options. The support workers are crucial in understanding the therapeutic orientations of Archway counselors and matching the client to the most appropriate counselor. The Archway counselors are a skilled team who work effectively with clients. It seems important that there is an opportunity to capture some of the client journeys, which clearly evidence both the importance of counseling and support but also how successful and necessary it is within Archway.

The link between PTSD and sexual health is recognized and is prevalent in the context of a SARC. PTSD is evidenced both in the immediate and the long-term aftermath of trauma. Adult attachment patterns can have an impact upon how someone recovers from trauma, and is a principal determinant of resilience to later trauma (Fonagy et al., 1991).

Such resilience is identified, but not often explored, as posttraumatic growth (PTG). "The topic of growth through adversity has become the concentrated focus of much empirical and theoretical work" (Joseph & Linley 2005, p. 262). Tedeschi, Park, and Calhoun (1998) refer to the approach of both psychiatry and psychology where the focus has been on the cause of disease and on the maladaptive behavior observed in those who have experienced traumatic events. In PTG, such traumas establish new psychological constructs that incorporate not only the possibility of such traumas but also better ways to cope. This presents an interestingly positive way to view the outcomes of trauma.

However, the impact of sexual assault is recognized as a significant trauma and one that might continue to impact on survivors for some significant period of time.

Long after the event, many traumatized people feel that a part of themselves has died. . . . Perhaps the most disturbing information on the long term

effects of traumatic events comes from a community study of crime victims including 100 women who had been raped. The average time elapsed since the rape was 9 years . . . the lasting destructive effects of the trauma were apparent. (Herman, 1997, pp. 49–50).

Frazier et al. (2001) investigated the timing and cause of PTG and the relationship between positive and negative life changes and posttraumatic distress among recent female sexual assault survivors who had counseling. Most of the participants reported positive change at 2 weeks. Positive change generally increased over time and negative changes decreased, although with significant individual variability in change patterns. Moreover, both positive and negative changes were associated with distress in expected ways although the relations with negative changes were stronger: "In addition to viewing posttraumatic growth as a long process, current theories contain the related assumption that the number of benefits survivors report generally increases over time" (Frazier et al., 2001, p. 1048).

Steve Retson Counseling

The Steve Retson Project (SRP) offers sexual health services to men who present as gay, bisexual, or who have had sex with other men. This is a well-established service and SCASS provides counseling to SRP clients. The SRP was established as a specialist sexual health clinic for men who have sex with men (MSM), in partnership with the gay community. At the time of its foundation in 1994, they wanted peers from the community to "meet and greet" clients accessing the service, in order to break down barriers and provide a safe and welcoming environment for service users. Host Helpers were initially used as volunteers, until the Health Board's policy on volunteering changed, at which point they became employees of Sandyford. They still provide a welcoming service to clients accessing the service. Since its inception, it has become the largest such service in the United Kingdom and is recognized internationally and nationally as a center of excellence in this field. It offers appropriate and accessible health services including advice and screening for sexually transmitted infections, hepatitis vaccination, HIV advice and testing, counseling, and other forms of support. CBT and person-centered counseling are available for clients who attend this service.

Steve Retson Project Choices

The importance of sexual health care for patients presenting with HIV is discussed elsewhere in this publication. The focus in this section will be on a specific therapeutic intervention. This is another innovative service and is again quite unique in offering CBT to MSM wishing to engage in exploring changes in behavioral patterns. It aims to reduce HIV-related sexual risk behavior among HIV-positive, HIV-negative, and untested MSM who are at risk of either HIV transmission or acquiring HIV.

Through the bloodborne virus (BBV) group, additional funding initially secured a 2-year cognitive behavioral therapist post to work with MSM who are engaged in high-risk sexual activities that place them at risk of HIV. This is a new project, and a cognitive behavioral therapist has been appointed who currently sees a number of male clients who can be referred through the SRP clinic or via Sandyford sexual health screening. Through such, men are identified who disclose MSM and have been diagnosed with a STI or report, for example unprotected anal intercourse (UAI) with two or more men, or UAI with a man of unknown HIV status or with a man of known discordant HIV status.

A specified CBT model is delivered for 10 sessions. The intervention is based on a study carried out in the United States between 1999–2001, 1999 and 2001, called EXPLORE (Koblin & the EXPLORE Study Team, 2004), which devised a 10-session model to be used with clients. The aim of therapy is to enable clients to make more positive healthy choices so that they engage with safe rather than unsafe sex. The cognitive behavioral therapist works with the client to identify risk-taking behaviors and any triggers. Known risk factors or triggers associated with unsafe sex among MSM clients include low self-esteem, poor assertiveness skills, and excessive alcohol consumption, and drug misuse. Therapy includes education on safe sex practices and risk factors. Therapists are trained to examine the client's attitude toward risk and enable him to discover why risk taking is such a factor in his experience as well as to consider attitudes toward what might be termed "safe risk taking." In therapy the client experience of communicating with a partner about sex will also be explored so that the client is able to develop the appropriate confidence to discuss with his sexual partner the importance of safe sex.

Figure 14-2 illustrates the client referral pathway and journey through SRP choices.

Transgender Counseling

There is a dedicated Gender team within Sandyford with two consultant psychiatrists, an associate specialist, a staff grade doctor, and two dedicated counselors. Anyone who is confused about their gender identity or their experience of their gender can refer to this service. However, it is primarily for transsexual people who wish to progress through the stages of transitioning. There is one person-centered counselor working with adult transgender clients in Sandyford who offers 10 client appointments each week. The main focus for therapy is coping with the significant life adjustments and family and other interpersonal relationships. The counselor works closely with the Gender Team. Again, this service is very much in demand and much of the client work is challenging. The Transgender Support Group for male-to-female clients meets in SCASS once a month. There is a cognitive behavioral therapist who provides counseling for young people under the age of 19. They are first seen for a full assessment by the consultant child and adolescent psychiatrist. The young person's family is invited to participate in discussions both with the psychiatrist and the cognitive behavioral therapist with the client's consent. Counseling for both adults and young people can often focus on the life adjustments, coping with the reaction of others, work, family, and relationships.

Working Therapeutically with Women in Prostitution: Base 75

Base 75 is a service for women involved in prostitution and Sandyford provides a 1-day walk-in sexual and reproductive health service as a joint-funding agreement with Glasgow City Council Community Safety Services. In January 2010, one of the person-centered counselors was appointed to work in Base 75 for 6 hours per week. This proved to be remarkably successful, as previous counseling input has not had the same level of success or impact.

Women who are involved in prostitution often have chaotic lifestyles and present with many complex needs. The model developed in Base 75 is a mix of Listening Ear appointments, counseling, and informal availability. Enabling the women to develop a sense of trust with the counselor has been a priority, and a number are now engaged in more formal counseling. This can help women in move out of prostitution and make important life changes. In 2013, this service became fully physically integrated within the Sandyford premises.

How Therapeutic Interventions Can Facilitate Improved Sexual Health

Sexual and emotional well-being are inextricably linked. In sexual health services, it is essential that sufficient attention be given to offering a holistic service to patients. There are numerous therapeutic modalities and interventions available; it is important to offer clients a range of options.

Psychodynamic Psychotherapy

Psychodynamic psychotherapy focuses on how unconscious desires drive our actions and experience. Freud identified the roots of depression in early relationships with parental figures. He further identified depression as a reaction to loss and grief, as well as unresolved resentments toward parental figures leading to guilt, which in turn can lead to depression. The tools might appear to explore complex concepts such as projective identification, splitting, and transference. It is, however, a therapy with a significant energy and places direct attention on the client–therapist relationship. It is often in this context that earlier relationships are acted out in the therapy room. The therapist is therefore constantly aware of transference. In sexual health therapy, it is important to address such concepts as unconscious desires and further the impact and relevance of emotional drives such as how guilt or guilty feelings (whether accurate or not) can impact sexual health.

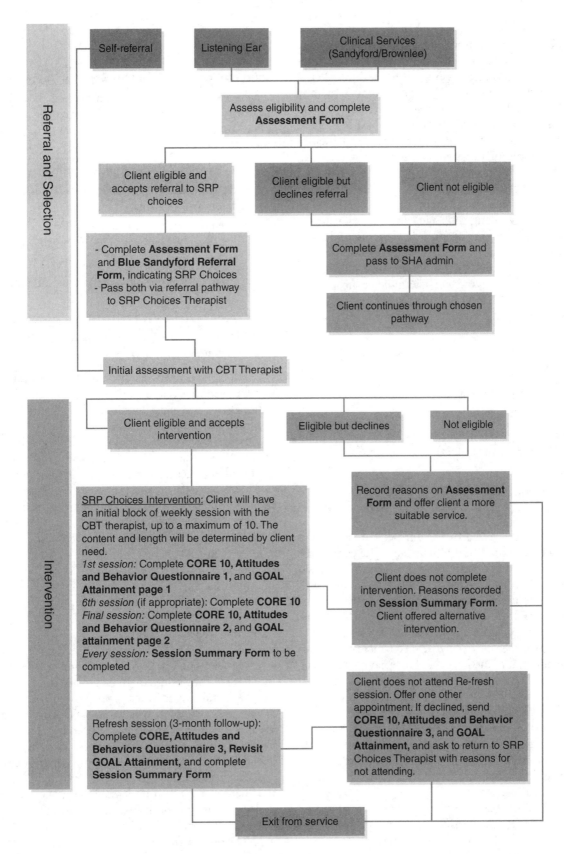

Figure 14-2 Client Referral Pathway and Journey Through SRP Choices
Reproduced from Steve Retson Project. SRP choices. Available at: http://www.steveretsonproject.org.uk/services/srp-choices/

Psychodynamic therapy is often regarded as a long-term intervention: "One common misconception is that a psychodynamic formulation is only indicated for those patients in a long-term expressive psychotherapy" (Perry, Cooper, & Michels, 2006, p. 297). Psychodynamic therapy does not necessarily have to be restricted to longer-term therapy, but the tools and concepts can enable a client to get in touch with very deep-rooted, often primal emotions. An example of psychodynamic therapy that can be used in a more time-limited way is psychodynamic interpersonal psychotherapy (PIPT), developed by Hobson in 1983. Hobson defined the main task of therapy as to develop a "mutual-feeling language" and a relationship of "aloneness-togetherness." Together, the therapist and client find a mutuality that is not necessarily defined by the use of specific psychodynamic terms (such as splitting), unless the client is able to grasp and work with such concepts and language. To that end, Hobson was determined to have a "jargon-free therapy."

Hobson's PIPT Model

The following components are part of Hobson's PIPT model:

- Exploratory rationale
- Shared understanding
- Staying with feelings
- Focus on difficult feelings
- Gaining insight
- Sequencing interventions
- Making changes

Hobson's model is clearly relevant to the management and treatment of sexual health problems. The concept of mutuality is also particularly valued by the client when so often sexual difficulties and problematic sexual health histories are intensely personal and often at the core of trauma seated in the past.

Another important construct of psychodynamic psychotherapy is the role of defense mechanisms. Defenses provide an important function in human behavior. However, in Psychodynamic Therapy it is important to name and explore these behaviors. Bond and Perry (2004) researched the use of defense mechanisms by using the Defence Style Questionnaire (constructed by Bond et al. in 1983). The findings indicate that those with a maladaptive style improved in time, and that in recovery from depression, patients used more mature defenses as their immature defenses gradually decreased.

Psychodynamic psychotherapy, either as it stands or in the form of PITP, can effectively help patients for whom their depression is linked to their early attachment figures, feelings of abandonment by an absent father or mother, and the desire to resolve these losses in therapy. For the psychodynamic therapist, the role of the unconscious and indeed the conscious are central to the therapeutic process and the use of good clinical supervision is essential to avoid counter-transference blocking the process.

Solution-Focused (Problem-Solving) Therapy

Steve de Shazer and Insoo Kim Berg of the Brief Family Therapy Center in Milwaukee are the founders of solution-focused therapy. The main determinants of this approach are the following:

- The focus is placed on the solution to the problem.
- Reaching the solution involves collaboration between client and therapist.
- Even relatively small changes are regarded as positive because they can enable further growth.
- The emphasis is on process.
- An eclectic approach is a main feature; the therapist makes full use of his/her skills.
- Although usually brief, it can also be longer term.
- There is a readiness to respond to diversity within the client's frame of reference.

Solution-focused therapy (SFT) uses a range of skills and interventions that include scaling, the miracle question, externalizing conversations, journals, the surprise tank, and mapping the influences of the problem.

In scaling, for example, the therapist might ask the client: "On a scale of 1 to 10, where 10 is that you feel well and 1 indicates that you feel despair, where might you rate yourself?" Scaling enables the client to self-assess their moods and responses. Scaling can also be used to explore the sexual health needs of a client, or any current difficulties that might be impacting their sexual functioning. The solution-focused therapist would endeavor to reinforce the positive from the client's self-assessment and might use questions such as: "So you place yourself at a 3 on the scale; perhaps you could tell me what is stopping you from being at a 2, because it sounds like there is something positive happening that is doing that."

SFT also uses narrative therapy and Guterman (2006) refers to the technique of Michael White called mapping the influences of the problem. In using this, the therapist helps the client understand how the problem (the depression) has influenced his/her life. The client is helped to map out the areas where the problem has had and still has influence. Throughout the therapy, the focus remains on the solution.

As a treatment for depression this therapy can be very successful. A helpful aspect of systematic therapy is using the client as expert in understanding their circumstances and identifying the problems. This approach moves beyond the medical model of a patient who needs treatment toward a deeper respect for the client and for the process.

The use of scaling for depression enables the client to have an increased awareness of their progress (or otherwise) in therapy and can provide some concrete indicators of what is working or not for the client. For some therapists, however, the use of solution-focused therapy would be too directed and not sufficiently client-led for their therapeutic approach.

Eye Movement Desensitization and Reprocessing

Eye Movement Desensitization and Reprocessing (EMDR) was discovered by Francine Shapiro in 1987. It is a well-researched intervention that treats psychological trauma with methods that enable bilateral stimulation of the brain. The methods can include asking a client to follow a moving light or to follow the therapist's hand movements. It is used for both emotional and physical trauma with people who have experienced abuse, disasters, accidents, conflict, traumatic injury, and so on. It is highly effective for both children and adults.

Sandyford is unique in having a number of trained therapists who are qualified to use EMDR with clients. EMDR is used frequently for clients who present with trauma related to sexual abuse, sexual assault, or rape.

Each EMDR session has eight phases:

- History and treatment planning
- Preparation
- Assessment
- Desensitization (during which the significant units of distress are measured or scaled by the client)
- Installation
- Body scan
- Closure
- Revaluation

Pre-Therapy Groups

The concept of pre-therapy is the work of American psychologist Garry Prouty. Prouty also referred to pre-therapy as "contact work," and it is essentially about enabling clients to regain contact at a psychological and emotional level. Prouty developed this for clients who would find contact difficult due to conditions such as dementia or psychosis, as well as for people with high levels of anxiety. Prouty described this difficulty with contact as "contact impairment." It seems a useful definition that encapsulates both the purpose and value of pre-therapy work. Training in pre-therapy focuses on how to talk and engage with people who are contact impaired. How this is implemented depends on the level of contact a healthcare professional has with patients. Contact might range from more enhanced communication between nursing and sexual health advisors to pre-therapy counseling work with individuals and groups. Pre-therapy is not only about the theory of psychotherapy and how to implement techniques, but also a way to understand psychological phenomena.

The Counseling Service has already developed and delivered a psycho-educational pre-therapy model. The benefits are the normalization of otherwise highly distressing symptoms and a reduction in the number of sessions required for individual therapy. Several pre-therapy groups have already addressed symptoms such as anxiety and PTSD in relation to historical sexual abuse. Two cognitive behavioral therapists have already received specialist training in delivering this model. Feedback from clients has been extremely positive and it has been possible to track the clients' progress through more time-limited therapy. There are important benefits to this form of service delivery—not least the impact this will have on the waiting lists. The clients who attend gain from the shared experience and normalization of symptoms. It is delivered as a psycho-educational rather than group therapy model with "homework tasks" agreed and shared on a weekly basis. The development of the group each time is evident in terms of increased confidence and the ability to manage what have been highly distressing and debilitating symptoms, which have previously prevented access to psychological therapies. In 2010, Sandyford took part in research through Napier University using a newly developed psycho-educational model of pre-therapy involving a group of female clients recovering from CSA. The same was replicated in North Glasgow, Lothian, and Lanarkshire. The research is due for publication. It is clearly a model that could be adopted by other counseling services in the future with very positive outcomes for clients. The impact for therapists is the satisfaction of enabling clients to manage symptoms as well as staff morale having an improved management of the waiting lists.

Current Developments in Psychological Therapy

Issues explored here in developments in psychological therapy are transferable across providers of most specialist and/or generic counseling services.

Mental illness causes considerably poor health in Scotland, where 1 in 4 people experience mental ill health. Suicide rates in Scotland, particularly among young men, are the highest in the United Kingdom. The work of Choose Life and NHS Scotland in the delivery of suicide intervention courses throughout the NHS, such as Applied Suicide Intervention Skills Training (ASIST), SafeTALK, Suicide TALK, and skills-based training on risk management (STORM), were challenged to meet the Health Improvement Efficiency, Access to Services Treatment (HEAT 5) target by December 2010. The HEAT 5 target was set in 2009–2010 as a Scottish Government initiative to address the high rates of suicide (National Health Service [NHS] Scotland, 2009). The target states:

Reduce the suicide rate between 2012–2013 by 20%.

Supported by 50% of by frontline staff in mental health and substance misuse services, primary care and accident and emergency, being educated and trained in using suicide assessment tools/suicide prevention training programmes by 2010. (NHS Scotland, 2009)

Sandyford met this target earlier in 2010 with all counselors trained in ASIST and an increasing number of medical and administrative staff trained in SafeTALK. Sandyford has three qualified ASIST Trainers within the Counseling Service. However, suicide intervention is not counseling although it uses counseling skills. The increasing awareness of suicidal risk has led to an increase in the number of people who seek counseling after they have experienced the extreme despair but, in surviving, realize that there are issues from the past/present that might be most appropriately addressed in counseling.

In 2009–2010, some 500 people were trained as trainers in ASIST, STORM, SafeTALK and SuicideTALK. By the end of 2010, 17,000 healthcare professionals and others had been trained. The training program continues to be delivered throughout Scotland.

Trainee Placements

Within the Counseling Service we regard placements for trainee therapists as being most important. A placement within sexual health can offer a trainee therapist a unique opportunity in two different ways. First, to work therapeutically with a range of psychological issues that are aligned to sexual health, and secondly to experience working in multdisciplinary teams. Trainees are given a placement for the academic year following a rigorous selection process. Students are accepted from a range of courses, including gestalt, CBT, person-centered therapy, psychodynamic therapy, and art therapy. Each student works for 1 day at SCASS and will see four or five clients a week. While there is no cost to SCASS for providing counseling, these trainees have to be both supported and managed. There is a structured mentor program in place managed by one of the team leaders. A Competency Record Book has also been produced and the expectation is that this is a point of focus for both the trainee and mentor. The Competency Record Book was piloted in 2010 and has been revised for this year. Students are also expected to attend mandatory monthly group supervision in Sandyford.

Taking the Sandyford Model into the Community: Counseling in Sandyford Hubs

Sandyford Hubs are located within areas of high deprivation across the NHSGG&C board area and provide full range of sexual and reproductive health services. Counseling is offered for 4.5 hours each week in all of the Hubs. Clients are seen for 6–8 appointments with awareness that if their issues are more complex they could be seen at Sandyford Central for further counseling. Counseling in the Hubs has enabled the model that was originally developed in the Center for Women's Health to be available within each community.

It was envisioned that offering counseling within the Hubs would reduce waiting lists at Sandyford Central; however, this is not the case, and there is an increasing number of clients seeking counseling for whom the journey into the center of Glasgow would be too difficult. Counselors use bibliotherapy to assist clients on the waiting list at each Hub. For the counselors themselves, working in a Hub allows them to be further integrated into Sandyford and they enjoy the opportunity to work within a multi-disciplinary team, as professional working relationships have been established. Referrals come from within the community and from the Hub staff as well as self-referrals. The waiting lists are monitored through Hub Counselors team meetings and attention is given to those Hubs where there is less demand. There are significant waiting lists at some Hubs that are either located in areas of higher deprivation or have links with vulnerable clients' groups, such as asylum seekers and minority ethnic groups.

Overview of Counseling Services in Sexual and Reproductive Health Care in the United States

An endorsed program for practitioners to undertake the role of counseling is the *Comprehensive Counseling for Reproductive Health: An Integrated Curriculum.* The program covers the following core elements (**Box 14-1**).

Other counseling programs are also available, designed for specific client groups such as adolescents. The U.S. Preventive Services Task Force (USPSTF) also advocates extensive programs designed to address specific issues. An example is the "Male Sexual and Reproductive Health Care: Recommendations for Clinical Practice" (Marcell, 2014).

In that program, the key SRH counseling components include the following:

- Condoms with demonstration/practice
- STD/HIV
- Pregnancy prevention including male and female methods and emergency contraception
- Preconception health
- Sexuality/relationships
- Sexual dysfunctions
- Infertility

This program is designed to improve delivery of family planning and preventive sexual and reproductive health care services for reproductive-aged males.

The Importance of Evidence-Based Therapies

As Quick (2008) noted, one of the most frequent complaints described by psychotherapy clients is depression. Many individuals seek therapeutic consultation following bereavement, relationship break-up, financial setbacks, health problems, and many other misfortunes (Quick, 2008).

The NICE Guidelines for the Treatment and Management of Depression are based on the best available research evidence and enable the identification of priorities. Overall, though, there is limited evidence for counseling and more research is needed on all therapeutic approaches, most specifically, short-term cognitive therapies.

There is currently a great interest—on both academic and practice level—in the effectiveness of therapeutic modalities. Great weight is given to cost-effective practices. Yet, exploring what might be both cost effective and evidence based is vital for any counseling service. Luborsky et al. (2002) found that person-centered/experiential therapies have been shown to be of equal effectiveness when compared to other forms of psychological treatment, including CBT.

> Two of the largest studies of the outcomes of psychological therapies (using 1309 and 5613 patients respectively). . . . found that person centered therapy was equivalent in effectiveness to cognitive-behavioral and psychodynamic therapies for clients with a range of mild, medium and severe psychological difficulties. (Cooper et al., 2007, p. 8)

It is worth noting that further national research (Stiles, Barkham, Twigg, Mellour-Clark, & Cooper, 2006) into the use of Clinical Outcomes Routine Evaluation (CORE) has identified those clients who have a planned allocation of 12 sessions commonly report significant improvement at sessions 9–10, regardless of therapy modality.

A recent review of the evidence for counseling and psychotherapy concludes that:

> There are only small difference in the effectiveness of different bona fide therapies . . . positive outcomes are associated with a collaborative, caring, empathic skilled way of relating. (Cooper, 2008, p. 156)

Sandyford has systematically developed an integrated service offering a mixed modality of therapies. Currently, the following are offered:

- Cognitive behavioral therapy
- Gestalt therapy
- Person-centered counseling
- Humanistic/integrative therapy
- Psychodynamic therapy
- Systemic therapy

Offering a range of therapeutic modalities within sexual health acknowledges what has become an increasing awareness of the range of modalities in those who seek counseling. Very often potential clients are clear about which modality they would prefer and will give examples of what has worked or not in previous therapy. Within the Social Model of Health, it seems appropriate to ensure that a range of modalities be offered.

Sandyford has developed its own assessment process, but it has evolved from assessments models used elsewhere in both primary care and community mental health teams. Assessment is primarily to determine if someone is suitable for counseling within SCASS—it does not automatically mean someone will be offered counseling. Consideration is always given to whether the potential client would benefit more from services within their local primary care mental health team. SCASS is also able to offer the Listening Ear and then suggest assessment to be seen for counseling. Essentially, assessment appointments are made by self-referral from the client and indicate how motivated the potential client might be to engage in a therapeutic relationship.

CORE is a good measurement tool for patient outcomes but can also be used as a viable measurement tool by individual staff. Clients are also asked to complete an evaluation that identifies the client's perception of counseling and also uses what Kirkpatrick (1959) (developed in 1975 and 1994) described as the four essential elements of evaluation:

1. Reaction
2. Learning
3. Behavior
4. Results

The design of this evaluation was a deliberate decision to move beyond what Bramley & Kitson (1994) would describe as 80% of evaluations being nothing more than "happiness sheets." It is essential that counseling, in order to be accountable, is subject to a robust evaluation process. Currently, completed evaluations are being collated and the information prepared for a report on counseling outcomes at Sandyford.

Sandyford has a particularly good working relationship with three of the most geographically close primary care mental health teams: Pathways, STEPS, and Riverside. By agreement, if a patient is referred to one of those teams and through assessment it is determined that the person would benefit from counseling at Sandyford (primarily because the issues are linked directly to sexual abuse), the assessment is sent to Sandyford and the client allocated to a waiting list rather than having to undergo a further assessment.

Improving Access to Psychological Therapy

The phrase *psychological therapies* is used to describe a wide range of practices, and there is a degree of confusion over the meaning of the term. At the higher tiers of the stepped-care system, staff may be accredited to a specialist level in one of the major therapeutic approaches. Further down the pyramid, they may simply be required to use circumscribed elements of any particular approach (Mental Health in Scotland, 2011).

The Matrix (Mental Health in Scotland, 2011) is intended to provide a summary of information on the effectiveness of specific psychological therapies for particular service user groups. The Matrix does not cover all conditions or mental health patient groups. It focuses on common mental health problems, the conditions covered by the Integrated Care Pathways, and other key Scottish Government priority areas.

The levels are outlined as follows:

- **"Low-Intensity" interventions:** Low-intensity interventions are aimed at transient or mild mental health problems with limited effect on functioning, time-limited, and normally lasting between 2–6 sessions.

- **"High-Intensity" interventions:** High-intensity interventions are secondary care based and are aimed at common mental health problems with significant effect on functioning, and normally lasting between 6 and 16 sessions.

- **Specialist Interventions:** Specialist interventions are most commonly accessed through secondary care and specialist services. They are aimed at moderate/severe mental health problems with significant effect on functioning (e.g., substance misuse, eating disorders, bipolar disorder) and normally last between 10 and 20 sessions.

- **Highly Specialist Interventions:** Highly specialist, individually tailored interventions based on case formulations drawn from a range of psychological models are aimed at service users with highly complex and/or enduring problems, and normally lasting 16 sessions and above.

Conclusion

There is significant evidence therefore for an integrated sexual health service that includes psychological support and evidence-based therapeutic interventions. Such a service must encompass a healthy attitude toward sexual health and emotional well-being, which must go beyond just responding to develop more of an attitude of proactive care. In turn, offering interventional therapy might ensure that later development of depression is minimal. Finally, the benefits for those working in such an integrated service are also important to recognize. Having professionals from different areas of the NHS working alongside each other has enabled a better understanding of expertise and how they can work together to ensure the best possible response to patient care.

••• REFERENCES

Bond, M., Gardiner, S. T., Christian, J., Sigel, J. J. (1983). Empirical study of self-rated defense styles. *Arch Gen Psychiatry.* 1983; *40*(3): 333–338.

Bond, M., Perry, J. C. (2004). Long-term changes in defense styles with psychodynamic psychotherapy for depressive, anxiety, and personality disorders. *Am J Psychiatry* 2004 Sept; *161*(9): 1665–1671.

Anderson, A. E. (Ed.). (1990). *Males with eating disorders.* Cleveland, OH: Therapeutic Resources.

Bramley, P., & Kitson, B. (1994). Evaluating training against business criteria. *Journal of European Industrial Training, 18*(1), 10–14.

Chambless, D. L., & Ollendick, T. H. (2001). Empirically supported psychological controversies and evidence. *Annual Psychological Review, 52,* 685–716.

Cooper, M. (2008). *Essential research findings in counseling & psychotherapy.* London, United Kingdom: Sage.

Cooper, M., McLeod, J., Elliott, R., Mearns, D., Hilton, J., McGinnis, S., . . . Gillon, E. (2007). *Widening and increasing access to psychological therapies proposed intervention: Person-centred/experiential psychotherapy and counselling.* Retrieved from https://www.researchgate.net/publication/237631099_widening_and_increasing_access_to_psychological_therapies_proposed_intervention_person-centredexperiential_psychotherapy_and_counselling

Fogany, P., Steele, M., Steele, H., Moran, G. S., & Haggitt, A. C. (1991). The capacity for understanding mental states: The reflective self in parent and child and its significance for security attachment. *Infant Mental Health Journal, 12*(3): 201–218.

Frazier, P., Conlon, A., Glaser, T. (2001). Positive and negative life changes following sexual assault. *J Consult Clin Psychol.* 2001 Dec; 69(6): 1048–1055.

Gilbert, M., & Shmukler, D. (1992). *Brief therapy in couples: An integrative approach.* Chichester, United Kingdom: John Wiley.

Gleaves, M. R., & Eberenz, K. M. (1994). Sexual abuse histories amongst treatment resistant bulimia nervosa patients. *International Journal of Eating Disorders, 15,* 227–231.

Guterman, J. (2006). *Mastering the art of solution-focused counseling.* Alexandria, VA: American Counseling Association, United States of America.

Herman, J. L. (1997). *Trauma and recovery: The aftermath of violence — from domestic abuse to political terror.* New York, NY: Basic Books.

Hobson, R. F. (1983). *A conversational model of psychotherapy: A teaching method.* (Three videotapes). London, UK: Tavistock Publications.

Hunt, R., & Fish, J. (2008). *Prescription for change: Lesbian and bisexual women's health check.* London, United Kingdom: Stonewall.

Joseph, S., & Linley, P. A. (2005). Positive adjustment to threatening events: an organismic valuing theory of growth through adversity. *Review of General Psychology, 9*(3), 262–280.

Kenny, S. (2010). *Young people: Alcohol & sexual risk taking. A literature review for the north east region.* Brantingham, United Kingdom: Claire Cairns Associates Ltd.

Kirkpatrick, D. L. (1959). Techniques for evaluating programs. *Journal of American Society of Training Directors, 13*(3), 21–26.

Koblin, B. A., & The EXPLORE Study Team. (2004). Effects of a behavioural intervention to reduce the acquisition of HIV infection among men who have sex with men: The EXPLORE randomised controlled study. *The Lancet, 364*(9428), 41–50.

Marcell, A. V. and the Male Training center for Family Planning and Reproductive Health. (2014). *Preventive Male Sexual and Reproductive Health Care: Recommendations for Clinical Practice.* Philadelphia, PA: Male Training Center for Family Planning and Reproductive Health; Rockville, MD: Office of Population Affairs.

Luborsky, L., Rosenthal, R., Diguer, L., Andrusyna, T. P., Berman, J. S., Levitt, J. T., . . . Krause E. D. (2002). The dodo bird verdict is alive and well—mostly. *Clinical Psychology: Science & Practice, 9*(1), 2–12.

McCormack, C., Buckeridge, S., Campbell, T., Cooper, M., Norton, S., Scheepers, D., & Broadberry, D. (2005; Revised 2008). *Standards framework for counsellors & counselling services.* Retrieved from http://www.nhsggc.org.uk/media/220580/nhsgg_standards_counselling_primary_care_summary.pdf

Mental Health in Scotland. (2011). *"The Matrix"—A guide to delivering evidence-based psychological therapies in Scotland.* Retrieved from http://www.nes.scot.nhs.uk/media/425354/psychology_matrix_2011s.pdf

National Health Service Scotland. (2009). *Public health HEAT targets 2009-10.* Retrieved from http://www.shb.scot.nhs.uk/board/publichealth/documents/phar10-heattargets.pdf

Palmer, R. L., Oppenheimer, R., Dignon, A., Chaloner, D. A., & Howells, K. (1990). Childhood sexual experiences with adults reported by women with eating disorders—an extended series. *British Journal of Psychiatry, 156,* 455–463.

Perry, S., Cooper, A. M., & Michels, R. (2006). The psychodynamic formulation: Its purpose, structure and clinical application. *Focus, 4*(2), 297–305.

Quick, E. K. (2008). *Doing what works in brief therapy.* Cambridge, MA: Academic Press.

Sanderson, C. (2008). *Counselling adult survivors of child sexual abuse.* London, United Kingdom: Jessica Kingsley.

Schwartz, M., Cohn, L. (1996). *Sexual abuse and eating disorders.* New York, NY: Brunner/Mazel.

Shorey, H. S., & Snyder, C. R. (2006). The role of adult attachment styles in psychopathology and psychotherapy outcomes. *Review of General Psychology, 10*(1), 1–20.

Stiles, W. B., Barkham, M., Twigg, E., Mellor-Clark, J., & Cooper, M. (2006). Effectiveness of cognitive-behavioural, person-centred & psychodynamic therapies as practised in UK National Health Service settings. *Psychological Medicine, 36,* 555–566.

Tedeschi, R. G., Park, C. L., & Calhoun, G. (1998). *Posttraumatic growth: Positive change in the aftermath of crisis.* Mahwah, NJ: Lawrence Erlbaum Associates.

Tice, L., Hall, R. C., Beresford, T. P., Quinones, J., & Hall, A. K. (1989). Sexual abuse in patients with eating disorders. *Psychiatric Medicine, 7*(4), 257–267.

Waller, G., Ruddock, A., & Cureton, S. (1995). Cognitive correlates of reported sexual abuse in eating disordered women. *Journal of Interpersonal Violence, 10*(2), 176–187.

● ● ● RECOMMENDED READING

Butt, A., & Wardle, D. (2007). Archway Glasgow: A first for Scotland. *British Medical Journal, 334,* 1154.

Haslam, S. (2006). *Evaluation of the Thrive service.* Glasgow, Scotland: FMR Research Ltd.

Kirkpatrick, J. D., & Kirkpatrick, W. K. (2016). *Kirkpatrick's Four Levels of Training Evaluation. Alexandria,* VA: ATD Press.

U.S. Preventive Services Task Force. (2013). U.S. Preventive Services Task Force screening and behavioral counseling interventions in primary care to reduce alcohol misuse. *Annals of Internal Medicine, 159*(3), 210–218.

Wortman, C. (2004). Posttraumatic growth: Progress & problems. *Psychological Inquiry, 5,* 1.

● ● ● **USEFUL WEBSITES**

British Association for Behavioural & Cognitive Psychotherapies: www.babcp.com

British Association for Counseling and Psychotherapy: www.bacp.co.uk

British Association for Sexual Health & HIV: http://www.bashh.org/

British HIV Association: http://www.bhiva.org/

COSCA - Counselling in Scotland: www.cosca.org.uk

Faculty of Sexual & Reproductive Healthcare: http://www.ffprhc.org.uk/

Family Planning Association (sexual health charity): http://www.fpa.org.uk/home

Health Protection Scotland: Blood Borne Viruses and STIs: http://www.hps.scot.nhs.uk/bbvsti/index.aspx

HIV drug interactions (also available as an app): http://www.hiv-druginteractions.org/

Medical Foundation for AIDS and Sexual Health: http://www.medfash.org.uk/

National AIDS manual public HIV website: http://www.aidsmap.com/

Sandyford Initiative: www.sandyford.org

Scottish HIV & AIDS Group (SHIVAG): http://www.shivag.co.uk/

United Kingdom Council for Psychotherapy: www.psychotherapy.org.uk

CHAPTER

15

Roles and Responsibilities of Sexual Health Advisers and Partner Services Providers

THEODORA D. KWANSA

Introduction

The aim of sexual health advising and partner services provision is to reduce the number of infected persons requiring treatment and to curtail transmission rates among high-risk social network groups. Professionals in sexual health advisory and partner services provision may play different roles. A public health partner services provider may undertake identification of needle-sharing sexual partners to offer them medical health assessment and authorized treatment, while clinicians in partner services provision may counsel index patients/clients and provide them with written information and medication for their sexual partners according to state regulations. The clinician provider may carry out direct assessment and treatment of the identified sexual partners with the aim of reducing reinfections and curbing transmission rates. Therefore, clinicians are required to encourage index patients/clients to advise and support their sexual partners to seek medical health assessment and treatment. Furthermore, the role also requires that the clinician providers should collaborate with the state and local health departments.

The U.K. Department of Health has advocated development of the role of sexual health advisers (SHA) to complement the implementation of the National Strategy for Sexual Health and HIV. Different countries undoubtedly use alternative titles for their equivalent of sexual health advising. With origins that derived from varied professional disciplines, sexual health advising encompasses elements from nursing, social work, and the medical, psychology, and counseling professions. Consequently, the role and responsibilities expected of these practitioners within different aspects of sexual health care may vary, although they are essential in the multidisciplinary context of care and service delivery.

In the United States, these roles and responsibilities may be performed by clinicians, public health nurses, and nurse practitioners. These roles may also fall under the broader umbrella of partner services provider or disease intervention specialist (DIS). However, the roles and responsibilities of DIS are not confined to the context of sexual and reproductive healthcare and incorporate supportive care and services for patients diagnosed with various infectious disease conditions, which include tuberculosis and hepatitis as well as sexually transmitted infections (STIs) and HIV/AIDS. Within the context of this chapter, the concept of partner services provision as described in the Centers for Disease Control and Prevention's (CDC's) recommendations for passport to partner services curriculum and clinical application (CDC, 2015a) is more applicable. The diverse roles and responsibilities of SHAs and partner services providers are explored in this chapter with emphasis on partner notification and the related processes.

Overview of Sexual Health Advising, Partner Services Provision, and Disease Intervention Specialism

Sexual health advising and provision of partner services are recognized as indispensable aspects of sexual and reproductive healthcare. Partner notification and management, contact tracing, and counseling feature as foremost in the focus of sexual health advising and partner services provision. Contraception services and young people and special client groups' services also benefit from the health adviser's professional expertise to various extents. SHAs practice in specialist clinical and community settings focused on genitourinary medicine (GUM) and STI/HIV care and services. The designated titles, roles, and responsibilities may vary between countries but the core principle of partner notification and contact tracing is the same.

The delicate and personal nature, sensitivity, privacy, and confidentiality of an individual's sexuality, sexual behavior, and health present complex moral and ethical challenges for sexual healthcare practitioners. Their encounters with individuals who present with complicated sexual health issues challenge them with a range of exacting dilemmas. Their professional duty of care and responsibility extends beyond the patients to the general public as a whole. They are expected to demonstrate appropriate commitment to professional accountability through compliance with relevant policies, guidelines, and regulations. They are also expected to respond appropriately to or act within the boundaries of complex legal and regulatory demands and obligations. The code of professional conduct, performance, and ethics with which practitioners from nursing, public health, and social work backgrounds embark on sexual health advising reinforces transferability of the required professional attributes.

Locating and Notifying Sexual Partners and Sexual Contacts

Partner notification and contact tracing aim to curb the transmission and spread of STIs and HIV. While these methods prevent reinfection by curable bacterial and parasitic organisms, viral infections are incurable (Turner et al., 2011). There is evidence to support an association between efficient implementation of partner notification procedures and decreased STI rates. Trelle, Shang, Nartey, Cassell, and Low (2007) reported improved effectiveness of partner notification among patients with STIs. Further, various studies have shown that reduction in STI transmission can be attributed to early detection and early treatment. Lanjouw, Ossewaarde, Stary, Boag, and Van Der Meijden (2010) noted that early detection and treatment is associated with avoidance of complications, achieving total cure where applicable, or curtailing ongoing spread and reduction of the viral load in viral STIs. Partner notification also allows provision of health promotion and education on safer sex practices among high-risk groups (Tiplica et al., 2015). Other, related findings reveal increased reporting of STIs, including HIV infection, and the benefit of more advanced diagnostic techniques ensuring correct identification and appropriate treatment of the specific infections (Du, Gerber, & McNutt, 2007; World Health Organization [WHO], 2009). Locating and notifying the sexual contacts of patients/clients who are diagnosed with HIV or other STIs is one of the fundamental duties of SHAs and counterparts. The key rationale for identifying and treating asymptomatic partners of patients with STIs is to minimize potential long-term complications. Turner et al. (2011) examined the economic benefits of different chlamydia screening and partner notification strategies, which have shown reduction in the rates of transmission and spread among different social groups. The CDC, 2015b) recommends that partner management be implemented as a component of the STI prevention programs.

The Joint United Nations Programme on HIV and AIDS (UNAIDS) and the World Health Organization (WHO) defined partner notification as including two key processes: (1) locating sexual partners of STI patients to inform them about exposure to the infection, and (2) providing partners as well as patients with treatment and advice toward prevention of further STIs (UNAIDS/WHO, 1999). This definition indicates that many sexual contacts may not be aware of their vulnerability and susceptibility to STIs or HIV infection. Other related terms used are *contact tracing* and *partner management* (Tiplica et al., 2015). A crucial element in the notification interaction is encouraging the individual to take advantage of available counseling, laboratory testing, preventive measures, and therapeutic services. Trelle et al.'s (2007) systematic review highlights potential advantages for more patient involvement in the partner notification process. Practitioners should recognize the factors that may deter individuals in order to provide support that recognizes the patient's perspective while upholding professional regulations. Practitioners have an obligation to respect privacy, confidentiality, and autonomy in the partner notification process and are expected to obtain the individual's consent for specific issues.

Although partner notification and contact tracing have recognizable health and economic benefits, some findings suggested that the overall positive impact within society might not be entirely observable (European Centre for Disease Prevention and Control [ECDC], Mathews et al., 2002). Therefore, there is a call for more extensive and detailed evaluative studies both locally and nationally to assess the effectiveness of this vital service. Hence, the national audit of HIV partner notification (British HIV Association/ BASHH, 2013) encourages sexual health practitioners to participate in such audit projects. Implementation of evidence-based national guidelines could prove invaluable in contact tracing and partner notification improvement, with more effective patient outcomes (Faldon, 2004a). Effective programs must consider individuals who are unaccounted for due to a patient's deliberate or inadvertent neglect to divulge them. Moreover, practitioners must acknowledge the changes and replacement of sexual partners, specific infections, and the period of active infection. Peterman et al. (2006) and Brunham, Porbohloul, Mak, White, and Rekart (2005) noted that index patients are more vulnerable to be reinfected or to contract other STIs if they engage with multiple sexual partners, new sexual partners, and frequent changes of sexual partners.

Impact of Social Network Analysis

Social network analysis is a technique for establishing patterns of infection through information obtained from the patients/clients and through the partner notification process. This allows for identification of population group clusters among whom the infection prevails. Helman (2007) maintains that social network analysis proves to be especially useful in contact tracing for studying patterns of spread of a specific infection during an outbreak. The survey may target population groups such as local communities, identified club members, college students, sexual partners, and commercial sex workers. The analysis may also help in establishing the nature of social support that affected individuals receive within their communities. Wylie, Cabral, and Jolly (2005) maintained that social network analysis proves to be useful in providing valuable information revealing localized HIV and STI transmission patterns among specific communities in given geographical areas. Moreover, they noted that the findings may also help to determine the kind of care and support required to meet the needs of groups considered to be at greatest risk. Risley et al. (2007) explored the geographical and demographic patterns of gonorrhea transmission among specific groups or social clusters in parts of London. Ward et al.'s (2007) social network analysis examined the patterns of lymphogranuloma venereum spread in the United Kingdom. Similarly, Tanser, Bärnighausen, Cooke, and Newell's (2009) study examined clustering of HIV infections among different communities across a wide area of South Africa and their findings revealed geographical and demographic transmission patterns. In a different context, Crawford, Bowser, Brown, and Maycock (2013) explored the assumption of social networks among migrant populations in relation to reduction of HIV and STI transmission.

The rationale for social network analysis is to locate the nuclear enmeshed groups and the specific individuals within the communities with endemic STI transmissions. The findings from such analysis may be useful for achieving more effective results from the partner notification process (Wylie et al., 2005). More insight and understanding of the factors associated with the spread of STIs should be continually explored in order to implement appropriate primary preventive measures.

Factors That Influence Partner Notification Procedures in Different Areas

Key factors influencing partner notification procedures include human rights and privacy laws and social, cultural, and religious values and beliefs, all of which can present various difficulties. Differences in partner notification practices in different health service organizations have been reported (Arthur, Lowndes, Blackham, Fenton, & the European Surveillance of STI, 2005) and inadequate records of certain national data and sexual-health-related statistics have been identified. These may be attributable to factors such as economic status, resource and financial allocation, and the types and characteristics of the specific STIs (Arthur et al., 2005; Lanjouw et al., 2010). The European Centre for Disease Prevention and Control's (ECDC) 2013 report highlighted variations in partner notification services that can be attributed to differences in policy regulations that guide practice in different healthcare organizations in different countries. Without a robust system of coordinated sexual health services as the United Kingdom and some other countries have established at the national level, disjointed and disorganized services become an additional factor influencing partner notification outcome evaluations. In such systems, he records of index patient with STI or HIV infections and those of their sex partners could be held in different departments, thus creating disruption of integrated care (Faldon, 2004a). However, ongoing reviews of sexual healthcare and service provision allow for continual improvements to be made (Trelle et al., 2007) and more recent changes, such as the 2013 Sexual Health Strategy in the United Kingdom, are intended to bring about improvement and satisfaction in patient outcomes.

Practitioners' Perceptions of Variations in Policy Regulation and Guidelines for Partner Notification and Partner Management

Faldon (2004a) draws attention to findings from a previous study that revealed concerns among sexual health practitioners in the United Kingdom. Practitioners had misgivings about the following:

- Intrusion on patient's/client's privacy and violation of trust
- Uncertainty and perceived defiance or inadvertent breaking of the law

- Misgivings about inadvertently deterring people from taking up the available services for testing STIs/HIV
- Processes that may cause unwarranted worry and apprehension for patients/clients
- Heavy work load and depletion of staffing levels in some health service areas
- Availability of sustainable funding and other resources

More recently, Theunissen et al. (2014) reported the views of healthcare professionals about barriers to partner notification for *Chlamydia trachomatis* that need to be removed and facilitating factors that should be supported and continued. They suggested introduction of an approved and endorsed partner-notification procedure. They also proposed a potential internet-based partner-notification arrangement along with a feedback mechanism reporting on the approaches employed and the opinions on the entire partner notification process. Another suggestion was to offer education and training opportunities to practitioners to develop or enhance their motivational interviewing skills. Lorimer, Martin, & McDaid, (2014) also explored the thoughts of professional practitioners regarding barriers and facilitators of internet-based chlamydia screening targeting young heterosexual men. They deduced that confidentiality, feasibility, and sociocultural factors influence implementation of an internet-based approach to screening. They pointed out that potential limitations include wider social and cultural issues, as well as the unpredictable attitudes of young people and the healthcare professionals towards screening. They proposed that a multifaceted approach incorporating innovative endeavors to achieve effective interventions be placed on the policy agenda. Bilardi et al. (2009) had previously observed that innovative resources could enhance partner notification for chlamydia in primary care.

It is important that policy decision-makers and practitioners explore and critically examine examples of best practice through systematic reviews, clinical audits, and research activities. In this way, possible consideration could be given toward improving the national and organizational policy guidelines and the procedures applied to the design and delivery of partner-notification and contact-tracing procedures.

The Requisites and Challenges of Implementing Guidelines for Partner Notification

The general opinion is that guidelines for partner notification should be recognized and implemented as an essential component of sexual health service provision. The guidelines should represent a system that provides all-embracing, interconnected, and well-organized HIV and STI prevention, intervention, guidance, and support. The British Association for Sexual Health and HIV (BASHH, 2015) *Standards of Management of STIs* provides explanation of the U.K.

regulations and national guidelines. The key requisites include knowledgeable and well-informed SHAs with appropriate level of experience, together with realistic and manageable workload allocation. Provision of appropriate education and training for practitioners is recommended to cover the current techniques of diagnosis and treatment as well as related ethical considerations (ECDC, 2013). The Society of Sexual Health Advisers (SSHA) current competency framework for SHAs (2013) outlines the required range of competencies that should be developed.

The ECDC (2013) maintains that policy makers need to understand ample resource provision. Resources include suitably furnished rooms with visual aids for patient consultations for partner notification interventions, interviews, discussion, and sexual risk-prevention counseling. The ECDC recommends standardization of national and international legal requirements and policy regulations, as well as evaluation of current laws. National partner notification policy guidelines should be flexible to adapt to different health service organizations and primary care settings, as well as different population groups. Bearing in mind copyright regulations UK practitioners are encouraged to explore details of the current SSHA *Guidance on Partner Notification, August 2015*, available at ssha.info /wp-content/uploads/ssha-guidance-on-partner-notification -aug-2015.pdf.

Alternative Systems of Referral Employed in Partner Notification

As in other healthcare settings, interchangeable use of terminology occurs in sexual health advising, and clarification of terms is necessary. Various authors have described referrals for partner notification as methods, approaches, or interventions.

Terms used include *patient or partner referral, provider or active referral,* and *conditional or contract referral.* Other, less commonly used terms include *negative referral, passive referral,* and *self-referral.* The referral pathways describe scenarios in which the index patient diagnosed with an STI or HIV is encouraged to communicate with or provide information about his/her sexual partners and contacts. The purpose is to inform the partners about their exposure to infection, and advise them about the availability of evaluation or assessment, testing, and treatment. The interaction between the sexual partners may occur without the direct involvement of the SHA, partner services provider, or a designated healthcare professional. Young et al. (2007) noted that appropriate communication is crucial in achieving effective partner notification. The health adviser may provide support to the index patient in deciding how best to go about this situation and what information to communicate to the sexual partner(s). Depending on the actions taken, the terms *simple, enhanced,* or *expedited partner therapy (EPT)* may be used (Ferreira, Young, Matthews, Zunza, & Low, 2013; Trelle et al., 2007).

Expedited Partner Therapy (EPT)

Evidence suggests that providing the index patient with written information and/or medication to be delivered to the sexual partner (where applicable) proves to be more effective (Golden et al., 2007; Kissinger et al., 2005; Trelle et al., 2007). In addition, the index patient may offer or be invited to accompany the sexual partner to the clinic (Faldon, 2004a; WHO, 2001). Alternatively, the index patient may supply the SHA or healthcare worker with the necessary details to develop a contact slip for notifying the sexual partner(s) and sexual contacts. Apoola et al. (2007) found differences in individuals' preference for partner notification while Brown et al. (2011) found that personal involvement in partner notification proves to be satisfying, practicable, and successful. Although index patients tend to express a preference for personally informing or notifying their sexual partners and contacts, certain circumstances may prevent them from doing so. In situations in which the index patient acquired the STI through forced or nonconsensual, unprotected sexual intercourse they may feel reluctant to divulge the necessary details for contact tracing. Likewise, in cases of sexual assault, sexual abuse, or concealed or repressed rape, the individual may not feel confident to share the necessary details for contact tracing. Provider notification may be an alternative pathway if the index patient consents with the assurance of strict confidentiality and anonymity by the sexual health professional, SHA, or partner services provider. Other modes that have been gaining increasing popularity include the internet, emails (Clark et al., 2014; Mark, Wald, Drolette, & Golden, 2008; Mimiaga, Tetu, et al., 2008; Vest, Valadez, Hanner, Lee, & Harris, 2007), and sex-partner websites (Levine, Woodruff, Mocello, Lebrija, & Klausner).

The Partner/Patient Referral Process

The partner/patient referral process has apparently proven to be favorable in many areas (Apoola et al., 2007; Mackellar et al., 2009). Indeed, some findings indicate that many individuals prefer to communicate with partners by telephone rather than impose on another's privacy through a healthcare professional. Moreover, many index patients express their preference for these modes of notification as being more compassionate, thoughtful, and supportive (Mimiaga et al., 2009; Newton & McCabe 2008). In this process, index patients communicate with their sexual partners regarding exposure to the specific infection, possibility of transmission, and availability of support services. In their systematic review, Ferreira et al. (2013) distinguished between simple patient referral and enhanced patient referral. Simple patient referral describes verbal advice given by the healthcare professional to the index patient to encourage their sexual partners to receive or present for treatment. Enhanced patient referral describes use of a combination of interventions to strengthen the effectiveness and success of the simple patient referral (as proposed by Trelle et al.,

2007). Thus, written information about specific STIs, home sampling kits for the sexual partners, preliminary risk prevention counseling, and reminders such as telephone calls and/or videos are suggested.

Provider Referral or Active Referral

Provider referral involves the practitioner notifying the index patient's sexual partner(s) using the details provided on a contact slip. Generally, within the United Kingdom, this duty is carried out by the SHAs in the GUM clinic settings (Faldon, 2012a), the partner services provider in the United States, or kurators in Sweden (CDC, 2012; Ferreira et al., 2013). The professional health adviser or delegated healthcare worker obtains the necessary details from the index patient. It is the health adviser who notifies the sexual partner(s) and sexual contacts in confidence, after obtaining the index patient's consent (ECDC, 2013).

Conditional Referral, Contract Referral, or Negative Referral

Conditional referral, contract referral, and negative referral describe an amalgam of actions. In this case, the initial patient or partner referral is supplemented by a provider referral after an agreed-upon period of time if the partner fails to attend the clinic (Faldon, 2004a). For that reason, as Ferreira et al. (2013) observed, the contract or conditional referral is usually employed as accompanying supportive intervention to back a simple patient referral. Healthcare professionals must demonstrate respect for patient confidentiality during the partner notification process. The process should be voluntary, with no coercion of individual patients.

Although research and advances in the methods of partner notification in HIV and STIs appear to be somewhat varied in different sexual health service organizations in different countries, recent approaches have claimed to be more effective. Bell and Potterat (2011) maintain that contemporary methods reflect new diagnostic and treatment procedures, and current modes and advances in communication technology. Crucially, application of any contemporary method must be appropriately controlled, regulated, and managed by approved evidence-based national guidelines (ECDC, 2013).

Referral services are most effective when all involved have a clear understanding of the process. A sense of personal responsibility by the index patient or sexual partner will also influence effectiveness. Referrals provided in more formal environments (e.g., hospitals, GUM clinics) may impact effectiveness due to organizational factors (Apoola et al., 2007; Ward & Bell, 2010; Woodward, Roedling, Edwards, & Armstrong, 2010). Readers are encouraged to explore the NAT (2012a) report, which examines key issues relating to HIV partner notification. The 2012 BASHH statement on partner notification for sexually transmissible infections is also highly recommended as further reading.

Management of Regular Sexual Partners: The Recommended Guidelines

Notification of regular sexual partners presents certain challenges where the practitioner is faced with the obligation to protect the index patient's identity. Thus a sexual contact may not have a full explanation regarding the purpose of their attendance at a clinic or the interview for their personal sexual history. The professional bodies emphasize compliance with the duty of confidentiality but recognize that this may have to be broken only in the interest of another person or the public (General Medical Coumcil [GMC], 2013, 2017). An explanation in such circumstances should be given to the individual.

The following WHO (2001) general proposals for the management and treatment of sexual partners are considered applicable and incorporated into the current guidelines:

1. Offering prompt or urgent epidemiological treatment based exclusively on the diagnosis of the index patient without laboratory investigations.

2. Offering prompt epidemiological treatment but also having to collect specimens for laboratory investigations to confirm the diagnosis.

3. Postponing treatment until confirmatory results from the laboratory investigations are available.

4. Choosing an appropriate partner notification and management strategy: Key determinant factors taken into account may include:

   ◆ Extent of vulnerability imposed by the infection

   ◆ Seriousness in terms of the degree of threat to life imposed by the disease

   ◆ Convenience of effective investigative tests

   ◆ Possibility of an individual going back for follow-up interventions

   ◆ Availability of effective medication and required therapeutic intervention

   ◆ Possibility of ongoing transmission if epidemiological treatment is not given

   ◆ Convenience and accessibility to an organized setup for following up with patients

The recommendation is that epidemiological treatment given to all sex partners should be the same as the treatment regimen prescribed for the index patient (CDC, 2012).

Patient-Delivered Partner Therapy

Patient-delivered partner therapy (PDPT) refers to an EPT practice designed to provide sexual partners of index patients with treatment as soon as possible (Kissinger et al., 2005). It was envisioned that this would increase the proportion of sexual partners and sexual contacts who receive treatment (2011, 2015a). The sexual health physician supplies the index patient with the prescribed medication, information about STIs, condoms, and the appropriate helpline contact number in a package to be given to the sexual partner. In this way, sexual contacts avoid delays caused by awaiting medical consultation, examination, and tests as well as the pressure of direct formal clinic attendance (Sutcliffe, Chaman, Cassell, & Estcourt, 2009). The benefits of this approach—improving the disclosure, early diagnosis and treatment for treatable STIs, frequency of uptake, the overall impact and effectiveness—have been reported from various studies (Mohammed, Leichtliter, Schmidt, Farley, & Kissinger, 2010). Hadsall, Riedesel, Carr, and Lynfield, (2009) implemented PDPT with a view to reducing STIs in Minnesota, and Shiely et al. (2010) also found this to be an especially beneficial intervention. Stephens, Bernstein, Katz, Philips, and Klausner (2010) reported on the effectiveness in association with chlamydial and gonococcal reinfections in San Francisco. Nonetheless, others emphasize that potential barriers must be thoroughly explored (Estcourt et al., 2012; Golden & Estcourt, 2011).

The CDC's (2012) recommendation is that, based on emerging evidence of gonococcal resistance to cephalosporins, routine prescription of oral intake of cefixime for treatment of gonorrhea is no longer considered. Instead, a combination therapy should be prescribed for the treatment of uncomplicated urogenital, anorectal, and pharyngeal gonorrhea. The recommended combined therapy comprises the following:

- Single-dose ceftriaxone intramuscular injection 250 mg together with

  ◆ Single-dose azithromycin 1 g orally, **or**

  ◆ Doxycycline 100 mg orally twice daily for 7 days

This treatment regimen is recommended for the index patient's sexual partners over the preceding 60 days following assessment and testing. Intramuscular injection is not used in EPT. Therefore, the CDC recommends that heterosexual partners of index patients diagnosed with gonorrhea could be considered for EPT if they are unlikely to seek assessment, diagnosis, and treatment in time (CDC, 2012). Men who have sex with men (MSM) are not considered for EPT due to the high risk of coexisting STIs, including HIV infection (CDC, 2012).

The CDC recommends that EPT should be provided with clear instructions for taking medication, warnings regarding pregnancy and allergy, health education, and risk-prevention counseling about gonorrhea. It is also recommended that sexual partners be instructed to have a test-of-cure performed approximately 1 week after completing the prescribed treatment regimen (CDC, 2012). Sexual partners with pelvic inflammatory disease (PID) should be advised to seek direct consultation for assessment, testing, and treatment without delay. The policy in the United Kingdom is that EPT without prior assessment of the sexual partner is illegal (Ward & Bell, 2014). In the United States,

Cramer et al. (2013) reported that provision of EPT was notably higher in those areas where legal and policy regulations permitted this practice. They also noted that EPT administration was higher where the professional boards had issued policy statements advocating EPT. Clearly, there is a need for practitioners to give careful consideration to the legal and ethical implications, organizational policy, and professional regulations pertaining to EPT at national and local levels.

Accelerated Partner Therapy

Accelerated partner therapy is another approach in partner notification in the United Kingdom. It refers to the practice of treating sexual partners following appropriate medical assessment conducted by an authorized pharmacist, sexual health adviser, or designated sexual health professional. The sexual partner is required to pick up the sampling kit and the medication from the prescriber following a telephone consultation (Ward & Bell, 2014). Shackleton, Sutcliffe, and Estcourt (2011) examined the suitability and practicality of this within the context of general practice. The attitudes of the patient/client group (Woodward et al., 2010) and the preferences for different partner notification methods (Apoola et al. 2007; Trelle et al. (2007); Bell & Potterat, 2011; Kissinger, 2009; Sven et al., 2007) are factors that may influence the effectiveness of these approaches. Careful examination may reveal the types of patient groups who may benefit from expedited and accelerated partner therapy.

Postal Home Sampling

Postal home sampling entails using a postal testing kit to collect the necessary sample within the individual's preferred private environment. This has the potential risk of delay, reinfection, and continuous transmission of STIs to other sexual partners. However, combined testing and treatment kits allow the sexual partner to get tested for an STI and receive the prescribed treatment immediately. This process seems to be more preferred by individuals who may be anxious to know if they have acquired the particular STI, while also having the reassurance of immediate treatment (Bell & Potterat, 2011).

Although no particular method or approach to partner notification is deemed as best or applicable to all patient case scenarios, there is some evidence that enhanced partner notification and EPT produce more positive outcomes. Thus, apart from acceptability of partner notification among particular patient groups, careful consideration should be given to the types of STIs in question and the processes involved in expedited, enhanced, and accelerated partner therapy.

Tracing and Managing Other Relevant Sexual Contacts

The 2014 European Guidelines on the management of sexual partners of patients diagnosed with STIs recommends that all related sexual contacts should also be tested for the infection to which they may have been exposed (Tiplica et al., 2015), followed by the recommended treatment of the specific infection right away. Depending on the type of infection, the contact may be prescribed epidemiological treatment before laboratory tests confirm positive infection. Infections for which this is recommended include chlamydia, gonorrhea, HIV, nonspecific urethritis, *Trichomonas vaginalis*, lymphogranuloma venereum, syphilis, pelvic inflammatory disease, ano-genital warts and chancroid, epididymo-orchitis, and donovanosis. Additionally individuals with a history of STIs and risky sexual behaviors should be tested for other STIs (Bignell & Fitzgerald, 2011; Kingston et al., 2008; Lanjouw et al., 2010). It is recommended that in confirmed cases of infection the secondary sexual contacts (other partners of the contacts) also be provided treatment if unable to present for clinical examination and serological tests (Kingston et al., 2008). Detailed information through interviewing is of crucial importance to achieve effective patient notification.

Processes in the Notification Interview
Arranging the Notification Interview

Notification interviews may be scheduled to follow the initial diagnostic consultation and treatment. However, the practitioner may realize that a particular client does not intend to wait to be interviewed after receiving treatment, and should thus schedule the interview to take place prior to treatment administration (or simultaneously with treatment administration if the practitioner is qualified). The index patient should be advised to avoid exposure to untreated partners through unprotected sexual intercourse (Bell, 2004a).

Functions of the Notification Interview: Obtaining Relevant Details

Bell (2004d) emphasizes the importance of gaining a patient's/client's confidence and readiness to work in partnership with the SHA or health professional. The General Medical Council (GMC) (Brook et al. 2013; GMC, 2008) and the National Institute for Health and Care Excellence (NICE, 2011) concur on the significance of efficient interviewing to obtain detailed, specific, pertinent general and sexual history. The benefit of skillful and competent communication cannot be overstated. The sexual health practitioner uses appropriate techniques to diminish the tendency to withhold pertinent information and to discourage concealment of important sexual health problems and needs. The aim is to foster patient/client empowerment.

Choice of Venue and Ambience for Effective Notification Interview

The notification interview environment should be warm and friendly to minimize anxiety, convey reassurance and support, and increase the individual's confidence for disclosing deeply personal matters. Practitioners must put out clear information while maintaining regard for privacy and respect. The interview room should be conducive to a successful and productive dialogue between the health professional or health adviser, and the patient/client. The room should be private and ideally in a sound-proof environment (Brook et al., 2013). Students may only observe an interview with the patient's consent.

Requests for a chaperone or for a preferred gender of the clinician or practitioner should be tolerated with understanding (Brook et al., 2013). The GMC's 2013 guidelines on intimate examination and chaperones (GMC, 2013b) provide a useful resource for U.K.-based clinicians and sexual health practitioners. Accessibility is crucial and maximum privacy with no interruptions should ensure that personal details and confidentiality are closely safeguarded. Moreover, confidential records should not be openly displayed or left exposed or unattended at any time. In escorting patients/clients to the interview room it is important to confirm the individual's identity by the correct name and clinic number. The Brook et al. (2013) recommends that the policy for safeguarding confidentiality should be openly publicized at the clinic. The regulations for safeguarding confidential information about patients/clients are explained in the service standards on confidentiality (Faculty of Sexual and Reproductive Healthcare, 2012). Various alternative interview approaches have been explored. Tideman et al. (2007) compared computer-assisted sexual history taking as an alternative to face-to-face interview while Koch et al. (2008) explored the impact of self-completed sexual history questionnaires on clinical outcome for HIV-positive MSM. These authors noted the usefulness of these alternative sexual history taking modes and maintain that they have a place in contemporary health care practice and could be considered in sexual healthcare. Previous studies had explored audio computer-assisted self-interviews compared to face-to-face interactions to assess the preferences among STI clinic patients. The findings suggested that it may be worthwhile to consider alternative contemporary modes to obtain the sexual history (Ghanem, Hutton, Zenilman, Zimba, & Erbelding, 2005; Kurth et al., 2004).

Rationale for Skillful Interviewing

The interview serves as a means of helping the patient/client to gain sufficient understanding about what infection they may have contracted. The aim is to foster an individual's motivation toward compliance with the treatment regime and fulfilment of the subsequent appointments for assessment of progress. Moreover, the interview allows the practitioner and patient to discuss effective and realistic measures for self-protection against recurrent infections or susceptibility to contracting and transmitting long-term STIs. The interaction provides an opportunity to establish and address the patient/client's perceived needs for support and further referral as necessary. Importantly, the interview

provides much-needed insight into sexual networks, the nuclear population groups amongst whom transmission of STIs is contained. This information can help shape policies aimed at the correct populations.

As part of the process of partner notification the practitioner aims to make certain that individuals who have been exposed by direct contact to STIs are advised either by the index patient voluntarily or by the SHA or designated healthcare worker.

The interview should not feel judgmental or daunting and should empower the patient/client with the confidence to divulge difficult and deeply personal problems. Unlike the standard health history, the probing method employed in sexual-health-related interviewing could prove to be embarrassing for both patient and practitioner alike. Appropriate training is required to achieve the competencies required for this process. This is clearly stipulated in the current competency framework for Society of Sexual Health Advisers 2013.

Gaining and Maintaining Patient's/Client's Full Cooperation

An individual's willingness to participate in the interviews may be influenced by positive atmosphere, approachability and support of the staff, and a serviceable and functioning referral system. This requires that all members of the team are clearly informed about the referral criteria for identifying when patients/clients should be interviewed. All relevant team members should have adequate knowledge and insight about what partner notification entails. Team members share a commitment to safeguard the patient's interests. The team should maintain efficiency in their management of patients/clients together with professional attitudes and short waiting times. The importance of patient/client motivation is a crucial incentive and personal control in the choice of referral system enhances this. Motivation can be influenced by emphasizing the potential risks of specific STIs, reinfection and possible long-term complications to current and future contacts (CDC, 2015a: Kingston et al., 2008). Information leaflets are also useful to reinforce the importance of partner notification.

Efficient preparation, organization, and progressive sequencing of the interview process are important. The practitioner's professionalism in the actual conduct of clinical interviews helps in obtaining informative and pertinent sexual or other health histories about the specific problems presented by the individual.

A familiar reminder to healthcare professionals is to be attentive, empathetic, and responsive to patients by listening carefully to what they convey. Something in the individual's communication may direct the practitioner to discover the particular condition and associated problems and needs. Gathering of health information—history taking—is a particularly responsible procedure which requires well-developed skills, efficiency and thoroughness. Effective verbal and nonverbal communication and practitioner-patient interactions form the basis for appropriate patient care. An excellent reference document is the guideline for interviews that entail sexual history taking formulated by the Clinical Effectiveness Group of the British Association for Sexual Health and HIV (BASHH) (Brook et al., 2013). The document incorporates recommendations for sexual risk assessment based on best practice and aims to ensure competent interaction with patients through skilful sexual history taking. The quality of the interview will depend in part on the practitioner's competence, level of education, qualifications, and practical experience. Staff education and training activities, supervision, and available resources also affect the interview.

The potential impact of differences in organizational structures, dissimilar contexts of sexual healthcare provision, and the needs of diverse population groups are highlighted in the ECDC's (2013) findings, which has been critically examined by Brook et al. (2013).

Identifying Interviewees with Serious or High-Risk STIs for Detailed Information

Due to the seriousness of certain STIs and the potential for long-term complications, individuals who acquire these infections are interviewed for sexual partner and contact notification. Generally all index patients who are diagnosed with gonorrhea, chlamydia, syphilis, PID, epididymitis, HIV, hepatitis B (HBV) and C virus (HCV), and nonspecific urethritis are invited for interview to obtain a detailed sexual history. The statement on partner notification for sexually transmissible infections (BASHH, 2010; McClean, Radcliffe, Sullivan, & Ahmed-Jushuf, 2013) provides a more comprehensive catalogue and guidance on the infections for which partner notification should be offered, taking account of look-back periods.

Competent Communication Techniques for the Notification Interview

Various factors may affect the quality and effectiveness of practitioner–patient communication, regardless of the practitioner's competency level. For example, patients may present with learning difficulties, hearing problems, or may be nonnative speakers. Clinics should have policies regarding provision of language interpreters (Brook et al., 2013).

Communication should begin with respect and approachability, with due attention paid to nonverbal cues throughout the consultation. The practitioner should be cordial, warm, and sincere in the way in which he/she receives the patient/client. Good eye contact and professionalism in body language may initiate an element of trust. Despite publicity about the services offered at the clinic, it is useful to review services and explain what the consultation would entail. The use of open questions helps to encourage the patient to talk about their most pressing concerns. It may help to explain the reason for asking certain questions in order to dispel doubt and put the patient at ease. Language use and word choice is important and must not embarrass or offend the patient. Together, the practitioner and patient should find the terminology and language most acceptable to the patient.

The practitioner should watch for signs of anxiety and distress in order to determine the cause and provide reassurance. If necessary, support services and the option for referral may be explained (Brook et al., 2013). Professional guidance bodies emphasize the importance of avoiding judgmental attitudes related to individuals' sexual orientation, cultural sexual practices, religious principles, or specific moral values (GMC, 2013a, 2017; Nursing and Midwifery Council [NMC], 2015).

Establishing the Reason for Clinic Attendance

Practitioners will need to establish the reason for attendance during the initial interview. Individuals may present to the clinic for a routine examination, because they experienced symptoms, in response to a partner's request, or on the advice of a health professional. Careful review of the sexual history is needed to establish the nature and length of the symptoms and what diagnostic tests have been performed. Any specific concerns expressed by the patient/client should be noted for careful consideration. Establishing the reason for attendance may reveal concern about having been exposed to an STI or to seeking medical treatment for the onset of symptoms. Where symptoms are experienced, specific closed questions can establish symptom characteristics and duration. It may also be necessary to inquire about direct sexual contacts. Questioning is meant to elicit the sexual contact's name, diagnosis (type of infection), prescribed treatment, and sexual history (if known).

Specific components of the history may be tailored to the specific services offered at that sexual health sector. The history of previous STIs and last sexual intercourse as well as the gender of sexual partner(s) should be established. Additionally, practitioners should clarify the date of last menstrual period and what contraception is used, if any, as certain infections can affect a fetus. Assessment and testing for blood-borne viruses such as HBV, HCV, and HIV as well as determining vaccination status may also be necessary if risk is indicated. This is particularly important if the history reveals high risk of drug misuse and needle sharing.

Opinions vary among clinicians regarding the practicality of routine symptom review. The rationale for doing so is that carrying out the symptom review may help to reveal problems that a patient may have disregarded or neglected to mention. Specific questions addressed to female patients that may indicate the presence of particular symptoms should focus on abnormal vaginal discharge, or change in the amount, color, or odor; any disorder or minor symptoms over the vulva; lower abdominal pain; dyspareunia; dysuria; or abnormal patterns of bleeding such as intermenstrual or postcoital hemorrhage.

Symptom review questions addressed to male patients may focus on dysuria; urethral discharge; swelling or discomfort in the testicles; discomfort or any disorders over the genital skin; and pain or discomfort indicating perianal and anal symptoms, particularly in MSM.

Details for Specific Purposes

The amount of detail obtained depends on the purpose and intended use of the information and the service to be provided. Interviewing prior to STI screening tends to require less detail, whereas more detailed information is obtained if the STI screening test reveals positive results. Additional details can help to determine geographic sites of direct sexual contacts, what specimens should be collected, and which tests to carry out. It also helps to identify patients who should be offered hepatitis screening and vaccination. It is important to establish the period of last sexual contact to assess risk of current infection, indications for emergency contraception, and postexposure prophylaxis for HIV infection. It is also important to assess for risk of blood-borne viruses via injection drug use or MSM activities. These risk factors would indicate vulnerability in sexual partners and need for appropriate diagnostic tests. Practitioners should document the number of sexual partners/contacts within the past 3 months (the look-back period) and indicate those known to have STIs.

Patients/clients who disclose having had unprotected oral, vaginal, and/or anal sex during the previous 3 months could be at risk of acquiring particular STIs. Those individuals require appropriate examination, testing, and treatment, and initiation of the partner notification process. It is important that the SHA or partner services provider has adequate insight of the core components of this interview to ensure appropriate referral.

Rationale for Establishing the History of Previous STIs

Practitioners should document history of previous STIs (including date contracted), especially history of syphilis to determine serology results. Comprehensive history should include risky lifestyle behaviors such as alcohol and drug use in order to offer appropriate help and support. The Clinical Effectiveness Group's full guidelines provide more information on these.

In clinics that offer integrated contraception and sexual healthcare services specific details obtained in the sexual history may focus on the individual's gender, current complaint and needs. For females, information from the reproductive health history, menstrual history, and contraception use may also be obtained where services involve integrated sexual and reproductive health. By exploring current use of contraception, compliance, satisfaction or problems such as discomfort and abnormal bleeding, risk of unintended and unwanted pregnancy, practitioners can offer appropriate guidance and support. Human papilloma virus (HPV) vaccination status is established to encourage completion or uptake.

The purpose of obtaining these details is to institute appropriate referrals within the organization for the required diagnostic assessments with tests, treatment, and support. The personal and family history is relevant to determine and manage specific risks appropriately as stipulated in the internal referral policy.

For male patients/clients, information about own use of contraception and the female partners' use of contraception are explored in the integrated contraception and sexual health clinic history. The symptoms review may reveal unreported or unrecognized lower urinary tract symptoms, so that appropriate assessments and tests and treatment interventions can be offered. This discussion draws on the U.K. National guideline for consultations requiring sexual history taking (Brook et al., 2013).

Policy Recommendations for Documenting and Storing Patient/Client Records

The importance of compliance with national and organizational policies regarding documentation of a patient's history is emphasized. Use of appropriate database systems for secure storage is also stressed. U.S.-based practitioners should be aware of both Health Insurance Portability and Accountability Act (HIPAA) guidelines and Centers for Disease Control and Prevention (CDC) STI reporting requirements.

Required Resources

Materials used during these interactions may include authorized forms, referral sheets, information documents, and leaflets. Patients may have seen and picked up sexual health information leaflets displayed at various places, such as their local general practitioner (GP) clinics, colleges, gyms, or social clubs. Therefore, additional material can be used during the consultation to clarify specific sexual health related issues and the role of the clinic. The range of visual aids may include poster diagrams, models, and demonstrators, with a selection of condoms for explanations and instruction. The room should be appropriately furnished, with a pleasant atmosphere and not be intimidating or daunting in any way. Safety measures should be functional and up to recommended standards. In many clinics, simple toys and games are provided for young children who accompany their parents.

Box 15-1 presents an outline of the key elements in the techniques to motivate patients to achieve effective and productive notification interviews.

Dealing with a Patient's Reluctance to Divulge Information: Alternative Actions

Reluctance to divulge the required information for partner notification and contact tracing should be addressed sensitively in an open minded manner by providing the index patient

---

BOX 15-1 Techniques for Motivating Effective Participation in the Notification Interview Establishing Rapport

- **The emphasis here is to establish effective dialogue** by encouraging the patient/client to feel at ease to engage in the discourse with confidence. The practitioner should show interest in the patient/client with courtesy and compassion to make him/her feel valued. Effective listening skills are crucial for this process and should be well developed. The patient/client's expressed intentions toward improvement and better sexual health behavior should be acknowledged and encouraged.

- **Fostering patient/client control** could be achieved through the assurance that the individual has freedom of choice to discuss issues. Coercion and forceful extraction of information is regarded as unprofessional, morally and ethically unacceptable, and should be avoided.

- **Testing resistance** involves the technique of using open-ended questions to enable the patient/client to divulge what they feel comfortable sharing with the practitioner without fear of recrimination or reproach. Whenever the individual demonstrates reticence to discuss a particular issue it could be postponed until he/she feels ready and comfortable to address that issue. This helps to foster a sense of personal control and a willingness to cooperate to achieve successful outcome in the partner notification process.

- **Inviting the patient/client to set the scene** should involve nonjudgmental discussion about shared values, attitudes, and behaviors among their social network groups. Use of familiar language and expressions may help the person to feel more at ease and empowered to share information.

- **Using the social context** in terms of identifying social connections and the main venues for social activities could be useful for targeting health promotion and on-site screening.

- **Encouraging disclosure** could prove to be difficult unless the patient/client feels unthreatened and not reproached. Therefore, the questions should convey acceptance without disapproval.

- **Use of memory prompts** as described by Brewer and Garrett (2001) enables the patient/client to recall the source of acquisition and probable timing of the infection. It also helps him/her to make connections to the nature of the relationship within which the infection may have been acquired. For example: regular partner relationship, casual relationships, one-night stand, or in connection with occupation as a sex worker. Additionally, location cues help to recall where and with whom the sexual contacts took place and personal timelines help to recall specific events and the individuals who were involved in recreational and sexual activities. Network cues are used to prompt recall about the sexual contacts known to each other. Finally, alphabetic cues may be used to prompt the patient to make the right connections by recalling the names of the sexual contacts using the letters of the alphabet as cues.

- **Obtaining detailed sexual history** serves the purpose of identifying sexual contacts who may have been deliberately omitted by the patient on the assumption that the degree of predisposition to the infection is insignificant. It is important to establish who else may have been exposed to the infection as a sexual contact. The patient's other assumptions regarding possible sources and timing together with appearance of symptoms should be thoroughly examined. Moreover, the types of sexual activities in terms of the mode of sexual intercourse with specific partners should be tactfully determined and use of vague and interchangeable terminology should be avoided. It is also important to establish the partners with whom condoms were used.

- **Avoiding and safeguarding sexual contacts from blame** can be achieved by tactful questioning including establishing how long since the infection was discovered and the fact that a particular sexual contact could have been asymptomatic and not aware of having acquired the infection.

Data from Bell, G. (2004a). 'Partner notification: Interviews' in *The Manual for Sexual Health Advisers.* London: Society of Sexual Health Advises (SSHA).

---

appropriate explanations and reassurance. Alam, Chamot, Vermund, Streatfield, and Kristensen (2010) reported that individuals' readiness and cooperation to divulge depends on the type of STI and the gender of the person. They noted wide variations in the process more often implemented for spousal partner notifications than for causal or commercial partner notifications. Barriers to successful implementation and outcomes include social/cultural factors, stigma, and fear of abuse for having acquired STI, and other related factors, including inadequate staffing resources, lack of training and counseling support, inefficient diagnostic techniques, and referral systems. These findings had been identified in studies of sexually active people living with HIV (Simbayi et al., 2007). Similar findings also emerged among female patients with chlamydia whose intention to divulge may be influenced by how important they consider this issue (Niccolai, Livingston, Teng, & Pettigrew, 2007). The impact of disclosure among people living with HIV was explored by Mayfield Arnold, Rice, Flannery, and Rotheram-Borus (2008) and Vu, Andrinopoulos, Matthews, Chopra, and Eisele (2012), which revealed the impact of stigma and antiretroviral therapy (ART) on sexual relationships. They noted a difference in disclosure of HIV status to regular sexual partners and to casual sexual contacts. They also reported the importance of increased access to ART and behavior interventions in reducing casual sexual relationships among HIV-positive individuals.

It is important for the index patient to understand that there is risk of infection from other STIs or reinfection of the initial STI if appropriate treatment is not provided. It is also important for patients to understand that the sexual contact may not develop symptoms, and therefore will remain unaware of having acquired the infection unless they are informed about having been exposed to it. The practitioner should explain the potential long-term complications that the sexual contact could develop if not notified, managed, and treated appropriately. Reassurance should be given regarding strict confidentiality and that no information about the patient's own diagnosis or his/her other sexual partner(s) would be divulged to that particular sexual contact. In the same way, the sexual contacts details should be kept strictly confidential.

The patient should feel empowered to take control in determining the preferred system of referral: patient referral or provider referral. It should be made clear to the patient that the sexual contact has a right to know that he/she has been exposed to an STI. The use of appropriate leaflets may help to provide additional pertinent information to confirm the purpose and significance of contact tracing and notification and what the procedure entails. The BASHH (2015) standards state that all patients/clients who access STI services should be provided with information and advice sensitively. Treatment and support should also be offered without disapproval, and the required care should be delivered fairly with an open mind. The method of partner notification should be carefully negotiated and the preferred choice respected.

Facilitating the Referral by the Index Patient

In the patient referral process, sensitivity and tact should be demonstrated by carefully preparing the index patient. The individual's direct participation in the decisions about timing, venue, and the method of communicating with the sexual contact should be encouraged. While confidentiality must be ensured, it is important for the index patient to understand the boundaries that protect his/her own diagnosis from being divulged to other sexual partners. Of equal importance, they should understand that the

boundary operates in the same way for the sexual partner in terms of safeguarding and holding in confidence that person's details. It should be made clear that the partner, too, has a right to be informed about his/her own diagnosis and given assurance about confidentiality.

Obtaining Details for Combined Testing and Treatment

Purposefully designed contact slips are found to be effective in inviting sexual contacts for diagnostic examination and testing and to ensure timely treatment to avoid potential complications. The goal is using a contact slip to arrange clinic attendance for STI management. Contact slip details should include clinic address, phone number, and clinic hours. In the United Kingdom sexual contacts are referred to the GUM clinic that is most easily accessible to them.

Choosing Effective Modes for Communicating with the Sexual Partners and Sexual Contacts

The provider referral process begins with a determination of an appropriate method to notify the sexual contact which may be by mail, telephone call, or personal visit. If the suggested means of contact proves unsuccessful, an alternative means may be used and the index patient may be able to help in determining which might be most effective. The boundaries of confidentiality would be similar to those applicable to patient referral. However, the index patient should be assured that his/her personal details including name, gender, type of relationship, area of residence, date of exposure to the infection, or unprotected sexual intercourse would be safeguarded with strict confidentiality. Similarly, the sexual contact's personal details would also be safeguarded with strict confidentiality. The index patient should be sensitively prepared for the conceivable reaction by the sexual contact, which may include anger, frustration, and/or embarrassment about a presumed act of deception. Thus, individuals may not feel very confident about partner notification for various reasons or may demonstrate resistance. In such scenarios, alternative methods may be needed to address the reasons for which individuals oppose to the notification.

Outline of Details Obtained for Provider Notification

Practitioners are encouraged to critically consider each of the following elements. These may vary in different areas based on policy guidelines.

- The individual's full name
- Date of birth
- Full address
- Date of first sexual contact
- Date of most recent sexual contact

- Type of sexual activities or practices, the nature of relationships
- Venues where the acquaintance or social contacts were made
- Pattern of condom usage

Additional information that may be required includes relevant telephone numbers, email address, current employment, work address, domestic circumstances, record of aggression or other forms of violence, abuse and record of addictive problems (Bell, 2004d).

These details may be obtained and stored in strict confidence. The SHA or partner services provider has the additional responsibility to provide required guidance and support toward reduction of index patient's susceptibility to reinfection and acquisition of other STIs following the current episode. Thus, risk prevention counseling may be justified.

Advice, Education, and Support Toward Minimizing Susceptibility to STIs

Advice, education, and support are essential to avoid ongoing exposure and acquisition of further infections. The individual's understanding and insight about the routes of acquisition and transmission of infections through different sexual activities should be reexamined to deal with misconceptions about genital, anal, and oral contacts. Evidence-based information should be provided regarding more effective use of condoms and potential limitations to condom protection. This information should be pertinent to the particular index patient's personal needs. It should include prevalence of specific STIs among relevant population groups (such as adolescents or commercial sex workers) as applicable. This allows for customization of the information about specific STIs and the most practical and effective preventive measures that the individual would be able to realistically practice (Bell, 2004d).

It is important to tactfully explore any hesitant confidence in a patient's claims about condom use, minimization of number of sexual partners, or types of sexual activities and contacts. The index patient should be encouraged to be more selective by choosing partners who have been screened and received appropriate treatment. Personal efforts should be encouraged, while providing the necessary education, guidance, and support. Other factors that contribute to sexual risk-taking activities should be explored and relevant guidance provided. Appropriate protective and preventive measures include vaccination against specific hepatitis viruses as indicated. Referral to agencies such as alcohol and/or drug rehabilitation may be required and the necessary arrangement made in the patient's best interest.

Importance of Accurate Recording/Documentation: the Details

Clear and meticulous documentation of the details about the sexual contact, consensus decisions, and planned actions are necessary. Accurate recording of all the necessary information relating to the interviews is a professional imperative. The decisions and actions taken should be documented in detail and the final outcomes recorded. Additionally, the sexual contact's details and any documented evidence that he/she has received treatment from his/her GP or elsewhere in another country should be recorded.

Advantages and Rationale for Evaluating the Notification Process

Tiplica et al. (2015) identified the general advantages of effective partner notification and management, which can be summarized as follows. The main advantages are as follows:

For the index patient:

- Avoidance of recurrence of the original infection
- Reducing the chances of frequent STIs by receiving evidence-based advice, health promotion/education, and sexual risk-prevention counseling

For the sexual contacts:

- Quick and timely treatment for those infected even if asymptomatic
- Limiting possible complications, screening, and treatment of coexisting STIs
- Reducing the chances of frequent STIs by receiving evidence-based advice, health promotion/education, and sexual risk-prevention counseling

For the general public:

- Curbing the frequency of outbreaks
- Reducing infectiveness and continuing transmission
- Curbing unsafe sexual behaviors among high-risk groups in the communities and among specific social groups
- Achieving possible cost effectiveness (Althaus et al., 2014; Turner et al., 2011)

In order to establish the benefits of evaluating the notification process in terms of patient outcomes and cost effectiveness, more evaluative studies and clinical audits of specific alternative methods are called for. Tiplica et al. (2015) propose that regular evaluative studies should be carried out to establish the effectiveness and outcomes of partner/contact notifications and management. These studies might explore the number of sexual contacts identified, actually traced, tested positive, and treated. Training staff to perform such studies should be an organizational priority.

Partner Notification in Confirmed HIV Infection

HIV partner notification is a public health initiative designed to prevent further spread of infection. While anti-retroviral drugs are effective in reducing HIV levels in vaginal secretions and seminal fluids, transmission to others can still occur and sexual contacts may not be aware of their vulnerability. Therefore, HIV partner notification should also be aimed at prevention of transmission to individuals who have not acquired the infection (Thirlby & Jarrett, 2004). These authors maintain that apart from the initial distress and personal life changes that individuals face when diagnosed with HIV, many patients cope with this news responsibly. The index patient is burdened with the responsibility of informing his/her current and previous sexual contacts about their exposure and susceptibility to HIV infection. The process enables individuals to make informed decisions and choices in important matters in their lives, such as having children.

Active partner involvement in the notification process has been reported as favorable for early referral and treatment (Brown et al., 2011). Nonetheless, variations have been reported in index patients' preferences of partner notification (Apoola et al., 2007).

Key Principles in HIV Partner Notification

A useful reference material is the current document on HIV partner notification by the National Aids Trust (NAT, 2012a). The key principles emphasize assurance of strict confidentiality during the pre-test consultation and discussions. Voluntary cooperation is crucial and the ethical obligation places the onus on the index patient to inform his/her sexual contacts and needle-sharing contacts. However, if the individual is reluctant to do so, the health adviser and relevant consultant may have to take appropriate action, albeit with sensitivity, making sure to avoid coercing index patients to notify their sexual partners. Current guidelines stipulate that index patients should not be forced to consent to provider referral because that could dissuade susceptible individuals from presenting for testing and appropriate management. The BASHH (2013) statement on partner notification highlights the need to support HIV-infected individuals and encourage involvement of their sexual contacts. New patients with HIV-positive diagnosis should be referred to the sexual health adviser. Compassionate follow-up with HIV-positive individuals transferred from other clinics is important (Thirlby & Jarrett, 2004). The guidelines on routine investigation and monitoring of adult HIV infected individuals (Asboe et al., 2012. See also: British HIV Association (BHIVA) Guidelines for the routine investigation and monitoring of adult HIV-1-positive individuals, 2016.) appropriately complement the U.K. national guidelines for HIV testing (British HIV Association; British Association of Sexual Health and HIV & British Infection Society, 2008).

Accurate record keeping is particularly crucial in HIV notification and index patient's disinclination to see the SHA should be recorded in the case notes. It is important that the assurance of confidentiality continues to be reaffirmed in the HIV pre-test counseling and during the HIV post-test counseling support sessions (Thirlby & Jarrett, 2004). The argument that "good quality partner notification should not compromise rights to confidentiality" (Radcliffe, 2013) poses an ethical dilemma and practitioners should consider it worthwhile to explore and reflect on the related challenges. The National AIDS Trust's (2012) HIV partner notification provides an important reference resource.

The problem of ongoing risk of HIV transmission to sexual contacts who are not aware of their vulnerability creates particular legal and ethical concerns. The risk to such individuals may outweigh safeguarding of index patient's confidentiality in certain circumstances, and the GUM clinician may implement the current recommendations in the GMC professional guidance. In this way, an appropriate course of action can be taken if the index patient cannot be persuaded to do so, but he/she is made aware of the need for disclosure (Thirlby & Jarrett, 2004). Practitioners should understand the guidelines that shape organizational confidentiality policies.

Ethical and Moral Challenges, Potential Legal Aspects Relating to Interviewing for HIV Partner Notification

Interviewing for notification is complex process that poses various moral, ethical, and legal challenges. The required competencies for these interviews are outlined in the current *Competency Framework for Sexual Health Advisers* (SSHA, 2013) and no doubt in the equivalent frameworks and manuals in other countries. An overview of specific ethical principles is presented in the ensuing sections. However, Rogers and Braunack Mayer's (2008) "Ethical Reasoning and General Practice" is also highly recommended.

Respect for the Patient's/Client's Autonomy

In practical terms, autonomy applies to truthfulness, informed consent, empowerment, independence, personal secrecy, and respect for personal choices. The health adviser may be confronted with difficult decisions during patient interactions where respect for the individual's autonomy could be threatened, creating tension. The autonomy of one person—the index patient—could result in disregard another person's autonomy, perhaps the sexual contact. Surrendering personal autonomy to the health adviser to make a decision for the patient creates difficulty when the professional is trying to foster empowerment. Tension also arises when the personal decision or choice made by a patient would have adverse consequences and not be to the best advantage of the individual. An individual's self-doubt and confused frame of mind when he/she expresses personal preference in decisions about care and treatment could pose difficulty for the health adviser and the multidisciplinary team. However, the WHO (2011) advocates professional decisions and actions aimed at achieving best possible outcomes for patients. The actions should be based on examples of excellence in practice supported by sound evidence. The practitioner's obligation in protecting the rights of the patient's requires that individuals be truthfully and honestly informed about their condition, treatment, and prognosis supported by best available evidence (WHO, 2011).

The Professional Obligation to Do Good and Not Cause Harm

These principles have been applied to sexual health practice as the obligations of beneficence and nonmaleficence. These concepts relate to the practitioner's duty of care and commitment to achieve the best possible outcomes in care delivery. They require that appropriate evidence-based measures be applied with the aim of avoiding harm to patients (WHO, 2011). This requires that in all interactions with patients practitioners recognize an individual's self-respect and self-worth, choice, and independence. It also requires that safe and efficient practice guided by evidence-based policies, protocols, and procedures within a safe environment are recognizable principles. Appropriate referrals to relevant experts in the multidisciplinary team and specialist consultations ensure that the patient receives all relevant care and services that are available to him/her. A difficult situation may arise when the professional's decision and action aimed at achieving positive outcome for one patient could worsen another individual's vulnerability to STIs and associated complications (Bell, 2004c). Providing information provision enables individuals to make informed independent decisions that they perceive to safeguard their personal best interest and safety rather than choices being made for them.

Professional Obligation Relating to Justice

In practical application justice requires that all patients/clients be treated with respect and fairness, including young people, as stated in the Faculty of Sexual and Reproductive Healthcare's (FSRH) 2012 Service Standards on Confidentiality. The application of standard protocols, specific recommendations, and stipulated procedural guidelines ensures that the care and service provision remains consistent for every patient. Justice should eliminate discrimination on the basis of gender, age, ethnicity, personal and/or religious values, beliefs and principles, and sexual disposition. This can be explained as implying equal opportunity for all patients and the right of access to consultations, care, and treatment together with clear awareness of the facilities available to them. A careful needs assessment is required to determine and provide appropriate evidence-based care with psychological and social support. As Bell (2004b) argued, justice becomes questionable when a specific policy stipulates that certain patients/clients be given priority access while imposing restricted access and delays for others.

Respect for Patient Confidentiality

Respect for confidentiality forms an important component of professional practice in healthcare. Suggested relevant documents include Health Insurance Probability and Accountability Act of 1996. U.K. practitioners are encouraged to explore the suggested documents listed in Appendix A at the end of this chapter for further reading.

In certain situations, however, public interest requires that particular infections be reported to the CDC through their National Notifiable Diseases Surveillance Systems. The rationale for this is to protect the public from the risk of acquiring the infections by putting in place measures to control the rate of spread and acquisition. Practitioners should be aware of which STIs are reportable and the consequence of not reporting them. Details of patient's sexual history should not be divulged to third parties and the preferred mode of correspondence should be respected and utilized as the individual requests. Furthermore, the health adviser should not inadvertently breach doctor–patient confidentiality by asking an individual's general practitioner to divulge specific personal details. The use of identifiable items including personal details and photographs must be consented to by the individual. Various dilemmas arise in relation to the duty of confidence and it is possible that protecting the confidentiality of one patient or the sexual contacts could have deleterious consequences for other individuals (Bell, 2004c), Bickley, Szilagyi & Hoffman (2017) also provide useful insight into the ethical issues relating to detailed health history taking. Practitioners may find it useful to critically analyze these to consider how best these can be interpreted and translated into practical application.

Box 15-2 provides an outline of the recommendations for STI screening and for notification actions for selected STIs and HIV infections. It is always useful to explore the relevant national policy documents that provide full details of the guidelines for the STIs. The BHIVA, BASHH, SSHA, and NAT *HIV Partner Notification for Adults: Definitions, Outcomes and Standards (2013)* is recommended here. It is particularly important to carefully note the current changes in such documents.

BOX 15-2 Recommendations for Notification of Partner and Sexual Contacts for Specific STIs and HIV Infection

Gonorrhea

It is recommended that the index patient should be encouraged to refer his/her sexual contacts for assessment and treatment. Where this is not acceptable to the individual the option of provider referral may be offered. The sexual contacts should be screened and treated for gonorrhea and chlamydia based on specific criteria related to the index patient.

- Men with urethral symptoms for 2 weeks before establishment of other characteristic symptoms.
- All women and men without symptoms—12 weeks prior to diagnosis of urethral, cervical, rectal, or throat infections.
- If last sexual intercourse more than 8 weeks prior to manifestation of symptoms or diagnosis, only the most recent partner should undergo the treatment intervention.

Chlamydia

It is recommended that the index patient be encouraged to refer his/her sexual contacts for assessment and treatment. Where this is not acceptable to the individual the option of provider referral may be offered.

- The recommendation for men is 4 weeks prior to onset of symptoms.
- For all women and men with no symptoms—6 months and until the last previous sexual contact.

Nonspecific Urethritis

It is recommended that the index patient/client should be encouraged to refer his/her sexual contacts for assessment and treatment. Where this is not acceptable to the individual, the option of provider referral may be offered. Screening and treatment for uncomplicated chlamydia infection is based on the specified criteria:

- In men 4 weeks prior to the onset of symptoms
- For men with established symptoms, 6 months or until last previous sexual partner

It is also recommended that correspondence details be obtained at the first visit and consent for communicating also obtained for notifying the index patient/client and sexual contacts if laboratory investigations for chlamydia and gonorrhea show positive results.

Trichomonas

It is recommended that the index patient/client should be encouraged to refer his/her sexual contacts for assessment and treatment. Where this is not acceptable to the individual the option of provider referral may be offered.

Genital Warts

There is insufficient evidence that screening and treatment reduces transmission and reinfection, therefore, they are not routinely recommended. However, screening of current sexual partners for STIs is considered beneficial.

Genital Herpes

There is insufficient evidence that screening and treatment reduces transmission and reinfection therefore, it is not routinely recommended. However, psychological support and health promotion/education may be offered.

Viral Hepatitis—Type B

- Options of patient and provider referrals offered for sexual contacts involving penetrative vaginal and anal sex, as well as needle sharing partners from 2 weeks prior to onset of jaundice until blood tests show negative surface antigen.
- For patients/clients without symptoms risk assessment may be conducted to inform partner notification.
- Children born to infectious women should be screened for HBV if the baby is not vaccinated at birth.
- Nonsexual contacts who may be vulnerable should be referred to the Public Health Authority or PHE centers as stipulated in the national and local policy guidelines.

Viral Hepatitis—Type C

- Options for patient and provider referrals offered for sexual contacts involving penetrative vaginal and anal sex, also needle sharing partners during the period of infectivity—2 weeks prior to appearance of jaundice.
- Screening of children born to women who are infected.
- Non-sexual contacts who may be vulnerable should be referred to the Public Health Authority or PHE as stipulated in the national and local policy guidelines.

HIV

- Patient and provider referrals offered to sexual and drug/equipment sharing partners.
- Thorough risk assessment informs look back period and partner notification.

Data from Faldon C. (2004b). 'Sexually transmitted infections' in *The Manual for Sexual Health Advisers*. London: Society of Sexual Health Advises (SSHA).

Important to refer to the current guidance from BASHH and the Expert Advisory Group on AIDS (EAGA) regarding HIV window period. A single HIV test performed 4 weeks after possible exposure to HIV infection is claimed to adequately detect or exclude infection. Further test only if categorized as high-risk exposure.

Application of Consultation Models to the Interviewing and Communication Interactions: Related Principles and Research

Because the notification interview involves sensitive questions about sexual history, it is useful to apply effective consultation models to information giving, health promotion, and counseling interactions. The dilemmas relating to privacy, moral, ethical, and legal issues also make it particularly important that practitioners can translate the different models and related theories correctly for efficient application.

The sensitivity of sexual health problems requires assurance of privacy during all interactions. Patients may experience exaggerated distress responses based on the emotional and psychological impact of the acquired STI. Patients may harbor fear, anxiety, and apprehension about possible complications and potential long-term effects.

Individuals may present feelings of embarrassment, guilt, anger, and frustration about their acquisition and possible transmission of STIs. As a result, sexual health practitioners are faced with diverse reactions. Therefore, their approach to the consultation and interview should be methodical and logical, without being rigid or inflexible, which could cause a patient to become nervous and reluctant to divulge information.

To gain the patient's trust and confidence, a practitioner must project respect, empathy, and nonjudgmental attitude. Silverman, Kurtz, and Draper (2005) emphasize the importance of applying good consultation and communication skills to strengthen patients, willingness to consider and act upon healthy lifestyle guidance. This helps in fostering compliance with prescribed medication. Simmons, Sharp, Fowler, and Singal (2013) examine the impact of implementing a novel communication tool to examine individuals' understanding of care and how they express their satisfaction. Practitioners have an obligation to aim to achieve better outcomes from the health care that they provide.

Practitioners should be ready to provide opportunistic health promotion information and education to address issues that the individual perceives to be important or perceives as a threat to their physical or mental health. In order to perform effective and productive consultation, it is crucial for the practitioner to carefully select and apply an effective model.

Determining an Appropriate Model to Achieve Effective Consultation Outcome

Various models for consultation have been proposed over the past few decades. While some of these may be rather dated, they do, nonetheless, form the theoretical basis for many more recent models. The differences tend to be the core assumption(s) on which the model focuses. The important thing for the clinician and other professional practitioners is to critically examine, evaluate, and compare existing models to determine which type would be realistically applicable to a specific context. Critical examination of a selection of models also allows the possibility of devising an in-house version that may be eclectic but purposeful and easy to implement. The skills required to achieve effective communication and a satisfying outcome for the patient and the professional practitioner need to be well developed.

The applied model must be suitable for exploring and addressing the particular patient's clinical problem and related personal circumstances and needs for care and support. **Box 15-3** presents brief descriptive overviews of the characteristic features of each consultation model such as the patient's perspective, the process, or behavior.

BOX 15-3 Concise Descriptive Overviews of Various Consultation Models: Exemplars

The **"folk model"** proposed by Helman (1981) explores the concerns of the patient/client regarding the presenting problem and provides answers to questions, seeking explanations about why that has happened, the implications, the required treatment, and possible complications.

The **"consultation model"** proposed by Pendleton, Schofield, Tate, and Havelock (2003) applies a patient-centered approach to the consultation interaction. Seven key tasks guide the progress of the interaction. These comprise establishing the reason for clinic attendance including the history, etiology, personal concerns, and expectations. The model explores related issues such as risk factors, and proposes involvement of the patient in determining appropriate actions for the identified problems, sharing an understanding, establishing clarifications, involving the patient in the management decisions, and encouraging him/her to accept personal responsibility, ensuring appropriate use of resources and realization of all objectives of the tasks, as well as establishing and maintaining a positive clinician or professional practitioner and patient relationship.

The **"inner consultation"** model proposed by Neighbour (1987, 2004) postulates five check points described as connecting, summarizing, handing over, safety net, and housekeeping. In essence these allow the clinician to establish rapport with the patient by determining and summarizing the reason for clinic attendance, the problem being presented by the patient, the concerns and expectations. Thus, an agenda can be negotiated from the perspective of each party, the doctor's and the patient's. The clinician or practitioner must consider alternative actions in the best interest of the patient in all possible eventualities. This outlines what could be done if the plan does not work and the need for maintaining professional efficiency, effectiveness, and alertness to carry on with other responsibilities.

(continues)

BOX 15-3 Concise Descriptive Overviews of Various Consultation Models: Exemplars *(continued)*

The three-function approach to the medical interview proposed by Cohen-Cole (1991) and Cohen-Cole and Bird (2000) focuses on understanding the patient's emotional responses. This model allows for managing communication challenges and overcoming cultural and language barriers while exploring specific disquieting concerns.

The comprehensive Clinical Method/Calgary-Cambridge Guide Mark 2 evolved from the work of Kurtz et al. (2003) combines the information gathered from the current clinical history, past medical history, social and family history, and drug history with the disease-illness model. The key elements of the comprehensive Clinical Method/Calgary-Cambridge model include initiating the session, gathering information, building the relationship, explanation, and planning and closing the session.

The disease-illness model given by McWhinney et al. (1985) represents the tasks in a consultation in two parallel frameworks. The patient presents a problem followed by information gathering and two parallel frameworks of tasks.

The Illness Framework

From the patient's perspective, this component of agenda represents the individual's ideas, concerns, expectations, feelings, thoughts, and effects that provide a basis for understanding the personal experience of the illness.

The Disease Framework

From the doctor's perspective this component of agenda represents the history obtained to establish the symptoms and the physical examination to establish the clinical signs. It also includes the diagnostic investigations performed. These provide the basis for determining the condition or pathology, ruling out the differential diagnosis, and confirming the specific diagnosis.

Integrating the information from the two frameworks allows for developing informed explanation and appropriate planning, which should involve shared understanding and joint decision-making.

Becker and Maiman's (1975) Health Belief Model of Consultation

The health belief model of consultation has been extensively adapted and used for several years. It focuses on the patient's perspective throughout the consultation process. This model allows for exploring the patient's thoughts, beliefs, feelings, and personal concerns about the effects of the illness and their expectations of clinical interventions. The information gained provides a better understanding of the patient's perspective and can help in developing an effective management plan to achieve better patient outcome. It is based on the rationalization that if an individual believes that taking a particular health-related action can prevent them from contracting a specific condition, they would be motivated to do that. Therefore, the healthcare professional has a responsibility to provide the individual with pertinent evidence-based information to enable them to make informed choices about what to do. For example, the individual would conscientiously and correctly use condoms to prevent STIs and unplanned pregnancy, and in addition to the provision of advice, the professional may also suggest follow-up support.

The main features of the model are the following:

- Perceived susceptibility in terms of vulnerability to develop the condition and the consequences of not receiving appropriate treatment.
- Perceived severity in terms of their idea of the seriousness of the condition and the advice provided.
- Perceived benefits in terms of the improvement and related advantages of taking the relevant course of action.
- Perceived barriers in terms of the financial implications of the advice, actions, and treatment.
- Cues to action in terms of what makes the individual decide to seek consultation, healthcare intervention, and treatment.
- Self-efficacy in terms of the individual's motivation about health and the extent to which they would strive to achieve good health.

The locus of control can be described at different levels:

1. Internal controller: Having personal control of own life and health
2. External controller: The individual's belief of being helpless and having no control over personal health
3. The powerful other: The patient's belief that the healthcare professional has the knowledge and expertise to take charge and deal with all their health problems and associated needs

Pendleton et al.'s (2003) patient-centered consultation model describes the essential actions for achieving successful interaction and effective outcome. This can be compared to Coulter and Collins's (2011) examination of the importance of shared decision-making in the consultation interaction between the professional and the patient.

Required Consultation Skills

To effectively implement these models, a range of specific skills are required for obtaining relevant information from the patient and providing education and explanation about the presenting problem while facilitating cooperation and compliance. Abdel-Tawab et al.'s (2011) useful framework for consultation concerning medication enables the practitioner to critically examine that interaction and personal consultation skills. While some models, such as the Calgary-Cambridge Guide to the Medical Interview, are accompanied by the required set of professional skills, others are not and may have to be implemented using generic skills. It is useful to pursue courses and workshop training activities that enable the practitioner to develop interviewing and communication skills for efficient consultation. **Box 15-4** below presents a set of generic skills applicable to different consultation models.

Required Skills for Application of the Calgary-Cambridge Model

The practitioner should be well prepared (e.g., materials, temperament) for the dialogue with the patient, and prior to the consultation should review specific details about the individual. Establishment of rapport should begin with self-introduction, a kind and polite welcoming. The practitioner then establishes the patient's reason for attending this consultation and what they anticipate to gain from it. Note that the patient's aim may be in conflict with that of the practitioner.

Information gathering involves use of effective questioning techniques, good listening skills, and appropriate responses to ascertain the patient's concerns, expectations, and ideas. The acronym ICE (ideas, concerns, and expectations) is often used.

Physical examination, such as recording of vital signs, basic screening tests, and obtaining specific specimens, could be performed as necessary in the context or sexual health care. Any information given to the patient should be accurate and easy for the patient to understand to be able to share in a joint decision-making with well-reasoned and consensus action plans.

The session should be closed with concise restatement of the main points discussed, confirming commitment to the action plan, and outlining an alternative action plan in case of unforeseen eventuality. The final interaction should involve confirmation that all issues have been addressed to the satisfaction of the patient and the practitioner.

The consultation should be well structured with a useful agenda and the progress of the interaction should be periodically summarized to encourage recall and clear understanding. Use of signposting and concise transitional statements may help to maintain structure and consistency throughout the progress of the consultation. The relationship between the practitioner and the patient should be properly

---

BOX 15-4 Generic Skills for Effective Consultation Interaction

In order to achieve effective consultation, specific skills must be developed. While some skills will further improve with practice, each professional practitioner is likely to make certain adjustments to achieve efficiency in practice. The following could be considered as generic skills that are applicable to most if not all consultation situations, though not necessarily in the same sequence.

- Drawing out the patient's problems and how the individual perceives these as well as how the problems, impact on himself/herself and the family in terms of the physical, social, and emotional repercussions.
- Providing pertinent information that is tailored to meet the patient's requirements and checking that this is clearly understood.
- Establishing the patient's reaction to the information provided and encouraging them to express their main concerns.
- Determining the patient's readiness to participate in the decisions about management and the treatment options if applicable.
- Examining with the patients the implications of each treatment option.
- Enhancing the patient's motivation to comply with the agreed decisions about the treatment and lifestyle changes.

---

built with sound rapport and accepting and approachable body language. The consultation should be supportive with empathy, genuineness, tolerance, and a balance of power in the partnership.

Essential Skills for Application of the Three-Function Model

The three-function approach devised by Cohen-Cole and Bird (2000) requires three sets of skills. **Box 15-5** presents an outline of the key elements. First, communication skills are needed to obtain information to help understand the patient's problems. The practitioner must recognize that accuracy and thoroughness are crucial to obtain all the relevant biological, social, and psychological information necessary for accurate diagnosis and for contextualizing the management and therapeutic interventions. Next, emotional skills are required to establish good rapport with the patient. Empathic responses are crucial and may be conveyed verbally or nonverbally. Finally, behavioral skills are required to establish shared decisions based on

---

BOX 15-5 Essential Communication Skills Applicable to the Three-Function Model of Consultation

Required skills for thorough, methodical, and accurate information gathering:

- Attentive listening skills, ability to frame/ask clear and concise open-ended questions, using simple language and understandable terms are important skills.

- Additional skills to facilitate and encourage the patient, checking for accuracy, survey/scanning of other problems, and thoroughly examining these include:

    - the skills for negotiating priorities, clarifying, directing, and summarizing;

    - the skill for exploring the expectations of patients, as well as their ideas about the etiology or cause of the problem; and

    - the impact that the illness has had on their quality of life.

Required skills for developing a rapport and responding to the related emotional element of the consultation interaction:

- The skills of reflection in recognizing and conveying a deep sense understanding of the emotion involved in the building of rapport convey expression of empathy.

- Legitimation as an element in the three-function model of consultation conveys acknowledgment of the patient's feelings while also facilitating or enabling trust in the rapport. The provision of support upholds the emotion.

- Establishing and maintaining partnership and collaboration helps in strengthening the relationship between clinician/professional practitioner and patient.

- The aptitude of conveying respect is demonstrated through genuine recognition as well as commenting appropriately when the patient has done well by providing positive reinforcement.

The behavioral skills applied in motivating and educating patients comprise:

- Establishing a clear and shared understanding of the problem, determining what needs to be done, and a shared commitment to bring about these to achieve the desired outcome. In fulfilling this element of the three-function model, the professional practitioner applies her knowledge and skills for assessing what the patient knows about the problem, how much understanding, and what views the patient holds about it.

- The practitioner educates the patient about the illness and provides advice and reasoning in a way that is comprehensible and also assesses that the patient understands.

- Practitioner and patient in collaboration negotiate and agree on a plan of management and treatment.

- In the case of nonadherence, the challenge is to use appropriate motivational skills to reinforce and further strengthen the partnership, and reestablish and corroborate the agreed plan, which they must try to achieve.

---

the specific problem, and to determine what actions should be employed to address the problem.

Barnett, Jbraj, and Varia (2013) suggest the health coaching approach, which gives recognition to the knowledge and expertise of the healthcare practitioner while also taking account of the patient's perspective. The healthcare professional provides information, advice, guidance, and support regarding the patient's condition and the therapeutic intervention. At the same time, the individual is encouraged to express their experiences with the condition, the medication, and the impact on their social circumstances and financial situation. Information sharing between the patient and the professional is done on a mutual basis as they examine the pros and cons of alternative options. The professional practitioner and the patient make joint

decisions and determine appropriate actions, then negotiate the action plans and the consensus agreement is recorded.

The Patient Recall System: Continuance of the STIs/HIV Consultation Interaction

Lee (2004) explains patient recall as a means of reminding individuals to return to the clinic for follow-up treatment or supplementary screening. Thus, the intervals for recall may vary, ranging from 4 months to 12 months, depending on the type and seriousness of the STI and the associated potential complications. The process of active recall involves reminding patients to return for retesting for HIV/STIs, which may be done via short message service (SMS), email, telephone call, letter, or by sending out a home sampling kit. Although as yet the most effective mode of active recall cannot be determined with confidence, emerging evidence seems to indicate that active recall is associated with increased rates of retesting for HIV and STIs. Nevertheless, Burton, Brook, McSorley, and Murphy (2014) reported that the use of SMS texts as a mode of recall to remind patients at higher risk of STIs and HIV did not increase the rate of reattendance. This was compared to the conventional modes of reminders.

Evidence from systematic reviews and various clinical surveys have shown that patients who present for STI and HIV testing could continue to be at risk of other sexually transmitted infections. Indeed, many patients continue to cause ongoing spread of infections. (Burton et al., 2014; NAT, 2013). Other evidence also reveals that acquisition of different STIs potentially increases an individual's vulnerability to HIV infection. This indicates apparent risk behaviors that promote ongoing HIV transmission (NAT, 2013). While genital ulcers associated with syphilis and herpes cause lesions in the genital tract allowing entry of HIV, inflammatory tissue damage from chlamydia and gonorrhea is also implicated as foci for HIV. The national guidelines for HIV testing propose that this should be performed for all patients diagnosed with STIs (NAT, 2013). These scenarios justify the need for implementing the patient recall system.

Generally, it is the health adviser's responsibility to remind patients about the need to return for retesting and required therapeutic interventions. Additional interventions include medication administration, diagnosis discussion, recovery assessment, repeat screening, hepatitis vaccination, post-vaccine serology, specialist diagnostic examinations such as cytology and colposcopy, and partner notification discussions.

The standard of good practice requires that accurate records be maintained that document all the relevant details about further actions and ongoing provision of support. The records should specify the purpose of the recall and the mode or method(s) employed, such as telephone, letters, email, or a visit to the individual's home. Documentation of the health adviser's actions should include when the communication was made, the information that was conveyed, and the reaction of the patient. The outcome of all recalls should also be documented and discussions with the medical consultant and/or the sexual health lead or nurse manager should be recorded dated and signed by the SHA or designated professional. Experts suggest that evaluation of the interviewing techniques may help in examining and improving the recall system for sexual and drug injecting partners (Brewer & Garrett, 2001).

The Triage Arrangement: A Supplementary Intervention

Limited capacity to provide timely consultations, preventive advice, guidance, diagnosis, and treatment for all patients who seek STI specialist and nonspecialist support justifies the establishment of a triage service. The triage arrangement allows for identification and prioritization of patients who require a medical or health professional's attention before the next unscheduled appointment. A key rationale for triage is that prolonged waiting could prove detrimental and increase the vulnerability of patients who need immediate attention. Bell (2004e) explains triage as a system of determining the need for an individual to receive attention before the next unfilled appointment.

The main principles guiding the precedence for treatment before the next due appointment or ahead of other patients are as follows:

- Patient at risk of developing preventable disorders or complications before the next appointment
- The level of incapacity associated with severe pain and tenderness, worry, and distress
- The possibility of untreated acute STI
- The possibility of spreading infection before the next vacant appointment
- The possibility of contributing to the control of STI

Hitchings and Barter (2009) examined the impact of self-triage and reported that apart from effectively reducing waiting times, duplication of work, and needless clinic visits, there was improvement of STI care pathways for the patients. These authors maintained that the process allows prioritization of urgent cases, improvement in the organization of resources, and patient satisfaction. Griffiths and Ahmed-Yushuf (2005) reported that the triage arrangement ensured that patients who required more immediate attention had access to the appropriate available services. Knight and McNulty (2006) reported that in addition to reducing patient waiting time by half, the triage process is associated with improvement in patient flow and diminished patient anxiety and aggression.

Sexual health organizations in different countries that offer triage services, such as the United Kingdom and Australia, convey common key elements in the principles of triage. These include proper selection of patients for specialist services guided by a set of approved criteria. They also emphasize optimization of access to other services and referral of non-priority patients to alternative services.

Applied Eligibility Criteria for Triage

Triage decisions should be managed based on specific criteria to indicate a patient's priority status. Criteria may encompass the following:

- Direct exposure to gonorrhea, chlamydia, syphilis, hepatitis, or HIV infection
- Severe abdominal, testicular, or genital pain
- Severe anxiety and distress
- Exposure to sexual assault

- Emergency contraception and postexposure to HIV prophylaxis
- Young person under 16 years of age
- Unwillingness to wait for the next appointment
- Difficulty with arranging appointment due to work demands and/or domestic commitments (Bell, 2004e; Griffiths & Ahmed-Yushuf, 2005; Hitchings & Barter, 2009; Knight & McNulty, 2006)

Overview of the Arrangement/Set-Up and Procedure

The triage procedure involves use of documentation form(s) for detailed assessment and recording of the following:

- Degree of distress and anxiety
- Past history of infections aimed at establishing associated severity and duration of STI symptoms including pain, discharge, and other characteristic signs and symptoms of specific STIs
- Sexual history aimed at establishing personal and partner's exposure to any particular STIs (and if any sexual contact has mentioned specific STI symptoms)
- Risk of transmission of STI if medical attention is delayed
- Ability and willingness to return for postponed appointment if not attended to immediately
- Eligibility for urgent (same-day) appointment
- Alternative arrangements within the health service organization including GP clinic, family planning clinic, local pharmacy, full documentation of all stipulated details, advice provided, and decisions made by senior staff (Bell, 2004e; Griffiths & Ahmed-Yushuf, 2005; Hitchings & Barter, 2009; Knight & McNulty, 2006)

As an exemplar of good practice, the New South Wales (NSW) Sexually Transmissible Infections Program Unit (2013), identifies different models of triage to meet the requirements of patients depending on the administration and involvement of designated staff. Thus, services may be provided within the context of community or primary health center by administrative staff who then triage the patient to the available physician or obtain patient contact details for a clinician to call him/her. A second triage model may involve sexual health service administrative staff, delegated and trained nonclinical staff who respond to patient phone calls or assist individuals who attend without appointment. Following the guidelines on establishing the reason for attendance, the process may involve triaging to the first available clinician, a qualified sexual health professional practitioner. If unavailable, the administrative staff may obtain the required details for the clinician to call him/her or they may be advised to make personal contact on-line. A third model involves triaging of individuals who fall into the category of priority population groups with high-risk

of susceptibility. These include the young age group, minority ethnic groups, MSM, commercial sex workers, and injection drug users (IDUs). Based on the relevant criteria, such clients would be referred to the first available clinician for assessment and treatment. Sivapalan, Dale, Brown, and Colley (2005) draw attention to the need for appropriate training of staff to implement the triage process; this is also emphasized by the NSW Sexually Transmissible Infections Program Unit (2013). These systems ensure that every effort is made to provide treatment and support to patients.

Incorporating Health Promotion into Notification Interactions

The following practical considerations draw on the key principles of the charter for health promotion. The main roles of the SHA in translating each of these into actions are summarized.

Establishing Liaison with Relevant Agencies: Building a Healthy Public Policy

Wilson (2004) identified certain policies as examples of systems with which the health adviser may have some involvement. Among these are the teenage pregnancy strategy, healthy schools scheme, condom distribution scheme among high-risk population groups including young people's support groups or youth clubs, the LGBT communities, and ethnic minority communities. The SHA or equivalent may establish liaison with the relevant coordinators or representatives and the public health sector in providing appropriate health promotion.

Contributing to the Establishment of Supportive Environments with Accessible Social Work Undertakings

The SHA may help meet community needs in STI prevention through establishing accessible care and services. These professionals may support social work undertakings in young people's clinics by providing health coaching activities toward improving their sexual health behaviors, practices, and lifestyle (Barnett et al., 2013). Practitioners may also promote health within youth clubs through drop-in centers with supportive environments. SHAs may collaborate with other healthcare professionals involved with outreach projects (Wilson, 2004).

Contributing to the Enhancement of Community Endeavors Through Self-Support, Empowerment, and Peer Education

Strengthening community action can be achieved by supporting commercial sex workers through fostering self-support, empowerment, and peer education. In this context, individual and community empowerment must be considered to be directly interlinked (Woodall, Raine,

South, & Warwick-Booth, 2010). These authors maintain that community empowerment emanates from individual empowerment. In turn, individual empowerment is pooled in the pursuit of change through collaboration, involvement, and shared activities within the community (Koelen & Lindstrom, 2005; Wallerstein, 2006). The involvement of supportive and like-minded parties evolve into community organizations. These work together to achieve desired social and political change with balanced distribution of resources and power Laverack, 2006; Wallerstein, 2002, 2006; Woodall et al., 2010).

Community engagement is the process of fostering active involvement of communities in decisions that directly impact them in terms of improvement and reduction of health inequality (National Institute for Health and Clinical Excellence [NICE], 2008). This may be considered as demanding involvement. Nonetheless, the outcomes have proven to be beneficial for individuals, their social network groups, and the wider community where trusting relationships can be established. Adoption of this initiative in the interactions with support groups and drop-in centers is therefore, recognized.

Fostering Development of Personal Skills, Confidence, and Autonomy for Making Informed Decisions and Choices

This role enables the SHA to address interventions such as condom use while promoting the importance of respect and responsibility between sexual partners. Apart from discussing safer sex, the professional is able to establish individuals' needs for teaching and instruction and provide accurate evidence-based explanation and correct demonstration of the required skills. The professional's responsibility to empower individuals allows for conveying an understanding and assurance that personal concerns are respected and taken into consideration. Thorough needs assessment, sensitivity, and a nonjudgmental attitude should be demonstrated at all times among the professional, individuals, social groups, and the community.

Individual empowerment refers to a person possessing control over their own life issues. This is noted to be crucial in improving mental and physical health (Koelen & Lindstrom, 2005). De Silva (2011) explored how worthwhile it is to foster self-management through the process of helping people to help themselves. By developing and enhancing personal skills and attributes of self-esteem, self-worth, coping mechanisms, and confidence in making health-related choices, individual empowerment enables a person to contribute to community endeavors (De Silva, 2011).

Conducting Detailed Needs Assessments to Inform the Refocusing of Required Services

The SHA may participate in facilitating workshop training sessions, and ongoing support for school nurses, youth leaders, and other youth workers to implement health promotion within those contexts. Within sexual health centers, there may be a need to reorganize specific arrangements such as fast tracking of appointments for patients with special circumstances, including children in residential homes and looked-after children. The supportive role providing health promotion in these situations is crucial.

Collaborating in Partnership with Other Professionals to Provide Health Promotion Activities

The Schools for Health in Europe (SHE) represents a network that provides support for organizations and professionals to develop health promotion in schools within each European country. The network is coordinated by a community-based organisation (CBO) in its capacity as a WHO collaborating center for health promotion. The concept of health promotion schools refers to schools that implement standardized and endorsed plans for the health and well-being of all pupils and both teaching and non-teaching staff.

Some health promotion schools focus on specific issues such as nutrition, psychological health, drug misuse, and sexual health. Peer education is advocated as a useful practice among the teachers, school nurses, parents, and among the students who constantly interact with peer groups. Designated professionals who may participate in these schools include health promotion specialists, health advisers, and their equivalents.

An additional role for professionals is delivery of student workshops on issues such as sexual health and contraception. Olsen and Nesbitt (2010) explored health coaching in interventions aimed at improving healthy lifestyle behavior and concluded that it is worth considering in supporting patients/clients, individuals, and social groups. They also suggest that more detailed research is needed. Unplanned pregnancies among young people, accessibility to services, and reduction of STIs are identified as important issues to explore through research in order to inform evidence-based policy, recommendations, and practice. In performing these roles it is important to avoid competing with other professionals who may be working on similar projects and to avoid repeating ongoing activities.

Additional Practical and Regulatory Considerations

The Guiding Principles and Related Quality Standards

Klien, Sawney, and Thirlby's (2004) standards and guidelines serve as an example of good practice in the development and implementation of sexual health promotion within genitourinary services and it is worth exploring in depth. The current framework of competencies for SHAs upholds the view of implementing evidence-based standards and guidelines in sexual health promotion (SSHA, 2013). Other useful standards and guidelines are worth exploring in more detail. These include Department of Health's (2013) framework for sexual health improvement, the National AIDS Trust (2015), HIV and Black African Communities in the United Kingdom the gay men's HIV prevention strategy, and the teenage pregnancy strategy (HIV Prevention England, 2017; The Scottish Government, 2016).

Quality standards for good practice include moral and ethical principles and ensure that all individuals have equal access to sexual health promotion. Ethical standards of practice should accommodate diversity in terms of sexual disposition, age, ethnicity, and capability. Standards should foster individual and community empowerment and respect individual and community rights. Individual experiences should be recognized and cultural perspectives taken into account. Partnership and collaboration between relevant agencies, organizations, and communities is suggested.

Rationale for Combining HIV Consultation with Health Promotion, Risk Prevention Counseling, and Testing

Realistically, this concept should entail evaluation of these two systems of practice among the population groups of MSM, commercial sex workers, and specific communities (e.g., black Africans in England; NICE [2011]) provides insight into the strategies, procedures, and related factors that influence favorable acceptance of services. Extensive research and systematic reviews findings have provided the sources of the current evidence-based national guidelines on the policy for HIV testing and counseling in the United Kingdom. The evidence reveals that successful health promotion requires efficient implementation of behavior change models that incorporate factual information about the risks of unprotected sexual intercourse and ways of avoiding risky behavior. The health belief model considers factors designed to influence behavior change. These include perceptions about the particular risks to personal health, the known or expected success of treatment interventions, the predictable effects, and eventual advantages (Sharma & Romas, 2012). Nevertheless others argue that it is not entirely practical to plan and develop interventions aimed at effecting behavior change (Webb, Sniehotta, & Michie, 2010). Successful development of persistent behaviors requires recognition of the individual as an autonomous decision-maker while taking account of their extended social context.

Various authors emphasize the importance of gaining appropriate insight into the circumstances, actions, values, and convictions about the risks that are inherent among identified population groups. Research application, peer education, and the implementation of multiple processes are considered as effective approaches to health promotion (Klien et al., 2004). For instance, McFarlane, Kachur, Klausner, Roland, & Cohen (2005) examined the successes and barriers to internet-based health promotion. They found that although some successes may be achieved, there is also evidence that policy-related barriers can prove to be a hindrance to implementing this mode in some areas. There is a need for more extensive research to support this strategy in the prevention of sex-related infections and disease.

Recording the Progress and Outcome of the Health Promotion Interaction

This is always crucial, and the key elements in the documentation of sexual health promotion should include discussion of safer sex issues, together with explanation of potential risks and the measures considered for risk reduction. The provision of condoms and lubricants should be recorded and the demonstrations noted. If the individual declines these, it should be documented that they are aware of the risks and the measures for risk reduction. Individual's concerns regarding condom failures or other reservations should be addressed sensitively and documented together with discussion about safer sex negotiation (Klien et al., 2004; NICE, 2007).

Referrals for Further Support and Specialist Counseling by Relevant Experts

Patient-centered referrals should also be documented. Details about injecting drug users, the specific local drug services, and needle exchange schemes that they use should be carefully documented. Specialist services for young people, refugees, and asylum seekers should be clearly held on record in order to implement appropriate patient-centered referrals (Klien et al., 2004). The importance of monitoring, evaluation, and auditing activities in sexual health promotion should be carefully considered.

Risk Prevention Counseling Intervention in the STI/HIV Notification Interaction: A Role Ambiguity?

The earliest and subsequent updated recommendations to integrate voluntary HIV testing and counseling led to the conduct of Project RESPECT (Kamb et al., 1998). The British Association for Counseling and Psychotherapy describes counseling as involving a methodical process that allows individuals to examine, learn, and establish more resourceful living and fulfilment of health and contentment. It also encompasses resolving difficulties, dealing with tragedies, and catastrophic situations as well as clearing up discords to improve interpersonal relationships (British Association for Counselling and Psychotherapy [BACP], 1987; Leach, 2004).

Specific patient circumstances may indicate a need for counseling that is apparent at the initial stage of consultation while the needs of others may become evident later during the intervention. Examples include concerns about sexuality,

HIV testing and specific STIs, pre- and post-termination of pregnancy (pre- and post-abortion), sexual abuse, and rape. Other patients may present a need for psychosexual counseling where irrational and unfounded anxiety and fearfulness manifest even in the absence of sexual health problems. Some individuals may present with multiple problems and need a more intensive level of counseling.

Alternative Arrangements for Implementing Risk Prevention Counseling in the Notification Interaction

Counseling may be offered as one-to-one, couple or group situations, face-to-face or telephone counseling, outreach, ward or clinic-based, the community healthcare context, and drop-in settings (Leach, 2004; McMahon et al., 2015; NICE, 2007).

Different Descriptive Terms Applicable to Specific Counseling Support

Different practices are employed based on specific circumstances and the choice of a particular practice should be appropriate to meet the specific need(s) of the individual, couple, or group. Depending on the specific circumstances, the required counseling may be any of the following:

- Crisis intervention counseling
- Contract-based time-limited counseling
- Ongoing, supportive counseling
- Intermittent counseling or interrupted supportive counseling

Other types include advocacy, case work, and referral. These are explored in more detail by Leach (2004) and the relevant processes employed in sexual health advising are also clarified.

As Rietmeijer (2007) noted, the main theories from which contemporary models of counseling incorporate various psychological elements designed to influence behavior change. The more universally applied proposals include the health belief model as already considered. The social cognitive theory, which is also universally applied, portrays the molding of behavior on particular peers or significant others and the individual's confidence in their own capacity to control personal behavior and achievement. Other comprehensively applied proposals include the theories of reasoned action and planned behavior which portray individuals' attitudes and perceived social norms as influencing the intention to adopt a particular behavior change and to embark on that challenge.

Critical examination of the Project RESPECT reveals a combination of elements from these and other models including the transtheoretical or stages-of-change model as well as the HIV/STD prevention counseling model. The common objective in the implementation of the different proposals is to encourage and provide support for the progression through the stages-of-change in behavior. Leach

(2004) provides detailed information about the theoretical elements, related models, and principles.

Brief and Enhanced Prevention Counseling Session

Two distinct prevention counseling sessions were implemented in the Project RESPECT study. A "brief prevention counseling" intervention involves two separate pre-test and post-test counseling sessions of 20 minutes duration. An "enhanced counseling" intervention was also implemented, involving a 20-minute pre-test prevention counseling followed by three consecutive counseling sessions of 1-hour duration each in the weeks that followed. Incorporating elements from the theories of reasoned action and the social cognitive theory, these sessions focused on attitudes, social norms, and self-efficacy in relation to condom use (Kamb et al., 1998). Findings from the Project RESPECT study revealed that brief counseling interventions involving an individualized risk-reduction approach can improve condom use and prevent acquisition of new STIs. Furthermore, they maintained that effective counseling is practical within the context of a busy clinic (Kamb et al., 1998).

Hogben, McNally, McPheeters, and Hutchinson (2007) noted that partner counseling and referral services represent a crucial component of the range of care and services available for HIV-positive individuals and their sexual or needle-sharing partners. Generally, referral entails informing partners of their exposure, followed by testing if possible, together with prevention or risk-reduction counseling or arrangement of therapeutic intervention if positive test result is confirmed. Their evaluation of the effectiveness of partner counseling and referral services with partner notification among the population group at high risk of HIV infection also aimed at increasing testing among those groups. They noted that partner counseling and referral services that involve provider referral proved to be effective among high prevalent HIV groups. However, due to insufficient evidence, it was not possible to establish the effectiveness of partner counseling and referral services together with partner notification in achieving behavior change and reduction in the transmission rate. Extensive systematic reviews would no doubt help to establish the effectiveness of these proposals.

Mackellar et al. (2009) evaluated patient partner notification and health professional partner notification to inform sexual partners of their possible exposure to HIV. They examined the counseling of sexual partners including prior exposure to partner counseling together with options of referral services. Their findings showed that a considerable proportion of locatable sexual partners do not receive notification of their possible exposure to HIV regardless of the potential advantage of being notified. They recommend routine partner counseling and referral services to all HIV infected patients to ensure that every locatable partner is notified and informed about their risk to exposure and current HIV status.

LeFevre (2014) also examined U.S. recommendations for all sexually active adolescents and adults who are at high risk of sexually transmitted infections to receive intensive behavioral counseling. The rationale for this was based on the CDC's estimate of the significant increases of new STIs, in the region of 20 million each year in the United States (LeFevre, 2014). Identified high-risk groups included all sexually active adolescents, all adults with current STIs or within the preceding year, adults involved with multiple sexual partners, and those who do not habitually practice condom use. The evidence showed positive outcomes when the contact time of the interventions range in intensity from 30 minutes to over 2 hours, with greater benefits associated with increase in intensity of the intervention. Interventions may be provided by primary care physicians or referral of the patient to appropriately qualified behavioral counselors. The best success has been associated with provision of information about STIs and the transmission patterns as well as assessment of the risk of transmitting the infections. Training and instruction of relevant skills should include correct and consistent use of condoms. Required communication skills should also be fostered in relation to the practice of safer sex, problem solving, and goal setting. The ultimate goals of risk-prevention counseling are to reduce the rates of STIs and HIV infections and to curb transmission and spread within endemic communities and among high-risk population groups.

Significance of Professional Competency and Expertise for Counseling in STI/HIV Notification Interactions

Counseling skills are utilized in partner notification, promotion of sexual health, patient education, and information provision (BHIVA/BASHH/SSHA?NAT, 2013; Leach, 2004). The intensity of the counseling that is provided depends on the requirement of the patient and the timeliness of the information needed. While SHAs may have the competence and expertise to provide intensive counseling, others may not be adequately qualified to do so. Many SHAs enter the post with relatively basic counseling knowledge and skills. Adequate education and training are vital for efficient performance of the counseling role. While many SHAs can and do apply counseling skills at certain levels according to the needs and particular patient care scenarios, this varies, depending on the health adviser's level of counseling competence. As Leach (2004) points out, although SHAs may utilize different domains of counseling skills in different interactions with patients, the practitioner's qualification and expertise determine what level.

Building expertise is a progressive process of professional and personal growth and is influenced by the practice opportunities for counseling available within the specific organization. It also reflects the complexity of the context of care and services provided in that field of sexual healthcare. The diverse range of patient problems and needs that the practitioner has to deal with may reflect the level of counseling qualification and expertise applied in any particular context. The SSHA competency framework for SHAs (SSHA, 2013) outlines the domains of the essential knowledge and skills for performing this role.

Role Ambiguity and Recognition of Specialist Expertise

There is no doubt that the sensitive nature, moral, ethical, and potential legal implications of patient concerns justify and confirm the significant role of counseling in this field. However, psychosexual counseling and therapy is a highly specialized field, and Lewington (2004) provides considerable insight into the broader concept. Sexual health clinicians and SHAs who have not attained full qualification in counseling should work within the boundaries of their professional practice. The specialist knowledge and expertise of other members in the multidisciplinary team should be recognized and respected to correctly implement the referral pathways to meet the needs of the patient. In compliance with professional regulations, practitioners should make appropriate referrals to more highly qualified and specialist counselors on the multidisciplinary team in accordance with internal policy.

To fulfill the requirements of their current posts, some SHAs may find it useful to explore counseling qualification programs offered by higher education institutions. Where the SHAs post requires them to gain counseling qualification that incorporates psychosexual therapy, they are likely to be given the necessary management support to undertake a particular program of study. Practitioners must comply with the professional regulations to function at appropriate levels of education and qualification and within the boundaries of their professional discipline.

Significance of Clinical Supervision in the Counseling for Partner Notification

Clinical supervision is a structured sequence of prescribed, organized, and frequent interactions between a proficient or specialist professional practitioner and one or more supervisees. It encourages for facilitating reflection in terms of contemplative practice toward development of practical competencies (Leach, 2004). The supervision support helps to nurture and further enhance the supervisee's regard and application of principles and standards in professional practice. It serves as a means to foster compliance with stipulated professional regulations, ethics, and principles. The health adviser is encouraged to critically examine personal strengths and weaknesses and to seek appropriate assistance and support to attain the attributes for efficient performance in quality care provision (Bambling, King, Patrick, Schweitzer, & Lambert, 2006; Bradshaw, Butterworth, & Mairs, 2007; Leach, 2004; White & Winstanley, 2010).

Despite these core elements, some experts argue that the definitions, choice of models, implementation, and evaluation of clinical supervision vary across different aspects of education and practice (Milne, 2007; Milne et al., 2008).

The good practice guidelines of the Society of Health Advisers in Sexually Transmitted Diseases (SHASTD) identify managerial, counseling, observation, and guidance as crucial qualities for efficient performance of the role of sexual health advising. The role requires application of counseling skills in dealing with patients who present with problems relating to HIV/AIDS sexual assault, sexual abuse, sexuality, and difficulties in relationships with sex partner(s). The SHASTD holds the view that all the elements of clinical supervision should be considered as crucial components of the education and support of SHAs. The SHASTD stipulates the requirement for all health advisers who undertake counseling roles to be provided with supervision and advisory assistance, to be provided separately from interactions with the person who holds managerial status (Leach, 2004).

Individual or group supervision is recommended at approximately monthly intervals by a qualified counselor with extensive experience in clinical supervision, such as a qualified psychotherapist (or clinical psychologist). In the United Kingdom accreditation of the British Association of Counselors (BAC) is highly recommended (Leach, 2004).

Rationale for Clinical Supervision

Clinical supervision provides the supervisee with the opportunity to examine performance matters, questions, and specific factors influencing his/her professional development and the capacity to keep abreast of his/her own professional practice. Supervision also provides an opportunity to reflect on the impact that difficult and emotionally challenging aspects of their roles and interactions might have on the practitioner. It is important to ensure that neither the patients nor the professional practitioner is inadvertently exposed to emotional trauma that could create further problems for others. Advantages of supervision include improvement in well-being, self-awareness, confidence, lessening of emotional stress, and exhaustion (Winstanley & White, 2011). By encouraging regular reflectivity, clinical supervision may help practitioners avoid problems of distancing from interpersonal interactions and harboring a sense of nonachievement (Leach, 2004). The supervision and reflective periods provide an ambience of safety for expressing stress while gaining the support of the supervisor in his/her work. Moreover, the supervisee develops a deeper understanding of his/her professional role and responsibilities and is better able to examine and analyze the complex issues encountered in practice. Various authors maintain that apart from the personal health and professional benefits, other benefits include high standard-of-care provision with better outcomes for the patients and enhancement of the supervisor's professional growth (Bambling et al., 2006; Bradshaw, et al. 2007; White and Winstanley, 2010). The

key elements of the professional and personal development of the SHA are detailed in the competency framework for SHAs (SSHA, 2013).

Three Key Functions of Clinical Supervision

White and Winstanley (2010) noted three key functions of clinical supervision:

- The formative function addresses the supervision and support provided for the development of professional knowledge and skills (White & Winstanley, 2010), which reflect the supervisee's capability in relation to the specific role being performed.

- The restorative/supportive function relates to measures to safeguard the personal well-being of the supervisee (White & Winstanley, 2010). It encompasses recognizing and providing appropriate support following intensive interaction with patient that may have resulted in emotional trauma and distress. The health adviser may require supervisory support to examine such personal reactions in order to deal with them.

- The normative function enables the supervisor to demonstrate his/her responsibility of ensuring that the supervisee's work complies with standards of professional practice, including ethical regulations (Leach, 2004; White & Winstanley, 2010).

Essential Attributes for Clinical Supervision: The Supervisor

There is no doubt that clinical supervision should be provided in the right environment, with ample time allocated for sessions. Supervisors must possess the appropriate education and clinical experience, as well as training in clinical supervision. Where stipulated, the supervisor's knowledge base and clinical practice background should be congruent with that of the supervisee, and therefore supervisors should have adequate insight and understanding of the role of health advising. They should also be familiar with the levels of qualification and clinical experience of the different grades of the practitioners whom they supervise (Leach, 2004; White & Winstanley, 2009; White & Winstanley, 2010).

Thus, in the context of partner notification interactions, the clinical supervisor should be familiar with the referral pathways as well as the systems and support services in place. Appropriate insight about HIV/AIDS and issues relating to genitourinary medicine, the related care interventions, and services is also essential. SHAs are encouraged to discuss with their managers other forms of support, including managerial and peer/colleague support.

In addition to the support and guidance provided by the managers, senior colleagues, and peers, clinical supervision of SHAs provides a supplementary support system for this group of professionals. Apart from reflecting on and discussing personal performance, personal reactions, and interpersonal interactions, clinical supervision provides the opportunity for appraising personal and professional development.

Rationale for Research Application to the Partner Notification Process

The rationale for application of research to the partner notification process should include careful examination of relevant studies as well as critique and appropriate utilization of the findings to substantiate evidence-based practice. The need for critical systematic reviews of published studies is recognized and requires team collaboration. Rigorous investigation of emerging issues in practice through empirical studies ensures that questions relating to policy, procedures, and patient concerns about aspects of care and services can be explored. Research also allows for exploring concerns about existing or emerging issues in the practice of sexual health advising.

The main problem regarding systematic reviews of sexual health advising might be the limited amount of published studies conducted by practicing SHAs. However, other types of sound evidence should not be disregarded. Thus, findings from studies that have evolved from quality care provision, standards of local or internal procedure guidelines, and care pathways may also prove be useful sources of evidence.

Furthermore, committee reports, meticulously developed descriptive accounts, the views of peers and colleagues, and the opinions of authorized bodies or organizations contribute invaluable forms of evidence. Importantly, the evidence-based clinical guidelines developed by recognized national organizations such as NICE and Scottish Intercollegiate Guidelines Network (SIGN) are invaluable for guiding evidence-based practice.

However, as Faldon (2004c) noted, many of the published studies on aspects of sexual health advising have been conducted by researchers with no professional background as health advisers. The main shortcoming, therefore, is the lack of empirical studies conducted by practicing SHAs.

Identified practical issues and topics for possible research investigations in sexual health advising may relate to policy guidelines or to the perceptions, attitudes, and preferences of patients/clients regarding particular aspects of care and service provision.

Box 15-6 lists suggested topics that SHAs may consider for possible research endeavors.

There is no doubt that practicing SHAs may identify other topics within their areas of practice. Discussions with colleagues in the multidisciplinary team may help clarify a particular topic, refocusing and formulating appropriate research questions or hypotheses for investigation. Ideas

---

BOX 15-6 Potential Topics for Possible Research Investigation and Evaluative Studies

- Evaluation of the effectiveness of the partner notification process and/or outcomes
- Exploration of how factors such as gender, age, sexual disposition, nature of sexual relationship, or the diagnosis of specific STIs/HIV impact partner notification and contact tracing
- Evaluation of the interviewing and communication interactions between the professional practitioner, the index patient, and sexual partners/sexual contacts
- Comparison of community-based sexual health advising and GUM clinic-based sexual health advising
- Comparison of acceptability of referral systems and referral preferences for partner notification and contact tracing among LGBT, commercial sex workers, and heterosexual patients/clients
- Evaluation of the existing policy and guidelines for patient recall
- Exploration of different triage arrangements in relation to the size of the sexual healthcare organization

---

for innovative practice to improve care and service provision could be shared with colleagues, explored through the literature, discussed, and developed for detailed research studies. Alternatively, extensive search of the literature could be a useful start to develop a critical appraisal of publicized studies.

Systematic reviews and consideration of the findings for possible implementation in evidence-based practice could prove to be an exciting and useful activity shared by members of the multidisciplinary team.

Significance of Clinical Audit Activities to Maintain High Standards in Partner Notification and Contact Tracing

Auditing forms a crucial component of clinical governance and provides a mechanism by which the team of sexual healthcare practitioners can enhance the effectiveness of the process and outcomes of partner notification. It provides a means to evaluate practice policies, procedures, and outcomes by comparing these to the stipulated standards in order to improve the care and services provided.

Overview of Related National and Local Audit Projects and the Reported Findings for Evidence-Based Partner Notification and Contact Tracing

To understand the importance of clinical audit evaluative studies in sexual health care and services, it is important that practitioners are aware of relevant projects conducted at national and local levels. It is particularly important for practitioners to be aware of the audit projects that their own multidisciplinary teams may be required to participate in. An exemplar of a national clinical audit of sexual health care and services in the United Kingdom is British HIV Association/ British Association for Sexual Health and HIV (BHIVA/ BASHH, 2013b) which identified four main improvement areas: (1) late or missed HIV diagnosis, (2) reducing new STIs by reducing the infectivity period, (3) partner notification, and (4) testing for all four main STIs when testing for any. Three levels of sexual health services were audited according to the nature of the sexual health problems and the therapeutic and care interventions provided.

Level 1 services that can be provided by all GPs and in other community settings comprise history taking, screening for STIs in asymptomatic patients, HIV testing, and provision of emergency contraception. Additional services include basic sexual health education, condom use, and other contraception, as well as vaccination.

Level 2 services provided by GPs who have acquired the relevant competencies for performing stipulated procedures in community settings with appropriate resources involve a higher level of care and services. These include STI testing in symptomatic patients, treatment of uncomplicated STIs and genital warts, and provision of long-acting reversible contraception.

Level 3 services represent integrated sexual health clinics located within the hospital or community settings. These provide specialist sexual healthcare and services for dealing with serious and complicated STIs in vulnerable patients with problematic sexual health issues. Additional services provided at level 3 include screening and provision of treatment for complicated gonorrheal and HIV infections as well as coordinated partner notification and difficult IUD insertion and removal.

The proposal was to conduct audit projects that extend from screening to diagnosis to treatment and outcomes. This means that sexual healthcare practitioners and multidisciplinary teams working in the hospital and community may be obligated to participate in such projects. It is important that practitioners be aware of the findings from national audits, the identified examples of good practice, and changes in policy regulations, recommendations, and procedure guidelines.

For instance, evidence from partner notification outcomes emphasizes the importance of implementing high standards in the notification process. Bell (2004d) outlines key indicators that characterize standards of good practice in partner notification:

- Immediate referral of patients who are diagnosed with specific STIs and HIV to the SHA on the day of diagnosis to discuss the importance of partner notification. The identified infections include gonorrhea, chlamydia, syphilis, HCV, and HIV.
- Interviewing the patient within 15 minutes, during which the options of referral are discussed and the outcomes recorded in terms of patient's acceptance or rejection and the reasons for acceptance or rejection.
- The health adviser is required to explain the availability of provider referral to all index patients/ clients who express reservation or concerns about patient referral. The decisions that are agreed for the provider referral should be acted upon without delay.
- Support may be sought from a clinic accessible to the sexual contact if he/she resides outside the geographical locality. Similar assistance is provided to other clinics who may refer other sexual contacts residing within the immediate locality.
- Patient referrals are followed up and provider referral offered repeatedly if the index patient has difficulty with the option of patient referral.
- The clinic attended by the index patient should be informed of the sexual contact's attendance. The acceptability of the partner notification process to the index patient and the sexual contact should be documented.

Auditing of effectiveness of policies, protocols, and procedures at local and national levels allows for identification and more efficient utilization of resources. An example of a relevant national audit was McClean et al.'s (2008) case note audit on chlamydial infection management which explored information-giving, partner notification, and follow-up. Clinical audits serve as a means to improve standards and achieve high-quality care and services for better sexual health outcomes for the general population.

Recall and triaging can also be audited to evaluate effectiveness of the related policies and procedures. Crucially, however, the success of any audit project depends on the collaboration of members of the multidisciplinary team. Therefore, the need for appropriate training at all levels should be addressed by policy makers.

Requisite Preparatory Programs for Sexual Health Advisers and Partner Services Providers

The scope of the role and responsibilities of sexual health advising and partner services provision may include elements of clinical assessment, counseling, simple diagnostic testing, and treatment. Variations in these depend on what is sanctioned by national or state regulations, department of health, or the sexual healthcare organization. Therefore, the requirement for undertaking a prescribed education/training program, such as the United Kingdom's sexual health advising program or the CDC's Passport to Partner Services training courses should be considered as mandatory. In the United States the Division of HIV/AIDS Prevention and STD Prevention collaborated with the National Network of STD/HIV Prevention Training Centers to create the Passport to Partner Services program to train disease intervention specialists.

Undoubtedly, there may be certain countries where health advising or partner services provision does not form an established component of the multidisciplinary team of sexual health professionals. For those countries, the policy and decision makers and indeed the sexual health practitioners may find this practice in the United Kingdom, United States, and other European countries worth exploring as examples of good practice.

Rationale for the Prerequisite Education and Training of SHAs/Partner Services Providers

Apart from fostering insight and understanding of the principles and practice of sexual health advising or partner services provision, preparatory education and training ensures that the practitioner is adequately knowledgeable and competent at the expected professional level. The education and training programs provide opportunities to enhance existing knowledge and diversify professional qualifications and competency.

The *Competency Framework for Sexual Health Advisers* (SSHA, 2013) identifies four domains with expected levels of proficiency:

- First domain—Legal requirements, professional regulations, ethical considerations
- Second domain—Patient-needs assessment, planning, and delivery of care
- Third domain—SHA roles and responsibilities within the wider public health context
- Fourth domain—Professional and personal development

Comparatively, the key elements indicated in these domains are not entirely dissimilar from the CDC's 2013 recommended curriculum for the Passport to Partner Services training courses, which focus on the following tracks:

- Track A—Core principles for partner services provision
- Track B—Interviewing skills, partner elicitation, and notification; focus on HIV-positive patients
- Track C—Expands Track B skills to gonorrhea, chlamydia, syphilis, and HIV
- Track D—Wider scope of partner services; includes syphilis case management and visual case analysis

A Hypothetical U.K. Exemplar of Essential Competencies for Sexual Health Advising

The key competencies required for performing the role and responsibilities of health advising encompass the ability to do the following:

- Apply the stipulated ethical principles and related legislation in healthcare professional practice and to demonstrate compliance with the professional regulations
- Demonstrate respect for the rights of individuals' privacy and confidentiality
- Perform efficient sexual history taking, demonstrating effective communication skills, and effective listening skills, sensitivity, respect, and confidentiality (essential components of the partner notification process)
- Demonstrate efficient interviewing skills in obtaining pertinent information for partner notification purposes and for post-notification discussion
- Conduct efficient partner notification processes and contact tracing when appropriate
- Support for index patients/clients, the identified sexual partners, and sexual contacts
- Provide evidence-based factual information about prediagnostic tests together with required encouragement, guidance, and risk-prevention counseling
- Competently identify and assess patient needs including assessment of the needs of the wider community
- Facilitate prioritization of the identified needs and coordinate effective planning of appropriate actions
- Establish and maintain stable and effective interpersonal relationships while working in partnership with patients
- Foster empowerment and autonomy in individuals, groups, and communities reflecting people centeredness and cultural sensitivity to enable informed decision-making and choices
- Liaise effectively and productively with other professionals in interagency and interprofessional interactions
- Carry out meticulous collection, organization, and documentation of information for developing detailed reports

These, together with the competencies for workload management and related essential skills, should be developed to a high level for professional practice. These are by no means exhaustive and are not derived from any specific source other than the envisioned characteristic roles and responsibilities of sexual health advising.

A Hypothetical Exemplar of Practice Placements for Acquisition of the Practical Competencies

Exposure to the environments of practice and involvement in the actualities of patient care situations provide experiential learning opportunities. Thus in addition to placements at STI/HIV, GUM clinics, and various community clinics, some exposure to gynecology and other special clinics and wards may be helpful.

Range of Practice Placement Opportunities

The following represent potential placement and population opportunities for practitioners in educational programs:

- STI or GUM clinics, the triage services, and placement opportunities in GUM wards
- Care of HIV/AIDS patients
- Hepatitis C patients
- Adolescent and youth initiative projects aimed at reducing sexual risk-taking behaviors and practices
- Involvement in sex and relationships education (SRE) programs in schools
- Development and implementation of community health promotion programs or involvement in SHE where applicable
- Young people's sexual health clinics
- Prison sexual health services (depending on the regulations)
- Prostitutes/commercial sex workers
- Homeless and hard-to-reach client groups
- Laboratory testing facility to learn about viral test specimens and correct interpretation of blood borne viral test results, HIV, HCV, and specific STIs

Hypothetical Exemplar of the Theory Components

Theoretical aspects of a hypothetical SHA education program should entail the following suggested topics:

- The principles of public health and the principles of sexual health advising
- The code of professional conduct, performance, and ethics
- Applied legal and ethical concepts in healthcare professional practice
- The concepts of morality, values, beliefs, and principles
- The concepts of health and the principles of the Ottawa Charter for health promotion together with the Jakarta Declaration

- Health promotion, the related principles, models, and approaches
- Overview of the different types of STIs together with HIV (this element enables the SHA to provide accurate evidence-based explanations about specific infections, the recognition and potential associated complications, the management and related services available to the patients/clients)
- Epidemiology of sexually transmissible infections in relation to the different STIs and HIV, and the patterns of prevalence, transmission, and course of the specific infections
- The principles and rationale for partner notification and contact tracing, related ethical implications, the value of contact slips, and options of referral
- Systems of recall and triaging
- Young people and special client groups
- Risk assessment in relation to sexual risk-taking behaviors, different types and levels of risk reduction, and types of preventive measures
- Overview of contraception services and methods (depending on the type and level of academic attainment and the practice requirements)
- Applied reproductive science
- Theories and models of consultation, communication, interviewing, theories, concepts, and principles of counseling
- Research utilization and clinical audit

Conclusion

Achievement of the desired outcomes of partner notification for maintaining better sexual health and well-being in individuals and the general public depends on certain factors. Standardization of good practice is influenced by factors including compliance to the related legal, ethical, and organizational policies. Clearly outlined procedures with stipulated clinical guidelines typify well-structured and efficient partner notification services. These should reflect the perspectives of the patients, the health service organization in its capacity as provider, and the practitioners. Processes must be underpinned by appropriately substantiated evidence of best practice to achieve effective partner notification outcomes.

The procedures employed in partner notification and contact tracing should be carefully designed, correctly implemented, and evaluated on a regular basis. The sexual health practitioners' responsibilities in partner notification should reflect a clear understanding of the referral systems of patient and provider options. The processes of recall and triage that form essential components of the notification process also require appropriate application of stipulated policy guidelines. Variations in practice have been reported based on different healthcare organizational and clinical practice policies. Consequently, the practitioner must be fully aware of national and local guidelines and standards for practice.

Interviewing patients and the techniques for motivating effective patient participation in the interviews are essential skills that should be properly developed. Attentive listening in professional practice has to be learned and practiced conscientiously to gain the patience, concentration, tolerance, and expertise to diagnose the health problem and determine appropriate therapeutic interventions. Because partner notification incorporates health promotion, counseling, and clinical supervision, the knowledge and skills required for carrying these out must be developed to the appropriate level for efficient role performance. Professional regulations must be conscientiously complied with to safeguard privacy, anonymity, and confidentiality of the patients.

The health adviser contribution to research activities is imperative for evidence-based implementation of partner notification processes. However, the level of research activity may depend on the level of academic and professional qualification, the scope of professional capability, and the range clinical expertise. Assessment of the effectiveness of policy, procedures, and interventional outcomes requires sexual health practitioners to demonstrate commitment to participate in clinical audit projects. Auditing of partner notification services, the policy, guidelines, methods, and procedures at national and local levels allows for determining examples of best practice by the degree of effectiveness. At the same time, it allows for ascertaining the strengths and limitations in the current practice that could be further enhanced or improved.

Sexual health advising/partner services education programs should be suitably designed to achieve efficiency in practice. The key components of the requisite theory, essential competencies, and required practice placements are carefully considered in the national programs for SHAs and partner services providers.

The need for appropriately trained and designated SHAs/partner services providers in the multidisciplinary team is recognized. Therefore, in organizations where the policy makers recognize a gap in the multidisciplinary team for sexual health advising/partner services provision, appropriate guidance could be considered. Guidance should also be sought regarding the requisite program validation process and approval for professional affiliations.

• • • REFERENCES

Abdel-Tawab, R., James, D. H., Fichtinger, A., Clatworthy, J., Horne, R., & Davies, G. (2011). Development and validation of the medication-related consultation framework (MRCF). *Patient Education and Counselling, 83*(3), 451–457.

Alam, N., Chamot, E., Vermund, S. H., Streatfield, K., & Kristensen, S. (2010). Partner notification for sexually transmitted infections in developing countries: A systematic review. *BioMed Central Public Health, 10*(19), 1–11. Retrieved from http://www.biomedcentral.com/1471-2458/10/19

Althaus, C. L., Turner, K. M. M., Mercer, C. H., Auguste, P., Roberts, T. E., Bell G., . . . Low, N. (2014). Effectiveness and cost-effectiveness of traditional and new partner notification technologies for curable sexually transmitted infections: Observational study systematic reviews and mathematical modelling. *Health Technology & Assessment, 18*(2), 1–100.

Apoola, A., Radcliffe, K., Das, S., Robshaw, V., Gilleran, G., Kumari, B., . . . Rajakumar, R. (2007). Preferences for partner notification method: Variation in responses between respondents as index patients and contacts. *International Journal of Sexually Transmitted Diseases and AIDS, 18*(7), 493–494.

Arthur, G., Lowndes, C. M., Blackham, J., Fenton, K. A., & the European Surveillance of Sexually Transmitted Infections (ESSTI) Network. (2005). Divergent approaches to partner notification for sexually transmitted infections across the European Union. *Sexually Transmitted Diseases, 32*(12), 734–741.

Asboe, D., Aitken, C., Boffito, M., Booth, C., Cane, P., Fakoya, A., . . . Yirrell, D. British HIV Association Guidelines for the routine investigation and monitoring of adult HIV-1-infected individuals 2011. *HIV Medicine* 2012, *13*, 1–44.

Bambling, M., King, R., Patrick, R., Schweitzer, R., & Lambert, W. (2006). Clinical supervision: Its influence on client-related working alliance and client symptom reduction in the treatment of major depression. *Psychotherapy Research, 16*(3), 317–331.

Barnett, N., Jubraj, B., & Varia, S. (2013). Adherence: Are you asking the right questions and taking the best approach? *Pharmaceutical Journal, 219*, 153–156.

Becker, B. H., & Maiman, L. A. (1975). Socio-behavioural determinants of compliance with health and medical care recommendations. *Medical Care, 13*(1), 10–24.

Bickley, L. S., Szilagyi, P. G., Hoffman, R. M. (2017). Interviewing and the health history. In *Bates' Guide to physical examination and history taking*. (12th ed, pp. 65–106) Philadelphia: Wolters Kluwer.

Bell, G. (2004a). Ethical issues in patient recall. In: Society for Sexual Health Advisers. *The Manual for Sexual Health Advisers*. (pp. 93–95). London, United Kingdom: AMICUS HEALTH Sector, Society of Sexual Health Advisers (SSHA).

Bell, G. (2004b). Partner notification: Audit. In: Society for Sexual Health Advisers. *The Manual for Sexual Health Advisers*. (pp. 55–60). London, United Kingdom: AMICUS HEALTH Sector, Society of Sexual Health Advisers (SSHA).

Bell, G, (2004c). Partner notification: Ethical issues. In: Society for Sexual Health Advisers. *The Manual for Sexual Health Advisers*. (pp. 51–54). London, United Kingdom: AMICUS HEALTH Sector, Society of Sexual Health Advisers (SSHA).

Bell, G. (2004d). Partner notification: Interviews. In: Society for Sexual Health Advisers. *The Manual for Sexual Health Advisers*. (pp.23–40). London, United Kingdom: AMICUS HEALTH Sector, Society of Sexual Health Advisers (SSHA).

Bell, G. (2004e). Triage. In: Society for Sexual Health Advisers. *The Manual for Sexual Health Advisers*. (pp. 96–99). London, United Kingdom: AMICUS HEALTH Sector, Society of Sexual Health Advisers (SSHA).

Bell, G., & Potterat, J. (2011). Partner notification for sexually transmitted infections in the modern world: A practitioner perspective on challenges and opportunities. *Sexually Transmitted Infections, 87*(2), 34–36.

Bignell, C., & Fitzgerald, M. (2011). Guideline Development Group; British Association for Sexual Health and HIV UK. UK national guideline for the management of gonorrhoea in adults 2011. *International Journal of Sexually Transmitted Diseases and AIDS, 22*(10), 541–547.

Bilardi, K. E., Hopkins, C. A., Fairley, C. K., Hocking, J. S., Tomnay, J. E., Pavlin, N. L., . . . Chen, M. Y. (2009). Innovative resources could help improve partner notification for chlamydia in primary care. *Sexually Transmitted Diseases, 36*(12), 779–783.

Bradshaw, T., Butterworth, A., & Mairs, H. (2007). Does structured clinical supervision during psychosocial intervention education enhance outcome for mental health nurses and the service users they work with? *Journal of Psychiatric and Mental Health Nursing, 14*(1), 4–12.

Brewer, D.D., & Garrett, S.B. (2001). Evaluation of interviewing techniques to enhance recall of sexual and drug injecting partners. *Sexually Transmitted Diseases, 28*(11), 666–677.

British Association for Counselling and Psychotherapy (BACP). (1987). *What is counselling?* Lutterworth, United Kingdom: Author.

British Association for Sexual Health and HIV (BASHH). (2010). *Standards for the management of sexually transmitted infections (STIs)*. London, United Kingdom: Medical Foundations for AIDS & Sexual health (MedFASH).

British Association for Sexual Health and HIV (BASHH). (2012). *Statement on Partner Notification for Sexually Transmitted Infections*. Retrieved from http://www.bashh.org/documents/4445.pdf

Brewer, D. D., Potterat, J. J.. Muth, S. Q., Malone, P. Z., Montoya, P., Green, D. L., . . . Cox, P. A. (2005). Randomized trial of supplementary interviewing techniques to enhance recall of sexual partners in contact interviews. *Sex Transm Dis.* 2005 Mar; *32*(3): 189–193

British Association for Sexual Health and HIV (BASHH). (2015). *HIV partner notification for adults: Definitions outcomes and standards*. Retrieved from http://www.bashh.org/documents/SSHA_National_Competency_Framework_Final_Jan13.pdf

British HIV Association/BASHH. (2013a). *Joint BHIVA/BASHH national clinical audit of HIV partner notification*. Retrieved from http://www.bhiva.org/National-Clinical-Audit-HIV-Partner-Notification.aspx

British HIV Association/British Association for Sexual Health and HIV. (2013b). STI/HIV National Clinical Audit and Patient Outcomes Programme (NCAPOP). Retrieved from https://www.hqip.org/NCAPOP/NCA/HIV-and-STI/National-Clinical_Audit_of_STIs_and_HIV_Feasibility_Study_Report_Annexv1.pdf

British HIV Associstion; British Association of Sexual Health and HIV & British Infection Society. (2008). *UK National Guidelines for HIV Testing 2008*. Retrieved from http://www.bhiva.org/documents/Guidelines/Testing/GlinesHIVTest08.pdf

BHIVA/BASHH/SSHA/NAT. (2013). *HIV partner notification for adults: Definitions, outcomes and standards*. Retrieved from http://www.bashh.org/documents/SSHA_National_Competency_Framework_Final_Jan13.pdf

British HIV Association (BHIVA). (2016). *Guidelines for the routine investigation and monitoring of adult HIV-1-positive individuals*. Retrieved from https://www.bhiva.org/monitoring-guidelines.aspx

Brook, G., Bacon, L., Evans, C., McClean, H., Roberts, C., Tipple, C., . . . Sullivan, A. K. (2013). U. K. National guideline for consultations requiring sexual history taking. Clinical Effectiveness Group, British Association for sexual Health and HIV. London: BASHH. *International Journal of Sexually Transmitted Diseases & AIDS, 25*(6), 391–404.

Brown, L. B., Miller, W. C., Kamanga, G., Nyirenda, N., Mmodzi, P., Pettifor, A., . . . Hoffman, I. F. (2011). HIV partner notification is effective and feasible in Sub-Saharan Africa: Opportunities for HIV treatment and prevention. *Journal of Acquired Immune Deficiency Syndrome, 56*(5), 437–442.

Brunham, R. C., Pourbohloul, B., Mak, S., White, R., & Rekart, M. L. (2005). The unexpected impact of a chlamydia trachomatis infection control program on susceptibility to reinfection. *Journal of Infectious Diseases, 192*, 1836–1844.

Burton, J., Brook, G., McSorley, J., & Murphy, S. The utility of short message service (SMS) texts to remind patients at higher risk of STIs and HIV to reattend for testing. *Sexually Transmitted Infections, 90*(1), 11–13.

Centers for Disease Control and Prevention (CDC). (2011). *Legal/policy toolkit for adoption and implementation of expedited partner therapy*. Retrieved from https://www.cdc.gov/std/ept/legal/legaltoolkit.htm

Centers for Disease Control and Prevention (CDC). (2012). *Expedited partner therapy*. Retrieved from http://www.cdc.gov/std/ept/default.htm

Centers for Disease Control and Prevention (CDC). (2015a). *Legal status of expedited partner therapy by jurisdiction*. Retrieved from http://www.cdc.gov/std/ept/legal/default.htm

Centers for Disease Control and Prevention (CDC). (2015b). Sexually transmitted diseases treatment guidelines. *Morbidity and Mortality Weekly Report: Recommendations and Reports, 64*(3), 1–137.

Clark, J. L., Segura, E. R., Perez-Brumer, A. G., Reisner, S. L., Peinado, J., Salvatierra, H. J., . . . Lama, J. R. (2014). Potential impact and acceptability of internet partner notification for men who have sex with men and transgender women recently diagnosed as having sexually transmitted disease in Lima, Peru. *Sexually Transmitted Diseases, 41*(1), 43–45.

Cohen-Cole, S. A. (1991). *The Medical interview: The three function approach*. University of Michigan, MI: Mosby Year Book.

Cohen-Cole, S., & Bird, J. (2000). *The medical interview: The three-function approach* (2nd ed.). St Louis, St Louis County, MO, U.S.A.: Mosby Publishing Company.

Coulter, A., & Collins, A. (2011). *Making shared decision-making a reality: No decision about me without me*. London, United Kingdom: The King's Fund.

Cramer, R J. D., Leichliter, J. S., Stenger, M. R., Loosier, P. S., Slive, L. J. D., & SSunN Working Group. (2013). The legal aspects of expedited partner therapy practice: Do state laws and policies really matter? *Sexually Transmitted Diseases, 40*(8), 657–662.

Crawford, G., Bowser, N. J., Brown, G. E., & Maycock, B. R. (2013). Exploring the potential of expatriate social networks to reduce HIV and STI transmission: A protocol for qualitative study. *British Medical Journal Open, 3*(2), e002581.

De Silva, D. (2011). *Helping people help themselves: A review of the evidence considering whether it is worthwhile to support self-management.* London, United Kingdom: The Health Foundation.

Du, P., Gerber, F. B., & McNutt, L. A. (2007). Effects of partner notification on reducing gonorrhoea incidence rate. *Sexually Transmitted Diseases, 34*(4), 189–194.

Estcourt, C., Sutcliffe, L., Cassell, J., Mercer, C. H., Copas, A., James, L., . . . Johnson, A. M. (2012). Can we improve partner notification rates through expedited partner therapy in the UK? Findings from an exploratory trial of accelerated partner therapy (APT). *Sexually Transmitted Infections, 88*(1), 21–26.

European Centre for Disease Prevention and Control (ECDC). (2013). *Public health benefits of partner notification for sexually transmitted infections and HIV.* Stockholm, Sweden: European Council for Disease Prevention and Control.

Faldon, C. (2004a). Sexually transmitted infections. In *The manual for sexual health advisers* (pp. 41–46). London, United Kingdom: Society of Sexual Health Advisers (SSHA).

Faldon, C. (2004b). Partner notification: An introduction. In *The manual for sexual health advisers* (pp. 67–82). London, United Kingdom: Society of Sexual Health Advisers (SSHA).

Faldon, C. (2004c). Partner notification: Further research. In *The manual for sexual health advisers* (pp. 61–65). London, United Kingdom: Society of Sexual Health Advisers (SSHA).

Faculty of Sexual and Reproductive Healthcare (FSRH). (2012). *Service standards on confidentiality: Setting standards, in contraception improving sexual health for all.* London, United Kingdom: Royal College of Obstetricians and Gynaecology.

Ferreira, A., Young, T., Matthews, C., Zunza, M., & Low, N. (2013). Strategies for partner notification for sexually transmitted infections including HIV. *Cochrane Database Systematic Review, 10*, CD002843.

General Medical Council (GMC). (2008). *Consent: Patients and doctors making decisions together.* LondonLondon, United Kingdom: General Medical Council. Retrieved from http://www.gmc-uk.org/guidance/ethical_guidance/consent_guidance_index.asp

General Medical Council (GMC). (2017). *Confidentiality: Good practice in handling patient information (2017).* Retrieved from http://www.gmc-uk.org/guidance/ethical_guidance/confidentiality.asp

General Medical Council (GMC). (2013a). *Good medical practice.* London, United Kingdom: General Medical Council. Retrieved from http://www.gmc-uk.org/guidance/good_medical_practice.asp

General Medical Council (GMC). (2013b). *Intimate examinations and chaperones.* Retrieved from http://www.gmc-uk.org/guidance/ethical_guidance/21168.asp

Ghanem, K. G., Hutton, H. E., Zenilman, J. M., Zimba, R., & Erbelding, E. J. (2005). Audio computer assisted self-interview and face to face interview modes in assessing response bias among STD clinic patients. *Sexually Transmitted Infections, 81*(5), 421–425.

Golden, M. R., & Estcourt, C. S. (2011). Barriers to the implementation of expedited partner therapy. *Sexually Transmitted Infections, 87*, ii37–ii38.

Golden, M. R., Hughes, J. P., Brewer, D. D., Holmes, K. K. Whittington, W. L. H., Hogben, M., . . . Handsfield, H. H. (2007).

Evaluation of a population based program of expedited partner therapy for gonorrhoea and chlamydial infection. *Sexually Transmitted Diseases, 34*(8), 598–603.

Griffiths V., & Ahmed-Yushuf I. H. (2005). Is triage an appropriate way of dealing with walk-in patients attending genitourinary medicine clinics? *International Journal of Sexually Transmitted Diseases and AIDS, 16*(12), 819–821.

Hadsall, C., Riedesel, M., Carr, P., & Lynfield, R. (2009). Expedited partner therapy: A new strategy for reducing sexually transmitted diseases in Minnesota. *Minnesota Medicine, 92*(10), 55–57.

Helman, C. G. (1981). Disease versus illness in general practice. *Journal of General Practice, 31*, 548–562.

Helman, C. G. (2007). *Culture, health and illness* (5th ed.). London, United Kingdom: Hodder Arnold.

Hogben, M., McNally, T., McPheeters, M., & Hutchinson, A. B. (2007). The effectiveness of HIV partner counselling and referral services in increasing identification of HIV-positive individuals: a systematic review. *American Journal of Preventive Medicine, 33*(2), S89–S100.

Hitchings, S., & Barter, J. (2009). Effect of self-triage on waiting times at a walk-in sexual health clinic. *Journal of Family Planning and Reproductive Health Care, 35*(4), 227–231.

HIV Prevention England. (2017). Key guidelines and reports. Retrieved from https://www.hivpreventionengland.org.uk/evidence-and-guidance/national-guidelines/

Kamb, M. L., Fishbein, M., Douglas, J. M. Jr., Rhodes, F., Rogers, J., Bolan, G., . . . Peterman, T. A. (1998). Efficacy of risk-reduction counselling to prevent human immunodeficiency virus and sexually transmitted diseases: A randomised controlled trial. Project RESPECT Study Group. *Journal of the American Medical Association, 280*(13), 1161–1167.

Kingston, M., French, P., Goh, B., Goold, P., Higgins, S., Sukthankar, A., . . . Young, H. (2008). Syphilis Guidelines Revision Group 2008, Clinical Effectiveness Group. UK National Guidelines on the Management of Syphilis 2008. *International Journal of Sexually Transmitted Diseases and AIDS, 19*(11), 729–740.

Koch, O., De Silva, S., Edwards, S., Peake, T., George, B., Brough G., . . . Benn, P. (2008). Does using self-completed sexual history questionnaires in HIV-positive men who have sex with men affect clinical outcomes? *International Journal of Sexually Transmitted Diseases and AIDS, 19*(3), 203–205.

Koelen, M. A., & Lindstrom, B. (2005). Making healthy choices easy choices: the role of empowerment. *European Journal of Clinical Nutrition, 59*(1), S10–S16.

Kissinger, P. (2009). Considering the patient-delivered partner therapy. *Sexually Transmitted Infections, 85*(2), 80–81.

Kissinger, P., Mohammed, H., Richardson-Alston, G., Leichliter, J. S., Taylor, S. N., Martin, D. H., & Farley, T. A. (2005). Patient-delivered partner treatment for male urethritis: A randomised controlled trial. *Clinical Infectious Diseases, 41*(5), 623–629.

Klein, D., Sawney, F., & Thirlby, D. (2004). Standards and guidelines. In *The manual for sexual health advisers* London, United Kingdom: AMICUS HEALTH Sector, Society of Sexual Health Advisers, 287–308.

Knight, V., & McNulty, A. (2006). Triage in a public outpatient sexual health clinic. *Sexual Health, 3*(2), 87–90.

Kurth, A. E., Martin, D. P., Golden. M. R., Weiss, N. S., Heagerty, P. J., Spielberg, F., . . . Holmes, K. K., (2004). A comparison between audio computer-assisted self-interviews and clinician interviews for obtaining the sexual history. *Sexually Transmitted Diseases, 31*(12), 719–726.

Kurtz, S., Silverman, J., Benson, J., Draper, J. (2003). Marrying content and process in clinical method teaching: enhancing the Calgary-Cambridge guides. *Acad Med.* 2003 Aug; 78(8): 802–809.

Lanjouw, E., Ossewaarde, J. M., Stary, A., Boag, F., & Van Der Meijden, W. I. (2010). European guideline for the management of chlamydia trachomatis infections. *International Journal of Sexually Transmitted Diseases and AIDS, 21*(11), 729–737.

Laverack, G. (2006). Improving health outcomes through community empowerment: A review of the literature. *Journal of Health Population and Nutrition, 24*(1), 113–120.

Leach, G. (2004). Counselling. In *The manual for sexual health advisers*. London, United Kingdom: AMICUS HEALTH Sector, Society of Sexual Health Advisers, 104–124.

Lee, K. (2004). Patient recall. In *The manual for sexual health advisers*. London, United Kingdom: AMICUS HEALTH Sector, Society of Sexual Health Advisers, 83–92.

LeFevre, M. L. (2014). Behavioural counselling interventions to prevent sexually transmitted infections: U.S. Preventive Services Task Force Recommendation Statement. *Annals of Internal Medicine, 161*(12), 894–901.

Levine, D., Woodruff, A. D., Mocello, A. R., Lebrija, J., & Klausner, J. D. (2008). inSPOT: The first online STD partner notification system using electronic postcards. *PLoS Medicine, 5*(10), e213.

Lewington, L. (2004). Psychosexual counselling and therapy. In *The manual for sexual health advisers*. London, United Kingdom: AMICUS HEALTH Sector, Society of Sexual Health Advisers,155–16

Lorimer, K., Martin, S., & McDaid, L. M. (2014). The views of general practitioners and practice nurses towards the barriers and facilitators of proactive, internet-based chlamydia screening for reaching young heterosexual men. *BMC Family Practice, 15*, 127. Retrieved from https://bmcfampract.biomedcentral.com/articles/10.1186/1471-2296-15-127

Mackellar, D. A., Hou, S. I., Behel, S., Boyett, B., Miller, D., Sey, E., Harawa, N., . . . Ciesielski C. (2009). Exposure to HIV partner counselling and referral services and notification of sexual partners among persons recently diagnosed with HIV. *Sexually Transmitted Diseases, 36*(3), 170–177.

Mark, K. E., Wald, A., Drolette, L., & Golden, M. R. (2008). Internet and email use among STD clinic patients. *Sexually Transmitted Diseases, 35*(11), 960–965.

Mathews, C., Coetzee, N., Zwarenstein, M., Lombard, C., Guttmacher, S., Oxman, A. & Schmid, G. (2002). A systematic review of strategies for partner notification for sexually transmitted diseases, including HIV/AIDS. *International Journal of Sexually Transmitted Diseases and AIDS, 13*, 285–300.

Mayfield Arnold, E., Rice, E., Flannery, D., & Rotheram-Borus, M. J. (2008). HIV disclosure among adults living with HIV. *AIDS Care, 20*(1), 80–92.

McClean, H., Crane, C., Bunting, P., Bhaduri, S., Fernandes, A., Dhar, J., . . . Daniels, D. (2008). UK National audit of chlamydial infection management in sexual health clinics. Case notes audit: Information-giving, partner notification and follow up. *International Journal of Sexually Transmitted Diseases and AIDS, 19*(7), 477–479.

McClean, H., Radcliffe, K., Sullivan, A., & Ahmed-Jushuf, I. (2013). 2012 BASHH statement on partner notification for sexually transmissible infections. *International Journal of Sexually Transmitted Diseases and AIDS, 24*(4), 253–261.

McFarlane, M., Kachur, R., Klausner, J. D., Roland, E., & Cohen, M. (2005). Internet-based health promotion and disease control in the 8 cities: successes, barriers, and future plans. *Sexually Transmitted Diseases, 32*(10), S60–S64.

McMahon, J. M., Pouget, E. R., Tortu, S., Volpe, E. M., Torres, L., & Rodriguez, W. (2015). Couple-based HIV counselling and testing: A risk reduction intervention for US drug-involved women and their primary male partners. *Prevention Science, 16*(2), 341–351.

McWhinney, I. R. (1985). Patient-centred and doctor-centred models of clinical decision making. In: Sheldon, M., Brook, J., Rector, A. eds. Decision Making in General Practice. London: Stockton. (pp. 31–46).

Milne, D. (2007). An empirical definition of clinical definition. *British Journal of Clinical Psychology, 46*(4), 437–447.

Milne, D., Aylott, H., Fitzpatrick, H., & Ellis, M. (2008). How does clinical supervision work? Using a 'Best evidence synthesis' approach to construct a basic model of supervision. *The Clinical Supervisor, 27*(2), 170–190.

Mimiaga, M. J., Reisner, S. L., Tetu, A. M., Bonafide, K. E., Cranston, K., Bertrand, T., . . . Mayer, K. H. (2009). Partner notification after STD and HIV exposures and infections: knowledge, attitudes, and experiences of Massachusetts men who have sex with men. *Public Health Reports, 124*(1), 111–119.

Mimiaga, M. J., Tetu, A. M., Gortmaker, S., Koenen, K. C., Fair, A. D., Novak, D. S., . . . Mayer, K. H. (2008). HIV and STD status among MSM and attitudes about internet partner notification for STD exposure. *Sexually Transmitted Diseases, 35*(2), 111–116.

Mohammed, H., Leichtliter, J. S., Schmidt, N., Farley, T. A., & Kissinger, P. (2010). Does patient-delivered partner treatment improve disclosure for treatable sexually transmitted diseases? *AIDS Patient Care and Sexually Transmitted Diseases, 24*(3), 183–188.

National Aids Trust (NAT). (2012a). *HIV partner notification: A missed opportunity?* London, United Kingdom: National AIDS Trust. Retrieved from http://www.nat.org.uk/publication/hiv-partner-notification-missed-opportunity

National AIDS Trust (2014). HIV and Black African Communities in the UK. http://www.nat.org.uk/sites/default/files/publications/NAT-African-Communities-Report-June-2014-FINAL.pdf

National AIDS Trust (2015). Preventing HIV in the UK heterosexual population. http://www.nat.org,uk/sites/default/files/publications/Het_HIV_prevention_July2015.pdf

National Institute for Health and Clinical Excellence (NICE). (2007). *One to one interventions to reduce the transmission of sexually transmitted infections (STIs) including HIV, and to reduce the rate of under 18 conceptions, especially among vulnerable and at risk groups*. London, United Kingdom: London: National Institute for Health and Care Excellence.

National Institute for Health and Clinical Excellence (NICE). (2008). *Community engagement to improve health*. NICE Public Health Guidance 9. London, United Kingdom: Author.

National Institute for Health and Clinical Excellence (NICE). (2011). *Increasing the uptake of HIV testing to reduce undiagnosed infection and prevent transmission among men who have sex with men.* Public Health Guidance, PH34—Issued: March 2011. London, United Kingdom: Author.

Neighbour R. The inner consultation: How to develop an effective and intuitive consultation style. (1987). Lancaster, England; Kluwer Academic Publishers.

Neighbour R. (2004). The inner consultation; How to develop an effective and intuitive consultation style. (2nd ed) Oxford: Radcliffe Medical Press.

New South Wales Sexually Transmissible Infections Programs Unit. (2013). *Standard operating procedures manual 2013.* NSW Health Sexual Health Services. Sydney, New South Wales, Australia: New South Wales Ministry of Health, Centre for Population Health.

Newton, D. C., & McCabe, M. P. (2008). Sexually transmitted infections: impact on individuals and their relationships. *Journal of Health Psychology, 13*(7), 864–869.

Niccolai, L., Livingston, K., Teng, F., & Pettigrew, M. (2007). Behavioural intentions in sexual partnerships following a diagnosis of chlamydia trachomatis. *Preventive Medicine, 46*(2008), 170–176.

Nursing & Midwifery Council (NMC). (2015). *The code: Professional standards of practice and behaviour for nurses and midwives.* London, United Kingdom: Nursing and Midwifery Council.

Olsen, J. M., & Nesbitt, B. J. (2010). Health coaching to improve healthy lifestyle behaviour: An integrative review. *The Science of Health Promotion, 25*(1), e1–e12.

Pendleton, D., Schofield, T., Tate, P., & Havelock, P. (2003). The new consultation: Developing doctor-patient communication. Oxford, United Kingdom: Oxford University Press.

Peterman, T. A., Tian, L. H., Metcalf, C. A., Satterwhite, C. L., Malotte, C. K., DeAugustine, N., . . . RESPECT Study Group. (2006). High incidence of new sexually transmitted infections in the year following a sexually transmitted infection: A case for re-screening. *Annals of Internal Medicine, 145*(8), 564–572.

Radcliffe, S. (2013). Good quality partner notification should not compromise rights to confidentiality in HIV. *British Medical Journal, 346,* f2148.

Rietmeijer, C. A. (2007). Risk reduction counselling for prevention of sexually transmitted infections: How it works and how to make it work. *Sexually Transmitted Infections, 83*(1), 2–9.

Risley, C.L., Ward, H., Choudhury, B., Bishop, C. J., Fenton, K. A., Spratt, B. G., . . . Ghani, A. C. (2007). Geographical and demographic clustering of gonorrhoea in London. *Sexually Transmitted Infections, 83,* 481–487.

Rogers, W., & Braunack-Mayer A. (2008). Ethical reasoning and General practice. In W. Rogers and A. Braunack-Mayer *Practical Ethics for General Practice* (2nd ed.). Oxford, United Kingdom: Oxford University Press. Oxford, United Kingdom: Oxford University Press, 9–26.

Scottish Government. (2016). *Pregnancy and parenthood in Young People Strategy 2016-2026.* Retrieved from http://www.gov.scot/Publications/2016/03/5858

Shackleton, T., Sutcliffe, L., & Estcourt, C. (2011). Is accelerated partner therapy partner notification for sexually transmissible infections acceptable and feasible in general practice? *Sexual Health, 8*(1), 17–22.

Sharma, M., & Romas, J. A. (2012). *Theoretical foundations of health education and health promotion* (2nd ed.). Sudbury, MA: Jones and Bartlett.

Shiely, F., Hayes, K., Thomas, K. K., Kerani, R. P., Hughes, J. P., Whittington, W. L., . . . Golden M. R. (2010). Expedited partner therapy: A robust intervention. *Sexually Transmitted Diseases, 37*(10), 602–607.

Silverman, J., Kurtz, S., & Draper, J. (2005). *Skills for communication with patients* (2nd ed.). Oxford, United Kingdom: Radcliffe.

Simmons, S. A., Sharp, B., Fowler, J., & Singal, B. (2013). Implementation of a novel communication tool and its effect on patient comprehension of care and satisfaction. *Emergency Medicine Journal, 30*(5), 363–370.

Simbayi, L. C, Kalichman, S. C., Strebel, A., Cloete, A., Henda, N., & Mqeketo, A. (2007). Disclosure of HIV status to sex partners and sexual risk behaviours among HIV-positive men and women in Cape Town, South Africa. *Sexually Transmitted Infections, 83*(1), 29–34.

Sivapalan, S., Dale, M., Brown, C., & Colley, L. (2005). Triage criteria in genitourinary medicine. *International Journal of Sexually Transmitted Diseases and AIDS, 16*(9), 630–632.

Society of Sexual Health Advisers (SSHA) (2013). *Competency framework for sexual health advisers.* London, United Kingdom: AMICUS HEALTH Sector, Society of Sexual Health Advisers.

Stephens, S. C., Bernstein, K. T., Katz, M. H., Philips, S. S., & Klausner, J. D. (2010). The effectiveness of patient-delivered partner therapy and chlamydial and gonococcal re-infection in San Francisco. *Sexually Transmitted Diseases, 37*(8), 525–529.

Sutcliffe L., Brook M. G., Chapman J. L., Cassell J. M., & Estcourt C. E. (2013). Is accelerated partner therapy a feasible and alternative strategy for rapid partner notification in the UK: A qualitative study of genitourinary medicine clinic attenders. *International Journal of Sexually Transmitted Diseases and AIDS, 20*(9), 603–606.

Tanser, F., Bärnighausen, T., Cooke, G. S., & Newell, M-L (2009). Localised spatial clustering of HIV infections in a widely disseminated rural South African epidemic. *International Journal of Epidemiology, 38,* 1008–1016.

Theunissen, K. A. T. M., Schipper, P., Hoebe, C. J. P. A., Crutzen, R., Kok, G., & Dukers-Muijrers, N. H. T. M. (2014). Barriers to and facilitators of partner notification for chlamydia trachomatis among healthcare professionals. *BMC Health Services Research, 14*(2), 647. Retrieved from http://www.biomedcentral.com/1472-6963/14/647

Thirlby, D., & Jarrett, S. (2004). Partner notification: HIV. In *The manual for sexual health advisers.* London, United Kingdom: AMICUS HEALTH Sector, Society of Sexual Health Advisers, 314–325.

Tideman, R. L., Chen, M. Y., Pitts, M. K., Ginige, S., Slaney, M., & Fairley, C. K. (2007). A randomised controlled trial comparing computer-assisted with face-to-face sexual history taking in a clinical setting. *Sexually Transmitted Infections, 83*(1), 52–56.

Tiplica, G.-S., Radcliffe, K., Evans, C., Gomberg, M., Nandwani, R., Rafila, A., . . . Salavastru, C. (2015). 2015 European guidelines for the management of partners of persons with sexually transmitted infections. *Journal of the European Academy of Dermatology and Venereology, 29*(7), 1251–1257.

Trelle, S., Shang, A., Nartey, L., Cassell, J. A., & Low, N. (2007). Improved effectiveness of partner notification for patients with sexually transmitted infections: Systematic review. *British Medical Journal, 334*(7589), 354–357.

Turner, K., Adams, C., Grant, A., Mcleod, J., Bell, G., & Clarke, J. (2011). Costs and cost effectiveness of different strategies for chlamydia screening and partner notification: An economic and mathematical modelling study. *British Medical Journal, 342*, c7250 2011.

UNAIDS/ World Health Organization. (1999). *Sexually transmitted diseases: Policies and principles for prevention and care.* Retrieved from http://www.who.int/hiv/pub/sti/pubstiprevcare/en/index.html

Vest, J. R., Valadez, A. M., Hanner, A., Lee, J. H., & Harris, P. B. (2007). Using e-mail to notify pseudonymous e-mail sexual partners. *Sexually Transmitted Diseases, 34*(11), 840–845.

Vu, L., Andrinopoulos, K., Matthews, C., Chopra, M., & Eisele, T. P. (2012). Disclosure of HIV status to sex partners among HIV-infected men and women in Cape Town, South Africa. *AIDS & Behavior, 16*(1), 132–138.

Wallerstein, N. (2002). Empowerment to reduce health disparities. *Scandinavian Journal of Public Health, 30*(59), 72–77.

Wallerstein, N. (2006). *What is the evidence on effectiveness of empowerment to improve health?* Copenhagen, WHO Regional Office for Europe. Health Evidence Network Report; retrieved from http://www.euro.who.int/Document/E88086.pdf

Ward, H., & Bell, G. (2010). Partner notification. *Medicine, 38*(5), 239–241.

Ward, H., & Bell, G. (2014). Partner notification. *Medicine, 42*(6), 314–317.

Ward, H., Martin, I., Macdonald, N., Alexander, S., Simms, I., Fenton, K., . . . Ison, C. (2007). Lymphogranuloma venereum in the United Kingdom. *Clinical Infectious Diseases, 44*, 26–32.

Webb, T. L., Sniehotta, F. F., & Michie, S. (2010). Using theories of behaviour change to inform interventions for addictive behaviours. *Addiction, 105*(11), 1879–1892.

White, E., & Winstanley, J. (2009). Clinical supervision for nurses working in mental health settings in Queensland, Australia: A randomised controlled trial in progress and emerging challenges. *Journal of Research in Nursing, 14*(3), 263–276.

White, E., & Winstanley, J. (2010). A randomised controlled trial of clinical supervision: Selected findings from a novel Australian attempt to establish the evidence base for causal relationships with quality of care and patient outcomes as informed contribution to mental health nursing practice development. *Journal of Research in Nursing, 15*(2), 151–167.

Wilson, H. (2004). Sexual health promotion: Theories and principles. In *The manual for sexual health advisers.* London, United Kingdom: Society of Sexual Health Advisers (SSHA). London, United Kingdom: AMICUS HEALTH Sector, Society of Sexual Health Advisers, 277–286.

Winstanley, J., & White, E. (2011). The MCSS 26©: Revision of the Manchester Clinical Supervision Scale© using the Rasch Measurement Model. *Journal of Nursing Measurement, 19*(3), 160–178.

Woodall, J., Raine, G., South, J., & Warwick-Booth, L. (2010). *Empowerment and health & well-being: Evidence review.* Leeds, United Kingdom: Centre for Health Promotion Research. Leeds Metropolitan University.

Woodward, C. L. N., Roedling, S., Edwards, S. G., Armstrong, A., & Richens, J. (2010). Computer-assisted survey of attitudes to HIV and sexually transmissible infection partner notification in HIV-positive men who have sex with men. *Sexual Health, 7*(4), 460–462.

World Health Organization (WHO). (2001). *Guidelines for the management of sexually transmitted infections.* Geneva, Switzerland: World Health Organization.

World health Organization (WHO). (2009). *WHO Technical working group on HIV incidence assays.* Cape Town, South Africa: World Health Organization.

World Health Organization (WHO). (2011). *Prevention and treatment of HIV and other sexually transmitted infections among men who have sex with men and transgender people: Recommendations for a public health approach.* Geneva, Switzerland: Author.

Wylie, J. L., Cabral, T., & Jolly, A. M. (2005). Identification of networking of sexually transmitted infection: A molecular, geographic and network analysis. *Journal of Infectious Diseases, 191*(6), 899–906.

Young, T., de Kock, A., Jones, H., Altini, L., Ferguson, T., & van de Wijgert, J. (2007). A comparison of two methods of partner notification for sexually transmitted infections in South Africa: Patient-delivered partner medication and patient-based partner referral. *International Journal of Sexually Transmitted Diseases & AIDS, 18*(5), 338–340.

● ● ● SUGGESTED FURTHER READING

For more detailed evidence-based information relating to partner notification the following documents are recommended. At the same time, respect should be given to the specified copyright regulations and appropriate permission should be sought if professional application of the recommendations and guidelines is considered.

Armstrong, H., & Fernando, I. (2012). An audit of partner notification for syphilis and HIV. *International Journal of Sexually Transmitted Diseases and AIDS, 23*(11), 825–826.

Brewer, D. D. (2005). Case-finding effectiveness of partner notification and cluster investigation for sexually transmitted diseases/HIV. *Sexually Transmitted Diseases, 32*(2), 78–83.

Burgher, M.S., Rasmussen, V. B., & Rivett, D. (2005). *The European network of health promoting schools (ENHPS): The alliance of education and health.* Copenhagen, Denmark: WHO Regional Office for Europe.

Bourne, C., Zablotska, I., Williamson, A., Calmette, Y., & Guy, R. Promotion and uptake of a new online partner notification and retesting reminder service for gay men. *Sexual Health, 9*(4), 360–367.

BASHH statement on partner notification for STI: McClean, H., Radcliffe, K., Sullivan, A., & Ahmed-Jushuf, I. (2013). 2012 BASHH statement on partner notification for sexually transmissible infections. *International Journal of Sexually Transmitted Diseases and AIDS, 24*(4), 253–261.

Centers for Disease Control and Prevention (CDC). (2010). *Sexually transmitted diseases surveillance 2010.* Retrieved from https://www.cdc.gov/std/stats10/surv2010.pdf

Centers for Disease Control and Prevention (CDC). (2011). *Legal/policy toolkit for adoption and implementation of expedited partner therapy.* Retrieved from https://www.cdc.gov/std/ept/legal/legaltoolkit.htm

Centers for Disease Control and Prevention (CDC). (2012). *Expedited partner therapy.* Retrieved from http://www.cdc.gov/std/ept/default.htm

Care Quality Commission. (2013). *Supporting information and guidance: Supporting effective clinical supervision.* Retrieved from http://www.cqc.ogr.uk/sites/default/files/documents/20130625_800734_v1_00_supporting_information_effective_clinical_supervision_for_publication.pdf

Centers for Disease Control and Prevention (CDC). (2015). Legal status of expedited partner therapy by jurisdiction. Retrieved from http://www.cdc.gov/std/ept/legal/default.htm

Department of Health. (2013). *A Framework for sexual health improvement in England.* Retrieved from https://www.gov.uk/government/publications/a-framework-for-sexual-health-improvement-in-england

European Dermatology Forum Guideline on the management of partners of persons with sexually transmitted infections: Tiplica, G.-S., Radcliffe, K., Evans, C., Gomberg, M., Nandwani, R., Rafila, A., . . . Salavastru, C. (2015). 2015 European guidelines for the management of partners of persons with sexually transmitted infections. *Journal of the European Academy of Dermatology and Venereology, 29*(7), 1251–1257. [Note that these guidelines are set to expire while this chapter is in revision; readers should seek out updated guidelines after October 1, 2017.]

Golden, M. R., Whittington, W. L., Handsfield, H. H., Hughes, J. P., Stamm, W. E., Hogben, M., . . . Holmes, K. K. (2005). Effect of expedited treatment of sex partners on recurrent or persistent gonorrhoea or chlamydia infection. *New England Journal of Medicine, 352*(7), 676–685.

Mir, N., Scoular, A., Lee, K., Taylor, A., Bird, S. M., Hutchinson, S., . . . Goldberg, D. (2001). Partner notification in HIV-1 infection: A population based evaluation of process and outcomes in Scotland. *Sexually Transmitted Infections, 77*, 187–189.

Munro, S., Lewin, S., Swart, T., & Volmink, J. (2007). A review of health behaviour theories: How useful are these for developing interventions to promote long-term medication adherence for TB and HIV/AIDS? *BMC Public Health, 7*, 104.

Mimiaga, M. J., Fair, A. D., Tetu, A. M., Novak, D. S., VanDerwarker, R., Bertrand, T., . . . Mayer, K. H. (2008). Acceptability of an internet-based partner notification system for sexually transmitted infection exposure among men who have sex with men. *American Journal of Public Health, 98*(6), 1009–1011.

Medical Foundation for HIV and Sexual Health (MEDFASH). (2014). *Standards for the management of sexually transmitted infections.* Retrieved from https://www.bashh.org/about-bashh/publications/standards-for-the-management-of-stis/

National Aids Trust (NAT). (2012b). *HIV testing action plan to reduce late HIV diagnosis in the UK* (2nd ed.). London, United Kingdom: National AIDS Trust.

National Institute for Health and Care Excellence. (2016). HIV testing: Increasing uptake in men who have sex with men. Retrieved from https://www.nice.org.uk/guidance/ph34

Radcliffe, K. W., Flew, S., Poder, A., & Cusini, M. (2012). European guidelines for the organisation of a consultation of sexually transmitted infections. *International Journal of Sexually Transmitted Diseases and AIDS, 23*(9), 609–612.

Seedhouse, D.F. (2001). *Health: The foundations for achievement* (2nd ed.). Chichester, United Kingdom: John Wiley & Sons.

The Schools for Health in Europe (SHE). *Health promoting schools.* Retrieved from http://www.schools-for-health.eu/she-network/health-promoting-schools

Woodward, C. L. N., Roedling, S., Edwards, S. G., Armstrong, A., & Richens, J. (2010). Computer-assisted survey of attitudes to HIV and sexually transmissible infection partner notification in HIV-positive men who have sex with men. *Sexual Health, 7*(4), 460–462.

Appendix A

Guidelines on Respect for Patient Confidentiality Relevant to U.K. Practitioners

- *National Health Service Confidentiality: NHS Code of Practice* (NHS, 2003) and *Confidentiality: NHS Code of Practice Supplementary Guidance: Public Interest Disclosure* (NHS, 2010). The latter provides supportive interpretation of the key principles specified in the code of practice to guide practitioners when faced with decisions of disclosure of patient confidentiality.
- Caldicott Principles of Confidentiality (Brook et al., 2013; FSRH, 2012)
- General Medical Council—*Regulating doctors ensuring good medical practice: Principles of confidentiality* (GMC, 2013, 2017)
- Nursing and Midwifery Council—*The Code: Standards of Conduct Performance and Ethics for Nurses and Midwives* (NMC, 2008, 2015)
- General Pharmaceutical Council—*Guidance on Patient Confidentiality* (GPhC, 2012)
- The *Code of Practice on Protecting the Confidentiality of Service User Information* issued by the Northern Ireland Department of Health Social, Services and Public Safety, January 2009.

CHAPTER

16

Health Promotion and Health Education: Integral Components of Excellence in Sexual and Reproductive Health Care

THEODORA D. KWANSA

CHAPTER OBJECTIVES

The main objectives of this chapter are to:

- Explore the global agreement and recognition of the Health for All objectives
- Identify the key components of the Ottawa Charter for Health Promotion and the Jakarta Declaration on Leading Health Promotion into the 21st Century
- Examine the rationale, principles, policy, and practices of health promotion and health education
- Examine selected health promotion models and approaches, including ethical implications
- Explore the characteristics of best practice in health promotion
- Describe the role and significance of research and evidence-based practice in health promotion
- Summarize the requisite competencies, education, and training to ensure efficient practice of health promotion
- Recognize the importance of policy evaluation and health impact assessment in health promotion

Introduction

There is a global consensus in the 21st century to prioritize health promotion, which calls for a review of public health strategies and coordination of health services to heighten recognition of health promotion. The World Health Organization's (WHO) Health for All goal, established in 1981, envisioned that people in all societies worldwide should have the capability to safeguard and maintain a state of health that enables them to achieve realistic economic and social benefits. The key factors that affect achievement of the desired health outcomes include living environments, social and economic means, and sustainable resources. Therefore, models for health promotion must take account of these factors. Though some of the health promotion models cited in this chapter seem dated, they represent the foundation upon which more recent models were built. There is a persistent emphasis on incorporating evidence-based principles into sexual and reproductive healthcare practice, which is in part related to the ongoing changes in modern society, complex lifestyles and behaviors influenced by religious and cultural values and principles, sexuality, and sexual inclinations. Consequently, health promotion threads through all aspects of sexual health care and other related aspects of health. While appropriately qualified health promotion specialists are the ideal coordinators of health promotion and education, other healthcare professionals also have an obligation to provide information and guidance for maintaining healthy lifestyles. This chapter explores the ways in which health promotion models and concepts have been translated and transformed into practical application.

The Concept of Health Promotion

Although there are different definitions of health promotion, they all indicate that people-centeredness with individual and community participation and empowerment are consistent, key elements (Ewles& Simnett, 2003; Nutbeam, Harris, & Wise, 2010; Scriven, 2010; World Health Organization [WHO], 1986, 2009). The WHO's definition of health promotion describes a process of enabling people to enhance personal control over their health to achieve improvement. Others emphasize the connection between health promotion and lifestyle improvement on both an individual and a societal level. In this regard, prioritization of health becomes an obvious cornerstone of personal and public health agendas (Ewles & Simnett, 2003; Scriven, 2010).

Building on the WHO's (1986) definition of health promotion Wilson, et al. (2004) conceptualizes health as dually embracing shared (community) resources and relying on personal resources and physical potential. Wilson, et al. (2004) draws attention to Seedhouse's (2001) theory of health as an ultimate condition of physical and mental capability to function socially, reflected by physical and intellectual well-being. Wilson (2004) mentions Tannahill's (2009) conceptualization of the three activities of health promotion as education, protection, and prevention. Health education is a fundamental component of health promotion as it enhances an individual's understanding of factors that influence well-being and ill health. Additionally, health education is a means to foster lifestyle and behavior modification skills. French (2006) sees health promotion as a means to make sense of the public factors that contribute to the improvement, advancement and safeguarding of health and wellbeing. It is apparent that each of these ideas echoes the key principles of the Ottawa Charter for Health Promotion and the Jakarta Declaration on Leading Health Promotion into the 21st Century (WHO, 1986, 1997).

Most definitions of health promotion derive from the WHO's (1986, 2009, 2013) clarification of health and many of the interpretations incorporate elements from factors that are perceived to affect health. Some see the key determinants of health to be individuals' or communities' ability to meet basic health needs and to achieve desired health goals. Physical capability to cope with or adjust to environmental factors is also considered. Thus, health is perceived as a resource for life (Ewles & Simnett, 2003; WHO, 1986, 2009, 2013). Factors that influence health, such as changes within health systems, hereditary status, personal conducts, and social, economic, and environmental factors must also be considered (Haggart, 2000). However, Ewles and Simnett (2003) assert that there seems to be no established mutually agreed-upon interpretation of precisely what health promotion entails.

The Essential Principles

Health promotion characteristically represents the following precepts:

- Targeting people in their normal daily life situations, engaging in their day-to-day activities as influenced by various life circumstances
- Acting on the causes of ill health
- Using varied operational strategies in terms of education; information provision; and developing, improving, and advancing the community through health campaigning and support
- Coordinating participation schemes; securing organizational, individual, and population group involvement
- Acknowledging statutory and legal regulations
- Accepting and valuing public participation
- Capitalizing on the commitment of health professionals, particularly the primary care sector, in developing, fostering, and supporting health promotion (Ashton & Seymour, 1988)

The Ottawa Charter and the Jakarta Declaration: Common Precepts

The Ottawa Charter for health promotion (1986) and the Jakarta Declaration on leading health promotion into the 21st century (WHO, 1997) advocate similar principles: that health promotion should exemplify equity and social justice for all members of the particular society. Both documents urge that health promotion should nurture lasting and sustainable changes that can be maintained by the people as a permanent ongoing pursuit rather than merely a temporary effort. It therefore requires multiple and practical approaches, including development of new policy or change in policy, possible organizational change, and suitable community structuring. Consideration should also be given to statutory and legal regulations that safeguard the welfare of the people. Further critical analysis of the tenets reveals that health promotion encompasses the following key components:

- Empowerment: Supporting and assisting people as individuals or groups, to assume more control over factors that influence their health state
- Participation: Maximizing involvement of groups, communities, and individuals from the initial stages throughout the different stages

- Holism: Consideration of the physical mental/psychological health state, social and cultural values and beliefs, and religious and ethical principles that affect aspects of their health
- Interagency cooperation: Collaboration among participating sectors, such as governmental, nongovernmental, voluntary, and other relevant organizations, to achieve multisector involvement

Eriksson and Lindstrom's (2008) critical examination of the Ottawa Charter presents clarification of the sociological perspective on the origins of ill health and disease as well as recovery. It is useful to explore this in more detail to gain better insight to what the charter actually represents in practical terms.

Current public health encompasses a community standpoint, and acknowledges governmental commitment to address inherent social and economic factors associated with ill health. Partnership and collaboration with local communities in consultations, provision of advice, policy, and decision-making in the development of services are also important components. There is emphasis on careful planning of coordinated activities at all levels (Ewles & Simnett, 2003). Additionally, interagency collaboration and involvement of the public are advantageous in devising measures toward accomplishing better health for the people. Current statutory and legal public health regulations recognize that building and supporting community confidence is essential. Support and assistance from governmental, nongovernmental, and voluntary organizations are likewise recognized as important (Ewles & Simnett, 2003).

The main task of health promotion encompasses policy development for supporting health in all the relevant contexts. Education and information provision is essential to encourage change of behavior, which requires community needs assessments. This should be undertaken through shared endeavors with appropriate organizational restructuring and improvement as necessary. Needs assessments should occur in every aspect of people's lives, work, and recreation, in all life situations, and the environments in which people live and function. Key objectives should reflect a collaborative approach characterized by partnerships that empower both individuals and communities.

The Ottawa Charter for Health Promotion: A Broad Overview

The main values outlined in the WHO's 1986 Ottawa Charter for Health Promotion embrace partnership, advocacy, mediation, and enablement. These are also conveyed in the principles of the Health for All initiative, which is derived from the charter. Further developments that followed the launching of the original charter can be obtained from the 7th Global Conference on Health Promotion (WHO, 2009) and the 8th Global Conference on Health Promotion (WHO, 2013) (see Recommended Readings).

Health for All: A Mutual Global Foresight and Prediction

The Health for All initiative encompasses the following specific key elements:

- **People-centered approach:** This principle requires that programs recognize the health needs of the population and should be realistic in terms of the particular country's social and economic circumstances.
- **Right to health:** This principle supports the idea that all individuals have the fundamental human right to their lives and fulfilment of their health potential.
- **Equity:** This principle urges for recognition of a balanced social justice that aims to eliminate health inequality without encroaching on people's personal rights and freedom.
- **Empowerment and participation:** This principle recognizes the benefits of nurturing and enhancing individuals' and communities' potential to have sufficient power. It encourages and supports shared ownership and control to influence and participate in their own health and social care decisions and actions (Eriksson & Lindstrom, 2008; McQueen & Jones, 2007; WHO, 1998, 2008).

McQueen's (2011) critical examination of advances in health promotion draws attention to certain essential strategies, such as comprehensive health promotion aimed at fostering and enhancing the capabilities of people to achieve better health. The context of evolving social, economic, and environmental circumstances is particularly crucial (McQueen & De Salazar, 2011). In addition to interventions focused on safer lifestyle behaviors, it is necessary to reexamine key factors like lack of education and lack of adequate health care. These must be recognized as factors that influence inequalities in the distribution of financial resources while also affecting fundamental human rights (McQueen, 2011). Clearly these components of the Ottawa Charter for Health Promotion derive from the general principles that underpin the Health for All Initiative. The importance of social justice is emphasized in the WHO's (DH, 2008) report, *Closing the Gap in a Generation: Health Equity Through Action on the Social Determinants of Health*. This concept is acknowledged by the Department of Health DH (2008). McQueen proposes prioritization and adequate funding with appropriate research to ensure effective health promotion outcomes (McQueen, 2011). The need for appropriately qualified health promotion practitioners with appropriate level of knowledge and competencies is emphasized. The ensuing examination of the Ottawa Charter for Health Promotion is intended to encourage practitioners to reflect more critically on the rationales and principles that direct its practical implementation.

The Practical Considerations: Main Components of the Charter

Launched in 1986, followed by further developments in 2009 and 2013, the Ottawa Charter explains health promotion as the means of empowering people to manage their general health and to enhance their well-being. Thus two predominant values of health promotion are personal control and the capacity to improve personal health regarding physical, mental, and social well-being. The operational guiding principles emphasize the following:

- Equity in health and healthcare provision
- The right to participate in policy decisions that concern their health
- Involvement of the public or the population in the planning and implementation of their healthcare service
- People knowing that the healthcare decisions, plans, and actions take account of their needs and are not perceived as an imposition

The Charter advocates the importance of individuals' and communities' determination, motivation, and commitment to fulfill their needs and make adjustments to their environments. In this way, the desired state of physical, mental, and social health and welfare is accomplished. The healthcare system has an obligation to, and must display, commitment and accountability in this collective social concern. As Kickbush (2010) points out, while the health service organization must bear the consequences of chronic disease, we must take account of the wider social and environmental impacts. Of equal importance is individual recognition of the need to take personal responsibility in pursuing and maintaining healthy lifestyles, personal welfare, and safety. Saans and Wise (2011) also explore the potential impact of enabling, mediating, and advocating which are constantly emphasized as key elements in the implementation of health promotion.

Identified Strategies, Intentions, and Directions for Action

Significance of Advocacy in Terms of Collaboration and Shared Support in Health Promotion One aim of health promotion is to favorably influence biological, cultural, and behavioral factors as well as social, economic, political, and environmental factors. Ultimately, health and well-being ensures a beneficial and positive resource for society (WHO, 1986, 1998, 2009, 2013). In practical terms, advocacy entails embracing, defending, and safeguarding the welfare and interests of an individual, patients, or a vulnerable population group. Problems that inhibit health and well-being may be related to age, gender, literacy or educational status, financial status, health status or physical ability, and social status. Therefore, interventions in health promotion should involve support and guidance of underprivileged groups as they strive to improve these situations. The WHO's (2009) *Milestones in Health Promotion* statements from international conferences are worth exploring in more depth.

Healthcare and social care practitioners, in particular, health promotion officers, must recognize their professional accountability and obligation to lobby for provision of adequate resources to meet identified needs. To do so successfully, professionals must clearly understand the nature and extent of the problems within the community. As Finlay and Sandall (2009) point out, having built a trusting relationship with the individual patient, client group, or community, the practitioner is in the best position to act as advocate. In their professional role they would have gained good insight and understanding of the particular needs of the people. Moreover, they would have established a sense of loyalty and responsiveness to address the needs of the individual client or the community. Crucially, the Right to Health of All People emphasizes the importance of national programs, facilities, and initiatives aimed at avoiding preventable infections, diseases, and disability that are associated with social circumstances; (Ewles & Simnett, 2003; Fry, 1996; Orme, Powell, Taylor, Harrison, & Grey, 2003; Scriven, 2010). Thus, health promotion should be supported at government level through national initiatives and policies focused on deprivation and specific social requirements (Ewles & Simnett, 2003; Scriven, 2010).

The challenge for the practitioners, however, is the importance of the target population recognizing their own risk for the identified health problem. The people's commitment to collaborate in partnerships with the professionals and relevant agencies is crucial. To achieve this, Townsley, Marriot, and Ward (2009) emphasize the importance of establishing a trusting relationship and continuity with effective advocacy.

Carey (2000) maintained that within the context of multidisciplinary professional practice, prerequisites toward effective advocacy should include evidence-based knowledge, effective interactions, information exchange, skills in critical examination and resolution of difficult and complex issues, and facilitation and evaluative skills to enable practitioners to support and empower patients in their personal responsibilities. Featherstone and Fraser (2012) examine the attributes for effective advocacy while Townsley et al. (2009) highlight the key elements of advocacy as previously mentioned. Newbiggins, McKeown, and French (2011) also point out the need for cultural sensitivity in advocacy.

The concept of advocacy also connotes fostering and supporting individuals in their autonomy and control over decisions and actions relating to their health (Carey, 2000; Featherstone & Fraser, 2012; Newbiggins et al., 2011). Various experts maintain that the process enhances self-confidence and ensures that those who access particular services are able to make their voices heard. Therefore, in their role as advocate, the professional practitioner must recognize the responsibility to motivate and inspire client empowerment (Featherstone & Fraser, 2012). Respecting and safeguarding the best interest of individuals and vulnerable groups while ensuring that people have appropriate choice in the health and social care provision is also emphasized (Action for Advocacy, 2011). A particular challenge is the need for careful evaluation of a new or emerging health policy that may illuminate limitations of existing organizational policies inevitably leading to change. Nevertheless, such evaluation is justified.

Essential Processes in the Provision of Information and Support

Amplification Carey (2000) considers amplification as a key element in information provision and support. Initial actions involve a two-way interactive process between the practitioner and the patient(s). The practitioner must be able to present well-reasoned and understandable yet succinct information that is presented to the client in a logical manner, allowing for a two-way interaction to examine the information (Featherstone & Fraser, 2012). Once patient awareness and understanding of the problem is established, the practitioner assesses the patient's needs. Further information should reflect these needs and take into account the patient's comprehension level. Moreover, information should be reinforced by using different modes and effective tools and materials to enhance the individuals' ability to digest it. Ethical consequences and potential financial implications related to the problem should be discussed so that the patient is aware of the consequences related to their health decisions. It is important that the practitioner acknowledges the client's viewpoint and preferences in order to establish a partnership in which beneficial support is provided.

Clarification Following the information provision, advocacy should proceed with clarification, in that the practitioner should allow the patient to reiterate their understanding of the information provided and seek further interpretation or explanation as necessary. The practitioner may use pertinent examples to facilitate the patient's understanding and must give the patient the opportunity to request additional information. Palmer et al.'s (2012) outcome measures for efficient advocacy provide useful insights.

Verification Clarification should be followed by identification of any misinformation through careful review of the facts (verification). This process may be influenced by prior personal experiences, prior knowledge, and perceived consequences (Carey, 2000). The practitioner and advocate should be familiar with the client's particular problem and needs and should be able to determine appropriate evidence-based ways of addressing them. This requires practitioner training, supervision, and support toward developing competencies to perform advocacy efficiently (Featherstone & Fraser, 2012; Palmer et al., 2012).

Supporting Supporting, another element in advocacy, is explained as protecting, safeguarding, and defending the rights of the patient group or individual to make personal choices and act on them. Practitioners should familiarize themselves with the guidelines regarding the rights and responsibilities of individuals as outlined in their code of professional practice and in national legislation (such as The Patient Rights [Scotland] Act 2011, the Patient Protection and Affordable Care Act of 2010 in the United States or equivalent laws).

Affirming Affirming refers to establishing that the decisions and choices made by the patient are based on ethical and moral values that are acceptable to the patient. Individual choices in response to health promotion should lead to improvement in the quality of life (Tengland, 2007, 2010). The practitioner should recognize that the patients' needs, expectations, and demands are liable to change based on variations in society and changes in personal circumstances (Carey, 2000; Tengland, 2012). Additionally, patient autonomy may be interpreted in different ways and may involve diverse choices and decision-making, influenced by differences in social context and cultural structure (Newbiggins et al., 2011; Tengland, 2007, 2008).

Clearly, advocacy is complex and should be critically examined when implementing health promotion (Featherstone & Fraser, 2012). The provision of reliable facts, resources, services, alternative options, and consequences is important to empower patients, families, communities, and identified population groups at risk of specific health problems (Carey, 2000). Essentially, advocacy should ensure that patients are made aware of ongoing changes in the healthcare and social care systems. They should also be made aware of the available facilities, services, opportunities, and the support to realize the benefits of health and well-being (Featherstone & Fraser, 2012; Finlay & Sandall, 2009; Newbiggins et al., 2011).

Practical Actions Relating to Mediation

In practical terms, mediation generally involves an intervention by an expert or third party to provide support and assistance to others who have difficulty accessing a particular service or facility. Agencies and organizations mutually interested in the health and well-being of the nation must work cooperatively. Such agencies include governmental agencies, the health service organization, social services, the economic sector, industries, local authorities, voluntary organizations, and the media. An example of excellence is the Commission of the European Communities' (2009) strategy, which aimed at reducing health inequalities throughout Europe. Moreover, it is crucial that individuals, families, communities, and people from all walks of life contribute to the endeavor to curb inequalities in health and social circumstances (Newbiggins et al., 2011). Health promotion programs should take account of social and cultural needs, as well as the assessed needs of the population and the economic status of the country (WHO, 1986, 1998, 2009, 2013).

In mediation the professional facilitates the decision-making interaction to achieve the required or preferred service or resources, and therefore prioritizes the rights and welfare of the client group. Establishing a partnership is of crucial importance in these processes. However, practitioners must recognize that patients may exercise their right to reject or decline the evidence-based information and advice that they may have provided. Patients should not be denied the professional's obligation and duty of care to provide efficient support despite their choice for less-favorable alternative interventions (Featherstone & Fraser, 2012). Such decisions may be influenced by a variety of factors, including personal, social, and environmental circumstances, and physical and psychological capabilities (Carey, 2000).

The Interrelated Concepts of Enabling and Empowerment

To truly empower all people to achieve their maximum health potential, health promotion programs should influence reduction of health status inequalities and the provision of facilities and resources for health and social care services. Programs and campaigns should influence creation of an environment that is supportive, promotes information provision, and allows facilitation and acquisition of basic skills (Eriksson & Lindstrom, 2008; Nutbeam et al., 2010) for maintaining a healthy lifestyle. Enabling connotes individuals' capacity to claim and command personal control in making informed choices and decisions about their personal health, lifestyle, and well-being. Crucially, this principle applies to all people in society irrespective of gender, ethnicity, cultural, religious, educational, social, and economic status (WHO, 1986, 1998, 2009, 2013). The significance of cultural sensitivity in health promotion cannot be trivialized (Newbiggins et al., 2011).

The concept of enabling encompasses two crucial elements: (1) the provision of materials, funding, and other supportive resources, and (2) identification and removal of factors that may hinder goal attainment (Saan & Wise 2011; Seedhouse, 2004). Whereas some treat enabling and empowerment as synonymous, the two concepts are complementary but distinct.

Varied Interpretations of Empowerment The general assumption in health promotion is that individual responsibility is a crucial component and that people would willingly want to change their lifestyles. This emphasizes individuals' need to improve their health and maintain what they perceive to be healthy lifestyles. However, as various experts argue, this assumption places the onus of responsibility (and accountability) on the individual regarding his/her health (Carey, 2000). The complexity of empowerment and varied interpretations of such is continually discussed in health promotion literature. The advocating

and fostering of empowerment might be seen by some as conflicting with political and/or organizational policies, professional regulations, and codes of ethics. Within the context of health promotion, and in this chapter, the concept of empowerment is based on Carey's (2000) observation that the solution to community empowerment is the nature and degree of its participation and commitment to the preferred methods and techniques adopted for utilization in health promotion undertakings.

The WHO's Ottawa Charter for Health Promotion (1986, 2009, 2013) draws attention to the importance of community participation to achieve effective health promotion. The recommended level of community participation requires active and continuous dialogues, and collaboration to prioritize actions, with policy makers and decision-makers. Participation in decision-making at organizational and local levels in the planning and implementation is strongly encouraged for successful health improvement.

Carey's (2000) adapted format of community participation indicates a continuum with minimal or low participation on one end and high participation on the other. The low end is characterized by nonexistence of community participation and little to no information shared about decisions made or actions taken. Community members are only reactive (not proactive). A bit further along the continuum the community may be consulted to a certain extent in order to gain its agreement and approval of action plans. Or community input may be sought to make adjustments to programs developed by health professionals. Even further along the continuum the community may be allowed some involvement in planning while recognizing its obligation to respond, to a greater extent, to the desired change envisioned by health-promoting professionals (Carey, 2000).

Nearer the high participation end of the continuum, the community may be allowed considerable influence from the initial stage of the decision-making and planning. Nonetheless, ultimate power and control over the health promotion process, related policy, and decisions remain with professionals. At the highest participation end of the continuum, the community identifies the problems and needs of the people. The community is empowered in its commitment and responsibility to deliberate on these and to determine the best possible resolutions and endeavors to achieve improvement in lifestyles and better health.

This continuum of levels of participation, power, and control demonstrates that programs that allow minimum or no participation while coercing or compelling compliance are likely to achieve minimal and unsustainable realization of the expected outcomes. Whereas the strategies that encompass maximum community participation are more likely to achieve more beneficial and sustainable outcomes for the people (Carey, 2000).

It is clearly important that communities be involved in all discussions involving the identification of problems and the prioritization, planning, and implementation of actions. Moreover, the communities' viewpoint should be respected regarding its cultural diversity, how it influences the community, and the health implications of that diversity. Full community involvement should be essential to thoroughly examine environmental factors that may be influencing particular health behaviors and lifestyles. The community should be fully involved in a thorough needs assessment and in determining the best possible and feasible local strategies. It should also be involved in discussions about the financial and other resource implications. Of equal importance, the community's acknowledgment of its commitment, responsibility, and ownership should be clear and unquestionable.

Significance and Implications of Decisions and Actions

Building a Healthy Public Policy Policy makers in all relevant sectors must consider the potential health implications of their decisions and actions. It is important that they recognize their obligation and accountability regarding the health of the nation. A successful public health policy should coordinate elements from different sectors and encompasses statutory requirements, regulations, and taxation. Ideally, multiparty collaboration will allow for equitable social policies, healthcare and social care facilities, and healthy public services and environments; however, both the health and non-health sectors must collaborate in their endeavors and commitment to the health of the population (WHO, 1986, 1998, 2009, 2013).

Creating a Supportive Environment The development and maintenance of healthy and supportive environments essentially starts in the homes, yet the responsibility for such extends to the wider community as well. Ongoing scientific and technological advancements and workplace environments should be on the agenda for health promotion. Of equal importance, the nation's leisure environment should also support healthy lifestyles. Furthermore, people's awareness should be raised that each society has a shared responsibility for preservation of natural resources throughout the world (WHO, 1986, 1998).

Fostering Development of Personal Learning Skills Development of specific personal skills enables individuals to lay claim on, and retain control over, issues relating to their personal health and the environments within which they live. It enables people to continually learn, adopt new skills, and to make sense of new and substantiated information to help them cope with health issues such as illness, injuries, and disabilities. Health promotion and education programs should be available to all individuals, families, and specific population groups. Social skills acquisition can occur at home, in schools, within the community, and in work settings so these sites should be developed accordingly (WHO, 1986, 1998, 2009, 2013).

Strengthening Community Actions The objective in this case is to inspire and encourage communities to recognize their ownership and control of their responsibility for making decisions, and planning and implementing actions for improving the health of the people. That includes measures to improve the environment as well as establishing self-help associations and special interest organizations to support vulnerable population groups. Liu et al.'s (2016) adaptation of health promotion interventions for ethnic minority groups recognized that health promotion should capitalize on the attributes, knowledge, and skills within the communities with involvement and support of local experts to address current recognizable internal/domestic health issues. Appropriate health-related information should always be accessible to all within the community (WHO, 1986, 1998, 2009, 2013).

Refocusing of the Health Service Provision This objective requires that health promotion be seen as the shared responsibility of the government, the communities, and individuals. This principle requires that, in addition to providing clinical care, healthcare professionals have an obligation to expand their roles by contributing to health promotion through research activities. Appropriate education and training is imperative and practitioners must be prepared to deal with changing requirements and to adopt a holistic approach to prevention as well as clinical care and support (WHO, 1986, 1998). Furthermore, health promotion must take account of the WHO's "conditions and resources for health" (1986), which include peace, shelter, education, food, income, sustainable resources, social justice, and equity. All of these factors can influence sexual health problems such as risk-taking behaviors, sexually transmitted infection (STI) transmission, related long-term complications, and sexual abuse.

The Jakarta Declaration: A Broad Overview

Launched in 1997, the Jakarta Declaration on Leading Health Promotion into the 21st Century emphasized that the strategies and key themes for action outlined in the charter are applicable to each country. The consensus was to urge for a more comprehensive approach to health promotions, based on the key themes for action outlined in the charter. It advocates a holistic, people-centered health promotion involving partnership in decisions, planning, and actions. Therefore, it should be essential that health literacy, through ongoing, accessible education and support, be incorporated in health promotion policies and actions.

Recommended Principles and Standards

- Advocating societal concern and conscientiousness for health
- Strengthening security and assurance for health improvement

- Augmenting and multiplying partnerships in health promotion
- Intensifying the scope of competence and power within the community through empowerment of individuals
- Establishing and safeguarding an organized structure for health promotion

Implications for Health Promotion

The principles of health promotion maintain the need to encourage individuals and communities to retain command over determinants of their health, which should reduce the threats to and hazards of ill health. The principles of people centeredness and collaborative partnerships thread through the various expositions of health promotion (Downie, Tannahill, & Tannahill, 1996; Ewles & Simnett, 2003; Nutbeam et al., 2010; WHO, 1986).

It is worthwhile to consider that there is no one singular, ethically correct aim, policy, or protocol for health promotion. Practitioners must determine which aims and objectives they perceive to be most pertinent and/or pragmatic. Practitioners are encouraged to reflect critically on their philosophy of health promotion in determining particular health and lifestyle improvement goals.

Applied Mechanisms

- Primary prevention refers to actions implemented in the absence of, or before the onset of, infection disease. Approaches largely entail health promotion and health education activities and processes, such as meticulous hand washing and immunizations.
- Secondary prevention involves diagnostic methods of early detection and early treatment of existing infection or disease. Examples include STI screening programs referrals for specialist interventions, patient education and support, treatment, and counseling.
- Tertiary prevention refers to measures employed to restore organ or structural body functions to minimize the impact of disease complications. The implementation of tertiary preventive measures usually follows detection and diagnosis of infections or disease conditions. Tertiary measures encompass specialist therapeutic interventions with appropriate supervision, treatment, counseling, education, and ongoing support (Kutash, Duchnowski, & Lynn, 2006).

Three Tiers of Prevention Applied in Health Promotion

The above mechanisms of prevention may occur in one of three tiers, including the following:

1. Universal prevention, which aims at targeting entire population groups, districts, communities, or schools.
2. Selective prevention, which targets vulnerable groups at high risk of a particular health-related problem.

This tier takes account of factors such as age, gender, social, and economic circumstances, family history and perhaps ethnicity, lifestyle, and sexual inclination.

3. Indicative prevention entails programs (such as screening) to identify people who are in the early stages of acquired conditions. This level of prevention also involves identification of individuals, families, communities, social groups, or ethno-racial population groups who engage in specific risk-taking practices associated with particular health problems. There are characteristic health-risk indicators that may be identifiable through social behaviors and networks whether at school, home, or within the community (Kutash et al., 2006). Other, more self-explanatory concepts applied to the tiers or levels of prevention are provided at national, local, work, and personal levels.

Screening as an Element of Health Promotion

As a crucial component within the three tiers of prevention, screening programs allow for identifying individuals who have developed specific conditions, infections, or particular health problems. The Public Health England (PHE) (2014) outlined specific criteria that should be fulfilled before implementation of a screening program for any condition. The stipulated prerequisites for assessing the validity, effectiveness, and justification for screening include the following:

- The condition or specific health problem should be a significant concern.
- There should be adequate knowledge and clear understanding about the condition, the epidemiology, and course of the condition from latent to the established disease.
- There should be indisputable evidence and noticeable risk factor, disease marker, or indicator with latent and early symptomatic manifestations.
- All the appropriate economical primary preventive measures should have been implemented.
- If carriers of a mutation are identified the psychological impact should be recognizable.
- The test should carry simplicity, safety, precision, authenticity, and approval.
- The test value distribution among the target population group should be confirmed.
- Acceptability of the test to the particular population should be clearly established.
- There should be an agreed policy on further diagnostic investigation and available alternative options for individuals with positive results.
- There should be clearly specified criteria for selecting subsets to be tested if all possible mutations are not being tested.

- Treatment of patients/clients identified through early detection should be effective and there should be evidence-based policy for determining who would best benefit from the treatment.
- The clinical management and patient outcomes should be of high standard and continually improved in all healthcare organizations participating in the screening program.

The guidelines emphasize that a screening program should be justified by sound research evidence that substantiates reduction in morbidity and mortality. It is important that all information provided about the test and outcomes are clear and simple for the patient to understand. Additionally, the test itself and the diagnostic procedures and treatment interventions should be clinically, socially, and ethically acceptable to the practitioners and the general public. The benefit of the test should outweigh potential physical and/or psychological damage caused to the patient by the test, investigative procedures, or treatment interventions. The related costs, including the administrative support, training, and quality assurance, should be economical and all alternative options for managing the condition should have been carefully examined to ensure cost effectiveness. It is also stipulated that there should be an agreed-upon policy for auditing and quality assurance standards. Of equal importance, staffing and resource facilities should be organized prior to commencement of the screening program. Patient welfare is vital; therefore, evidence-based information regarding the consequences of the testing, diagnostic investigation, and treatment should be provided to enable the individual to make an informed choice. Where genetic mutation is concerned, the screening should be clearly explained to the carriers and their families and should be acceptable to the affected individuals (PHE, 2014).

The main drawbacks are errors, such as false positive results, that lead to individuals being informed that they have tested positive for a condition. False negative results lead to individuals being informed that they do not have the condition, when in fact they do (PHE, 2014).

An Exemplar of Health Promotion Screening Program in Sexual Health Care

An exemplar of a health promotion screening program is the United Kingdom's National Chlamydia Screening Programme (NCSP) aimed at reducing the prevalence of chlamydia. Since implementation, there has been an increase in testing and uptake of sexual and reproductive health clinic services. It is recognized that the inclusion of chlamydia testing in the prevailing contraception and STI consultations delivers more thorough and all-encompassing sexual health service provision. Moens, Baruch, and Fearon (2003) reported high uptake of chlamydia screening with high treatment compliance among young women who attended contraception clinics. However, they also noted a need for more committed effort in contact tracing of the male partners of women who tested positive for chlamydia.

In order to improve uptake, the guidance outlined by the National Health Service (NHS, 2010) emphasizes staff training to ensure that all relevant practitioners are competent to provide chlamydia testing and treatment. Protected learning time is recommended for practitioners, with use of competency structure, objectives, and indicators to support the acquisition of knowledge and skills relating to chlamydia management. Additionally, staff training in STI testing and management could form part of the career development process.

Staff involvement is also recommended to raise awareness among young people about the benefits of the screening program. Suggestions include "one-stop" STI clinics, use of leaflets, advertisements in the waiting rooms, opt-out rather than an opt-in approaches, and diligent record keeping of first appointments, screening services, reasons for refusal, and solutions employed (NHS, 2010).

Practitioners in other countries are encouraged to explore the screening services available nationally and locally within their particular country and the related policy, regulations, and procedures that guide these.

Health Promotion: Characteristic Elements

Health and social care practitioners who are faced with the challenge of developing health promotion programs would find it useful to understand the different types of models. In the multidisciplinary team context, practitioners working together on health promotion projects can jointly determine appropriate models presented as exemplars or archetypes that fulfil the purpose of their particular programs. The important thing is to recognize and distinguish between different types of models. As Noar and Zimmerman (2005) observed, psychological models designed to clarify, predict, and assist health-related behavior have widely varied components and some are considered as distinctive to individual models. However, the general view is that many of the components are common to most models and overlaps are frequently observed. See also Ybara, Korchmarcos, Kiwanka, Bangsberg, and Bull 2013 exploration of applicability of the information, motivation behavioral skills model (IMB), in predicting the use of condoms among secondary school students.

Examples of Health Promotion Models

Models can be understood as paradigms, blueprints, or exemplars to develop and implement specific programs. Essentially, models should represent application of ideas, theories, and concepts that are based in research (Van den Broucke, 2012; Weinstein & Rothman, 2005). Health promotion models should represent evidence-based guidelines as well as relevant policy and strategies.

Generally, health promotion research tends to focus on changing people's attitudes and behaviors and hence there is an emphasis on attitudinal change and behavior modification in various models. However, the outcomes and benefits are intended for the best interest and welfare of population groups, communities, or individuals. Each specific model and the accompanying approach should serve as a framework that explains in simple terms the links between the underpinning theories, related concepts, and the methodological approaches to implementation. The following models have been proposed in the field of health promotion.

The Medical Model

The medical model embraces a "paternalistic" approach of preventing or eliminating disease within the context of primary prevention. The approach is directed and controlled by the "expert," because this person is a knowledgeable and proficient practitioner. The main emphasis is primary prevention of disease with the assumption that the individual would demonstrate readiness to cooperate in this process. Therefore, the model requires that healthcare professionals, in particular medical, nursing, and allied health practitioners, comply with their professional responsibility and accountability by integrating prevention in their consultation interactions as appropriate. This suggests that the professionals should develop and implement the health promotion program that they perceive to be best for the patient or the target population group and the target group is expected to respond appropriately. The process involves coaxing and influencing tactics as well as campaigns and policies to achieve compliance by the patient, group, or community. Which preventive interventions are employed depends on the nature of problem, the prevalence, assessed needs, and the perceived impact. Thus, the intervention may be in the form of immunization or screening programs. Examples include breast awareness, cervical screening, and testicular screening. The main flaws and disadvantages of this model lie in its paternalistic connotation with emphasis on physical health while failing to take account of the mental, psychological, social, and economic repercussions of disease and ill-health (Ewles & Simnett, 2003; Scriven, 2010).

The Health Belief Model

The health belief model (HBM) assumes that people's decisions and motivation to change their lifestyles and behaviors to adopt preventive actions for better health depends on their personal beliefs, reasoning, and interpretations. These include perceptions of how severe and life threatening they consider the condition and its associated complications to be; the impact on their health; the perceived difficulties that these can create in their personal lives, work, and income and on their families; and how vulnerable and predisposed to the particular condition they consider themselves to be.

It is postulated that the stronger the perceived vulnerability and predisposition, the more inclined people are to adopt risk-reducing lifestyle behaviors.

Motivation to adopt appropriate preventive lifestyle behavior becomes even stronger when the perception of the vulnerability and predisposition is combined with perceived severity of the condition and threat to life. Perceived risk and vulnerability to HIV/AIDS and serious STIs may enhance the motivation to adopt healthier sexual health behaviors, safer sex, and preventive measures, including conscientious and correct use of condoms and/or other barrier methods. Perception of the value, advantages, and usefulness of the lifestyle modification strongly influences personal decision for behavior change. Anticipated health benefits are crucial factors that influence change in behavior and adoption of specific preventive measures involved in the HBM (Carpenter, 2010; Haggart, 2000; Janz & Becker, 1984).

Examples include an individual's conscientious practice of breast awareness and uptake of a cervical screening program. Perceived barriers relate to individuals' conviction and understanding of the physical, psychological, and financial burdens that hinder them from adopting preventive measures and behavioral change. For example, in cervical screening the barriers may be fear of pain and/or embarrassment with the procedure. Financial implications could also hinder uptake (Haggart, 2000; Janz & Becker, 1984).

The concept of "cues to action" in the HBM involves incidents, circumstances, or occurrences that trigger the adoption of a particular action or change in behavior. These are motivators that inspire individuals to take appropriate preventive actions or utilize available screening services. Examples may be serious illness or death of a much-loved family member, or a popular celebrity, as a result of a particular condition. Cues to action can be internal (personal physical signs and symptoms) or external (encouragement by family and friends, or information gained through media campaigns) (Janz & Becker, 1984). Practitioners would find it useful to read Carpenter's (2010) examination of the effectiveness of different applications of the health belief model in predicting behavior.

The Health Promotion Model

An elaborate model devised by Pender (1996) encompasses specific human characteristics as people live and function within the environment and strive for improved health. This health promotion model (HPM) is considered an accompaniment to the models of health protection.

Three integral components of the HPM are the following:

- Individual attributes (characteristics and experiences)
- Intellect, reasoning, and feelings that influence behavior (behavior-specific cognition and affect)
- Consequences of specific conduct and actions (behavioral outcomes)

Multiple influencing factors highlighted in the model include the following:

- Personal characteristics and circumstances, including gender, age, psychological, social, cultural, and economic elements
- Perceived advantages and the perceived constraints associated with the health behavior action
- Perceived personal capability and feelings relating to the adoption of the health-promoting behavior
- Expectations and influences of other people
- Influences of the individual's current state
- Dedication and enthusiasm for the plan of action
- Equivalent pressures, desires, and preferred choices
- Attainment of positive health outcomes in terms of improved health, personal satisfaction, and contentment (Pender, 1996)

These key elements persist in other models that have evolved from this model.

Theories

Theories put forward logical explanations to show the interconnections and make predictions about occurrences and relationships (Naidoo & Wills, 2005; Polit & Beck, 2013; Van den Broucke, 2012). In essence, theories evolve from sets of integrated ideas that provide the reasoning for occurrences or events and must be testable to be recognized as scientific theories. In that sense, a theory can be explained as a set of assumptions or hypotheses linked by logical reasoning. Therefore, experts argue that the hypotheses, conjectures, and/or assumptions conveyed by the interconnected concepts have to be tested, explained, and confirmed through research (Jones, 2007; Nutbeam et al., 2010; Robson, 2011).

Health Promotion Theories Examined

Human beings are assumed to be rational decision-makers and are therefore inclined to prefer healthier lifestyles because people's thoughts, intellect, and reasoning direct their actions. Individuals' behaviors are determined not only by what beliefs they hold but are also influenced by what they perceive their significant others may think or say in terms of approval or disapproval. Two fundamental theories integral to the approach of behavior change are explored.

The Theory of Reasoned Action

The theory of reasoned action (TRA) claims that an individual's attitude toward a specific behavior depends on the beliefs they hold about the consequences of that behavior and their evaluation of those beliefs (Ajzen & Dasgupta, 2015; Fishbein & Ajzen, 2010). In this case, the individual considers the potential effects, and the value and significance

of the outcome of the adopted behavior, whether desirable or undesirable. The intention to adopt the behavior is also influenced by the subjective norm, which entails the opinions of significant others, sociocultural norms, peer pressure, societal expectations, and the individual's desire to conform. Another influencing element is the motivation to comply, whereby the individual deliberates whether or not to comply with the behavior change and why. Thus, the individual questions his/her willingness to do what others expect, and assesses why and how strong the motivation is to do so. This theory assumes that human behaviors are under personal, voluntary control. Moreover, it assumes that individuals normally contemplate on the consequences and implications of their actions and behaviors before they make a decision to embark on such actions (Ajzen & Fishbein, 1980; Fishbein & Ajzen, 2005, 2010; see also Ajzen & Dasgupta, 2015).

The Theory of Planned Behavior

The theory of planned behavior (TPB) is said to be an expansion on the TRA (Ajzen, 2012; Ajzen & Dasgupta, 2015). This theory takes into account that people may or may not consider themselves to have the power or control over a particular behavior. Therefore, behavior control comprises the resources available to the individual, including personal capabilities, skills, and opportunities. The individual's perception of the value or importance of achieving the particular outcome from the behavior also operates strongly in perceived behavioral control. Self-efficacy assumes that an individual's choices and preferences for particular activities, their diligence in preparation, and the effort put into the performance of those activities are influenced by perception of one's own self-efficacy. This concept postulates the influence of human cognition, motivation, affective processes, and selection of behavior (Ajzen & Sheikh, 2013, 2016). Therefore, personal feelings, how people think and motivate themselves, and how they behave are interdependent (Bandura, 2004). Thus, perceived behavioral control evidently influences how hard an individual thinks about a particular change in behavior. It also influences how willing they are to change and how much determination and hard work they decide to put into adopting the particular behavior (Ajzen, 2012; Ajzen & Sheikh, 2013, 2016). The TPB encompasses all the concepts of the TRA and incorporates the concepts of control, beliefs, and the individual's perception of the importance of control (Ajzen & Klobas, 2013; Klobas & Ajzen, 2015; Liefbroer, Klobas, Philipow, & Ajzen, 2015). Together with attitude and subjective norm, these influence the behavioral intention and ultimately the adoption of the behavior (Ajzen, 2012; Ajzen & Dasgupta, 2015).

Although intention should lead to adoption of behavior, the reality is that the longer the delay between the intention and actual behavior change, the less likely it is the individual will actually adopt the healthier lifestyle. What kind of predictions can be made from examining these behavior change theories? Although arguments have been put forward that behavioral intention can be predicted through the theories of reasoned action and planned behavior the debate still continues.

The Transtheoretical Model

The transtheoretical model (TTM) draws on theories that underpin other models to form a comprehensive theory, in essence a biopsychosocial model that is applicable to a diversity of behaviors, population groups, and situations. However, Taylor et al. (2006) commented that TTM also incorporates a sequence of events described as the stages of change (Van Wormer, 2008). These form the elements that facilitate change of health behavior as described by Burkholder and Nigg (2002) and Adams and White (2003). The theory originated from elements of psychotherapy, such as techniques of managing emotional and behavioral problems and psychiatric disorders through verbal and nonverbal communication (Markowitz & Weissman, 2004). This therapeutic method is intended to help the individual to determine what helps them to feel confident, bright, and cheerful and what causes them to experience anxiety attacks and psychological distress (Markowitz & Weissman, 2004). Thus, psychotherapy involves interactive interventions rather than drug treatment. By learning to understand personal thoughts and feelings, the individual comes to accept personal strengths and weaknesses (Markowitz & Weissman, 2004). Social cognition involves individuals' attitudes, behaviors, and reaction to other people, influenced by their ability to process, store, and apply information about those people (Bandura, 2004; Martin Ginis et al., 2011). Critics argue that some elements in TTM are, in fact, the same as those of models based on social cognition (Noar & Zimmerman, 2005).

The stages TTM are as follows:

- Precontemplation stage occurs when there is no intention to change.
- Contemplation indicates the individual is thinking about health behavior change within the next 6 months.
- Preparation refers to the individual considering preliminary arrangements in the immediate month.
- Action refers to the behavior change during the past 6 months.
- Maintenance describes sustained behavior change over a minimum period of 6 months.
- Termination describes fully established behavior change for 5 years or longer (Burkholder & Nigg, 2002; Adams & White, 2003).

Van Wormer (2008) demonstrates application of the stages of change model in the context of counseling toward health behavior change. Experts observe that the stages evolve in a spiral manner in which the individual's progress may go in either direction (make good progress or fall back).

The stages of TTM occur due to the patient's experiences and behavior. The stages of precontemplation and contemplation help a patient to develop new awareness, emotional expression, and consideration of social circumstances. These are also described as consciousness raising, dramatic relief, and reevaluation of the environment (Adams & White, 2003; Mace, 2007; Van Wormer, 2008). The change from contemplation to preparation is described as self-reevaluation and is due to intellectual and emotional acceptance. The phase of preparation and action is described as social and self-liberation. These processes are presumed to strengthen awareness of other lifestyles while enabling and fostering the commitment and ability to change. The phase of progressing from action to maintenance involves adopting alternative behaviors and forming helping relationships, reinforcement, management, and stimulus control (Adams & White, 2003; Mace, 2007; Van Wormer, 2008). Despite the apparent popularity of the TTM, various critics suggest a need to further enhance this model through more extensive research (Weinstein & Rothman, 2005).

Di Noia and Prochaska's (2010) application of the transtheoretical model for understanding the decision making process in dietary behavior change and Nigg et al.'s (2011) examination of the mechanisms for behavior change in tailored interventions consider the TTM as a framework for conceptual clarity and measurement of behavior change as well as for facilitating and promoting strategies that are easily adaptable for individuals and groups. Kroll, Keller, Scholz, and Perren (2011) maintain that interventional programs can be developed to take account of the needs of the specific group by fostering the most important pros and decreasing the cons or disadvantages. These authors recognize that the stages of change involve multiple factors.

Velicer et al. (2012) recognize the TTM as an integrative model of behavior change which encompasses emotions, cognition, and behavior and also provides a conceptual basis for improving implementation of effective interventions. These authors suggest application of the TTM to a wider population for health behavior interventions such as sexual risk reduction counseling. Horwath, Schembre, Motl, Dishman, and Nigg (2013) maintain that the processes of change, in particular the self-liberation process, may help to predict effective behavior change. The question, however, is whether the core constructs of the TTM (the stages of change and the related processes of change, decisional balance, self-efficacy) differ between those who achieve successful and unsuccessful stage transition.

The Integrated Theory of Health Behavior Change

Health promotion necessitates that people take responsibility to change existing unhealthy behaviors in favor of healthy lifestyle behaviors. Prevention is crucial, and thus precautionary and protective actions are a necessary part of a healthy lifestyle. These actions must be based on accurate and well-substantiated information. It is important to raise people's awareness about the relevance of screening programs, immunization, and vaccination programs through primary health promotion and education endeavors. For example, sexual healthcare practitioners have an obligation to continually encourage uptake of STI screening, cervical screening, and other preventive services.

The integrated theory of behavior change (ITBC) is rather eclectic in that it merges and assimilates certain core elements from different models, such as the health belief model (Carpenter, 2010; Haggart, 2000; Janz & Becker, 1984), the theory of reasoned action (Ajzen & Fishbein, 1980; Ajzen et al., 2007; Fishbein & Ajzen, 2005), the theory of planned behavior (Ajzen, 1988; Taylor et al., 2006), and concepts from the social cognitive theory (Ashford & LeCroy, 2013; Glanz, Rimer, & Viswanath, 2015; McAlister et al., 2008; Usher & Pajares, 2008). Moreover, the ITBC model elaborates on prediction of behavior (Ajzen et al., 2007; Fishbein & Ajzen, 2010). The assumption is that people act on their intentions when they have the necessary skills to do so and when their performance of the behavior would not be impeded by environmental factors.

Thus, assimilation of the core elements in ITBC allows further enhancement of the TRA and TPB by considering the knowledge and skills required for performing the desired behavior. Individuals' intention to perform particular behaviors follow from the reasoned beliefs that people hold about those behaviors, and therefore, the ITBC takes a reasoned action approach to understand human behavior (Fishbein, 2008; Fishbein & Ajzen, 2010). Nevertheless, researchers such as Bodenheimer (2005) noted that factual information on its own may not necessarily influence change in behavior (Paasche-Orlow & Wolf, 2007). Others argue about the uncertainty regarding the extent to which social and demographic factors impact on an individual's intention to change behavior, although the potential impact of social facilitation is recognized (Ryan et al., 2009).

Demographic, cultural, and socioeconomic factors as well as media interventions and the differences in human characteristics are all contexts that influence human behavior and intention to change (Ryan et al., 2009). Evaluation of outcome beliefs influences attitude. Normative beliefs, together with the motivation to comply, influence the perceived norm, while held beliefs about efficacy also influence self-efficacy. Thus, these interconnected influences are considered determinants of intention to perform a particular behavior. The assumption is that intention, which is dependent on acquired relevant skills and environmental constraints, determines whether the behavior is performed or not (Ryan et al., 2009).

Self-efficacy relates to the individual's belief in his/her ability and the capacity to perform the desired behavior successfully and efficiently (Ajzen et al., 2007; Fishbein & Ajzen, 2005, 2010). This is determined by the individual's self-confidence of having the specific skills for performing the behavior. Personal agency refers to individual's capability to originate and direct their actions for given purposes, whether a person feels motivated enough to initiate the desired

behavior change. Perceived control relates to the perception of how various factors within the environment facilitate or constrain performance of behavior (Ryan, et al. 2009).

A three-step approach is applied to identifying personal belief and can be used as a guide to design integrated model-based health messages (Bruce et al., 2013; Ryan et al., 2009) in the following ways:

- Defining the behavior to be changed should address the action, target, and the relevant context context (Fishbein & Ajzen, 2010).
- Identifying salient beliefs determining the belief system underlying that behavior (Fishbein, 2008; Fishbein & Ajzen, 2010).
- Determining which of the significant beliefs should be addressed in the message (Ryan et al., 2009).

Ryan (2009) notes two routes to behavior change:

- Use messages to change those beliefs most strongly related to intention to perform the behavior.
- Use messages to reinforce those beliefs that favor the recommended behavior and are already held by most members of society.

For example, Bruce et al.'s (2013) study of sexual risk behavior and risk-reduction beliefs revealed a belief that undetectable viral load reduces infectivity, which affects risk behavior associated with unprotected anal intercourse.

Ryan's et al. (2009) integrated theory of health behavior change proposes that an individual's enhanced (fact-based) knowledge, coupled with personal values, about a specific condition or behavior leads to a better understanding of that behavior. Moreover, as a person's belief in self-efficacy grows, so too does their confidence to change behavior, even under stress. The individual develops an expectation of positive outcome (related to the health benefit) from undertaking the behavior change (Ryan et al., 2009).

Ryan's theory also notes that self-regulation, as a factor in goal-setting and decision-making, is influenced by social determinants, such as an influential person inspiring the individual to change his/her behavior. Other social influences include the healthcare practitioners, family, friends, colleagues, the media, articles, leaflets, and other printed materials. Emotional support, information provision, and essential tools for bringing about change in behavior also form part of these social influences (Ryan et al., 2009). The combination of factors arouses the individual's motivation to exercise self-management to accomplish and maintain the desired behavior.

Related Research and Practical Application of ITBC As a basis for developing an intervention the application of ITBC aims at promoting and nurturing change in health behavior through increasing and improving the knowledge and beliefs held by the individual, group, or community. Another aim is to assist and empower development of self-regulation nenting and strengthening social support. ...ge base about the identified condition ...is assessed together with the perception ...risk factors. Depending on the findings ...assessment, specific, evidence-based information is provided to address the particular problem of the identified patient group. Through self-regulation individuals are able to apply the acquired knowledge, skills, and the modified beliefs toward adoption of improved lifestyle and change of a specific health behavior (Ryan et al., 2009). The process may be gradual, yet it can be maintained through self-monitoring, social support, and encouraging feedback.

Motivational Interviewing in Health Promotion Toward STI Prevention

This section presents a brief overview to contextualize motivational interviewing (MI) as part of the intervention for STI and HIV prevention. Motivational interviewing is a form of patient-centered counseling designed to guide and strengthen motivation toward change in health-related behavior (Miller & Rollnick, 2009; Miller et al., 2003; Treasure, 2004).). The technique is useful in encouraging an individual at the precontemplative stage who is starting to consider adopting healthier lifestyle behavior. As Treasure (2004) emphasized, the essential process involves partnership and collaboration as opposed to argument and confrontation. The aim of the technique is to help the individual through compassion, sensitivity, and understanding to examine and overcome their uncertainty about the change in behavior. The individual receives guidance and support to recognize the health benefits and how economical the health behavior change might prove to be. Treasure (2004) proposed the following key guidelines:

- Convey empathy with deep and thoughtful listening to appreciate the individual's point of view and ambitions.

- Establish inconsistencies between the individual's inherent values and the current lifestyle behavior.

- Avoid disagreement with the individual for refusing to comply, but instead employ tactful negotiation with kindly understanding.

- Encourage the individual that the change is achievable, while fostering realization of self-efficacy and development of self-confidence.

Rubak, Sandboe, Lauritzen, and Christensen (2005) noted that this approach does not necessarily take longer than giving advice to the patient during the consultation interaction. They also observed that the effect increases with longer duration and additional sessions and that a single intervention may have some lingering effect after 12 months of follow up. Various findings from studies in sexual health care have revealed some reduction in the rate of HIV acquisition among HIV-negative MSM (Koblin et al., 2004). These authors described 10 sessions of one-to-one counseling over a period of 6 months using MI intervention techniques. Moreover, the authors noted reduction in the rate of self-reported practice of unprotected anal sex among MSM sexual partners and contacts over a 48-month follow-up period. Clutterbuck et al. (2012) proposed that intensive individualized multi-session interventions focusing on skills acquisition, communication improvement, and strengthening of motivation to adopt safer sexual behaviors should be considered. They also suggest application of MI techniques in intensive counseling of MSM who are at high risk of contracting HIV infection (Clutterbuck et al., 2012). Moreover, they suggest incorporating 15- to 20-minute MI sessions during the GUM clinic consultation interactions for patients who are at high risk of STIs and HIV; this also reflects the view of Crosby et al. (2009).

The benefits of well-conducted MI by appropriately trained professionals have been reported. Evidence indicates that MI can be incorporated into a health coaching intervention to encourage change in lifestyle behavior (Rubak et al., 2005). Various authors also uphold the benefit of helping individuals explore their perceptions and feelings about their existing situation and identified problem and note the benefit of helping individuals to consider the personal advantages from the change in lifestyle (Rollnick, Butler, Kinnersly, Gregory, & Mash, 2010; Shannon & Davies, 2010). However, an individual's readiness to change is crucial and the practitioner must stimulate the individual's personal interest and motivation to change. The practitioner should be able to persuade and support the individual to talk about their desire to change and to anticipate successful outcome.

The general view is that in many cases, advice giving by healthcare professional proves to be unproductive. However, MI involves an active partnership between patients and practitioners, in which they are both engaged in discussing, clarifying, assessing, and establishing the individual's problem, needs, and wishes (Miller & Rollnick, 2009). These processes help to arouse the individual's motivation to change while fostering self-confidence and independence in their decision-making and actions. The key processes in motivational interviewing involve purposeful and constructive guidance and support through a dialogue rather than instructions, orders, directives, or dictates with little or no consideration given to the individual's involvement. The objective is to arouse the individual's willingness to change and to encourage him or her to determine the preferred ways of working toward achievement of the change. It is important for the individual to feel empowered and allowed to carefully examine the necessary health behavior change. A crucial attribute of the practitioner is to project genuine interest and deep empathetic listening skills. These elements are found to improve the practitioner-patient relationship.

Social Change Theory: The Stages of Change

Social change theory emphasizes readiness to adopt behavior change that is influenced by the individual's or community's perception of their vulnerability to an identified health problem. Other influencing factors are the held beliefs and perceived value of the change in health behavior. Stages of change embedded in this theory are decision, determination, and action (U.S. Department of Health and Human Services, 2010).

Approaches to Implementation of Health Promotion Models

In health promotion, the term *approaches* refers to the pathways or the strategies to accomplish something (Seedhouse, 2004). They represent the ways and means of implementing the selected models. Tones and Green (2004) explore the practicalities of the planning and related strategies for implementation of health promotion.

The Health Behavior Change Approach: Related Interventions

This approach embraces specific techniques employed to foster change in people's thoughts and reasoning in relation to particular lifestyles. The aim is to modify conduct and activities in aspects of daily lives and practices in order to maintain healthier lifestyles, continual improvement, and better health (Ewles & Simnett, 2003; Scriven, 2010). In relation to sexual health, respect and responsibility should be fostered by self-confidence and self-esteem among sexually active young people. The intention is to discourage unwary and irresponsible drinking and sexual risk-taking behaviors that lead to unprotected sexual intercourse, STIs, unintended pregnancies, abortions, and the associated complications of ill health. Crucially, the healthy lifestyle behavior should be emphasized by processes that are realistic, achievable, and acceptable to the target population group. These processes should be effective alternative distractions that are preferred to the negative attitudes, careless activities, and risk-taking behaviors. For example, raising awareness of the potential health risks of certain STIs along with knowledge of how STI transmission occurs should be key elements of this approach. From there, the benefits of healthier options should become integral to this approach. The strategy of involvement and partnerships with relevant parties, patients, and communities should be carefully considered and applied (Carey, 2000; WHO, 1986).

The Educational Approach

This approach aims to provide well-substantiated, evidence-based information about an identified health issue. Individuals are likely to willingly consider changing their behavior for adoption of a healthier lifestyle if they have knowledge and understanding about the nature of the problem. Motivation to change is strengthened by factual information about the prevalence of the condition, perceived personal vulnerability, and how worthwhile the behavior change would be. Therefore, the educational approach aims to foster confidence in individuals to make

appropriately informed decisions about identified health issues in their lives, in order to improve and maintain better health. The challenge for the professional is to support the individual to examine what beliefs they hold regarding the particular health problem. It is also important to examine personal attitude, other influencing factors and the potential hindrances, perceived personal control, and the advantages of the behavior change. Long-term practical guidance and support should be provided to ensure realization of the individual's choices and decisions about the options available to them. Whether applied to groups (e.g., schools and colleges) or social community groups, information provision should have a client-centered focus. The professional's responsibility is to address pertinent health issues and provide appropriate support with the patient's best interest and welfare as key priorities (Ewles & Simnett, 2003; Scriven, 2010).

Information should be provided in comprehensible language in the form of a two-way dialogue to allow for clarification, personal decision-making, and personal choices without imposition from the professional. While the professional has the responsibility to determine much of the educational content by providing pertinent, evidence-based information, the individual's right of choice should be respected (Ewles & Simnett, 2003; Scriven, 2010). In addition to education, the individual's capability to develop the required skills is crucial and should be carefully considered. Moreover, availability of appropriate resources, support, and opportunities invariably influence perception of personal control. There is no doubt that partnerships and collaborations are fundamental for successful implementation of the educational approach.

The Client-Centered or Self-Empowerment Approach

This approach concentrates on health issues of personal concern to the patient. The core theme of client-centeredness requires that the patient is allowed to retain maximal control in a partnership with the professional in the facilitative role. Therefore, the practitioner fosters client confidence in determining personal learning needs. This approach allows the individual to identify and examine their health concerns, personal values, beliefs, and choices and the factors that influence these. It also enables the individual to examine perceived capabilities and the skills that they may need to develop to make effective lifestyle change. Thus, respect for personal rights is maintained in all aspects of this approach and the two parties cooperate with each other on an equal level throughout the interactions.

Participatory learning is a component of this approach and requires flexible learning context with actively engaging learner(s) who participate in active dialogues and communication. The learning climate should convey an ambience of collective or social sharing of concerns, intentions, and goals. The learning process should be adaptive and tailored to the individual's or group's progress and learning needs. This necessitates their full engagement in determining the desired goals and developing the required learning activities in collaboration with the professional facilitator. Learning through small group interactions provide a social element and enhances communication skills (Quinn & Hughes, 2007).

While effective communication, assertiveness, and problem-solving skills can be acquired through interactions with the professional on a one-to-one basis, the small group context provides more favorable opportunities for skills acquisition.

The Societal Change Approach

The societal change approach emphasizes joint or collective action. It aims at dealing with health-related issues in the natural environment while addressing the social and economic factors that adversely affect the health of the community, specific groups, or the entire society. Joint governmental and social action through partnerships and collaborative initiatives are required to achieve the desired outcomes of healthier societal lifestyles and better health. This approach requires that the people have ownership of their collective decisions about what information they need on which aspects of their lives and health. They should also feel empowered to fully participate in determining what facilities and resources would enable them to make the desired changes (Ewles & Simnett, 2003; Scriven, 2010).

Involvement should include community and youth group leaders as well as key persons within the different communities. This ensures that representation comprises people appointed and delegated by the society or the population groups themselves. They should be committed to the best interest of the people and are therefore responsible and accountable to them. Examples of societal change or collective approach strategies include national policies on sexual health screening programs, condom distribution programs, and HIV-control policy.

Exemplars of Practical Application in Sexual Health Promotion

The fundamental aims of sexual health promotion include encouraging effective contraception use to avoid unintended and unwanted pregnancies; fostering conscientious use of suitable, functional barrier methods to prevent STIs; and empowering autonomous decision-making, personal choices, and behaviors in sexual activities (Barnes, 2009). This author argues that the present situation of ever-increasing rates of STIs, unwanted pregnancies, and abortions justify the need for efficient health promotion in this field. Arguing against the top-down process of the medical model, Barnes (2009) challenges the emphasis on the professional agenda implicated in the behavior change approach with questionable degree of patient involvement. The point is made that this conflicts with the principle of fostering patient empowerment, self-confidence, and self-esteem to make independent choices. Another point of argument is

that it also conflicts with the concepts of self-efficacy and the rights of individuals (Barnes, 2009).

To determine appropriate models applicable to health promotion in sexual health care, Barnes (2009) identifies the importance of empowerment, independence, information provision, and motivation enhancement. The challenge is finding a model that embraces empowerment, education, and behavior change. Different models, theories, and approaches confirm the lack of clarity of these terms in health promotion (Barnes, 2009).

An Exemplar of Good Practice: Application of Health Promotion

In recognition of the risk of infections and potential vulnerability of its employees, a reputable international board consulted experts to devise a comprehensive policy and guidelines for hygiene, prevention, and control of infection. Unquestionably, this represents an example of good practice for health promotion. The policy guidelines are underpinned by specific factors:

- Individual close interactions, direct and indirect encounters with several people such as colleagues, staff, and members of the public in different situations and venues during various aspects of their careers
- The communal use of facilities and equipment
- International travel and exposure to indigenous bacterial organisms, diseases, and infections for which individuals may not have acquired immunity
- Sexual risk-taking behaviors and other unsafe recreational activities
- Varied modes of acquisition and spread of infections including tissue damage
- Vector-borne infections (Horgan & Bergin, 2010).

In terms of sexual health promotion, STIs were considered to pose a particular challenge for health professionals due to lifestyle behaviors that potentially put the employees at risk for example, young sexually active individuals whose careers invariably entail national and international trips that potentially lead to unpredictable and impulsive social activities. Therefore, information provision, education, and communication approaches were incorporated into the health and safety guidelines developed for these professionals. Regular consultations with medical professionals were considered as opportunities for individuals to privately discuss any sexual health concerns. The program incorporated cautionary guidance regarding abstinence from sexual activities with individuals who might be carrying active infection or receiving treatment for specific STIs (Horgan & Bergin, 2010).

Elements of the health promotion program include pre-exposure hepatitis A virus (HAV), HBV, and human papilloma virus (HPV) vaccinations; guidance on safer sex practices; screening and identification of asymptomatic individuals; raising awareness of STI transmission; condom use; and the importance of tracing sexual partners for diagnosis and treatment. Moreover, individuals have the right to request screening tests for STI infections and specific blood-borne viral infections.

Primary prevention is emphasized through promoting standard hygiene precautions that are applicable to all. Additionally, immunization and vaccinations are offered as necessary. Prevention of secondary spread is also advocated to curb recurrence of infections (Horgan & Bergin, 2010). A particular strength of these health promotion guidelines is that they were developed by infectious disease experts.

A Hypothetical Exemplar: Information, Education, and Communication Approach

Drawing on various examples of good practice, a hypothetical higher academic institution may also devise a policy of sexual health promotion for their student population that emphasizes the information, education, and communication (IEC) approach. The policy requires that the population group be provided with comprehensive information on STIs through appropriate education and training with ongoing communication, support, and counseling. Therefore, the students receive factual information about specific infections, the mode of transmission of each infection and the associated potential complications. Additionally, information about symptoms, diagnostic tests, preventive measures, available screening programs, and treatment interventions is also provided. The information is intended to raise the students' awareness about the different STI infections and allow individuals to reflect on their personal beliefs about the consequences of sexual health problems. This also encourages reflection on personal values, motivation, control, and the perceived benefits of the change of lifestyle behaviors. The objective is to foster empowerment and encourage not just intentions, but actual *actions* to adopt healthier lifestyle behaviors. Such a hypothetical policy of sexual health promotion could foster individual empowerment, yet the choice of health promotion model and determination of the appropriate approach may prove to be a challenge for the health professionals.

An Example of Health Promotion Aimed at Prevention of STIs/Disease: The U.K. Government

The U.K. government emphasizes the importance of prevention due to the persistently high incidence of STIs and HIV infection. The principal aims are to curb the prevalence of undiagnosed cases, reduce the spread of HIV and STIs, and reduce unintended pregnancy rates. These clearly confirm the need for health promotion, education, and support. Information provision is key component of these efforts, as are network development comprehensive service provision and integrated services. Examples of these include chlamydia screening programs, open access to GUM clinics, and contraceptive services. Research is also a priority, to strengthen the evidence basis for good practice in sexual and reproductive health and HIV care.

Importantly, the healthcare organization advocates consumer participation in services planning and delivery and recognizes the need for effective partnerships and collaboration to achieve effective patient-centered services. Factors associated with sexual risk-taking behaviors such as misconceptions, social deprivation, and age (e.g., adolescence), must also be addressed.

Various issues of contention emerged from the earlier DH (2001) strategy:

- A medical model of health promotion (paternalistic approach)
- Nationwide information campaign in which health practitioners convey specific messages (not patient centered)
- Sexual health promotion as an integral part of school education was not addressed
- Lack of emphasis on ethical issues
- Little attention to cultural or ethical diversity, sexual health inequalities, or poor uptake of services
- Impact of personal, social, and community circumstances

Positive Ongoing Endeavors

The Department of Health's (2013) Strategy for Sexual Health and HIV recognizes the need to develop more effective safer sex campaigns. Helplines providing evidence-based guidance on HIV and STI prevention through a range of media also serve to disseminate sexual health information to target audiences. The National Institute for Health and Care Excellence (NICE) proposed evidence-based guidelines for health promotion endeavors to address issues relating to young people. NICE (2007, 2016) outlines six key recommendations on STIs and adolescent conceptions. Each of the recommendations considers the identified target, the appropriate practitioners to address the problem, and the recommended actions to take. For example, in Recommendations 1, the identified target population includes groups at high risk for STIs: MSM, people from high HIV-prevalence areas and recent visitors to those areas, people who practice STI-risk-related behaviors, alcohol/substance abuse, early onset sexual activities, unprotected sex, frequent changes of sexual partners, and multiple sexual partners. The professionals and other relevant collaborators who should take action include general practitioners, GUM clinics, representatives from the community, voluntary organizations, and schools. The recommended actions include identifying those at high risk through sexual history, carrying out risk assessment, STI testing, smear test, and travel immunizations, and discussion of STI risks with a trained sexual health practitioner.

One goal of sexual health promotion is to create lasting mechanisms to address sexual health problems. Community-based endeavors (peer education programs, outreach work) are important cornerstones to achieve this goal. However, contracting for and authorization of sexual health promotion programs is the responsibility of the primary care sector. Thus, the Department of Health developed a sexual health promotion toolkit to assist organizations with guidelines on adequate resourcing, recommendations to achieve standardization, and specifications for conducting sexual risk assessments.

Sensitive dilemmas may relate to particular sexual health problems, target audience, and specific health promotion models. The topic of ethics has been explored in a separate chapter. Therefore, practitioners are encouraged to explore potential ethical implications in the implementation of sexual health promotion programs and examine each analytically. The related moral and ethical controversies should be examined in detail.

The preceding sections reveal that in addition to the complexity of sexual health promotion various ethical debates persist regarding the implementation of the programs and campaigns. Ewles and Simnett (2003), also Scriven (2010), argue about the ethical implications of control and power, widening inequality, the health promoter as personal example, and inconsistencies in health and lifestyle messages due to varied evidence from research findings. They also query the lack of clarification and differing interpretations of the concept of health. Another issue of argument is the lack of sensitivity to the diversity of social, cultural, economic, and ethnic circumstances in society and within communities. The potential problem of professional exclusion of health promotion within the healthcare profession could create a hindrance. Moreover, potential oversight of the real purpose of health promotion while campaigns and programs become engulfed in marketable money-making business ventures are also considered as issues of contention.

Social Marketing Integrated into Health Promotion

The ethical implications of social marketing should be carefully considered in the context of STI and HIV prevention and sexual health promotion. To the extent that social marketing incorporates mixed approaches with the intent of influencing behaviors to benefit individuals, target groups, communities, and the general public social marketing campaigns should integrate theories, research, and evidence of best practice; identify appropriate audiences; and establish effective partnerships. These campaigns must be feasible, sustainable, and acceptable to all concerned. The International Social Marketing Association, European Social Marketing Association & Australian Association of Social Marketing (2013) provide more insight about social marketing.

Examples of integration with other approaches relevant to sexual health include the following. Publicity of STI and HIV prevention measures is commonly linked to practices such as condom use and contraception methods (Eloundou-Enyegue

et al., 2005; Rojayapithayakorn, 2006), which is intended to achieve the dual benefit of STI prevention and prevention of unplanned and unwanted pregnancies. Newton et al. (2013) consider that selection of target audiences may be necessary and feasible in the social marketing of health-related issues. As Kotler et al. (2007) maintain, by helping to raise awareness about the consequences of identified health problems, social marketing may have a positive impact on behaviors. However, Guttman and Salmon (2004) highlight potential hindrances relating to self-reproach, apprehension and perhaps trepidation, stigma, indignity, and disparity in knowledge as ethical concerns that should be carefully considered. Therefore, scrutiny is important in monitoring compliance to the related ethical regulations (Guttman & Salmon, 2004), which should be a standard requirement in the development and implementation of health promotion programs (Guttman & Salmon, 2004; Loss & Nagel, 2010; Parker et al., 2007). It is particularly necessary to consider these ethical concerns in the development, implementation, and evaluation of social marketing, health promotion, and health education programs for STIs and HIV.

Target marketing is another issue that requires careful ethical consideration. It is particularly important that targeted population groups not be misled by specific messages aimed at them. Integrated social marketing and health promotion programs have been subject to criticism of the methods employed when targeting specific groups. These groups may include adolescents/teenage and young adult population groups, MSM, migrant population groups commercial sex workers, sexual network groups, and long-distance truck drivers. Guttman and Salmon (2004) urge carrying out thorough critical assessment of campaigns to determine inadvertent stigmatization or further widening of existing social gaps. Potential impact of messages must be examined to avoid unnecessary distress, dissatisfaction, and even rejection of the messages (Guttman & Salmon, 2004; Newton et al., 2013). Ethical concerns include unintended misleading information about risky sexual practices, omission of elements from evidence-based information, promotion of products that may not have been adequately tested, and potential adverse effects of recommended behaviors (e.g., not addressing latex allergies when promoting condom use).

The Role of the Social Cognitive Theory in Facilitating Health Communication

The theory of social cognition is particularly useful for the facilitation and implementation of health communication through health promotion and education. Health communication involves using communication strategies to inform and guide individual's decisions that enhance health (Centers for Disease Control and Prevention, 2017; The Community Guide, 2004; National Cancer Institute). The following components apply:

1. Reciprocal determinism refers to the predictable and potent interaction of three main determinant

factors: the person, the behavior, and the environment in which the behavior is performed (Bandura, 2004). Consideration of behavior change must take account of the continuous interplay among these three factors. Reciprocal determinism maintains that observational learning alone is not likely to lead to change in behavior unless the environment supports the acquired behavior (Usher & Pajares, 2008).

2. The environment represents factors that are physically external to the individual (the social environment) and that provide opportunities and social support. Thus, relevant facilities with appropriate and adequate resources, such as STI and contraception clinics with supportive services, are crucial. Environmental opportunities and support also include provision of evidence-based information, availability of protective products (e.g., condoms), and appropriate instruction for correct application.

3. Situation describes individuals' perceptions of the environment. Therefore, misperceptions or uncertainties can be corrected and healthy behavior promoted. While expectations describe the anticipated outcomes of a particular behavior, the concept of social outcome expectations refers to an individual's expectation of how others may judge his or her behavior (Anderson et al., 2007). Self-evaluative outcomes expectations are the individual's expectations of how he or she expects to feel about him/herself on performing a particular behavior. A related concept is expectancies, which describes the value the individual places on certain outcomes (which essentially constitutes incentive) (Ashford & LeCroy, 2013; McAlister et al., 2008).

4. Behavioral capability encompasses the knowledge and skills to perform a particular behavior (McAlister et al., 2008). Reinforcements are the responses a person receives for performing of a particular behavior. Reinforcement can be direct, vicarious, or self-reinforcement. Moreover, depending on the nature of behavior, the reinforcement might reward positive behaviors or sanction negative behaviors. Thus, the particular reinforcement may strengthen or weaken the likelihood of repeating the behavior (Nabi & Clark, 2008).

5. Personal control in this instance relates to self-regulation, which requires self-monitoring (evaluating personal behavior, goal setting). Feedback and self-reward are both important to encourage positive behavior change. Other processes of self-regulation involve self-instruction, in which one employs self-talk to maintain one's inspiration, and enlistment of social support (obtaining encouragement from others who approve the effort to achieve change). Emotional coping responses relate to personal devices employed by an individual to manage and cope with emotional influences. This is applicable to problem solving and stress management scenarios (Ashford & LeCroy, 2013; McAlister et al., 2008).

6. Observational learning represents a core component of the social cognitive theory (SCT) and relates to the suggestion that an individual's acquisition of behavior occurs by watching the way other people act and behave. Additionally it involves development of the skills to perform the modeled behavior (Pajares, 2009; Pajares et al., 2009). The observed outcomes and the reinforcement given for the particular behavior influence the observational learning and acquisition of behavior. However, this notion assumes that there must be a credible role model to be observed.

Observational learning encompasses five key concepts: modeling, outcome expectations, self-efficacy, goal setting, and self-regulation (Ashford & LeCroy, 2013; McAlister et al., 2008; Pajares et al., 2009).

Self-efficacy refers to an individual's belief in their ability to accomplish a task, which in this instance may be changing undesirable behaviors. In such situations, the practitioner might help the patient to break down the behavior into manageable stages of change. Slowly and progressively, the individual develops self-direction to manage the behavior by himself or herself (Anderson et al., 2007). Self-efficacy is considered to be most important prerequisite for behavior change (Pajares, 2009; Williams & Williams, 2010).

Identified Limitations of the Social Cognitive Theory

Social cognitive theory (SCT) has its limitations. One is that it is broad with multiple components. Rather than representing a unified theory with interlinking concepts there seems to be a lack of cohesiveness to the elements. Another limitation is that evaluative studies of the entire theory seem to be lacking although the evidence suggests that self-efficacy has been extensively investigated (Williams & Williams, 2010). SCT puts across the supposition that environmental changes are inevitably associated with changes in people's behaviors, although in reality that does not happen in all situations. Moreover, the theory seems to place strong emphasis on the dynamic interplay between person, behavior, and the environment. However, it fails to clearly demonstrate the extent to which each element contributes to actual behavior in people. It also fails to demonstrate which element has the strongest influence on behavior and in what way (McAlister et al., 2008; Schunk et al., 2014). It is also obvious that while many studies have concentrated on activities of learning, little attention has been given to hormonal and biological predispositions that potentially influence behaviors. The theory does not give much attention to emotion or motivation. It only makes vague implications to emerging incentives and the need for managing emotional stress associated with some aspects of behavior change. Applicability of all the constructs to one public health problem proves to be difficult where intensive public health programs are concerned. In view of the emphasis on the individual person and the environment, SCT continues to be widely used in health promotion. This is because the environment seems to be a major issue of focus in current health promotion programs and activities (Ashford & LeCroy, 2013).

Health Education: Concept Clarification

The WHO's (1998) definition of health education includes learning experiences that help an individual to improve their health through knowledge acquisition or influencing attitudes. Essentially, the key components of the health education programs comprise information provision, assessment of moral and ethical beliefs and principles; health decision-making, and development of the capabilities for modifying lifestyle behavior. The assumption is that health education programs should foster enhancement of self-worth and confidence building to enable people to adopt appropriate actions for improving their lifestyles for better health (Ewles & Simnett, 2003; Scriven, 2010).

The common threads in different conceptions of health education are the processes of information acquisition, awareness, and comprehension and competencies for taking health-related decisions and actions. Within the context of contemporary health care, health education is broadly construed as a system by which individuals, communities, and groups are provided pertinent, evidence-based information to improve their health and lifestyle behaviors. Thus, health education represents a means by which people are informed about healthy lifestyles and better health, through improved health knowledge, behavior modification, and acquisition of appropriate skills.

Health education derives from and therefore comprises biomedical, psychological, and environmental theories with its main emphasis on prevention. Hence, the assumption that health information provision alone should be an adequate motivator to inspire individuals to change their behaviors and adopt healthier lifestyles. However, as Whitehead (2001) argued disillusionment of that strategy stems from the practitioner's unrealistic expectation and misconception of the complexity and potential difficulties associated with such demands on individuals. The claim that exploration of the underlying reasons for adopting particular health and lifestyle behaviors provides more useful evidence for facilitating behavior modification. The approach to health education that focuses on simply providing health information has been contended as being rather narrow for addressing health and lifestyle issues adequately. That notion of health education fails to address the broader scope of information provision, competence acquisition, support, empowerment, and enabling.

Contrarily, health education is seen by some as representing the paternalistic and authoritarian elements of the medical model. Application on an individual basis or to varied group sizes through the media systems, road shows, and health conference exhibitions (Ewles & Simnett, 2003; Institute for Work & Health, 2015), fails to allow scope for productive participation. This fails to take account of the social, economic, and political implications of health and the facilitation and supporting of health behavior change.

There has been interchangeable use of the terms *health education* and *health promotion* with no clear distinction between them. However, in current practice, health education is recognized as a fundamental component of the all-embracing concept of health promotion. The broader concept of health promotion/education encourages individuals, groups, and communities to make educated and competent decisions about health-related issues in their lives. It also recognizes the importance of active participation and partnerships between the target groups, their representatives, relevant agencies, organizations, stakeholders, and practitioners.

Primary health education is directed at individuals who are free from infirmity and therefore, the focus is on prevention of infection, disease, injuries, and disability. General health issues remain consistently topical for young people and generally encompass hygiene, cleanliness, social skills, and interpersonal interactions. Of equal importance, advice and guidance on sexual health-related issues, safer sex practice, and contraception should also be emphasized. The aim is to nurture development and enhancement of self-esteem, with a sense of personal responsibility for maintaining healthy lifestyle behaviors and well-being.

Secondary health education is mainly directed at people who are experiencing ill health. The aim in this case is to curtail and counteract the disease or state of ill health from progressing to cause long-term complications and disability. Furthermore, secondary health education involves enhancing the knowledge to make necessary lifestyle modifications and providing the guidance and support for patients to do so. This also requires nurturing self-motivation, self-discipline, and cooperation to adhere to the course of treatment.

Tertiary health education is directed at patients with chronic illnesses and various forms of incapacities. The aim is to nurture survival and coping mechanisms. It requires provision of evidence-based information about alternative ways to reduce discomfort. At the same time, it aims at enhancing the individual's potential and motivation to maintain an achievable state of health with lessening of incapacity and helplessness.

Determining the need for a particular form of health education may not always be straightforward due to varied perceptions of an individual's state of health (Ewles & Simnett, 2003; Scriven, 2010). Clearly, the more beneficial approach is establishing effective communication, partnership, and active participation with patient cooperation at all stages, including determining the most feasible and achievable health education for that individual.

Information, Education, and Communication

Naidoo and Wills's (2005, 2009) explanation of IEC suggests a composite approach that encompasses and utilizes health education and actions toward behavior change. The WHO recommends that IEC considers what behavior needs to be changed, the target audience recognition of the problem to be addressed, and a time frame in which the behavior change should occur. Moreover, it should be economical, practical, and realistic for accomplishing the desired behavior or lifestyle change. The phases of IEC are establishment of awareness, augmentation of knowledge, attitude modification, and inspiring people to change and adopt or maintain healthier lifestyles. The WHO emphasizes the importance of identifying barriers to the success of IEC and the enabling factors in the evaluation.

Techniques for implementing IEC include mass media campaigns (television, radio, poster advertisements, flyers, leaflets, etc.) and one-on-one or group interactions (Naidoo & Wills, 2005, 2009).

Significance of Communication

Communication is a fundamental and crucial component of health education. As such, it is important to identify the elements that constitute effective communication. Naidoo and Wills (2005, 2009) identified the following key elements: integrity and knowledge of the communicator (including proficiency and dependability); nature of the message (format used, quality of information); readiness of the target audience (held beliefs, values, literacy level); and source of the information. The context and setting within which the message is delivered is also important.

The authors advocate a public health system that includes a detailed needs assessment that involves identification of the population group at risk, their perceptions and reactions to the problem, considerations of appropriate actions to take, and deliberation about alternative options. Objectives should be formulated with full participation of the patient group. It may be necessary to determine the differing population subgroups in order to sensitively devise and test the health messages. Such a system should also include a robust mechanism for evaluation and feedback (Naidoo & Wills, 2005, 2009).

Clearly, health education cannot be separated from the broader concept of health promotion. Findings from the literature substantiate that effective implementation of health promotion requires the combination of efficient provision of information, education, and communication. It also requires establishment of partnerships and dialogues among practitioners, the patients, and the community. It is important to gain deeper insight of people's conception of well-being, and their perception of health protection, health improvement, and maintenance of good health. It is also equally important to gain insight about the actions that they take to achieve what they perceive as better health.

Essential Competencies Employed in the Implementation of Health Promotion

The diversity of health promotion activities is illustrated by Ewles and Simnett (2003) in their framework of health promotion activities.

Preventive health services in the framework focuses on immunization programs, sexual health preventive measures including condom usage, contraception, and other forms of prevention. Health promotion activities in community-based work involve collaboration with community members in the planning and development of health programs and services. Such collaboration aims to foster patient and community empowerment. It is absolutely important that the resource provision is responsive to the expressed and assessed needs of the people and reflects the cultural, social, and economic circumstances, and the environmental conditions.

Organizational development activities include policy development and implementation of programs. Environmental measures are directed toward improving the environment in order to establish and maintain healthier living conditions. Economic and regulatory activities occur at the governmental level (Ewles & Simnett, 2003; Scriven, 2010).

Significance of Evidence-Based Practice in Health Promotion

In response to the emphasis on evidence-based practice, there is an ongoing effort to ensure that health promotion incorporates research, includes program and process evaluation, and that systematic reviews of relevant research are performed. The challenge for the health promotion practitioner is to conduct extensive literature search to identify and select appropriate studies that have relevance to the problem of interest.

The 51st World Health Assembly advocated that all the member states should utilize an evidence-based approach to the policy and practice of health promotion. Moreover, it stressed the importance of applying a range of qualitative and quantitative methodologies (Potvin, Haddad, & Frohlich, 2001). As Ewles and Simnett (2003) noted, while research allows for developing new knowledge and innovative mechanisms and procedures for clinical application, evaluation is equally crucial. The benefits of combined methods for policy evaluation and assessment of the quality and effectiveness of health promotion programs are recognized (Jolley, Lawless, & Hurley, 2008; Nutbeam, 1998; WHO, 2001).

Evaluation of Health Promotion Policy, Guidelines, and Effectiveness

Milio (2001) proposed very useful questions for evaluating an applied policy in health promotion, which examined the following:

- How the problem for the policy was defined
- The different options in aims and processes that were considered and examined

- The rational for selecting specific options
- The criteria and selection process utilized
- The type and range of resources (funding, staffing, equipment, facilities, and technical support systems) that were allocated and earmarked for the undertaking
- The assessment of progress
- The type of proactive executive or administrative group appointed and its function

Undoubtedly, these are pragmatic issues to address in most, if not all, health promotion policy evaluations. O'Connor-Fleming, Parker, Higgins, and Gould (2006) also explore very useful and popular planning/evaluation frameworks and is a highly recommended reading for additional information. Additionally, Jolley et al.'s (2008) framework and tools for planning and evaluating community participation in health promotion is recommended. The WHO (2001) also provides useful practical considerations.

Speller, Wimbush, and Morgan (2005) provide recommendations made by three national agencies: the Health Development Agency in England, the Health Improvement Agency in Scotland, and the Netherlands Institute of Health Promotion and Disease Prevention. These agencies propose ideas for implementing continually emerging new research evidence. The ongoing expansion of the scope and depth of professional knowledge and the accumulating evidence in health promotion and public health all contribute to the realization of efficient evidence-based health promotion. The authors posit that accomplishing an efficient evidence-based health promotion system requires systematic review of the evidence, creation and distribution of evidence-based guiding principles, policies and regulations, and a system for disseminating new evidence and best practices (Speller et al., 2005).

Health Impact Assessment (HIA)

Health impact assessment (HIA) refers to the process of establishing the potential health effects of a particular intervention, policy, or program on a community or identified population group. HIA takes into account the group's circumstances, genetic profile, social status, economic status, and environmental factors. Together, these serve as the basis to predict the potential effects. Implementation and process decisions can be made based on the findings from an HIA. While HIA is applicable before implementation of a health promotion policy, it could also be applicable afterward.

The main stages of HIA include the following:

- Choosing and critically examining the policy or program to be assessed
- Carrying out detailed assessment of the identified population in terms of circumstances and related attributes
- Documenting the perceptions of relevant parties regarding the potential effects of the policy and program

- Assessing the significance, extent, or degree of impact and the chance occurrence of the predicted impacts
- Developing a report and formulating proposals for managing, dealing with, or controlling any adverse effects (Ewles & Simnett, 2003; Frankish, Green, Ratner, Chomik, & Larsen, 2001; Scriven, 2010)

The WHO notes that many useful HIA guidance documents are currently available for conducting detailed work. These share common core elements although intermingling and overlaps occur in the theoretical stages. Nevertheless, while there are no significant differences between the methods, the number of stages may vary (4, 5, or 6). Related guidance documents published by the WHO include *The HIA Procedure*; *Toolkits, guides* and *overviews*; and *Evaluating your HIA*. The latter provides guidance on process evaluation to examine progress of the activities (whether the components are practicable); impact evaluation guidance to measure the immediate effects (the project objectives); and outcome evaluation guidance to measure the long-term effects (the project goals). The important thing is correctly identifying and implementing an appropriate tool for a specific purpose to achieve useful information for policy decisions.

HIA provides a useful mechanism to raise awareness of policy makers and decision-makers at the organizational level, when they are considering new health promotion policies. Heller et al.'s (2014) 'Promoting Equity Through Health Impact Assessment' provides an excellent resource that explores all the essential elements and practical applications of HIA. Practitioners are encouraged to learn how to conduct health impact assessments for predicting or evaluating relevant programs.

Conclusion

The scope of this chapter does not allow for exhaustive exploration of health promotion in its broader context. The sources of the health promotion principles from the Health for All initiative and the Ottawa Charter for Health Promotion were examined with particular reference to the requisites for action, including advocacy, mediation, enabling, and empowerment. The guiding principles urge for all health-promoting practitioners in all countries to campaign for and endeavor to accomplish specific key objectives. These include building healthy public policies and supportive environments, developing personal skills, strengthening community actions, and refocusing health services provision as outlined in the Jakarta Declaration. These principles affirm international recognition of the importance of the consensus initiatives for health promotion.

A clear understanding of the rationales for health promotion and health education, the related principles and mechanisms of prevention and screening is important. Collaboration with different sectors and endorsement of the relevant regulatory bodies is envisioned to accomplish integrated and interagency provision of health promotion.

Empowerment of patients, their representative groups, the communities, and their cooperation with professional practitioners ultimately lead to active participation in various aspects of health promotion.

This chapter explored the different definitions of health promotion and provided overviews of the related key components. The complexity of health promotion is apparent not only from the definitions and interchangeable usage of terminology but also in the multiplicity of models and approaches. Some of these are not entirely distinguishable from one another due to considerable overlap. Nevertheless, it is important for practitioners to recognize and understand the different models.

Specific concepts applied in the implementation of health promotion such as social marketing and health communication were reviewed and the concept of social cognitive theory was also examined. The related ethical issues are particularly complex and require thorough exploration to ensure appropriate safeguarding of patient welfare with regard to professional accountability. The role of health education and the significance of health impact assessment were explored as well as the need for deeper exploration of equity in care provision, information provision, education, and communication.

Ongoing research activities nurture efficiency in professional practice in terms of evidence-based health promotion with continuous improvements in the health of individuals and communities. Development of the requisite competencies, together with clear insight of the regulatory requirements and the code of professional conduct and ethics, help to guide and enhance practitioners' personal and professional growth.

● ● ● REFERENCES

Action for Advocacy. (2011). *Advocacy in a cold climate: study of the state of services that ensure people are listened to, safeguarded, respected and have choice in health and social care.* London, United Kingdom: Action for Advocacy.

Adams, J., & White, M. (2003). Are activity promotion interventions based on the transtheoretical model effective? A critical review. British *Journal of Sports Medicine.* 37(2): 106–114.

Ajzen, I. (2012). The theory of planned behaviour. In P. A. M. Lange, A. W. Kruglanski, & E. T. Higgins (Eds.), *Handbook of theories of social psychology* (Vol. 1, pp. 438–459). London, United Kingdom: Sage.

Ajzen, I., & Dasgupta, N. (2015). Explicit and implicit beliefs attitudes, and intentions: the role of conscious and unconscious processes in human behavior. In: P. Haggard & B. Eitam (Eds.), *The Sense of Agency* (pp. 115–144). New York: Oxford University Press.

Ajzen, I., & Fishbein, M. (1980). *Understanding attitudes and predicting social behaviour.* Englewood Cliffs, NJ: Prentice Hall.

Ajzen, I. (1988). *Attitudes, personality and behaviour.* Maidenhead, United Kingdom: Open University Press.

Ajzen, I., & Klobas, J. (2013). Fertility intentions: An approach based on the theory of planned behaviour. *Demographic Research,* 29(8), 203–232.

Ajzen, I., & Manstead, A. S. R. (2007). Changing Health-related behaviors: An approach based on the theory of planned behavior. In: Hewstone, M., Schut, H. A. W., de Wit, J. B. F., van den Bos, K., & Stroebe, M. S., (Eds.) *The Scope of Social Psychology: Theory and applications. (A Festschrift for Wolfgang Stroebe)* (pp. 43–63) Psychology Press: Festschrifts, Hove: Psychology Press,

Ajzen, I. & Sheikh, S. (2013). Action versus inaction: Anticipated affect in the theory of planned behaviour. *Journal of Applied Social Psychology, 43*(1), 155–162.

Ajzen, I. & Sheikh, S. (2016). Erratum: Action versus inaction: Anticipated affect in the theory of planned behaviour. *Journal of Applied Social Psychology, 46*(5), 313–314.

Anderson, E. S., Winett, R. A., Wojcik, J. R. (2007). Self-regulation, self-efficacy, outcome expectations, and social support: Social cognitive theory and nutrition behavior. *Ann Behav Med.* 2007 Nov-Dec; *34*(3): 304–312.

Ashford, J. B., & LeCroy, C. W. (2013). *Human behavior and the social environment: A multidimensional perspective.* Belmont, CA: Brooks/Cole, Cengage Learning.

Ashton, J. & Seymour, H. (1988). *The 'new public health' and health promotion agendas.* Buckingham, United Kingdom: Open University Press.

Bandura, A. (2004). Health promotion by social cognitive means. *Health Education and Behaviour, 31*(2), 143–164.

Barnes, J. (2009). Health promotion in sexual health: Different theories and models of health promotion. *Nursing Times, 105,* 18.

Bodenheimer, T. (2005). Helping patients improve their health-related behaviors: What system changes do we need? *Dis Man. Oct; 8*(5): 319–330.

Bruce, D., Harper, G. W., Suleta, K. (2013). and The Adolescent Medicine Trials Network for HIV AIDS Interventions. (ATN) Sexual risk behavior and risk reduction beliefs among HIV-Positive young men who have sex with men, *AIDS Behsv.* 2013 May; *17*(4): 1515–1523.

Burkholder, G. J., Nigg, C. R. (2002). Overview of the transtheoretical model. In: Burbank P., Riebe D. (Eds.) *Promoting exercise and behavior change in older adults: Interventions with the transtheoretical model* (pp. 57–84). Springer Publishing Company.

Carey, P. (2000). Community health and empowerment. In J. Kerr (Ed.)., *Community health promotion: Challenges for practice* (pp. 27–47). Edinburgh, United Kingdom: Baillière Tindall.

Carpenter, J. (2010). A meta-analysis of the effectiveness of health belief model veraibles in predicting behaviour. *Health Communication, 25*(8), 661–669.

Centers for Disease Control and Prevention. (2017). *Gateway to Health and Social Marketing Practice.* Retrieved from www.cdc .gov/healthcommunication

Crosby, R., DiClemente, R. J., Chamigo, R., Snow, G., Troutman, A. (2009). A brief clinic-based, safer sex intervention for heterosexual African American men newly diagnosed with an STD: A randomized controlled trial. *Am J Public Health.* 2009; 99(Suppl 1): S96–S103.

Clutterbuck, D. J., Flowers, P., Barber, T., Wilson, H., Nelson, M., Hedge, B., . . . Sullivan, A. (2012) UK National Guideline on safer sex advice. *Int J STD AIDS* 2012; 23(6): 381–388.

Department of Health (DH). (2001). *Better prevention, better services, better sexual health: The national strategy for sexual health and HIV.* London, United Kingdom: Department of Health.

Department of Health (DH). (2008). *Health inequalities: Progress and next steps.* London, United Kingdom: Department of Health.

Department of Health (DH). (2013). *A framework for sexual health improvement in England.* London, United Kingdom: Department of Health.

Di Noia, J., & Prochaska, J. O. (2010). Dietary stages of change and decisional balance: A meta-analytic review. *American Journal of Health Behavior, 34*(5), 618–632.

Downie, R. S., Tannahill, C., & Tannahill, A. (1996). *Health promotion: models and values* (2nd ed.). Oxford, United Kingdom: Oxford University Press.

Eriksson, M., & Lindstrom, B. (2008). A salutogenic interpretation of the Ottawa Charter. *Health Promotion International, 23*(2), 190–199.

Eloundou-Enyegue, P. M., Meekers, D., Claves, A. E. (2005). From awareness to adoption: The effect of AIDS education and condom social marketing on condom use in Tanzania (1993-1996). *J Biosoc Sci.* 2005 May; *37*(3). 257–268.

Ewles, L., & Simnett, I. (2003). *Promoting health: A practical guide* (5th ed.). Edinburgh, United Kingdom: Baillière Tindall.

Featherstone, B., & Fraser, C. (2012). I'm just a mother. I'm nothing special, they're all professionals: Parental advocacy as an aid to parental engagement. *Child & Family Social Work, 17*(2), 244–253.

Finlay, S., & Sandall J. (2009). Someone's rooting for you. Community advocacy and street-level bureaucracy in UK maternal healthcare. *Social Science and Medicine, 69*(8), 1228–1235.

Fishbein, M., & Ajzen, I. (2005). Theory-based behaviour change interventions: Comments on Hobbis & Sutton. *Journal of Health Psychology, 10*(1), 27–31.

Fishbein, M. (2008). A reasoned action approach to health promotion. *Med Decis Making. 2008 20*(6): 834–844.

Fishbein, M., & Ajzen, I. (2010). *Predicting and changing behaviour: The reasoned action approach.* New York, NY: Psychology Press (Taylor & Francis).

Frankish, C. J., Green, L. W., Ratner, P. A., Chomik, T., & Larsen, C. (2001). Health impact assessment as a tool for health promotion and population health. In I. Rootman, M. Goodstadt, B. Hyndman, D. V. McQueen, L. Potvin, J. Springett, & E. Ziglio (Eds.), *Evaluation in health promotion: Principles and perspectives.* pp. 405–437). Geneva, Switzerland: WHO.

Fry, S. T. (1996). Ethics in community health nursing practice. In M. Stanhope & J. Lancaster (Eds.), *Community health nursing: Promoting health of aggregates, families and individuals* (4th ed., pp. 93–116). London, United Kingdom: Mosby.

Glanz, K., Rimer, B., & Viswanath, K. (2015). *Health behaviour: Theory, research and practice* (5th ed.). Hoboken, NJ: John-Wiley & Sons.

Guttman, N., & Salmon, C. T. (2004). Guilt, fear, stigma, and knowledge gaps: ethical issues in public health communication interventions. *Bioethics.* 2004 Nov; *18*(6): 531–552.

Haggart, M. (2000). Promoting the health of communities. In J. Kerr (Ed.), *Community health promotion: Challenges for practice.* Edinburgh, United Kingdom: Baillière Tindall.

Heller, J., Givens, M. L., Yuen, T. K., Gould, S., Jandu, M. B., Choi, T. (2014). Advancing efforts to achieve health equity: equity metrics for health impact assessment practice. *Int J Environ Res Public Health.* 2014 Oct 24; *11*(11): 11054–11064.

Horgan, M., & Bergin, C. (2010). *Putting players first: International Rugby Board Policy on hygiene infection control and prevention of infection.* Retrieved from http://tekobooks.com/downloads /international_rugby_board_putting_players_first/

Horwath, C. C., Schembre, S. M., Motl, R. W., Dishman, R. K., & Nigg, C. R. (2013). Does the transtheoretical model of behaviour change provide a useful basis for interventions to promote fruit and vegetable consumption? *American Journal of Health Promotion, 27*(6), 351–367.

International Social Marketing Association, European Social Marketing Association, and Australian Social Marketing Association (The iSMA, ESMA and AASM). (2013). *Consensus Definition of Social Marketing.* Retrieved from http://www.i-socialmarketing .org/assets/social_marketing_definition.pdf

Janz, N. K., & Becker, M.A. (1984). The health belief model: A decade later. *Health Education Quarterly, 11*(1), 1–47.

Jolley, G., Lawless, A., & Hurley, C. (2008). Framework and tools for planning and evaluating community participation, collaborative partnerships, and equity in health promotion. *Health Promotion Journal Australia, 19*(2), 152–157.

Jones, K. (2007). Doing a literature review in health. In M. Saks & J. Allsop (Eds.), *Researching Health: Qualitative, quantitative and mixed methods.* London, United Kingdom: Sage Publications.

Kickbush, I. (2010). *Implementing health in all policies: Adelaide 2010.* Adelaide, Australia: Department of Health, Government of South Australia.

Klobas, J., & Ajzen, I. (2015). Making the decision to have a child. In D. Philipov, A. C. Liefbroer, & J. E. Klobas (Eds.), *Reproductive decision-making in a macro-micro perspective* (pp. 41–78). Amsterdam, Netherlands: Springer.

Koblin B., Chesney M., Coates T., EXPLORE Study Team. (2004). Effects of a behavioural intervention to reduce acquisition of HIV infection among men who have sex with men: The EXPLORE randomised controlled study. *Lancet* 2004 Jul 3-9; *364*(9428): 41–50.

Kotler, P., Burton, S., Deans, K. R., Brown, L., Armstrong, G. M. (2007). Marketing | Kotler, Burton, Deans, Brown, Armstrong. (9th ed.). Freinchs Forest, New South Wales: Pearson Australia.

Kroll, C., Keller, R., Scholz, U., & Perren, S. (2011). Evaluating the decisional balance construct of the transtheoretical model: Are two dimensions of pros and cons really enough? *International Journal of Public Health, 56*(1), 97–105.

Kutash, K., Duchnowski, A. J., & Lynn, N. (2006). *School-based mental health: An empirical guide for decision-makers.* Tampa, FL: University of South Florida. Retrieved from http://rtckids .fmhi.usf.edu/rtcpubs/study04/default.cfm

Liefbroer, A. C., Klobas, J., Philipov, D., & Ajzen, I. (2015). Reproductive decision-making in a macro-micro perspective: A conceptual framework. In D. Philipov, A. C. Liefbroer, & J. E. Klobas (Eds), *Reproductive decision-making in a macro-micro perspective* (pp. 1–16). Amsterdam, Netherlands: Springer.

Liu, J. J., Davidson, E., Bhopal, R., White, M., Johnson, M., Netto, G., & Sheikh, A. (2016). Adapting health promotion interventions for ethnic minority groups: A qualitative study. *Health Promotion International, 31*(2), 325–334.

Loss, J., & Nagel, E. (2010). Social marketing - seduction with the aim of healthy behavior? *Gesundheitswesen.* 2010 Jan; 72(1): 54–62.

Mace, C. (2007). Mindfulness in psychotherapy: An introduction. *Advances in Psychiatric Treatment, 13*(2), 147–154.

Markowitz, J. C., & Weissman, M. M. (2004). Interpersonal psychotherapy: Principles and applications. *World Psychiatry, 3*(3), 136–139.

Martin, Ginis, K. A., Latimer, A. E., Arbour-Nicitopoulos, K. P., Bassett, R. L., Wolfe, D. L., & Hanna, S. E. (2011). Determinants of physical activity among people with spinal cord injury: A test of social cognitive theory. *Annals of Behavioural Medicine, 42*(1), 127–133.

McQueen, D., and Jones, C. (2007). *Global Perspectives on health promotion effectiveness.* New York: Springer.

McQueen, D. (2011). A challenge for health promotion. *Global Health Promotion 18*(3).

McQueen, D. V., & De Salazar, L. (2011). Health promotion, the Ottawa Charter and 'developing personal skills': a compact history of 25 years. *Health Promotion International, 26*(2), ii194–ii201.

Miller, W. R., & Rollnick, S. (2009). Ten things that motivational interviewing is not. *Behavioural and Cognitive Psychotherapy.* 37(2): 129–140.

Milio, N. (2001). Evaluation of health promotion policies: Tracking a moving target. In I. Rootman, M. Goodstadt, B. Hyndman, D. V. McQueen, L. Potvin, J. Springett, & E. Ziglio (Eds.), *Evaluation in health promotion: Principles and perspectives* (pp. 365–385). Geneva, Switzerland: WHO.

Miller, W. R., Yahne, C. E., Tinigan, J. S. (2003). Motivational interviewing in drug abuse services: A randomized trial. *Journal of Consulting Clinical Psychology.* 71(4): 754–763.

Moens, V., Baruch, G., & Fearon, P. (2003). Opportunistic screening for chlamydia at a community based contraceptive service for young people. *British Medical Journal, 326*(7401), 1252–1255.

Naidoo, J., & Wills, J. (2005). *Public health and health promotion: Developing practice* (2nd ed.). Edinburgh, United Kingdom: Baillière Tindall.

Naidoo, J., & Wills, J. (2009). *Foundations for health promotion* (3rd ed.). Edinburgh, United Kingdom: Baillière Tindall, Elsevier.

National Cancer Institute. (n.d.). *Publications.* Retrieved from www.cancer.gov/cancertopics/cancerlibrary

National Health Service (NHS). (2010). *Towards best practice for chlamydia screening in reproductive and sexual health services.* London, United Kingdom: Health Protection Agency.

National Institute for Health and Care Excellence (NICE). (2007). *Prevention of sexually transmitted infections and under 18 conceptions.* Retrieved from http://www.nice.org.uk/guidance/ph3

National Institute for Health and Care Excellence. (NICE). (2016). *Harmful sexual behaviour among children and young people. (NICE Guidance NG55)* Retrieved from https://www.nice.org.uk/guidance/ng55

Newbiggins, K., McKeown, M., & French, B. (2011). Mental advocacy and African and Caribbean men: Good practice principles and organisational models of delivery. *Health Expectations, 16*(1), 80–104.

Newton, J. D., Turk, T., Ewing, M. T. (2013). Ethical evaluation of audience segmentation in social marketing. *European Journal of Marketing.* 47(9) 1421–1438.

Nigg, C. R., Geller, K. S., Motl, R. W., Horwath, C. C., Wertin, K. K., & Dishman, R. K. (2011). A research agenda to examine the efficacy and relevance of the transtheoretical model for physical activity behaviour. *Psychology in Sport and Exercise, 12*(1), 7–12.

Noar, S. M., & Zimmerman, R. S. (2005). Health Behavior Theory and cumulative knowledge regarding health behaviors: Are we moving in the right direction? *Health Educ Res.* 2005 Jun; 20(3): 275–290.

Nutbeam, D. (1998). Evaluating health promotion–progress, problems and solutions. *Health Promotion International, 13*(1), 27–44.

Nutbeam, D., Harris, E., & Wise, M. (2010). Theory in a nutshell: A practical guide to health promotion theories. North Ryde, Australia: McGraw-Hill.

O'Connor-Fleming, M. L., Parker, E., Higgins, H., & Gould, T. (2006). A framework for evaluating health promotion programs. *Health Promotion Journal of Australia, 17*(1), 61–66.

Orme, J., Powell, J., Taylor, P., Harrison, T., & Grey, M. (2003). *Public health for the 21st century: New perspectives on policy, participation and practice.* Maidenhead, United Kingdom: Open University Press.

Ottawa Charter for Health Promotion. *First International Conference on Health Promotion.* November 21, 1986, Ottawa, Canada. Retrieved from http://www.who.int/healthpromotion/conferences/previous/ottawa/en/

Paasche-Orlow, M. K., & Wolfe, M. S. (2007). The causal pathways linking health literacy to health outcomes. *American Journal of Health Behavior.* 31(1) S19–S26.

Pajares, F. (2009). Toward a positive psychology of academic motivation: The role of self-efficacy beliefs. In: R. Gilman, E. S. Huebner, & M. J. Furlong (Eds.), *Handbook of Positive Psychology in Schools* (pp. 149–160). New York: Taylor Francis.

Pajares, F., Prestin, A., Chen, J., Nabi, L. R. (2009). Social cognitive theory and media effects. In: L. R. Nabi, M. B. Oliver (Eds.), *The SAGE Handbook of Media Processes and Effects* (pp. 283–297). Los Angeles: Sage.

Palmer, D., Nixon, J., Reynolds, S., Panayiotou, A., Palmer, A., & Meyerowitz, R. (2012). Getting to know you: Reflections on a specialist independent mental health advocacy services for Bexley and Bromley residents in forensic settings. *Mental Health Review Journal, 17*(1), 5–13.

Pender, N. J. (1996). *Health promotion in nursing practice* (3rd ed.). Stamford, CT: Appleton & Lange.

Polit, D. F., & Beck, C. T. (2013). *Essentials of nursing research: Appraising evidence for nursing practice* (8th ed.). London, United Kingdom: Lippincott Williams &Wilkins.

Potvin, L., Haddad, S., & Frohlich, K. L. (2001). Beyond process and outcome evaluation: A comprehensive approach for evaluating health promotion programmes. In I. Rootman, M. Goodstadt, B. Hyndman, D. V. McQueen, L. Potvin, J. Springett, & E. Ziglio (Eds.), *Evaluation in health promotion: Principles and perspectives* (pp. 45–62). Geneva, Switzerland: WHO.

Public Health England. (2014). *Evidence and recommendations: NHS population screening.* Retrieved from https://www.gov.uk/guidance/evidence-and-recommendations-nhs-population-screening

Quinn, F. M., & Hughes, S. (2007). *Quinn's principles and practice of nurse education* (5th ed.). Cheltenham, United Kingdom: Nelson Thornes Ltd.

Robson, C. (2011). *Real world research* (4th ed.). Chichester, United Kingdom: John Wiley and Sons Ltd.

Rojanapithayakorn, W. (2006). The 100% condom use programme in Asia. *Reproductive Health Matters.* 2006 Nov; *14*(28): 41–52.

Rollnick, S., Butler, C., Kinnersley, P., Gregory, J., & Mash, B. (2010). Motivational interviewing. *British Medical Journal, 340,* 1242–1245.

Rubak, S., Sandboek, A., Lauritzen, T., & Christensen, B. (2005). Motivational interviewing: A systematic review and meta-analysis. *British Journal of General Practice, 55*(513), 305–312.

Ryan, R. M., Williams, G. C., Patrick, H., & Deci, E. L. (2009). Self-determination theory and physical activity: the dynamics of motivation in development and wellness. *Hellenic Journal of Psychology. 6*(2): 107–124.

Saan, H., & Wise, M. (2011). Enable, mediate, advocate. *Health Promotion International, 26*(2), ii187–ii193.

Schunk, D. H., Meece, J. L., & Pintrich, P. R. (2014). *Motivation in education: Theory, research, and applications.* (4th ed.). Boston, MA: Pearson.

Scriven, A. (2010). *Promoting health: A practical guide.* (6th ed.). Edinburgh, United Kingdom: Bailliere Tindall, Elsevier.

Seedhouse, D. F. (2001). *Health: the foundations for achievement* (2nd ed.). Chichester, United Kingdom: John Wiley & Sons.

Seedhouse, D. (2009). *Ethics: the heart of healthcare* (3rd ed.). Chichester, United Kingdom: Wiley-Blackwell.

Shannon, R., & Davies, E. (2010). How motivational interviewing can help patients change their lifestyles. *Clinical Pharmacist, 2,* 28–30.

Solidarity in Health: Reducing Health Inequalities in the EU. (2009). *Commission of the European Communities. Communication from the Commission the the European Parliament the Council, the European Economic and Social Committee and the Committee of the Regions.* Retrieved from http://www.ec.europa.eu/health/ph_determinants/socio_economics/documents/com2009_en.pdf

Speller, V., Wimbush, E., & Morgan, A. (2005). Evidence based health promotion practice: How to make it work. *Promotion & Education, 12*(1),15–20.

Tannahill, A. (2009). Health promotion: The Tannahill model revisited. *Public Health, 123*(5), 396–399.

Taylor, D., Bury, M., Campling, N., Carter, S., Garfield, S., Newbould, J., & Rennie, T. (2006). *A review of the use of the health belief model (HBM), the theory of reasoned action (TRA), the theory of planned behaviour (TPB) and the trans theoretical model (TTM) to study and predict health related behaviour change.* London, United Kingdom: NICE.

Tengland, P.-A. (2007). Empowerment: A goal or a means for health promotion? *Medicine, Health Care and Philosophy, 10*(2), 197–207.

Tengland, P.-A. (2008). Empowerment a conceptual discussion. *Health Care Analysis, 16*(2), 77–96.

Tengland, P.-A. (2010). Health promotion and disease prevention: Logically different conceptions? *Health Care Analysis, 18*(4), 323–341.

Tengland, P.-A. (2012). Behaviour change or empowerment: On ethics of health promotion strategies. *Public Health Ethics, 5*(2), 140–153.

The Community Guide. (2004). *What Works.* Retrieved from https://www.thecommunityguide.org/sites/default/files/assets/What-Works-Health-Communication-factsheet-and-insert.pdf

Tones, K., & Green, J. (2004). Health promotion: Planning and strategies. London, United Kingdom: Sage.

Townsley, R., Marriot, A., & Ward, L. (2009). *Access to independent advocacy: An evidence review.* London, United Kingdom: Office for Disability Issues.

Treasure, J. (2004). Motivational Interviewing. *Advances in Psychiatric Treatment.* 2004; *10*(5): 331–337.

Usher, E., & Pajares, F. (2008). Self-regulated Learning; A validation study. *Educational & Psychological Measurement.* 68(3): 443–463.

Van den Broucke, S. (2012). Theory-informed health promotion: Seeing the bigger picture by looking at the details. *Health Promotion International, 27*(2), 143–147.

Van Wormer, K. (2008). Counselling family members of addicts/alcoholics: The stages of change model. *Journal of Family Social Work, 11*(2), 202–221.

Velicer, W., Prochaska, J. O., Fava, J. L., Rossi, J. S., Redding, C. A., Laforge, R. G., & Robbins, M. L. (2012). Using the transtheoretical model for population-based approaches to health promotion and disease prevention. *Homeostasis in Health and Disease, 40*(5), 174–195.

Weinstein, N. D., Rothman, A. J. (2005). Commentary: revitalizing research on health behavior theories. *Health Education Research, 20*(3): 294–297.

Whitehead, D. (2001). Health education, behavioural change and social psychology: Nursing's contribution to health promotion? *Journal of Advanced Nursing 34*(6), 822–832.

Wilson, H. (2004). Health Promotion: theories and Principles. In Society of Sexual Health Advisers. (SSHA) *The Manual for Sexual Health Advisers* Self-determination theory and physical activity: The dynamics of motivation in development and wellness. *Hellenic Journal of Psychology.* London, United Kingdom: AMICUS HEALTH Sector, Society of Sexual Health Advisers.

Williams, T., & Williams, K. (2010). Self-efficacy and performance in mathematics: Reciprocal determinism in 33 nations. *Journal of Educational Psychology.* 102(2):453–466.

World Health Organization (WHO). (1986). *The Ottawa Charter for Health Promotion: First International Conference on Health Promotion.* Geneva, Switzerland: Author.

World Health Organization (WHO). (1997). *The Jakarta Declaration on Leading Health Promotion into the 21st Century.* Geneva: WHO.

World Health Organization (WHO). (1998). *Health promotion glossary.* Geneva, Switzerland: Author.

World Health Organization (WHO). (2008). Closing the gap in a generation: Health equity through action on the social determinants of health. WHO Global Commission on Social Determinants of Health. Geneva, Switzerland: Author. Retrieved from http://whqlibdoc.who.int/publicactions/2008/9789241563703_eng.pdf

World Health Organization (WHO). (2009). *Milestones in health promotion: Statements from global conferences.* Geneva, Switzerland: Author.

World Health Organization (2013). 8th Global Conference on Health Promotion. *The Helsinki Statement on Health in all Policies.* Helsinki, Finland: World Health Organization.

Ybara, M. L., Korchmaros, J., Kiwanuka, J., Bangsberg, D. R., & Bull, S. (2013). Examining the applicability of the IMB model in predicting condom use among sexually active secondary school students in Mbarara, Uganda. *AIDS & Behavior, 17*(3), 1116–1128.

••• SUGGESTED FURTHER READING

The following references may also be beneficial further reading for policy makers and decision-makers as well as practitioners regarding evaluation of health promotion programs.

Abraham, C., & Sheeran, P. (2005). The health belief model. In M. Conner & P. Norman (Eds.), *Predicting health behaviour: Research and practice with social cognitive models* (pp. 28–80). Maidenhead, United Kingdom: Open University Press.

American Congress of Obstetricians and Gynecologists (ACOG), (2009). Motivational interviewing: A tool for behavior change. Committee Opinion Number 423 January 2009 (Reaffirmed 2016).

Boamah, G. (2011). *Concepts and dimensions of health and health beliefs.* Motec LIFE-UK. Retrieved from https://www.pdffiller.com/269277407-Concept-of-Healthpdf-CONCEPTS-and-DIMENSIONS-of-HEALTH-and-HEALTH-BELIEFS-Various-Fillable-Forms

Department of Health and Children & the Health Service Executive. (2008). *National strategy for service user involvement in the Irish Health Service.* Retrieved from www.hse.ie/eng/publications/Your_Service_Your_Say_Consumer_Affairs/Strategy/Service_User_Involvement.pdf

French, J. (2006). Targets, standards and indicators. In M. Davies & W. McDowall (Eds.), *Health promotion theory: Understanding public health* (pp. 77–90). Maidenhead, United Kingdom: Open University, McGraw-Hill.

Gold, R.S. (2001). Report on the 2000 Joint Committee on Health Education and Promotion Terminology. *American Journal of Health Education 32*(2), 89–103.

Glanz, K., Rimer, B., & Viswanath, K. (2015). *Health behaviour: Theory, research and practice* (5th ed.). Hoboken, NJ: John-Wiley & Sons.

Greene-Moton, E. (2010). Exploring the role of partnerships for health promotion. Invited presentation, Australian Health Promotion Association Conference.

Health Education Authority (HEA). (1999). *Promoting the health of the homeless.* London: HEA.

Institute for Work and Health. (2015). *What researchers mean by primary, secondary and tertiary prevention.* Retrieved from https://www.iwh.on.ca/wrmb/primary-secondary-and-tertiary-prevention

Jacobs, J. A., Jones, E., Gabella, B. A., Soring, B., & Brownson, R. C. (2012). Tools for implementing an evidence-based approach in public health practice. *Prevention and Chronic Disease, 9,* 110324. doi: http://dx.doi.org/10.5888/pcd9.110324

Johnson, B. T., Scott-Sheldon, L. A., Huedo-Medina, T. B., & Carey, M. P. (2011). Interventions to reduce sexual risk for human immunodeficiency virus in adolescents: A meta-analysis of trials 1985–2008. *Archives of Pediatric and Adolescent Medicine, 165*(1), 77–84.

Prochaska, J. O., Butterworth, S., Redding, C. A., Burden, V., Perrin, N., Leo, M., . . . Prochaska, J. M. (2008). Initial efficacy of MI, TTM tailoring, and HRIs in multiple behaviors for employee health promotion. *Preventive Medicine, 46*(3), 226–231.

Mace, C. (2007). Mindfulness in psychotherapy: An introduction. *Advances in Psychiatric Treatment, 13*(2), 147–154.

Manson, H. M. (2012). The development of the CoRE-Values framework as an aid to ethical decision-making. *Medical Teacher, 34,* e258–e268.

McAlister, A. L., Perry, C. L., Parcel, G. S. (2008). How individuals, environments, and health behaviors interact: Social cognitive theory. In Glanz K., Rimer B. K., Viswanath K. (Eds.). *Health behavior and health education: Theory, Research, and Practice* (4th ed, pp. 169–188). San Fransisco, CA: Jossey-Bass.

Naidoo, J. & Wills, J. (2000). *Health promotion: Foundations for practice* (2nd ed.). Edinburgh, United Kingdom: Baillière Tindall.

Nutbeam, D. (1996). Achieving 'best practice' in health promotion: improving the fit between research and practice. *Health Education Research, 11*(3), 317–326.

Nutbeam, D. (2006). Using theory to guide changing communities and organisations. In M. Davies & W. MacDowell (Eds.), *Health promotion theory: Understanding public health series* (PP. 24–36). Maidenhead, United Kingdom: Open University Press, McGraw-Hill.

Polit, D. F., & Beck, C. T. (2011). *Nursing research: Generating and assessing evidence for nursing practice* (9th ed.). London, United Kingdom: Wolters Kluwer Health | Lippincott Williams &Wilkins.

Prochaska, J., & Velicer, W. (1997). The transtheoretical model of health behaviour change. *American Journal of Health Promotion, 12*(1), 38–48.

Prochaska, J. J., Prochaska, J. M., & Prochaska, J. O. (2013). Building a science for multiple-risk behaviour change. In S. Shumaker, J. Ockene, & J. Riekert (Eds.), *The handbook of health behaviour change* (4th ed. pp. 245–276). New York, NY: Springer.

Protogerou, C., & Johnson, B. T. (2014). Factors underlying the success of behavioural HIV-prevention interventions for adolescent: a meta-review. *AIDS & Behavior, 18*(10), 1847–1863.

Rootman, I., Goodstadt, M., Hyndman, B., McQueen, D. V., Potvin, L., Springett, J., & Ziglio, E. (Eds.). (2001). *Evaluation in health promotion: Principles and perspectives.* Geneva, Switzerland: WHO.

Saks, M., & Allsop, J. (2007). *Researching health: Qualitative, quantitative and mixed methods.* London, United Kingdom: Sage.

Seedhouse, D. (2004). *Health promotion: Philosophy, prejudice and practice* (2nd ed.). Chichester, United Kingdom: John Wiley & Sons Ltd.

Seifer, S. D., & Gottlieb, B. (2010). Transformation through partnerships: Progress in community health partnerships. *Research Education and Action, 4*(1), 1–3.

Seifer, S. D., & Sgambelluri, A. (2008). Mobilising partnerships for social change: Progress in community health partnerships. *Research Education and Action, 2*(2), 81–82.

U.S. Department of Health and Human Services. (1989). *Making health communication programs work.* Washington, DC: U.S. Government Printing Office.

U.S. Department of Health and Human Services (DHHS). (2010a). *Healthy People: Understanding and improving health* (Vol. 1; 2nd ed.). Washington, DC: U.S. Government Printing Office.

U.S. Department of Health and Human Services (DHHS). (2010b). *Healthy People: Objectives for improving health* (Vol. 2; 2nd ed.). Washington, DC: U.S. Government Printing Office.

von Sadovszky, V., Drauott, B., & Boch, S. (2014). A systematic review of reviews of behavioural interventions to promote condom use. *Worldviews Evidence-Based Nursing, 11*(2), 107–117.

World Health Organization (WHO). Short Guides. Geneva, Switzerland: Author. Retrieved from http://www.who.int/hia/about/guides/en; for WHO Publications guidance and tools, see: http://www.who.int/hia/tools/toolkit/en/

World Health Organization (WHO). (1998). *Health promotion evaluation: Recommendations to policy-makers: Report of the WHO European Working Group on Health Promotion Evaluation.* Copenhagen, Denmark, Author.

World Health Organization (WHO). (2009). *Milestones in health promotion: Statements from global conferences.* Geneva, Switzerland: Author.

World Health Organization (WHO). (2012). *Health education: Theoretical concepts, effective strategies and core competencies.* Cairo, Egypt: Regional Office for the Eastern Mediterranean, WHO.

World Health Organization (WHO). (2013). *8th Global Conference on Health Promotion, Helsinki 2013,* Switzerland: Author. Retrieved from. http://www.who.int/healthpromotion/conferences/8gchp/outcomes/en/

The Wider Context of Sexual and Reproductive Health Care: Workforce Development and The Significance of Research and Clinical Audit

17

Developing a Competent and Capable Sexual and Reproductive Workforce

LORRAINE FORSTER

CHAPTER OBJECTIVES

The main objectives of this chapter are to:

- Explore the sexual and reproductive health services provided within the largest health board area in Scotland
- Promote nurse leadership as a key driver for change
- Explain the complexities of service integration and management
- Examine specific competency development
- Explore subject areas for future consideration and possible development

Introduction

The aims of this chapter are to demonstrate the scope for developing multidisciplinary, integrated sexual and reproductive health services in the United Kingdom and to provide a service and governance framework for nursing leadership and staff role development to support the delivery of these services.

The National Health Service of Greater Glasgow and Clyde (NHSGGC) is the largest of 14 health boards in Scotland; with a staff of 44,000, it delivers services to a population of 1.1 million. There are significant issues affecting the health of the population with respect to deprivation, low educational attainment, low income, addiction to drugs and alcohol, unintended pregnancy, and poor mental health that increase the complexities inherent in service delivery. High rates of sexual risk-taking (e.g., men who have sex with men [MSM]) with resultant increases in sexually transmitted infection (STI) rates and complexity of presentation presents challenges to healthcare

providers to maximize risk-reduction approaches and improve patient outcomes.

Sandyford is a part of NHSGGC and provides integrated specialist sexual and reproductive health services on behalf of the National Health Services (NHS) board. It was formed in 2000 through the co-location of community-based family planning services, hospital-based genitourinary medicine (GUM) services, and the Center for Women's Health—a women-only service providing counseling and support services. Services are aimed at promoting positive sexual health and reflect the objectives contained in national policies and strategies. Health statistics indicate that in 2016, the Glasgow and Clyde Health Board area had the highest number of HIV-infected persons of any area of Scotland (Health Protection Scotland, 2017).

Evidence suggests that people in the health inequalities groups and in disadvantaged communities experience the greatest barriers to health (Gravelle & Sutton, 2003). Sandyford, unlike many other sexual health centers, operates within a social model of health framework that recognizes the significant impact of health inequality and operates in a gender-sensitive and non-discriminatory way. A person-centered approach to health risk assessment is essential to ensure that individuals attending the center are afforded every opportunity to have their individual needs met. The importance of maximizing opportunistic health improvement or health-promoting activities is fundamental to all consultations, with brief interventions where appropriate (see the Appendix at the end of this chapter for the alcohol brief intervention as an example of good practice).

Integrated Sexual Health Services in the United Kingdom

The major driver for integration of sexual health services in Scotland was concern among public health practitioners and government health departments about increasing rates of STIs (including HIV), unintended pregnancy, and pregnancy termination in young people. Another major consideration was the recognition of significant inefficiencies in the way health services were delivered across Scotland as evidenced by long waiting times and treatment delays (Djuretic et al., 2001; National Health Services Scotland, 2017; Woods, 2001). Identifying robust leadership across the specialties of community-based family planning and hospital-based GUM services was the first stage of the process. Improvements were needed to clinical leadership, interagency communications, patient and clinician information availability, service access, and most important, ways of working in partnership to deliver these. There was an appreciation of the impact that effective clinical leadership can have on service organization and delivery approaches and the need for these individuals to lead on the development of a much-needed sexual health strategy for Scotland, Respect, and Responsibility (Scottish Executive, 2005b). This was an innovative policy supported by the national government, which recognized the need for a multidisciplinary approach to tackling the health services problems in Scotland. Significant resources, including appropriate funding, were made available.

Staff, key partners, and stakeholders affected by the proposal were engaged in the early stages, which helped to build secure relationships that enabled some of the integration work to move forward. Some of these key partnerships are described later in the chapter. Once the decision had been made to integrate family planning and GUM services and a suitable venue had been found, these services co-located with the Center for Women's Health. The process of integration followed the initial co-location of family planning and GUM services to a large city center location in 2000. This was a slow process that resulted in the full integration of family planning and GUM staff and services, which included access to counseling and support services for men. This integration was necessary to achieve a person-centered approach to service provision with a one-stop shop for individuals attending the service. Staff across nursing and medical disciplines had to acquire the competencies to support such integrated care. The majority of nursing and medical staff now have dual competence in both specialty areas (GUM and reproductive health). Service integration supported the development of professional leadership roles for both medical and nursing staff, including the development of advanced nurse practitioner roles as outlined in the National Career Framework for Sexual Health Nursing.

The need to ensure effective clinical practice throughout all areas of the service was achieved through shared protocols and guidelines that met the needs of both clinical and administrative staff. Existing policies and protocols were updated to reflect the change in clinical practice, with in-house teaching sessions on the changes. In addition, paper and electronic versions of documents were made available for ease of reference.

Integration is a particularly challenging process, as individuals with responsibility for clinical practice decisions need to work together to effect a change in practice. The decisions and resultant changes may be questioned by staff at all levels and from all disciplines. It is important that respected individuals from all parts of the organization be engaged in the change process to help garner widespread staff support. Major redesign of staffing and services is a challenging time for an organization. Staff are not yet familiar with new protocols and guidelines; they may be inexperienced in managing patients who present with specific conditions, and there may be communication delays and misunderstandings. All of this can create stress for the staff and affect productivity. Staff need time to familiarize themselves with their new roles and responsibilities; ideally this should be done in a supportive way that maximizes the skills of staff (e.g., through the use of shadowing and mentorship). Unfortunately, the process of change can increase both waiting times and patient complaints in the short term. Although these effects are time-limited, they should be identified clearly in the planning arrangements.

Visible and resilient nursing leadership is an essential part of any organizational governance framework to ensure practice is safe, effective, and within the professional scope and range. This can be achieved through placing senior nurses in supportive or leading roles in such areas as clinical governance and practice development. There is also an opportunity to develop new nursing roles to support organizational change, and these can be used to promote nursing leadership within the new organization. Respecting the role of senior nurses within senior management positions, such as a head of nursing role, ensures professional values and governance processes are recognized and inherent in all service planning and delivery.

Prior to the service integration, all specialist areas had previously worked well as independent units within their respective locations and many found it difficult to accept the rationale for integrating services. For many staff, there was a perceived loss of professional identity and integrity. In addition, there was some difficulty in making changes to the women-only space, with a perception by many counseling staff that men should not be able to utilize the existing counseling services. There were fears that women would not attend if men were present, and this took some time to resolve. Many medical and nursing staff expressed concern about the competence and effectiveness of staff from other disciplines undertaking an integrated role. This was a major barrier to service change. The leaders gave reassurance that no staff would be expected to undertake a role for which they had not been fully prepared and that all staff would be expected to work within the limits of their competence. Individual teams had developed strong bonds over time and these were exposed to significant change.

Cultural differences also had to be addressed. For example, one culture difference was that GUM staff wore uniforms and family planning staff wore civilian clothes.

This was a major issue for some staff, as there was a perceived loss of professional respect from patients if they were not allowed to wear their uniform. However, a short audit of patient preference showed that uniforms were seen as presenting a barrier to open communication, and patients preferred staff to be professionally dressed and to identify themselves by name and title (i.e., doctor or nurse). There were also staff concerns about maintaining infection control standards out of uniform, yet wearing civilian clothing does not present an identified infection-control risk, assuming all staff observe universal infection-control precautions and wear single-use plastic aprons and/or single-use gloves when undertaking procedures that may involve exposure to body fluids.

There were different patient confidentiality processes: GUM services utilized numbers to identify patients at clinics, whereas family planning would use patient names; one system used electronic clinical records and the other used paper forms. This generated many issues for the new service with respect to specimen and form labeling and obtaining results. In addition, the family planning service had mixed waiting areas where both men and women could be seated, while GUM had designated male and female waiting areas. This generated difficulties, as family planning patients were used to open waiting areas and did not want to be "segregated." The community access coordinator interviewed patients to ascertain what form of waiting space would be preferred. The majority of patients indicated a preference to sit in a mixed waiting area and be called by their first name.

These differences between each service area may not seem important, but were stated by many staff as reasons why full integration could not take place. There was a significant amount of time and energy expended exploring and negotiating these and other issues, which posed a significant risk of detracting from patient care issues. It is important to carefully consider and respect these differences in patient culture and to develop opportunities to work through concerns. Use of short-life working groups with staff representation from different disciplines can help manage the process. Patient questionnaires and focus groups will provide patient viewpoints on experiences of other service areas where successful service integration has taken place. The resulting service at Sandyford was unique in being the only integrated sexual and reproductive health service in the United Kingdom.

Sandyford Services Overview

Sandyford services are delivered on a hub-and-spoke model with its main base at Sandyford Central in West Glasgow. This allows a tiered service delivery model:

- **Tier One** includes formal and informal sources of information and advice, which individuals may access directly.

- **Tier Two** covers services not specifically focused on sexual health and includes community groups, youth clubs, and community pharmacies.

- **Tier Three** includes services providing a range of contraception and specialist testing provided by primary care practitioners, specialist voluntary organizations, and sexual health drop-in services.

- **Tier Four** includes contraceptive services, sexually transmitted infection and blood-borne virus testing, and treatment provided in specialist sexual and reproductive health clinics by primary care teams with a special interest in sexual health.

- **Tier Five** combines the provision of Tier Four specialist services with HIV treatment and care, contraception and reproductive health, coordination of partnership notification and elements of sexual and reproductive health needs assessment, psychosexual medicine, termination of pregnancy, clinical governance, and quality assurance of all tiers of service.

Sandyford Hubs provide a Tier 4 service and have formal links with the local government sexual health planning groups, ensuring targeted access to local services for individuals within each area. Each hub is led by a specialist sexual health nurse with responsibility for ensuring that clinical services meet a range of local and national standards. They also have responsibility for promoting the service to designated populations within their own geographic area (e.g., patients with learning disabilities, homeless, young people, and MSM). The lead nurses develop effective strategic links with key health and social care professionals such as specialist community public health nurses, school nurses, primary care physicians, community mental health counselors, and community addictions staff. This role is supported by a multidisciplinary team of medical, nursing, and healthcare assistant staff. Satellite services within the community and aligned to each hub provide a Tier 3 service with a move to provide intrauterine contraceptive devices where possible. These services are led by either a specialist nurse or an advanced nurse practitioner. The services are all supported by Sandyford Central Tier 5 service, where consultant-led specialist advice and services are available by telephone or to facilitate patient transfer when needed.

In addition to a full range of sexual and reproductive health care, the main Sandyford service also provides termination of pregnancy and referral services, community gynecology (e.g., hysteroscopy and hysteroscopic sterilization), a range of community colposcopy treatments, and local anesthetic vasectomy operations. The Steve Retson Project was established in 1994 to meet the specific sexual health and well-being needs of gay men, many of whom are at risk for HIV, syphilis, and other STIs. Although a majority of gay men access mainstream sexual health clinics, there is a significant number who prefer and benefit from access to a designated clinical service. Nurse-led community outreach services are provided to individuals who are homeless and living in hostels, individuals with addictions under court supervision orders, and women involved in prostitution. An extensive range of sexual and reproductive health services are provided within these outreach sites; where this is not possible, assisted attendance at a mainstream Sandyford clinic is ensured. These nurse-led services enable access to sexual and reproductive health care for individuals who find it particularly difficult to access mainstream health services.

Accredited counselors provide a substantial range of therapeutic interventions to patients through Sandyford Counseling and Support Services. This counseling service is unique in that individuals can self-refer, although many clients are referred by other healthcare professionals. Counselors with specific competence in psychological therapies provide support through a "Listening Ear" service for patients in crisis. This is a one-off session to establish a patient's needs and provides an opportunity for assessment or referral to other services such as community mental health teams or psychiatrists as appropriate. Their work is aligned to that of other professionals working within community mental health teams.

The addition of an open-access library and information center with computer access within Sandyford Central provides a source of up-to-date literature in a variety of formats and can also be accessed by the general public, even if not attending specific health services. The library is staffed by professional librarians who ensure a range of materials is available in a variety of formats within Central and each Hub. This supports integration of sexual health services within the local communities and provides a robust platform for dissemination of public health and well-being materials.

Sandyford's suite of service provision includes the Glasgow Archway, the rape and sexual assault center in Scotland. Opened in 2007, 10 years later it remains the only such center in Scotland. This service provides forensic medical examination to individuals reporting rape or sexual assault within the past 7 days and is supported by a team of experienced sexual health nurses. Support workers and counselors are available to provide support to victims of rape or sexual assault to facilitate recovery, extending that support through court hearings, as necessary.

Workforce and Workforce Development

Sandyford services are led by a general manager and supported by a small senior management team that includes the head of nursing and the clinical director. The unit is consultant-led with service design and delivery supported by a large team of senior nurses and doctors, administrative staff, and allied health professionals. The role of some staff groups is described here.

Medical consultants are supported by a range of doctors with specialist qualifications in GUM and reproductive health. The service participates in medical faculty training programs as an approved training institution, providing a range of opportunities for medical staff to achieve specialist qualifications.

Nursing staff are well represented and are the largest workforce in Sandyford, working across a wide range of professional roles. Training and experience is provided for undergraduate pre-registration nurses and postgraduate registered nurses undertaking specialist qualifications.

Clinical biomedical scientists at Sandyford Central provide accredited laboratory services, such as immediate reporting on prepared slides and can support differential diagnoses with a high level of accuracy (e.g., the presence of gram-negative diplococci in the diagnosis of gonorrhea). This can improve patient care through reducing the time treat patients from first presentation. Laboratory staff are trained to national standards and are professionally managed by senior staff employed within NHS hospital-accredited laboratories.

Uniquely, Sandyford employed a community access coordinator to work with service users and would-be service users to improve access; in particular, those who have difficulty accessing sexual health services. In addition, the role facilitates service evaluations and contributes to equality impact assessments within the service. No service would be complete without a range of administrative support, such as medical secretaries, information technology, receptionists, and telephone answering staff. These roles all complement the work of the clinical staff and provide a valuable front-line service to the public.

In building an integrated service, it was apparent that some medical and nursing staff had worked exclusively within one service area and therefore were not likely to have the necessary clinical knowledge and skills to work within and across both disciplines. Staff development was supported through the creation of knowledge- and skills-based competency frameworks. Staff were encouraged to complete a skills audit via an anonymous paper-based survey, although response rates varied due to reluctance of some staff to identify areas of needed development. Questions ranged from competence to perform speculum examination and cervical smear tests to venipuncture and eliciting a sexual history. Additional questions explored staff confidence in sexual history taking, as many family planning staff would not have had experience in seeing male patients, let alone asking detailed and explicit questions about an individual's sexual activity. The audit results were very helpful in establishing that a substantial investment in education and in-house training/ shadowing programs would be necessary for all staff to develop the necessary competence to successfully run an integrated service.

The organization provided training sessions on "attitudes and values," facilitated by members of the Sexual Health

Improvement Team and designed to explore individual clinicians' own perceptions and encourage reflection. All clinical and administration staff were invited to attend these sessions, and the majority found the experience enlightening and very positive. Some staff found the experience challenging, as they had not been exposed to this type of learning environment before and found it difficult to have long-standing personal beliefs questioned and challenged in a supportive way. Despite this, the values and attitudes training proved to be a fundamental part of the workforce development applied across all staff groups, supporting the required behavior changes necessary to integrate the services.

Another area of change was role development. The goal was to allow patients to be seen by the most appropriate practitioner at the time of presentation. From that goal, new workforce roles emerged. One example of this is the healthcare support worker role, where individuals with a minimum educational qualification of Scottish Vocational Qualification level 2 or 3 will undertake specific tasks that have been delegated by a registered nurse or doctor. This may or may not involve direct patient contact. Within Sandyford, this role is called a "healthcare assistant" and was developed from one of no direct patient contact to the provision of one-to-one patient care supporting asymptomatic sexual health testing. A major concern with the development of these roles has been one of public protection and accountability, as until now, they have not been required to register with a professional body such as the Nursing and Midwifery Council (NMC) in the United Kingdom. This accountability for practice was the responsibility of the individual head of service and led to much variation in practice and responsibility. Healthcare support workers are currently going through a process to provide the public and employers with reassurance that robust systems are in place to ensure high standards of conduct similar to registered staff. In Scotland, all sexual healthcare staff sign a code of conduct contract. There are associated mandatory induction standards that all employers are required to adhere to as an assurance of quality. It is anticipated that this will provide employees with a sound measure of what is expected of them and should be used within the context of existing job descriptions and employer's policies and protocols. Not all staff working within health care are appropriately supported by their employers; however, the legal framework is being reinforced to protect the public.

The process of regulation and working to professional codes is well established for nurses, medical staff, and some allied health professionals; however, the NMC is currently reviewing its code of conduct and ethics and is likely to produce documentation to provide more robust guidance to directors of nursing to support professional decision-making with respect to accountability in practice.

Exemplar of Good Practice

Capacity building within the workforce through the development of specific competencies to support existing nursing roles, and new roles such as healthcare assistants, allowed registered staff to undertake more direct patient care. Improving the skill-mix of staff can increase productivity through allowing patients to be seen by the most appropriate practitioner and can provide opportunities for role and career development, such as advanced nurse practitioners.

Partnerships

All the healthcare interventions provided at Sandyford are done in partnership with colleagues across many disciplines within health and social care. Strategic planning frameworks to facilitate this are developed with local community health partnerships and local government planning groups.

There are multiple partnerships involved in the development and sustainability of an integrated sexual health service. Some involve financial support or accommodation; others involve decisions on meeting the specific sexual health needs of a local population. These relationships vary in their complexity; some can be extremely productive, others can be difficult to sustain, and still others may be subject to inequitable decision-making. The most productive partnerships are those in which there is a common purpose and agreement about what is to be achieved. The nursing leadership has been at the center of a partnership developed through the identification of gaps in service provision. This leadership has enabled the nursing profession to influence service design and delivery, which is important, as the majority of specialist sexual and reproductive health care is undertaken by nurses and healthcare support workers.

The strategic vision for professional nursing in Scotland comes from the chief nursing officer (CNO) who is a key member of the Scottish government's Health Directorate. As a direct report to the Cabinet Secretary for Health, this post holder is in a highly influential position and as head of profession is directly responsible for ensuring that the nursing and midwifery workforce is fit to undertake the roles required within health policy. The CNO is responsible for developing strategic nursing initiatives and ensuring that nursing and midwifery professional practice is modernized to keep pace with economic priorities and challenges.

The strategic vision for public health, including sexual health, blood-borne viruses, and HIV, is led by the Scottish Government, and the National Sexual Health and HIV Committee is chaired by the Minister for Public Health. The lead clinicians for sexual health and HIV were appointed following a recommendation made within Respect and Responsibility 2005 (The Scottish Government, 2008). The lead clinician and lead nurse roles make an important multidisciplinary partnership and an opportunity to provide strong strategic leadership to promote sexual health and well-being.

In Scotland, lead medical and nursing colleagues from across different health board areas meet regularly to discuss and agree on how best to deliver the government's strategic vision in relation to sexual health. Having this solidarity and consensus of senior colleagues is a very powerful tool to utilize when undertaking local negotiations. Having the ability to share ideas and good practice in a formal and constructive way has led to significant improvements in sexual health care throughout Scotland and has been well supported by the Scottish Government Health Directorate, ensuring a direct link between policy development and policy implementation. Clear evaluation measures developed in partnership with the lead clinicians and lead nurses demonstrate where there has been successful modernization of sexual health services.

U.K. countries have policy documents that should include recommendations to support nursing leadership being at the forefront of service modernization. Nursing is the largest workforce within the National Health Service, and as such, nursing leadership should be fully represented at all levels of the organization.

Patients are our most important partners and it is important to seek the views of service users and potential service users. National patient experience programs, such as Better Together (Bruster, 2008), were designed to ensure that patient experience was used across services to provide a benchmark of acceptability and performance. Sandyford has a long tradition of seeking users' views on service provision, which has informed many developments and service changes. Input is collected in a variety of ways, including comment cards, compliments, complaints, user surveys, and focus groups. Proactively asking for user feedback and not relying on reactive responses to complaints is important in any organization. The relationship with service users can be difficult due to the balance of maintaining service provision within a financial framework and meeting user expectations of what the service should provide.

Exemplar of Good Practice

At the start of integration there were difficulties with patients being seen by one clinician for their sexual health testing and treatment and having to see another clinician for their contraceptive needs. This generated long waiting times and treatment delays. Feedback from patients suggested that if possible, they would prefer to see one clinician who could deliver all the services they required at one visit. They had no preference for whether this was a doctor or a nurse, as long as they were professional in approach, competent, and showed respect for the individual patient's needs. This patient feedback was valued and underpinned some of the work to support staff competence development.

The fundamental principle underpinning all nurse, midwife, and allied health professional (NMAHP) practice is the acquisition of evidence-based knowledge and skills. This may be achieved in a variety of ways, including through formal educational courses. Sexual and reproductive health is one of many specialty areas available through university study at the post-graduate and master's level. Foundation sexuality modules have also been incorporated into some undergraduate nursing courses, which is an important step in "normalizing" sexual health.

Close multidisciplinary partnerships with the Faculty of Sexual and Reproductive Healthcare (FSRH) and the British Association for Sexual Health and HIV (BASHH) have supported educational development. These two bodies are responsible for ensuring national standards in relation to medical training and clinical practice, which in turn supports the development of nurse training and clinical practice. Both organizations provide accessible learning options for nurses, including some accredited distance learning modules with a nursing diploma award. This new development has come about through the persistent lobbying and influence of professional nursing leaders across the United Kingdom.

The Royal College of Nursing published Sexual Health Competencies (Royal College of Nursing, 2004) and the British HIV Nurses Association published HIV Nursing Competencies (National HIV Nurses Association, 2007). Both documents are extremely useful and have the capacity to inform sexual health nursing practice across a range of specialist and non-specialist settings. These should be used within the context of local protocols and guidelines. Individual nursing roles and practice may differ according to the country and area of practice, but this should not be fundamentally different from published practice.

Partnership work with NHS Education for Scotland (NES) has facilitated the development of a career framework for nurses providing sexual health care. It has also provided an opportunity to showcase the work of sexual health nurses in Scotland and the range of new roles they have developed. Successful lobbying of NES has resulted in the inclusion of competence standards for a sexual health advisor within the existing sexual health nursing competency framework, which further supports the work of integrated services and workforce development.

Within health care in Scotland, there are shared governance systems to ensure that services (including sexual health care) are appropriately designed and delivered within a local area. Services like Sandyford provide services in many different local government areas on behalf of the area health board. This involves multiple partnerships with staff within local health areas to ensure that sexual health service delivery in their area meets local population needs. There will usually be a local strategic decision-making group consisting of representatives from local government and education, as well as a range of health providers. This group will interpret guidance and standards from strategic documents and develop services designed for local populations. Not all local governments will have an approach, with some being more progressive and others more reluctant to change.

There can be challenges made from locally elected representatives to local councils and members of parliament when service changes are made and constituents make complaints. Although the changes may be in line with current strategy and serve the greater good, and may have been made following consultation with community groups, these changes may conflict with what an individual within a local community may expect. Elected representatives can be very supportive and provide a more positive approach to service provision. Their networking skills and influencing can be beneficial in promoting change either locally or at a national level, such as lobbying for a change in national policy to support the development of sexual assault and referral centers.

A small but significant amount of sexual health care is delivered by non-NHS voluntary agencies and this should complement the work of established healthcare services by establishing access to vulnerable individuals and allowing for a more tailored approach within communities. British Pregnancy Advisory Service (BPAS) is one such organization, providing a range of contraception and termination of pregnancy services. Sandyford has a long-established partnership with BPAS to support women who present for termination of pregnancy and require referral to services in England. This nurse-led arrangement supports access to a service not currently provided within Scotland due to late gestational age. The numbers of women accessing late termination of pregnancy in Scotland are currently low (Information Services Division Scotland, 2011). There has been significant work done over the past 10 years to support improved access to contraception, including long-acting methods and improved access to early termination of pregnancy. This has been achieved through significant investment in the education of healthcare professionals to facilitate early access to appropriate information, advice, and referral. These are all thought to be contributory factors to the low levels of women requesting late termination of pregnancy. Sandyford works with partner agencies across area health boards to ensure that services are accessible to patients and has developed referral pathways between primary care and hospitals, utilizing early medical discharge following termination of pregnancy and provision of specific medical expertise where required.

Clinical priorities in sexual health are developed in partnership with public health practitioners who have overall responsibility for population based-health initiatives. They are informed by data published by the information statistics division of the Scottish Government who are in turn informed by services such as Sandyford. There is a close correlation with harm-reduction work within sexual health and addiction services working to reduce transmission of blood-borne viruses, particularly HIV and hepatitis B and C. Sexual health improvement specialists provide

a valuable support to Sandyford staff, delivering clinical services through asset-based and targeted sexual health prevention and education programs. They also provide training and support materials to education partners, teachers and residential care home staff as part of the collaborative approach to improving sexual health through the provision of sexual health education in schools.

Local hospital services are essential partners in the provision of sexual health services and integrated care pathways have been developed with respect to termination of pregnancy referral. This enables a streamlined approach to care of women requesting termination of pregnancy and ensures a high standard of communication between services. HIV services are provided in partnership with staff at the Brownlee Infectious Diseases Unit. Medical and nursing expertise is provided to individuals diagnosed with HIV and requiring treatment or ongoing care. Primary care physicians and nurses providing sexual and reproductive health care are supported by Sandyford through the development of specific competencies, such as contraceptive implant fitting and removal, and the appropriate management of clients with STIs.

Strong working partnerships have been established with clinicians who care for people with learning disabilities, physical disabilities, addictions, and young people, including those in foster care or group homes. Interdisciplinary communication helps support continuity of care for the most vulnerable in society. A Managed Clinical Network for Sexual Health was established to support cooperation and collaboration between NHS health boards. This has supported the development of shared clinical protocols that are used across health board areas which helps to reduce variation in patient care.

Nursing Policy

The development of a workforce that can meet the challenges of today's complex sexual healthcare environment is ongoing. Modernizing Nursing Careers (Department of Health, 2006; Scottish Government, 2006) provided a national framework to support NMAHP leadership across healthcare services and positions this leadership concept as a central theme within health service structures. This framework was developed across all four U.K. countries and can be used to evidence the need for new and existing nurse leadership roles and influence change. It also recognizes a role for nurses with advanced practice skills and competencies to undertake a range of client care and emphasizes that opportunities should be developed within organizations to support this.

In Scotland, key documents such as *Delivering for Health* (Scottish Executive, 2005a) and *Better Health, Better Care* (Scottish Government, 2007), were published to support the leadership role of nurses and midwives and asserted the belief that this leadership is fundamental to care delivery. The plethora of policy documents to support this fundamental principle were summarized in *Curam*

(Scottish Government, 2009), a publication designed to reinvigorate the nursing profession across all disciplines and realign the key nursing principles of care and compassion. Within sexual health these policy documents were utilized to strengthen the arguments for nursing leadership and develop new roles, such as lead nurses, clinical governance, and practice development nurses. Advanced practice roles that facilitate greater involvement in the clinical care of patients with complex conditions further strengthen the leadership role of nurses in sexual health services. The Scottish Sexual Health Strategy, Respect and Responsibility (Scottish Executive, 2005b) advocated for nurse leadership to have a central role in sexual and reproductive health initiatives designed to improve the patient journey and experience.

Educational Preparation

Historically, the National Board for Nursing and Midwifery Scotland ratified courses in family planning, but there was no equivalent for GUM nursing. This was a predecessor to the United Kingdom Central Council, started in 1983, which then became the Nursing and Midwifery Council in 2002. Nurses and midwives providing sexual and reproductive health services within the United Kingdom must be registered with the NMC. The NMC has a statutory responsibility to ensure appropriate preregistration education standards for nursing and midwifery, but not for post-registration standards.

Lead nurses for sexual and reproductive health across Scotland lobbied for formal recognition of the leadership provided by senior nurses through strategic planning arenas arguing that they should be an integral part of local service developments and delivery, leading on service design and workforce planning. The publication of *A National Career Framework for Nurses Working within Sexual and Reproductive Health Services* (NHS Education for Scotland, 2009), which was developed by members of the Scottish Lead Nurse Group and NHS Education for Scotland, helped to articulate the differences in educational level and suggested scope of competence expected across a nurse's career in the specialty. Each level was linked to the national nursing pay scales. This provides a toolkit for nurses and managers to benchmark roles and career pathways throughout a range of services, ensuring standards are consistent with agreed professional and educational standards. The document can be used by nurses working across a range of settings (e.g., school nurses, practice nurses, and specialist and public health nurses). It is not prescriptive, and local variation in service delivery models will inform specific competences required. What is particularly important about this document is that it is the first published career framework for sexual health nursing. It recognizes the diversity within sexual health nursing, the scope and range of nurse involvement in sexual health care, and the need to provide a supportive and robust framework to support service and workforce planning. This framework puts nurses at the forefront of care planning and delivery and as such requires strong leadership within the profession to ensure its implementation. It also requires nurses to have the confidence to take the lead in patient care, which can only be achieved through demonstrating they are highly educated and appropriately skilled to undertake the necessary care of clients.

Professional Nursing Leadership

There has always been a clearly defined nursing leadership position central to Sandyford that was embedded in the organization's senior management structure. This arrangement ensures strategic authority and autonomy in addition to operational management responsibility. The head of nursing role has strategic links to the nurse director of the NHS board and the service general manager. Leadership development and succession planning within the nursing team has created a strong culture of maximizing each nurse's leadership capability, instilling the importance of nurse leadership at all points of the patient journey to ensure excellence in care. Nurses are encouraged to take responsibility for their own actions and to challenge the actions and behaviors of their colleagues where they are not in keeping with the organization's leadership culture.

The head of nursing provides strategic leadership to all nurses and allied health professionals and is supported by a team of senior nurses. The nurses have delegated responsibility to ensure appropriate line management, staff development, and performance and have regular communication with the head of nursing.

The following senior roles support the work at Sandyford:

- The *clinical governance coordinator* role is central to ensuring Sandyford meets all aspects of governance, such as health and safety, risk management, and clinical effectiveness. The coordinator works with service managers and senior managers to ensure a proactive approach to risk management. The role also supports the development and implementation of a robust audit framework to help provide an evidence base for service effectiveness.

- It is the responsibility of each *senior nurse* to ensure that principles of the governance framework are embedded across nursing and clinical practice.

- Workforce development is an essential component of any service area, and in Sandyford this is supported by the *practice development nurse*. The nurse in this role translates workforce development plans into action. It is essential to have a motivational leader in this type of post, someone who has enthusiasm for change and who can engage staff to learn new skills and translate them into practice.

- The *clinical coordinator* supports the day-to-day operational management of the service, including pharmacy budgeting, stock and equipment ordering, and ensuring health and safety and infection control measures are implemented and high standards maintained. Ensuring an appropriate skill mix of staff within each clinical location is a major part of this role.

- The *senior sexual health advisor* supports adherence to public health standards and partner notification and provides training to staff from other disciplines across health services as well as medical students.
- The *Archway Glasgow lead nurse* ensures nurse delivery of elements of the forensic medical examination, maintaining forensic integrity of the environment and samples obtained and ensuring appropriate professional standards and behaviors of nurses working within the sexual assault referral center. This is a very challenging environment to work in due to the complexity and frequently distressing nature of the cases.

All senior nurses maintain specialist clinical skills through face-to-face patient consultations. They provide line management to a group of staff ensuring appropriate staff governance across the service, address staff performance issues, and support staff recruitment and retention. Some specific leadership responsibility is delegated to a small team of nurses who provide a range of services to specific client groups (e.g., homeless individuals, women requesting termination of pregnancy, young people, and individuals in prison). These nurses provide specific expertise and leadership to the wider clinical team members and ensure that organizational objectives are translated into clinical practice. Nurses are all encouraged to demonstrate leadership skills in all aspects of clinic and client management, with some undertaking further leadership competencies. Senior nurses continue to lead on all aspects of service development and provide guidance and support to the wider nursing team.

Leadership is provided in all Sandyford Hubs through designated nurses who are actively involved in promoting Sandyford services within their local communities, sit on local planning groups, and participate in service design. Part of their leadership role is to support members of the community to learn more about sexual health services. This might be done by inviting individuals from groups with known access needs to tour the services and learn about how the staff can make a positive impact on sexual health and well-being. These nurses work in close partnership with key staff in the community health centers.

Professional Considerations

The following section discusses some fundamental principles to support clinical practice that should be considered as essential requirements.

It is imperative that nurses are adequately supported when working within the complex environment of sexual health. Issues that arise include undertaking face-to-face consultations to explore an individual's sexuality and sexual behavior, both past and present, to effectively assess their risk of sexually transmitted infection and blood-borne virus. Disclosures of sexual abuse and/or assault can add to the complexity of the relationship. There is a relatively short time available within the consultation in which to build a trusting therapeutic relationship with patients, and this can make it increasingly difficult for nurses to make appropriate decisions. There is often conflict between time management and meeting patients' needs. The added conflict of knowing that some questions, no matter how essential to ask, may cause distress to the patient when they recall events that were previously "forgotten" may add to the nurse feeling less effective and perhaps question the validity of the consultation process. Professional differences are also a consideration, particularly if the patient's needs cannot be met by the individual nurse, who may feel disempowered when passing care to another clinician.

Clinical supervision is an effective means of providing a robust framework for nurses to face their own prejudices and share their experiences of client and peer interactions and reactions. Nurses are human beings who have personal and emotional experiences of their own that may impact their ability to do their job well. They need to be able to recognize when factors prevent them from communicating well with and showing care and compassion toward their patients. Nurses who have traditionally been seen as taking charge of a situation and providing "care and support" to individuals can find it difficult to accept that it is neither appropriate nor possible to meet the needs of all patients all of the time. Nurses must be supported to prevent emotional burn-out. A confident nurse who has been appropriately educated and well supported at work will often be less affected by patient trauma than a nurse who is poorly prepared for the role and who feels underequipped to deal with the challenges of patient stories. Having an opportunity to "debrief" either with a supportive partner/friend or colleague at work before they leave will minimize the long-term effects of stress.

Peer supervision should be provided by those who have undertaken specific training in supervision counseling or by counselors accredited by the British Association of Counselors and Psychotherapists. It is useful but not essential for the supervisor to have direct experience of the specialty. Supervision is a supportive process and should not be confused with line management and case load supervision, and where possible should be kept separate and undertaken by different individuals. Individual supervision sessions should take place in a private environment free from noise and interruptions, ideally within the workplace. This protected time should be valued by managers and service providers as an essential and fundamental part of the nursing role.

Nursing supervision at Sandyford is based on an internally designed model that meets the needs of a large and diverse workforce in which individual staff deal with conflict, complexity, and trauma differently. Healthcare assistants are included in the supervision process, particularly as their role becomes more developed and more involved in direct patient care. They were encouraged to participate in group supervision to provide a forum to validate their concerns and articulate frustrations through facilitated peer discussion. This was successful, as it allowed the group to explore and find solutions to benefit the whole team, and team members felt the process was positive and supportive.

Nurses may be suspicious of supervision if they have never been offered it before, and some may say they don't need it. It is essential to articulate properly what the framework would look like, why it is being offered, and what the perceived benefits might be to the individual and to the organization. Aligning the supervision model to an existing development plan, strategic framework, or policy plan will help support access to the necessary funding. Personal experience of having participated in clinical supervision will vary widely within staff groups and it is important to publicize the benefits to nurses and nursing. It is also important to articulate how it can improve patient care and benefit patients.

Exemplar of Good Practice

The individual responsible for the professional nursing leadership within the organization, no matter how small or large, should ensure that clinical supervision is provided within their service area. There is a small financial cost attached to providing supervision, but this can be minimized if there is investment in peer education through attendance at a recognized post-graduate certificate level course.

Peer support is interpreted here as provision of encouragement to others in a supportive environment, whether on an individual basis or in a group setting. In a group setting, there should be a clear focus for discussion, a group leader, and a framework for how the group will be run. It may be necessary to have different peer support groups for nurses in the different service areas. These groups allow nurses to share practice issues and ensure they are up to date with new developments. Peer support can also be provided ad hoc through debriefing with colleagues at the end of a clinical session or over a cup of coffee in the staff base. It should be provided by the individual with the most relevant experience in the field to avoid confusion and conflicting messages to staff. Consultant staff, where available, or senior nursing or clinical staff should be encouraged to provide accessible peer support to junior staff. Senior clinical staff should be encouraged to ask individual clinical staff how they feel about the patient cases they may have seen that day and to provide an opportunity for reflective discussion. This

allows staff to highlight concerns or questions that they might not have thought important or relevant. Clinical case review and case-based discussions can also form part of the peer support process, either in a group or one-on-one, with cases presented anonymously so as to adhere to data protection and confidentiality legislation. This can be a good forum for discussion and clarification.

Exemplar of Good Practice

Practitioners seldom work in isolation; instead, they work increasingly as part of a multidisciplinary team. It is still possible for these individuals to feel professionally isolated and find it difficult to identify where support might be needed. It is important for nurse leaders to ensure that opportunities for peer discussion and review are promoted in the workplace. Organizations should promote and support a culture of lifelong learning.

Job descriptions are a vital tool in ensuring staff members have a clear understanding of what is expected of them. Articulating the level of practice required of the post will enable the post holder to evaluate what their learning needs are and gain the necessary skills and competence to achieve what is required. Nurses might not have a job description or might have one that is so outdated that it fails to reflect the role that is required of them. Service delivery models will change over time and so must job descriptions. This can be a lengthy, but rewarding process. Where there is to be a significant role change (i.e., taking more responsibility for more complex client presentations), the senior medical staff of the area should be involved in deliberating the rationale for the decision, the benefits for the patients, service improvement, and team motivation. Expanded nursing roles with more responsibility may challenge medical staff, who might feel concern about erosion of their role within the clinical service. Nurses may be nervous but excited by the prospect of undertaking more complex patient management and should be supported within the appropriate governance framework and with appropriate nursing leadership.

Different disciplines within healthcare have different arrangements for personal development planning and appraisal. Nurses and healthcare assistants working in the National Health Service have a clearly articulated framework for appraisal and development planning. It is an essential requirement for all staff working within healthcare to undertake a meaningful development review each year with a senior staff member. This individual needs to be aware of how to access training and development opportunities and possible funding sources to support these (e.g., training budgets).

Independent nurse prescribing (non-medical prescribing) is an additional qualification within the Nursing and Midwifery Council and is being taken up by a number of sexual health nurses across Scotland, giving nurses the scope to prescribe within their specialist area (Tyler & Hicks, 2001). This qualification has contributed to improved access to services and reduced waiting times for clients. Independent nurse prescribing has provided a robust framework for the provision of nurse-led services (Scottish Executive, 2006). Nurses working in sexual health should be actively encouraged and supported to undertake this qualification, as it can be used to further support autonomous decision-making in practice. Non-medical prescribers are also a more cost-effective prescribing resource than doctors, due to the significant pay differential. Sandyford has a long and safe record of medicines management, with nurses being well informed about the medicines they provide and having robust protocols to inform decision making. The use of Patient Group Directions (Nursing and Midwifery Council, 2007) has supported Sandyford nurses initiating and completing a range of episodes of care including contraceptive provision, oral postcoital contraception and contraceptive implants, and the provision of treatments for a range of infections. Patient Group Directions (documents that allow healthcare professionals to administer medication to groups of patients, without individual prescriptions) are developed locally and are subject to a rigorous, peer-reviewed validation process within the NHS Board Drug and Therapeutics Committee. They enhance nurses' decision-making capacity and capability and will often reduce waiting times and improve access to services for patients. Medical and nurse prescribers support decision-making and prescribing capacity when required, although by nature Patient Group Directions are limited in their scope and range and are not a substitute for nurses undertaking non-medical prescribing courses.

Scotland has been promoting access to long-acting reversible methods of contraception such as implants and intrauterine devices for some time. In an effort to improve access and reduce waiting times, nurses were invited to undertake faculty-approved training to develop competence in contraceptive implant fitting and removal. This was a quantum leap for the profession, as this had always been a medically led initiative and many medics questioned whether nurses would have the ability to perform this service safely. Training sessions were initially led by a medical consultant and process evaluations indicate nurses have had a positive experience. Patients appreciate the improved access to service and have confidence that the practitioner is highly skilled and qualified to undertake the role. This training has been provided to nurses working in gynecology services and to some community nurses. Intrauterine contraceptive device removal is a core competence for all Sandyford nurses; however, this is not true of national practice. This is a simple procedure and one that can easily be undertaken by a competent nurse.

In order to provide an efficient service to patients and reduce waiting times, nurses have led the development of competencies to support testing for and management of STIs and blood-borne viruses. Patients at increased risk of HIV or hepatitis B are excluded from nurse-led testing and instead are seen by a nurse with sexual health–advising competencies or a sexual health advisor. Patients with symptoms outside the scope of the nurse-led protocol or patients requesting to see a doctor will be seen by a member of the medical staff. Asymptomatic testing competencies were developed to support nurses to undertake individual patient risk assessment prior to testing. Nurses receive additional training in supporting and protecting sexually active young people to ensure a risk-based and appropriate response to requests for sexual health information or contraception.

The public health role of sexual health nurses is key to ensuring appropriate follow up where STI is suspected or diagnosed, through activities such as partner notification and delivery of risk-reduction strategies. Uncomplicated partner notification refers to individuals diagnosed with one infection who have one sexual partner within the partner notification period. Training for this core competency is delivered by nurses with sexual health advising competence and is followed through with supervised practice sessions. Nurses are signed off through a peer-review process and ongoing competence is assured through case-based discussion and audit. Cervical screening competence is assessed by a mix of theoretical learning, supervised practice, and review of sample results. This skill supports a national screening program to increase the detection of cervical cancer. Nurses must meet an agreed standard to maintain competence and are required to undertake further training and supervised practice if their individual rate of unsatisfactory smear results exceed the target.

Venipuncture was not previously a requirement for family planning staff, as there was no opportunity to use and maintain the skill. In a service as large as Sandyford that undertakes thousands of blood tests per year, it was determined that venipuncture should be a core competency for all staff in order to reduce waiting times. An in-house training program was developed by the senior nurse team and practice sessions were supported by a GU consultant. This simple skill has improved Sandyford's capacity to provide effective and efficient testing for blood-borne viruses.

In response to long waiting lists for patients accessing human papilloma virus (HPV) treatment, nurses were trained in the use of liquid nitrogen cryotherapy. This is currently a first-line therapy at Sandyford due to the relatively high cost of other topical treatments and requires multiple attendances to affect visible symptom reduction.

Healthcare assistants currently undertake a range of duties that were previously undertaken by registered nurses, including venipuncture, setting up and clearing sterile trolleys, and assisting at minor operations (e.g., local anesthetic vasectomy). This extended role has been very successful and has grown to incorporate patient-facing opt-in asymptomatic testing clinic duties. A short questionnaire is completed by the patient, and if all questions are answered "no," then the healthcare assistant can proceed to test. This has been well evaluated by patients and staff and has made a significant contribution in improving access and reducing waiting times for patients wanting asymptomatic testing.

The importance of attitude and values training for individuals undertaking a patient contact role cannot be underestimated. The role of chaperone is crucial within sexual health services and must be taken seriously by all staff involved. Chaperones must understand that they are there to protect the patient and act as patient advocate if required. The importance of body language and subtle nonverbal cues are particularly relevant within the context of genital examination. On successful completion of the competency framework, there is a letter sent from the Head of Nursing confirming their achievement and providing evidence for their personal development portfolio and CV, if required. Career development should be supported across all grades of staff, as it engenders a culture of investment in staff, succession planning, and leads to greater autonomy and, one would hope, job satisfaction.

Sandyford nurses have expanded their role through education and training and the demonstration of competence through utilizing competency-based workbooks. Appropriately skilled nurses undertake a range of clinical activity, supported by independent nurses, including vaccination, onward referral of clients, and partner notification. Nurses are fully involved in contraception planning and provision, including subdermal implant insertion and removal. Nurses have demonstrated competence in all aspects of client management with particular regard to showing sensitivity to vulnerable individuals. All nurses are required to undertake appropriate training and skills building to support the patient journey through an integrated sexual and reproductive health service. For example, many nurses who had worked in family planning services had little or no experience in working with male patients and were not comfortable with making enquiries about gay men's sexual behavior. This was addressed with staff on an individual basis where required before embarking on competency development training.

Following the successful implementation of asymptomatic testing competencies by nurses, symptomatic testing competencies were developed to support nurses in further expanding their role. Testing excluded complex medical conditions such as syphilis and HIV, recurrent infection, and dermatological conditions. Nurses may undertake a full sexual history and symptomatic testing according to protocol. If the findings are within the nurse-led protocol, then treatment may be given; however, if the findings are inconclusive or fall outside of protocol, the nurse will seek advice of a senior colleague. This initiative again improved access to services for patients and reduced waiting times. It has provided nurses with a robust governance framework to participate more widely in client management and is an excellent example of nurse-led safe and effective person-centered practice within a multidisciplinary environment.

Sandyford provides an accessible termination of pregnancy and referral service to women upon request. An integrated care pathway was developed with local gynecology services to facilitate improved access to termination services. Women attending nurses have undertaken FSRH-approved ultrasound training to support access and reduce waiting times. This imaging is for pregnancy confirmation and dating purposes only. There is no diagnostic component, and medical ultrasonographers are available in the department at all times, if required.

Barriers to Nursing Role Development

Barriers to role development may come from the individual, within the profession, other professional groups or the organization. This is one of the most challenging areas, and one that takes careful planning and organization. It is important to communicate clearly what any role change might be and "sell it" to the staff who might be subject to the change. There has long been a drive in the health service to improve capacity and build capability within the workforce. This has never been more evident than in the past few years with a plethora of new roles being developed along with education and leadership programs to support these individuals. The move to graduate-level exit awards for registered nurses has made it even more important that nurses already working in all areas of sexual health care have the knowledge and skills to ensure a capable and confident workforce.

The nursing profession has an established tradition of role development and growth. This has for the most part been a successful evolution and one that has seen nurses take responsibility for a greater amount of patient care. This has been to some extent an ad hoc development without clear strategic vision and planning. Local initiatives have supported the development of some roles, some have been developed due to a reduction in resource for other staff groups or change in terms and conditions, and some based on an individual nurse's willingness to undertake a particular role or task. Responsibility for patient management provides nurses with an opportunity to develop a clear strategic vision and multidisciplinary partnership approach to role expansion.

Best practices for role development based on the Sandyford model include the following:

- Encouraging nurses to delegate tasks where appropriate within local protocols
- Networking with peers to share good practices, service models, guidelines, and protocols
- Spending quality time developing working action plans and documents to reflect planned changes

U.S. Initiatives Toward Development of Knowledgeable and Competent Sexual and Reproductive Health Workforce

In the United States, recognition of the deficient number of appropriately trained and competent sexual and reproductive health (SRH) practitioners resulted in the 2012 RAND Corporation study. This project was conducted to analyze the demand, supply, and employment of adequately trained and qualified health professionals competent to deliver SRH care and services, with particular emphasis on nurse practitioners (NPs). The evidence showed definite increase in demand for SRH services since implementation of the Affordable Care Act (ACA) (Auerbach et al., 2012).

Specific Factors Associated with Deficient Preparatory Programs and Limited Employment of SRH NPs

- Inadequate theory and clinical practice experience provided to nursing students on sexual and reproductive health care in pre-licensure RN programs
- Emphasis on generic nursing education and training programs
- Lack of standardization for implementation of core competencies and curricula content
- Limited opportunities for clinical training in SRH
- Lack of loan repayment options
- Fragmented nature of SRH care delivery and disconnection from primary care (Auerbach et al., 2012)

The RAND Corporation study (Auerbach et al., 2012) recommends policy interventions to align SRH education, practice, and credentialing to meet workforce needs. The need for pre-licensure competency-based SRH education, continuous professional development and service delivery is acknowledged. In the 2008 report, "From Education to Regulation: Dynamic Challenges for the Health Workforce," Dower (2008) pointed out that licensure on a state-by-state basis hinders mobility of appropriately qualified health professionals and explores the feasibility of workforce capacity expansion by aligning practice activities more closely with competencies. In the same report, Collier (2008) noted ongoing concerns that education and workforce distribution have not been addressed appropriately in the United States.

Summary of the RAND Corporation's Recommendations

- Adopting a unified and standard definition of SRH as advocated by the WHO. Thus, the previous narrow definition encompassing maternal–child, family planning and women's health care now acknowledges the reproductive health of men and women throughout the lifespan. Additional elements in this comprehensive definition are preconception, contraception, pregnancy, women's health and common gynecological routine care, men's genitourinary conditions, infertility, and sexual health promotion. These should be provided within the contexts of public health and primary care.
- Another recommendation is to implement a standardized, interprofessional curriculum for teaching required SRH core competencies. The World Health Organization's (WHO, 2011) standard set of domains and core competencies for SRH provides a basis for competency-based SRH education, practice, and credentialing within a coordinated system of primary care and public health.

The model employed in the U.K. NHS sexual health system illustrates an interpretation and translation of the WHO's recommended comprehensive integrated SRH services. The following 10 areas of competence are stipulated:

- Basic skills and services for sexual and reproductive health care
- Contraception
- Unplanned pregnancy
- Women's health and common gynecological problems
- Assessment of specialist gynecological problems
- Pregnancy
- Genitourinary conditions of men
- Sexual health promotion
- Public health, ethical, and legal issues
- Leadership, management, health technology, quality assurance (Faculty of Sexual and Reproductive Healthcare [FSRH], 2010; Royal College of Nursing, 2009; Royal College of Obstetricians and Gynaecologists [RCOG], 2009)

Models for SRH Implementation in the United States

In the United States, different models have been proposed to achieve effective implementation of the SRH core competencies. The exemplars noted by the RAND Corporation include the Arizona State University (ASU) College of Nursing and Health Innovation, the RN–APRN Team Model of Family Planning and Public Health Services (Southeastern Department of Public Health), and the Urban Northeastern area. A brief outline is provided here as described by RAND Corporation (Auerbach et al., 2012).

- Model I. Aligning clinical practice and education (ASU College of Nursing and Health Innovation model): This model aligns primary care delivery and family planning services with education.
- Model II. The RN–APRN Team Model of Family Planning and Public Health Services: This is a preventive health integrated-services model that merges family planning, STD/HIV, immunization, adult, and adolescent services as an integrated

clinical program for men, women, and adolescents. The team-based workforce comprises public health nurses and advanced practice registered nurses (APRNs).

- Model III. Adolescent reproductive health service delivery: This model portrays two approaches to adolescent reproductive health service delivery.
  - A health system-affiliated center that partners with local community school-based health center.
  - Family planning services that partner with a community nonprofit youth organization and health system–affiliated health centers and academic partners. This healthcare system integrates primary and specialty care, community hospitals, academic medical centers, specialty facilities, community health centers, community health improvement, and health professional training programs (Auerbach et al., 2012).

There is no doubt that interdisciplinary learning has the potential advantage to foster more meaningful clinical and professional learning among students in different of professional disciplines. Additionally, addressing the impact of the fragmentation of SRH services requires strong dedication, continuity of care, and management commitment (Wisby & Capell, 2005). Collaboration is crucial in terms of interdisciplinary, interprofessional, and interagency alliance and partnerships. A standard competency framework for SRH allows for benchmarking roles and responsibilities and can also be useful to define job specifications and career planning. Furthermore, the competency framework provides a basis for education and training requirements. Managers and clinical educators are able to review their own strengths and identify gaps in their professional capacity as they apply the framework to SRH care. The framework is also useful for informing the commissioning, development, and delivery of training and education, as well as supervision, recruitment, and selection procedures (Wisby & Capell, 2005).

Conclusion

Sandyford presents as an exemplar of best practice and readers can learn from the lessons of staff leadership and staff development there. Individuals with professional leadership responsibility or those aspiring to lead the profession in the provision of clinical services should themselves be aspirational and inspirational. Having a vision for the future delivery of services and a keen eye to identify improvements or efficiencies in provision is helpful. Recognizing what is appropriate development of a nurse role will ensure safe practice for the public and the professional. It is important to staff to believe that nursing leaders have a true understanding of the challenges facing them in their everyday working environment. It is also useful to have a sound

practical knowledge of the clinical service and its delivery model in order to identify opportunities for change.

Succession planning is fundamental to service progress and the professional development of others should be seen as a core part of any nurse leader's role. It is very satisfying to see individuals learn and gain confidence to manage more and more complex situations and problems.

Change within an organization can present opportunities that may not have been expected. There are many resources available to explain and support the management of change and leadership development. In addition to academic learning and resources, coaching and mentorship should be considered sources of support. Change management is an art form, do it well and it will create something beautiful.

• • • REFERENCES

Auerbach, D. I., Pearson, M. L., Taylor, D., Batistelli, M., Sussell, J., Hunter, L. E., . . . Schneider, E. C. (2012). Nurse practitioners and reproductive health services: An analysis of supply and demand. Santa Monica, CA: RAND Corporation. Retrieved from https://www.rand.org/pubs/technical_reports/TR1224.html

Bruster, B. (2008). *Better together: Scotland's patient experience programme: building on the experiences of NHS. Scottish Government Social Research*. Retrieved from http://patientperspective.org/wp-content/uploads/2014/10/Scottish-Government-Building-on-the-Experience-of-Patients.pdf

Collier, S. N. (2008). Changes in the health workforce: Trends, issues, and credentialing. In D. E. Holmes (Ed.), *From education to regulation: Dynamic challenges for the health workforce* (pp. 1–20). Washington, DC: Association of Academic Health Centers. Retrieved from http://www.aahcdc.org/Portals/41/Publications-Resources/BooksAndReports/From_Education_to_Regulation.pdf

Djuretic, T., Catchpole, M., Nicoll, A., Hughes, G., Bingham, J., Robinson, A., & Kinghorn, G. (2001). Genitourinary medicine services in the United Kingdom are failing to meet current demand. *International Journal of Sexually Transmitted Diseases & AIDS, 12*(9), 571–572.

Dower, C. (2008). Pulling regulatory levers to improve healthcare. In D. E. Holmes (Ed.), *From education to regulation: Dynamic challenges for the health workforce* (pp. 47–62). Washington, DC: Association of Academic Health Centers. Retrieved from http://www.aahcdc.org/Portals/41/Publications-Resources/BooksAndReports/From_Education_to_Regulation.pdf

Faculty of Sexual & Reproductive Healthcare (FSRH). (2010). *Training curriculum plan*. London, United Kingdom: Author.

Gravelle, H., & Sutton, M. (2003). Income related inequalities in self assessed health in Britain: 1979-1995. *Journal of Epidemiology & Community Health, 57*, 125–129.

Health Protection Scotland. (2017). Surveillance Reports. HIV Infections and AIDS: Quarterly report to 31 December 2016. *HPS Weekly Report, 51*(11). Retrieved from http://www.hps.scot.nhs.uk/ewr/article.aspx#

Information Services Division Scotland. (2011). Abortions Statistics - Year ending 31 December 2010. Retrieved from http://www.isdscotland.scot.nhs.uk

National Health Services Scotland. (2017). *Termination of pregnancy statistics*. Retrieved from https://www.isdscotland.org

/Health-Topics/Sexual-Health/Publications/2017-05-30/2017-05-30-Terminations-2016-Report.pdf

NHS Education for Scotland. (2009). *A career framework for nursing in sexual and reproductive health*. Edinburgh, United Kingdom: Author.

Nursing and Midwifery Council. (2007). *Standards for Medicine Management* United Kingdom: Author.

Royal College of Nursing (RCN). (2004). *Sexual health competencies: an integrated career and competency framework for sexual and reproductive health nursing*. London, United Kingdom: Author.

Royal College of Nursing (RCN). (2009). *Sexual health competencies: An integrated career and competency framework for sexual and reproductive health nursing across the UK*. London, United Kingdom: Author.

Scottish Executive. (2005a). *Delivering for health*. Edinburgh, United Kingdom: Scottish Government.

Scottish Executive. (2005b). *The Scottish sexual health strategy: Respect and responsibility*. Edinburgh, United Kingdom: Scottish Government.

The Scottish Government. (2006). *Modernising nursing careers: Setting the direction*. Edinburgh, United Kingdom: Scottish Government.

The Scottish Government. (2007). *Better health, better care: Action plan for NHS Scotland*. Edinburgh, United Kingdom: Author.

The Scottish Government. (2008). *Supporting the Development of Advanced Nursing Practice-A Toolkit approach*. Edinburgh: Scottish Government.

The Scottish Government. (2008). *Respect and Responsibility: Delivering improvements in sexual health outcomes 2008-2011. Action 3.6*. Edinburgh, United Kingdom: Author.

The Scottish Government. (2009). *Curam: Nurses, midwives and allied health professionals working for Scotland's health*. Edinburgh, United Kingdom: Author.

Tyler, C., & Hicks, C. (2001). The occupational profile and associated training needs of the nurse prescriber: An empirical study of family planning nurses. *Journal of Advanced Nursing, 35*, 644–653.

Wisby, D., & Capell, J. (2005) Implementing change in sexual health care. *Nursing Management, 12*(8), 14–16.

Woods, K. J. (2001). The development of integrated health care models in Scotland. *International Journal of Integrated Care, 1*, 1–10.

World Health Organization (WHO). (2011). *Sexual and Reproductive Health Core Competencies in Primary Care: Attitudes, Knowledge, Ethics, Human Rights, Leadership, Management, Teamwork, Community Work, Education, Counselling, Clinical Settings, Service, Provision*. Geneva: Author. Retrieved from http://apps.who.int/iris/bitstream/10665/44507/1/9789241501002_eng.pdf

Appendix A

Alcohol Screening and Brief Interventions in Sexual Health

It is generally recognized that patients attending sexual health clinics have higher levels of alcohol consumption, making the clinical setting perfect for the delivery of alcohol screening and brief interventions (SBI). These are very effective health interventions that can reduce and moderate drinking among users attending sexual health services, thereby minimizing sexual health risks associated with excessive and heavy drinking. Many people are unaware they are drinking at dangerous levels and introducing screening can benefit all aspects of their health. Many of those individuals seen within sexual health clinics are hazardous binge drinkers and, through the introduction of screening, this group is encouraged to self-monitor and increase awareness of their alcohol consumption. Integrating screening and brief interventions can strengthen the link between alcohol use and risky sexual behavior, encouraging a more preventative approach with wider health implications and reduced costs to services.

Alcohol Screening

Alcohol screening is an early preventative measure, with evidence showing it is sufficient to influence behavior change. Alcohol screening will identify the early stages of problem drinking before behavior becomes problematic and ingrained, it will provide staff with a legitimate opportunity to intervene and offer support and influence behavior change. Wider integration of alcohol screening and brief intervention sits comfortably within a person- centered care approach offered within sexual health (WHO, 2009). The process of screening increases awareness of an individuals' drinking and encourages self-assessment and regular monitoring, resulting in a reduction in alcohol use, with individuals taking a more responsible approach towards their sexual health. Evidence is available showing the delivery of SBI in sexual health setting to be effective (Lane, Proude, Conigrave, de Boer, & Haber, 2008).

There are many different screening tools that will identify different stages of drinking, for example hazardous, harmful, and dependent drinkers. The AUDIT screening tool used within Sandyford services is the gold standard and is recommended within the SIGN Guideline 74 (Scottish Intercollegiate Guidelines Network, 2003). Research shows the AUDIT to be especially useful when screening women and minorities, also showing promising results when tested in adolescents and young adults. The FAST screening tool detects hazardous risky drinkers and is a shorter and less robust version of the AUDIT tool.

Alcohol Brief Intervention

A brief intervention is usually delivered when the screening tool score identifies drinking at a hazardous level and is delivered by a trained member of staff when clients consent and it feels comfortable for staff to intervene and discuss alcohol further. The aim of the brief intervention is to motivate and support clients to think about their drinking and decide to change or modify their behavior; it is not to tell them or to direct them. The intervention is supportive, non-confrontational, ideally using a motivational style.

Acknowledgments

With thanks to Patricia Keogh, Young Persons Drugs and Alcohol Support, Sandyford, Glasgow.

● ● ● **REFERENCES**

Lane, J., Proude, E. M., Conigrave, K. M., de Boer, J. P., & Haber, P. S. (2008). Nurse-provided screening and brief intervention for risky alcohol consumption by sexual health clinic patients. *Sexually Transmitted Infections, 84*(7), 524–527.

Scottish Intercollegiate Guidelines Network. (2003). *The management of harmful drinking and alcohol dependence in primary care* (updated December 2004). Retrieved from http://www.care inspectorate.com/images/documents/3210/SIGN_74_The_management _of_harmful_drinking_and_alcohol_dependence_in_primary_care _-_Amended.pdf

World Health Organization (WHO). (2009). *Evidence for the effectiveness and cost effectiveness of interventions to reduce alcohol related harm.* Retrieved from http://www.euro.who.int /en/publications/abstracts/evidence-for-the-effectiveness-and -costeffectiveness-of-interventions-to-reduce-alcohol-related -harm-2009

Significance of Research and Clinical Audit in Sexual and Reproductive Health Care

THEODORA D. KWANSA

CHAPTER OBJECTIVES

The main objectives of this chapter are to:

- Critically examine the research governance framework (RGF), ethical principles, role of research ethics committees, ethical regulations, and guidelines and protocols
- Explore sources of professional knowledge and the significance of research in contributing to the development of professional knowledge
- Explore the logical progression of the research process
- Explore qualitative and quantitative designs, development of different research instruments, and the conduct of pilot study
- Explore methods of data collection and analysis
- Consider reasoned discussion of the findings from research and the making of inferences and recommendations
- Discuss research findings and research critique
- Explore what clinical audit involves
- Explore the significance of clinical audit within the framework of governance
- Identify the key components of the audit cycle and what each element represents
- Establish the links in the stages of the cycle to the implementation and evaluation of audit projects
- Establish the impact of recommendations and guidelines from audit projects on the effectiveness of change and improvement in professional practice. the effectiveness of change and improvement in professional practice

Introduction

Healthcare research plays a vital role in evidence-based healthcare practice. By substantiating decisions and actions with evidence from research, healthcare professionals are able to assure patients that the care and information provided is accurate and sound. The challenge for practitioners is to determine credible research through efficient critique and correct and competent application to practice. Arguably, not all practitioners have the knowledge and competence or the capability to conduct substantial research studies. Nevertheless, application of research evidence is considered an imperative professional requirement. Qualified practitioners are expected to have the competence to conduct or participate in research and to critique, interpret, and translate pertinent and seminal research findings to practical situations.

This chapter provides a useful fundamental basis for clinical managers and sexual health multidisciplinary team leaders who are committed to establishing an environment of research and evidence-based culture. Clinical and academic research in health care is regulated and directed by national and international frameworks or research governance. The ensuing section examines the research governance frameworks (RGF) of the United Kingdom and United States as exemplars of good practice.

The Research Governance Framework

Research is defined in the Department of Health (DH, 2005) research governance framework as: "the attempt to derive generalizable new knowledge by addressing clearly defined questions with systematic and rigorous methods" (DH, 2005, p. 3). The research governance framework for health and social care launched by the Department of Health (DH, 2001a, 2005) encompasses principles of excellence in practice. It also considers clinical and nonclinical research activities within the National Health Service (NHS) and adult social care. The core standards ensure consistency in application of research principles across the healthcare organizations and social care.

Thus the governance is designed to maintain ongoing improvement and innovation in research. The RGF is applicable to all staff who may be involved directly or indirectly with research activities in healthcare professional practice and therefore include the following:

- Experts who design research
- Establishments that host research
- Organizations that fund research
- Authorities that manage and monitor the research ventures
- Those parties who undertake to conduct research projects/studies
- Managers and different grades of staff in all professional disciplines who participate in different forms of research
- Staff working in health and social care research contexts
- The primary, secondary, tertiary, social, and public health sectors
- Academic establishments, staff and research students (DH, 2005; HRA, 2016)

Principally, the research governance serves as a standard mechanism by which the quality of research can be substantiated while ensuring that the safety, rights, and dignity of all concerned are safeguarded. That includes the study participants, other consumers of the health service, the researchers and other practitioners, the stakeholders, and the general public, who may be directly or indirectly involved. It is crucial that all parties concerned in the fields of health and social care are aware that the new research framework applies to all. This implies the expectation of responsibility and accountability of all interested parties including the following:

- Research participants
- General public
- Research staff
- Academic institutions
- Research students and their supervisors
- Research ethics committees
- Research councils
- Research sponsors/funders
- Health and social care professionals and their professional organizations
- Pharmaceutical and related industries

- Local authorities
- Department of Health (DH, 2005; HRA, 2016)

The framework outlines the essential requirements, principles, and standards that should be met in relation to research. Furthermore, the RGF safeguards public interest by highlighting and clarifying the key domains of ethics, science, information, health and safety, finance, and intellectual property in terms of sponsorship. These domains are explored in the ensuing sections.

Related Legislation, Regulations, and Required Standards

The Ethical Domain: The Rights, Dignity, and Safety of Participants

The ethical domain addresses respect for the rights, dignity, and safety of the research participants. The ethical requirement places particular emphasis on informed consent and seeks to ensure that the measures and procedures that are used to obtain informed consent are rigorous, trustworthy, and unambiguous. Therefore, a crucial legal requirement stipulated in this domain is that researchers in the United Kingdom should comply with the Mental Capacity Act of 2005. The terms and conditions of this legal regulation protect the rights of individuals who may have lost, or who never developed, the cognitive ability to make or express their personal wishes, choices, and decisions. The RGF requires that there should be clearly defined appropriate alternative formats in language and pictorial images that can be used to obtain consent from mentally challenged persons. Additionally, there should be clearly defined custodian responsibilities that legitimize specific caregivers, parents, or identified significant others to give consent on behalf of the mentally incapacitated person. Where applicable, they may convey an individual's previous wishes.

The terms and conditions of the Human Tissue Act of 2004 require that the research ethics committee approves and confirms the use of the specific tissue samples for the research study. Individual anonymity should be protected and appropriate disposal regulations and procedures should also be fulfilled by all researchers. The Human Tissue Authority regulates the storage, utilization, and disposal of human tissue and organs. The RGF requires researchers to comply with appropriate confidentiality regarding sources of data and to recognize the concern of consumer representatives regarding the design, conduct, analysis, and reporting of research. For that reason, it is recommended that relevant NHS research committee should include at least two consumer representatives in their membership.

Diversity is also addressed in the RGF, and researchers are required to take into account gender, age, race, culture, religion, disability, and sexual orientation. Of equal importance, related social diversities should be reflected, as appropriate, in the research studies. The RGF stipulates that where applicable, potential risks should be clearly documented for the research ethics committee and clearly explained to the participants. Any potential risks, such as pain and discomfort, must be kept to a minimum. Compensation arrangement for unforeseen nonnegligent disadvantage, harm, or impairment should also be made clear to participants (DH, 2005).

Justification for the Ethical Domain in the RGF

Strategies employed in certain types of research methodology could potentially expose the participants and the researchers themselves to various consequences and risks. Therefore, the research governance framework stipulates that there should be an acceptable balance between those risks and the ultimate overall benefits of study findings. Moreover, by regulating, scrutinizing, and monitoring the process of research studies, the framework is dedicated to averting unethical practices and potential disadvantages to the study participants and other concerned parties.

The research governance framework serves as a mechanism to carefully determine the following:

- The practicality of the research topics that are put forward
- How robust, trustworthy, and thorough the research methods are
- Adequacy of resources and competence of researchers
- Respect for the dignity, autonomy, privacy, confidentiality, and anonymity of research participants (DH, 2005)

In the United Kingdom specific regulatory control in place at national and local levels occurs in the forms of the National Research Ethics Service (NRES), the National Health Service Research Ethics Committee (NHS REC), and the local research ethics committee. The Health Research Authority (HRA) Approval, launched in England in 2016, is the current process to apply for approvals for project-based research approval led from England within the NHS.

Academic institutions also have research ethics committees and these collaborate with the NHS REC whenever applicable. At each level, appropriate guidelines, protocols, and policies are provided that stipulate research requirements. Therefore, researchers are required to submit detailed proposals that are thoroughly examined before permission is granted to conduct the study. The professional statutory and regulatory bodies of the medical and nursing professions also provide regulatory guidance for practitioners in regard to codes of conduct and ethics in all aspects of professional practice, including research.

The Scientific Domain

The scientific domain emphasizes the quality and integrity of the research. Researchers are required to conduct meticulous systematic reviews of all relevant studies to avoid obvious duplication. Peer reviews are also recommended. National and international regulations for the use of human embryos for research are in place. Researchers are

expected to carefully explore these regulations and seek appropriate clarification and guidance to act on them. Collected data can only be stored for a stipulated period of time and consent must be obtained for further analysis or for future monitoring processes as recommended by the relevant regulating authorities (DH, 2005).

Information

Based on the recognition that research should benefit the particular target population, the framework stipulates certain requirements.

Researchers are required to make the main study findings accessible to all concerned following meticulous scientific review. This requirement applies whether the findings proved to be favorable or unfavorable and the report should be in simple language, free from technical jargon and ambiguity. Researchers are required to submit their work for formal, professional scientific examination of the findings and related data. The information should then be made accessible to the participants and those who may benefit from it. Thus, dissemination of the findings should be given careful attention (DH, 2005; HRA, 2016).

Health and Safety

The RGF emphasizes strict controls and conscientious compliance with all aspects of research study health and safety regulations. Appropriate measures and procedures should be clearly outlined regarding provision of information, containment, shielding, and monitoring (DH, 2005).

Financial Implications

The RGF ensures that justifiable financial remuneration be honored by the organizations that employ researchers. This should be carefully considered whether the cause of any harm sustained by participants as a direct result of the study is deemed to be negligent or nonnegligent. Additionally, the related HM Treasury (U.K. Treasury) rules and requirements must be honored while giving careful consideration to exploitation of the funding and sponsorship rights (DH, 2005; HRA, 2016). The overall research expenditure should be carefully calculated and accounted for, including disbursement of funds. The RGF requires measures to avoid, detect, or address potential or inadvertent misappropriation of funds. Where research findings have commercial implications, the RGF requires that the healthcare organization and the relevant commercial organization collaborate as partners in taking appropriate actions (DH, 2005). **Box 18-1** lists key elements specified in the RGF.

Practitioners in the United Kingdom are advised to further explore the Department of Health Governance Arrangement for Research Ethics Committees (DH, 2011) and the current related Annex for full details of the principles, requirements, and regulations. Similarly, practitioners in the United States are advised to explore the Institutional Review Boards (IRBs) requirements and current regulations,

---

BOX 18-1 Key Elements Specified in the RGF

- The scientific quality and integrity of the research

- Enhancement and excellence in research practice

- Compliance with the requirements and specifications for rigorous ethical reviews

- Adequate and comprehensive information regarding the research findings and related data

- Monitoring in terms of regulating and supervising all activities involved in the research endeavors

- Preempting and averting poor performance and professional misconduct, adverse incidents, and fraud in order to protect the public

- Protecting the well-being and safety of the public by reducing adverse consequences in innovative research practices while ensuring that lessons are learned and near misses are avoided

- Health and safety in terms of exposure of participants, researchers, and other relevant participating staff to harmful substances, potentially risky equipment, or exposure to organisms

- Careful consideration of the financial implications (draws on DH, 2005)

Data from Health Research Authority. (2017). UK policy framework for health and social care research. Retrieved from https://www.hra.nhs.uk/planning-and-improving-research/policies-standards-legislation/uk-policy-framework-health-social-care-research/

BOX 18-2 Key Benefits of the Research Governance Framework

- The RGF ensures that clinical and other healthcare decision-making are guided by high-quality research.

- Of equal importance, the RGF ensures that professional practitioners can realistically engage in collaborative research ventures to avoid superfluous investigations.

- The mechanism of the RGF provides the public with a way of ascertaining the accountability and transparency relating to the research projects in which they are approached to participate.

- The RGF enables the healthcare organizations to protect members of the general public for whom they have a legal, ethical, and moral responsibility and duty of care. The mechanism enables the organizations to safeguard the public from potential harm or impairment that individuals may be caused as a result of their participation in any health and social care research. (DH, 2005)

Data from Department of Health. (2005). Research governance framework for health and social care (2nd ed). Department of Health. Retrieved from https://www.medschl.cam.ac.uk/wp-content/uploads/2013/12/research-governance-framework-for-health-and-social-care.pdf

---

which are still in discussion as of this writing (Department of Health and Human Services [DHHS], 2017; Food and Drug Administration [FDA], 2016a). See **Box 18-2** for key benefits of the RGF.

The RGF requires that every study specifies appropriate measures to identify and avert or address potential risks associated with the conduct of the study. It also requires that there be clear agreement regarding the roles and responsibilities of all parties involved. Additionally, the governance emphasizes the legal and ethical prerequisites, professional obligations, high-quality practice, and excellence in research (DH, 2005).

The Federal Office of Human Research Protections (OHRP): The Role of Institutional Review Boards (IRBs)

Regulations Relating to Patient Safety Research in the United States

Institutional review boards are recognized by the federal Office of Human Research Protections (OHRP) within the Department of Health and Human Services (DHHS)

and have the responsibility to critically examine all health research proposals. IRBs and other formally authorized research ethics committees in the United States may also be known as research ethics boards (REB), ethical review boards (ERB), and independent ethics committees (IEC). Comprising scientists, doctors, and nonscientists, these committees have the responsibility to scrutinize, monitor or oversee, and review biomedical and behavioral research involving humans. In that way, the committees ensure standardization of ethical conduct of research. The process usually involves a risk–benefit analysis to establish whether the proposed study is permissible. The function of IRB is to ensure that appropriate measures are taken to safeguard the fundamental human rights and welfare of research subjects/participants. See **Box 18-3** for a list of the IRB's main requirements.

Requirements for Research Education and Training

Practitioners in the United States are strongly advised to carefully explore IRB regulations, policies and procedures, and guidelines. An IRB will stipulate that all personnel who participate in any aspect of human subject research must undertake appropriate training in the protection of human subjects. Training and education programs on the protection of human research subject are available and

---

BOX 18-3 The IRB's Main Requirements

- Respect for all the research participants
- Minimal risks—ensuring independent review of risks and potential benefits (reasonable risks in relation to potential personal and societal benefits)
- Voluntary informed consent
- Making research inclusive while protecting individuals categorized as vulnerable
- Compensating for harm directly relating to research participation
- Establishing comprehensive effect and modernizing the system
- Protecting participants from avoidable harm whether the research is publicly or privately financed

---

initial training should be followed by continuing education updates. Furthermore, funding agencies and certain research sponsors may also require that the researchers undertake additional training in the responsible conduct of research (RCR). The U.S. Office of Good Clinical Practice (GCP) provides training in clinical research (FDA, 2016b). Of particular importance, practitioners embarking on research should familiarize themselves the guidelines and procedures of the particular state or academic institution with which they are directly affiliated.

Influence of the RGF on the Enhancement of Evolving Professional Knowledge

The term *knowledge* as used in different contexts of personal and professional life represents a multifaceted concept that is perceived, interpreted, and applied in different ways. Indeed, Nickols' (2010) observation of different forms of knowledge is presented here describing in particular, tacit, explicit, declarative, and procedural forms of knowledge (Nickols, 2000, 2010). The concept has different connotations, one of which in professional practice refers to the specialized intellectual learning and acquired explicit information in a given field of practice, subject area, and specialism. An apt description proposed for that type of knowledge is "knowing about" (Nickols, 2000). The broader concept of knowledge within the context of professional practice represents the "professional body of knowledge" that is formally endorsed by the professional organizations of the relevant disciplines both nationally and internationally. In the United States the Agency for Healthcare Research and Quality (AHRQ) stipulates its three key objectives in its model of knowledge transfer as (1) development and refinement of knowledge, (2) dispersal and distribution, and

(3) organizational adoption and implementation (Nieva et al., 2005). The Patient Safety Research Coordinating Committee plays a particularly important role in accomplishing these objectives.

Thus, knowledge can represent the prescribed set of theories, principles, specialist methods and techniques, prescribed formulae, and procedural specifications contained in the official documents of a given professional discipline, together with the related policies and regulations (Cortada & Woods, 2001; Nickols, 2000). Indeed, Nickols (2010) cited Davenport and Prusak's (1998) view of knowledge, which is construed here as an imprecise and indefinite mix of accumulated learning. It describes professional experience and insight that forms the basis for processing new learning and integrating new competencies. They suggest that these occur in the individual's intellect and are applied as necessary (Davenport & Prusak, 1998). In the context of healthcare organizations, knowledge can be interpreted as the prescribed essential information that is communicated through organizational documents, policy recommendations and guidelines, protocols, practices, and procedure manuals.

It is important that the practitioner demonstrates the ability to apply learning gained through formal and informal education and training activities. Nickols (2000) described this ability to utilize acquired knowledge as a state of "knowing how." An individual's capability to interpret and translate information—to learn theory, concepts, and principles and effectively and appropriately apply them to practical situations—sums up the processes of knowledge acquisition and utilization. The states of intellectual acquisition—"knowing about" and the state of utilization—"knowing how" should be regarded as compatible in professional practice. This denotes knowledge as the basis for professional decision-making and problem solving, and as a source of reasoning for taking professional actions (Slevin, 2002).

Healthcare practitioners have an obligation to continually update and enhance their acquired specialist knowledge through continuing education and personal professional development.

Various distinctions of knowledge have been proposed, yet it is beyond the scope of this chapter to explore them all in extensive detail. Nonetheless, the ensuing section provides an overview of explicit knowledge, tacit knowledge, and implicit knowledge. These are considered to have practical relevance to sexual and reproductive health care.

Although some may consider Nonaka and Takeuchi's (1995) theory on the creation and building of knowledge as somewhat dated, their explanations are, nonetheless, noteworthy. Also of relevance is Nonaka and Nishiguchi's (2001) notion of the knowledge development and the advancement of the scope of knowledge creation.

Explicit Knowledge

Explicit knowledge refers to knowledge that has been formally endorsed and communicated in various forms such as documents, manuscripts, numerical/statistical formats, diagrammatic illustrations, and other specifications (Nickols,

2016). This is formal knowledge that has been systematically and scientifically tested. This is clearly applicable to healthcare practice within the NHS organization where documented standards for best practice are continually developed and launched. Criteria for professional performance are considered explicit knowledge, as described by experts (Nickols, 2010; Nonaka & Von Krogh, 2009).

Tacit Knowledge

Tacit knowledge is personal, deep seated, and ingrained in an individual's life experiences. Tacit knowledge is essentially imperceptible and integrates personal beliefs, principles, perceptions, and moral, ethical, and cultural values (Nonaka & Nishiguchi, 2001; Nonaka & Takeuchi, 1995). From the tacit state of knowing the authors posit that knowledge conversion encompasses the interchange of experiences and observations among colleagues. Externalization then evolves whereby new concepts, theories, and initiatives are expressed through articulation and documentation. Substantiation of this emerging knowledge occurs through systematic exploration, hypothesizing, and testing through investigative research to arrive at its validation as explicit knowledge. The newly formed explicit knowledge is then assimilated with the pre-existing explicit knowledge resources (Nonaka & Nishiguchi, 2001; Nonaka & Takeuchi, 1995), which could represent the existing body of professional knowledge. Others concur with the element of socialization in the process of building explicit knowledge from tacit knowledge via shared problem solving, testing and trialing, operationalization, and assimilation of new information.

Implicit Knowledge

Implicit knowledge is knowledge that although unarticulated, can in fact be expressed in recognizable forms. Essentially, this reflects the intuitive knowing demonstrated by expert practitioners in their professional competence and proficiency. The process of conversion from implicit to explicit knowledge may involve expert task analysis or meticulous practical skills analysis (Nickols, 2016). It can be construed, therefore, that the transition of knowledge from tacit to implicit to explicit encompasses processes of informal and formal interchange of thoughts and ideas through critical discussions. It also encompasses brainstorming and problem-solving activities among colleagues. These have practical implications for research in terms of the preliminary activities of problem identification and exploration through literature reviews to confirm a particular clinical issue of concern.

Research as the Basis for the Development and Ongoing Enhancement of Professional Knowledge and Practice

Many advocates of the positivist perspective of research maintain that the soundness of explicit theoretical knowledge can only be justified by rigorous investigative processes, objective testing, and validation. That view influences the tendency to reject forms of knowledge that are not considered substantiated and validated through empirical research. The post-modernist perspective, however, draws attention to the human element in social research. The participants around whom the studies evolve present distinctive behaviors that reflect their unique interpretations, values, reasons, and incentives (Holland, 2010).

By using different approaches in conducting research and providing detailed descriptions of specific care and therapeutic interventions, practitioners substantiate not only the accuracy of the professional knowledge but also the standard and quality of practitioner performance. In order to become a recognizable professional resource, tacit knowledge must be articulated and translated through implicit to explicit forms. However, relevance is crucial in this context, and the evolving knowledge must be deemed pertinent to fulfilling professional and academic requirements. The newly developed explicit professional knowledge must withstand critical examination for accuracy and thoroughness (See recommended reading: Basford, L., & Slevin, O. (Eds.). (2003). *Theory and practice of nursing: An Integrated Approach to Caring Practice.* (2nd Ed.). Cheltenham, UK: Nelson Thornes.).

The preceding explanations of knowledge taxonomies highlight the reality that professional knowledge is acquired from various sources in different forms. Knowledge goes through processes of sharing, discussion, interchange, empirical exploration, testing, and validation to be implemented in actual professional practice. These are processes in the evolution and enhancement of professional knowledge.

Following the processes of validation and approval, knowledge becomes integrated with confidence into professional practice as a basis for solving clinical problems and making clinical decisions.

The Role and Significance of Research for Substantiating Clinical Practice

Practitioners apply meticulously tested theories as the basis for performing practical procedures in care and service provision. It is therefore crucial to recognize that practitioners have a responsibility to contribute to the existing body of knowledge in their particular field or professional discipline. The processes of testing, refining, and confirming emerging new knowledge are necessary to enhance not only the scope, but also the trustworthiness and depth of what is already known in the field of professional practice (Polit & Beck 2011, 2013; Rees, 2010a).

Thus, the role of research in developing new procedures, and confirming and guiding the development of new skills must be recognized. Indeed, at international and national levels, various frameworks, policies, recommendations, and guidelines are described as being research and evidence based. These include the clinical interventional and procedural guidelines published by the World Health

Organization (WHO), as well as major national organizations such as the National Institute for Health and Care Excellence (NICE) and the Scottish Intercollegiate Guidelines Network (SIGN). The different statutory professional bodies associations and societies of medical, nursing, and allied health disciplines all advocate ongoing research activities in professional practice and this is concurred by the NHS organizations, which emphasize the role and significance of research in healthcare professional practice. Evidence-based practice is rooted in ongoing research activities and cannot be implemented any other way (Polit & Beck, 2011, 2013, Rees, 2010a).

The rigorous and systematic stages involved in research enable professional practitioners to explore difficult and complex clinical questions and to solve puzzling clinical problems. Practitioners are able to make sound and trustworthy clinical decisions for the improvement of care and service provision. No single research study can provide all the answers that the researcher(s) set out to explore, hence the need for establishment of proactive research cultures in the multidisciplinary team contexts.

Sources of Research Ideas, Problems, Questions, and Topics

Personal interest and creativeness, recurrence of topical issues in the professional literature, and specific internal and external organizational occurrences consistently influence emergent research ideas and questions. Experts such as Polit and Beck (2011, 2013) describe triggers that arise from knowledge gained from the literature concerning issues in professional practice. The foci of personal interest for practitioners are likely to differ and depend on the clinical specialism, background of professional discipline, subject area, and the setting in which the practitioner functions.

A clinical teacher or mentor of students of varied professional disciplines may have personal interest in the way they learn. Thus, a potential research topic may relate to development of specific clinical competencies that create a particular common problem or are difficult for the students to grasp. Another topic may relate to the professional socialization of new students to particular clinical situations such as the genitourinary medicine clinics or contraception clinics. Other sexual health professionals may identify specific clinical programs such as screening for HIV or sexually transmitted infections (STIs), to investigate the trends in uptake among specific social network groups or high-risk population groups.

These issues may trigger specific questions or hypotheses that lead the practitioner to ascertain how significant, how prevalent, and how researchable the identified problem is. In the performance of professional duties, practitioners invariably encounter ideas that trigger questions about why things are done in certain way. Other questions may relate to the cause of identified situations and consider investigating what might be the outcome if a particular

change or intervention was implemented (Polit & Beck, 2011, 2013).

Professional journals provide an additional source of potential topics or questions of practical interest and significance requiring further investigation. This seems to be the case when systematic reviews of published studies reveal specific gaps that require further research (Burns, Grove, & Gray, 2012).

The practice environment may be another source for research topics. Questions to investigate may be based on the level of patient dependency or the impact of the internal and external demands and expectations on staff. Observable and measurable patient outcomes or patient satisfaction or dissatisfaction may also trigger questions for investigation. Sexual abuse among identified vulnerable client groups poses a significant problem that colleagues in a multidisciplinary team may consider for research investigation. That kind of study could examine specific multiple factors of gender, age, culture, ethnicity, religious influences, and values, together with the psychological, social, and economic implications and support systems.

Staff morale and level of satisfaction and the impact on the rate of staff turnover of particular groups of practitioners could emerge as a cause of concern, necessitating research investigation. The trend of these problems might be considered a common occurrence across particular areas of the health service organization such as the STI and HIV outpatient departments and clinics. Conversely, the overall performance of the multidisciplinary team and/or the attitude of specialist staff may reveal protracted/intrinsic problems, questions, or topics.

Therapeutic interventions, specific aspects of care provision, measurable patient outcomes, or variations in patient outcomes linked to specific therapeutic interventions may all provide questions, hypotheses, or problems for possible research investigation.

The equipment used for specific therapeutic procedures could reveal questions for research investigations. In particular, if similar problems are reported by different units or departments within a healthcare organization, an extensive investigation may be required at an organizational level. It may become necessary to reexamine the usefulness, effectiveness, and safety of the particular equipment, even through retrospective evaluative studies.

The implementation of recommended guidelines, policies, and protocols could also raise questions for detailed examination of their impact in a given clinical area.

Confirming a Recognizable Problem for Research Investigation

It is important to ensure that the identified issue is recognizable as a significant problem of concern shared by the other members of the team. Depending on the incentive for investigating the particular problem, the researcher(s) must determine exactly what needs to be investigated about the problem. The initial topic is likely to be broad and unfocused, but asking a series of questions may help the team arrive at consensus on what should be the focus of the study (Parahoo, 2014).

Open communication with team members and extensive exploration of the relevant literature are meant to confirm that the problem is recognized as a shared concern among the team of professional practitioners in that area of practice. The aim is to implement effective evidence-based practice to achieve improvement in care and service provision with better outcomes and satisfaction for the patients/clients. Nonetheless, it is also important to avoid unnecessary repetition of research studies (Polit & Beck, 2011, 2013; Rees, 2010b; Robson, 2011).

Consideration of the Significance of the Problem from Different Perspectives

Practitioners are encouraged to consider a series of concerns related to the significance and feasibility of the research question.

One topic to consider is the inconsistent translation of policy guidelines in relation to a particular professional discipline. The question that could be pondered is: How do the findings from the study contribute toward further improvement of the practice of the particular discipline? For example, the investigation might focus on sexual healthcare within public health services or primary care. It is important to establish the magnitude and wide-ranging implications of the identified research problem or topic. This may depend on the clinical context and the source of incentive for the study and the envisioned benefits (Parahoo, 2014; Rees, 2010b; Tappen, 2011).

Careful consideration should be given to the impact of the problem on current practice, the reason for the investigation, and the potential implications to the field if not investigated. Experts emphasize the importance of establishing a clear purpose for the study. This means considering which patient group or practitioners would benefit from the evidence that emerges from the study and the application to clinical practice. Whether or not the problem or topic is suitable for research investigation should be carefully considered (Parahoo, 2014; Tappen, 2011).

Potential time limitations are important to consider when examining the feasibility of the study. The available time for the study may be influenced by various factors (Tappen, 2011). In a large and complex organization, the available time for the study may depend on prioritization of other issues on the healthcare agenda. The time needed or available could also be influenced by the size and scope of the study, which should be carefully considered beforehand.

Thus, assurance of ample time, availability of adequate funding, and other essential resources should be given careful consideration. Accessibility to the appropriate target population with the required characteristics is also an important and requires careful consideration. Equally important, the principal investigator must have appropriate level of professional knowledge and practical expertise in the specific subject area and clinical field (Melnyk & Fineout-Overholt, 2014).

Regulations That Guide Implementation of the RGF Requirements

Other relevant details may be sensibly included as required. The additional obligations are also stipulations in the research governance framework and clearly intrinsic in the clinical governance. It is required that all healthcare researchers and practitioners familiarize themselves with the content of the research governance framework and clinical governance to be adequately informed about the recommendations and guidelines for clinical research. The measures designed to fulfill these requirements should be incorporated in the research proposal. Researchers are required to comply with these statutory and organizational regulations and all the related ethical issues to demonstrate their professional responsibility and accountability.

The research requirements may depend on the size of the study and the source of sponsorship. Therefore, careful consideration should be given to achievability of the project by assessing realistically the resources required to conduct of the study (Rees, 2010b; Tappen, 2011). These may include technical and specialist assistance such as statistical support, specialist laboratory support, IT technical support, and delegated research clerical assistance. To protect the research data, confidential materials, and any special equipment, it may be necessary for restricted admittance and/or a security system to be installed. In small-scale studies at ward or departmental levels, the required facilities and equipment may be limited.

Funding support may prove to be a determinant factor for conducting the research study. The RGF emphasizes the importance of establishing the availability of adequate allocated budget to support a high-quality study to its completion (DH, 2005). A carefully calculated budget should be submitted with the research proposal. Practitioners may find the National Institute for Health Research (NIHR) 2014 useful to seek information on funding for research in healthcare professional practice.

Successful research projects depend to a great extent on the researcher having adequate knowledge of the subject and specialist area. Moreover, familiarity with the clinical context and the field of practice within which the identified problem exists is particularly advantageous and the professional expertise of the researcher(s) is invariably crucial (Holland & Rees, 2010; Tappen, 2011). Moreover, motivation and personal incentive sustain researchers in their diligence in conducting the study to a successful completion.

The use of specific interviewing or observational techniques may require particular skills. Of equal importance, researcher(s) must understand statistical analysis and interpretation of the results. These and other technical skills enable the researcher to present and discuss the findings clearly and competently and to develop an efficient report (Polit & Beck, 2011, 2013).

Application of the Research Process to Sexual and Reproductive Health Care

While different approaches exist, the research process embraces a logical sequence and organization of components that are applicable to all the different types of research (Gerrish & Lathlean, 2015; Parahoo, 2014).

Stages of the Research Process

Identification of the Research Problem, the Topic, and Title of Study

Research topics could originate from many places, including the following:

- Shared ideas among colleagues in the multidisciplinary team and from team meetings
- Continuing professional development education and training events, conferences, seminars, study days, and workshops
- The implementation of internal policy guidelines
- Specific procedural intervention or use of specific equipment
- Critical incident occurring in the situation of care provision
- Findings from extensive systematic review of the professional literature
- The complaints system and general comments by patients/clients, their relatives, and other stakeholders of the particular health service
- Demographic events in society, the general population, or local communities
- The practitioner's unarticulated intuitive knowledge, personal interest, personal ambition, and motivation (Gerrish & Lathlean, 2015; Rees, 2010b)

Extensive Search of the Literature and Focusing of the Research Problem

The literature search should be meticulous and systematic. Practitioners who require appropriate training and guidance are advised to consult academic or relevant institutional subject librarians and IT technicians for help and support.

Critical Appraisal of Previous Research Reports

This stage of the research process is crucial for examining what is known and has been published about the topic. The review enables the researcher(s) and colleagues to gain deeper understanding of the topic. The appraisal enables the researcher(s) to find out what kinds of studies have been carried out on the particular topic and what methodological strategies have been applied in the previous studies. Moreover, the researchers are able to examine the findings, claims, inferences, and recommendations that have previously been made about the topic. The literature review and appraisal may reveal gaps in the professional knowledge. It may also help to confirm the researcher(s') and the team's concerns about the problem. The review and appraisal allow for refining and refocusing the issue to be investigated and the potential scope of the study (Aveyard, 2014; Gerrish & Lathlean, 2015; Polit & Beck, 2013; Rees, 2010e).

Preliminary Note Taking—Critical and Strategic Reading

Preliminary note taking should be logically organized and comprehensive, with the appropriate references cited correctly. Critical reading of each selected paper should always be considered as an essential preliminary component of the literature review.

Note the author(s') name(s) and background(s) and the date. These may give indication of the authenticity, level of knowledge, and professional and research expertise. From the executive summary or abstract and introduction determine whether the problem has been explored from specific viewpoints, such as educational, clinical, social, or psychological perspective(s). Read critically and pay particular attention to how well substantiated are the claims made by the researcher(s) (Rees, 2010e; Robson, 2011).

Writing Up the Findings from the Literature

Writing up the findings from the literature review should show a logical organization. Aveyard (2014) provides excellent detail on this process and is highly recommended.

Introduction This opening section should expound the nature and background of the research problem. It is also useful to explain the motivation for this research undertaking. It is useful to outline the key issues to be addressed and the appropriate logical sequence in which they will be examined (Aveyard, 2014; Caldwell, Henshaw, & Taylor, 2011).

The Main Body of the Review In writing up the literature review, organize the themes and address each separately (e.g., clinical perspective, social perspective, national and local guidelines, recommendations, and related policy regulations). It is important to demonstrate the ability to synthesize key elements of the findings from different studies.

The style of writing is equally crucial. Develop a comprehensive critical discussion starting with a balanced argument about the findings from the seminal or influential studies that have direct relevance to the research problem. Be sure to include the study sample characteristics and system of sample selection, statistical methods and techniques employed, the researchers' assumptions, rationalizations, main claims, conclusions, and recommendations (Aveyard, 2014; Rees, 2010e).

The above is followed by review of the secondary studies. Competent cross referencing is effective in the development of cohesive critical discussion and this should finish with a balanced and realistic conclusion. It is useful to reiterate the identified gaps and the research questions at this stage. The critical appraisal of the selected studies should show use of a well-developed and validated set of criteria (Caldwell et al., 2011).

Statement of the Aim The aim should be clearly formulated to indicate the ultimate goal or the specific issue under study in terms of exactly what factor is being studied. Moreover, the aim should be formulated to convey how the researcher intends to investigate, such as assessing, explaining, measuring, examining, exploring, or evaluating the identified factor.

Essentially, the aim should convey the focus of the research study and the possible course of actions that might be taken in the investigation. Crucially, the statement of the aim should tell the means by which it might be achieved (Gerrish & Lathlean, 2015; Parahoo, 2014).

Statement of the Purpose The purpose statement generally conveys the researcher(s') intention to describe, explore or explain (Robson, 2011). The statement of purpose often mirrors the aim, creating unnecessary confusion. Therefore, many researchers tend to state one or the other rather than both. However, an elaborate example of a statement of the purpose may read as follows:

Example

The purpose of this study is to explore what factors influence the common practice of unprotected sexual intercourse among adolescents and young adults: A comparative exploration of the beliefs, attitudes, and ideas about sexual risk-taking behaviors among adolescents of 13–16 years of age and young adults of 17–20 years of age.

This statement of purpose conveys the problem to be investigated, the target population and the sub-groups to be studied, and the course of actions that will be taken for the exploration. However, the statement could be more concise than this or it may be split into two separate statements of purpose.

Formulating Researchable Questions

Formulating a research question requires critical reflection on the topic and the purpose of the study. The researchers must provide a concise clarification of the key variables, which form the basis of the questions. Each question is then justified by the underlying rationale.

Usefulness of Research Questions The practicality of formulating and applying research questions is that they help to highlight and summarize the main concerns about the problem of the study.

The research questions help to confine the investigation within the limits of theory and practice. Apart from focus

and scope of the literature search, research questions guide the researcher(s) to collect pertinent data. The researcher(s) are able to determine an appropriate research method and an effective technique to analyze the data (Gerrish & Lathlean, 2015; Parahoo, 2014; Robson, 2011).

Types of Research Questions Different research questions generate specific types of information. The type of question enables the researcher to devise the appropriate research design and process for collecting pertinent data. Essentially, different types of questions enable the researcher(s) to determine what design to employ, what methods, what type of information to collect, and what technique(s) to use for the data analysis (Blankenship 2010; Newman, 2011; Robson 2011). Question types include the following:

- Explanatory, or change. In these cases, the types of questions require answers to *what*, *why*, and *how* enquiries for investigations (Blaikie, 2007, cited by Robson, 2011).
- Descriptive, evaluative, narrative, causal, and effects.
- The types of questions for the descriptive enquiries would be phrased using *what*, *who*, *where*, and *when* (Knight, 2002, cited by Robson 2011).
- Enquiries relating to evaluative, narrative, causal and effects would be phrased using *what*, *why*, and *how* types of questions.

When formulating research questions, it is important to bear in mind the direct relevance to the problem under investigation. Therefore, the main question(s) and the sub-questions that derive from them should reflect the title of the research study. While the main research question could be formulated at an earlier stage to guide the review of the literature, sub-questions may evolve at varying stages as the review progresses. As the researcher(s') knowledge about the problem increase, they may decide to investigate the problem from different perspectives to address all the relevant dimensions.

A practical advice is that the questions must be clear, concise, and relate directly to the statement of purpose. Furthermore, as Robson (2011) suggests, they should be explicit, unequivocal, and not disconnected.

Formulating Hypotheses

Research hypotheses indicate the likelihood of interconnection between one factor and another.

Sources and Applications of Hypotheses Hypotheses may derive from research questions in the form of anticipated answers.

Deductive hypotheses are those that arise from research findings or from other published work that a researcher may set out to test with a view to proving or disproving it. Inductive hypotheses are observations of a link between different trends or incidents occurring in clinical practice situations.

Different Formulations, Different Predictions The key elements in the formulation of hypotheses include the population or subjects; the causal, manipulated, or treatment variable; the outcome variable; and the projected correlation between them. Directional hypotheses explicitly state the occurrence of a connection between the variables and indicate the probable direction of the outcome. By contrast, nondirectional hypotheses state the occurrence of a connection between variables, but do not stipulate one way or another what the outcome might be (Rees, 2010b; Tappen, 2011).

Essentially, research hypotheses convey the occurrence of connections between variables and state the predictable options. Null hypotheses uphold the perspective that there is no connection between the variables. They therefore predict that no difference in outcome can be expected (Newman, 2012; Tappen, 2011).

In considering whether to formulate research questions or research hypotheses, it is important that the researcher(s) have a clear understanding of what each of these involves. While the formulation of research questions is generally applicable to quantitative and qualitative research studies, the formulation and testing of hypotheses more appropriately apply to quantitative and empirical or experimental research studies.

Determining the Research Approach—Quantitative or Qualitative

Characteristics of Quantitative Research

- Quantitative research in the clinical context typically involves factors from the outcomes of care, therapeutic, and/or procedural interventions that can be observed and measured objectively in quantifiable figures and be systematically recorded.

- Characteristically the statistical methods employed in quantitative research require thoroughness in measurement of the observed outcomes. The data have to be presented in statistical or numerical format.

- Quantitative research embraces the principles of the positivist paradigm and the objectivity in the data collection, processing, and analysis are perceived as particular strengths of the integrity of this approach.

- Quantitative research requires that the instruments used for the data collection are both reliable and valid. This assures credibility and generalizability of the results.

- The stages of a quantitative study should be repeatable to reproduce similar results. Therefore, documentation and the final report should provide all the necessary details of the study.

- The technique of sampling the identified target population should be clear, explicit, and unambiguous.

- Characteristically, the principles of the positivist paradigm allows for hypothesis testing in quantitative

research (Blankenship, 2010; Newman, 2012; Robson, 2011).

Polit and Beck (2013) describe the five phases of quantitative research as follows:

1. A conceptual phase involving determining and focusing the problem, exploration of the literature and the clinical context, development of the conceptual framework and hypothesis.

2. Design and planning phase involving choosing an appropriate study design, protocol development, identification of the target population, devising an appropriate strategy for the sampling of participants, devising the measurement processes, determining safeguarding systems to protect the study participants, and confirming the plan for the investigation.

3. An empirical phase involving collecting and processing the data.

4. An analytic phase involving breakdown and examination of the data, making appropriate calculations, and interpreting the results.

5. The dissemination phase, involving distribution of the findings and application of the pertinent key discoveries to professional practice as approved and recommended (Gerrish & Lathlean, 2015; Tappen, 2011).

Designs Employed in Quantitative Research

- True experimental designs—randomized controlled/ clinical trials (RCT)—involve random assignation of the study participants to either the experimental group or the control group. Manipulation of the treatment intervention administered to the experimental group enables the researcher to observe, measure, and record the effects of the intervention on those participants. Comparison is then made to the control group and the researcher attempts to establish a causal effect.

- Quasi-experimental designs (nonrandomized trial) allow the researcher to measure the outcome of the treatment intervention administered to a sample group. However, in this case the researcher does not employ the process of random assignation of participants to the experimental or control groups.

- Nonexperimental designs may involve correlational or observational designs to establish associations between variables and to measure the nature and magnitude or degree of association between the variables (Blankenship, 2010; Parahoo, 2014; Tappen, 2011).

Researchers are likely to employ a nonexperimental design if the feasibility to conduct a randomized controlled trial is questionable, for example, where manipulation of the specific variables or the characteristics under investigation would be unacceptable or questionable. Therefore, careful consideration should be given to all relevant details when faced with the challenge of determining between experimental and nonexperimental designs.

Characteristics of Qualitative Research

- Qualitative research embraces inductive reasoning in the strategy for gathering the required information followed by unraveling and extracting key concepts to formulate theories.
- This approach emphasizes the expressed meanings, values, and importance that individuals place on specific life experiences, personal circumstances, events, phenomena, and the context of their day-to-day existence. Therefore, it requires that a great deal of confidence be placed on the lived experiences, perceptions, personal views, and concerns of the study participants who represent the identified target population.
- Moreover, qualitative research requires that the particular social context within which the phenomenon occurs must be considered as crucial.
- Because of the inevitable subjectivity in the information obtained in qualitative studies absolute objectivity is not deemed to be a critical requirement. However, researcher reflexivity is considered to be important.
- Rather than numerical data, the information gathered in qualitative studies involves verbal and narrative formats. Generally, nonnumerical methods are used to analyze the data.
- Although pertinent to the study group, generalizability of the findings tends not to be a critical requirement.
- As compared to quantitative research studies, the number of study participants or sample size tends to be comparatively smaller (Holland, 2010; Holloway & Wheeler, 2010; Newman, 2012; Streubert & Carpenter, 2011).

Suggested Sequence of Actions in a Qualitative Study

- Develop the plan for the study.
- Review the relevant literature.
- Determine a broad research approach.
- Seek permission for access to study settings.
- Establish precautionary measures to protect the safety and well-being of the study participants.
- Develop the data collection method.
- Identify the specific source from which to obtain the information.
- Collect, manage, process, and analyze the data.
- Disseminate the findings through appropriate channels.
- Consider making recommendations for further research.
- Construct a conceptual framework.

Usefulness of Conceptual Frameworks Conceptual frameworks help researchers to selectively determine significant meanings that evolve from the interconnected concepts.

Moreover, a conceptual framework instigates critical thinking whereby the researcher(s) reflect on their decisions in developing strategies for their research design. This aids in planning the data collection in terms of what kind of information to gather, what process to employ, and how to analyze the data (Parahoo, 2014; Streubert & Carpenter, 2011).

Key Elements of Conceptual Frameworks Robson (2011) advocates a practical guide to develop a conceptual framework comprising the following key elements:

- Develop the full diagrammatic illustration on the same page to show the interconnections.
- Establish and utilize different sources for the framework in terms of research, pilot studies, or preexisting theories pertinent to the central theme. Consider personal intuitions, practitioners, the patients, and representative groups and possibly relevant stakeholders as applicable.
- Careful examination of the evolving framework helps to identify and eliminate similarities, discrepancies, and inconsistencies that may cause confusion and ambiguities. The emerging framework may represent a descriptive model or reflect a specific theory or other particular model.
- It is useful to submit the evolving framework to the scrutiny of colleagues for their constructive comments. It is also useful for a team of researchers to attempt individualized models then review each one and produce a final mutually agreed-upon framework.
- Ensure that each of the interconnected concepts is appropriately supported by reasoned justification or rationale.
- The framework should be thoroughly reviewed either after the pilot testing in a fixed design study or at various stages of the data collection, depending on the nature of a flexible design study (Holloway & Wheeler, 2015).

Developing Qualitative Research Design: Key Considerations Robson's (2011) model for the development of research design encompasses five key elements with questions to guide researcher(s):

1. The purpose of the study—what is the study intended to accomplish?
2. The conceptual framework—what is the researcher(s) theory about the problem?
3. The research question—exactly what issues are the researchers seeking answers to?

4. The methods—what is the best data collection process and analysis technique for this study?

5. The sampling procedures—what are the potential sources for obtaining information?

Establishing the link between the purpose of the study and the conceptual framework enables researchers to formulate appropriate researchable questions. It also enables them to devise the strategies for the data collection and the sampling of study participants (Tappen, 2011).

Phenomenological Research Design

Phenomenological research embraces an interpretive stance.

The researcher explores and provides an interpretation of the lived experiences of the particular target population (Newman, 2012; Parahoo, 2014). The emphasis is on the personal views that humans hold about themselves and the social world within which they live and function. Therefore, the researcher attempts to delve into and uncover the deeply held, even obscure, meanings that people hold about their routine day-to-day experiences. Crucially, the researcher attempts to gain thorough understanding with empathetic and sympathetic awareness of the perspective of the particular people (Robson, 2011). This qualitative research design enables the researcher to develop a detailed descriptive account of how people interpret their experiences of a particular phenomenon that is affecting their lives. Therefore, the identified sample group or participants represents the authentic provider of the required information. A concise outline of the main stages is presented in **Box 18-4.**

Ethnographic Research Design

The key features of ethnographic research involve a researcher's exploration of an identified population group to gain insight about the way they behave and act in given situations. The researcher attempts to discover the circumstances in which particular behaviors are demonstrated and how that population perceives and interprets those circumstances. Moreover, the researcher sets out to learn from the people the inherent cultural meanings that they attach to their ethnic and social conducts, performances, and behaviors.

The researcher must gain an insider's perspective, and therefore sets out to learn about the cultural group from themselves. This requires that the researcher seeks direct involvement in the form of social contacts to join, share, and fully partake in the cultural happenings. This insider's viewpoint is described as the emic perspective (Newman, 2012; Parahoo, 2014). Conversely, the etic perspective refers to the researcher's attempt to study and interpret the cultural affairs and the people's conducts and behaviors from the professional perspective without directly mingling or having any social involvement with them (Newman, 2012; Parahoo, 2014; Streubert & Carpenter, 2011).

> **BOX 18-4 Concise Outline of the Main Stages of Phenomenological Research**
>
> - Identification of the phenomenon of interest or concern.
> - Identification of the source and context within which the phenomenon occurs.
> - Identification of the particular population group that represents the source of the study participants.
> - Data collection involving the use of varied methods including deep searching, interviewing technique, written accounts obtained from the individual participants, observation, or videotaping.
> - Analysis of the data begins from the outset when the data are being collected.
> - As the analysis progresses the nature and quality of the emerging information helps to guide subsequent data collection to gain the full scope, richness, and depth of the lived experiences portrayed by the population. The researcher should explain unexpected findings that emerge from the data collected and from the analysis.
> - The researcher uses theoretical statements to present his/her interpretation of the lived experiences from the perspectives of the participants. A useful suggestion is that the researcher should ascertain the extent to which the findings from the review of the literature actually substantiate the findings from the study.
> - Further validation can also be established by the use of direct quotes from the responses. Therefore, the format of the analysis tends to be narrative, although thematic content analysis could be employed involving a combination of narrative and numerical format.

Types of Information Obtained and the Different Processes Employed Polit and Beck (2011, 2013) describe the types of information obtained from ethnographic studies as focusing on the specific cultural behavior of interest, the cultural artifacts, and cultural expressions. Effective means of obtaining information include participant observation, in-depth interviewing, cultural records, photographs, and other written documents. Another potentially rich resource is tacit cultural knowledge that has not been articulated or formally recorded.

Practical Actions in Ethnographic Research In ethnographic studies, it is considered more practical for the researcher to enter and conduct the study within the actual environment in which that population exists. Importantly, this enables the researcher to realistically describe their habitual behaviors and natural social patterns. Prolonged direct involvement with that cultural group may be required. This allows the researcher to observe behaviors and events that occur regularly in order to gain an awareness and insight about the meaning and importance that are put to these events.

Inevitably, the data collection is likely to be a lengthy process that may involve a series of stages. Researchers may decide to conduct macro or micro ethnographic studies. However, that decision depends on whether they intend to study the target population in the wider social context or intend to focus on an identified small group (Newman, 2012; Parahoo, 2014; Streubert & Carpenter, 2011).

Box 18-5 presents a broad but useful outline of the stages employed in ethnographic research studies.

Grounded Theory

Grounded theory embraces the identification of theory that emerges from the data. This design involves the coordinated and simultaneous processes of observation, data collection, data processing, and theory development. The data collection includes in-depth interviewing with audio recording and transcribing.

The data analysis involves coding and categorization. Robson (2011) describes the sequences as open coding in which the researcher creates categories from the information obtained.

This is followed by identification of subcategories to establish the different dimensions of the issue.

Axial coding follows the open coding and involves reorganization of the data and development of a coding paradigm or logical diagram depicting the key factors as summarized in **Box 18-6**.

Selective coding involves an amalgamation of the categories in the axial coding, thus enabling the researcher to postulate hypotheses. It also involves identification of emerging themes to generate theories that are substantiated by excerpts from the data.

Thematic content analysis provides some quantitative element to qualitative data analysis. In the report, the researcher presents a narrative account of the stages of developing the study. The process of generating theory and the final outcome and recommendations from the findings are also reported. (Newman, 2012; Parahoo, 2014)

Observational Designs

Observation may be used in the exploratory phase of a study to determine specific activities in an identified situation. In a multi-strategy design, the initial data may be quantified, but could be followed by qualitative data collection. Therefore, while observation can be implemented as the primary research method, the data collected may also be useful to supplement and support data from other sources (Robson, 2011). Other advantages are that watching and

---

BOX 18-5 Concise Outline of the Main Stages of Ethnographic Research

- Careful consideration should be given to the identification of the cultural group to be studied.
- The specific factors or variables of interest to be observed and studied should also be carefully determined.
- A thorough systematic search and meticulous review of the relevant literature is particularly important and should be conducted as for conventional research studies.
- In compliance with ethical requirements, appropriate measures should be taken to seek permission for access to enter the cultural group's social environment and other related ethical considerations should be conscientiously acknowledged and taken into account.
- The need for immersion into the cultural setting and the social affairs of the people should be carefully considered and arranged to ensure adequate involvement of the researcher with the people.
- Selection of the "Informants"—the information providers should be given careful thought and the right decision made regarding who to approach for information.
- The collecting of information should be done methodically and accurate documentation, recording and storage carefully considered. It is important to conduct this efficiently.
- The data analysis tends to be narrative, however content analysis could also be applied. The analysis involves the identification of the meanings that the cultural group assign to particular behaviors, actions, events, and objects that they produce and utilize.
- Validation is achieved by exposing the information to the "informants" before the final refinement is carried out for the report.
- The report should provide a detailed accurate description of the culture.
- Theory development could prove to be a challenge for the novice researcher. Nonetheless, this process should relate directly to the findings from the study. (As construed from various sources)

---

listening to the study participants' activities minimizes exaggeration while enhancing trustworthiness of the findings. Inconspicuous observation in experimental studies by watching the behaviors of participants in experimental conditions can provide significant information and understanding of specific reactions to particular situations. However, the effects that the observer may have on the

---

BOX 18-6 Key Elements of Axial Coding

- The core category derived from the phenomenon—central phenomenon
- The related influencing conditions—causal conditions
- The interrelated activities emanating from the core phenomenon category—strategies
- The conditions that impact on the strategies—context and intervening conditions
- The effect of the strategies—the consequences regarding the phenomenon

Data from Robson, C. (2011). Real world research: *A resource for users of social research methods in applied settings* (3rd ed.). London, United Kingdom: John Wiley and Sons.

---

situation and on the study participants could be difficult to determine and control. Moreover, the time commitment required to achieve adequate immersion into the social or tribal context can, over a prolonged period, prove to be exacting, lengthy, and exhausting (Robson, 2011).

Types of Observational Studies Participant observation is characterized by the degree of the observer's involvement with the social group under study. The observer has to physically move into the communal and symbolic domain of the group to exist with and share their lived experiences. In this way, the observer is able to learn, comprehend, and gain insight into the participants' communal customs, rules and practices, traditions, lifestyles, and linguistic and nonverbal communications. The observer may require taking on or accepting a particular role within the group (Robson, 2011).

1. Complete participant observation allows the observer to conceal the fact that he/she is conducting an observational study. However, participant-as-an-observer requires that the observer makes known to the group his/her specific role right from the outset. Nevertheless, it is important that he/she establishes a close relationship with the members of the group. The observer participates in the group's activities while asking members to explain specific goings-on. The double role could prove to be difficult and factors such as differences in age, gender, and ethnicity could create hindrances in the observation.

2. Marginal participant observation allows the observer to assume a passive role. This should be acceptable to the group and they should feel comfortable with that situation. It is important that the observer is familiar with the role and conducts the observation with an open mind.

3. Observer-as-participant enables the researcher to make known his/her role as observer within the group. The observer's role as researcher is perceived as one of the roles within the larger or extended group. However, it is also questioned as to whether anyone in that position can be considered as taking no part in the group's activities (Robson, 2011).

In each of these roles detailed, careful preparation is crucial if the observational study is to be properly conducted.

Recording in Participant Observational Studies When recording in participant observational studies, the emphasis is to ensure that the data obtained are unequivocal. Instantaneous observation and recording is found to be most beneficial. However, it is important that the researcher reexamines the recorded information within a short time to incorporate additional detail in a reliable and comprehensible way. Forgotten information that is recalled should be carefully recorded, as should any deductions from the initial analysis of the situation. Personal impressions, subjective feelings, and reactions should be carefully noted.

Observational Biases Observational biases may involve selective attention to detail that may be influenced by the researcher's personal interest, expectations and experience. Selective encoding may occur inadvertently with the researcher not being entirely conscious of this. Selective memory recall could occur due to prolonged delay in recording and the suggestion is to write a narrative account of field notes immediately. Interpersonal factors, sentiments, or outlooks between the researcher and members of the group could affect the data collection. Adequate training is recommended prior to embarking on observational studies to put measures in place to avoid or minimize these biases (Robson, 2011).

Technique of Structured Observational Data Collection This technique of data collection involves prescribed instruments with protocols, sets of rules, and guidelines. The procedures stipulate what to observe, over what period of time, and the manner of recording the required information. The researcher functions as a detached observer in collecting quantitative data such as noting and recording specific elements in a particular behavior. Development of the coding system requires predetermining the categories to be observed. Categories may involve simple or multiple systems and tend to be quite broad. Alternatively, checklists represent rather longer series of items that should be observed and recorded.

Reliability testing is crucial and may involve reliability testing.

The coding system employed in structured observation in experimental studies commonly involves measures of dependent variables and tends to employ simple coding methods (Parahoo, 2104; Robson, 2011).

Determining a Coding System Determining a coding system should be done at the exploratory stage of unstructured observation. Adoption of an existing coding system requires careful consideration of the research question. Pilot testing should always be carried out (Parahoo, 2014). **Box 18-7** details points to consider in devising a new coding system.

Data Collection Instruments

In addition to structured observation, there are two other popular instruments for data collection to consider.

Questionnaires

Questionnaires may consist of closed-ended question items or statements and include the following examples:

- Dichotomous questions ask the respondents to make one of two choices in the answers.
- Multiple-choice questions ask the respondents to determine their personal views or preferences from different choices.
- Rank-order questions ask respondents to determine and organize responses from most least important.
- Forced-choice questions ask respondents to choose between two contending viewpoints.
- Cafeteria questions ask respondents to select from a list of responses, the one that closely relates to their personal view.

BOX 18-7 Main Considerations in Devising a New Coding System

- The categories developed should generate information that is pertinent and directly related to the research question.
- Each category should be described in detail and clearly distinguished.
- The categories should encompass all possibilities.
- They should be mutually exclusive and exhaustive while at the same time being easy to record. Therefore, it is important that the observer is conversant with the system of categorization employed for the data collection.
- Carefully selected aspects of the occurrences in the situation under observation should be thoroughly examined to establish the usefulness of the information that may yield from that.
- Objectivity should be demonstrated, and speculations by the researcher/observer should be avoided.

Data from Robson, C. (2011). Real world research: *A resource for users of social research methods in applied settings* (3rd ed.). London, United Kingdom: John Wiley and Sons.

- Rating questions ask respondents to make a choice by indicating on a horizontal scale or continuum showing two polar extremes.
- Other scales may be employed for specific measures, including a Likert scale for attitudinal tests.
- Visual analogue scales allow for assessing sensations, subjective physiological experiences, or clinical symptoms such as pain.
- Open-ended questions may be used to give the respondents the opportunity to convey their responses in their own words. These are more applicable to qualitative research. (Gerrish & Lathlean, 2015; Polit & Beck, 2013)

Interview Schedules

- Structured interview schedules allow all study participants to be asked exactly the same questions in the same sequence.
- Unstructured interview schedules allow for further probing and the use of prompts to encourage respondents to clarify or elaborate on particular issues. These may comprise concise conversational statements used as memory aids.

Considerations for Sampling the Study Participants

- Researchers should ensure that the population chosen for the study represents the relevant traits or specific factors that the research problem and hypothesis are designed to investigate.
- There should be clearly defined and precise criteria to guide the sample selection in terms of inclusion and exclusion. The technique for selecting the treatment and control groups should be unbiased, while ensuring appropriately balanced and thorough investigation.
- The sample size should be adequately representative and adequate enough to allow for accurately carrying out the required tests/measurements and to ensure confidence in generalizing the findings to similar population groups (Gerrish & Lathlean, 2015).

The selection process and the criteria used, the sample size, appropriateness of this to the scope and depth of the information gathered, and related rationales should be carefully considered. Importantly, researchers should be able to consistently apply and clearly describe the criteria for inclusion and exclusion and the measures to ensure correct selection of the study participants. The means of seeking access and the process of approaching potential participants should be carefully planned and clearly described. Individuals' reasons for declining to participate in the study should also be documented.

Ethical Considerations

Specific measures should be taken by the researcher(s) to protect the welfare and rights of the study participants. The study participants' confidentiality, anonymity, autonomy, and informed consent should be obtained with clear explanation given to each participant. It is the responsibility of researcher(s) to guard against any form of possible harm, criminal act, ill-treatment, or any form of abuse to participants as a direct result of participating in the research study. Researcher(s) are expected to strictly adhere to the stipulated policy regulations for gaining access to the study setting and the patients/clients. Importantly, the requirements of the relevant data protection act should be adhered to (Blankenship, 2010). The risk of role conflict should be taken into account in situations where study participants may be their own professional colleagues. Researcher(s) should consider appropriate measures to deal with such potential tensions.

Considerations Relating to the Process of Data Collection

Researchers are expected to provide clear explanation and their reasoning regarding the stages of development and testing of the data collection instrument(s). These should be clear and unambiguous. The techniques used to test for validity and reliability of the instrument(s) should be detailed, and the actual process of collecting the data should be consistent and thorough. Unexpected complications, if any, should be noted to devise appropriate means for dealing with them effectively (Blankenship, 2010; Gerrish & Lathlean, 2015; Parahoo, 2014).

Considerations Relating to the Techniques of Data Analysis

- Data processing and analysis should be determined by the nature of the problem under investigation. The techniques for data analysis should be appropriate and applicable to the problem/phenomenon under investigation.
- All coding and categorization systems developed for the analysis should be reliable and a means of testing for consistency should be carefully devised.
- If the researchers plan to use independent validators, it is important to give careful thought to the extent of their involvement. Researchers should outline clear and unambiguous instructions to guide the validators.
- Researcher(s) should provide clarification of the emerging themes from the responses.
- Researchers should explain if and how they use direct quotations from the responses.
- It is important that researcher(s) substantiate or verify the emerging themes from the responses and their interpretations of these.

Researchers may verify the emerging themes by using narrative accounts and interpretive processing and if so they should provide clear justifications for using excerpts from the respondents' accounts of their experiences (Holloway & Wheeler, 2010; Newman, 2012).

Key Elements in the Presentation of the Results and Discussion of the Findings

- In order for practitioners and stakeholders to understand and have confidence in the findings from the study, it is important that researchers provide clear and comprehensive explanation regarding presentation of the results.
- Presentation of the results should be easy to read, understand, and interpret.
- All figures, tables, and graphs representing specific data sets should be realistic and accurate.
- Narrative presentation of the data should make sense to all concerned, without vagueness or confusion (Gerrish & Lathlean, 2015).

The Role of Pilot Studies

Apart from testing the precision and reliability of the data collection instrument(s), pilot studies serve the purpose of identifying practical problems before proceeding with the main study. Pilot studies are useful to prevent any unnecessary and potential waste of funding and may be referred to as "feasibility studies" (Polit & Beck, 2011, 2013; Rees, 2010b; Robson, 2011). Some elements in the research process such as structured questionnaire formulation and the process of preparing instruments for direct structured observations incorporate pilot testing procedures.

Usefulness of Pilot Studies

Pilot studies enable researchers to ascertain the following:

1. The appropriateness and effectiveness of the study design and the procedures involved before implementing these in a larger-scale study
2. The thoroughness and conscientiousness of the participant selection process
3. Suitability and robustness of the instruments
4. The extent of relationship between the key variables to guide correct calculation of the required number of participants for the study
5. Identification of confounding variables in order to devise measures to manage and suppress these
6. Effectiveness of the resources and the strategy for research staff training
7. Potential problems relating to shortfalls in the study participants following commencement of the study

8. The extent to which the initial evidence favors subsequent more rigorous study
9. The need to test, refine, and improve interventions before implementation of the full interventional study

The Research Proposal

A research proposal is a written description articulating the researcher's plan for a research project. The proposal provides a succinct version of the research process delineating each component of the study. The research questions, the rationale and timeliness of the study, and the expediency of the investigation should be clear in the proposal (Rees, 2010b; Robson, 2011). The proposal should be clear and unambiguous.

Utility of research proposals includes the following:

- Approval for the research study from the relevant authorized committee(s) in particular the ethics committee of the organization's research and development sector
- Permission for access to participants and facilities, confidential documents, and specific information.
- Present clarity of thoughts and ideas about the strategies the researchers plan to implement

Essential Components of Research Proposals

Researchers should formulate an abstract to provide a concise overview of the problem and its significance. A brief explanation should be provided about the reason conducting the study. The proposed methods to be used should also be indicated briefly (Polit & Beck, 2011, 2013; Robson, 2011).

The background and purpose of the study should be provided and should convey findings from the literature review. The researcher(s) should try to convince the review committee that there is an identified gap that the proposed study is intended to fill. A plan of work and timetable may be required and this should incorporate clear and unambiguous explanation of the elements outlined in **Box 18-8**.

It is likely that repeated attempts may have to be made in writing the proposal to an acceptable standard (Gerrish & Lathlean, 2015; Parahoo, 2014).

Submission

The submission of the proposal should be done formally and professionally. Appropriate advice should be sought from the research ethics committee regarding the correct format of the proposal document. It is also important to establish the correct procedure to be followed for the submission in terms of the number of copies required and other additional enclosures to be submitted. A copy of the participant information sheet and a copy of the letter or form to obtain consent from each of the study participants, where applicable, should also be enclosed with the proposal. The ensuing sections explore the processes

---

BOX 18-8 Concise Outline of the Plan of Work in a Research Proposal

Details of the plan of work should include the following:

- Study design
- Key variables to be studied or tested
- Methods developed for measuring and recording the specific outcomes
- Strategy for selecting the study participants, and the technique to be used or the process of sampling should be clearly explained
- Choice of study setting supported by a convincing justification
- Ethical considerations outlining the measures designed to address each of the potential ethical issues
- Process to be employed for collecting the data
- Statistical techniques that the researcher(s) intend to employ for analyzing the data
- How they intend to present the results in the report

Where a timetable is required, this should be clearly presented, indicating the anticipated time frame for the different stages of the study (as construed from Robson, 2011)

---

involved in clinical audit applicable to sexual and reproductive health care.

Clinical Audit

The interventions, procedures, and patient/client outcomes from the care and service provision in sexual and reproductive health care necessitate regular evaluations. The main purpose of clinical audit is to thoroughly examine the current practices of care and service provision in order to identify and/or verify issues of particular concern. The process allows for establishing the specific factors associated with the particular shortfalls together with high performance and quality care delivery. The intention is to effectively deal with identified limitations relating to a specific clinical procedure, policy recommendation, professional practice, or team performance. The means of achieving this is through systematic evaluation processes together with effective management of change. Clinical audit provides the mechanism to observe and measure performance to assess improvement in quality of care and service provision. It also allows for identifying performance strengths and comparing these to other settings with commendable standards or excellence in clinical performance. The policies and guidelines, therapeutic and procedural interventions that exemplify excellence or best practice provide criteria and/or benchmarks with which to compare high performing settings or teams. Implementation of evidence-based quality enhancement processes ensures that best practice and improvement of outcomes can be accomplished. Clinical audits are obligatory and all healthcare practitioners are required to participate in audit activities at varying levels in their areas of practice.

The Healthcare Quality Improvement Partnership (HQIP) is an independent organization in the United Kingdom led by the medical royal colleges, the RCN, and National Voices. Their aim is to promote excellence in health care and to strengthen the impact that clinical audit has on healthcare quality improvement. Thus, HQIP collaborates with patients and healthcare professionals to influence and improve all levels of healthcare practice.

The National Clinical Audit and Patient Outcomes Program (NCAPOP) commissioned by HQIP is a U.K. exemplar of extensive clinical audit projects. It comprises several national audits relating to commonly occurring conditions. The program involves collecting and analyzing data obtained from local clinicians in order to provide a national depiction of care standards for specific conditions.

Clinical Audit: Clarification of the Concept

Clinical audit has been defined as a mechanism to enhance the quality of care provision. It involves examination of the current systems, policies, and procedures in order to implement change as necessary (DH, 1989). Clinical audits encompass methodical assessment or examination of practice against benchmarks of approved standards. Clinical audits may assess specific components of the structure, policies, procedures, and the effects of care interventions. The importance of ascertaining ongoing enhancement of care delivery has been consistently emphasized and endorsed (DH, 2001b; Ellis, 2000; Flottorp, Jamtvedt, Gibis, & McKee, 2010; National Institute for Health and Care Excellence [NICE], 2002; Scally & Donaldson, 1998).

Clinical audits comprise a cycle of evaluation, application of explicit criteria, and implementation of change at different levels. Ongoing monitoring and feedback are necessary to confirm that the desired improvement has been accomplished (Burgess, 2011; Gifford et al., 2012; QPSD, 2013). The cycle of events in a clinical audit are designed to improve clinical care from different perspectives (Esposito & Dal Canton, 2014). Thus, clinical audits also provide a standardized process to evaluate day-to-day patient care. As such, clinical audits ensure recognition of good practice, comparisons through benchmarking, and necessary ongoing improvements in care delivery (Health Service Executive [HSE], 2008; National Health Service [NHS] Executive, 1999a, 1999b). HSE 2008).

From a government standpoint, clinical audit is required to ascertain compliance to the standards of "best practice." In the United Kingdom there are government reports, such as the Standards for Better Health (2004) and the Current Statutory and Mandatory Requirements (2016), that serve to guide healthcare practitioners. These emphasize the professional obligation to partake in national and local clinical audits. Internationally, the World Health Organization (WHO) published *Using Audit and Feedback to Health Professionals to Improve the Quality and Safety of Health Care* (Flottorp et al., 2010), which readers are encouraged to explore.

Rationale for Clinical Audits

The principles of best practice in clinical audit launched by NICE, and the new principles of best practice in clinical audit and HQIP (Burgess, 2011; NICE, 2002) provide adequate resources. The ultimate rationale for clinical audit is to improve the quality of care and service provision (Ashmore & Ruthven, 2008; Benjamin, 2008; Currie, Morrell, & Scrivener, 2003). The findings from clinical audits provide invaluable source of information on the basis for decisions to implement change and to raise standards of care. Findings from audits may also help to outline recommendations toward more effective use of resources (Baker et al., 2010; HSE & Quality and Patient Safety Directorate [QPSD], 2013; Flottorp et al., 2010; Jamtvedt, Young, Kristoffersen, O'Brien, & Oxman, 2003).

From the organizational perspective clinical audits may be conducted as a means to verify that the existing levels of performance meet stipulated expectations (Bullivant & Corbett-Nolan, 2010; Bullivant, Godfrey, Thorne, Sutton, & Baltruks, 2015; Gifford et al., 2012; HSE & QPSD, 2013). From the perspective of clinical practitioners, audits serve as a means to substantiate that the level of professional practice complies with the expected regulations, standards, and stipulated criteria (Fereday, 2015; General Medical Council [GMC], 2013; NICE, 2002; NMC, 2015).

The Related Principles and Types of Clinical Audits

It is important that healthcare practitioners are familiar with the national and organizational standards on which clinical audits will be based, and implement these standards in clinical practice. Moreover, practitioners should become accustomed to and compliant with the need for and the process of periodic monitoring.

Practitioners' involvement in the interpretation and translation of standards into practical terms ensures ownership and increases compliance. Monitoring serves the dual purpose of establishing areas of excellence in performance as well as areas that require improvement (Bullivant & Corbett-Nolan, 2010; HSE & QPSD, 2013).

Clinical audits vary in scope depending on the level at which the event is conducted. Thus, audits may be conducted on a specific issue or aspect of care provision by colleagues from a particular professional discipline or as a multidisciplinary venture. Alternatively, the audit could be conducted at the level of a cross-boundary venture to assess a particular clinical event or compare differences between specific intervention outcomes (Bullivant & Corbett-Nolan, 2010; Gifford et al., 2012).

Communication, ownership, and consensus are all crucial for a successful clinical audit. The team of practitioners should have a clear understanding of the audit process and be familiar with the audit tool. Organizational and managerial support will enhance the team's ability to implement the audit, as well as their motivation and interest (Gifford et al., 2012).

Potential Challenges in Clinical Audit within Sexual Health Care

Sexual health practitioners are urged to familiarize themselves with the key principles of clinical audit. It is to an individual's advantage to participate in audit workshops to gain adequate insight and understanding of the stages involved in conducting a clinical audit. Professionals of varied backgrounds functioning at different levels within the field of sexual health care present a particular challenge for audits and implementation of change. The complexity of the structure and broad context of sexual health service provision could make the conduct of clinical audit quite complicated. Different services being delivered from different locations by different teams may create inevitable tension and potential barriers against change to achieve the desired improvements in patient care (Gifford et al., 2012).

The current initiative is the provision of comprehensive, integrated sexual and reproductive health care and service. However, actual translation of this ideal into practice lacks clarity. This is evident in the variations of sexual healthcare structures with uncertainties about role definitions. In view of these issues, the conduct of clinical audit within the context of sexual health care requires careful detailed preparation.

The Main Prerequisites for Embracing Clinical Audit Projects

- Effective and overt communication with the relevant teams of practitioners.
- Practitioners should be provided with clear and transparent information about the intended audit, the aim, and the objectives.
- The concept of "good practice" criteria should be thoroughly discussed and understood.
- Establish the knowledge and clinical expertise in the field within which the audit is to be conducted.
- Careful selection of an audit team is crucial. Appoint an audit team lead with prior experience and proven competence in conducting a clinical audit.
- Effective collaboration and respectable interpersonal working relationships among the members of the audit team.
- Appropriate consideration of training requirements to ensure that team members and all participating staff are adequately informed about the nature and purpose of the audit, the scope, general principles, process, and techniques involved.
- Transparency is important to boost practitioner motivation and commitment.

- The clinical leads' and ward managers' commitment, facilitative, and supportive roles provide encouragement for the staff's preparation and participation.
- Relevant materials and supportive resources should be appropriately secured.
- The audit program should be presented as a comprehensive formal protocol. This should include a clear outline of the stages, as summarized in **Box 18-9**.
- Confirm approval of the organization and management.
- Carefully examine potential ethical implications and measures to address them.
- Determine the time needed for the audit within each unit of practice and area of care provision. (Copeland, 2005; HSE & QPSD, 2013; Potter, Fuller, & Ferris, 2010)

Various clinical audit designs have been proposed, some of which are less comprehensive than others. Excellent examples include the University of Bristol's (2009) series of clinical audit guidelines and the HSE and QPSD (2013) practical guide. These documents provide comprehensive and detailed step-by-step guidelines and explanations on all the key aspects of clinical audit. They also represent useful resources for those in managerial positions, and policy makers and decision-makers to better understand clinical audits.

A clearly structured template is useful for documenting the required details. If an organization chooses to develop an independent template, they should be sure it is clearly laid out and reflects the necessary details. Pilot testing the template is recommended. The final report should be detailed and formal and it is advisable that the template has been approved and endorsed by the relevant authorities (Gifford et al., 2012).

Box 18-10 presents an outline of the stages of conducting an audit within a unit of care provision (Ashmore & Ruthven, 2008; Benjamin, 2008; Potter et al., 2010).

Planning and Organization

An audit should begin with a convincing proposal with a clearly outlined protocol. It should include a well-designed audit tool that is relevant and applicable to the specific context of care provision. Other essential factors such as a supportive environment, appropriate education and training, resource availability, and motivation of staff invariably impact on the successful implementation of clinical audits (Ashmore & Ruthven, 2008; Ashmore, Ruthven & Hazelwood, 2011a; Benjamin, 2008; Bullivant et al., 2015).

Key Elements in the Planning

Communication, staff commitment, and management support are important factors. The purpose of the audit should be made clear and necessary support secured. Staff should be encouraged to further their training in clinical

---

BOX 18-9 Key Elements of a Clinical Audit Design

- The title of the audit
- The date of commencement and the date completion
- Name and title of the coordinator or lead of the audit
- Names and titles of other practitioners involved
- Name and address of the healthcare unit
- The health service organization / NHS Trust as applicable and the contact details
- The background and rationale for the audit
- The overall aim should convey, for example, that the audit is intended for the proposed for the purpose of
  - ascertaining if the current practice meets the pre-specified criteria of excellence in performance
  - improving care provision practices,
  - assessing specific outcome of an intervention, or
  - evaluating the patterns of uptake of a specific service by identified group(s) of patients/clients.
- Clear objectives of what actions would be required to achieve the aim
- Exploration of the relevant literature, critical appraisal, and statement of the key findings from the review
- The sources of the standards:
  - National guidelines and recommendations

- Organizational stipulations
- Professional organizations
- Internal protocols and policy guidelines
- Systematic reviews of research evidence and exemplars of excellence in professional practice
- The team's shared principles and standards
- Sources of the data to be collected
- The process of data collection
- The sampling techniques
- The identified collectors of the data
- The techniques of data analysis
- Outline of the key findings
- The proposed mechanism for feedback, including the nature of information and the process employed
- Considerations of the specific aspects for change in professional practice
- The implementation of the change strategy, the date of commencement, and the date of completion
- Consideration of re-auditing and related details
- The anticipated resource and cost implications
- Reflective evaluation of the strengths and limitations of the audit
- Recommendations for future audit

BOX 18-10 Concise Outline of the Stages of Clinical Audit at Local Level

- Communication, support, and commitment of the team of colleagues
- Identification of the area of practice and the particular aspect of care or topic that requires to be audited
- Identification of the audit team comprising staff with a mix of background knowledge, prior experience in clinical audit, specific skills including statistics, IT and development, testing and correct application of data collection questionnaires, and other data collection instruments
- Exploration of the relevant literature sources for evidence-based practice and examples of excellence in the particular aspect of care provision

- Setting of clear objectives
- Development of the standards for measuring the current performance
- Collection and collation of the data
- Analysis, interpretation, and review of the results
- Identification of specific limitations in the care provision requiring improvement
- Feedback and development of an appropriate action plan
- Implementation of the action plan
- Evaluation and writing up of the detailed audit report for feedback and dissemination

---

audit practices (Ashmore et al., 2011a; HSE & QPSD, 2013; University Hospitals Bristol, 2009, 2010).

The Function of Audit Cycles

Audit cycles provide a summary of the stages involved in conducting an effective clinical audit project. The cycles ensure a logical process in a multidisciplinary team context and can help to achieve standardization in a multicenter audit undertaking (Gifford et al., 2012). It may be necessary to remind staff about the organizational and professional mandate regarding compliance with participation. Suggested resources include the NICE (2002) publication *Principles*

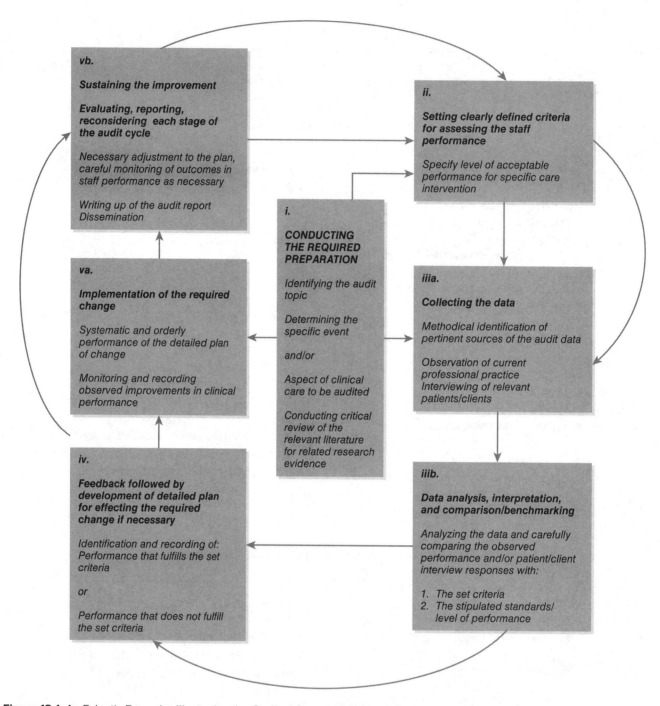

Figure 18-1 An Eclectic Exemplar Illustrating the Cyclical Stages of Clinical Audit

for Best Practice in Clinical Audit, Burgess (2011), and HSE and QPSD (2013).

The audit cycle comprises a spiral representation of audit events, with each successive event progressing to the next stage. Proposed audit cycles comprise differing number of stages depending on how the processes are organized (Bullivant & Corbett-Nolan, 2010; HSE & QPSD, 2013). A relatively generic staged progression involves a series of events from observation of current practice to the setting standards for performance assessment. Successive stages involve comparing current to expected standards and implementing change. Others are more detailed and comprise a series of 10 stages: topic selection, literature review, setting standards, designing the audit, collecting data, data analysis, feedback of the findings, changing practice, reviewing the set standards, and re-auditing. **Figure 18-1** shows a rather eclectic version of the cyclical stages of clinical audit. An attempt has been made to present a version that is relatively simple and easy to follow. However, practitioners are encouraged to critically examine and adapt this cycle.

The Initial Stage of Identification and Prioritization of the Audit Topic

A team approach to identifying the audit topic encourages practitioners to identify and report issues they think could benefit from an audit. Feedback from consumer groups could also be used to identify an audit topic. An effective complaint system, critical incident reports, and observational reports from the day-to-day aspects of care provision represent additional sources of audit topics (Ashmore et al., 2011a).

Related Challenges and Practical Considerations

Audit considerations include cost, amount of work entailed, and potential risk to patients and staff. Other considerations include evidence to justify the audit topic, current standards of performance, scope of the audit, and relevance to national policy (Bullivant & Corbett-Nolan, 2010; HSE & QPSD, 2013).

Statement of the Purpose

Topic identification should be accompanied by statement of the purpose, which conveys the audit aim and objectives. Indicators of success should be clearly stated to define expected performance standards. Clear criteria should be set to indicate which aspects of care will be examined. Identifying the type of data to be collected and the appropriate data collection tool is equally important.

Setting the Criteria

This stage of the audit cycle requires an extensive literature search focused on the particular audit topic. Specifications from relevant clinical guidelines on particular aspects of patient care or a clinical procedure can also serve as a useful source of information to develop audit criteria. The criteria should be measurable and specify an expected level of performance (Wollersheim et al., 2007). Formally approved professional benchmarks also prove to be useful in setting the criteria (Healthcare Quality Improvement Partnership [HQIP], 2009, 2016; HSE & QPSD, 2013; Regulation and Quality Improvement Authority [RQIP], 2015).

The Structure

The structure comprises the knowledge and expertise of practitioners, the organizational set-up, and the required equipment and space (Bullivant et al., 2010)

The Process

The process should be clearly explained and may involve procedural or therapeutic interventions, prescribing, assessment, investigations, education, communication, and evaluation activities. Explicit guidelines are important and accurate detailed documentation is required for the final audit report (HQIP, 2009, 2016; HSE & QPSD, 2013; Wollersheim et al., 2007).

BOX 18-11 Concise Outline of the Key Elements in the Audit Protocol

- Topic identification and formulation of a clear aim and objectives for the audit
- Identification of key elements of the care provision and specification of criteria/indicators for each element
- Thorough search of the relevant literature and systematic review reports
- Prioritization of the criteria and incorporating these into the details of the protocol
- Enclosure of a detailed audit design indicating the audit topic, participants, specific aspect of care, the sites or units of care provision to be to be audited, and the logical outline of the stages of the proposed audit
- Enclosure of the selected formal or new purposefully developed data collection pro-formas or templates with the detailed strategy and clear instructions for application of the instrument
- Submission of the protocol for external peer review followed by submission for management and/or organizational approval

---

The Outcomes

Expected outcomes must be stated and could include physical, mental, and psychological health benefits; anticipated improvement in patient outcomes; or patient (or other service user) satisfaction. The anticipated cost effectiveness should also be justified in a convincing statement and made clear to all concerned (HQIP, 2009, 2016; HSE & QPSD, 2013; Wollersheim et al., 2007). **Box 18-11** presents a concise outline of the key elements in the audit protocol.

Data Collection and Collation for Assessing the Level of Performance

The data collection process allows for refinement of the criteria and definition of the benchmarks. This forms the basis for comparing the level of performance in current practice to the expected level of excellence stipulated in the criteria (HSE & QPSD, 2013; Potter et al., 2010).

- Sources of data include interviews, observational records of practitioner actions patients' clinical documents, and statistical records.
- An appropriate sampling technique should be applied to achieve a realistic representation of the population. The system of selection should be randomized and unbiased and the sample size should be carefully calculated to achieve meaningful inferences from the data (Potter et al., 2010).

- The data collection may be an internal process (conducted by a practitioner) or an external process. Regardless of process, the data collected provides feedback on provision of care and clinical performance.

- The templates for collecting the audit data: Ideally, formally developed and tested data collection templates should be used. However, if newly developed instruments are to be used they should be rigorously pilot tested for validity and reliability. Data collection instruments should be clear and logically structured. Carefully consider who will be collecting the data and provide appropriate training.

- Data entry should be carried out by personnel with the skills to process and manage the data for effective reporting. Ethical considerations should be clarified and confidentiality should be ensured at all times. In the United Kingdom compliance to the Data Protection Act and all related regulations should be clearly demonstrated (Burgess, 2011; HSE & QPSD, 2013; Potter et al., 2010). In the United States compliance with the Healthcare Insurance Portability and Accountability Act of 1996 (HIPAA) is required.

Data Analysis and Interpretation

In audits at local levels, data analysis may involve relatively basic calculations of frequencies, means, standard deviations, and percentages with graphical illustrations of the results. However, larger scale audits at regional, area, or national levels require qualified statisticians to employ more sophisticated statistical techniques.

The important thing is to ensure that the analysis and presentation of the data is clear enough for practitioners to recognize what it represents. The results should indicate whether the current practice meets the standards that were set for the audit.

Usefulness of Performance Indicators and Benchmarking

Performance indicators are supported both nationally and internationally. See, for example, the WHO's program on the performance of healthcare systems, which proposes assessing performance against specific goals. In the development of the Quality and Outcomes Framework (QOF), NICE advocates the benefit of performance indicators.

At local levels performance is viewed in terms of clinical and patient outcomes as a direct consequence of the practitioners' overall quality of care provision. Evidently, these include the quality of outcome in relation to the quality of procedural and therapeutic interventions employed (Hogg & Dyke, 2011).

Benchmarking has been interpreted in various ways, yet within the context of healthcare provision certain common elements persist in the proposed explanations. Essentially, benchmarking is measuring the performance of a team of practitioners in a particular clinical setting against the best clinical performance in a high-performing similar setting. Performance measurement may focus on the standard and quality of care and service provision, positive outcomes, the patient/client satisfaction with recovery, or follow-up care (Wollersheim et al., 2007). Hogg and Dyke (2011) examined benchmarking for improving measurement of primary care systems performance while Schechter (2012) applied benchmarking to improve the quality of cystic fibrosis care. Fereday's (2015) guide to quality improvement methods is another useful reference.

Benchmarking enables the low-performing teams to assess what they can do to improve their current practices to achieve a higher level performance, with continuous quality improvement. The comparison should be on a specific aspect of patient care and the observation, benchmarking, and monitoring should occur over a given period. Wollersheim et al. (2007) demonstrate the importance of developing pertinent indicators that can be applied to particular aspects of care provision toward achievement of the expected outcomes. The experts identify certain key elements of benchmarking principles; in particular, determining the point of comparison of the high-level performance against which to measure and evaluate. Of equal importance is determining the exact level of performance that is realistically achievable and how much improvement can be feasibly accomplished. Thus, benchmarking provides opportunities for learning from excellence in practice, determining specific needs for change, implementing the required change, and monitoring achievement. **Box 18-12** presents a simple narrative outline of benchmarking principles (Hogg & Dyke, 2011; HSE & QPSD, 2013; Wollersheim et al., 2007).

These elements are not too dissimilar to some of the key principles in the stages of clinical audit.

Developing and Implementing the Required Change for Improvement

Critical examination of the range of potential barriers to change should be the starting point at this stage of the cycle. Appropriate supportive measures should be put in place to encourage the practitioners to recognize and confidently reveal the perceived threats and barriers to the anticipated change (Ashmore et al., 2011c).

Potential Hindrances to Change

Certain barriers to change emerge at different stages in the process of change implementation. An extensive review by Baker et al. (2010) reported interventions employed to specifically remove or overcome barriers to change. The review also reported on the effects on professional practice and related outcomes.

Potential barriers include lack of practitioner knowledge about what needs to change and for what reason. Another potential barrier is practitioners being uninformed about what the latest evidence-based guidance and recommendations

---

BOX 18-12 Key Elements in the Rationales and Principles of Benchmarking

Key elements in the rationales for benchmarking:

- Providing opportunities for sharing knowledge and expertise
- Facilitating improvement of the quality of care provision
- Acknowledging change to improve clinical practice
- Promoting reflectivity in practice
- Minimizing disjointed systems of care provision and services
- Effecting systematic assessment of practice
- Fostering multidisciplinary team building
- Enhancing the justification for additional resources while ensuring effective utilisation of the available resources
- Supporting substantiated innovative practice

12 stages of the principles in a model of benchmarking:

- Identifying the area of practice that is considered to require improvement
- Determining expert input from the available evidence-based practice
- Specifying patient focused outcomes that reflect the care provision
- Indicating the specific measurement factors— stipulated indicators that reflect patient focused outcome(s)
- Distinguishing the point of comparison (i.e. the benchmark of best practice) and exploring the

substantiating evidence by clarifying what actually represents best practice and to what extent this is realistically achievable

- Devising a scoring system or adopting an existing formally tested and approved system. The scoring may involve numeric or precise statements of best practice
- Scoring the existing or actual current practice as a starting point or base line, substantiating with relevant evidence, and comparing to the proposed best practice statement
- Comparing with the best practice score by obtaining the relevant details from the identified leading area of excellence in practice, arranging visits, networking, and sharing of ideas and expertise
- Sharing the commendable knowledge and expertise through use of exemplars of practice procedures, internal policies, and guidelines
- Devising an action plan to improve practice, specifying the envisaged dates for evaluation/reviews
- Updating the benchmark statements based on emerging new evidence in the area of practice and the specific aspect of care provision or intervention
- Determining the accuracy of rescoring to ascertain the improvement achieved, the extent of progress made, and aspects that still require further improvement (Hogg & Dyke, 2011; Royal College of Nursing ([RCN], 2007; Wollersheim et al., 2007)

---

are and/or what measures are needed to make the necessary change (Baker et al., 2010; NICE, 2007). Resource constraints, heavy workloads, and time constraints also create resistance to change, as well as indifferent attitudes and/or reluctance to participate in clinical audit projects and related activities.

Perceived Threat to Professional Authority, Uncertainty About Applicability

In situations where individuals or a team of practitioners perceive that a particular guidance that has been issued would undermine their authority, they may be inclined to resist the implementation of the change. Conversely, practitioners are unlikely to readily embrace and apply a set of guidelines if they are not confident that it would be applicable to the patient population they serve.

Regulation and national target setting, mandatory reporting, and Continuing Professional Developments are factors that influence implementation of change for improved patient care (Iles & Cranfield, 2004). Professional values and beliefs could pose threats to change if

the practitioners' perceptions of the benefits of the proposed change are negative or uncertain. Additionally, if the proposed change conflicts with other guidance issued by professional bodies it can create potential barriers. Similarly, resistance to change emerges when there is doubt regarding achievement of better patient care (Baker et al., 2010; NICE, 2007). Change in organizational leadership might also be a barrier to change.

Availability of the required resources, new equipment, and the organizational structure can also factors that could have various degrees of impact (Baker et al., 2010; NICE, 2007). External barriers beyond the control of practitioners are usually financial and/or political, and tend to be associated with resource and funding constraints.

Practical Considerations for Identifying Potential Barriers

Establishing the gaps between the current and the recommended practice helps to identify actual and potential barriers. The methods to identify and address specific barriers should be practical and realistically applicable. Baker et al. (2010) reported that interventions employed to overcome particular barriers to change can have positive effects on professional practice and healthcare outcomes. Nonetheless, they also argued that it is necessary to conduct appropriate research studies to test the degree of effectiveness.

The use of a questionnaire is an effective way of identifying inherent barriers. A well-developed questionnaire helps to explore the personal beliefs and attitudes of the staff. Questionnaires allow for rapid collection of an extensive amount of data from a large number of respondents. The process gives the opportunity to acknowledge the need for change. Additionally, depending on the structure and content of the questionnaire, statistical data can be generated.

Measures for Managing and Controlling the Barriers The measures for dealing with identified barriers may be specific and designed to target the particular problem (Baker et al., 2010). Educational materials are beneficial to provide basic information on the issue at hand; Baker et al. (2015) explored "tailored interventions to address determinants of practice." In this case, the authors emphasize the need to examine the components of the interventions to determine which ones most affect the professional practice.

Purposeful outreach visits are effective for certain types of change in care and/or service provision, such as the pharmacy services, preventive services, and in general practice. Outreach activities should address individual barriers to achieve more effective outcome. However, the cost implications of visits by external experts should also be carefully considered. Opinion leaders who portray and are perceived as well-respected role models for junior colleagues may be delegated to undertake outreach visits. This is an effective means of disseminating information. A particularly useful reference resource is the NICE (2007) detailed examination of how to implement change in clinical practice aimed at the level of clinical managers.

Consideration of Clinical Audit Feedback and Implications for Professional Practice

A clinical audit serves as a means of communicating to practitioners or the organization about their practice. As Flottorp et al. (2010) reported, this can prove to be an effective motivational strategy to urge practitioners to take appropriate actions to improve practice. Jamtvedt et al. (2003) explored the effects of audit feedback on professional practice and the outcomes of the care provision. Audit feedback may focus on outcome of care, costs, or other elements of performance and may include comparison against peers.

Reporting by a member of staff who holds a respected position is usually more effective particularly if additional education materials are provided and financial incentive is also made available. Reminders are beneficial if delivered at frequent intervals and focused on specific actions. In particular, reminders are found achieve more beneficial effect for healthcare trainees of varied backgrounds when timed with the point of decision-making. Jamtvedt et al. (2003) and Ivers et al. (2012) provide detailed reports on professional practice of audit and feedback and their recommendations to incorporate feedback into audit projects are particularly useful. **Box 18-13** presents an outline of strategies and measures for managing and controlling identified barriers to change.

Key Elements in the Action Plan for Improvement

Within the multidisciplinary context it is useful to designate specific roles and responsibilities to individuals who will coordinate aspects of the change implementation. Therefore, discussions about the resource allocation and cost implications should involve all the relevant parties, including those identified to take the action plans forward in the implementation of change. There should be clear timetables for the implementation of the change (Ashmore et al., 2011c; HSE & QPSD, 2013).

As change evolves during the implementation of the action plans, every detail should be systematically recorded on an ongoing basis. At completion of the change, each of the comprehensive records of the results should be methodically reexamined. This ensures that information is communicated to all concerned including the patients who receive the care and services. Review of the documented results should be undertaken by an identified group from the multidisciplinary team of practitioners to ensure thoroughness and consistency. **Box 18-14** outlines questions to explore when developing an audit plan. The questions can prove to be useful for monitoring and evaluating the audit project.

Reporting and Evaluating the Audit

A detailed comprehensive report should be written at completion of the audit. The report should incorporate preparatory measures that were undertaken at the initial stage as well as the information from the audit design as presented in Box 18-9, the stages outlined in Box 18-10, and the protocol as summarized in Box 18-11. The report should include an explanation of identified barriers and how they were addressed (as shown in Box 18-13).

Feedback of the results and any re-auditing that became necessary at any stage should all be documented and expounded in the audit report. Any refinements or adjustment made to the design, protocol, or stages should be appropriately justified in terms of the reason why the modifications became necessary and what difference was achieved by the adjustment. The final report should be clearly structured and thoroughly reviewed by the audit team before being submitted to the relevant authority. Additionally, pertinent content of the report should be made available to the members of the participating team of practitioners and the stakeholders (Ivers et al., 2012; Jamtvedt et al., 2003).

BOX 18-13 Outline of Strategies and Measures for Managing and Controlling Identified Barriers to Change

Awareness and knowledge

Educational materials and meetings

- Necessary for the purpose of raising awareness and informing about what the guidance says and what needs to change.
- The gaps between the current practice and the recommended practice can be highlighted.
- Practitioners have to know what exactly needs to change and in which aspect of care.
- Educational meetings and outreach visits by opinion leaders for the purpose of emphasizing the required change in practice.

Motivation

Reminders

- Helps in establishing a patient feedback system. Positive feedback informs practitioners about patient satisfaction with the care provided and can prove very encouraging.
- Comparison with another clinical practice setting that has benefited from a similar change can boost motivation to embrace and implement the change.
- Identification of good examples of clinical practice across the organization can provide an effective incentive.
- Keeping up-to-date with emerging new developments.
- Financial incentives to reward good practice, and recording of noncompliance with national standards and recommendations.

Skills

Clinical audit and feedback

- Educational workshops and work-based learning with peer and mentoring support enable the team to assess their own practices, procedures, and performance. This could be conducted by a team member on the basis of an internal audit or in the form of an external audit by a non-team-member, a peer, or from another health professional team. The information enables the practitioners to recognize the areas of strengths and weaknesses in their practice and to invest time for developing the required skills to improve the care provision.

Acceptance and beliefs

Educational outreach visits

- If the guidance is found to be in conflict with the guidance issued by the different professional bodies appropriate clarification should be sought to resolve the conflict. Practitioners' misgivings about the robustness of the recommendations as being evidence based and any skepticism or lack of confidence that the change will effectively achieve better care should be carefully addressed by motivational outreach visits.

Practicalities

Patient-mediated strategies

- Careful consideration should be given to the structure, facilities, equipment, staffing, and financial resources, as well as the potential impact of the guidance for change on local priorities.
- A creative and constructive strategy to sustain the change should be put in place.

Re-Auditing and Sustaining Change

The cyclical progression of the audit allows for confirming that the standards that were set in the audit continue to be complied with. Re-auditing allows for ascertaining the extent to which the recommendations from the audit are being implemented. It also allows for the aspects of care or performance that do not meet the criteria for the stipulated standards to be re-examined in more detail. This is followed by redesign of a more specific and realistically achievable audit plan that focuses on the identified shortfall.

Where it is found that standards are not complied with it may be necessary to review to ensure that they are realistic and achievable. It may also be useful to reexamine the related resources in order to make any necessary adjustments to effect compliance. Similarly, where the recommendations from the audit are found not to be adequately or efficiently implemented, thorough re-examination and appropriate re-adjustments are considered and a re-audit carried out (Ashmore et al., 2011d; Burgess, 2011; Flottorp et al., 2010; Potter et al., 2010).

Conclusion

This chapter explored the research governance framework and the relationship between the RGF and clinical audits. Inasmuch as clinical audits represent one of the key pillars of clinical governance, the relationship between these is obvious. Both address improvement of practice and patient care.

This chapter provided an overview of the research process. The logical stages of quantitative research were followed by the logical stages of qualitative research.

BOX 18-14 Questions for Monitoring and Evaluating Performance and Identifying Need for Change

---

Identification of the need for audit and change involves purposeful examination of these questions:

- In what ways are the standards being met and in what ways are they not being met?
- What specific issue or aspect of care currently shows shortfalls in performance?
- What is or are the potential causes of the shortfalls?
- What change(s) in practice could be implemented to resolve the underperformance in order to improve the care provision and patient outcome?
- To what extent are recommendations from previously completed audit been applied?
- What are the observed results?
- If not applied what explanation can be provided?
- What resources would be required to effect implementation of the required change and relevant recommendations?
- From what sources should support be sought for provision of the required resources?

The plan for the audit should involve purposeful examination of the following questions:

- What aspect of care or performance necessitates change for improvement?
- What measures should be taken to effect the change?
- Who should take joint responsibility or who should jointly participate in taking those measures to bring about the desired change?
- What time frame is envisaged from the commencement to the completion of the project?
- What strategies would be employed for monitoring the progress of the audit?
- How would the audit be evaluated?
- When would the evaluation be scheduled to take place?

Concise summary outlines of the main features of qualitative research designs were presented to provide a snap-shot of the particular structures.

Additionally, overviews of the different types of participant observation studies were outlined and the usefulness of unstructured and structured observational data collection considered in terms of the degree of actual immersion of the researcher. The key elements of pilot studies and the main components of research proposals were also considered.

As previously explained it was not the intention to present a comprehensive description of the stages of the research process. Rather, the intention was to pragmatically explore the fundamental elements of problem identification and to provide reasonable basis of what is involved in different methodological strategies and different methods employed. Practitioners undertaking CPD research courses may complement this by exploring more detailed books on research in the relevant modules. Readers are encouraged to explore the original works of the expert authors cited in this chapter as these provide excellent reference resources for more detailed information.

Clinical audits allow for periodic reviews to evaluate and compare the care and service provision against specific standards in order to effect appropriate changes toward improvement. The service providers and the practitioners who deliver the actual patient care have an obligation to comply with this core principle that is largely influenced by the principles of clinical governance, the NHS and National Service Framework (NSF), and NICE.

This chapter examined clinical audit in a pragmatic and easily translatable way. The key elements of an audit begin with identifying an appropriate audit topic, performing an extensive literature search, setting clearly defined criteria, and collecting the relevant data for correct analysis and interpretation.

Benchmarking and comparisons form crucial components in the audit cycle to apply the standards to current practice for better healthcare outcomes. The main objectives of benchmarking are to determine what and where improvements are called for, analyze how other organizations achieve their high performance levels, and use this information to improve performance. Feedback and development of a plan for implementation of the required change also form important stages in the cycle. Furthermore, the processes of evaluation, reporting, and constant reviews of the stages allow for sustaining the improvement with re-auditing activities as deemed necessary.

It is always useful to ask questions and seek clarifications from relevant experts. It is also useful to undertake audit training and workshop activities as part of personal and continuing professional development. These enable practitioners to not only participate actively in in-house audit projects, but also enable individuals to contribute to ongoing improvement to achieve high quality care provision and enhanced team performance.

● ● ● REFERENCES

Ashmore, S., & Ruthven, T. (2008). Clinical audit: a guide. *Nursing Management, 15*(1), 18–22.

Ashmore, S., Ruthven, T., & Hazelwood, L. (2011a). Stage 1: Preparation planning and organisation of clinical audit. In

R. Burgess (Ed.), *New principles of best practice in clinical audit* (pp. 23–58). Oxford, United Kingdom: Radcliff Medical Press.

Ashmore, S., Ruthven, T., & Hazelwood, L. (2011c). Stage 3: Implementing change. In R. Burgess (Ed.), *New principles of best practice in clinical audit* (pp. 81–92). Oxford, United Kingdom: Radcliff Medical Press.

Ashmore, S., Ruthven, T., & Hazelwood, L. (2011d). Stage 4: Sustaining improvement. In R. Burgess (Ed.), *New principles of best practice in clinical audit* (pp. 93–106). Oxford, United Kingdom: Radcliff Medical Press.

Aveyard, H. (2014). *Doing a literature review in health and social care: A practical guide* (3rd ed.). Berkshire, United Kingdom: Open University Press.

Baker, R., Camosso-Stefinovic, J., Gillies, C., Shaw, E. J., Cheater, F., Flottorp, S., & Robertson, N. (2010). Tailored interventions to overcome identified barriers to change: Effects on professional practice and health care outcome. *Cochrane Database Systematic Reviews, (3)*, CD005470.

Baker, R., Camosso-Stefinovic, J., Gillies, C., Shaw, E. J., Cheater, F., Flottorp, S., ... Jäqer, C. (2015). Tailored interventions to address determinants of practice. *Cochrane Database Systematic Reviews, (4)*, CD005470. doi: 10.1002/14651858.CD005470.pub3

Benjamin, A. (2008). Audit: How to do it in practice. *British Medical Journal, 336*(7655), 1241–1245.

Blaikie, N. (2007). *Approaches to social enquiry: Advancing knowledge* (2nd ed.). Cambridge, United Kingdom: Policy.

Blankenship, D. (2010). *Applied research and evaluation methods in recreation*. Champaign, IL: Human Kinetics.

Bullivant, J., & Corbett-Nolan, A. (2010). Clinical audit: A simple guide for NHS Boards and partners. London, United Kingdom: HQIP. Bullivant, J., Godfrey, K., Thorne, D., Sutton, D., & Baltruks, D. (2015). *Clinical audit: A guide for NHS boards and partners*. London, United Kingdom: Healthcare Quality Improvement Partnership (HQIP).

Burgess, R. (2011). *New principles of best practice in clinical audit*. Oxford, United Kingdom: Radcliffe.

Burns, N., Grove, S., & Gray, J. R. (2012). *The practice of nursing research: Appraisal, synthesis and generation of evidence* (7th ed.). Edinburgh, United Kingdom: Elsevier.

Cortada, J.W., & Woods, J.A. (Eds.). (2001). *The knowledge management yearbook 2000-2001*. Boston/Woburn, MA: Harvard University Business School Press/Butterworth-Hienemann.

Currie, L., Morrell, C., & Scrivener, R. (2003). *Clinical governance toolkit: An RCN resource guide*. London, United Kingdom: Royal College of Nursing.

Copeland, G. (2005). *A practical handbook for clinical audit*. Wales, United Kingdom: NHS.

Caldwell, K., Henshaw, L., & Taylor, G. (2011). Developing a framework for critiquing health research: an early evaluation. *Nurse Education Today, 31*(8), e1–e7.

Davenport, T. H., & Prusak, L. (1998). *Working knowledge: How organizations manage what they know*. Boston, MA: Harvard University School Press.

Department of Health. (1989). *White paper: Working for patients*. London, United Kingdom: HMSO.

Department of Health. (2001a). *A commitment to quality, a quest for excellence*. A statement on behalf of the Government, the medical profession and the NHS. Retrieved from http://webarchive.nationalarchives.gov.uk/+tf_/http://www.dh.gov.uk/en/Publications andstatistics/Publications/PublicationsPolicyAndGuidance/DH_4007446

Department of Health. (2001b). *The essence of care. Patient-focused benchmarking for health care practitioners*. London, United Kingdom: Department of Health.

Department of Health (DH). (2005). *Research governance framework for health and social care* (2nd ed.). Retrieved from https://www.gov.uk/government/uploads/system/uploads/attachment_data/file/139565/dh_4122427.pdf

Department of Health (DH). (2011). *Governance arrangements for research ethics committees: A harmonised edition* (updated April 2012). Retrieved from https://www.gov.uk/government/publications/health-research-ethics-committees-governance-arrangements

Department of Health and Human Services (DHHS). (2017). *Minutes of the Institutional Review Board (IRB) meetings guidance for institutions and IRBs*. Retrieved from https://www.hhs.gov/ohrp/minutes-institutional-review-board-irb-meetings-guidance-institutions-and-irbs.html-0

Ellis, J. M. (2000). Sharing the evidence: Clinical practice benchmarking to improve continuously the quality of care. *Journal of Advanced Nursing, 32*, 215–225.

Esposito, P., & Dal Canton, A. (2014). Clinical audit: A valuable tool to improve quality of care: general methodology and applications in nephrology. *World Journal of Nephrology, 3*(4), 249–255.

Fereday, S. (2015). A guide to quality improvement methods. Healthcare Quality Improvement Partnership (HQIP) Programme. Retrieved from http://www.hqip.org.uk/resources/guide-to-quality-improvement-methods/

Flottorp, S. A., Jamtvedt, G., Gibis, B., & McKee, M. (2010). *Using audit and feedback to health professionals to improve the quality and safety of health care*. Copenhagen, Denmark: WHO.

Food and Drug Administration (FDA). (2016a). *Institutional Review Board (IRB) written procedures: Guidance for institutions and IRBs. Draft Guidance*. Retrieved from https://www.fda.gov/downloads/regulatoryinformation/guidances/ucm512761.pdf

Food and Drug Administration (FDA). (2016b). *Office of Good Clinical Practice*. Retrieved from https://www.fda.gov/AboutFDA/CentersOffices/OfficeofMedicalProductsandTobacco/OfficeofScienceandHealthCoordination/ucm2018191.htm

General Medical Council (GMC). (2013). *Good medical practice*. London, United Kingdom: Author. Retrieved from https://www.gmc.uk.org/guidance/good_medical_practice.asp

Gerrish, K., & Lathlean, J. (2015). *The research process in nursing* (7th ed.). Oxford, United Kingdom: Wiley Blackwell.

Gifford, J., Boury, D., Finney, L., Garrow, V., Hatcher, C., Meredith, M., & Rann, R. (2012). *What makes change successful in the NHS? A review of change programmes in NHS South of England*. Horsham, West Sussex: NHS South of England.

Gormley, K. (1995). From theory to practice. In L. Basford & O. Slevin (Eds.), *Theory and practice of nursing: An integrated approach to patient care*. Edinburgh, United Kingdom: Campion Press.

Healthcare Quality Improvement Partnership (HQIP). (2009). *Criteria and indicators of best practice in clinical audit*. Retrieved from http://www.hqip.org.uk/public/cms/253/625/19/186/HQIP-Criteria%20and%20indicators%20of%20best%20practice%20in%20clinical%20audit-March%202012.pdf?realName=JlO6ff.pdf

Healthcare Quality Improvement Partnership (HQIP). (2016). *Best practice in clinical audit guidance.* London, United Kingdom: HQIP. Retrieved from http://www.hqip.org.uk/resources/best-practice-in-clinical-audit-hqip-guide/

Health Service Executive (HSE). (2011). *National Clinical Programmes: checklist for clinical governance.* Retrieved from http://www.hse.ie/eng/about/Who/QID/Quality_and_Patient_Safety_Documents/checklist.pdf

Health Service Executive (HSE) & Quality and Patient Safety Directorate (QPSD). (2013). *A practical guide to clinical audit,* V.1. Retrieved from http://www.hse.ie/eng/about/Who/QID/MeasurementQuality/Clinical-Audit/practicalguideclaudit2013.pdf

Hogg, W., & Dyke, E. (2011). Improving measurement of primary care system performance. *Canadian Family Physician, 57*(7), 758–760.

Holland, K., & Rees, C. (2010a). The professional and practical context of research and evidence-based nursing practice. In K. Holland (Ed.), *Nursing: Evidence-based practice skills.* Oxford, United Kingdom: Oxford University Press.

Holland, K. (2010). Research evidence: Qualitative methodologies and methods. In K. Holland & C. Rees (Eds.), *Nursing: evidence-based practice skills.* (pp. 68–106). Oxford, United Kingdom: Oxford University Press.

Holloway, I., & Wheeler, S. (2015). *Qualitative research in nursing and healthcare* (3rd ed.). West Sussex, United Kingdom: Wiley Blackwell.

Ivers, N., Jamtvedt, G., Flottorp, S., Young, J. M., Odgaard-Jensen, J., French, S. D., ... Oxman, A. D. (2012). Audit and feedback: effects on professional practice and health care outcomes. *Cochrane Database Systematic Reviews,* (6), CD000259. DOI: 10.1002/14651858.CD000259.pub3.

Jamtvedt, G., Young, J. M., Kristoffersen, D. T., O'Brien, M. A., & Oxman, A. D. (2003). Audit and feedback: Effects on professional practice and health care outcomes. *Cochrane Database Systematic Reviews,* (3), CD000259.

Knight, P. T. (2002). *Small-scale research: Pragmatic inquiry in social science and the caring professions.* London, United Kingdom: Sage.

Melnyk, B. M., & Fineout-Overholt, E. (2014). *Evidence-based practice in nursing and healthcare: A guide to best practice* (3rd ed.). Philadelphia, PA: Lippincott Williams & Wilkins.

National Health Service (NHS) Executive. (1999a). *Clinical governance: quality in the new NHS.* London, United Kingdom: Department of Health.

National Health Service (NHS) Executive. (1999b). *Quality and performance in the NHS: Clinical indicators.* London, United Kingdom: Department of Health.

National Institute for Health and Care Excellence (NICE). (2002). *Principles for best practice in clinical audit.* Oxford, United Kingdom: Radcliffe Medical Press.

National Institute for Health and Care Excellence (NICE). (2007). *How to change practice. Understand, identify and overcome barriers to change.* London, United Kingdom: NICE.

Newman, L. (2012). *Basics of social research: Qualitative and quantitative approaches* (3rd ed.). Upper Saddle River, NJ Pearson.

Nickols, F. (2000). The knowledge in knowledge management. In J. W. Cortada & J. A. Woods, (Eds.), *The knowledge management yearbook 2000-2001* (pp. 12–21). *Waltham, MA:* Butterworth Hienemann.

Nickols, F. (2010). *A model of helping people hit their performance targets. Performance Improvement.* 49(8): 21–26. San Francisco, CA: International Society for Performance Improvement (ISPI)/Wiley.

Nickols, F. (2016). *Change management 101: A primer.* Retrieved from http://www.nickols.us/change.pdf

Nieva, V. F., Murphy, R., Ridley, N., Donaldson, N., Combes, J., Mitchell, P., ... Carpenter, D. (2005). From science to service: A framework for the transfer of patient safety research into practice. In K. Henriksen, J. B. Battles, E. S. Marks, et al. (Eds.), *Advances in patient safety: From research to implementation: Vol. 2 Concepts and methodology* (pp. 441–453). Rockville, MD: Agency for Healthcare Research and Quality.

Nonaka, I., & Nishiguchi, T. (Eds.). (2001). *Knowledge emergence: Social technical and evolutionary dimensions of knowledge creation.* New York, NY: Oxford University Press.

Nonaka, I., & Takeuchi, H. (1995). *The knowledge creating company: How Japanese companies create the dynamics of innovation.* New York, NY: Oxford University Press.

Nonaka, I., & Von Krogh, G. (2009). Perspective tacit knowledge and knowledge conversion: Controversy and advancement. *Organisation Science, 20* (3) 635–652.

Parahoo, K. (2014). *Nursing research: Principles, process and issues.* Basingstoke, United Kingdom: Palgrave McMillan.

Polit, D. F., & Beck, C. T. (2011). *Nursing research: Generating and assessing evidence for nursing practice* (9th ed.). London, United Kingdom: Wolters Kluwer Health | Lippincott Williams & Wilkins.

Potter, J., Fuller, C., & Ferris, M. (2010). *Local clinical audit: Handbook for physicians.* London, United Kingdom: HQIP.

Quality and Patient Safety Directorate (QPSD). (2013). *A Practical Guide to Clinical Audit.* QPSD-D-029-1 V.1. Retrieved from www.kznhealth.gov.za/family/practical-Guide-Clinical-Audit.pdf

Rees, C. (2010a). Understanding evidence and its utilisation in nursing practice. In K. Holland & C. Rees (Eds.), *Nursing: Evidence-based practice skills.* (pp. 18–38). Oxford, United Kingdom: Oxford University Press.

Rees, C. (2010b). Understanding the research process for evidence-based nursing practice. In K. Holland & C. Rees (Ed.) (Ed.), *Nursing: Evidence-based practice skills.* (pp. 39–67). Oxford, United Kingdom: Oxford University Press.

Rees, C. (2010c). Searching and retrieving evidence to underpin nursing practice. In K. Holland & C. Rees (Eds.), *Nursing: evidence-based practice skills.* (pp. 143–166). Oxford, United Kingdom: Oxford University Press.

Rees, C. (2010d). Research evidence: Quantitative methodologies and methods. In K. Holland & C. Rees (Eds.), *Nursing: Evidence-based practice skills.* (pp. 106–142). Oxford: Oxford University Press.

Rees, C. (2010e). Evaluating and appraising evidence to underpin nursing practice. In K. Holland & C. Rees (Eds.) *Nursing:*

Evidence-based practice skills. (pp. 106–142). Oxford, United Kingdom: Oxford University Press.

Regulation and Quality Improvement Authority (RQIA). (2015). *The 5 stages of audit.* Retrieved from https://rqia.org.uk/what-we-do/rqia-clinical-audit-programme/clinical-audit-resources/clinical-audit-resources/the-5-stages-of-audit/

Robson, C. (2011). *Real world research: A resource for users of social research methods in applied settings* (3rd ed.). London, United Kingdom: John Wiley and Sons.

Royal College of Nursing (RCN). (2007). *Understanding benchmarking: RCN guidance for nursing staff working with children and young people.* London, United Kingdom: Author.

Scally, G., & Donaldson, L. J. (1998). Clinical governance and the drive for quality improvement in the New NHS in England. *British Medical Journal,* (4 July 1998), 61–65.

Schechter, M. S. (2012). Benchmarking to improve the quality of cystic fibrosis care. *Current Opinion in Pulmonary Medicine, 18*(6), 596–601.

Slevin, O. (2003). Theory, Practice and Research. In L Basford & O Slevin (Eds.) *Theory and Practice of Nursing: An Integrated Approach to Caring Practice* (Campion Integrated Studies), (2nd Ed). (pp. 141–282; 328–360). Cheltenham, United Kingdom: Nelson Thornes Ltd.

Streubert, H. J., & Carpenter, D. R. (2011). *Qualitative research in nursing: advancing the humanistic imperative* (5th ed.). Philadelphia, PA: Lippincott, Williams & Wilkins.

Tappen, R. M. (2011). *Advanced nursing research: From theory to practice.* Sudbury, MA: Jones & Bartlett (2009).

University Hoapitals Bristol NHS Foundation Trust. (2010). *Clinical Audit Policy Version 2.2.* Retrieved from www.uhbristol.nhs.uk/files/nhs-ubht/ClinicalAuditPolicy-2_2.pdf

Wollersheim, H., Hermens, R., Hulscher, M., Braspenning, J., Ouwens, M., Schouten, J., ... Grol, R. (2007). Clinical indicators: Development and applications. *Netherlands Journal of Medicine, 65*(1), 15–22.

⦁ ⦁ ⦁ SUGGESTED FURTHER READING

Ashmore, S., Ruthven, T., & Hazelwood, L. (2011b). Stage 2: Measuring performance. In R. Burgess (Ed.), *New principles of best practice in clinical audit* (pp. 59–79). Oxford, United Kingdom: Radcliff Medical Press.

Baker, R., & Fraser, R.C. (1995). Development of audit criteria: Linking guidelines and assessment of quality. *British Medical Journal, 31,* 370–373.

Basford, L., & Slevin, O. (Eds.). (2003). *Theory and practice of nursing: An Integrated Approach to Caring Practice.* (2nd Ed.). Cheltenham, UK: Nelson Thornes.

Betts, C., & Lawrence, E. (1996). Standard setting: A joint venture. *Nursing Standard, 10*(38), 26–27.

Bland, M. (2000). Producing benchmarks for clinical practice. *Professional Nurse, 15*(12), 767–770.

Burgess, R. (2010). *Criteria and indicators of best practice in clinical audit.* London, United Kingdom: Healthcare Quality Improvement Partnership Ltd.

Connorl B. T. (2014). Differentiating research, evidence-based practice, and quality improvement. *American Nurse Today, 9*(6).

Denscombe, M. (2010). *The good research guide for small scale social research projects* (4th ed.). Oxford, United Kingdom: Open University Press.

Department for Education. (2015; updated 2017). *Working together to safeguard children.* London, United Kingdom: DoE. Retrieved from https://www.gov.uk/government/publications/working-together-to-safeguard-children--2

Department of Health (DH). (2004). *Standards for better health.* London, United Kingdom: Author.

Ellis, P. (2016). *Understanding research for nursing students.* (Transforming Nursing Practice Series). London, United Kingdom: Sage.

Fitzpatrick, J. (2007). Finding the research for evidence-based practice. Part one: The development of EBP. *Nursing Times, 103*(17), 32–33.

Godwin, R., de Lacey, G., & Manhire, A. (Eds.). (1996). *Clinical audit in radiology: 100+ recipes.* London, United Kingdom: The Royal College of Radiologists.

Healthcare Commission. (2004). *Standards for better health.* London, United Kingdom: Department of Health.

Health Information and Quality Authority. (2010). *Guidance on developing key performance indicators and minimum data sets to monitor healthcare quality.* Retrieved from https://www.hiqa.ie/system/files/KPI-Guidance-Version1.1-2013.pdf

Health Information and Quality Authority. (2012). *Guidance on information governance for health and social health service in Ireland.* Retrieved from https://www.hiqa.ie/reports-and-publications/health-information/guidance-information-governance-health-and-social-care

Health Information and Quality Authority. (2012). *National standards for safer better healthcare.* Retrieved from http://www.hiqa.ie/standards/health/safer-better-healthcare

Health Service Executive (HSE). (2013). *National Consent Policy.* Retrieved from https://www.hse.ie/eng/health/immunisation/hcpinfo/conference/waterford9.pdf

Health Service Executive (HSE). (2014). *Checklist for quality and safety governance.* Retrieved from http://www.hse.ie/eng/about/who/qualityandpatientsafety/Clinical_Governance/CG_docs/NCPchecklistclgov.html

Health Research Authority (HRA). (2016). *UK Policy Framework for Health and Social Care Research.* Retrieved from https://www.hra.nhs.uk/planning-and-improving-research/policies-standards-legislation/uk-policy-framework-health-social-care-research/

Health Service Executive (HSE). (2008). *Healthcare Audit, Criteria and Guidance.* Retrived from http://www.hse.ie/eng/about/Who/Quality_and_Clinical_Care/Quality_and_Patient_Safety_Documents/guid.pdf

Human Tissue (Scotland) Act 2006: A guide to its implications for NHS Scotland. (2004). Retrieved from https://www.hta.gov.uk/sites/default/files/Information_about_HT_(Scotland)_Act.pdf

Irvine, D., & Irvine, S. (1991) *Making sense of audit.* Oxford, United Kingdom: Radcliffe Medical Press.

Iles, V. & Sutherland, K. (2001). *Managing change in the NHS: Organisational change, a review for health care managers, professionals and researchers.* London, United Kingdom: Service Delivery and Organisation Network.

Iles, V., & Cranfield, S. (2004). *Managing change in the NHS: Developing change management skills.* London, United Kingdom: Service Delivery and Organisation Network.

Lernard-Barton, D. (1995). *Wellsprings of knowledge: Building and sustaining the sources of innovation.* Boston, MA: Harvard Business School Press.

L. Basford., & Oliver Slevin (Eds.). (2003). *Theory and practice of nursing: An Integrated Approach to Caring Practice.* (2nd ed.). Cheltenham, UK: Nelson Thornes.

Mateo, M., & Foreman, M. D. (Eds.). (2013). *Research for advanced practice nurses: From evidence to practice* (2nd ed.). New York: Springer.

McCrea, C. (1999). Good clinical audit requires teamwork. In R. Baker, H. Hearnshaw, & N. Robertson (Eds.), *Implementing change with clinical audit* (pp. 119–132). Chichester, United Kingdom: Wiley.

Murray, C. J. L., & Frenk, J. (2000). A framework for assessing the performance of health systems. *Bulletin of the World Health Organisation, 78* (6). Geneva, Switzerland: WHO.

Mental Capacity Act: Code of practice. (2005). Retrieved from https://www.gov.uk/government/publications/mental-capacity-act-code-of-practice

National Health Service Health Research Authority. (2013). *Interest in good research conduct: Transparent research.* Retrieved from http://www.fdanews.com/ext/resources/files/archives/10113-01/09-11-13-HRA.pdf

Nursing and Midwifery Council (NMC). (2008). *The code: Standards of conduct, performance and ethics for nurses and midwives.* London, United Kingdom: NMC.

Nursing and Midwifery Council (NMC). (2015). *The code: standards of conduct, performance and ethics for nurses and midwives.* London, United Kingdom: NMC.

Patel, S. (2010a). Achieving quality assurance through clinical audit. *Nurse Manager (Harrow), 17*(3), 28–35.

Patel, S. (2010). Identifying best practice principles of audit in healthcare. *Nursing Standard 24*(32), 40–48.

Rees, C. (2016). *Rapid research methods for nurses, midwives and health professionals.* Oxford, United Kingdom: Wiley-Blackwell

Robertson, N. (1999). A systematic approach to managing change In R. Baker, H. Hearnshaw, & N. Robertson (Eds.), *Implementing change with clinical audit* (pp. 37–56). Chichester, United Kingdom: Wiley.

Royal College of Nursing (RCN). (1990). *Quality patient care—the dynamic standard setting system.* Harrow, United Kingdom: Scutari.

Royal College of Nursing (RCN). (2009). *Research ethics: RCN guidance for nurses* (3rd ed.). London, United Kingdom: Author

Royal College of Nursing (RCN) (2011). *Informed consent in health and social care research: RCN guidance for nurses* (2nd ed.). London, United Kingdom: Author.

Royal College of Nursing (RCN). (2013). *Developing an effective clinical governance framework for children's acute healthcare services.* London Royal College of Nursing.

Saks, M., & Allsop, J. (2007). *Researching health: Qualitative, quantitative and mixed methods.* London, United Kingdom: Sage.

Sanders, P., & Wilkins, P. (2010). *First steps in practitioner research: A guide to understanding and doing research in counselling and health and social care.* Ross-on-Wye, Herefordshire, United Kingdom: PCC Books Ltd.

Scottish Government. (2012). *National guidance for child protection in Scotland: Guidance for health professionals in Scotland.* Edinburgh, Scotland: Author. Retrieved from http://www.gov.scot/Publications/2012/12/9727

Swonnell, C. (2014). *Clinical audit policy.* University Hospitals Bristol NHS Foundation Trust. Version 3.1 Retrieved from http://www.uhbristol.nhs.uk/media/985118/clinicalauditpolicy-3_1.pdf

Tantrige, P. M. (2014). *Clinical audits must improve to benefit patients, providers and doctors.* BMJ Careers. Retrieved from http://careers.bmj.com/careers/advice/view-article.html?id=20018442

Tuomi, I. (1999). Data is more than knowledge: Implications of the reversed knowledge hierarchy for knowledge management and organisational memory. *Journal of Management Information Systems, 16*(3), 107–121.

University Hospitals Bristol NHS Foundation Trust. (2009). How to guides. Retrieved from http://www.uhbristol.nhs.uk/for-clinicians/clinicalaudit/how-to-guides

Other useful information and guidelines accessible from HQIP audit resource materials:

Criteria for high quality clinical audit

Guide to carrying out clinical audits on the implementation of care pathways

Guide to ensuring data quality in clinical audit

Ethics and clinical audit and quality improvement

Patient and public engagement in clinical audit

Clinicians and Clinical Audit homepage

Copyright regulations should always be respected and readers are strongly urged to explore the current versions of all the relevant documents.

19

Ethical, Moral, and Legal Quandaries in Professional Practice in Sexual and Reproductive Health Care

THEODORA D. KWANSA

CHAPTER OBJECTIVES

The main objectives of this chapter are to:

- Examine the interrelated concepts that derive from moral and ethical theories
- Identify the potential legal and moral challenges that practitioners may encounter
- Examine how these challenges relate to patient presentations
- Summarize the professional codes and regulations, as well as national and organizational policies, and the impact on practitioner compliance and behaviors
- Explore the potential implications of misdemeanors

Introduction

Individuals enter their professional careers already possessing personal values, principles, and attributes, such as compassion, sympathy, empathy, respect, honesty, a sense of privacy, personal sense of freedom, and autonomy. People also hold perceptions about quality of life, faith hope, integrity, discretion, justice, and fairness. Most of our moral values and principles are acquired very early in childhood. They are influenced by family values, cultural beliefs, and ideals passed down through generations and may be held consciously or in the subconscious state. Invariably, moral values, beliefs, and principles influence an individual's attitude, behavior, and reactions to situations encountered in different aspects of life. An individual can,

however, make a conscious effort to withhold, disallow, or reject specific influences.

The field of sexual and reproductive health care is fraught with ethical and moral issues, dilemmas, and conflicts. This chapter explores the impact that ethical issues encountered in professional practice can have on particular aspects of care and service provision.

Ethics: Key Components of the Definitions

While there are various definitions of ethics, the recurring theme is rules or codes of conduct that reflect notions of right and wrong (Hawley, 2007; Robson, 2011). Therefore, the term is often used interchangeably with the concept of morality, which refers to honesty, integrity, rightness, values, and principles in the more abstract sense. Generally, however, the term *morality* tends to engender connotations of the inherent values that an individual upholds and therefore is perceived as uniquely personal.

Within healthcare practice, *ethics* represents a broader concept that includes professional standards, principles, and codes of conduct in clinical practice and research. This chapter focuses on the principles of ethics that influence professional practice in day-to-day care provision.

Ethical Obligations: Expectations in Professional Practice

Practitioners are expected to display respect for all persons in their relationships and interactions with patients throughout care provision situations (Gabel, 2011; World Health Organization [WHO], 2011). In their duty of care, every sexual and reproductive health (SRH) practitioner has a fundamental obligation to provide the patient with all necessary information about his/her condition and the related treatment interventions. Moreover, the practitioner has a duty to respect each individual's autonomy and personal choices regarding the care that he/she is being provided. The practitioner is expected to demonstrate careful thought and sensitivity in the care and support of individuals with diminished capacity for autonomy when faced with personal choices and informed decisions. The best interest and welfare of the patient should be the practitioner's primary objective. Therefore, appropriate consultations with other relevant experts are expected.

Beneficence

Beneficence relates to the practitioner's commitment to act in ways that would achieve the best possible outcomes for the patient. The practitioner must endeavor to apply the best available evidence in making decisions and in providing quality care with the best possible outcome. The health and welfare of the patient should be the ultimate goal.

Nonmaleficence

The nonmaleficence principle requires that the practitioner applies appropriate measures to avoid causing harm to the patient. The practitioner has an obligation to ensure to the best of his or her capacity, potential sources of harm to the patient are effectively averted. These include clinical assault, damage, injury, or impairment that may be caused as a result of the care provision.

Proportionality

Proportionality refers to the notion of balancing carefully considered and reasoned decisions in care provision. Thus, decisions about the anticipated benefits of an intervention for the patient should be balanced against the potential associated risk of side effects, negative outcome, or harm. Ultimately, practitioners have an obligation to ensure that the intended benefits and positive outcomes of therapeutic interventions outweigh the unintended negative effects. In essence, this principle ensures that the care provision, decisions, and actions involve the minimum chance of harm or disadvantage but best possible outcomes for the patient. Childress et al. (2002) explain this concept as balancing the positive aspects of an intervention or policy against the negative features in deciding to implement or not.

Ethical Theories: Utilitarianism and Consequentialism

Acting ethically implies doing the right thing and that depends on how the outcome of the action is perceived by others within the particular context. Utilitarianism emphasizes actions that benefit the majority or are done for the greater good. However, consequentialism focuses on assessing actions independent of the outcome. An action may be deemed right or wrong regardless of the consequences.

Reflective Considerations

Rule Utilitarianism

- Consider the concept of rule utilitarianism, whereby a set of specific rules may be applied. This concept justifies withholding a particular action if the potential outcome of that action could result in more harm and unhappiness than achieving the greatest good for the greatest number of people.
- Discuss the pros and cons of this principle of rule utilitarianism.

The Principle of Justice

Justice links to utilitarianism in terms of the greatest good, right, happiness, or pleasure for the greatest number in a society or population group. Orb (2007) related this to equal opportunities in terms of equal access to facilities and services, and equal distribution and utilization of resources. However, there are conflicting views about what might be perceived as justice and fairness. For this chapter, we assume justice to reflect the fundamental rights of people to the greatest contentment and in terms of the right of people to food, shelter, health care, and employment.

Reflective Considerations

The Principle of Justice and Fairness

- Consider the accessibility of certain healthcare modalities or therapeutic resources such as drugs or specialist procedures. Is it justifiable for access to be withheld or restricted due to cost implications for the taxpayer and the wider society?
- Consider HIV treatment, free contraception, and outreach programs in response to the global agenda for sexual health care. How justifiable is it for any government in developing countries to restrict or withhold resources for the economic justification of the "greatest good for the greatest number" in those societies?
- Consider the justification of preventive and screening initiatives, vaccination and immunization programs for sexually transmitted infections (STIs) and reproductive tract diseases to limit transmission and spread and to protect the general public. Are restrictions of specific vaccines for specific population groups justified on the basis of the cost, or even because of the indifference of particular population groups to uptake of services? If these are not ethically justifiable, what national initiatives might prove to be effective and beneficial, just, and fair to the general population?

Deontology: Does Acting Fulfill Moral Duties?

The theory of deontology proposes that actions are right if carried out to fulfill particular duties or commitments. Unsurprisingly, the notion that actions can be determined through intuitive reasoning as being morally right, and therefore justifiable (DeWolf Bosek & Savage, 2007; Orb, 2007), raises various questions. Healthcare practitioners are considered to have an obligation to preserve life and to respect a patient's confidentiality (General Medical Council [GMC], 2016; Nursing and Midwifery Council [NMC], 2015). The practitioner faces the challenge of acting knowledgeably and caringly while at the same time demonstrating sensitivity and sympathy.

For example, a woman insists that her HIV-positive diagnosis should not be divulged to her husband, who is keen that they should start a family. The practitioner must consider that while he/she may want to consider this request with sensitivity and sympathy in respect of patient confidentiality, they are also expected to fulfill professional obligation to preserve the baby's welfare in pregnancy, during labor, and possibly breastfeeding. Therefore, this principle may present a dilemma that would require careful examination of the particular moral duty within the context of professional and organizational regulations and requirements.

The Principle of Categorical Imperative

The principle of categorical imperative derives from deontology and refers to the idea of acting out of moral obligation, regardless of intent. In health care, this could refer to the practitioner's sense of duty and commitment in delivering care, not merely as a means to an end but also as a vocation (Nelson, 2007). In situations where the practitioner encounters the dilemma of divulging patient confidentiality, this principle becomes demonstrable only if the action is deemed to be acceptable within the wider context of that professional practice. In these viewpoints, respect for the dignity of the individual should be the determinant factor that influences the action taken by the practitioner (Newham & Hawley, 2007).

Actions based on the assumption of universal law reflect the principle of respect for the patient's rights, dignity, confidentiality, and autonomy regardless of the individual's social and economic status. The practitioner has an obligation to act in the best interest and welfare of the patient. Such actions are deemed to be good despite any potential consequences (Newham & Hawley, 2007).

Reflective Considerations

Respect for Confidentiality

- Consider the situations in sexual health care where a spouse, partner, parent/guardian, or a friend or colleague asks to know details of the patient's condition. Consider the principles of professional obligation and duty, respect of patient confidentiality, and the individual's fundamental human rights.

- What issues should be taken into consideration in making a decision about how best to handle this scenario?

Rights, Duties, and Responsibilities

The concept of rights relates to entitlement to a particular justified option. Rights can be construed as implying that an individual should have the freedom to take a particular action or not and feel no guilt or fear about consequences of recrimination or punishment. The individual can demand or claim that right or decide not to take advantage of it. Categorizations of rights include human rights, legal or statutory rights, as well as welfare rights such as the statutory benefits and entitlements, and moral and ethical rights (Maude & Hawley, 2007). While human rights have become a global and international concern, legal rights may vary depending on the type of right and a particular country's legislative system. Readers would find the American Nurses Association's (2015a) position statement on ethics and human rights' an excellent resource and highly recommended reading.

The Rights of Patients/Clients

Healthcare practitioners are expected to protect the rights, interests, and welfare of patients. Generally, patients have three fundamental rights in health care: the right to treatment, the right to privacy, and the right to know. Thus, in fulfilling the obligation to protect those patient rights, healthcare professionals must provide information truthfully and honestly to the individual about his/her condition, prognosis, and the medical and nursing therapeutic decisions and interventions. The rights of patients embrace the tenet of the patients' charter or rights, which have evolved over more than four decades (Maude & Hawley, 2007). In the broader context those rights include:

1. Access to healthcare facilities and treatment
2. Informed consent to treatment
3. Acceptance or refusal of treatment and procedural interventions
4. Information about own health, the treatment, and care provision
5. Privacy, confidentiality
6. Informed decision and choices (Maude & Hawley, 2007)

The underlying theme of these rights is ensuring public protection, which is accomplished in the standards that relevant healthcare organizations and the statutory professional bodies set for guiding practitioners. The concept of moral rights and ethical behavior in professional practice is evident within the professional code of standards of practice and behavior. Maude and Hawley (2007) identify ethical and moral duties and behaviors of practitioners in protecting the dignity of patients and in the supportive duty of patient advocacy. They also identify practitioner accountability in care provision and the mutuality of the practitioner–patient relationship as partners in care.

Reflective Consideration

Conflict of Values and Principles

- Consider the hypothetical scenarios in which the practitioner's professional duty and the related ethical principles conflict with the personal rights that the patient wishes to exercise.

- How best can this be dealt with by the practitioner? How are practitioners expected to react when they encounter such situations?

The Rights of the Practitioner

Practitioners have rights as well. Practitioner rights include individual autonomy, the right to professional support, and the right to decline to participate in specific treatment or therapeutic procedures (Maude & Hawley, 2007). Reasons for declining may relate to the individual's religious, cultural and/or personal beliefs, values, and principles. While the professional code of standards of practice and behavior may override the personal values, practitioners can exercise certain personal rights.

The right to exercise conscientious objection as incorporated in the professional codes of the medical and the nursing and midwifery professions allow individuals the right to decline to participate in specific therapeutic interventions. An example of this is termination of pregnancy, in which a practitioner may exercise their personal, cultural, religious, ethical, and moral perspectives. It is crucial, however, that practitioners critically examine the conscientious objection statement in the code and carefully note specific clauses. Notably, this right is only applicable *except* where the priority is saving the life of the pregnant woman or to prevent serious permanent complications or damage to her physical or mental health. The practitioner is required to notify an appropriate person in authority of his/her decision to exercise the right of conscientious objection. The code stipulates that this should be done in advance, so that the employer and all relevant parties are aware of the objection. Thus, the lead clinician, nurse, or midwife manager, or other identified senior staff, should have time to put alternative arrangements in place.

These requirements are important, as they raise practitioner awareness of their duty to comply with the code of conduct and professional standards of practice and behavior. Practitioners should recognize that noncompliance with these requirements could essentially constitute professional negligence. Further, noncompliance could lead to disruption of care provision for the patients, additional workload for other members, and potential risk of harm to patients. Such scenarios necessitate emergency decisions to secure appropriate backup and alternative rearrangement, swapping, reallocation, and remedial delegation of duties to other staff to avoid undesirable consequences. Maude and Hawley (2007) advocate the use of an ethical grid for making a clear and reasoned assessment from the perspectives of the patient, healthcare professional, the organization, and the relevant authority in control of decisions about actions.

Duties

The concept of duty is connected to the concept of rights in that one person's rights require that another person has a duty to ensure respect, protection, and fulfilment of that right. The National Health Service organization (NHS), the current clinical commissioning groups (CCGs), and the service providers have a duty to meet the healthcare needs of the patients/clients. In their professional capacities, healthcare professionals have specific duties to patients to implement high standards in the provision of evidence-based quality care. Moreover, practitioners have a duty to promote patient recovery from the state of ill health. The public has an expectation of these duties, and the professional regulatory bodies provide guidance to ensure that these expectations are fulfilled. Patients have a right to claim and demand those rights and expect them to be met. Therefore, negligence on the part of the healthcare professional may be pressured by patients through the complaint system or even litigation proceedings. Healthcare professionals also have a duty to inform the patients about their rights within the context of the healthcare provision. The individuals should be made aware of how they can exercise their rights within that care situation. As part of their duty of care, practitioners are expected to act in ways that would benefit and not cause harm to patients.

The Duty to Protect

This principle extends the practitioner's duties to a third party identified by the patient. The duty to protect requires the healthcare professional to take appropriate actions to protect an individual toward whom the patient — normally owed full confidentiality — has expressed an intention to take a potentially harmful action (DeWolf Bosek, 2007). This may be an active threat of physical injury, or it may be an expressed wish to pursue a course of action that would prove harmful (e.g., refusing to allow partner notification after a diagnosis of a STI). The practitioner should advise that third party that he/she may be in danger or at risk of real harm.

The practitioner has a duty to act in order that the individual would not be exposed to that harm. Nevertheless, the issue of breaching patient confidentiality must be carefully considered. Alternative approaches involving educative and supportive strategies as part of the therapeutic intervention might help the patient avert the risk of harm to the identified third party (DeWolf Bosek, 2007).

In the context of sexual health care, it is important that the practitioner does not misconstrue what a patient may have divulged. Therefore, to avoid causing unnecessary distress to any third party, the information should be carefully clarified and the identity of the third party tactfully and sensitively confirmed. It may be useful to consult with a specialist and involve the patient in sharing information to seek clarity on this issue.

Reflective Considerations

Breaching Patient Confidentiality

- Consider the scenario of a patient who is confirmed as having human immunodeficiency virus (HIV) positive infection or even confirmed as having developed acquired immune deficiency syndrome (AIDS).
- The patient admits to being sexually active and having multiple sexual partners.
- The patient forbids the sexual health practitioner from divulging this information to his/her spouse, partner, or the sexual partners. Disregarding that would constitute breaching the patient's right to confidentiality.
- Consider carefully and discuss these scenarios with colleagues in the multidisciplinary team regarding what actions should be taken.

Responsibilities

The concept of responsibility is rather vague and remains undefined. Savage and Moore (2004) noted various connotations of the term that suggest an individual's moral accountability for their own decisions and actions and the ability to fulfill expected obligations. Other connotations suggest answerability to a charge entrusted on an individual and the capability to function and conduct oneself in a rational manner. There are various alternative interpretations such as credibility and trustworthiness.

However, within the context of health care, responsibility and accountability appear to be used synonymously (Savage & Moore, 2004). Nonetheless, the perceived level of professional knowledge and expertise along with competence, are considered to be at a higher level in relation to accountability than they are in relation to responsibility. Therefore, accountability is assumed to embrace responsibility (Savage & Moore, 2004).

Reflective Considerations

Ethical Dilemmas

- Consider carefully and critically analyze the rights, duties, and responsibilities of the autonomous practitioner in midwifery where a woman presents with STI, rape, or other significant sexual abuse. Discuss the actions that should be taken and carefully examine the ethical principles of rights, duties, and responsibilities from the perspectives of the patient, and the practitioner(s) in relation to sexual healthcare.
- Also consider whether a third party might be involved in any of these scenarios and what actions might be best to deal with the related ethical dilemmas.

Religious Values and Principles: Implications and Dilemmas in Professional Practice

The following brief overview of religious and cultural beliefs and principles may serve to raise the awareness of practitioners who have difficulty dealing with certain patient reactions and behaviors in the care setting. In the following sections, principles and ideals held by different cultural and religious faiths are considered with reference to the moral and ethical values relating to contraception and abortion. Practitioners should reflect on the related moral and ethical debates about the issues that influence the attitudes, behaviors, and decisions that patients may hold and how these affect certain clinical care interventions.

Anglicanism (Church of England and the Episcopal Church)

The Anglican communion's perspective on contraception is that while its use is acceptable within the marital relationship, both parties should agree on the use or avoidance of particular contraceptive methods. Additionally, the welfare of existing children is strongly emphasized. While termination of pregnancy (abortion) is strongly disputed and rejected, it is nonetheless recognized that moral consideration of the situation may allow termination of pregnancy in some specific circumstances (The Church of England, 2017).

Catholicism

The perspective of Catholicism is that by and large, the contraceptive practices—particularly those methods considered as artificial means of preventing conception—dispute what human sexuality entails. However, conventional, evidence-based, natural family planning techniques are considered as a respected approach to contraception, and therefore are more acceptable. Abortion is regarded as cessation or ending of human life, and the repercussion could be exclusion from the church if the individual is deemed to be knowingly seeking termination. Moral and ethical considerations designed to help women include being pardoned and supported while the lives of their unborn children are also protected (Catholic Bishops' Conference of England and Wales [CBCEW], Hirsch, 2008).

A moral and ethical dilemma arises when the principles of the double effects doctrine challenge the concept of therapeutic abortion. The double effects doctrine recognizes acts that achieve good or beneficial outcome but also cause harm as a consequence of the good. While the decision to terminate a pregnancy may be taken in the best interest of a mother carrying a fetus with severe congenital abnormalities that are incompatible with life, the actual act of abortion violates Catholic moral values. While the termination serves as a means to achieve good in the interest of the mother, it constitutes to a violation the double effects doctrine (Nelson, 2007). The moral wrong of terminating the pregnancy and the harm caused by ending the life of the fetus are not deemed as justifiable in resolving the maternal problem and therefore violate Catholic moral values. The Catholic religion advocates involvement of the husband in decisions about pregnancy termination and in pre- and post-abortion counseling. Moreover, the Catholic religion emphasizes that every effort should be made to safeguard the interest of the woman and her unborn child and protect both their lives (Lewis & Ward, 2007).

Islam

Islam upholds that while sexual needs in a legitimate marital relationship should be satisfied, premarital sex is forbidden—presumably for moral and ethical reasons. Contraception use is allowable to space childbearing, protect and safeguard the mental and physical well-being of the mother, and for reasons inspired by personal principles, moral values, and beliefs. Furthermore, coitus interruptus, condoms, cervical caps, and IUDs/IUS are acceptable methods of contraception on the basis that these are only temporary methods of avoiding conception. However, while vasectomy is strictly disallowed, female sterilization is permissible if the woman's life would be jeopardized or if her mental health would be seriously damaged by a pregnancy that is not preventable by other recognized lawful methods. Thus, in essence, so long as the method of birth control is unlikely to result in permanent sterilization or cause any harm to either member of the couple, it is acceptable to Islamic religion.

Regarding abortion, Islam strictly forbids abortion after the fourth month (120 days) except when necessary to save the mother's life (Hedayat, Shooshtarizadeh, & Raza, 2006). Termination of pregnancy is allowable before 120 days of gestation in the interest of maternal health, for reasons of rape, or if the termination is carried out to enable the woman to continue breastfeeding an existing baby, but is generally forbidden for non-therapeutic reasons (Hedayat et al., 2006). The Islamic religion requires that the husband be involved in decisions about termination of a pregnancy (Blake & Katrak, 2002; Doctor, Phillips, & Sakeah, 2009; Hawley & Landsdown, 2007; Lewis & Ward, 2007).

Beyond the abortion issue, Islamic moral principles advocate modesty in safeguarding and respecting a woman's femininity. A female doctor or specialist is considered more acceptable for women who must expose themselves for medical reasons, particularly gynecological examinations. Decisions relating to contraception, pregnancy, and abortion or termination of pregnancy should have the joint agreement of the woman and her husband. Matters relating to sexual intercourse are considered to be so private between the couple that the patient may appear to be uncooperative or reluctant to divulge any related information, even at gynecological consultations.

Sikhism

Sikhism professes sexual morality in terms of decorum dignity and modesty and therefore espouse monogamy and contraception as an acceptable practice to limit the size of the family. Abortion, however, is only accepted in dire circumstances to save the woman's life or in cases of rape.

Hinduism

The principles and ideals of Hinduism are perceived as rather complex. The fundamental moral values are underpinned by the pursuits of karma, artha, dharma, and moksha, which denote pleasure, material wealth, moral lifestyle or duty, and emancipation through self-denial, respectively. Hinduism advocates practices of sexuality that are deemed within that culture to be morally and ethically positive and therefore acceptable to the Hindu religion. While contraception is acceptable, there is a strong Hindu belief in the duty to produce sons or male offspring, which creates tension in their values. Thus, there is a moral conflict of disallowing use of contraception until that duty has been fulfilled.

Hindu disapproval of abortion is based on the belief that spiritual and physical life begin at conception. Nevertheless, in cases of rape, incest, or potential risk of harm to the woman's mental health, abortion may be permissible on ethical grounds (BBC, 2009; Crawford, 1995; Damian, 2010). It is worth noting, however, that uncertainty or indecisiveness on the part of a Hindu patient about such an issue may emerge during clinical consultation or care provision. The dilemma may be based on the fundamental principles of Hinduism, which give no exemption to rape or fetal malformations (Hawley & Lansdown, 2007).

Judaism

Judaism dictates that contraceptive use by men is not acceptable. However, this implies that the use of contraception by women is allowable. Nevertheless, surgical techniques (e.g., male and female sterilization) perceived as causing impairment of the structures and physiological function of the reproductive system are not acceptable. The oral contraceptive pill, however, is not considered to interfere with the natural process of sexual intercourse and therefore is acceptable, yet coitus interruptus or withdrawal is unacceptable by Jewish moral principles and belief. Contraception use is allowable when safeguarding the physical and psychological health of the woman in whom the pregnancy could cause detrimental effect. While abortion is not permitted, it may be allowable to save the life of the mother or prevent risk of harm to her mental and physical health. In other special cases such as rape, the rabbi may sanction termination of the pregnancy (Friedman, Labinsky, Rosenbaum, Schmeidler, & Yehuda, 2009; Lewis & Ward, 2007).

Buddhism

Buddhists believe that conception occurs at fertilization and therefore methods and contraception that act prior to this stage are allowable. The Buddhist view that human life begins at conception protects the human rights of the fetus. Nevertheless, a particular issue of sensitive ethical debate is that Buddhism also holds the view that all beings are not equal. For that reason abortion is allowable if the pregnancy would pose detrimental risk to the health of the woman, because the fetus is not considered to be of equal human status as the mother (Damian, 2010).

These concise overviews are meant to convey some of the moral and ethical issues that practitioners may encounter. Gaining some insight into the moral and ethical values and principles of various religions can help to deal with conflicts and dilemmas that may be encountered during consultations and care provision interactions. Frequently, culturally driven morals and/or religious principles are demonstrated in the behaviors, decisions, and actions of a patient and could impact the care that is provided to one or both members of the couple. While some religious and cultural principles forbid most if not all the conventional contraceptive methods other than abstinence, others permit only the methods that prevent fertilization of the ovum. Practitioners are required through the code of conduct and ethics to support and educate the woman or the couple to enable them to make informed decisions (Savage, 2007). Practitioners are expected to perform this duty sensitively, without judging the patient and despite the personal moral and ethical values and principles with which they may have entered their professional career. Rather than enforcing one's personal values on the patient, the professional code stipulates that practitioners base their judgments, decisions, and actions in care provision on best available evidence.

The issue of abortion raises moral dilemmas and ethical debates about the rights of the woman or couple, the timing and stage of viability, the human rights of the fetus, and the circumstances or reason for the termination. A woman's choice to terminate a pregnancy as a method of contraception is a moral and ethical concern that can have political ramifications (Savage, 2007). Using abortion simply as a means to achieve personal control or fulfill one's own motives may lead to dilemmas, conflicts,

and repercussions in the clinical care situation. These may conflict with the rights of the patient and the rights of the practitioner, as well as compliance with the professional code of conduct and the related professional obligations of duty and responsibility.

Reflective Considerations

Moral and Ethical Conflicts in Clinical Consultations

- In what ways might the practitioner react to situations that compromise his/her personal values, principles, and rights? Consider encounters with the different personal, religious, cultural, and moral values and principles that patients/clients of diverse backgrounds present to the practitioner–patient relationships.

- Consider a particular patient's apparent lack of interest to engage in any form of dialogue or interactions relating to sexual risk-taking behaviors and unprotected sexual intercourse. The underlying reason for the disinclination, unwillingness, or nervousness may be because of personal values, misconceptions, belief in specific sexual myths, or cultural and religious principles that probably put the onus for safer sex on the women.

- Discuss the most effective consultation interaction for supporting such a patient.

- It may be useful to review the models of consultation explored earlier in this text.

Female Genital Mutilation (Female Circumcision)

Female circumcision, also known as female genital mutilation (FGM), involves partial or total removal of the external genitalia with other associated injuries (WHO, 2000). **Figure 19-1** shows an image of normal female genitalia before circumcision is performed. The procedure is usually carried out for cultural rather than medical reasons and may not necessarily represent religious principles (Rahman & Tuobia, 2000). The broad definition of this genital impairment encompasses additional injuries that may have been intentionally or unintentionally inflicted on the genital structures. **Figure 19-2** shows an image of the circumcised genitalia following healing of the sutured wound. While FGM has provoked attention throughout the world, the practice tends to be prevalent among specific population groups in Africa, the Middle East, and Asia. For instance, it is estimated that 98% of Somali women undergo an FGM procedure (Danish Immigration Service, 2004). FGM is also practiced in Latin America, Malaysia, and Indonesia with an estimated incidence of 50% to 98%

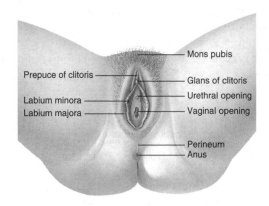

Figure 19-1 Female Circumcision: Before

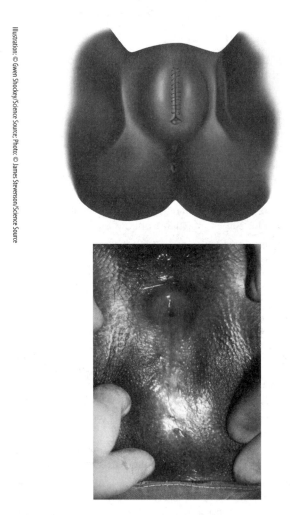

Figure 19-2 Female Circumcision: After

(Momoh, 2005). The World Health Organization (WHO) noted in 2000 that 100 million to 140 million females are exposed to this practice worldwide (WHO, 2000). Of that number, Powell, Lawrence, Mwangi-Powell, and Morison (2002) estimated that 86,000 young women in Britain have undergone some form of FGM.

Although commonly performed on young girls between 4 and 13 years of age, there is evidence that this cultural rite is performed on females outside of this range. It may be performed on infant girls or the procedure may be delayed until the girl is a young woman, just prior to marriage (United Nations Children's Fund [UNICEF], 2013, 2016; United Nations Population Fund [UNFPA] & UNICEF, 2015; WHO, 2017). The practice is vigorously opposed by the WHO and by pressure groups in several countries around the world. Yet, rather than judgmentally condemning what certain cultures value and uphold as morally and ethically acceptable, carefully considered and evidence-based critical examination and discussion are needed. Such evidence may help at the international level to find some sort of compromise in addressing FGM sensitively and efficiently.

FGM is generally performed by tribal circumcisers in the specific cultures (WHO, 1996). However, worldwide influences and emerging pressure groups have gained some success in imposing some changes. For example, while extensive efforts are being made to eliminate the practice throughout the world (United Nations General Assembly, 1993), the question arises: Is there ever any justification for a healthcare professional to perform FGM/C? It has been argued that FGM/C may be permissible to safeguard the welfare and interest of a young girl or woman if her mental health is deemed to be at risk if denied, as argued in Serour (2013). That rather controversial, sympathetic sanctioning does not appear to be advocated by authorized professional bodies and organizations. The main concerns regarding FGM focus on the complex effects on the young girl or young woman's physical and mental health, including possible complications associated with this practice. Of equal importance, the complexity of the moral, ethical, and legal implications should be given careful consideration.

Related National, Professional, and Organizational Policy Regulations

The Royal College of Nursing's (RCN) (2015) guidelines have similar components to the national and international framework on FGM to guide nursing, midwifery, and public health practitioners. The CCGs of the NHS organization's policies and protocols also derive from the international framework and require that healthcare practitioners gain adequate familiarity with the complications of FGM to ensure efficient evidence-based care provision.

Sexual healthcare and midwifery practitioners should explore and understand FGM, the associated complications, and the potential effects on young girls and women and their female infants. Practitioners will benefit from enhancing their professional knowledge and proficiency. **Figure 19-3** illustrates the extent of incision and suturing of genital structures which determines the specific FGM Type. Evidence-based knowledge will help provide a holistic approach to care for such patients within the multidisciplinary context. It is also worthwhile for practitioners to understand the practical implications of FGM within sexual health care, gynecological, obstetric/midwifery, and maternal child care statutory regulations and guidelines.

Further, gaining insight about this practice and its implications may help to establish better practitioner–patient relationships and create more effective partnerships in care provision. Three key recommended readings are Royal College of Midwives (RCM), RCN, and Royal College of of Obstetricians and Gynaecologists (RCOG) (2013); RCN (2015); and UNICEF (2016).

Some Cultural Values and the Underpinning Moral and Ethical Principles

Although FGM is condemned in many countries across the world, and the practice is perceived by global governments and NGOs as a physical assault and a human rights violation, that perception is not held in communities that practice FGM. Instead, the procedure is upheld as an important cultural rite to signify a young girl's acceptance into her society or transition to womanhood. In some cases, it is the family's way of declaring the young girl's eligibility for marriage. It is perceived as preserving and protecting the family's honor while upholding a cultural tradition (Mc-Cafferty, 2005; U.S. Dept. of Health and Human Services Office on Women's Health, 2017).

Healthcare practitioners have a professional responsibility to ensure they are adequately informed about FGM. Different types of FGM techniques are performed and practitioners should understand each of them for the related clinical care that the patients will require. **Box 19-1** presents concise descriptions of the different FGM techniques (**Figure 19-4**).

BOX 19-1 Concise Descriptions of the Types of FGM Techniques

FGM is classified according to the extent of excision of structures from the external genitalia.

- Type I – (FGM I) Excision of the prepuce (circumcision). This may or may not involve excision of the clitoris (clitoridectomy). This type constitutes the most minor form of the procedure. Figure 19-3 B.
- Type II – (FGM II) The "Sunna circumcision" (Arabic for traditional) involves excision of the clitoris with partial or total excision of the labia minora. Figure 19-3 C.
- Type III – (FGM III) The pharaonic circumcision, known as infibulation, involves excision of part of or the entire structures of the external genitalia followed by suturing to leave only a small opening for menstrual flow. This is considered as a very extensive form of FGM. Figure 19-3 D.
- Type IV – (FGM IV) refers to all other types including piercing, pricking, scraping, or cauterization of the clitoris and its surrounding tissue.

Data from World Health Organization (WHO). (2017). Female genital mutilation. Fact Sheet No. 241. Geneva, Switzerland: Author. Retrieved from http://www.who.int/mediacentre/factsheets/fs241/en/

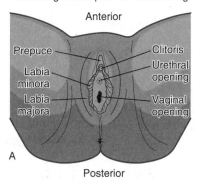

Normal genitalia prior to FGM/Cutting

Anterior

Prepuce — Clitoris
Labia minora — Urethral opening
Labia majora — Vaginal opening

A

Posterior

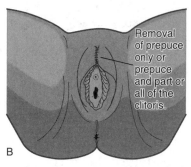

Type I - (FGM I) Circumcision

Removal of prepuce only or prepuce and part or all of the clitoris.

B

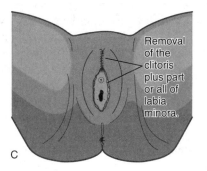

Type II - (FGM II) Sunna circumcision

Removal of the clitoris plus part or all of labia minora.

C

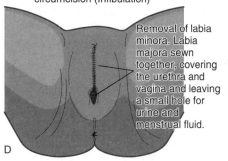

Type III - (FGM III) Pharaonic circumcision (Infibulation)

Removal of labia minora. Labia majora sewn together, covering the urethra and vagina and leaving a small hole for urine and menstrual fluid.

D

Figure 19-3 Three Types of FGM: I, II, & III

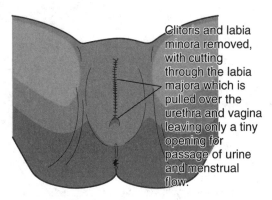

Figure 19-4 Type IV - (FGM IV) Varied Excisions of Clitoris and Surrounding Tissues

Complications Associated with FGM: Immediate and Long Term

The ongoing debates about and opposition to FGM are largely based on the mounting evidence of complications that can arise based on ways in which the procedure may be performed.

Immediate and intermediate complications include devastating pain, hemorrhage, shock, and infection, possibly with septicemia and even the risk of tetanus. The latter is attributed to the variety of instruments used without proper sterilization techniques (Denholm, 1998). The infection has been known to spread to other pelvic structures, which can in turn cause recurrent and chronic problems such as obstruction or difficulty with passage of urine, obstruction to menstrual flow, hematocolpus, and pelvic inflammatory disease. Recurrent vaginal and urinary tract infections, mainly cystitis, are common occurrences (RCN, 2006). Other complications include abscesses, benign nerve tumors, cysts, and abnormal scar tissue formation (U.S. Dept. of Health and Human Services Office on Women's Health, 2017).

The long-term complications include post-traumatic stress disorder, and the structural tissue damage can result in extensive scarring with the risk of adhesions. Moreover, extensive damage to reproductive structures can lead to infertility. Sexual complications include dyspareunia, and this, together with other associated problems, can lead to the phenomenon described by Delvin (2015) as "lack of sex drive in women." In this case, the flashbacks and permanent pain result in loss of libido, causing tension, bitterness, resentment, or even breakdown of the relationship between a couple. A lack of confidence in healthcare professionals as supportive and a lack of dependable caregivers have also been highlighted (RCN, 2006).

Potential Complications Associated with Childbirth

Impairment of the genital structures and the associated scar tissue (which may be extensive, depending of the type of FGM technique) can lead to greater risk of childbirth complications. The complications may occur because scar tissue does not stretch in the same way as healthy, uninjured tissue, thus the extensive scarring can result in not only delay in the second stage of labor, but also the risk of lacerations at the perineum with considerable hemorrhage. The available evidence showing that operative deliveries/cesarean sections are performed more frequently among women with FGM due to second-stage complications cannot be disregarded (Banks, Meirik, Farley, & Akande, 2006; Reisel & Creighton, 2015; WHO, 2000b). Wuest et al. (2009) noted that considerably more often, FGM patients had emergency caesarean section and third-degree vaginal tears. Postpartum hemorrhage and prolonged hospital stay are also reported (Banks et al., 2006). Additionally, the neonate may require considerable or mechanical resuscitation due to asphyxiation from the delayed second stage of labor (Kaplan et al., 2013). Stillbirth, early neonatal death, fetal distress, and low birth weight have also been reported (Kaplan et al., 2013; WHO, 2000). The indication for episiotomies should be promptly recognized to minimize such risks when attending to laboring women with FGM (Daley, 2004).

Ongoing Debates: Cultural Justifications, Moral, Ethical, Legal, and Governmental Acts

While the reasons for FGM may be unacceptable among those societies not practicing the procedure, there is a belief among societies that do practice FGM that it has hygienic benefits in that it prevents offensive genital odor. Additionally, the act is seen as a way to ensure the maidenhood, modesty, and dignity of the society's young virgins and to safeguard them from promiscuity. These benefits are strongly held and are considered culturally justified. The challenge for practitioners is to provide culturally competent care (Settelmaier & Nigam, 2007), while at the same time complying with professional ethical regulations.

The Joint Initiative to Minimize the Potential Risks

The opponents of FGM argue that it is nothing more than gender stratification and a violation of gender-specific human rights. There is an inherent element of powerlessness in the social control of a young woman's sexual pleasure by the removal of her clitoris (U.S. Dept. of Health and Human Services Office on Women's Health, 2017). Other opposition arguments emphasize discrimination against women, human rights abuses, and suppression of women's position within the cultures supporting the practice (McCaffrtey, 2005).

These debates led to the consideration in 1958 of FGM in the United Nations' (U.N.) agenda (Sigal & Denmark, 2013; see also Universal Declaration of Human Rights, 1948; United Nations General Assembly, 1993; United Nations Human Rights, 2014). The concern became recognized within a working group set up by the United Nations during 1975 to 1985 charged with the task of examining harmful traditional practices affecting the health of women and children. This was followed in 1997 by a joint initiative of the WHO, the United Nations' Children's Fund (UNICEF), and the U.N. Population Fund aimed at significantly reducing FGM within 10 years and to eradicate the practice completely within three generations (UNFPA & UNICEF, 2015). Practitioners are urged to read the RCM, RCN, and RCOG (2013) intercollegiate recommendations.

Related Acts and Protocols: Guiding Principles and Procedures

Within the United Kingdom and other western countries, concern about FGM in clinical care seems to coincide with increases of migrant groups and refugees. FGM became a criminal offense in the United Kingdom under the Prohibition of Female Circumcision Act of 1985. The Female Genital Mutilation Act of 2003 replaced the previous act, making it a criminal offense for the procedure to be performed on any U.K. nationals or citizens and permanent U.K. residents. That stipulation applies even when the individuals travel abroad. Furthermore, the act stipulates that aiding, abetting, and counseling or securing the performance of FGM within the United Kingdom constitutes a criminal offense. Likewise, involvement in any of these activities while visiting other countries where the practice is acceptable is also deemed a criminal offense (Department of Health, 2003). In the United States, FGM was made illegal under the Federal Prohibition of Female Genital Mutilation Act in 1977. Twenty-four U.S. states have separately enacted legislation prohibiting FGM, and other states lacking specific legislation targeting the practice may use more general statutes, such as child abuse legislation, to pursue criminal charges. The United States also passed the Transport for Female Genital Mutilation Act in 2013, making it illegal to transport a girl out of the country with the intent to have her undergo FGM elsewhere. Healthcare practitioners are urged to be vigilant in protecting young girls.

The Prohibition of Female Genital Mutilation (Scotland) Act 2005 stipulates that it is not an offense for a registered medical practitioner, a registered midwife, or a person undergoing training to perform certain operative procedures on women who have undergone FGM. Surgical operation on such women during any stage of labor (including just after) or just after the birth for therapeutic purposes should specifically relate to safeguarding the welfare and safety of the patient. However, it is an offense for any practitioner to perform re-infibulation following delivery. The stipulations are rather complex and the importance of being adequately informed about the related policies and protocols cannot be disregarded.

Current Regulations and Guidance

The Female Genital Mutilation Act (2003) has since been amended by the Serious Crime Act of 2015, which includes an FGM protection order. This act allows actual or potential victims protection under the civil law. Protection can be applied for through a family court and can be done on behalf of a victim by teachers, healthcare professionals, the police, or family members. The multi-agency practice guidelines on female genital mutilation stipulate job-specific guidance for health, education, police, and children's services. Furthermore, it provides step-by-step actions, advice on what to do, a list of points to consider, and legal guidance. The proceedings are unique to each case and comprise legally binding conditions, prohibitions, and restrictions to protect the person at risk of FGM.

The London Safeguarding Children Board (2009) published the "London Female Genital Mutilation" resource pack. More recently, the Home Office (2014) published a free e-learning package "Recognising and Preventing FGM," which provides information for professionals who need to find out more about identifying and responding to FGM. In 2014, the U.K. government (Department of Health, 2014) published the Anti-FGM Declaration, stipulating the following:

- Hospitals are required to provide information on patients who have been subjected to FGM.
- The launching of a community engagement initiative.
- Appointment of a consortium of leading FGM campaigners to deliver a global awareness campaign.

Mandatory Reporting of FGM

Professionals in the United Kingdom are required to make a report within one working day if they are informed by the FGM victim or observe signs of FGM in a girl under 18 years of age. Importantly, this is not considered a breach of confidentiality. A maximum time frame of 1 month is allowed for reporting in exceptional cases. The mandatory reporting duty (Mandatory Reporting of FGM) stipulates when and how to make a report, next steps following a report, and the consequences for failure to comply with the duty.

Care interactions with women who have had FGM should show appropriate sensitivity and compliance with professional duties, regulations, and legal requirements. Sexual health nurses and midwives should enquire about FGM during the history taking from women and young girls who hail from practicing cultures. Where applicable, it is necessary to explain to the patient the procedures that could be implemented to achieve the best possible outcomes. This is particularly important if the woman presents with type III FGM (see Box 19-1). It may be necessary to refer her to an obstetrician to discuss reversal or de-infibulation. The procedure may be performed under local or general anesthetic around 20 weeks' gestation and, ideally, not delayed until the onset of labor (RCM, 2006, 2015). Similarly, in sexual health care, a woman's privacy and confidence in her caregivers are crucial and should be respected. It is also important to use inoffensive language to avoid humiliating or emotionally upsetting patients when addressing this sensitive issue.

Midwives should be particularly vigilant during the care of women in labor who have had FGM, which is the period of highest risk to the mother and her baby. In some units, the policy may require that the obstetrician be alerted about a woman with FGM type III. If not already performed, the de-infibulation may be carried out under an epidural block during labor (Hindlay & Montagu, 1997). If the clitoris appears to have been buried under scar tissue during the initial procedure, it may have to be exposed in the reversal procedure (Momoh, 2000).

Women who have undergone FGM may experience emotional and psychological trauma during the postnatal period. The long-term impact of her FGM may be a sensitive and difficult issue for her. Moreover, the process of de-infibulation could prove to be emotionally overwhelming. Sexual health problems could also result from extensive stretching, lacerations, and damage to the perineal and genitourinary structures. Therefore, the midwife, sexual health nurse, and other members of the healthcare team should be particularly observant and supportive to the patient. If required, referrals for specialist care and counseling should be made available.

Some Germane Issues for Consideration

FGM is endemic among some ethnic groups in Africa, the Middle East, and Asia. While it is not necessarily legal, the practice is culturally acceptable to the specific ethnic groups for reasons that are considered justifiable to them. In particular, these reasons are related to cultural values, beliefs, and moral and ethical principles rather than medical or legal reasons. The age group at which FGM is performed varies and ranges from infancy to women of childbearing age.

National and international frameworks provide guidelines to raise the awareness of healthcare practitioners regarding their professional responsibilities for safeguarding children and young girls who may be exposed to FGM. Sexual health nurses, midwives, public health and community nurses, and neonatal and other pediatric nurses have a professional obligation to be vigilant about this procedure. The morbidity and mortality associated with FGM remain a constant concern in professional practice and in the wider society. Potential complications include hemorrhage, infections of the sexual and reproductive tracts, septicemia, and possibly tetanus.

In the United Kingdom, the NHS Boards and clinical commissioning groups provide guidelines and protocols to inform and guide practitioners. Nevertheless, appropriate training is also required to enhance the practitioner's competence in recognizing FGM. Sexual health nurses and midwives would particularly benefit from training programs that emphasize visual images of FGM. Critical incident analysis, exemplars of best practice, and case study discussions may prove to be effective modes of sharing views and experiences. These are also useful for identifying appropriate models of consultation, care provision, and support for such patients. Efficient referral systems are crucial to ensure that appropriate multidisciplinary care is provided.

Ethical Regulations That Guide Professional Practice

While each professional healthcare discipline is guided by its own code and set of standards, common elements are found in all healthcare professions. These include the following:

- Protecting the interest of the public
- Safeguarding the welfare of patients as primary concern
- Respecting the individual's dignity
- Demonstrating openness, honesty, and accountability as expected
- Providing high quality care based on best available evidence
- Maintaining cooperative relationships with colleagues and coworkers

It is important to acknowledge and respect differences in the professional codes of other disciplines. Reel and Hutchings (2007) proposed effective measures to combat potential ethical conflicts such as a sense of belonging, enthusiasm, joint pursuit of the same goals in care provision, directness, trustworthiness, candor, and dependability. Mutuality of respect and support among team members are also desirable.

As part of the professional socialization, individuals learn the professional code of conduct and related ethical principles through both theory and practical components of their education and training programs. Practical application through critical incident scenarios, case studies, and vignettes enable novice practitioners to understand the importance of the statutory regulatory requirements with which they must comply. Because these are underpinned by specific moral codes and ethical principles, part of the learning process should involve self-reflection. In this way, the novice practitioner is able to examine the extent to which the personal values and principles with which she/he entered the profession compare to the moral and ethical principles of the code of professional standards of practice. It is important to be able to partition one's personal moral values and principles in order to appropriately respond to the professional code. Not only does this help to avoid inner conflicts, but ensures professional integrity. This includes respect for individual's rights and the choice to exercise the conscientious clause if necessary in specific clinical situations.

Reel and Hutchings (2007) identified various models of intervention used to address differences in individuals' values and ethical principles among practitioners in a multidisciplinary team. Realistically, colleagues may find it useful to share information and advice which allows one another to recognize their alternative perspectives. Moreover, confronting beliefs and attitudes and expressing emotions about specific issues or incidents in clinical practice enables colleagues to support one another (Reel and Hutchings (2007). No doubt this makes it more acceptable for colleagues to encourage each other to seek professional counseling if necessary.

The American Nurses Association (ANA), the American Medical Association, and the healthcare professional disciplines also maintain their dedication to standards, guidelines and principles, ethical codes, and regulations. For example, the ANA works to elevate the nursing profession through its stipulation of values and priorities for registered nurses throughout the United States. Furthermore, the ANA provides direction on relevant legislation together with implementing a framework for objective evaluation of excellence. Its position statement (2016) outlines professional role competence.

The ANA Code of Ethics issues guidelines for carrying out nursing responsibilities in a manner consistent with quality nursing care and ethical obligations of the profession. The new *Code of Ethics for Nurses with Interpretive Standards* (ANA, 2015b) provides appropriate clarification on the key ethical requirements to guide professional practice; "Practical Clinical Application Part I" and the New "Code of Ethics for Nurses Practical Clinical Application Part II" are accessible online to practitioners. Additionally, "Leading from Middle to Ethical Climate and Safety" addresses issues relating to the following areas:

- Patient Safety: The Ethical Imperative
- Social Media: Managing the Ethical Issues
- Whistleblowing: Role of Organizational Culture in Prevention and Management
- Conscientious Objection in Nursing: Defining the Criteria for Acceptance (June 2014)
- Ethical Challenges in an Era of Health Care Reform
- Applying the Ethical Code of Care to your Nursing Practice

The ANA also outlines its recognition of a nursing specialty in its "Specialty Nursing Scope Statement." Practitioners in the United States are strongly encouraged to obtain the appropriate documents to comply with professional regulations and guidelines.

Significance of the Professional Codes

Professional councils provide guidance to practitioners regarding their professional duties and obligations. Professional codes represent prescribed guidance on the required standards and behavior expected of particular groups of practitioners. These are designed to regulate and control professional practice in terms of practitioners' actions, conduct, and performance. The individual's level of accountability also falls the standard of performance. Furthermore, the codes provide guidance on moral and ethical principles in professional practice. The International Council of Nurses' (ICN, 2015a, 2015b) *Code of Ethics for Nurses* stipulates

the fourfold fundamental responsibilities of the nurse. These are very useful references for nursing practitioners. All practitioners are advised to familiarize themselves with their national regulations and code of professional standards and conduct.

Reflective Considerations

Possible effects of personal values on practitioner–patient interactions:

- What moral and ethical values and principles may individuals bring into their professional career?
- How might these personal values conflict with the principles that underpin the professional code of conduct and ethics?
- The clinician or practitioner may be faced with situations in professional practice that conflict with her/his personal values, beliefs, and principles. Consider the following scenarios in which the practitioner may face the dilemma to uphold his/her personal values:
  - the patient who seems to be consistently neglectful of his/her health, and is constantly deliberately irresponsible and uncooperative
  - the patient who intentionally fails to take the prescribed medication
  - the patient who is constantly careless and unconcerned to comply with the treatment regimen or inconsistent with the medication
  - the patient who ignores the health promotion/education, advice, and support that would encourage self-protection, control deterioration, or enhance healing and full recovery

---

Settelmaier and Nigam's (2007) exploration of the origins of an individual's values and beliefs examines these issues. They also present an analysis of the health professional's values, together with the expectation of responsible ethical behavior and the potential implications for professional development. **Box 19-2** summarizes possible reactions to moral and ethical conflicts encountered in professional practice.

The Regulatory Code of Standards and Guidance for Medical Practice

The following reflective considerations could be used in group interactive exercises for junior doctors or student doctors to reflect deeply and gain adequate familiarity with the guidance on their professional standards. Consider carefully what your professional body requires of you regarding specific key duties.

BOX 19-2 Possible Reactions to Moral and Ethical Conflicts Encountered in Professional Practice

Possible reactions to ethical and moral dilemmas:

- Anger, frustration, disillusionment
- Disinclination to continue providing the required standard of care and support
- Providing substandard or relatively poor quality of care
- Inclination to exercise the right to conscientious objection

Particular reactions may be linked to the individual's set of values and moral and ethical principles but may also reflect compliance with other standards, including the following:

- The code of professional standards of practice and behavior
- The regulations stipulated by the employing organization
- The stipulated policy of the specific area of care and service provision

Dealing with personal moral dilemmas and conflicts:

- Introspection—carefully examining and clarifying own personal values
- Identification of the values and principles that are particularly important to one's self
- Reflection on own personality
- Determining own strengths and further improving as necessary
- Determining and dealing with personal weaknesses

Possible explorations and reflections:

- Increasing own awareness by talking about ethical issues
- Actively participating in ethical decision-making (moral agent)
- Seeking appropriate consultation, counseling, and support as necessary

Compliance with the code of professional standards and conduct:

- At all times remembering the moral and ethical duty of care
- Complying with the principles of the professional code
- Reflecting on the requirement of ethical behavior expected of practitioners

These could be used in group interactive workshop activities as part of enhancement of professional socialization of registered practitioners.

Reflective Considerations

Duties of the Medical Practitioner

- What is the guidance of your regulatory council regarding the doctor's primary concern in patient care?
- How should you deal with an individual's attitude, principles, and preferences that may be impacting on their current health state?
- What does the guidance stipulate about discriminating against patients based on personal assumptions or opinions?
- How might these affect your rapport with patients, the therapeutic care that you provide, prescribe, or organize for them?
- What is the stipulation regarding conflicts with own religious or moral principles in terms of professional candor in the performance of particular procedures or provision of required advice?
- What are you expected to do if personal conflict might have a negative impact on the performance of your professional duties regarding the treatment and/or provision of advice? Consider the patient's right to seek the required medical care and advice elsewhere. Consider the guidance on appropriate referral.
- What is the stipulation regarding expressing personal principles, political, religious, or moral values?
- Consider the potential impact on the patient by causing humiliation, insult, and dismay.
- What additional cautionary statement is provided to remind the medical professionals about the potential consequences of persistent non-compliance and avoidance of inadvertent violation of the regulations designed to guide "Good Medical Practice"?

It is important to explore guidance regarding the potential impact of personal beliefs on doctor–patient relationships. It is particularly important to understand ways that individuals cope with the pain and distress that may accompany their illness. Examine the guidance carefully to be aware of conflicts that may occur when patients reject therapeutic interventions that are prescribed in their best interest. Additionally, examine the guidance on conflicts that could arise when a patient asks for treatment or a procedure that the professional considers to be inappropriate for him/her. Critically examine the guidance on effective means to address such scenarios.

The importance of a trusting doctor–patient relationship, and effective consultation with truthful, non-judgmental, rational, and honest dialogues necessitates mutual respect for the conscience and integrity of both the doctor and the patient. Some patients may find it sensitive to talk about their deeply held cultural and religious beliefs and principles. However, others may consider that dialogue as salutary and calming in the holistic care intervention and healing process. Therefore, in partnership with the patient these may be addressed cautiously in a sensitive manner. The guidance provides useful practical examples in the care of patients pre- and post-termination of pregnancy, FGM, or circumcision, and special clothing worn in compliance with cultural and religious principles.

Some patients trust the doctor to use his/her professional knowledge and expertise to make appropriate decisions that ensure he/she will receive quality care. The doctor's personal opinion regarding a patient's characteristics and circumstances such as age, gender, ethnicity, cultural background, nationality, color, lifestyle, or sexual orientation should not adversely influence his/her decisions about care provision. Similarly, the marital, social, and economic status of the patient should not distort or create bias in a doctor's valuation of the patient's clinical needs. None of these characteristics should be allowed to hinder or limit the patient's access to any aspect of the medical care that he/she requires. Conscientious objection should be divulged to the health service employing organization or contracting body. The doctor has a responsibility to establish what alternative arrangements are in place and the organizations' terms and conditions on this issue in order to carefully comply with the requirements.

Readers with medical backgrounds who are involved in clinical teaching and facilitating the professional and personal development of junior colleagues may consider encouraging students to explore the full details in the current updated guidelines. Similarly, practitioners engaged in continuing professional development activities may consider exploring the full details for enhanced insight about addressing various ethical dilemmas. Critical evaluation of elements in the guidance may even generate ideas for systematic reviews, research, or clinical audit projects.

The Regulatory Code of Professional Standards for Nursing and Midwifery Practice

Similar to the medical profession, nursing and midwifery practice is guided by stipulated code and principles. This Nursing and Midwifery Council (NMC) also profiles its corporate plan and its regulatory capacity. These are the goals that are of public interest: assurance of public protection through maintaining high standard of education and practice and keeping a register of qualified practitioners who are deemed to be fit to practice; dealing promptly and justly with individuals whose professional integrity, quality of care provision, and performance in practice and safety of care provision are deemed to be unacceptable, or questionable; and establishing practical, receptive, and open communications to ensure that the public is constantly aware of the expected standards of care that should be provided by nurses and midwives (NMC, 2015).

The NMC declares its regulatory duties, responsibilities, and accountabilities regarding standards of education and training, rules, and guidance to ensure that all practicing nurses and midwives are deemed to be safe practitioners. It also declares its commitment to investigate and deal justly and fairly with allegations of noncompliance with the professional code (NMC, 2015).

Duties and Responsibilities Expected of Nursing and Midwifery Practitioners

The obligations and duties with which nursing and midwifery practitioners are expected to comply in their everyday work are clearly outlined in their professional code of standards of practice and behavior. The following reflective considerations may be useful to encourage practitioners and students to critically consider and discuss the requirements with colleagues. Practitioners have a duty to ensure that patients are able to trust them with their health and well-being. To justify that trust, practitioners are expected to collaborate with professional colleagues and other relevant parties to ensure provision of high quality care. Professional integrity should be demonstrated in every aspect of their duties by behaving and conducting themselves with honesty and openness. They are also expected to respect human dignity, avoid bias, show sensitivity and kindness, and help individuals to access pertinent information, required support, and beneficial health and social care resources and facilities (NMC, 2015). Consider the following issues carefully.

Nursing and midwifery practitioners are urged to keep up-to-date with the current *Code: Professional Standards*

Reflective Considerations

Provision of Evidence-Based Information

Utilization of best available evidence ensures delivery of a high standard of care. Practitioners are urged to ensure that the advice they provide is appropriately substantiated by sound evidence. The expectation to establish partnership in care with patients requires that practitioners be attentive to individuals' concerns, needs, and preferences. Effective practitioner–patient dialogues at appropriate levels of communication can be linked to health promotion and effective self-care.

Practitioners are expected to provide patients with the information they request regarding their own condition and the treatment interventions. However, a particular request may conflict with appropriate professional judgment, safe practice, evidence-based quality care provision, or positive outcome.

- How is the professional practitioner expected to deal with such a scenario?
- What caution does the Council emphasize about patient information and provision of advice?

Reflective Considerations

Consent and the Mental Capacity to Concede or Refuse

The emphasis on confidentiality—the need and reasons for information sharing, protection of an individual from potential risk of harm, and disclosing particular details should be in accordance with the legal requirements, expectations, and principles of the particular country within which the professional is practicing.

- What does the professional code require of you? These issues require respect of the fundamental human right and personal preferences. Regarding the requirement for obtaining patient consent:

- What are the guidelines on the timing of obtaining consent for the specific care and treatment procedure? Consider carefully the individual's right to concede or the right to refuse to allow or permit the prescribed treatment or procedure.

- What are the guidelines regarding the legal conditions and stipulations designed to safeguard the interest of individuals who lack competent decision-making ability? Consider the rationales for patient involvement in decisions about their personal care.

- How important is the guideline regarding assessment of the mental capacity of the patient and actions taken in emergency situations?

Reflective Considerations

Accurate Recording and Safeguarding of Authenticity of Original Records

Accurate record keeping is emphasized as another requirement in professional practice.

- How does the Council emphasize the recording of dialogues with patients about the therapeutic interventions that they may receive?

- Discuss the importance of maintaining the authenticity of original details of patient records, including electronic records and safeguarding of detailed confidential documents.

- What are the implications of noncompliance or misdemeanor with the related stipulated guidance?

Reflective Considerations

Team Leadership Expectations and Consequences of Misconducts

Effective team leadership in terms of well-judged delegation ensures that required standards for high quality care are met.

- What is the expectation of lead practitioners toward realization of this responsibility?

Practitioners are expected to take immediate action if an individual puts themselves at risk or someone may be at risk because of colleagues or other people.

- What action are individuals expected to take if they feel that they are unable, for one reason or another, to fulfill any component of the professional standards of practice and behavior?

- How are practitioners expected to demonstrate that they are accountable for their decisions and actions that may be associated with any oversight in their practice, or inadvertent or deliberate errors?

The consequences of risking the fitness to practice or jeopardizing the legitimacy to remain on the professional register as a result of failure to comply with the duties and expectations must be clearly understood by all practitioners.

- In what situations might it be necessary for a practitioner to seek guidance and clarification on indemnity insurance?

Reflective Considerations

Ensuring Safety and Quality Care Provisions

Monitoring each other's work in a multidisciplinary team in terms of quality care provision and compliance with stipulations ensures protection and safety of the patients.

- What is the guidance regarding the sharing each other's professional knowledge and expertise within the multidisciplinary team?

Consider the requirement for consultations among colleagues and appropriate referrals in the best interest of the patient and the implications of prejudicial attitudes and intolerance.

- What are the expectations regarding support for junior colleagues and students and facilitation of their professional knowledge and competencies?

- What is the Council stipulation for post registration, continuing education, and training?

- What are the stipulations in terms of absolute professional imperative in certain unacceptable behaviors? Consider professional boundaries, involvement in any form of arrangements with patients in your care, and maintaining clear sexual limits with patients or their relatives.

of Practice and Behaviour (NMC, 2015) to help them fulfill the expectations of the statutory professional body. **Box 19-3** provides a concise outline of key elements in the expectations of practicing nurses and midwives for reflective exercises.

BOX 19-3 Concise Outline of Key Elements in the Expectations of Practicing Nurses and Midwives

The Professional Standards

Professional standards represent the expected performance which practitioners such as nurses and midwives are required to achieve in their professional practice. Six key elements that underpin the NMC's professional standards are as follows:

- Specialized body of knowledge
- Code of ethics
- Provision of high quality service in the interest of the public
- Competent application of the relevant professional knowledge
- Revalidation requirements
- Responsibility and accountability

Main Stipulations

- Making the care of patients the foremost and principal concern
- Treating people as individuals
- Respecting patient dignity
- Working with others to protect and promote the health and well-being of those being cared for, their families and caregivers, and the wider community
- Providing a high standard of care and practice at all times
- Demonstrating trustworthiness, decency, and uprightness and safeguarding the status of the profession

Four Fundamental Requirements Emphasized

- Duty of care to patients
- Cooperative relationship with colleagues/coworkers
- Responsibility and accountability in maintaining high professional values and principles
- Acting with integrity and upholding the reputation of the profession

Data from Nursing & Midwifery Council. (2015). The code: Professional standards of practice and behaviour for nurses and midwives. Retreived from https://www.nmc.org.uk/globalassets/sitedocuments/nmc-publications/nmc-code.pdf

---

U.K. practitioners are urged to familiarize themselves and comply with the detailed stipulations in the regulations that are sent to them. Similarly, practitioners in other countries are also urged to comply with the national regulations of the countries in which they currently practice.

Obligations of the Health Service Organization

The health service organization has an obligation to ensure equal opportunities in the provision of health care and health services to all citizens regardless of age, gender, or ethnicity. The Race Relations Amendment Act of 2000 makes this duty a statutory requirement which the health service organization must respond to. An important component of this act is to create a service that meets the needs of the cultural and linguistic diversity, differences in lifestyle, and religious beliefs and principles of the people served. Another component is to tackle problems among population groups of varied ethnic origins; in particular, inequalities in health and healthcare access with poorer quality of services. Thus, the department of health is committed to reducing the gap in patient satisfaction, health inequalities, and the inequities in access.

Arguably, broad categorizations can conceal diversity within the ethnic groupings and differences in health problems. Cultural differences can be quite intense and religious differences quite profound with very diverse principles. Broad categorizations often lead to stereotyping and disregard of diversity.

Broad Categorizations and Potential Implications

1. Cultural insensitivity in the provision of health care
2. Discrimination
3. Deprivation
4. Poverty
5. Poor social and economic status
6. Low income

Inevitable Differences in the Healthcare Experience

As a result, differences exist in the experiences of healthcare services among the different population groups. These may relate to issues such as the following:

1. Not getting timely access
2. Not being allowed to make informed choices in their treatment options
3. Not being involved in decisions about different aspects of their personal care

Related Influencing Factors and Potential Repercussions

Moral and ethical conflicts between patient and practitioner are a frequent dilemma. Individuals may demonstrate strong reservations to discuss certain issues. Others may only consider some sort of compromise to allow certain healthcare interventions, guidance and education. The point of the issue is how best the practitioner can deal with issues sensitively and effectively when providing care.

Similar to the United Kingdom's professional regulatory bodies, the American Nurses Association (ANA) also provides regulations to guide nurses. The current versions of the ANA Position statements on ethics and human rights (ANA, 2015a) and *Code of Ethics for Nurses with Interpretive Statements* (ANA, 2015b) are highly recommended reading. Another highly recommended reading is "Ethics and Health" by Kurtz and Burr (2016), who examine ethics in healthcare practice in greater detail.

Conclusion

Moral values, beliefs, and ethical principles should always be carefully considered in all aspects of SRH care and service provision. The potential impact on the progress and outcome of any intervention presents a challenge in professional practice. The cultural beliefs and religious principles relating to sexual health care, abortion/termination of pregnancy, and contraception create additional complexity to the challenges faced by practitioners during their interactions with patients. Therefore, it is important to carefully consider these within the context of actual care provision.

Despite the ongoing controversy, strong debates, and campaigns, the practice of FGM persists. The current movement of migrant populations justifies the need for enhancing practitioners' understanding of FGM with appropriate provision of evidence-based guidance, through regulations and recommendations. It is important that culturally sensitive care is provided, giving due respect to the patient's deeply held beliefs while dealing with the associated challenges in clinical practice.

Readers are encouraged to further explore the ethical issues in health and social care with particular attention to the context of SRH care. Medical, nursing, and midwifery practitioners are encouraged to read their professional codes with critically reflective minds and seek clarifications as necessary regarding the components of the regulations and guidelines.

• • • REFERENCES

American Nurses Association (ANA). (2015a). *American Nurses Association position statements on ethics and human rights*. Retrieved from www.nursingworld.org/MainMenuCategories/EthicsStandards /Ethics-Position-Statements

American Nurses Association (ANA). (2015b). *Code of ethics for nurses with interpretive statements*. Retrieved from http:// www.nursesbooks.org/Main-Menu/Ethics/Code-of-Ethics.aspx

Banks, E., Meirik, O., Farley, T., & Akande, O. (2006). Female genital mutilation and obstetric outcome: WHO collaborative prospective study in six African countries. *The Lancet, 367,* 1835–1841.

BBC. (2009). *Hinduism and abortion*. Retrieved from http://www .bbc.co.uk/religion/religions/hinduism/hinduethics/abortion_1.shtml.

Blake, S., & Katrak, Z. (2002). *Faith values and sex and relationships education*. London, United Kingdom: National Childrens' Bureau Sex Education Forum.

Catholic Bishops' Conference of England and Wales (CBCEW). (2004). *Cherishing life*. London, United Kingdom: The Catholic Truth Society and Colloquium (CaTEW) Ltd.

Childress, J. F., Faden, R. R., Gaare, R. D., Gostin, L. O., Khan, J., Bonnie, R. J., . . . Nieburg, P. (2002). Public health ethics: Mapping the terrain. *Journal of Law and Medical Ethics, 30*(2), 170–178.

Church of England. (2017). *The Church of England medical ethics and health and social care: Contraception*. Retrieved from http:// www.churchofengland.org/our-views/medical-ethics-health-social -care-policy/contraception.aspx

Crawford, S. C. (1995). The ethics of abortion. In *Dilemmas of life and death: Hindu ethics in a North American context* (pp. 11–36). Albany, NY: State University of New York Press.

Daley, A. (2004). Female genital mutilation: Consequences for midwifery. *Journal of Midwifery, 12*(5), 292–296.

Damian, C.-I. (2010). Abortion from the perspective of Eastern religions: Hinduism and Buddhism. *Romanian Journal of Bioethics, 8*(1), 125.

Danish Immigration Service. (2004). *Human rights and security in Central and Southern Somalia: A joint Danish, Finnish, Norwegian and British fact finding mission to Nairobi and Kenya*. Copenhagen, Denmark: Danish Immigration Service.

Delvin, D. (2015). *Lack of sex drive in women (lack of libido)*. Retrieved from http://www.netdoctor.co.uk/sex_relationships /facts/lackingsexdrive.htm

Denholm, N. (1998). *Female genital mutilation in New Zealand: Understanding and responding: A manual for health professionals*. Auckland, New Zealand: FGM Education.

Department of Health. (2003). *Female Genital Mutilation Act 2003* (c31). Retrieved from http://opsi.gov.uk/acts/acts2003 /ukpga_20030031_en-1

Department of Health. (2014). *The anti-FGM declaration*. Retrieved from https://www.gov.uk/government/news/new-government -measures-to-end-fgm

DeWolf Bosek, M. S. (2007). Mental health nursing. In M. S. DeWolf Bosek & T. A. Savage (Eds.), *The ethical component of nursing education: integrating ethics into clinical experience* (pp. 311–346). Philadelphia, PA: Lippincott Williams & Wilkins.

DeWolf Bosek, M. S., & Savage, T. S. (2007). Ethical standards of practice. In S. M. DeWolf Bosek & T. A. Savage (Eds.), *The ethical component of nursing education: integrating ethics into clinical experience* (pp. 45–66). Philadelphia, PA: Lippincott Williams & Wilkins.

Doctor H. V., Phillips, J. F., & Sakeah, E. (2009). The influence of changes in women's religious affiliation on contraceptive use and fertility among Kassena Nankana of Northern Ghana. *Studies in Family Planning, 40*(2), 113–122.

Friedman, M., Labinsky, E., Rosenbaum, T. Y., Schmeidler, J., & Yehuda, R. (2009). *Observant married Jewish women and sexual life: An empirical study*. Retrieved from https://www.jewishideas.org /article/observant-married-jewish-women-and-sexual-life-empirical -study

Gabel, S. (2011). Ethics and values in clinical practice: Whom do they help? *Mayo Clinic Proceedings, 86*(5), 421–424.

General Medical Council (GMC). (2016). *Good medical practice: Standards and ethics guidance for doctors.* Retrieved from http://www.gmc-uk.org/guidance/index.asp

Hawley, G. (2007). Start at 'Go.' In G. Hawley (Ed.), *Ethics in clinical practice: An interprofessional approach* (pp. 3–14). Essex, United Kingdom: Pearson Education Limited.

Hawley, G. & Lansdown, G. (2007). Eastern philosophical traditions. In G. Hawley (Ed.), *Ethics in clinical practice: An interprofessional approach* (pp. 101–136). Essex, United Kingdom: Pearson Education Limited.

Hedayat, K. M., Shooshtarizadeh, P., & Raza, M. (2006). Therapeutic abortion in Islam: Contemporary views of Muslim Shiite scholars and effect of recent Iranian legislation. *Journal of Medical Ethics, 32,* 652–657.

Hindlay, J., & Montagu, S. (1997). Midwifery care and genital mutilation. In I. Kargar, & S. C. Hunt (Eds.), *Challenges in midwifery care* (pp. 63–75). London, United Kingdom: Macmillan.

Hirsch, J. S. (2008). Catholics using contraceptives: Religion, family planning, and interpretive agency in rural Mexico. *Studies in Family Planning, 39*(2), 93–104.

Home Office. (2014). *Free e-learning package: Recognising and preventing FGM.* Retrieved from http://www.safeguardingchildrenea.co.uk/resources/female-genital-mutilation-recognising-preventing-fgm-free-online-training/

International Council of Nurses. (2006). *Code of ethics for nurses.* Geneva, Switzerland: Author. Retrieved from www.icn.ch/images/stories/documents/about/icncode_english.pdf

International Council of Nurses. (2012). *The ICN code of ethics for nurses.* Geneva, Switzerland: Author. Retrieved from www.icn.ch/images/stories/documents/about/icncode_english.pdf

Kaplan, A., Forbes, M., Bonhoure, I., Utzet, M., Martín, M., Malick, M., & Ceesay, H. (2013). Female genital mutilation/cutting in The Gambia: Long-term health consequences and complications during delivery and for the newborn. *International Journal of Women's Health, 5,* 323–331.

Kurtz, P., & Burr, R. (2016). Ethics and health. In K. S. Lundy & S. Janes (Eds.), *Community health nursing: Caring for the public's health* (3rd ed., pp. 249–269). Burlington, MA: Jones & Bartlett.

Lewis, B., & Ward, C. (2007). Sexuality: Masculine and feminine ethical issues. In G. Hawley (Ed.), *Ethics in clinical practice: An interprofessional approach* (pp. 319–347). Essex, United Kingdom: Pearson Education Limited.

McCafferty, C. (2005). Foreword. In C. Momoh (Ed.), *Female Genital Mutilation* (pp. vi–vii). Oxford, United Kingdom: Radcliffe Publishing Ltd.

Maude, P., & Hawley, G. (2007). Clients' and patients' rights and protecting the vulnerable. In G. Hawley (Ed.), *Ethics in clinical practice: An interprofessional approach* (pp. 54–75). Essex, United Kingdom: Pearson Education Limited.

Momoh, C. (2000). *Female genital mutilation also known as female circumcision: Information for health care professionals.* London, United Kingdom: Guy's and St. Thomas' Hospital Trust.

Momoh, C. (2005). *Female genital mutilation: Awareness and management in the UK.* London, United Kingdom: King's College.

Nelson, K. (2007). Ethical theories and principles. In M. S. DeWolf Bosek & T. A. Savage (Eds.), *The ethical component of nursing education: Integrating ethics into clinical experience* (pp. 1–30). Philadelphia, PA: Lippincott Williams & Wilkins.

Newham, R. A. & Hawley, G. (2007). The relationship of ethics to philosophy In G. Hawley (Ed.), *Ethics in clinical practice: An interprofessional approach* (pp. 76–100). Essex, United Kingdom: Pearson Education Limited.

Nursing and Midwifery Council (NMC). (2008). *The Code: Standards of conduct performance and ethics for nurses and midwives.* London, United Kingdom: Author.

Nursing and Midwifery Council (NMC). (2015). *The Code: Professional Standards of practice and behaviour for nurses and midwives.* London, United Kingdom: Nursing and Midwifery Council. Retrieved from https://www.nmc.org.uk/globalassets/sitedocuments/nmc-publications/nmc-code.pdf

Orb, A. (2007). Who gets what? In other words, the allocation of resources. In G. Hawley (Ed.), *Ethics in clinical practice: An interprofessional approach* (pp. 300–318). Essex, United Kingdom: Pearson Education Limited.

Powell, R. A., Lawrence, A., Mwangi-Powell, F. N., & Morison, L. (2002). Female genital mutilation, asylum seekers and refugees: The need for an integrated UK policy agenda. *Forced Migration Review, 14,* 35. Retrieved from http://www.fmreview.org/sites/fmr/files/FMRdownloads/en/FMRpdfs/FMR14/fmr14.14.pdf

Rahman, A., & Tuobia, N. (2000). *Female genital mutilation: A guide to laws and policies worldwide.* London, United Kingdom: Zed Books.

Reel, K., & Hutchings, S. (2007). Being part of a team: Interprofessional care. In G. Hawley (Ed.), *Ethics in clinical practice: An interprofessional approach* (pp. 137–153). Essex, United Kingdom: Pearson Education Limited.

Reisel, D., & Creighton, S. M. (2015). Long term health consequences of female genital mutilation (FGM). *Maturitas.* 2015 Jan; *80*(1): 48–51.

Robson, C. (2011). *Real world research* (3rd ed.). West Sussex, United Kingdom: John Wiley & Sons Ltd.

Royal College of Midwives (RCM). (1998). *Female genital mutilation (female circumcision).* Position Paper 21. London, United Kingdom: Author.

Royal College of Midwives, Royal College of Nursing, & Royal College of Obstetricians & Gynaecologists (RCM, RCN, & RCOG). (2013). *Tackling FGM in the UK: Intercollegiate recommendations for identifying, recording, and reporting.* London, United KIngdom: Royal College of Midwives.

Royal College of Nursing (RCN). (2006). *Female Genital Mutilation: An RCN educational resource for nursing and midwifery staff.* London, United Kingdom: Author.

Royal College of Nursing (RCN). (2015). *Female genital mutilation. An RCN resource for nursing and midwifery practice* (2nd ed.). London, United Kingdom: Author.

Savage, T. (2007). Women's health nursing. In M. S. DeWolf Bosek & T. A. Savage (Eds.), *The ethical component of nursing education: integrating ethics into clinical experience* (pp. 281–310). Philadelphia, PA: Lippincott Williams & Wilkins.

Savage, J., & Moore, L. (2004). *Interpreting accountability: An ethnographic study of practice nurses, accountability and multidisciplinary team decision-making in the context of clinical governance*. London, United Kingdom: Royal College of Nursing.

Serour, G. I. (2013). Medicalization of female genital mutilation /cutting. *African Journal of Urology, 19*(3), 145–149.

Settelmaier, E. & Nigam, M. (2007). Where did you get your values and beliefs? In G. Hawley (Ed.), *Ethics in clinical practice: An interprofessional approach* (pp. 15–34). Essex, United Kingdom: Pearson Education Limited.

Sigal, J. A., & Denmark, F. L. (2013). *Violence against girls and women: International perspectives*. Santa Barbara, CA: Praeger.

The London Safeguarding Children Board. (2009). *London female genital mutilation resource pack*. Retrieved from https:// www.reducingtherisk.org.uk/cms/sites/reducingtherisk/files /folders/resources/fgm/resource_pack.pdf

United Nations Children's Fund (UNICEF). (2013). *Female genital mutilation/cutting: A statistical overview and exploration of the dynamics of change*. Retrieved from http://www.unicef.org /health/files/FGCM_Lo_res.pdf

United Nations Children's Fund (UNICEF). (2016). *Female genital mutilation/cutting: A global concern*. New York, NY: Author.

United Nations General Assembly. (1993). *Declaration on the elimination of violence against women* (A/RES/48/104). Retrieved from http://www.un.org/documents/ga/res/48/a48r104 .htm

United Nations Human Rights. (2014). *Women's rights are human rights*. HR/PUB/14/2. New York, NY and Geneva, Switzerland: United Nations. Retrieved from http://www.ohchr.org/Documents /Events/WHRD/WomenRightsAreHR.pdf

United Nations Population Fund (UNFPA) and United Nations Children's Fund (UNICEF). (2015). 2014 annual report of the UNFPA-UNICEF joint programme on female genital mutilation/ cutting: Accelerating change. New York, NY: Authors.

U.S. Dept. of Health and Human Services Office on Women's Health. (2017). *Female genital cutting*. Retrieved from https:// www.womenshealth.gov/a-z-topics/female-genital-cutting

World Health Organization (WHO). (1996). *Regional plan of action to accelerate the elimination of female genital mutilation in Africa* (AFR/WAH/97.1). Brazzaville, Republic of Congo: WHO Regional Office for Africa.

World Health Organization (WHO). (2000a). *Female genital mutilation: A handbook for frontline workers*. WHO/FCH/ WMH/005 Rev.1. WHO, Geneva, Switzerland: Author.

World Health Organization (WHO). (2000b). *A systematic review of the health complications of female genital mutilation including sequelae in childbirth*. WHO/FCH/WMH/00.2 Geneva, Switzerland: Author.

World Health Organization (WHO). (2011). *Sexual and reproductive health: Core competencies in primary care*. Retrieved from http://www.who.int/reproductivehealth/publications /health_systems/9789241501002/en/

World Health Organization (WHO). (2014). *Global health ethics: Key issues*. Geneva, Switzerland: Author.

World Health Organization (WHO). (2017). *Female genital mutilation*. Fact Sheet No. 241. Geneva, Switzerland: Author. Retrieved from http://www.who.int/mediacentre/factsheets/fs241/en/

Wuest, S., Raio, L., Wyssmueller, D., Mueller, M. D., Stadlmayr, W., Surbek, D. V., & Kuhn, A. (2009). Effects of female genital mutilation on birth outcomes in Switzerland. *British Journal of Obstetrics & Gynaecology, 116*(9), 1204–1209.

• • • SUGGESTED FURTHER READING

For more information, practitioners would find it useful to explore this topic in more comprehensive resources.

Epstein, B., & Turner, M. (2015). The nursing code of ethics: Its value its history. *The Online Journal of Issues in Nursing, 20*(2).

Family Planning Association. (2011). *Religion, contraception and abortion factsheet*. Retrieved from http://www.fpa.org.uk /factsheets/religion-contraception-abortion

Fowler, M. (2015). *Guide to the code of ethics for nurses: Development interpretation and application* (2nd ed). Silver Spring MD: American Nurses Association.

Gyimah, S. O., Takyi, B., & Tenkorang, E. Y. (2008). Denominational affiliation and fertility behaviour in an African context: An examination of couple data from Ghana. *Journal of Biosocial Science, 40*(3): 445–458.

Kridli, S. A., & Libbus, A. (2001). Contraception in Jordan: A cultural and religious perspective. *International Nursing Review, 48*(3):144–151.

Mulongo, P., Hollins, Martin, C., & McAndrew, S. (2014). The psychological impact of female genital mutilation/cutting (FGM/C) on girls/women's mental health: A narrative literature review. *Journal of Reproductive and Infant Psychology, 32*(5), 469–485. Serour, G. I. (2010). The issue of reinfibulation. *International Journal of Gynaecology and Obstetrics, 109*(2), 93–96.

United Nations Population Fund (UNFPA). (2015). *Female genital mutilation (FGM) Frequently asked questions*. Retrieved from www.unfpa.org/frequently-asked-questions

United Nations General Assembly. (1993). Declaration on the Elimination of violence against women (A/RES/48/104). Retrieved from http://www.un.org/documents/ga/res/48/a48r104.htm.

United Nations Initiatives. *AI index 77/15/97 female genital mutilation*. Retrieved from https://www.amnesty.org/download /Documents/156000/act770151997en.pdf

Utz-Billing I. I., & Kentenich H. H. (2008). Female genital mutilation: An injury, physical and mental harm. *Journal of Psychosomatic Obstetrics and Gynecology, 29*(4), 225–229.

Other sources for further information relating to FGM

Children's Act 1989: Retrieved from https://www.legislation.gov .uk/ukpga/1989/41/contents

FGM Scotland Act 2005: Retrieved from https://www.legislation .gov.uk/asp/2005/8/contents

Serious Crime Act 2015: Retrieved from http://www.legislation .gov.uk/ukpga/2015/9/contents/enacted

The FGM Act 2003: Retrieved from http://www.legislation.gov .uk/ukpga/2003/31/pdfs/ukpga_20030031_en.pdf

V

Providing Sexual and Reproductive Care and Services in Resource-Constrained Developing Countries

CHAPTER

20

Providing Sexual and Reproductive Care and Service in Resource-Constrained Countries: Sub-Saharan Africa—Lesotho

PHILIP OKAI ODONKOR, REGINA M. MPEMI, AND MASEABATA V. RAMATHEBANE

CHAPTER OBJECTIVES

The main objectives of this chapter are to:

- Identify policies, guidelines, and procedures for establishing and providing efficient, cost-effective, and culturally acceptable sexual and reproductive health services
- Assess sexual health with respect to sexuality and sexual practices, sexual dysfunction and sexual disorders, HIV/AIDS, and sexually transmitted infections, with a focus on prevention, treatment, and care
- Determine the availability and utilization of family planning services
- Identify and highlight best practices for providing sexual and reproductive health care
- Evaluate research, education, and training initiatives as well as support services for sexual and reproductive health care
- Determine challenges in the provision of sexual and reproductive health services
- Explore knowledge, attitudes, and practices that influence the provision, acceptance, and utilization of sexual and reproductive health services

Introduction

This chapter provides an overview of how HIV services have been evolving in a resource-constrained, developing country in sub-Saharan Africa. Lesotho represents an example at one end of the spectrum typifying the complexity of multiple resource constraints with regard to economic privation, deficient staffing and levels of professional expertise, poor infrastructure and organization, inefficient diagnostic procedures, lack of established referral systems, and inadequate specialist treatment, follow-up, and support service availability. The chapter provides insight into the origin of situations in which indigenous and migrant patients live and the consequential impact on their sexual health. Practitioners in developed countries will be able to compare and better understand the influences of diverse cultural principles and the impact of economic and religious constraints, which result in limited access to sexual healthcare facilities. The structure and organization of sexual health care and services in Lesotho will be outlined and family planning services, sexually transmitted infection (STI) and genitourinary services, and HIV/AIDS prevention and treatment options will be addressed in detail. A selection of national and international policies, recommendations, regulations, and guidelines will be analyzed and discussed. There will also be a discussion about ongoing efforts to improve and maintain standards of sexual and reproductive health care and service provision.

A wide variety of international development partners support the government of Lesotho in the health sector. The Health Development Partners Forum, co-chaired by the World Health Organization (WHO) and the U.S. President's Emergency Plan for AIDS Relief (PEPFAR) facilities coordinator, support the government from the partners' side (Elizabeth Glaser Pediatric AIDS Foundation, 2013).

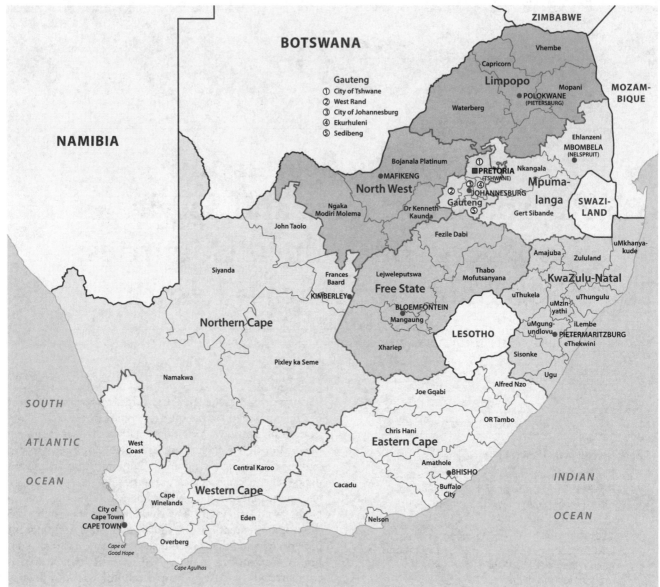

Figure 20-1 Lesotho

Background

Lesotho is a small, mountainous country surrounded by the Republic of South Africa (**Figure 20-1**). Due to its high altitude and mountains, it is often called "the kingdom in the sky." It is divided into 10 administrative districts, which differ in terms of topography, size, climate, and stage of development (United Nations Population Fund, 2012). As the historic homeland of the Basotho people, it is almost a purely monoethnic, monolinguistic society. Most Basotho are Christians, and the dominant denominations are the Catholic, Lesotho Evangelical, and Anglican churches. Lesotho has a total population estimated at 1.89 million (52% female), with a low annual economic growth rate. Three-quarters of the population lives in rural, rugged areas, but urbanization is slowly on the rise. Only 10% of the land is arable. The country is vulnerable to

disasters, particularly floods, drought, and disease outbreaks. Exposure to natural hazards is aggravated by chronic food insecurity, low agricultural productivity, poverty, malnutrition, and the impact of HIV/AIDS.

Many sub-Saharan African countries like Lesotho have limited reports on mortality because of unreliable vital registration systems of births and deaths, the usual source of accurate information sufficient to calculate demographic estimates (Bureau of Statistics, 2013). The statistics used in this chapter, though in some cases are over 5 years old, are the latest available. Sixty four percent of funding for HIV prevention, care, and treatment has come from international sources (U.S. President's Emergency Plan for AIDS Relief [PEPFAR], 2016). Statistics are drawn from the reports of the sponsoring bodies as well as Lesotho government sources (PEPFAR, 2016).

The Healthcare System in Lesotho

Lesotho adopted primary health care (PHC) as a strategy to deliver healthcare services at the community level. The reason for the adoption of PHC was to enhance equitable access to health services in the spirit of social justice. With the support of the World Bank, the Ministry of Health and Social Welfare (MoHSW) embarked on health sector reforms to improve service delivery and increase access to such services.

There are 22 hospitals in the country and over 170 health centers, most of which are situated in the rural areas. The government of Lesotho, through MoHSW, works in partnership with the Christian Health Association of Lesotho (CHAL) to deliver healthcare services. Nongovernmental organizations (NGOs) and international development partners support the activities of both the MoHSW and CHAL.

Lesotho is a signatory to several international declarations and conventions aimed at improving access to, and provision of, quality healthcare services to the population, as well as reducing morbidities and mortalities. Lesotho is committed to achieving the U.N. Millennium Development Goals (MDGs) and has put in place measures to accelerate maternal and newborn health, including a commitment to reduce child mortality by 66% and maternal mortality by 75% by the year 2015. These goals were not met, but in 2016 the United Nations Population Fund Representative to Lesotho applauded the commitment of a joint United Nations Family Planning Association (UNFPA) venture to join with the business community in Lesotho to reduce the HIV and maternal mortality rates there. This advocacy and outreach campaign is expected to reach all the districts and regions of Lesotho (United Nations Population Fund, 2016).

Maternal and newborn morbidity and mortality is a global concern. Maternal mortality is particularly high in Africa, where the maternal mortality rate is estimated to be about 1,800/100,000 live births. According to the 2014 Lesotho Demographic Health Survey (Ministry of Health and ICF International, 2016), Lesotho had a maternal mortality ratio for the 7-year period before the survey of 1,024 deaths per 100,000 live births. The maternal mortality ratio is not significantly different from the estimates from 2004 and 2009 and has shown little improvement.

The global concern has led to various global and regional declarations, aimed at eliciting commitments from governments and their health authorities to develop strategies and action plans geared toward reducing maternal and newborn morbidity and mortality by 2015 (Ministry of Health and Social Welfare, 2012). On realizing that African countries are not likely to achieve the MDGs without significant improvements in the sexual and reproductive health (SRH) of the people of Africa, the African Ministers of Health adopted the continental policy framework on Sexual and Reproductive Health and Rights in October 2005. This was endorsed by the African Union (A.U.) Heads of State in September 2006, and the A.U. Health Ministers

developed the Maputo Plan of Action to operationalize the Continental Policy Framework on Sexual and Reproductive Health and Rights. Ten years later, the Maputo Plan of Action 2016–2030 urges all governments and civil societies to double their efforts to implement the sexual reproductive health policies (African Union Commission, 2016). These aspirations ride on the 10 strategic interventions of the Continental Policy Framework on Sexual and Reproductive Health and Rights:

- Increase resources to SRH and rights programs
- Translate the International Conference on Population and Development (ICPD) commitments into national legislation and SRHR policies
- Continue to reduce maternal mortality and morbidity as well as infant and child mortality
- End all preventable deaths of mothers, newborns, and children
- Continue efforts to combat HIV/AIDS
- Expand contraceptive use
- Reduce levels of unsafe abortion
- End early and forced child marriage
- Eradicate female genital mutilation
- Prevent gender-based violence
- Ensure access of adolescents and youth to SRH care (African Union Commission, 2016)

Infant Mortality Rates

According to the 2011 Lesotho Demographic Survey (Bureau of Statistics, 2013), the level of infant mortality increased from 74 deaths per 1,000 live births in 1996 to 94 deaths per 1,000 live births in 2011. The Bureau attributes this continuing rise to the high unemployment rate that is prevailing in the country. Poverty is strikingly high, hence food shortage results in exposure of children to the risk of dying. The increase in infant mortality rates is associated with the high prevalence of HIV and AIDS especially among young women.

Total Fertility Rates

The Bureau of Statistics (2013) has noted that total fertility rates have declined over the last 3 decades. The data indicates a total fertility rate of 3.4 children per woman, and this is reported to be one of the lowest rates in sub-Saharan Africa (Ministry of Health and Social Welfare, 2010). The factors that influence total fertility rate include place of residence and educational status; total fertility rate is high among women who reside in rural areas and whose educational status is low. The figures depict a decline in fertility among female youth in Lesotho with a peak fertility at the ages 25–29 years (Bureau of Statistics, 2013). This demonstrates that women are now commencing childbearing at a much later age than was previously the case.

Table 20-1	Regional and International Declarations and Lesotho National Policies and Guidelines at a Glance	
National Policies and International/Regional Declarations		**Year**
Social Welfare Policy		2002
Lesotho National Sexual and Reproductive Health Policy		2009
Reproductive Health Policy Implementation Strategic Framework		2010
Gender and Development Policy		2003
Lesotho National Adolescents Health Policy		2006
Health Sector Policy on Comprehensive HIV Prevention		2010
National Population Policy		2011
The Child Protection and Welfare Act 2011		2010
Lesotho Blood Transfusion Service Policy		2006
MoHSW: Continuing Education Strategy for Workers in the Lesotho Health and Social Welfare Sector		2009
Millennium Development Goals		2000
Paris Declarations		2005
Gaborone Declaration (SRH Policy Framework)		2005
Southern African Development Community (SADC) SRH Strategic Plan		2006
Abuja Declaration		2011
Maputo Plan of Action		2006
Ouagadougou Declaration		2008
Data from Family Health Division, MoHSW-Lesotho.		

Pregnancy and Childbirth

The number of women using contraception has showed a steady increase since 2001 and has continued to rise in the most recent survey available (Bureau of Statistics, 2013). Compared to previous data, there is a significant increase in the number of women who attend the prenatal clinic in Lesotho. Most women seek prenatal care from health facilities, where they are attended to by trained healthcare providers. In 2011, 75% of births were delivered in a health facility, the majority in public sector health facilities. However, the remainder of infants are delivered at home. Delivery assistance from a skilled provider has increased from 55% in 2004 to 78% in 2014, yet only 62% of women received a postnatal check-up within 2 days of delivery, while 26% had no postnatal check-up within 41 days of delivery (Ministry of Health and ICF International, 2016).

International, Regional, and National Declarations and Policies

Based on its commitment to combating maternal and neonatal morbidity and mortality, Lesotho has developed several policies and guidelines with the aim of facilitating implementation of measures to address the SRH needs of the country (Table 20-1). The policies and guidelines provide a framework for the realization of the international and regional declarations that Lesotho has signed.

Ouagadougou Declaration 2008

The Ouagadougou Declaration on Primary Health Care (PHC) and health systems in Africa was a response to a global movement to reactivate and redirect PHC. The commitment of member states to the values of equity solidarity and social justice, as well as the PHC principles in the Alma-Ata Declaration of 1978, has been echoed at many international and regional as well as national conferences, including the WHO Regional Committee meetings.

Despite the policy's progress in service, development has been slow (World Health Organization, 2008). The Ministry of Health and Social Welfare (2012) provided an update of the implementation of a Lesotho project linking HIV and SRH in 2011. Lesotho had committed to implement the project in 2 years from 2011. Significant activities planned for 2011 were not realized. The study found strong support for strengthening SRH and HIV linkages in Lesotho. However, there was a need to streamline policy and strategic direction and strengthen leadership on integration.

At the policy level, the report found that integration commitments were fragmented in various documents. The country lacked a universal national SRH and HIV integration policy. The study also found that there was a lack of leadership to champion the integration concept and coordinate integration activities.

At the systems level, the report found that existing systems on planning, funding, human resource capacity and development, procurement, supplies, and logistics for commodities, and monitoring and evaluation did not effectively support integration.

At the service delivery level, the report found that some level of integration of HIV and SRH services was occurring, but not in a structured manner due to lack of service and supervision guidelines. The challenges included staff shortages and inadequate skills, poor infrastructure, weak referral systems, and logistical challenges in ensuring consistent availability of SRH and HIV commodities. A further report released in 2013 (Ministry of Health and Social Welfare, 2013) identified some progress that had been made in the supply of commodities. Gaps identified included uncoordinated data requests from several donors which were thought to be time-consuming and limited the practical time available for supervisors who are required to collate this data. There was unsustainable reliance on donor-funded staff. Significant equipment and infrastructure challenges continued, particularly for facilitating integration in remote areas, including a lack of accessible laboratory services, a lack of storage facilities, substandard examination and delivery rooms, poor lighting, and poorly maintained facilities.

A number of Lesotho legal requirements were either confusing or hindering service delivery. For example, women who wished to receive tubal ligation required their husband's consent. For young people, there were different minimum legal ages for marriage (16 years of age for girls and 18 for boys), whereas voting was permitted at the age of 18. To receive HIV testing and counseling, a young person could consent at the age 12, whereas consent to undergo medical procedures could not be given until age 21 (Ministry of Health and Social Welfare, 2013).

Plan of Action 2016–2030

The goal of the Maputo Plan of Action is to attain universal access to comprehensive SRH services in Africa by 2030. Table 20-2 identifies the strategic focuses, and gives examples of interventions with indicators for monitoring progress.

National Policies and Guidelines on Sexual and Reproductive Health in Lesotho

The government of Lesotho, through the MoHSW, with technical and financial assistance from international development partners, has developed several policies and guidelines that are used as tools to address SRH problems and issues in Lesotho.

Roadmap for Accelerating Reduction of Maternal and Newborn Morbidity and Mortality in Lesotho

During the 54th meeting of the WHO Regional Committee (RC 54), the MDGs were presented and discussed by the Ministers of Health of the African region. The committee unanimously adopted the generic roadmap for accelerating the attainment of MDGs that relate to maternal and newborn health, through Resolution AF/RC/54. The resolution urges

member states to adopt it and commence implementation. The roadmap follows the adoption of the MDGs in 2000 by the United Nations. MDGs 4 and 5 call for the reduction of child mortality by 66% and maternal mortality by 75% of the 1990 levels, respectively, by 2015. Countries were subsequently urged to develop country-specific roadmaps based on the findings of an emergency obstetric care (EmOC) needs assessment. The first Lesotho EmOC study was conducted between March and June 2005. The Roadmap for 2007–2015 was launched in 2006, and it aimed at achieving MDGs 4 and 5 (Ministry of Health and Social Welfare, 2012). The Lesotho roadmap gave direction for implementing comprehensive integrated maternal and newborn health interventions in the context of the National Sexual and Reproductive Health Policy.

A review of progress undertaken in 2010 indicated the following: The support of local councilors, chiefs, parliamentarians, and other decision-makers had been solicited. Healthcare personnel had been trained on the management of sexual abuse survivors. The national health sector budget had been increased to 11% (the Abuja Declaration recommends 15%). Advocacy for sexual and reproductive health/rights and nutrition programs was accomplished. Behavior change communication education materials on maternal and newborn health and nutrition were developed in both Sesotho (the primary language) and English and were distributed to health facilities. Health professionals were trained on EmOC, prevention of mother-to-child transmission of HIV (PMTCT), resuscitation of the newborn, integrated management of childhood infections (IMCI), baby-friendly health initiatives, infection prevention and control, reproductive tract cancer screening, and procurement, supply, and management of commodities.

All doctors were trained on manual vacuum aspiration, and there had been a training of trainers for health workers on family planning methods. Community-based distributors as well as family planning and community health workers were trained on PMTCT. Further, there were trainings to increase coverage, utilization, and quality of essential maternal and newborn care.

The following public policies were developed: the National Adolescent Health Policy (2006), blood transfusion policies, National Reproductive Health (2009), Infant and Young Child Feeding (IYCF) policy (2010), and the code on breast milk supplements. Reproductive health equipment, including manual vacuum aspiration kits, cancer screening equipment, and family planning commodities, were procured. The Nurses and Midwives Act was reviewed to increase the scope of practice of midwives.

EmOC training manuals and guidelines on IYCF, IMCI, and management of survivors of sexual abuse were developed and distributed to health facilities. The curriculum for General Nursing and Midwifery programs were reviewed to accommodate emerging reproductive health issues. Doctors and nurses were trained on confidential enquiries into maternal deaths. Nurses were trained in

Table 20-2	Examples of MPOA for Implementing the Continental Sexual and Reproductive Health and Rights Policy Framework, 2016–2030	
Strategic Focus	**Example of Priority Interventions**	**Indicators for Monitoring Progress**
Improve Political commitment, leadership and Governance for reproductive, maternal, newborn, child, and adolescent health (RMNCAH)	Removal of user fees for SRH/MNCAH services and institution of innovative social protection schemes	• Patient/household out-of-pocket expenditures of accessing or obtaining services (collected intermittently) • Fraction of the population protected against catastrophic/impoverishing out-of-pocket health expenditure
Institute health legislation in support of RMNCAH	Implement policies, strategies, and action plans to reduce unintended pregnancies and unsafe abortions	Proportion of unsafe abortions performed
Gender equality, female empowerment, and human rights	Eradicate female genital mutilation/cutting (FGM/C) and other harmful traditional practices	Percentage of girls and women aged 15–49 years who have undergone FGM/C, by age group
Improve SRH information, education, and communication	Promote community involvement and participation in RMNCAH, with a special focus on the involvement of men	Percentage of men accompanying spouses, children, and adolescents for RMNCAH services
Invest in adolescents, youth, and other vulnerable and marginalized populations	Improve access to and uptake of quality SRH services for youth and adolescents, including human papillomavirus (HPV) vaccination	• Proportion of young people accessing SRH services • Adolescent birth rate (10–14 years and 15–19 years) • HIV prevalence among young people aged 15–24 years • Proportion of girls vaccinated with 3 doses of HPV vaccine by age 15 years • Contraceptive prevalence rate
Optimize the functioning of health system and improve human resource for RMNCAH	Expand access to high-impact health interventions such as immunization, skilled attendance at birth, and quality care, including emergency care	• Maternal mortality ratio per 100,000 live births • Neonatal mortality rate per 1,000 live births • Stillbirth rate (and intrapartum stillbirth rate) • Mortality rate of children under age 5 years per 1,000 • Prevalence of wasting in children under 5 years • Percentage of births attended by skilled health personnel • Number of facilities per 500,000 providing basic and comprehensive emergency obstetric care
Improve partnerships and collaborations with private sector, communities, other extra-health sectors, CSO, and other partners	Develop policies that promote involvement of civil society, private sector, and communities in RMNCAH service delivery within national programs	Proportion of countries implementing policies on public–private partnership on sexual and reproductive health/rights
Ensure accountability and strengthen monitoring and evaluation, research, and innovation	Develop/strengthen civil registration and vital statistics systems	Percentage of children under 5 whose births have been registered with civil authority Birth [and death] registration
Increase health financing and investments	Identify and institute budget lines and budgetary allocations for essential and cost-effective SRH interventions and programmes	Existence of budget lines for essential/cost-effective interventions within the SRH/MNCAH budget

Data from African Union Commission. (2016). Maputo Plan of Action 2016 - 2030. Retrieved from https://www.au.int/web/sites/default/files/documents/24099/

integrated management of childhood diseases, integrated management of acute infections, and infant and young child feeding in the context of HIV/AIDS.

Family Planning

Family planning plays a key role in improving the quality of health of couples. Access to family planning and other reproductive health services are essential in reducing the personal, family, and societal costs associated with high fertility rates, unplanned pregnancies, and increased prevalence of sexually transmitted infections (as well as their sequelae). To strengthen family planning services, the government of Lesotho is committed to ensuring provision of family planning services to clients with emphasis on the following:

- Protection against unintended pregnancies
- The use of condoms for prevention of STIs, including HIV
- Ensuring provision of family planning services to adolescents in accordance with the National Adolescent Health policy
- Strengthening community-based distribution of family planning commodities
- Ensuring protection of the rights of individuals, women, and couples, including people living with HIV and AIDS (PLWHA) to make an informed choice on the methods of contraception they want, including surgical-based contraception
- Ensuring provision of various contraceptive methods at all levels of the health system
- Ensuring that HIV-positive clients make an informed choice on their preferred method of contraception
- Ensuring availability of all essential family planning commodities
- Strengthening implementation of the Reproductive Health Commodity Security Strategic Plan
- Ensuring integration of family planning into PMTCT of HIV services and relevant PHC services

Enshrined in the family planning guidelines are the rights of women and men as agreed to in the 1994 International Conference on Population and Development (ICPD) held in Cairo. In order to ensure that healthcare providers offer appropriate and quality services, both the rights of the clients and of healthcare providers have been addressed (**Table 20-3**).

To enforce these reproductive rights, Lesotho has developed policies, guidelines, pieces of legislation, programs, and strategies, yet due to cultural, economic, and religious constraints, not all reproductive rights are met. For instance, a male partner, as a right, can accompany his spouse when going for reproductive health services such as family planning, prenatal care, labor, and delivery. However, this right is not exercised because facilities have not been

Table 20-3	Clients' Rights and Healthcare Providers' Needs
Client's Rights	**Healthcare Provider's Needs**
Information	Training
Access	Information
Choice	Infrastructure
Confidentiality	Supplies
Privacy	Guidance
Dignity	Back-up
Comfort	Encouragement
Continuity	Self expression
Opinion	Feedback

Data from Government of Lesotho. (2011). National Family Planning Guidelines. Maseru, Lesotho: MoHSW.

built to accommodate or serve the needs of male spouses. Furthermore, even though there is legislation to protect the rights of people with different sexual orientations, there are still varying degrees of discrimination and stigmatization against gay and lesbian people. There are no reproductive healthcare services specifically designed for people who engage in sexual practices other than penile–vaginal intercourse. For instance, health facilities, both private/ NGO and governmental, do not offer oral condoms/dental dams or unlubricated condoms for individuals who wish to engage in protected oral sex. Additionally, there are no health education materials on various sexual practices, nor do healthcare professionals address them when they offer health education, even though it could help individuals avoid HIV/AIDS. For instance, individuals who practice oral sex may not be aware that they can still acquire STIs, including HIV, if they fail to protect themselves. They also need to know that sexual practices other than penile–vaginal sex do not contribute to pregnancy.

There are no sex therapists or urologists in Lesotho from whom individuals with sexual problems can obtain advice/help. Most of the time, clients who present with sexual disorders are referred to psychologists or general counselors who may not be knowledgeable about such disorders. Also, these professionals are concentrated in the urban Maseru and are not available to the rural population.

Contraceptive Use in Lesotho

Sixty percent of married women age 15–49 use any method of family planning; nearly all of these women use modern methods of family planning. The most popular methods are injectables, the male condom, and the pill. More than 70% of sexually active, unmarried women age 15–49 use modern methods of family planning, and 1% use traditional methods. The most popular modern methods are the same as those reported that married women use. Married women living in urban areas are slightly more likely than married women living in rural areas to use modern methods. Use of modern methods increases with household wealth. The use of modern methods of family planning by married women has increased steadily over the last decade. The use of traditional methods has declined over the same period. The use of male condoms has more than tripled since 2004. The use of injectables has also increased in this time (Ministry of Health [Lesotho] and ICF International, 2016).

In order to increase access to family planning commodities, there are community-based distributers of contraceptives (male and female condoms and combined oral contraceptives) who serve areas where local health centers or hospitals do not provide contraceptives due to religious restrictions (e.g., facilities owned by the Roman Catholic Church).

Age of First Sexual Intercourse

While it is normally expected that individuals would commence sexual activities only after marriage, it is not unusual to find many men and women engaging in sexual activities before marriage. Women and men in Lesotho begin sexual activity at approximately the same age. The median age at first sexual intercourse for men and women is 18 years. Women with more than secondary education wait longer to initiate sexual intercourse than less educated women. In contrast, men with no education begin sexual activity later than men with higher levels of education. The median age at first birth for women is 20 years. In Lesotho, once married, the societal expectation is that women should bear a child within the first year of marriage. This means that without the use of contraceptives, a couple would be likely to have 7–12 births during the woman's entire reproductive life (Ministry of Health [Lesotho] and ICF International, 2016).

Lesotho has aligned itself with the 1995 International Planned Parenthood Federation (IPPF) Charter on Sexual and Reproductive Rights, which is based on international human rights instruments. While there is a will to observe all the rights, Lesotho has considerable work to do to guarantee these rights. The issue of wife beating, for example, has been studied nationally. Women and men were asked if they agreed that a husband was justified in beating his wife for at least one of the following reasons: if she burnt the food, argued with him, went out without telling him, neglected the children, or refused to have sex with him. One-third of women and 40% of men agreed that a husband is justified in beating his wife for at least one of those reasons. While a quarter of women studied were most likely to believe that a husband was justified in beating his wife if she argued with him, more men were most likely to believe wife beating was justified if she neglected the children or argued with him.

Often, women must seek permission to use any form of family planning commodity, including condoms to protect themselves against unwanted pregnancy and STIs (Ministry of Health [Lesotho] and ICF International, 2016). Benefits of family planning include delaying or avoiding pregnancies, child spacing, and deciding on the timing of birth and the number and frequency of pregnancies (**Table 20-4**).

Table 20-4	Benefits and Advantages of Family Planning		
Women	**Family**	**Community**
• Protection from unplanned and unwanted pregnancies; enforces right to determine the spacing and number of children • Reduces the need for unsafe abortions • Reduction of maternal morbidity and mortality by avoiding high-risk pregnancies (too early, close, late, many) • Opportunity to decide when and how often to become pregnant • Time for professional development • Increased educational, employment, and economic opportunities and development • May prevent sexually transmitted infections, including HIV/AIDS • Empowers women to have control over their own fertility • May prevent reproductive cancers	• Give the family freedom to decide when and how many children to have • When the family has few children, they are more able to take care of their children and provide them with basic needs, provide better life and education for them • Career development for prospects of better financial position for now and in the future; help to increase educational, employment, and economic growth and opportunities • Helps postpone having children in the event of disease or financial challenges • Encourages healthy sexual relationships between couples by removing fear of pregnancy with every sexual encounter	• Prevent overpopulation, enhancing opportunity for economic growth and development; people can obtain jobs more easily, with limited competition for the available resources • Future demands on available economic resources are reduced • Reduction in environmental pollution • Every person will have a better opportunity for a good life, education, and employment, and in turn, reduce poverty • Reduces the incidence of teenage pregnancies, street children, and crime rate

Data from WHO, Family Planning and Population Division of Family Health. (1995). Health benefits of family planning. Retrieved from http://apps.who.int/iris/bitstream/10665/62091/1/WHO_FHE_FPP_95.11.pdf

Family Planning Services in Lesotho

Family planning services are integrated into other SRH services, including STIs and HIV/AIDS services. While there are stand-alone family planning clinics, family planning services are also offered at all levels of care. The stand-alone family planning services are provided by Lesotho Planned Parenthood Association (LPPA), which has satellite clinics in the various districts of the country. LPPA also runs men's clinics, where male circumcision services, HIV/AIDS services, and cancer screening are offered. An estimated 75% of LPPA's clients are poor, marginalized, socially excluded, and/or under-served. Target groups include cattle herders, prisoners, rural populations, factory workers, university students, police trainees, and people living with HIV and AIDS (International Planned Parenthood Federation, 2017). The methods of contraception commonly found in all levels of care are hormonal, intrauterine, emergency, barrier method, lactation amenorrhea method, and fertility awareness–based methods. Female and male sterilization is mainly done at the hospital level. However, for doctrinal reasons, the Catholic Church does not allow its health facilities to provide artificial methods of family planning. The only approved methods are the fertility awareness–based method and lactation amenorrhea. With the advent of HIV/AIDS, condom use is being advocated even in Catholic facilities, albeit only as a prevention method for HIV/AIDS. Community pharmacies provide hormonal contraceptives, including emergency contraception.

Condoms: Distribution and Use

Condoms are recommended for the prevention of STIs and HIV/AIDS and as barrier methods of family planning. Condoms are given free of charge at the health facility level. Some are distributed to institutions of higher learning. Both male and female condoms are also available for sale in shops and community pharmacies. While condoms are available in a variety of colors, textures, and fragrances, there are no condoms for oral sex. It is perceived that there is a thin line between providing services and promoting a behavior. There is an assumption that if such condoms are made available, these will perpetuate the behavior.

Abortion

In Lesotho, abortion is defined as termination of pregnancy before 28 weeks' gestation. Abortion may be spontaneous or induced. Induced abortion may be obtained for therapeutic purposes or for personal and/or social non-therapeutic reasons. In Lesotho, induced abortion, other than induced therapeutic abortion, is illegal. The Penal Code Act (Penal Code Act 2012) a Lesotho Statute, does not provide for abortion on social grounds. Thabane and Kasiram (2015) argue that the repercussion of such a law has led to an increase in unplanned and unwanted babies, many of whom may ultimately be neglected or abandoned. The children who end up in care facilities, fostered, or adopted are most likely to have been neglected and/or variously maltreated, as their study in Lesotho suggests.

Prenatal Care

The government of Lesotho recommends that a pregnant woman should attend prenatal care as soon as pregnancy is confirmed. The government has adopted the WHO recommendation of focused prenatal care, which advocates for a minimum of four visits. Currently, there are no prenatal care guidelines. However, because HIV/AIDS services, including PMTCT, are integrated into all reproductive health services, there are components of prenatal care in the PMTCT guidelines. These have indicated the activities to be performed at each visit for both HIV negative and positive clients.

The first prenatal care visit is between 0–16 weeks of pregnancy, the second between 20–24 weeks, the third between 24–32 weeks, and the fourth between 36–38 weeks.

The first prenatal care visit is recommended to commence at least during the first trimester. This is the period of organogenesis, when the growing fetus is highly susceptible to environmental hazards/insults. There is a need to educate the clients on dietary needs, lifestyle modification, and assessment of potential teratogenic medications. According to policies and guidelines of the MoHSW, (1) pregnant women are expected to obtain prenatal care and deliver in health facilities; (2) primigravida and multiparous women are urged to give birth in the hospital; and (3) health facilities should provide "waiting mothers' lodges" for expectant mothers who live far away from the health facilities. Pregnant women are expected to notify the shelters/waiting mothers' lodge at least a month before expected date of delivery. The deliveries at the health center are free.

Although prenatal care attendance and facility-based deliveries have improved over the years, some women do not use health facilities. Nearly all (95%) women age 15–49 received prenatal care from a skilled provider, while 5% of women received no prenatal care. Reasons may be due to long distances between places of residences and the health facility; lack of transport due to poor road infrastructure and bridges; lack of money to rent vehicles; negative attitudes toward health professionals; and absence of delivery services at nearby facilities (Ministry of Health [Lesotho] and ICF International, 2016).

Reproductive Tract Disease Screening and Treatment

Sexually Transmitted Infections

Sexually transmitted infections (STI) are among the top 10 causes of outpatient department attendance in Lesotho, with an incidence rate of 7%. This concurs with the high incidence of sexual activity among both men and women, non-monogamy among married couples, and low condom use with high prevalence of HIV.

Treatment of Sexually Transmitted Infections

STI case management in Lesotho is based on the WHO's recommended syndromic management approach. All health facilities (including health centers and hospital outpatient departments) in Lesotho offer STI services. The components of case management include history taking, clinical examination, correct diagnosis, early and effective treatment, advice on sexual behavior, promotion and/or provision of condoms, partner notification and treatment, case reporting, and clinical follow-up as appropriate. Treatment guidelines for STI are available in the form of posters placed on the consulting room walls. Similarly, STI information leaflets are distributed to patients.

Cervical Cancer and HPV

Cervical cancer is the most common cancer in Lesotho, and the leading cause of cancer death among women in the country—particularly for women living with HIV, who are four times more likely to develop cervical cancer than women who are HIV-negative (Elizabeth Glaser Pediatric AIDS Foundation, 2013).

The Ministry of Health, in partnership with the Elizabeth Glaser Pediatric AIDS Foundation and with funding from the U.S. Agency for International Development, helped to launch services at Lesotho's first organized cervical cancer screening and prevention facility. The center now offers comprehensive gynaecological services, with an emphasis on cervical cancer screenings, diagnoses, pre-cancer treatment services, and referrals to facilities for cancer treatment.

Human papillomavirus (HPV) infection is the cause of most cervical cancers. The immunization of girls against HPV types 16 and 18 is considered the most cost effective method of managing the occurrence of cervical cancer, and the Ministry of Health has implemented a number of vaccination campaigns over the past 5 years (Elizabeth Glaser Pediatric AIDS Foundation, 2013).

HIV/AIDS

Lesotho is one of the countries hardest hit by HIV, with the second highest HIV prevalence after Swaziland (UNAIDS, 2014). The MDG goal is to combat HIV/AIDS, and other diseases, such as malaria. The targets were to reverse the spread of HIV/AIDS by 2015 and to achieve universal access to HIV/AIDS treatment by 2010. The main targets for Lesotho's HIV prevention strategy are to reduce sexual transmission of HIV by 50% and eliminate mother-to-child transmission (MTCT). However, Lesotho's 2015 UNAIDS Country Progress Report, which contains 2014 data, indicated the country was not on track to meet either target. Overall, 25% of Basotho women and men age 15–49 are HIV-positive. HIV prevalence is higher among women (30%) than among men (19%). Basotho women and men living in urban areas are more likely to be HIV positive than those in rural areas (30% versus 22%) (Ministry of Health [Lesotho] and ICF International, 2016).

HIV/AIDS Prevalence

The HIV/AIDS pandemic continues to be a public health and socioeconomic problem in many countries around the world. The most affected countries are mainly found in sub-Saharan Africa. Recent figures indicate 13% of young women and 6% of young men (aged 15–24) were living with HIV. Prevalence has been rising among young women, as it stood at 10.5% in the 2009, but has remained stable among young men. Currently 310,000 of the total population of just over 2 million people live with HIV in Lesotho (Ministry of Health [Lesotho] and ICF International, 2016).

The main drivers fueling the HIV epidemic in Lesotho are multiple and concurrent sexual partnerships, and low levels of consistent and correct condom use. Debilitating poverty and unemployment, challenges for adolescents and youth to change patterns of sexual behavior, high rates of alcohol use, and low rates of male circumcision also contribute to the epidemic. In addition to women, young girls, orphans, and children, key affected populations are prison inmates, prison staff, and men who have sex with men.

While there are social and cultural factors affecting women and girls, there are also social and cultural inhibitions around open discussion of sex and sexuality, as well as income inequalities and disparities.

HIV Testing and Counseling

Prevention remains the key strategy in the fight against HIV. HIV testing and counseling (HTC) is important for determining the magnitude of the HIV infection among the population. This benefits public health workers for planning purposes, and individuals for their own future planning purposes. For instance, a pregnant woman can use this information to prevent passing HIV infection on to her unborn child.

Considerable progress has been made with HTC in Lesotho. The Know Your Status campaign was launched in 2004, and between 2006 and 2008 the number of individuals in Lesotho seeking HTC had increased significantly on a yearly basis. In 2014, the country-wide survey found 63% of men and 84% of women had tested for HIV (Ministry of Health [Lesotho] and ICF International, 2016). These were highest ever figures recorded in Lesotho. Community councils are currently involved in increasing the number of people who know their HIV status through community mobilization by facilitating training of community health workers in testing and counseling people about the test. All pregnant women are requested to undertake HIV testing at prenatal clinics. Mobile clinic testing was more appropriate for detecting new infections and home-based testing was more appropriate for children and those who had never been tested before. More and more people know their HIV status, and this augurs well for planning further action. The service has been compromised by frequent HIV test kit shortages and a lack of health staff, particularly in remote areas.

Behavior Change Communication

Even though behavior change communication is a necessary intervention, it is probably the most difficult to achieve. A variety of campaigns have been launched to reach 15- to 24-year-olds across the country. For example, the Kick 4 Life campaign, which uses football to bring HIV prevention messages to young people, has had country-wide viewing.

Various communication platforms such as television and social media are also being utilized. As an example, the television drama *Kheto ea ka!* (*Your Choice!*) has been produced by Lesotho's Ministry of Health and Social Welfare and in collaboration with a community group to target students with messages of HIV risk and prevention.

HIV stigma and discrimination remain major barriers to accessing vital treatment, prevention, and support services. Gossip, verbal as well as physical abuse, and exclusion from social, religious, and family gatherings or activities were found to be the main forms of HIV-related stigma and discrimination. Lesotho Network of People Living with HIV and AIDS (2014) report that a total of 4% of people living with HIV were reported to have been denied access to healthcare services over the previous 12 months. Despite this, the Ministry of Health [Lesotho] and ICF International (2016) found attitudes toward people living with HIV to have improved slightly.

HIV Prevention and Care

Disadvantaged Groups

Sex Workers Transactional sex is understood to be sex in exchange for money, favors, or gifts. Similar to other countries, there is limited research on female sex workers in Lesotho, which has resulted in little understanding of the HIV epidemic among this population. The Ministry of Health [Lesotho] (2015) reports that many female sex workers have reported experiences of sexual violence and harassment including rape and physical aggression. Many had also experienced police harassment and were too afraid to access health services. Statistics indicate in this report that 79% of sex workers are HIV seropositive (Ministry of Health [Lesotho], 2015).

Herd Boys Herd boys are among the most disadvantaged young people in Lesotho. Poverty encourages many to take up herding livestock as a full-time occupation, meaning many are deprived of formal education and lack access to health services, treatment, and care.

Condom Use for HIV Prevention and Knowledge of HIV Prevention Methods

The use of male condoms in Lesotho has more than tripled since 2004 (Ministry of Health [Lesotho] and ICF International, 2016). The majority (86%) of women and 81% of men age 15–49 know that using condoms and limiting sex to one uninfected partner can reduce the risk of HIV. Seven percent of women and 27% of men had two or more sexual partners in the past 12 months. Women and men who reported having two or more sexual partners in the past year were asked about condom use at their last sexual intercourse; 54% of women and 65% of men reported using a condom at last sexual intercourse (Ministry of Health [Lesotho] and ICF International, 2016). HIV prevalence is higher in females who did not use condoms in their first sexual encounter.

The United Nations Population Fund (2012) in its 5-year plan for Lesotho has identified targets for the development of HIV prevention revitalization plan that includes the scale-up of innovative prevention initiatives such as condom programming. Part of the plan includes strengthening the Logistics Management Information System that enhances non stock-out of condoms. Another part of the plan is to expand condom distribution channels to community level nationwide with a target of 20, 000 young people per year, 1,500 herd boys, and 60 sex workers.

Medical Male Circumcision

Voluntary medical male circumcision (VMMC) is a cost-effective, one-time intervention that provides lifelong partial protection against female-to-male HIV transmission (UNAIDS, 2016). Lesotho's VMMC program was launched in 2011. In 2014, the number of men receiving VMMC had roughly tripled to 36,200. VMMC in Lesotho has experienced challenges in scaling-up due to traditional methods of circumcision, a common feature of Lesotho culture. Predominantly in rural areas of Lesotho, boys are more likely to be circumcised during initiation rituals (Ministry of Health [Lesotho], 2015). Ritual circumcision does not achieve the same preventative impact in relation to HIV transmission, as many virgins who had undergone circumcision were found to be HIV positive (Brewer, Potterat, Roberts, & Brody, 2007). Currently, VMMC is only offered in hospitals and few other health facilities. Government plans include scaling up the number of safe community health facilities to offer adult male circumcision.

Prevention of Mother-to-Child Transmission of HIV

HIV may be transmitted from a mother to a child during pregnancy, delivery, or through breastfeeding. HIV prevalence is approximately 27% in pregnant women in Lesotho. Viral load at birth determines the rate of infection. Mother-to-child transmission (MTCT) can be prevented through antiretroviral therapy (ART) during pregnancy/delivery or breastfeeding. Exclusive breastfeeding has been found to reduce the rate of transmission.

The Millennium Development Goals (MDGs) adopted by the U.N. General Assembly in 2000 committed the international community to reducing child mortality, improving maternal health, and combating HIV/AIDS, malaria, and other diseases by 2015. The UNAIDS target is to eliminate HIV transmission from mother to child, aiming at the transmission rate dropping below 5%. While Lesotho's MTCT rate stood at 3.5%

in 2012, progress has now reversed, with MTCT standing at 5.9% in 2014 (Ministry of Health [Lesotho], 2015).

The PMTCT guidelines (Elizabeth Glaser Pediatric AIDS Foundation, 2013) inform health professionals about the management and prevention of HIV in children from various categories. The guidelines specify HTC for pregnant women and indicate how to address pregnant women who are already on highly active antiretroviral therapy (HAART), those who have never been exposed to HAART, and what medication to give to an infant from birth until a week after breastfeeding cessation. The guidelines also specify which HIV tests to carry out and when.

PMTCT involves a comprehensive approach that must all be implemented to optimize the program's effectiveness. The four prongs of PMTCT are the following:

1. Primary prevention of HIV among sexually active men and women. This is aimed at preventing new HIV infection.

2. Prevention of unintended pregnancies among HIV-positive women by addressing their family planning and contraceptive needs.

3. Prevention of HIV transmission from women to their infants. This will be achieved through the following:

   • Enhancing access to HTC during pregnancy, labor, and delivery

   • Providing ART drugs to mothers and infants

   • Instituting safer delivery practices to decrease the risk of infant exposure to HIV

   • Providing infant feeding education and support

4. Provision of treatment, care, and support to HIV-infected women, their infants, and their families.

5. With the help of the Clinton Foundation, a mothers-to-mothers program was also introduced. These are HIV-positive childbearing and rearing women who are stationed at various facilities to provide counseling on ARVs prophylaxis, treatment, adherence, and infant feeding for women who test HIV positive at the prenatal care.

Infant-feeding guidelines were developed in the context of HIV and AIDS (Ministry of Health and Social Welfare, 2010a):

   • Lay HIV counselors were introduced at the facility levels both at MCH and maternity units responsible for pre- and post-test counseling during prenatal care, labor, and delivery

   • Community health workers were involved in client follow-up

   • Prenatal, labor and delivery, and postnatal registers were developed

   • Infant tracking tools for babies born to HIV-positive mothers were introduced

Clinical staging is done at every visit, as such women are urged to bring their Mother Baby Packs for review, to monitor their adherence and to reinforce health education given during the initial visit. Nationally, Lesotho has made advances to prevent mother-to-child transmission, and nearly four-fifths of HIV-positive pregnant women receive antiretroviral drugs (United Nations Population Fund, 2012).

Workplace Programs

Employers are faced with high rates of absenteeism due to HIV-related diseases. Employees can be absent because they are sick or because they are taking care of sick family members. Therefore, companies play a role in the management of HIV/AIDS. Companies have to provide a nondiscriminatory environment for workers with HIV, and allow them to have some time off in order to attend their monthly medical check-ups. Companies must facilitate the provision of HIV/AIDS education and HIV prevention strategies for their employees. The Apparel Lesotho Alliance to Fight AIDS (ALAFA) is a good example of how companies can take care of workers in all aspects of HIV, including research, peer education, HTC, treatment, care, and support.

The National AIDS Commission (NAC) commissioned a situational assessment of public and private sector workplaces to better understand the state of workplace policy and program development related to HIV/AIDS. To address the gaps in workplace programs for the public sector, NAC conducted a series of training sessions to capacitate government ministry focal points with basic HIV/AIDS competencies and to provide them with technical skills to support workplace policy and program development.

Upon release of the WHO programmatic update in April 2012, Lesotho's Ministry of Health and HIV/AIDS services implementing partners initiated discussions weighing the benefits and challenges of implementing Option B+, in which ART to all HIV-positive pregnant women, regardless of CD4 count, would be initiated. They agreed to implement this strategy. Updated guidelines are available in most health facilities (Elizabeth Glaser Pediatric AIDS Foundation, 2013).

HIV/AIDS Treatment, Care, and Support

Each year more people are gaining access to ART in Lesotho with 41% of eligible adults on treatment in 2015. In June 2016, Lesotho became the first African country to implement a "Test and Treat" strategy. This means every person who tests HIV positive will be offered ART regardless of their CD4 count. HIV care, and treatment makes up the largest proportion of spending on HIV/AIDS in Lesotho. Consistent with the 2006 Brazzaville commitment, the aim is to achieve universal access to comprehensive HIV prevention, treatment, care, and support for all. To achieve this goal, scaling-up of HIV care was required. MoHSW adapted the provider-initiated model for HTC at all health facilities; decentralization of care and treatment initiation were devolved to the health center level. HIV services were rolled out to the rural communities in the highlands. Human resource capacity was increased by mobilizing lay counselors and expert patient and community health workers, expanding the role of nurses, and improving strategies for recruitment and retention of clinical staff. Finally, public–private partnerships were implemented, which improved access to HIV care and treatment and support throughout the country. There is a memorandum of understanding between the MoHSW and private sector practitioners that allows private practitioners to provide free ART services to HIV/AIDS patients. This has not only increased access to treatment, but has reduced overcrowding at public health facilities.

Earlier diagnosis and ART initiation has an impact on the incidence and intensity of opportunistic infection. This has led to improved quality of life of HIV/AIDS patients, reduced multiple-medication treatments, and as a result, reduced the cost of HIV/AIDS patient treatment. However, Lesotho has also had to contend with a second epidemic, tuberculosis (TB), which spreads rapidly and easily infects patients whose immune systems are already weakened by HIV. In 2014, 74% people living with TB in Lesotho tested positive for HIV. One of the ministry's targets is to increase the proportion of health facilities providing integrated TB/HIV services (Ministry of Health [Lesotho], 2015; United Nations Population Fund, 2012).

HIV treatment guidelines of 2010 offer a guide for who can take both HIV rapid tests and dry blood spots (DBS) for DNA PCR (**Box 20-1**).

Training of personnel to carry out HIV testing (**Table 20-5**) and DBS has a significant impact on HTC. This means that tests can be carried out easily from the community levels in the rural and most inaccessible places (by road), achieving the goal of early diagnosis, early referral, and treatment of HIV/AIDS.

BOX 20-1 Persons Who Can Perform HIV Rapid Tests and Take DBS for DNA PCR

- Laboratory technicians and technologists
- Counselors (including lay counselors and expert patients under close supervision)
- Midwives
- Nurses / nursing assistants
- Doctors
- Pharmacists / pharmacy technicians
- Social workers
- Ward attendants (under close supervision)
- Community health workers (under close supervision)

Data from Government of Lesotho Ministry of Health. (April 2016). National guidelines on the use of antiretroviral therapy for HIV prevention and treatment (5th ed). Maseru: Author. Retrieved from https://aidsfree.usaid.gov/sites/default/files/lesotho_art_2016.pdf

---

Besides HIV testing through the Know-Your-Status campaign and testing events through Kick for Life and other organizations, there were still some populations that could not be reached, yet they were still presenting to health facilities. Testing for HIV in children under 18 months will be done through rapid test and in conformity with DNA PCR after 6 weeks from birth if not breastfeeding, and a week after breastfeeding ceases.

Children who are exposed and test positive are taken as exposed children and enrolled for care until they stop breastfeeding and are confirmed HIV negative through DNA PCR protocol a week after cessation of breastfeeding.

Table 20-5	Recommended HIV Testing for Pregnant Women, Children, and Adults	
Pregnant Women	**Children**	**Adults**
During prenatal visit	Children who are admitted to hospital	Adults admitted to hospital
During labor, if not previously tested	Children diagnosed with TB and malnutrition	Adults diagnosed with TB, malnutrition, or STI
Those who tested negative after 36 weeks	Orphans or abandoned children	Adult receiving community home-based care
	Children receiving home-based care	Survivors of sexual assault
	Children with failure to thrive	Adults seen at outpatient clinics
	Children with contact with health facilities	Any caregiver of a child receiving chronic HIV care or receiving HAART
	Children who present in the under-5 clinic with diseases	Healthcare providers
	Children with HIV-positive mother and/or father	
	Victims of sexual abuse	
	Children receiving immunization who have not been previously tested	
	Children of parents who are on HAART	

Data from Government of Lesotho Ministry of Health. (April 2016). National guidelines on the use of antiretroviral therapy for HIV prevention and treatment (5th ed). Maseru: Author. Retrieved from https://aidsfree.usaid.gov/sites/default/files/lesotho_art_2016.pdf

HIV Care and Treatment Package

Clinical evaluation consists of WHO clinical staging, diagnosis, and management of current and acute infections/opportunistic infections, and screening and treatment of TB, STI, and pregnancy. Clinical evaluation also includes immunizations, and monitoring growth and development, primary care, and nutrition evaluation and counseling for children established at this stage: initiation of cotrimoxazole and isoniazid prophylaxis, taking samples for baseline laboratory investigations, and primary and supportive care.

Clinical evaluation also includes education and counseling to ensure adherence, readiness assessment, prevention counseling, and community linkages. The HIV care and treatment package is intended to assist in the provision of care at any level, from health center up to tertiary level. Patients will be provided with prophylaxis with the aim of reducing the incidence of opportunistic infections such as TB. Baseline laboratory tests will help clinicians choose the best treatment for the patient. Children infected with HIV come to the health facilities challenged with nutritional problems that may affect their growth. One of the ministry's targets is to make provisions for all people living with HIV and on ART get their daily minimal nutritional intake. It is important to monitor growth and also to carry out nutritional assessment and counseling (Ministry of Health [Lesotho], 2015).

Education and counseling prepares patients for life-long treatment. Patients should be made aware of support initiatives within their communities. These initiatives may assist patients with adherence monitoring, testing of family members, and support groups for people living with HIV.

Medication

Currently, HAART regimens include zidovudine as the first-line drug of choice for children, which can be replaced by abacavir in cases of anemia, while adults are given tenofovir, which replaces stavudine.

There should be an established reason to move to second-line treatment. Adherence should always be monitored and should not be the reason for treatment failure. If it is, this should be addressed before the patient is moved to second-line ART. Treatment failure in children and adults may be defined based on clinical, immunological, and/or virological criteria.

The decision to move to second-line ART depends on various factors, such as previous exposure to certain antiretroviral drugs, adherence to ART, toxicity of the drug, and resistance to the class of antiretroviral drugs. The decision is normally made by a multidisciplinary team at the central level. Once approval is given, the patient can be given second-line therapy. After 6 to 7 years of ART in Lesotho, the majority of HIV/AIDS patients are still on first-line ART, with only a few patients on second-line ART.

Because Lesotho is a developing nation, the cost difference between first- and second-line ART is an important limiting factor. Therefore, it is advisable that HIV/AIDS patients be kept on first-line therapy for as long as possible. This can be achieved through intensive patient adherence, counseling, and monitoring. HIV/AIDS patients have to be followed closely and pill counts must be monitored; any adherence issues must be addressed quickly and fully. Patients with adherence problems should be followed up closely, and patients who default on treatment should be tracked and be brought back to care and treatment. Resistance/susceptibility testing should ideally be carried out before the patient is moved to second-line therapy. However, because resistance/susceptibility testing cannot be done locally in Lesotho, other criteria for identification of treatment failure must be used in order to move patients into second-line ART.

There are some patients who have genuinely failed on second-line treatment and these patients must continue taking antiretroviral drugs for their HIV treatment. The following antiretroviral drugs have been approved as third-line treatment in Lesotho: darunavir, ritonavir, rotogravure, and etravirine. The procedure for moving patients from second-line to third-line is the same, and is done at the central level.

Toxicity of Antiretroviral Medicines All the drugs used for treatment may have side effects or adverse effects. Antiretroviral drugs have both adverse effects and toxicities that are well identified, and, when they occur in a patient, there is always an intervention intended to alleviate the adverse effect. The following guiding principles are used to manage toxicities and determine whether to continue using the drug or change to the next alternative drug (**Box 20-2**).

Monitoring of Patients on Antiretroviral Drugs Clinical and laboratory monitoring of patients on HAART is important, especially in the beginning of treatment. Once the patient has stabilized on treatment, the frequency of monitoring can be reduced.

Clinical Monitoring of the Patient

Monitoring the patient before and after initiation of treatment highlights any problems early to allow for timely intervention. After starting ART, clinical monitoring should be scheduled at 2 weeks, 1 month, 2 months, 3 months, and 6 months thereafter. This can be done by a doctor or a nurse under the supervision of a doctor. Frequent appointments can be made for patients with poor adherence and those who develop adverse effects to medication. Both children and adults should be clinically monitored. Weight, height, head circumference, and developmental and nutritional status of a child are monitored. New diseases such as opportunistic infections, TB, STI, substance abuse, and psychiatric diseases are diagnosed and managed. Medications, including incidence of side effects, adherence and dosing, drug interactions with other medicines, or treatment of other existing diseases are

---

BOX 20-2 Guiding Principles for Managing ART Toxicity

1. Determine the seriousness of the toxicity.

2. Evaluate concurrent medication and establish whether the toxicity is attributed to an antiretroviral drug or non-antiretroviral drug.

3. Consider other disease processes.

4. Manage adverse events according to severity:

   a. For grade four (severe life-threatening reaction) immediately discontinue all antiretroviral drugs, manage the medical event, reintroduce antiretroviral drugs using a modified regimen when the patient has stabilized.

   b. For grade three (severe reactions), substitute the offending drug without stopping treatment.

   c. For grade two (moderate reactions), consider continuation of ART for as long as feasible, if the patient does not improve on symptomatic therapy, consider single-drug substitution.

   d. For grade one (mild reaction), do not change treatment, reassure the patient.

5. Stress maintenance of adherence despite toxicity for mild and moderate reactions.

6. If there is need to stop ART due to life-threatening toxicity, stop all antiretroviral drugs at the same time until the patient is stabilized.

Data from Government of Lesotho Ministry of Health. (April 2016). National guidelines on the use of antiretroviral therapy for HIV prevention and treatment (5th ed). Maseru: Author. Retrieved from https://aidsfree.usaid.gov/sites/default/files/lesotho_art_2016.pdf

reviewed. Other issues, such as early diagnosis of pregnancy, that may affect adherence to medication are reviewed.

Laboratory Monitoring

Laboratory monitoring is very important even before initiation of ART. It helps in deciding the best drug for the patient, and when to change it if the need arises. Laboratory monitoring should complement clinical monitoring. Lesotho is a resource-limited country with a high prevalence of HIV. It is therefore important to note that there will be situations in which treatment can be started without the benefit of laboratory results. There may be a switch from one ART level to the next without the use of laboratory findings. At the moment, while CD4 cell count is part of routine testing, viral load is not routine.

Baseline laboratory investigations consist of CD4 cell count (or percentage for children), full blood count (where zidovudine is used), alanine aminotransferase (ALT), serum creatinine (where tenofovir is used), and pregnancy test to all females of childbearing age (where efavirenz is used).

Routine laboratory tests are based on the specific treatment and specified intervals are strictly followed. For example, hemoglobin concentration should be measured in patients receiving zidovudine at 1 month, 2 months, 3 months, and every 6 months thereafter. ALT should be checked in patients receiving nevirapine at 1 month, 2 months, and every 6 months thereafter. If on tenofovir, serum creatinine should be checked every 6 months, Hepatitis B surface antigen (Haig) should be performed to identify HIV/HBV co-infection, and to identify who should be put on tenofovir. The CD4 count should be checked every 6 months to determine treatment success or failure.

Measuring the Efficacy of Antiretroviral Treatment

Goals of ART include reduction of HIV-related morbidity and mortality, improvement of quality of life, restoration and preservation of immune function, maximal and durable suppression of HIV replication, and accelerated growth in children.

Efficacy of these goals can be measured in the following ways:

1. Clinically, by a reduction in the number and frequency of opportunistic infections

2. Immunologically, by gradual and steady rise in CD4 cell count

3. Biologically, by a fall in the viral load to undetectable levels 6 months after initiation of ART

Challenges of HIV/AIDS Treatment

Patient adherence to HIV/AIDS treatment is one of the major challenges for clinicians in Lesotho and elsewhere in the subregion. Patients adhere to treatment better when they are sick, but when they feel better they forget to take their medications. HIV/AIDS treatment requires a long-term commitment on the side of both the patient and the health professionals. Some patients may adhere to their regimen but when they come to the facility for a refill, they may find the medications out of stock due to supply-chain problems. Continuous supply of antiretroviral drugs should therefore be ensured.

Several countries with a high prevalence of HIV do not manufacture antiretroviral drugs, and price negotiations and supply may not be under their control. For example, pediatric ARV drugs are made into fixed-dose combinations and are supplied through one charity, the Clinton Foundation. In the Continental Policy Framework for Sexual and Reproductive Health and Rights (United Nations Population Fund, 2012), the problem of the stability of supply is identified and a target is local manufacturing of medicines and health equipment. The presence of the Clinton Foundation ensures a current supply of pediatric antiretroviral drugs, but with no future in terms of skills transfer for negotiating prices or procurement. Even though patients may be motivated and willing to adhere to HIV treatment, supply-chain management continues to be a challenge.

Treatment adherence monitoring should include an agreement wherein the patients sign a form to show that they agree to take their medication for life. Adherence monitoring and counseling should be continuous, so that if the patient who was adhering well to treatment in the beginning begins to show poor adherence, contributing factors may be identified and addressed immediately. Monitoring of treatment includes pill counts and liquid measurements.

The adherence percentage has to be calculated and entered into the patient's medical record. If adherence is lower than 95%, the patient should be referred for adherence counseling. However, if the patient has a valid reason for the lower adherence percentage and had been adhering well previously, counseling may not be required. Other methods, like signing an adherence card each time the patients take medicines, can be used. However, their value as a method of adherence monitoring is diminishing, as some patients fill the adherence card on the day they come to the facility. Honest reporting should be encouraged for this method of monitoring to be dependable.

When first initiated, HAART treatment adherence posed challenges for both patients and healthcare providers. Healthcare providers took a harsh approach to patient education, meaning to stress the importance of medication adherence. However, this was unnecessary, as there is no one more invested in treatment adherence than the patients themselves. The role of the healthcare professional is to provide the patient with relevant information and support; the patient will make an informed decision about whether to continue with treatment or not.

There are three adherence sessions before the patient is initiated on HAART. The sessions cover basic HIV/AIDS knowledge such as, what is HIV, what is AIDS, how HIV is transmitted, signs and symptoms of the infection, and the significance of CD4 count. HIV treatment literacy covers ARV drugs, importance of adherence, and adverse effects. Treatment literacy also explains how to take ARV medicines, to bring all medicines each time they come to the health facilities, and what to do if they forget to take their medication. Guidelines dictate that patients should take the medicines if they remember within 6 hours of the scheduled dose. Other general information is given to the patient about nutrition, opportunistic infection, TB and its treatment, what to do if they lose medicines, and concurrent use of traditional medicines with ARV drugs, which is a common practice in Lesotho.

Barriers to adherence should be identified and addressed appropriately; major adherence issues emanate from poverty, such as not enough food or no money for transport to the health facility. Such barriers can be addressed by referring the patient to the Department of Social Welfare for temporary financial assistance. Other barriers may be lack of education of HIV issues or alcohol abuse.

Another important barrier is lack of disclosure to family members. When family members are around, the patient may skip a dose because communities often know that patients who are on HAART take medicines at 7 pm.

Some patients ask for plain medication labels so that family members cannot identify the medicines as antiretroviral drugs; others ask for repacking of medicines because they say containers are well known. Nonetheless, it is important to address these issues.

There are couples in which one member does not disclose their HIV status to the other for fear of fighting, mistrust, and rejection. Patient disclosure should be encouraged to avoid secrecy and suspicion. If relatives and family members know about the patient's HIV status, they may eventually accept and provide support when the patient is on treatment. In turn, this may improve treatment adherence. Disclosure may also prevent HIV transmission from an HIV-positive spouse to an HIV-negative one.

HIV/AIDS Policy and Barriers in the Delivery of HIV/AIDS and SRH Services

HIV and AIDS is a serious challenge in sub-Saharan Lesotho. As such, Lesotho has put in place measures to curb the pandemic. There are several challenges to success in the reproductive health programs and activities. Some of these challenges were identified during the review of the Know Your Status campaign; the development of the Strategic Plan for Elimination of Mother-To-Child Transmission of HIV and for Pediatric HIV Care, and the treatment review 2011/12 – 2015/16 (**Box 20-3**).

Broader Economic Tests to Lesotho Strategic Plans

With the second highest HIV prevalence rate in the world among adults and the highest TB incidence, and low efficiency and effectiveness of public spending, the government regards HIV/AIDS as one of its most important development issues, which is evident in its HIV/AIDS National Strategic Plan. Between 1990 and 2005, life expectancy at birth declined from almost 60 years to 47 years, and currently stands at 49 years (World Bank, 2017). However, several logistical challenges exist to progress. Inefficient management of public spending is impairing the development. Public spending stands at 50% of the gross domestic product in 2016–2017. The high public wage bill is one of the highest in the world and is the biggest contributor to public spending. Unemployment remains high at estimated levels between 24% and 26%. There is a need to promote private sector jobs. Recently, the retrenchment of male mine workers and the absence of local economic opportunities led Lesotho women to migrate to the export garment factories in urban Lesotho. Currently, one-third of households have a member living somewhere else. The gender balance of households is altering with females moving away. Another government target is improving public sector and fiscal management, particularly contract management of the Queen Mamohato Memorial Hospital, which is one of the main modern Lesotho hospitals, under

---

BOX 20-3 Challenges and Bottlenecks in the Provision of SRH and HIV/AIDS Services

- Shortage of health workers, burnout, frequent rotation of health workers, and effective delivery of quality health services. There are also challenges with the consistent supply and procurement of basic medications and other medical supplies.

- The tough physical terrain in the rural areas and the cultural beliefs and traditions limit the access and use of healthcare facilities. Low access rates and utilization of health facilities result in low access to skilled attendants. These issues contribute to high maternal mortality and low coverage of PMTCT.

- Weak involvement of men on reproductive health issues. This not only limits their utilization of MCH and SRH services in general, but impedes women's access and utilization of services as well.

- Regular supportive supervision is a challenge, attributable to lack of finances and transport, especially for hard-to-reach facilities. Recruitment, deployment, retention, and training of skilled health personnel are central elements in the provision and access of quality healthcare services. These are challenges because of limited pool of skilled personnel, poor working conditions, unfriendly deployment policies, and uncoordinated trainings that are offered by the government of Lesotho through MoHSW.

- Strengthening and improving the functions of monitoring and evaluation and the Health Management Information System units in the health facilities, in order to improve availability of information in the MoHSW, still poses a challenge. However, data clerks are gradually being deployed in all health facilities.

- In Lesotho, there is no center for research. However, within the MoHSW, there exists a National Ethics Review Board that is made up of different stakeholders representing the government, professional councils and organizations, development and implementing partners, NGOs, civil society, and the Christian Health Association of Lesotho. This board has advocated for the establishment of institutional review boards in the various organizations and institutions.

- Research that needs to be conducted in the country has to first be approved by the National ethics review board, in the MoHSW. There have been several studies focusing on maternal and child health as well as reproductive health issues. These studies have helped to inform development and reviews of policies, guidelines, and protocols related to HIV and AIDS and SRH issues.

---

private–public partnership. The World Bank has endorsed a new Country Partnership Framework (CPF) 2016–2020 to support the Lesotho government in its long-term strategic plans (World Bank, 2016). The CPF is expected to deliver $154 million in financial support. Threats to the plan include food and oil price variability, climate change, weaknesses in private sector development, a decline in donor funding and insufficient HIV/AIDS and tuberculosis treatment coverage to reverse the epidemics (World Bank, 2017).

Conclusion

In conclusion, Lesotho has come a long way in addressing the pertinent issues regarding SRH. However, there is still more to be done through legislation and policies to address some of the remaining issues, while others could be changed through behavior and attitudes. Even though international and national efforts are being made, rigorous internal implementation, monitoring, and evaluation tools have to be in place to measure and effect real progress on the ground.

● ● ● **REFERENCES**

African Union Commission. (2016). *Maputo plan of action 2016–2030.* Retrieved from https://www.au.int/web/sites/default/files/documents/24099-poa_5-_revised_clean.pdf

Brewer, D. D., Potterat, J. J., Roberts, J. M., & Brody, S. (2007). Male and female circumcision associated with prevalent HIV infection in virgins and adolescents in Kenya, Lesotho, and Tanzania. *Annals of Epidemiology, 17,* (3), 217–226.

Bureau of Statistics [Lesotho]. (2013). *Lesotho demographic survey, 2011* (Vol. 1). Maseru, Lesotho: Author. Retrieved from http://www.bos.gov.ls/nada/index.php/catalog/6

Elizabeth Glaser Pediatric AIDS Foundation. (2013). *Assessment of prevention of mother-to-child transmission of HIV services in Lesotho.* Retrieved from https://www.unicef.org/evaldatabase/files/EGPAF_GF_PMTCT_evaluation_report.pdf

Government of Lesotho. (2011). *National family planning guidelines.* Maseru, Lesotho: Ministry of Health and Social Welfare.

International Planned Parenthood Federation. (2017). *Lesotho Planned Parenthood Association.* Retrieved from http://www.ippf.org/about-us/member-associations/lesotho

Lesotho Network of People Living with HIV and AIDS (LENEPWHA). (2014). *The people living with HIV stigma index, Lesotho.* Retrieved from http://www.stigmaindex.org/sites/default/files/reports/Lesotho%20Stigma%20Index%20draft%20report%206-%20L.pdf

Ministry of Health [Lesotho]. (2015). *Lesotho country progress report: January–December 2014.* Retrieved from http://www.unaids.org/sites/default/files/country/documents/LSO_narrative_report_2015.pdf

Ministry of Health [Lesotho] & ICF International. (2016). *Lesotho demographic and health survey 2014*. Maseru, Lesotho: Author.

Ministry of Health and Social Welfare. (2006). *National Adolescent Health Policy*. Maseru, Lesotho: Author.

Ministry of Health and Social Welfare (Lesotho). (2010a). *Infant and Young Child Feeding Participant's Manual*. Maseru, Lesotho: Author. Retrieved from http://www.iycn.org/files/Lesotho-Infant-and-Young-Child-Feeding-Participant-Manual-Part-1.pdf

Ministry of Health and Social Welfare (MoHSW). (2010b). *National guidelines for HIV/AIDS care and treatment* (3rd ed.). Maseru, Lesotho: Author.

Ministry of Health and Social Welfare. (2010c). *National guidelines for the prevention of mother to child transmission of HIV*. Maseru, Lesotho: Author. Retrieved from: https://aidsfree.usaid.gov/sites/default/files/tx_lesotho_pmtct_2010.pdf

Ministry of Health and Social Welfare (MoHSW). (2012). *Linking HIV and sexual reproductive health and rights in Southern Africa 2011–2012*. Retrieved from http://www.integrainitiative.org/blog/wp-content/uploads/2012/09/Lesotho-Annual-Performance-Report-2011.pdf

Ministry of Health and Social Welfare (MoHSW). (2013). *Rapid assessment of sexual and reproductive health and HIV linkages*. Retrieved from http://srhhivlinkages.org/wp-content/uploads/2013/04/ras_lesotho_en.pdf

Thabane, S., & Kasiram, M. (2015). Child abandonment and protection of abandoned children in Lesotho: Prevention strategies. *Social Work, 51*(1), 45–62.

UNAIDS. (2014). *The gap report*. Retrieved from http://www.unaids.org/en/resources/campaigns/2014/2014gapreport/gapreport

UNAIDS. (2016). *Global AIDS Progress Report*. Retrieved from http://www.unaids.org/sites/default/files/media_asset/2016-prevention-gap-report_en.pdf

United Nations Population Fund. (2012). *Lesotho United Nations Development Assistance Plan (LUNDAP), 2013–2017*. Retrieved from https://www.unfpa.org/sites/default/files/portal-document/Lesotho_UNDAP%202013-2017.pdf.pdf

United Nations Population Fund (UNFPA). (2016). *UNFPA and business community tackle HIV and maternal health issues*. Retrieved from http://lesotho.unfpa.org/en/news/unfpa-and-business-community-tackle-hiv-and-maternal-health-issues

U.S. President's Emergency Plan for AIDS Relief (PEPFAR). (2016). *Lesotho country operational plan (COP) strategic direction summary*. Retrieved from https://www.pepfar.gov/documents/organization/257640.pdf

World Bank. (2016). *Kingdom of Lesotho: Country partnership framework 2016–2020*. Washington, DC: World Bank Group. Retrieved from http://documents.worldbank.org/curated/en/987971467293534846/Kingdom-of-Lesotho-country-partnership-framework-2016-2020

World Bank. (2017). *The world bank in lesotho overview*. Retrieved from http://www.worldbank.org/en/country/lesotho/overview

World Health Organization (WHO). (1995). *Health benefits of family planning; family planning and population division of family health*. Retrieved from http://apps.who.int/iris/bitstream/10665/62091/1/WHO_FHE_FPP_95.11.pdf

World Health Organization (WHO). (2008). *Ouagadougou declaration on primary health care and health systems in Africa: Achieving better health for Africa in the new millennium*. Regional Office for Africa. Retrieved from http://ahm.afro.who.int/issue12/pdf/AHM12Pages10to21.pdf

21

Providing Sexual and Reproductive Health Care and Service in Resource-Constrained Countries: Ghana

SALLY-ANN OHENE

CHAPTER OBJECTIVES

The main objectives of this chapter are to:

- Consider the global and in-country context within which the Ghana national program evolved

- Explore the steps and strategies adopted to implement the health sector response

- Examine the relevant prevention, treatment, care, and support services delivered through the health sector

- Explore the relevant policies guiding their operations

- Describe the role of research monitoring and evaluation in HIV/AIDS service provision

- Identify the successes, achievements, and lessons learned in the process of providing services

- Examine the challenges and barriers to providing standardized care

Introduction

When faced with the first case of acquired immunodeficiency syndrome (AIDS) in 1986, Ghana—like many countries in sub-Saharan Africa—had to rise to the task of addressing the human immunodeficiency virus (HIV) epidemic. Because most HIV infections are being sexually transmitted, a key aspect of tackling the HIV epidemic involves addressing sexual and reproductive health (SRH) care, including sexually transmitted infection (STI) management. Other interventions

include preventing new infections, vertical mother-to-child HIV transmission, lifelong care of HIV-infected persons, and building the capacity of the health service to cope with these new programs.

This chapter provides an overview of evolution of SRH care and HIV services in resource-constrained developing countries. Adequate insight of backgrounds from which migrant patients come and awareness of problems and needs presented enable practitioners in developed countries to better understand the influences of cultural sexual practices such as female genital mutilation (FGM), religious restrictions, poor literacy, and limited access to high-standard sexual healthcare facilities. Ghana (**Figure 21-1**) typifies a sub-Saharan country with relatively complex limitations in economic, professional expertise, diagnostic procedures, and referral systems for high-quality SRH/HIV specialist interventions, follow-up, and support services. The purpose of this chapter is to raise awareness among practitioners in developed countries how multiple limitations impact patient outcomes in poorer countries.

This chapter highlights the initiatives and services implemented in Ghana to address HIV/AIDS care from the health sector perspective. The initial section gives insight into the global picture of HIV, then transitions into the experience of an HIV-related service delivery program in a resource-limited setting. This experience can serve as a resource for planning and implementation of HIV-related services.

Context of the Global HIV Epidemic: The Epidemiology, Impact, and Global Response

Ghana's response to HIV did not evolve in isolation, but rather developed and progressed within the global milieu of a complex and multifaceted pandemic. To gain

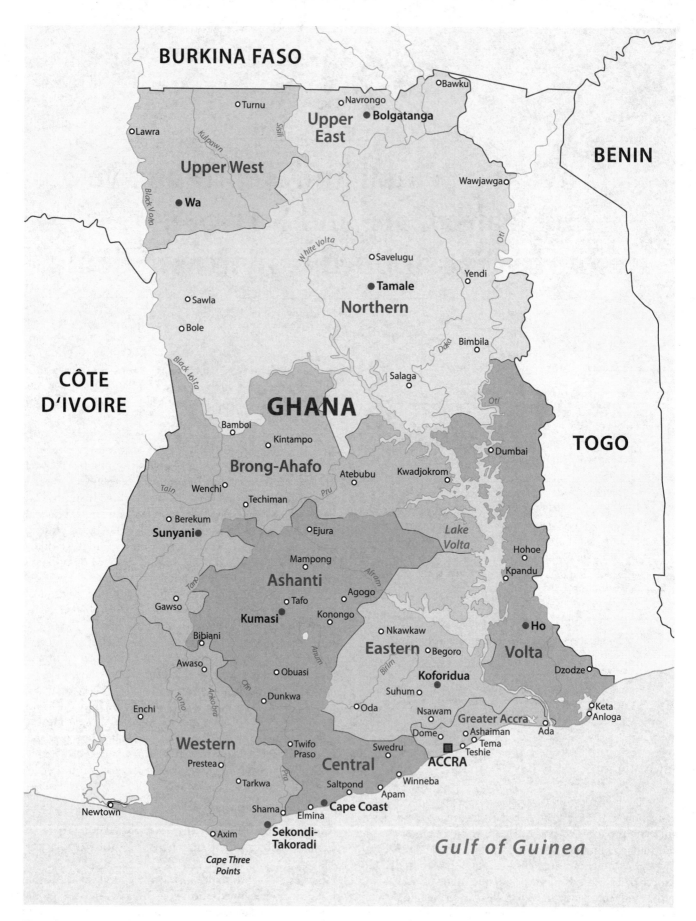

Figure 21-1 Ghana
© Rainer Lesniewski/Shutterstock

a better perspective of Ghana's HIV program, it is useful to understand the context of the global HIV epidemic: its epidemiology, impact, and the global response.

Global HIV Epidemiology

More than 3 decades after the initial recognition of AIDS, the HIV epidemic continues to be a major global healthcare priority, with a large population of people living with HIV (PLHIV). It is estimated that in 2009 there were about 33.3 million PLHIV worldwide, a 27% increase over the 1999 figure (Joint United Nations Programme on HIV/AIDS [UNAIDS], 2011); this number has risen to an estimated 34 to 39 million PLHIV worldwide in 2015 (World Health Organization [WHO], 2015b). Even though the spread of HIV is estimated to have peaked in 1997 with 3.2 million new infections, HIV transmission through sexual contact and other means still occurs, with UNAIDS (2016) estimating 1.8 to 2.4 million newly infected individuals in 2015. About 370,000 out of these new infections occurred among children via mother-to-child transmission in pregnancy, childbirth, and breastfeeding; an estimated 150,000 children under age 15 were newly infected in 2015. AIDS-related illnesses continue to be one of the leading causes of global mortality, accounting for 1.8 million deaths in 2009 (UNAIDS, 2011) and 1.1 million deaths in 2015 (WHO, 2015b).

Sub-Saharan Africa (SSA) is the most heavily affected region, with an estimated 23.1 to 28.5 million PLHIV in 2015 (WHO, 2015b). In this area, unprotected heterosexual contact with an HIV-positive partner is the main mode of transmission. Unfortunately, knowledge gaps about the mode of transmission, ignorance about vulnerability, and inadequate access to prevention, treatment, and care services have contributed to fueling the epidemic in this region. Other contributing factors include a high burden of sexually transmitted infections, seasonal labor migration, an active commercial sex industry, and cultural practices that allow for multiple sexual practices and intergenerational sex (UNAIDS & WHO, 2009; UNAIDS 2011). SSA, with an estimated 12.5% of the world's population, accounted for 66% of HIV infections worldwide in 2015, including 91% of the 150,000 new infections in children under 15 worldwide (U.S. Department of Health and Human Services [DHHS], 2017). In addition, 72% of the world's AIDS-related deaths in 2008 occurred in SSA (UNAIDS, 2016; UNAIDS & WHO, 2009; United Nations, 2010). Women and girls in SSA are disproportionately affected by HIV making up 76% of all HIV-positive women globally.

The Impact of the HIV/AIDS Epidemic

In the absence of both global and national responses, HIV places an enormous burden on human populations, with mortality from AIDS and ill health playing very significant roles. From 1993, when AIDS-related deaths among adult and children were estimated to be 500,000, there was a consistent rise in AIDS mortality over the ensuing years, peaking at 2.1 million in 2004 (UNAIDS, 2011). Though in recent years there has been a decline in the number of AIDS deaths, the high mortality from HIV has had devastating effects, with life expectancy falling to below 51 years in the worst affected countries in SSA (United Nations, 2010). In six sub-Saharan Africa countries, life expectancy has fallen below 1970 levels, a decline attributed to the HIV epidemic (United Nations Development Program [UNDP], 2010). The lowered immunity associated with HIV infection predisposes PLHIV to recurrent opportunistic infections, the upsurge of previously rare infections and malignancies, and a resurgence of tuberculosis—including drug-resistant strains—to epidemic proportions (Lamptey, Wigley, Carr, & Collymore, 2002). Particularly in low-income countries, this increases the workload on health staff who are already stretched because of inadequate staffing. To make matters worse, HIV infection among health personnel, especially in high HIV-burden countries, further limits the number of staff providing care (Lamptey et al., 2002). In addition to the public health burden, the HIV epidemic has a negative socioeconomic impact. People in the productive and reproductive age group are the most affected, resulting in a depletion of the workforce. Consequently, practically all sectors (education, agriculture, commerce, and governance) are adversely affected by the loss of manpower, resulting in reduced income, poverty, and food insecurity. Individuals, families, and communities are affected by HIV-associated stigma, the problem of AIDS orphans—many of whom become heads of households—and the breakdown of the social fabric. Indeed, practically every aspect of life and society is one way or the other deleteriously affected by HIV. By the mid-1980s, the severity of the HIV epidemic and the potential magnitude of negative future consequences had become evident, demanding an effective strategy to address the situation (Quinn, 2001).

The Global Response and Initiatives

In 1987, the World Health Organization (WHO) established the Global Program on AIDS, which led the way for coordinating the global response (Merson 2006; WHO 2010b). This involved working with ministries of health of low- and medium-income countries to create awareness about the epidemic, develop evidence-based policies and programs to limit the spread of the disease, and promote the participation of nongovernmental organizations (NGOs) in the global and national response to HIV. With the establishment of the Joint United Nations Programme on HIV/AIDS (UNAIDS) in 1996 to lead the coordinated, multisector global response, there was a move toward a multifaceted approach beyond the health sector to manage the national response to HIV. At the turn of the millennium, several initiatives boosted the commitment to address HIV, some of which are shown in **Figure 21-2**.

The sixth of the Millennium Development Goals (MDG), which evolved from the United Nations Millennium Declaration Framework for Development, called for a halt and reversal of the spread of HIV/AIDS and universal access to HIV/AIDS treatment by 2010 (WHO,

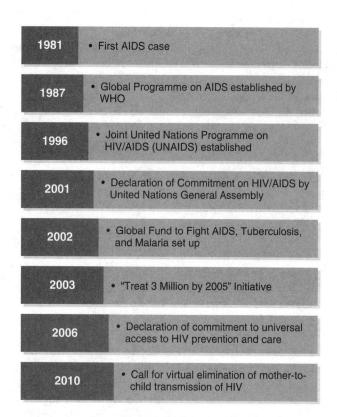

Figure 21-2 Chronology of Selected Global HIV-Related Initiatives

2010a). The 2001 Declaration of Commitment on HIV/ AIDS from the United Nations Special Session on HIV/ AIDS set program and funding targets for countries and donor partners, respectively (United Nations, 2001). Subsequently, in addition to the World Bank directing funds to HIV/AIDS, the multilateral Global Fund to Fight AIDS, Tuberculosis, and Malaria (GFATM) and the U.S. President's Emergency Plan for AIDS Relief (PEPFAR) were launched to support country-led HIV response initiatives in the areas of prevention, treatment, care, and support (Merson, 2006). Against this backdrop of unprecedented funding sources, the WHO and its partners launched the "Treat 3 Million by 2005" Initiative, with the global target of treating three million people with antiretroviral therapy (ART) by the end of 2005 (WHO, 2003b). Other, related initiatives include the declaration of commitment to universal access to HIV prevention, treatment, care, and support services and the call for virtual elimination of mother-to-child transmission of HIV (UNAIDS, 2009, United Nations, 2006).

The earlier global response and calls to action to address HIV/AIDS and subsequent ongoing initiatives have been instrumental in guiding countries as they tackle this complex epidemic. This has been especially true in the health sector response, with WHO being the lead agency in the establishing evidence-based policies, guidelines, and recommendations to support country response. The following historical perspective of HIV in Ghana in the early years highlights some of the links with the concurrent global trend.

HIV in Ghana: The Early Picture in the 1980s and 1990s

In March 1986, some 5 years after the identification of the initial AIDS cases, Ghana reported its first case (Amofah, 1992; Merson, 2006). By the end of that year, 26 AIDS cases had been confirmed. This increased to 227 reported cases (192 females and 35 males) by October 1988 Ministry of Health Ghana [MOH], 1988). It was reported that among the initial cases identified, three-fourths acquired HIV outside Ghana. Most of them were believed to be female commercial sex-workers (CSW). HIV prevalence was reported to be 2.5% among CSW in Accra, 4.6% among patients of a sexually transmitted disease clinic, and 0.5–1.5% among blood donors (Amofah, 1992).

In the late 1980s, HIV-related studies in Ghana shed light on the epidemiology and sociocultural factors of the HIV epidemic. In one such study of 1,330 pregnant women attending four prenatal clinics in the eastern region of the country in 1987, HIV prevalence ranged from 0.6% to 10.3% in the Manya Krobo District (MKD) (Neequaye et al., 1997). As women from the MKD had a tradition of working throughout West Africa as traders and/or commercial sex workers, and because MKD is a rural area away from major travel routes, the authors hypothesized that the high HIV prevalence likely reflected the tendency for pregnant or ill women to return to their home villages to be cared for by their families. A 1989–1990 community-based HIV seroprevalence survey conducted in rural and urban southern Ghana also indicated that, among 1,329 adults sampled, 1% of the men and 1.5% of the women were HIV infected (Neequaye et al., 1997). None of the 906 children tested were HIV positive, including six born to HIV-infected women.

Between 1987 and 1989, a series of surveys examined factors related to the spread of HIV infection, including knowledge about AIDS, sexual habits, use of CSW, traditional healer practices, and skin-piercing customs (Neequaye, Neequaye, & Biggar, 1991). Interesting findings included 55% of married men having concurrent sexual partners in addition to their wives, and limited use of condoms, with 66% of customers of high-class CSW refusing to use a condom even after a request to do so by the CSW. Among 74 rural traditional healers interviewed, many of whom had several clients a day, 39% performed skin piercing, including scarification, using unsterile instruments. The above data clearly indicated that there was an emerging HIV problem in Ghana that was challenged by sociocultural attitudes and practices. Fortunately, even before the first AIDS case was reported, the country had taken initial steps that eventually would lead to a national HIV response.

Early HIV/AIDS Program Management Summary

Most likely out of foresight, the Government of Ghana had set up the National Technical Committee on AIDS in October 1985, months before the initial AIDS case was identified in the country (Ghana AIDS Commission [GAC], 2004). The mandate of this committee was to advise the government and implement measures to contain the epidemic. The National AIDS Control Program (NACP), under the jurisdiction of the Ministry of Health (MOH), was established in 1987, followed by the appointment of the AIDS Control Manager in September of the same year (MOH, 1988). The AIDS prevention and control activities were governed initially by a Short-Term Plan 1987–1988 developed in July 1987 and subsequently, by the Medium-Term Plan 1 (MTP 1) 1989–1993 and the Second Medium-Term Plan (MTP 2) after 1993. Having taken the lead in coordinating the global AIDS response the WHO (through its Global Program on AIDS) was very instrumental in assisting countries' MOH develop these plans. Countries were also offered technical support for program management, surveillance, data management, clinical care, and HIV testing World Health Organization Regional Office for Africa [WHO AFRO], 2015).

The plans spelled out the objectives, strategies, and activities for the following program areas:

- Epidemiological surveillance, including AIDS surveillance, international notification using WHO clinical definition of AIDS, and sero-surveillance
- Prevention of HIV transmission through the provision of information, education, and communication materials; safe injection and other skin-piercing practices; the prevention and control of sexually transmitted diseases; and safe blood transfusion
- Prevention of sexual and maternal transmission of HIV by PLHIV
- Diagnosis, clinical management, and support of HIV-infected and AIDS patients

It is significant to note that even though the MOH/ NACP was the lead agency initially, multiple stakeholders were involved in various aspects of implementing the national response. They included representatives from other government sectors, academia, private sector, multilateral organizations, bilateral organizations, and international and local NGOs.

Despite the MTP 2 and the involvement of multiple players, it appeared that the national response was health-sector focused and not sufficiently catering to other aspects of HIV prevention and care (GAC, 2004). There was a growing recognition that the complex nature of the HIV problem required a more multidisciplinary strategy, which included the use of social-based approaches such as peer counseling and mass media campaigns. This inclination was actually in tandem with the global perspective. From 1996, UNAIDS took over from the Global Program on AIDS with a mandate of leading an expanded, coordinated, multisectoral global response (Merson, 2006). The eventual establishment of the Ghana AIDS Commission (GAC) in May 2000 as a supra-ministerial and multisectoral organization to coordinate

HIV-related activities by all stakeholders therefore did not come as a surprise. Several stakeholder consultations and advocacy from both local and international partners were involved in its formation. Following the assumption of GAC as the overall coordinating agency for HIV activities, the MOH through the NACP was now able to focus on implementing health-sector based HIV prevention, treatment, care, and support interventions. Previously, the health sector response had been limited to HIV prevention activities and supportive care for PLHIV. The MOH needed to be well positioned to take on the demanding role of planning and implementing a comprehensive HIV care program that would make a meaningful impact on the thousands of people infected and affected by HIV in Ghana.

HIV in Ghana in the New Millennium: Epidemiology, Trends, and Projections

A graphical presentation of the number of AIDS cases officially reported to the MOH from 1986 to the end of 2003, with a total of 76,139 persons, is shown in **Figure 21-3** (National AIDS/STI Control Program Ghana [NACP], 2003a). Much as the total figure of AIDS cases was thought to be underestimated and represented 30% of the actual number of cases in the country, the data provided useful information. More than 90% of the AIDS cases fell within the range of 15 to 49 years, about two-thirds were females and the most affected age groups were 25 to 34 for females and 30 to 39 for males.

In 2003, the nationwide Ghana Demographic and Health Survey (GDHS) included HIV testing among survey participants. The estimated HIV prevalence was 1.5% among men and 2.7% among women. This female-to-male ratio of 1.8:1 was reported to be higher than what appeared in

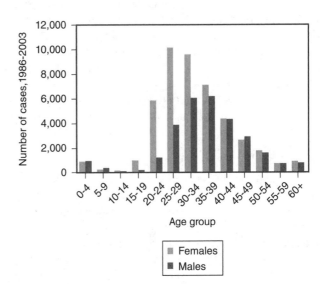

Figure 21-3 Cumulative Number of Reported AIDS Cases 1986-2003 By Age and Sex

Reproduced from National AIDS/STI Control Program, Ghana Health Service, Ghana AIDS Commission. (2004a). *HIV/AIDS in Ghana: Current situation, projections, impacts, interventions.* Accra, Ghana: Author.

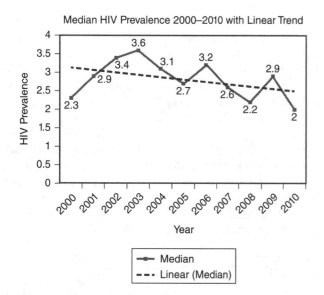

Median HIV Prevalence 2000–2010 with Linear Trend

Figure 21-4 HIV Sentinel Survey Results in Ghana 2000–2010
Reproduced from Ghana AIDS Commission. (2012). *Ghana country AIDS progress report.* Accra, Ghana: Author.

most population-based surveys in Africa (Ghana Statistical Service [GSS], 2004). Since the 1990s, the annual HIV Sentinel Survey (HSS) has measured HIV prevalence among pregnant women 15 to 49 years from both rural and urban areas in Ghana (NACP, 2011c). The results over the years have provided a proxy indication of HIV prevalence in the general population of Ghanaians. **Figure 21-4** shows the median HIV prevalence from the HSS from 2000 to 2010.

The highest HIV prevalence recorded in the history of the HSS was 3.6% in 1992 and 2003, and the lowest was 2% in 2010. It is, however, important to note that hidden behind the median values is a picture of varying rates, depending on the age group and locality.

For most of the surveys, the highest prevalence is recorded in the 25- to 29-year-old group while the 15- to 19-year-olds traditionally records the lowest prevalence. The 2006 figures for the two age groups were 4.2% and 1.4%, respectively, while the median prevalence that year was 3.2% (NACP, 2007a). In the 2007 HSS, the median HIV prevalence was 2.6%, however, there was a range of 0.3% in Krachi in the Volta Region to 8.9% in Agomanya in the Eastern Region of Ghana (NACP, 2008b). Urban women tend to have a higher HIV prevalence than those in the rural areas; 2.4% and 1.6%, respectively, were reported from the 2010 HSS (NACP, 2011b). Overall, the HSS results indicate a declining trend in HIV prevalence over the course of the last decade.

Over the years, the Estimations and Projections Package and Spectrum projection package software have been used to project national HIV prevalence, PLHIV population figures, number of childhood infections occurring through maternal transmission, estimates of PLHIV needing treatment, and AIDS deaths (NACP, 2004a). The modeling package utilizes data from demographic surveys, census, and other surveys (such as the HSS) to make these projections. According to these methods the number of PLHIV was approximated to be 118,000 in 1994 and 404,000 in 2004 (NACP, 2004a). Estimated rate in 2015 was; 270,000 PLHIV in Ghana (UNAIDS, 2015). Since the beginning of the epidemic in Ghana, about 200,000 people were estimated to have died from AIDS by 2004. Estimated number of deaths due to AIDS in 2015 was 13,000. In 2010, with the HSS indicating a 2.0% HIV prevalence in pregnant women, and 2.1% in 2011 and 2012, and 1.9% in 2013, the estimates from the modeling were as follows: adult national HIV prevalence was 1.5% in 2010, but 1.4% in 2012. Estimated number of PLHIV in 2010 was 221,941 and 150,000 in 2014. In 2010, new HIV infections in children 3,476; AIDS-related deaths 2,581 for children under 15 years, and 13,738 among those 15 years and above (NACP, 2011c). Estimated numbers in 2014 indicated 11,356 newly infected adults; and 9,246 AIDS-related deaths; newly infected adults in 2015 were 10,624 (GAC, 2014; NACP, 2016).

Epidemiological data and projections show the magnitude of the issues to be addressed in a health sector response. This epidemiological picture conveys the situation faced by the MOH in relation to planning for HIV services and programs in the new millennium. The following sections explore Ghana's health sector response and the provision of comprehensive care for HIV.

Health Sector Response to HIV: Mandate and Guiding Principles

In line with the care, support, and treatment elements outlined in the U.N. General Assembly Declaration of Commitments on HIV/AIDS ((United Nations, 2001), the MOH pursued its mandate of tackling health aspects of the epidemic. The WHO, which had been tasked by the World Health Assembly to develop the Global Health Sector Strategy (GHSS) for HIV/AIDS, was instrumental in supporting the health ministry in Ghana and other countries to carry out this mandate (WHO, 2003b). This was done by supporting capacity building and providing technical advice, including promoting the adaptation and use of evidence-based care guidelines that endorsed high standards of care, even in resource-constrained settings.

As stipulated in the National HIV/AIDS and STI Policy, the MOH was tasked with addressing medical aspects of the epidemic, including the following:

- Leading in the development and revision of counseling and testing guidelines, prevention of mother-to-child transmission (PMTCT) of HIV, management of opportunistic infections, home-based care
- Providing technical support to GAC and other ministries and sectors in their development and implementation of AIDS prevention and care activities

- Implementing health-sector-based intervention to prevent sexual, blood-borne, and maternal transmission of HIV, as well sexually transmitted infections
- Providing the appropriate health facility-based care for PLHIV, including counseling and home-based care and support (GAC, 2004)

The prevailing Ghana HIV/AIDS Strategic Framework (2001–2005) developed by the GAC and referred to as the National Strategic Framework I (NSF I) was the guiding document for the national response at the beginning of the millennium. It has been followed by the National Strategic Framework II 2006–2010 (NSF II) and the National Strategic Plan 2011–2015 (NSP). These documents reiterate the MOH's objectives of improving health service delivery for HIV/AIDS, mitigating its impact on individuals and families, and strengthening the capacity of health service personnel to provide HIV care (GAC 2001). The MOH 2002–2006 HIV/AIDs Strategic Plan aptly captures this mandate by stating the broad principles and goals for MOH HIV/AIDS activities (GAC 2002).

The following are the key components:

- Increasing access to quality HIV/AIDS/sexually transmitted infection (STI) prevention and care services to all clients through strengthening the technical and operational capacity of the MOH and other stakeholders to deliver quality HIV/AIDS and related services
- Reducing the vulnerability and susceptibility of employees to HIV and AIDS by establishing workplace HIV/AIDS programs for all health workers
- Strengthening the collaboration between the MOH and other sectors and providing technical support to other sectors and stakeholders involved in HIV/AIDS
- Creating an enabling policy environment for the HIV/AIDS response within the health sector

This culture of implementing programs within a structured framework in which goals and objectives are stated, targets are set, and strategies and activities for achieving the goals are outlined, facilitates prioritization, organized operationalization, and evaluation of progress (United Nations, 2001). MOH took steps to develop/adapt and use guidelines for the core components of the health sector. Other components of program development included establishing a framework for working with partners, capacity building, and resource mobilization (**Figure 21-5**). This set the framework for implementing and rolling out services in a robust and harmonized national program that aimed to promote high-quality interventions with consistent standards irrespective of where in the country the services were accessed.

Guidelines, Manuals, and Plans

In resource-constrained settings, as anywhere else, provision of the highest attainable standards of HIV treatment and

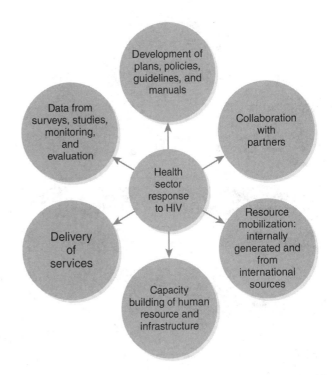

Figure 21-5 Key Components for Implementing the Health Sector Response

care requires planning and the use of evidence-based policy documents, guidelines, and training manuals. Drawing from documented experiences from both developed and developing countries, WHO/UNAIDS, and other international governmental and nongovernmental organizations, with the help of experts in the field of HIV, developed various guidelines and materials that were available for adaptation.

For the most part, Ghana took advantage of available resource materials and adopted and or adapted them to country settings without losing the core evidence-based components of the recommended standards. Ghana recognized that there were certain local approaches that would enhance service delivery or outcomes. For example, at the time the first edition of Ghana's ART guidelines was developed, the WHO guidelines suggested that a PLHIV who was newly started on ART should be followed up 1 month later. In Ghana's guidelines, however, it was stipulated that a person put on ART should be seen a few days, but certainly not more than 14 days, after initiation. This first post-ART initiation follow-up visit was to enable service providers assess for adherence to treatment, tolerance, and efficacy of treatment (MOH, 2002a, MOH, 2006).

Document adaptation was undertaken by a working group of experts and stakeholders who brought their experiences and local research evidence to bear in the process. Depending on the document or guideline being adapted or developed, team members were drawn from practicing service providers, academia and research institutions, public health specialists, laboratory, pharmacy and reproductive health personnel, international and nongovernmental

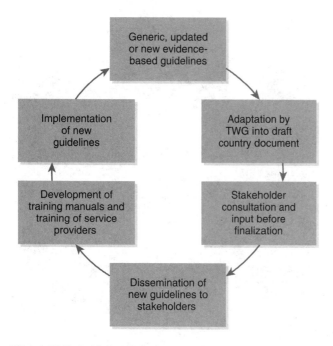

Figure 21-6 Guideline Development Process

organizations, development agencies and appropriate government and MOH institutions such as the Procurement Unit and the Food and Drugs Board.

Generically, the core working group, which would typically also include international experts, came up with a draft document that then received input from a larger group of people in a stakeholder consultative meeting before being finalized for implementation (**Figure 21-6**). There was also the expectation that documents would be updated periodically in ensuing years as new evidence-based information and recommendations became available. The adaptation and consensus building meetings frequently had the benefit of both technical and financial support from multiple agencies including WHO, UNAIDS, United Nations Children's Fund (UNICEF), Family Health International (FHI), and U.S. Centers for Disease Control and Prevention (CDC).

Some of the documents developed include the following:

- *Guidelines for Management of Opportunistic Infections and other Related HIV Diseases* (MOH, 2002b)

- *National Guidelines for the Development and Implementation of HIV Voluntary Counseling and Testing in Ghana* (GAC/MOH, 2002)

- *Guidelines for Antiretroviral Therapy in Ghana* (MOH, 2002)

- *National Guidelines for the Clinical Use of Blood and Blood Products* (MOH/National Blood Service 2013)

- *Prevention of Mother-to Child Transmission of HIV in Ghana: A Manual for Health Workers* (MOH, 2003)

- *Towards Universal Access to Antiretroviral Therapy: Ghana National ART Scale Up Plan: 2006–2010* (MOH, 2006).

Working with Partners

The pervasive nature of HIV/AIDS demands partnerships to collectively support the national program. Ghana's multisectoral response and certainly the health sector component benefits from various collaborations (**Box 21-1**). It is estimated that 40% of HIV/AIDS services are delivered by the government, 30% by nongovernmental partners, and 30% by the private sector (MOH, 2006). Some of the various collaborators are shown in **Table 21-1** and include community, faith-based, and civil-society organizations as well as the private sector. Some agencies provide funding for various aspects of the response, while others both implement programs and provide financial support.

Partnerships have the advantage of tapping into the various strengths of the agencies to maximize impact. This approach has been successful in mass media campaigns, community mobilization to undertake testing and counseling, peer counseling for CSWs and men who have sex with men (MSM), workplace and youth-based programs, condom promotion and distribution, and treatment for STIs.

One concern regarding the partnership was having one cohesive program with set standards and benchmarks. To achieve this, Ghana pushed for national guidelines and regulations to minimize situations where entities might use

---

BOX 21-1 Working with Partners in HIV Care

The District Response Initiative (DRI) was a Dutch Embassy-funded venture involving Ghana Health Service and Ministry of Local Government and Rural Development (MLGRD) with technical support from the WHO. This decentralized local level initiative was implemented in 40 districts in the Eastern and Ashanti Regions with the aim of building capacity of health workers, the district assemblies, communities, family members, and PLHIV for effective collaboration.

The objective was to establish linked networks that would increase the quality and coverage of the continuum of care from the district and health facilities through communities to the homes of those infected and affected by HIV. Another objective was to strengthen families and communities affected by HIV to care for orphans and vulnerable children.

Notable achievements included strengthened health systems through the training of 381 service providers and the establishment of well-equipped 51 voluntary counseling and treatment (VCT) and PMTCT centers, 780 trained community counselors who served as first-level support for people affected and infected by HIV in the community, formation of 66 PLHIV associations with the benefit of accessing micro-credit schemes, and training to engage in income-generating activities.

Data from World Health Organization (WHO). (2003a). Global health-sector strategy for HIV/AIDS: 2003-2007: Providing a framework for partnership and action. Geneva, Switzerland: Author.

Table 21-1	Multisector Response to HIV/AIDS	
Bilateral Agencies	**United Nations Agencies**	**Nongovernmental Organizations**
European Union	UNAIDS	Ghana Social Marketing Foundation (GSMF)
Danish International Development Agency (DANIDA)	United Nations Development Program (UNDP)	Family Health International (FHI)
Japanese International Cooperation Agency (JICA)	World Bank	
British Department for International Development (UKDID)	United Nations Fund for Population Activities (UNFPA)	
German International Cooperation (GIZ)	World Health Organization (WHO)	
Royal Netherlands Embassy (RNE)	International Labor Organization (ILO)	
United States Agency for International Development (USAID)	United Nations Children's Fund (UNICEF)	

unproven or suboptimal protocols in care provision (WHO, 2003b). Negotiating with partners to agree on a coordinated system of rolling out services aimed at improving access to comprehensive care became a necessity.

Resource Mobilization

As recognized in the UNGASS declaration, the magnitude of the HIV epidemic was such that particularly in low-income countries, national resources were not commensurate with the level of funding needed for an effective national response. Clearly, resource mobilization from multiple channels was essential for funding the HIV program.

In Ghana, funding for the comprehensive HIV/AIDS response over the years has come from both local and international resources (MOH, 2006). These include internally generated funds such as the Government of Ghana funding, development partners' budgetary support to the MOH, and the Ghana AIDS Respond Fund (GARFund) obtained under the World Bank's Multi-country AIDS Project. The World Bank through the Treatment Acceleration Program (TAP) provided funding to facilitate the roll out of ART through private–public partnerships and strengthen the capacity of the MOH for HIV service delivery. USAID, through support of bilateral projects is another source of funding for HIV activities. Through three successful proposals so far, the Global Fund to Fight AIDS, Tuberculosis, and Malaria has been one of the biggest contributors to Ghana's HIV response. The fifth replenishment was launched in December 2015. A total signed amount of US$161 million was obtained from the Rounds 1, 5, and 8 proposals submitted in 2002, 2005, and 2008 respectively and US$30 billion disbursed as of 2016 (**Box 21-2**; Global Fund to FIght AIDS, Tuberculosis, and Malaria [GFATM], 2017).

Several other organizations have also contributed resources through implemented programs and the donation of drugs, equipment, and other logistics.

BOX 21-2 Round 1 Grant from the Global Fund

In 2002, Ghana was among the first countries to be awarded money from the Global Fund. The overall goal of the program supported by this grant was to increase access and generate greater demand for both prevention and care services for groups vulnerable to HIV infection and to improve care and support for those already living with the virus (GFATM, 2017).

The total grant funding of US$14,170,222 was disbursed over a 5-year period starting January 2003. Activities funded by the grant included training of health personnel in HIV care, setting up PMTCT and VCT centers, and putting PLHIV on treatment. Seventy percent of expected targets were met or exceeded and overall the grant received an A rating.

Capacity Building

In resource-constrained settings, health personnel who are already limited in number and overstretched have to contend with the increased demand for services that comes with HIV care. Especially in the high HIV-burden areas, the loss of healthcare personnel to AIDS complicates matters further. Strengthening human resource capacity is imperative for effective comprehensive HIV care, especially with the introduction of ART management.

In the earlier days of HIV in Ghana, a major component of capacity building was educating health staff members to know more about HIV transmission and prevention to serve as resources to patients and local AIDS education activities (MOH, 1988). There was also training for different categories of health personnel on STI prevention and management, injection safety, safe blood transfusion, HIV diagnosis and related laboratory, counseling on nutrition and healthy living, and voluntary counseling and testing. This was the era when treatment was not available and HIV services consisted of prevention activities and supportive care only. Subsequently, formal training was organized for opportunistic infection management and ultimately, with the advent of antiretroviral drugs, PMTCT, post-exposure prophylaxis, and ART management training workshops were also organized.

In view of the scope of training to be undertaken, the initial strategy was to build the capacity of a core group of trainers, many of whom benefitted from training in other countries with established HIV programs. This core group then conducted a training of trainers in-country, with the assistance of WHO-supported international experts in the initial stages. These trainers then trained regional trainers from the 10 regions of the country who in turn cascaded the training at the district and lower levels, as illustrated in **Figure 21-7** (NACP, 2005). The development of guidelines and training manuals went a long way in setting and maintaining standards in these training programs in both private and public sectors. After the training, monitoring and supervisory visits to facilities from which the trainees came from also helped to reinforce acquired knowledge and correct deviations from the national guidelines.

Capacity building also involved setting up certain logistics and infrastructure standards according to the guidelines. This translated to a health system strengthening mechanism that also sought to improve healthcare delivery in general. One example was a situation in which laboratory equipment procured to facilitate laboratory monitoring of PLHIV on ART was made accessible to all patients with other ailments seen at the facility.

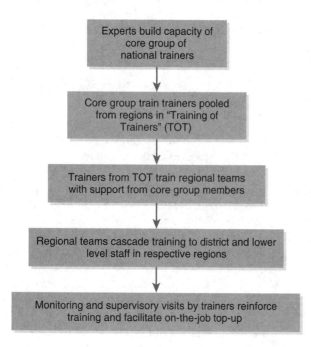

Figure 21-7 Strategy for Scaling Up Training for HIV Programs

Delivery of Relevant Services

The following sections focus on key components of the health sector response linked to HIV prevention, health promotion, and treatment. It is, however, important to consider the preceding section, as it provides the context and concepts underlying service delivery in general. Because the entire range of HIV health services is beyond the scope of this chapter, the emphasis will be on aspects that are closely linked to SRH care.

Prevention of New Infections

Due to the focus on prevention, it is not surprising that prevention of HIV and other STIs and health promotion targeting safer, more responsible sexual behavior and practices are core components of the health-sector response to HIV. This is particularly so in sub-Saharan Africa where the vast majority of new HIV infections are contracted through heterosexual intercourse (UNAIDS, 2011).

HIV health education among health sector clients complemented other multisector response such as mass media campaigns. Information was provided on the modes of transmission; risk factors for transmission; prevention methods, including condom use demonstration; and the package of health service interventions available. Various channels were used to convey these messages including health talks to waiting patients at the outpatient departments, community outreach programs, and one-on-one interactions with persons seeking care in health facilities.

STI prevention and management, HIV counseling and testing, and PMTCT services are among significant prevention interventions offered by the health sector.

STI Prevention and Management

STI prevention and management has always been known as an important weapon in the armoury of HIV prevention strategies. Results of the HIV sentinel survey (HSS) showed that the HIV prevalence among STI clinic clients was always higher than that among the general population of pregnant women. In the 2007 HSS, the rates in the two groups were 5.1% and 2.6%, respectively, while for the 2010 they were 5.3% and 2% (NACP, 2008b, 2011b). It was therefore imperative to adopt approaches that would effectively address STI control with the expectation that this would ultimately contribute to reduced transmission of HIV, particularly in the era before HIV treatment.

Earlier plans for HIV prevention and control recognized the importance of a formal STI control program with specific strategies to strengthen diagnosis and management. The Medium-Term Plan I (MTP I) developed in 1988 noted that the two STI clinics at that time (both of which were in Accra) had diagnostic challenges and medication for treating patients with STIs was not guaranteed. Some of the proposed activities to improve STI prevention, control, and management were the appointment of an STI manager who would serve as the deputy to the program manager of the National AIDS/STI Control Program (NACP), setting up STI clinics in the other nine regional hospitals, development of diagnostic and treatment protocols and algorithms for distribution to health facilities, training staff in the use of these tools, provision of laboratory commodities to strengthen diagnosis, and the procurement and distribution of drugs for treatment at facilities.

The insufficient laboratory infrastructure and manpower, coupled with the delays and the high expense associated with routine etiologic case diagnosis called for another approach of diagnosing STIs. This was imperative, given the need to integrate STI management into routine health services (GAC, 2002; NACP, 2008c).

Adapting the syndromic approach to managing STIs as proposed by the WHO, NACP developed technical guidelines for STI management in 1993. The guidelines utilized algorithms for the treatment of urethral discharge, vaginal discharge, genital ulcers, and lower abdominal pain. The unavailability of appropriate drugs for treatment and not having the recommended drugs on the MOH Essential Drug List (EDL), however, limited effective management. This was remedied with the introduction of the drugs on the EDL in 1996. Subsequent expansion of the guidelines in 1996 saw the inclusion of other STI-related syndromes such as inguinal buboes, scrotal swellings, and neonatal conjunctivitis. The 2001 revision of the guidelines added recurrent urethral discharge and other STI-related conditions.

These guidelines enhanced STI management training of health workers in both the private and public sectors down to the primary care levels (NACP, 2005). This was complemented at a point by the promotion of prepackaged STI kits that included drugs and condoms to simplify management. Equipping the health staff with the ability to provide expedient and inexpensive diagnosis and management of patients with STIs and their partners expanded access to STI care. It also afforded providers the opportunity to educate patients on STI prevention and safer sexual practices and pave the way for partner notification and treatment.

STI guidelines were revised in 2008, triggered by the new treatment updates in the Ghana essential drug list and new algorithms for the treatment of vaginal discharge adapted from the second edition WHO training modules for syndromic management of STIs (NACP, 2009c; WHO, 2007); see also NACP, 2013). Ongoing healthcare staff training, including primary healthcare workers, enhances accessibility to STI management irrespective of the level at which the patient presents. This effective treatment limits the cycle of STI transmission and ultimately reduces HIV spread. For the long term, the integration of syndromic management of STI into the curricula of all health training institutions is being strengthened. Consequently, graduating health service providers will be equipped with skills to prevent and manage STI in care delivery, further enhancing STI control as a strategy to reduce HIV transmission.

One of the key groups targeted for intervention under STI prevention and management was CSW. A 2001

> **BOX 21-3 HIV Program for Most At-Risk Populations**
>
> SHARP, in collaboration with the Ghana Health Service and other civil society organizations, reached more than 25,000 female commercial sex workers (CSW) with HIV/STI services including training peer counselors to educate their colleagues on HIV prevention and condom use and provision of treatment for STI, HIV counseling, and treatment.
>
> The initiative also identified nonpaying partners (NPP) of CSW as another high-risk group and was able to reach over 16,000 NPP with targeted HIV prevention interventions.
>
> About 7,500 MSM in 5 regions in Ghana were also reached with HIV information, referrals, and counseling services. (See also *Ghana National HIV and AIDS Strategic Plan 2016–2020* [GAC, 2016])

article on HIV infection reported an HIV prevalence of 50% among CSW in Accra, Ghana (Asamoah-Adu et al., 2001). By virtue of having multiple sexual partners and therefore sexual networks linking the general population, CSW not surprisingly were considered to play a significant role in HIV transmission in Ghana (Côte et al., 2004). Implementing interventions that promoted the adoption of safer sexual practices including the correct and consistent use of condoms in this group was a very important step in interrupting the cycle of HIV transmission. Among the organizations that took up this mandate was the Strengthening HIV/AIDS Response Partnerships (SHARP) Project, which was implemented from 2004 to 2009, led by the Academy for Educational Development and funded by USAID (**Box 21-3**) (Academy for Educational Development [AED], 2009).

Health Sector Condom Promotion Activities

The MOH has been complementing the efforts of other agencies that raise public awareness on the importance of correct consistent condom use as an effective means of reducing HIV transmission. Procurement and distribution of both male and female condoms through NGOs, social marketing agents, and community-based organizations have been ongoing for several years (GAC, 2002). In 2010, the National AIDS Control Program procured 50,000,000 condoms through the Global Fund in line with efforts to make condoms affordable and available to people in Ghana (NACP, 2011a; **Box 21-4**).

Condoms have been made increasingly accessible in the health facilities by expanding distribution outlets beyond the reproductive health units to other areas such as the counseling and testing centers. Health workers have also been at the forefront of educating attendants at health facilities, the general public, and training peer counselors on

BOX 21-4 Condom Promotion Initiative

Ghana Social Marketing Foundation (GSMF), a non-governmental organization in collaboration with the Ministries of Health and other partners, launched the "Stop AIDS, Love Life" campaign in 2000. The objectives were to increase HIV risk perception among Ghanaians, mobilize social support for HIV preventive behaviors, and increase condom sales, among others.

Interventions included mass media campaigns focused on the ABCs of prevention (**A**bstinence, **B**eing faithful to one's partner, and **C**ondom use) and condom promotions. Condom sales doubled from 18.8 million to 34.8 million during the 2-year period following the intervention (GSMF, 2003).

the proper use of condoms through condom demonstration campaigns using dummies.

Counseling and Testing

HIV testing is virtually the only means of knowing one's HIV status and is an entry point into accessing care should the test result be positive. Voluntary counseling and testing (VCT) has long been recognized and proven as an important HIV prevention strategy. Among others, it is an avenue through which people are empowered with useful information on how to reduce risky sexual practices, adopt safer ones, and facilitate behavior change. Easier acceptance of HIV serostatus and coping are enhanced through psychological and emotional support, early referral for opportunistic infection, and STI management and ART. VCT also facilitates social support and reduction in stigmatization (UNAIDS, 2002).

HIV testing was long noted to be an important component of the national response. One of the strategies stated in MTP I was to encourage individuals with high-risk behaviors to voluntarily come forward for free HIV testing. In the proposed testing policy, high-risk groups (identified as CSW, police and armed forces recruits, tuberculosis patients, and patients requiring repeated transfusions) would also be offered the opportunity for testing to facilitate early detection and counseling. It was stressed that human rights would be respected, confidentiality would be ensured, and pre- and post-test counseling would be provided.

To make blood transfusions safer, HIV testing became increasingly available in public health facilities in the 1990s. This also created the opportunity to test patients whose symptoms were suggestive of HIV infection; however, a nationally structured system of offering HIV testing with appropriate counseling had not yet been established.

By the year 2000, the need to increase public awareness about susceptibility to HIV became clear. With formal voluntary counseling and testing services nonexistent, the NSF I

deemed the initiation of VCT services an important strategy (GAC, 2001). This was reiterated in the Health Sector HIV Plan 2002, which included finalization of National VCT Guidelines and the capacity building of health institutions to provide VCT services as key activities (GAC, 2002).

In 2001, Family Health International, in collaboration with the Government of Ghana and multiple agencies, initiated the START program with a structured VCT service as one of the components (MOH, 2006). The first two VCT centers were strategically set up in Manya Krobo district, Eastern Region, an area that had consistently recorded the highest HIV prevalence in the country. In the following year, two more VCT centers were established in the teaching hospitals in Accra and Kumasi. Subsequently, Global Fund Round 1 resources were leveraged to increase the number of VCT centers from 4 to 24 across the country including the 10 regional capitals (GFATM, 2017).

The *National Guidelines for the Development and Implementation of HIV Voluntary Counseling* in Ghana were finalized in 2003 in a participatory process in partnership with FHI. Training manuals were subsequently developed (GAC & MOH, 2002). The guidelines covered the organization and operations of the VCT services, counseling related to HIV testing and HIV testing itself, quality assurance, and referrals. The guidelines with underlying principles of confidentiality, counseling, and consent emphasized setting up of the VCT center in an area that ensured privacy and confidentiality. Maintenance of confidentiality by VCT counselors was also stressed in their training. Components of the counseling included an assessment of HIV/AIDS and STIs knowledge, personal risk assessment and risk-reduction plan, demonstration of condom use, explanation of the HIV test and its implications, assessment of coping capacity and ability, notification of results, psychological and emotional support, and referral as indicated. VCT counselor training typically lasted 10 days.

With ART services set up in 2003 and the expansion of VCT centers, increasingly more people accessed the services. From a reported 15,490 people counseled and tested by 2004, the number increased exponentially, with 161,903 Ghanaians tested in 2007 (NACP, 2008d) and 798,763 in 2014 (GAC, 2014).

The *2004 UNAIDS/WHO Policy Statement on HIV Testing* recognized a low reach of HIV testing in low- and middle-income countries and noted that the primary model for HIV testing had been the provision of client-initiated voluntary counseling and testing services (UNAIDS & WHO, 2004). Consequently, the following four types of HIV testing were recommended:

- Voluntary counseling and testing as initiated by a client to learn his or her HIV status

- Diagnostic HIV testing, indicated whenever a person showed signs or symptoms that were consistent with HIV-related disease or AIDS to aid clinical diagnosis and management

- Routine offer of HIV testing by healthcare providers to be made to all patients being assessed in situations such as in a sexually transmitted infection clinic, prenatal clinic clients (to facilitate PMTCT services), and those who are asymptomatic but are being seen in clinical and community-based health service settings where HIV is prevalent and antiretroviral treatment is available
- Mandatory screening for HIV and other blood-borne viruses of all blood that is destined for transfusion or for manufacture of blood products

There was emphasis on ensuring an ethical process for conducting the testing, addressing the implications of a positive test result, reducing HIV/AIDS-related stigma and discrimination, safeguarding the human rights of people seeking services and ensuring that there were sufficient trained staff to cope with the ensuing increased demand for testing, treatment, and related services.

The 2008 revision of Ghana's guidelines adopted these recommendations in consideration of the fact that VCT uptake had been hampered by many of the same factors that hamper uptake of other HIV-related services. These included stigma, discrimination, and limited access to treatment care and health services in general, as well as gender issues (NACP, 2008e; see also NACP, 2013). In addition to the traditional VCT, which was termed client-initiated counseling and testing (CICT), provider-initiated counseling and testing (PICT) by health service providers was urged. In PICT, all clients who utilized health services irrespective of the reason for doing so were to be offered HIV testing. This would create the opportunity for HIV to be diagnosed more systematically and hopefully early to enable patients access to needed HIV prevention, treatment, care, and support services. The three types of PICT described were routine offer, diagnostic, and mandatory as per the UNAIDS/WHO recommendations. Also included in the new guidelines were procedures for conducting outreach testing and counseling services in the communities with the stipulation that the nearest accredited health facility was to serve as the referral site for follow-up services (**Box 21-5**).

To reduce bottlenecks in the HIV testing procedure and delays in receiving results, the use of simplified HIV testing algorithms and procedures involving two different rapid test kits was adopted. There was also a shift from limiting HIV testing to only laboratory personnel to involve other service providers such as nurses, midwives, and HIV counselors who were trained to do testing. The VCT training was subsequently modified to accommodate practical sessions in which counselors were trained to conduct HIV testing using the rapid test kits. The directive from the MOH to provide HIV testing free of charge in public health facilities removed the barrier of cost, which may have been a disincentive for testing. Compare to the WHO's 2012 Universal Strategy. (**Figure 21-8**; NACP, 2009a).

BOX 21-5 "Know Your Status" Campaign

With the 2008 Voluntary Counseling and Testing (VCT) guidelines in operation, the National AIDS/STI Control Program launched the "Know Your Status" campaign in 2008 with the exercise really taking off in 2009. The objective was to shift the concentration of HIV testing in health facilities to the community level. By sending VCT services to the doorsteps of the people, hard to reach groups such as rural communities with poor roads and persons who would not ordinarily access VCT in a health facility could now take advantage of the service. The campaign was carried out during community and outdoor events, in churches and educational institutions to name a few (NACP, 2009a).

The "Know Your Status" campaign was very effective and was noted to contribute to the phenomenal numbers of people being tested. The reported 467,935 tested for HIV in 2008 almost doubled in 2009 to 865,058. In 2010, over a million Ghanaians (1,063,058) were tested for HIV within a calendar year, 21% of whom were male (NACP, 2011a).

As the "Know Your Status" campaign was underway there was advocacy by a public health consultant to change the slogan from "Know Your Status" to "(KYS)^2", translated as "Know your status and keep your status!" Rightly so, because whether one tested positive or negative, there was a need to maintain that status—even those who tested positive for HIV needed to avoid risky sexual behaviors to avoid reinfection with other strains of HIV, which could lead to a deterioration of their status to AIDS (NACP, 2010b).

As at 2010, almost 1200 VCT centers (most of them set up through GFATM funding) were in operation throughout the country (NACP, 2011a). The majority are in public health institutions and the rest run by the private health sector and NGOs, but all were governed by the same guidelines. Because most of the VCT sites were not in locations where ART was available, there was an emphasis on systematic referral of all HIV-positive clients identified through VCT to appropriate facilities for clinical care, including opportunistic infection management and ART (Centers for Disease Control and Prevention [CDC], 2016; Dapaah, 2016a, 2016b; UNAIDS, 2016).

Prevention of Mother-to-Child Transmission of HIV (PMTCT)

In Ghana's MTP 1, it was indicated that only a small number of infants with AIDS had been reported, with the speculation that most of them died from childhood illnesses and their HIV status had gone unrecognized. The proposed strategy to tackle mother-to-child transmission

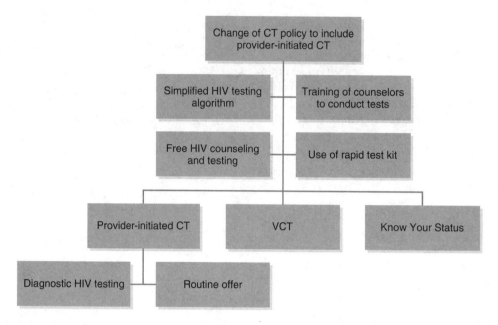

Figure 21-8 Strategy for Making HIV Counseling and Testing More Accessible
Reproduced from WHO. (2012). Service delivery approaches to HIV testing and counselling (HTC): A strategic HTC programme framework. Geneva, Switzerland: WHO Document Production Services. Retrieved from http://apps.who.int/iris/bitstream/10665/75206/1/9789241593877_eng.pdf

of HIV (MTCT) included development of guidelines to educate and counsel HIV-positive women of child-bearing age and their spouses and encourage contraception use. Beyond counseling there did not seem to be much to offer by way of PMTCT. By about the year 2000, it was estimated that MTCT accounted for 15% of new cases of HIV infections in Ghana (GAC, 2001). Recognizing the absence of a PMTCT policy and a structured PMTCT program, the NSF 1 included an objective to initiate a PMTCT program and a target to reduce mother-to-child vertical HIV transmission by 30% by the year 2005 (MOH, 2014). The impetus for this objective was the proven reduction of MTCT from the prophylactic use of antiretroviral drugs (UNAIDS, 2002). Though the use of antiretroviral prophylaxis for pregnant women to prevent MTCT has been the better-known aspect of PMTCT, in reality the updated comprehensive PMTCT program has four prongs (UNAIDS, 2016; WHO, 2010b, 2017):

- Primary prevention of HIV among parents-to-be
- Prevention of unintended pregnancies among HIV-positive women
- Prevention of HIV transmission from women living with HIV to their children
- Provision of treatment, care, and support to women living with HIV, their children, and families.

In the first prong there is emphasis on health services instituting interventions to reduce the risk of contracting HIV, particularly during pregnancy and breastfeeding. The second stresses the need for HIV-positive women to be supported in the choices they make for their reproductive lives.

They are to be provided with the necessary knowledge, skills, and commodities that will enable them to avoid unintended pregnancies and they are to be given support for planning a pregnancy. In the third prong, all HIV-positive pregnant women are required to receive lifelong ART if eligible for treatment, or prophylaxis to reduce MTCT. In addition, the essential package of services during childbirth, including skilled birth attendance, are to be made available to them. Finally, the fourth prong requires that infants born to HIV-positive mothers are to be given antiretroviral prophylaxis and follow-up care. Their mothers are to be supported to make infant feeding safe to reduce HIV transmission and promote child survival. **Figure 21-9** presents a synoptic outline of the recommended MTCT prevention program.

Ghana's PMTCT program is skewed towards the third prong. The Health Sector HIV Plan 2002 proposed the integration of PMTCT into existing maternal and child health services and the development of PMTCT guidelines and protocols. Keen on building capacity of health workers to implement PMTCT services across the country, a training manual that provided guidance on PMTCT implementation in Ghana was developed in 2003, but with a focus on pregnant women. Areas covered included VCT for pregnant women, the service package provided during prenatal care with the inclusion of information on PMTCT, management of labor and delivery for HIV-positive mothers, infant feeding options, and organization of services (MOH, 2003). Ghana's initial PMTCT intervention was more or less directed primarily at pregnant women coming for prenatal care. The strategy was more of an "opt-in" approach in which pregnant women who came for prenatal

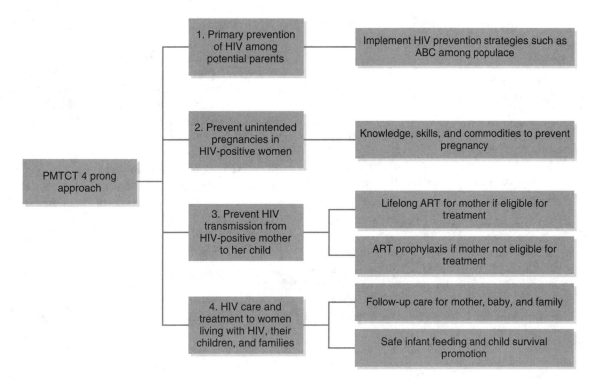

Figure 21-9 Preventing Transmission of HIV from Mother to Child

care were counseled on the benefits of HIV testing. Those who opted to get tested gave their consent for the test to take place. Initially, Ghana opted for the nevirapine regimen in which the HIV-positive mother in labor was given a single dose of nevirapine. Her baby was also given a single dose of nevirapine within 72 hours of birth. Nevirapine was selected due to its demonstrated efficacy in clinical trials in reducing MTCT, the relatively low cost, and the simplicity of its use in PMTCT programs.

Through the FHI START program mentioned earlier, PMTCT services had been piloted concurrently with VCT in the same two facilities in the eastern region in 2001. Lessons learned from the pilot informed the development of the PMTCT manual used for training. From the beginning, the direction was for PMTCT centers to be set up in the same institutions and concurrently as VCT services were being introduced. Naturally, the condition that had to be met was the availability of prenatal clinic services in the health facility. Consequently, with the exception of a few stand-alone VCT centers run by NGOs and clinics without prenatal clinics, practically all the facilities that have VCT sites also offer PMTCT services.

VCT training was later combined with that of the PMTCT (NACP, 2006a). Not only did the two curricula have a lot in common, some health personnel who provided PMTCT services were the same people who ran the VCT centers in their facilities.

This is especially true in maternity homes run by private midwives. In the spirit of private–public partnerships, the NACP collaborated with the Ghana Registered

Private Midwives Association to train 32 private midwives in the combined PMTCT/VCT curriculum. The trained midwives were then supplied with the necessary tools and equipment to support the provision of both these services.

In 2006, in the light of evidence showing the superiority of combination highly active antiretroviral drugs over the monotherapy regimen in reducing MTCT, the WHO and CDC came up with new guidelines for PMTCT (NACP, 2007b). Aligning itself with this new global direction, the country came up with a new policy, the summary of which is as follows:

- HIV-positive women who were eligible for treatment because of specific criteria, including a low level of immunity, were to be put on the three-drug ART combination as any PLHIV who qualified for treatment as per national guidelines discussed here.

- Those pregnant women who were not eligible for ART were to be offered a prophylaxis regimen consisting of two antiretroviral drugs (zidovudine and lamivudine), starting from 28 weeks or thereafter if she was identified later. The single dose of nevirapine was still given in labor.

- The infant also benefitted from a combination of zidovudine and lamivudine with the duration dictated by how long the mother had been on treatment or prophylaxis before delivery.

- It was clear that the implementation of this new policy was going to be a challenge given the following issues:

+ The relative complexity of the regimen as compared to the single-dose nevirapine
+ The associated increased workload on the prenatal clinic personnel
+ The logistical management issues related to the antiretrovirals
+ The unavailability of laboratory testing in the majority of PMTCT centers required to distinguish which pregnant women were eligible for antiretroviral prophylaxis from those needing treatment.

Not with standing these issues, steps were taken to eventually roll out the new policy. Teams of trainers from all the regions underwent training. These trainers, many of whom were hands-on VCT/PMTCT service providers subsequently facilitated regional trainings. In 2008, sites started to transition from the nevirapine-based PMTCT regimen to the combination regimen, and by 2009, many sites had implemented the change. As expected work overload is frequently raised as an issue of concern at review meetings and there are challenges with logistics management of ART. One attempt to address this concern has involved working with the regions to facilitate training midwives so that the workload is spread across more people and not limited to only a handful of trained personnel. Another solution has been to introduce a simple pharmacy software to help pharmacy staff keep track of antiretroviral supplies.

It is interesting to note that the policy document that outlined the new combination PMTCT direction was eventually finalized as a hard copy and printed in 2008. Incorporated in this document was the combination antiretroviral regimen for PMTCT previously described and other updated guidelines including the routine offer of HIV testing for all pregnant women. In effect, the testing mechanism shifted from the "opt in" to an "opt out" approach. In other words, HIV testing was included in the routine tests offered and carried out during prenatal care. Unless women specifically opted out of having the HIV test, it would be done followed by counseling and other appropriate steps, depending on the results. There were also updates on safer infant feeding practices for babies born to HIV-exposed mothers and prophylactic medication against opportunistic infections. At the end of 2009, new evidence emerged that warranted a change in the guidelines that would reduce MTCT even further. These new WHO guidelines involved the use of three drugs for prophylaxis during pregnancy starting at 14 weeks' gestation and continuing after delivery during the period of breastfeeding.

In prong 3 of the PMTCT program, it is instructive to note that the entry point for the intervention is HIV testing of pregnant women. With the exception of those who already know their HIV status, HIV-positive pregnant women are identified through HIV testing in the prenatal clinic. Therefore, the more pregnant women tested, the greater the likelihood of identifying those who are HIV-positive status.

From very few pregnant women (only 8,576 in 2004), the number of pregnant women tested annually increased dramatically (NACP, 2006a). In 2005, the figure was 20,296 and 2 years later there was a fivefold rise to 104,045 (NACP, 2008d). In 2010, a record 520,090 pregnant women, representing more than half of the expected pregnancies for the year, were tested (NACP, 2011a). The increasing numbers of pregnant women tested for HIV can be attributed to several factors. One of these is likely the introduction of routine countrywide HIV testing. There are, however, reports of individual facilities adopting approaches that have increased HIV testing of pregnant women in their prenatal clinics (**Box 21-6, Box 21-7**).

BOX 21-6 The Use of Prenatal Clinic Motivators in PMTCT

The Edwin Cade Memorial Hospital, located in Obuasi, a mining town in the Ashanti Region of Ghana in the bid to increase the number of pregnant women tested for HIV, came up with the idea of using prenatal clinic motivators.

These prenatal clinic motivators are pregnant women who have themselves undergone an HIV test in the current pregnancy. They are encouraged to talk to their counterparts at the prenatal clinic on the importance and benefits of having an HIV test during pregnancy. Equipped with the necessary information, they are able to answer the frequently asked questions put to them by their peers.

Not only did this method reduce the stigma associated with HIV testing at the facility, it also increased the uptake of HIV testing with 100% of the 559 prenatal clinic registrants in 2007 being tested WHO Country Office in Ghana [WCO], 2009a.

BOX 21-7 Outreach PMTCT Service

To increase the number of pregnant women benefitting from their underutilized PMTCT service, staff of Bomso Clinic, a private facility also in the Ashanti Region, innovated the idea of an outreach PMTCT service. This was implemented by networking with 4 maternity homes within their catchment area, training their staff and providing HIV testing to pregnant women on selected days.

In 2007, of the 1,434 prenatal clinic registrants seen at the Bomso Clinic and the 4 facilities, 94% were from the outreach maternity homes. Approximately 80% of these pregnant women were tested. Out of the 54 identified as HIV positive, 83% received antiretroviral prophylaxis to reduce MTCT. Without this outreach service many of these PMTCT beneficiaries would not have had the advantage of this opportunity (WCO, 2009b).

With an increasing number of pregnant women being tested, more HIV-positive pregnant women are being identified and will benefit from the PMTCT intervention. The 2010 WHO PMTCT guidelines recommended that HIV-positive mothers continue to take antiretroviral prophylaxis as long as they are breastfeeding (MOH, 2010). This has the benefit of reducing the risk of HIV transmission through breast milk and also reduces stigma from an HIV-positive mother not breastfeeding her baby for fear of passing on the virus. Ultimately, the PMTCT intervention should translate into a reduced number of children contracting HIV from their mothers. Monitoring the outcome of the PMTCT has been difficult because using the available antibody testing method, children born of HIV-positive mothers who benefitted from PMTCT intervention had to be followed up until 18 months of age before their HIV status could be verified. The challenge of loss to follow up has meant that the program does not have a complete record of the serostatus of the babies benefitting from PMTCT services (AVERT, 2017; Reece, Norman, Kwara, Flanigan, & Rana, 2015).

The Ghana guidelines and protocols for early infant diagnosis (EID) were developed in 2009 with training of health staff beginning thereafter. Essentially, the EID of HIV exposed infants involves using a test that is able to detect viral components of HIV as early as 6 weeks and therefore establish whether the child has HIV or not. This has the potential of reducing losses to follow up as one does not have to wait until the infant is 18 months old to establish whether HIV transmission occurred. Another important advantage of EID is being able to start HIV-positive infants on ART within the first year of life, as recommended in the ART guidelines. This increases the child's chances of survival.

In 2010, UNAIDS called for the virtual elimination of mother-to-child transmission of HIV, which translates to an MTCT rate below 5% (UNAIDS, 2016; WHO, 2015b). In demonstration of the country's commitment toward this vision, a PMTCT Scale up Plan 2011–2015 was developed to spell out the strategies, targets, activities, and a budget outlining the required resources for achieving this feat. The goal of Ghana's plan is the virtual elimination of HIV transmission from mother to child and to improve family health—especially maternal, newborn, and child health—within the context of the HIV and AIDS response in Ghana. The key modality is the assimilation of PMTCT services into maternal, nutrition, neonatal, child, adolescent health and other HIV-related services (MOH, 2010). In addition to planned operational research to assess implementation, midterm and final program reviews were scheduled in the third and fifth years, respectively, to assess the impact of the PMTCT program.

Clinical Services for Persons Living with HIV

Before the availability of ART on a programmatic level in Ghana, delivering clinical care services for PLHIV was a challenge. Having a disease that had neither cure nor treatment seemed to fuel denial as well as stigma and discrimination. There was certainly no motivation to get tested. Notwithstanding these issues, clinical services were offered to PLHIV. This mainly centered on the treatment of opportunistic infections such as tuberculosis (TB), counseling on good nutrition, psychosocial support, and education on other preventive measures such as maintenance of good hygiene, reduced alcohol intake, and safe sex to reduce HIV transmission and reinfection. Methods of using male and female condoms were also taught. These services were useful particularly for PLHIV who were in the earlier stages of the disease. For those who were in later stages and were quite ill, institutional care was available. It was, however, fraught with challenges and put a strain on health facilities. Home-based care programs ran by MOH, nongovernmental and faith-based organizations played a key role in the continuum of care for PLHIV and took some of the burden off the health facilities. The National Catholic Health Service, one of the pioneers in home-based care, provided palliative care through mobile nursing and clinic services, spiritual and psychosocial counseling, and nutritional support to both PLHIV and their families in their homes (GAC, 2001, 2002; WCO, 2009a).

To introduce standardization in the clinical care of PLHIV, the National AIDS Control Program produced the *Guidelines for Management of Opportunistic Infection and Other Related HIV Diseases* in 2002 (MOH, 2002b). This was accomplished with the help of a task team consisting of representatives from the medical, pediatric, and pharmacy departments of the teaching hospitals, research institutions, reference laboratories, WHO, FHI, and NACP. They made use of reference materials from UNAIDS and Médecins Sans Frontières (known in English as Doctors Without Borders), to develop the guidelines, which were also informed in part by the experiences from FHI implementation of clinical services in the START program. Technical and financial assistance was provided by WHO (MOH, 2002b).

The guidelines provided a practical approach to managing HIV-related illnesses, bearing in mind the potential absence of laboratory infrastructure to facilitate appropriate diagnosis. Various conditions were addressed under the respective systems, including genital and sexually transmitted conditions, respiratory disorders, skin conditions, and malignancies in HIV disease. General and specific measures that safeguard against opportunistic infections, including prophylaxis with certain drugs, were also highlighted. The guidelines have subsequently been used to train service providers to manage opportunistic infection in PLHIV in facilities with and without ART. In 2008, the document was revised in light of new knowledge and the introduction of newer medications and formulations for opportunistic infection management.

Antiretroviral Therapy (ART)

There is a plethora of reasons why the advent of antiretroviral drugs made a dramatic difference to the threat posed by HIV. The reduction in mortality and the prolongation of lives are clear advantages. The decline in AIDS-related mortality, from a peak of 2.1 million in 2004 to an estimated 1.8 million in 2009 globally and dropping to 1.1 million in 2015, is attributed in part to the availability of ART (UNAIDS & WHO, 2009, 2015b).

Estimates also point to 14.4 million life-years gained from the provision of ART. These global figures trickle down to individual countries. At the country level this increasing survival means fewer teachers, health workers, civil servants, and a myriad of other professionals succumb to HIV infection. This ultimately reduces the threat posed to education, health service provision, the economy, the political and governance fabric of society, and all the other areas that were under siege from HIV. The reduction of stigma, the uptake of VCT, and even the HIV prevention prospects from the effect of reducing HIV transmission are also definite indications for making treatment as widely available as possible to all eligible for ART.

With the progression of the HIV epidemic in Ghana, the burden on the health sector kept growing. The additional hospital bed occupancy due to HIV-related illness was estimated at about 20% in 1995 and about 40% in 2000, with AIDS reported as the leading cause of death from infectious disease in the teaching hospital (GFATM, 2017).

The NSF 1, recognizing the need to expand HIV services, highlighted strategies to make ART accessible to PLHIV, in addition to strengthening opportunistic infection management and the other components of care and support already being provided. In synchrony, the Health Sector HIV/AIDS Strategic Plan outlined activities to make programmatic provision of ART a reality. Up until then, antiretrovirals had been imported into the country by the private sector but the medications were too expensive for most (MOH, 2002a). Although a few individuals had also been sent drugs by friends and family abroad, this did not begin to address the need. Consequently, several initiatives were set into motion including development of guidelines, description of the drug management systems, resource mobilization arrangements, and piloting of ART service.

In a similar process to the development of the opportunistic infection management guidelines, the National AIDS Control Program developed Guidelines for Antiretroviral Therapy in Ghana also with the help of the Technical Working Group (TWG). The TWG also had representation from the drug procurement unit, food and drugs board, and reproductive health unit of the Ghana Health Service. Technical assistance was provided by WHO and FHI. The ART guidelines covered recommended ART regimens, initiation and exclusion criteria, switching and stopping of ART, management of OIs, clinical and laboratory monitoring, ART counseling on issues such as adherence and drug information, post-exposure prophylaxis for healthcare workers, and antiretroviral drug procurement, storage, and distribution. The resolve to have one national program in which both public and private providers agreed on ART management

was strong. As such, the document was also submitted to a consultative stakeholders' meeting to solicit and incorporate their input before finalization. Subsequently, the national guidelines were also used to train ART management teams in all sectors. In keeping with updated evidence for ART management, the guidelines were revised in 2005, 2008, and 2010 (WHO, 2015a).

ART management for PLHIV is a lifelong commitment, yet nonadherence and development of HIV-drug resistance still occur. Consequently, issues pertaining to drug supply, management systems, and quality assurance are concerning. It was recognized that while drugs for palliative care, STI, and opportunistic infection management could be part of the existing MOH drug-supply mechanism, special arrangements had to be made for antiretrovirals. The stipulation was that antiretrovirals would be procured centrally into the public drug supply system and would not be for sale in the open market. The guidelines spelled out conditions to be met by manufacturers, regulations for registration, and monitoring and evaluation. Thus, the policy directive that addressed the importation, stocking, and supply of antiretroviral drugs was issued to guarantee the quality of products imported and streamline procurement from accredited sources.

Obviously, the provision of ART comes at a cost but it was decided to subsidize that cost for PLHIV. The overall cost of care was estimated to be US$5 per month (NACP, 2003b). This included laboratory investigations, 1 month's supply of antiretrovirals, and drugs for opportunistic infections. Regional estimates of care and ART coverage for PLHIV ranged from $14 to $71. Regional estimates of units cost in 2014 ranged from US$107 to US$126 for CSW and MSM respectively (U.S. Department of State, 2015). The actual annual cost per person for all these services, however, was estimated to be US $630 (MOH, 2006). In addition, there were several other related costs such as strengthening health and community systems. This involved training for health workers, infrastructural development, and community-level capacity building to set up linkages and referral networks and support the continuum of care in the community. Thus the establishment of the Global Fund for AIDS, TB, and Malaria in 2002 could not have come at a better time (Merson, 2006). Ghana was one of the first countries to submit a successful proposal to the fund. In this Round 1 proposal, the third objective was to establish and make operational at least three centers providing comprehensive care, including opportunistic infection management and ART for PLHIV by December 2003. The strategy was to strengthen existing centers with high patient load to provide quality services.

The proposed activities included:

- Training approximately 30 doctors and 100 other relevant staff from public, private, and mission sectors on ART for 3 days
- Refurbishing and supplying basic equipment (laboratory included) to the three centers

- Procuring and distributing opportunistic infection and ART drug supplies for 18 months for three centers targeting 2,000 patients

- Producing and distributing information, education, and communication materials

In addition to the GFATM funding, other partners provided technical and financial support in diverse ways toward the establishment of ART management.

Family Health International (FHI), an HIV/AIDS technical assistance agency that had successfully introduced ART into existing HIV/AIDS programs in Rwanda and Kenya, was one such organization. In partnership with the Government of Ghana and other collaborators, FHI (funded by the U.S. Agency for International Development) consolidated the previously established VCT, PMTCT, and clinical care services by piloting ART management. This pioneering feat was undertaken in June 2003 in two district facilities in the Manya Krobo district, the area worst affected by HIV in Ghana.

Embarking on the pilot ART program turned out to be a wise decision because the lessons learned helped inform the eventual scale up of ART to other facilities in the country. Before the launch of the program, community sensitization in the Manya Krobo district was undertaken. This education addressed misconceptions about HIV as well as stigma and discrimination. The process proved to be a catalyst for patronage of VCT and other clinical services, including ART, as the prospect of hope was kindled in the community (NACP, 2004b). The need for counselors to be equipped with enhanced counseling skills beyond what was provided at VCT was also identified. It is instructive to note that Ghana's ART guidelines stipulated that a person initiating ART had to disclose his or her HIV status to a family member or friend to galvanize support for adherence to lifelong treatment. Consequently, counselors were tasked with guiding the PLHIV to disclose their status and the confidence to effectively take up the supportive role.

The pilot ART program was also useful in documenting the the ART regimen, side-effect profile, how those side-effects were managed, and the adherence counseling strategy adopted. The concerted effort for structured implementation of the ART program and its success demystified HIV treatment and paved the way for more sites to come on board. With additional resources from the U.K. Department of International Development (UKDID), two teaching hospitals in Accra and Kumasi soon took up the challenge and joined the rank of "learning sites" (MOH, 2006).

In 2003, WHO launched the "3 by 5" initiative, which had the goal of putting 3 million people on ART by 2005 (WHO, 2003b). The declared ART target for Ghana, which was one of the 49 "3 by 5" focus countries, was 30,000 by the end 2005 (WHO, 2004)—a very ambitious target. In March 2004, the Government of Ghana exhibited its commitment in working toward this target by formally requesting support from the WHO to scale up ART access. Unlike in the pioneer sites, which had initiated ART under "controlled project conditions," the rollout to other facilities nationwide would be under a programmatic setting. This required proper planning optimize the benefits to be gained from providing treatment while simultaneously minimizing the emergence of HIV-drug resistance. Thus, the *Ghana National ART Scale-Up Plan 2006–2010* (MOH, 2006) was developed to guide the scale up of comprehensive HIV services, ART included. The various guiding principles, strategies, activities, and budgetary implications highlighted were in tandem with the National Strategic Framework (NSF).

The proposed ART delivery model would be hospital-based with multiple entry points such as testing and counseling, PMTCT, TB, and community home-based care services (**Figure 21-10**).

A multidisciplinary team approach comprising clinicians, nurses, pharmacy staff, counselors, nutritionists, and laboratory and social workers would be adopted. With ART being part of a continuum of care, there would be a linkage structure with community support systems and organizations.

The scale up would initially be a phased approach to regional hospitals and subsequently to district level facilities. The proposed sites were to be assessed using the National Criteria for Accreditation to identify readiness to initiate ART. The assessment consisted of evaluating several areas, including the presence of a leader with experience and training in managing antiretroviral programs at the site, model of HIV care available, and the use of protocols for delivery of care including antiretroviral management, physical space, availability of HIV-related care services on site or linkages to VCT, PMTCT, opportunistic infection, TB, and STI management. Other domains assessed were the level of community involvement, human resource capacity to manage HIV services, laboratory capacity, appropriate health management

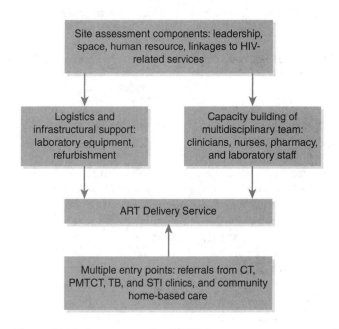

Figure 21-10 Components for ART Delivery

information systems, and drug procurement and supply management systems. The purpose of the assessment was identification of gaps to address such issues as inadequately trained staff or lack of laboratory equipment, so that the site could meet accreditation standards to manage ART.

The scale-up plan outlined a host of other approaches, including the adaptation and use of WHO's integrated management of adult/adolescent illness (IMAI) guidelines and training modules. The IMAI concept facilitates rapid training of a large number of health staff to provide basic community and clinical care in the continuum of comprehensive HIV care, including ART management.

Following the piloting of ART in the two district facilities and two teaching hospitals, the regional hospitals were next. Not surprisingly, the Eastern Regional Hospital was the first to come on board in 2005, as this was the region with the highest HIV prevalence. Subsequently, ART clinics were set up in each of the remaining regional hospitals as well as selected district hospitals. The main source of funding was the GFATM. Other resources came from the World Bank-supported Treatment Acceleration Program (TAP), the UKDID, the German Development Agency (GTZ), and the Japanese International Cooperation (NACP, 2007b).

As at the end of 2010, there were a total of 150 ART centers set up across the country. One of the objectives of the plan was to put 71,000 persons living with HIV on ART by 2010. In reality, two-thirds of this target was achieved with 47,559 PLHIV cumulatively initiated on treatment at the end of 2010. About a third (32%) were male. Children under 15 years constitute less than 6% of those initiated on ART. Among all persons ever started on treatment, 85% of them were still on ART by December 2010 (NACP, 2011a) and 95% by end of December 2014 (GAC, 2014).

With the expected evolution of HIV-drug resistance, and with so many people are on treatment, a surveillance and monitoring system for HIV drug-resistance emergence was set up in conjunction with the ART program.

Private Sector Involvement in HIV Service Delivery

In Ghana, the private health sector (all nongovernmental health services) is estimated to contribute to about a third of healthcare delivery in the country (NACP, 2006b); 30% to 40% of health service delivery in 2014 (Bjerrum, 2016). **Figure 21-11** shows a snapshot of a Private Sector HIV Care Facility. So, in the quest to scale up ART service, ignoring the private sector would not be in the best interest of the national response. It is against this background that private–public partnerships were leveraged to facilitate the involvement of private facilities in comprehensive HIV care. The World Bank-supported Treatment Acceleration Programme (TAP), operating within the context of the WHO's 3 by 5 initiative, was one such partnership (WCO, 2008). A key objective of the TAP was to derive lessons from the

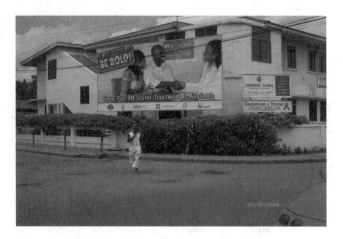

Figure 21-11 Odorna Clinic, A Private Sector HIV Care Facility

BOX 21-8 Private Sector HIV Care: The Odorna Clinic Experience

Odorna Clinic, a private for-profit facility was one of the FHI protégé health institutions supported by TAP to provide ART. The management and staff embraced the concept of providing comprehensive HIV care and wholeheartedly underwent the processes involved in achieving accreditation.

By 2006, services being provided included VCT, opportunistic infection management, TB care, and provision of ART. Though lack of a labor ward and in-patient services limited the full range of PMTCT services, pregnant women seeking care in Odorna could access all other HIV care services. By 2008, there were 260 PLHIV enrolled in care with 110 on ART. The clinic set up a psychosocial HIV support group for the PLHIV accessing care and also linked up with some NGOs in their community who offered nutritional support for patients.

A useful lesson learned was the need to innovate to accommodate private sector needs. Instead of the hitherto usual 1 week of blocked time dedicated for training in HIV care, the training for the Odorna personnel was sequenced over evenings and weekends. With this strategy, the situation of the private clinic grinding to a halt during the day when the clinic was busiest and revenue highest was avoided.

With a minimum package of laboratory services onsite while relying on an offsite public sector facility to provide specialized tests, Odorna Clinic was able to initiate ART services demonstrating the feasibility of private–public partnerships in ART care (WCO, 2008).

experience that would inform the future expansion of HIV care to other private health institutions (see **Box 21-8**).

In Ghana, this initiative was executed through Family Health International and the National Catholic Health Service in collaboration with NACP, the designated public sector partner. The capacity of 10 private health facilities in 4 regions was built to provide comprehensive HIV care, including ART services STI management, and PMTCT/VCT. Training and service delivery were as per national guidelines and the supply of drugs and other HIV commodities followed the same supply chain as for public sector facilities. This was in line with the plan to have one national program with the same standards. In so doing, Ghanaian PLHIV could be assured that the same national protocols of care practiced in the public sector would be available to them regardless of the facility in which care was sought.

The Role of Surveillance, Research, Monitoring, and Evaluation

To optimize planning for programs, reliable data is needed to inform the framework of the plan and prioritization of strategies and activities. During implementation, data also helps in evaluating progress and outcomes and can help decision making on cost-effective approaches and innovations

(WHO, 2003a). This is particularly so for the HIV epidemic, given the magnitude of its impact, especially in the milieu of limited resources. Consequently, surveillance, research, and monitoring and evaluation activities are key sources of information that assist the health sector to respond responsibly to HIV (**Figure 21-12**). Monitoring and evaluation also play important roles in promoting quality standards in clinical care, prevention programs, and other interventions. In recognition of these advantages, surveillance, monitoring and evaluating structures, and research have always been key components of Ghana's HIV program.

Surveillance and Research: AIDS and STI Surveillance

From when the first AIDS case was identified, the MOH recognized the need to set up an AIDS surveillance data gathering system (NACP, 2003a). The objective was to monitor the nature of the HIV epidemic, the character of the HIV infections, and the impact on the general population. This was always in consideration of the fact that the AIDS cases represented the visible portion of the HIV epidemic iceberg. AIDS case reporting evolved from an already

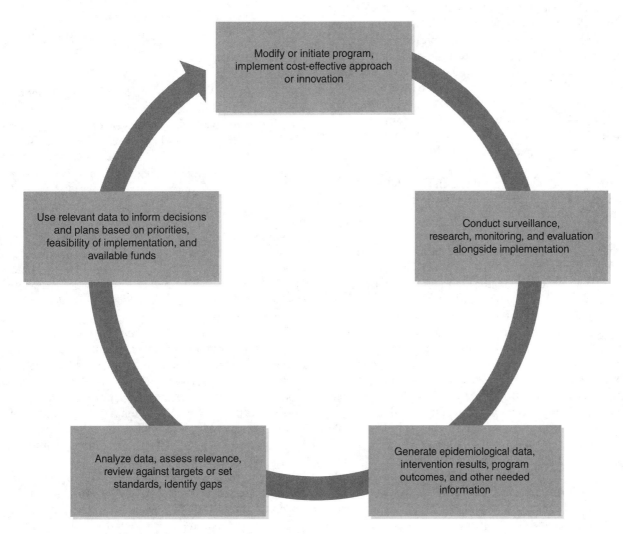

Figure 21-12 Role of Surveillance, Research, Monitoring, and Evaluation in Service Delivery

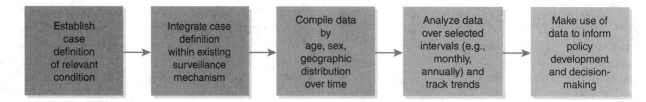

Figure 21-13 Utilization of Surveillance Data

existing surveillance system, in which institutional health data was methodically collected, analyzed, disseminated, and utilized by health providers (**Figure 21-13**).

The AIDS case definition consisted of clinical signs and symptoms and a positive HIV test. This was used to compile AIDS surveillance data that painted a picture of Ghana's epidemic by showing the distribution of those affected by age, sex, and geographic regions and the trends over the years. This helped to identify high-risk areas and informed the sequential selection of medical services to provide care for those infected, as well as suggest potential areas for epidemiological research. AIDS surveillance data therefore will always be viewed as one of the earlier important sources of information for policy decisions. In recent times, many more HIV-positive persons are being picked up in earlier stages, and with the advent of ART, progression to AIDS is not as likely as before. Nevertheless, AIDS surveillance is still ongoing, and the Integrated Disease Surveillance Report (IDSR), sentinel surveillance system, and Ghana AIDS Control program compile this information annually.

Each year STI surveillance data is obtained through the IDSR/sentinel survey, which reports on three STI syndromes: female genital ulcer, male genital ulcer, and urethral discharge. This data gives an indication of the burden of STI and is useful for tracking trends over time.

Surveys and Research

Another key data source is the HIV Sentinel Survey (HSS), initiated by the MOH in 1992 with the objective of providing HIV prevalence data for planning, monitoring, and evaluation of HIV prevention and care activities. In this annual cross-sectional HIV prevalence survey conducted among pregnant women, the results are viewed as proxy indicator of the spread of HIV infection among the Ghanaian population.

From 8 sites in 1992, the number of sentinel sites increased over the years to 40 sites in 2005 and has remained so since then (Addo , Yawson, Addo, Dornoo, & Seneadza, 2014). The survey is also conducted among male and female patients seeking treatment for STI in two STI clinics. During the survey period, which usually starts in September and lasts 12 weeks, blood is collected from survey participants using an anonymous unlinked method and tested for HIV and syphilis. This has provided HIV and syphilis prevalence data among prenatal clinic and STI clients and trends over the years. The HSS data is also used for the estimation and

---

BOX 21-9 Survey Findings and Decision-Making

An example of survey findings contributing to decision making can be seen in the selection of a particular HIV test kit. The HSS findings demonstrated that HIV subtype I was the dominant strain accounting for more than 90% of circulating viruses.

There was also the small but notable minority of PLHIV with HIV type II or dual infection who would be missed and lose the opportunity for tailored management unless the appropriate test kit was used.

This contributed to the change in the use of one rapid test kit for another kit that could detect and distinguish between both strains at a go (NACP, 2007a, 2008a).

---

projections of HIV prevalence in the general population and has been used to inform intervention programs. In addition, the HSS makes available information on the proportions of circulating HIV subtypes I and II over the years. **Box 21-9** presents key findings that influenced the decisions made.

A myriad of other surveys and studies have been undertaken or commissioned through multiple collaborations involving NACP, Noguchi Memorial Institute for Medical Research, the Ghana Statistical Service, the Health Research Unit of the Ghana Health Service, the WHO, and the CDC, among others. These collaborations have yielded the nationwide HIV Prevalence Survey, alongside the Ghana Demographic and Health Survey in 2003, the Behavioral Surveillance Survey (BSS) in 2006, and the ongoing HIV drug resistance monitoring survey initiated in 2007 and HIV-incidence survey. The BSS was a cross-sectional survey conducted in 35 districts across the country to obtain baseline information on HIV-related behavior to help track and monitor risk behaviors among adults, in and out of school youth, and military personnel and their families within the age group 15 to 49 years. Another objective of the survey was to obtain data to guide program planning and review. The findings revealed a high level of HIV awareness (over 95%) but lower in-depth knowledge, particularly related to HIV transmission. Condom use with multiple partners was low (less than 50%). Uptake of counseling and testing was rather low (9%); more than half were uncertain about the cost, availability, and accessibility of HIV/AIDS services; and only 6% of respondents indicated a nonstigmatizing attitude toward HIV. These findings added impetus to the repackaging of HIV messages to highlight the reduction of risky sexual behaviors, the benefits of preventing and treating STIs, the uptake of VCT, the modes of HIV transmission, and to address the problem of stigma against PLHIV (NACP, 2008a).

The importance of research and its findings is the provision of strategic information and evidence-based data to inform policy and programming. For example, it is not by chance that comprehensive HIV care on a programmatic level began in the Manya Krobo District in the Eastern Region. Neither is it coincidental that the Eastern Regional Hospital was the first among the regional hospitals to initiate ART services. Surveillance and research data pointed out these areas as the worst hit by HIV in Ghana and guided policy decisions on the setting up and rolling out of services while being cognizant of equity and accessibility issues.

One of the HIV drug resistance surveys investigated whether HIV drug-resistant strains were being transmitted in those newly infected with HIV. The results showed that the prevalence of HIV drug-resistant strains among the population surveyed was less than 5%, which is interpreted as low. In other words, the drug regimens being used for the PLHIV on treatment in the ART program (over 30,000 people in 2009) were still effective as the viral resistance to these drugs was low. If the converse had been true, there would have been a need to change the ART guidelines to include drugs that were more effective against the resistant strains found. This was great news for the program because the ART regimens were relatively cheaper compared to newer drugs for drug-resistant viruses. The research showed the program to be on the right track, as the limited antiretroviral options in use had not yet been jeopardized as a result of resistance. Considering the important role played by research, it continues to be high on the HIV program agenda (NACP, 2010a).

Program Monitoring and Review

For effective implementation of the several ongoing HIV programs, there is a need for regular monitoring and evaluation to assess the progress, identify and address challenges, verify reports submitted, inspect infrastructural developments, provide hands-on training as necessary, and reinforce national guidelines. As part of the quarterly and periodic monitoring and supervisory visits instituted by the National AIDS Control Program, a range of these activities are undertaken by different groups of people both national and international. At the regional level, teams made up of the regional HIV coordinator and other relevant personnel, such as the regional laboratory technologist and data managers, conduct monitoring visits to sites offering different HIV-related services. When and where indicated, they also supervise activities within their jurisdiction, such as the HIV Sentinel Survey (NACP, 2009b). National teams consisting of the various categories of staff from NACP including the program manager and members of the Technical Working Group on ART complement the monitoring undertaken by regional teams with supervisory

visits to verify adherence to guidelines and provide onsite mentoring of service providers. Due to the support of the Global Fund, various categories of GFATM staff and ambassadors periodically come to pay official visits to verify first hand that activities are implemented. The visits undertaken by both in-country and international monitors have proven to be useful, as they contribute to keeping the program on track. The visits are well received by the service providers on the ground, who are motivated by the support and appreciation shown them by the visiting teams (NACP, 2004c, 2009a).

Prevention, Treatment, Care, and Support (PTCS) Stakeholders Meeting

To enable the various stakeholders from the regions involved in HIV prevention, treatment, care, and support to compare regional efforts and peer-review their performance, the NACP instituted the PTCS stakeholders' meetings. This forum, held twice a year in January and August since 2006, creates a platform for the regional teams to share experiences, progress made, achievements, good practices, challenges, and planned activities related to HIV service delivery. It is also an opportunity for NACP to disseminate service delivery targets set for the year and progress made toward achieving them, new policy directions and guidelines and updates on research to stakeholders. Other participants at the PTCS meetings include the HIV care providers from law enforcement agencies health facilities and the private health sector, development partners, and PLHIV representatives. The uniformed service health personnel at the forefront of HIV prevention treatment and care also get the opportunity to share ongoing activities in their respective domains.

The PTCS meetings have been very successful in helping to improve service delivery (**Box 21-10**). For example,

---

BOX 21-10 Motivated to Improve PMTCT Services

In the area of PMTCT, the Komfo Anokye Teaching Hospital (KATH) is an example of a facility that was noted to improve its services dramatically in the course of successive PTCS meetings. PMTCT services were virtually nonexistent (only 4% of pregnant women were tested for HIV in 2007) as a result of various challenges and this consistently drew queries from PTCS participants.

This triggered a resolve from the team from KATH to work on their bottlenecks including dedicating HIV counselors to the PMTCT service and identifying doctors to champion the course of PMTCT in the obstetrics and gynecology department. This resulted in a marked improvement in their PMTCT uptake, with 98% of pregnant women being tested to the admiration of all during the January 2010 PTCS meeting (NACP, 2009d, 2010b).

in earlier PTCS very few regions reported on outcome of HIV-exposed babies whose mothers had benefitted from the PMTCT intervention. It was reiterated that the continuum of PMTCT services necessitated follow-up of the babies until their HIV status was determined at 18 months (NACP, 2009d). Subsequently, the regions improved on the follow up of the mother-baby pair and began reporting on the number of babies testing positive at 18 months (NACP, 2010c). In January 2011, the PTCS meeting began to award prizes through a peer-selection mechanism, for the best-performing region. These PTCS meetings continue to be a useful tool to help the program motivate stakeholders to collectively work towards achieving the program goals. Regions that are not performing well benefit from the innovations that others are using to achieve results. Those that are doing well are motivated to do better in order to hold on to the enviable position of being best-performing regions.

The Program in Retrospect

It is clear that much has been achieved as far as the health sector's responsibility of setting up and implementing HIV care services, including an STI prevention and management component (**Figure 21-14**). More and more Ghanaians know their HIV status, and PMTCT services are being promoted with virtual elimination of MTCT in mind. Increasingly, ART is becoming more accessible for those who are eligible and STI services have been decentralized.

A host of other complementary activities that support the implementation of these services were set up.

Strengths

Looking back, the strengths of the program include the following:

- Setting up well-defined governing systems guided by plans, policies, and guidelines according to international standards to promote quality HIV products and services
- Having one strong national leadership under the National AIDS Control Program to coordinate the health sector response and promote uniformity of services in both the public and private sector
- Fruitful collaborations with multiple stakeholders, including development partners, civil society, and NGOs and PLHIV associations, which have enhanced synergism in contributing to HIV prevention, treatment, and care services
- The hardworking health personnel running the HIV services who, despite having to go the extra mile to cater for an ever-increasing number of people seeking services, do so with dedication
- The use of data generated from research, surveillance, and other multiple sources to guide policy, planning, and decision-making
- Documentation and dissemination of program activities through multiple channels such as the NACP bulletin and annual reports

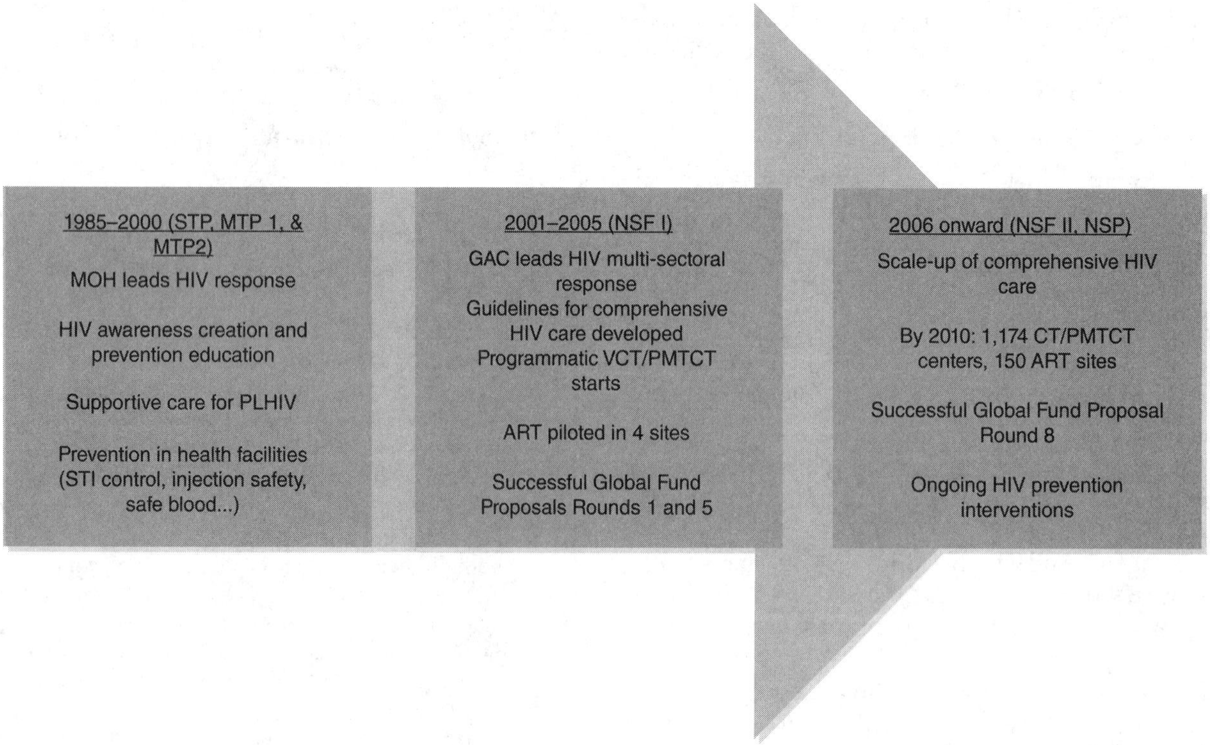

1985–2000 (STP, MTP 1, & MTP2)
MOH leads HIV response

HIV awareness creation and prevention education

Supportive care for PLHIV

Prevention in health facilities (STI control, injection safety, safe blood...)

2001–2005 (NSF I)
GAC leads HIV multi-sectoral response
Guidelines for comprehensive HIV care developed
Programmatic VCT/PMTCT starts

ART piloted in 4 sites

Successful Global Fund Proposals Rounds 1 and 5

2006 onward (NSF II, NSP)
Scale-up of comprehensive HIV care

By 2010: 1,174 CT/PMTCT centers, 150 ART sites

Successful Global Fund Proposal Round 8

Ongoing HIV prevention interventions

Figure 21-14 Ghana Health Sector HIV Response at a Glance

Challenges

The program has faced multiple challenges, some of which are ongoing while others that may be faced in the future are looming ahead.

Due to human resource constraints, there is a limited number of personnel providing HIV services. In some situations, the same personnel have other responsibilities and end up working longer hours than their counterparts not involved in HIV care. This precipitates burnout that may end up affecting quality of care. Task shifting, in which some tasks are taken on by other categories of staff and full integration of HIV care as done for other conditions, can help to take some of the pressure off the overworked staff.

Bureaucratic bottlenecks and inefficiencies in logistics management of HIV commodities have sometimes affected procurement and supply management, occasionally leading to supply shortages. Continuous advocacy is needed to avoid procurement delays and assure the continuous supply of commodities to avoid the unnecessary emergence of HIV drug-resistant strains.

Delays in submitting narrative and financial reports on funded activities undertaken and indicators may compromise data quality ultimately affecting planning and disbursement of funds to undertake other needed activities. The engagement and capacity building of data managers and the use of simplified data collection tools help improve on data reporting and timely submissions of reports.

Reliance on external sources of funding creates problems as far as sustainability is concerned, especially in an era of a global economic downturn and donor fatigue. In country generation of funds and increasing government support for HIV care will lessen dependence on external funding.

The relatively low proportion of private sector health facilities offering HIV services despite the success stories of private–public partnerships in HIV care is a problem. Persistent advocacy and the active engagement of the private sector through private medical associations are channels to draw these providers on board.

Other challenges include the low level of integration between HIV services and sexual reproductive health services, low uptake of HIV services by men, and competing activities and expectations of health workers. Documentation and dissemination of best practices provides opportunities for learning from innovative ways others have addressed these constraints.

Lessons Learned

The promotion of innovative strategies to improve uptake of services and improve delivery helps to achieve targets and implementation schedules. The launch of the "Know Your Status" campaign and the training of counselors in HIV testing instead of reliance on the laboratory personnel reduced delays in obtaining HIV test results and facilitated taking services to the doorstep of the populace. More people were able to access VCT.

Cascading training of personnel enables more people to be trained in a shorter period thereby enhancing scale up of service. Conducting training of trainers for regional teams paved the way for decentralizing training. This increased the number of people acquiring essential HIV-related skills in a shorter period to keep up with service rollout.

Peer review of work being done and learning from others' strategies and innovations motivates performance. With the institution of the prevention, treatment, care, and support fora, regional teams were challenged to improve their effort when their performance was compared to that of their counterparts.

Regular monitoring and supervision present the opportunity to promote standardized service provision as well as energize staff. During monitoring visits, adherence to national protocols and guidelines were verified and onsite training was conducted when shortfalls were identified. This sent a message to the personnel that there was an interest in the service they were providing, which motivated them.

Coordinating the contribution and work of partners enhances the concept of having one program and minimizes duplication.

The involvement of civil society and PLHIV in care provision as well as task shifting lessens the burden placed on health staff.

Looking Ahead

With HIV requiring lifelong treatment and in the absence of a cure, the health sector has the responsibility of providing HIV treatment, care, and support services for PLHIV integrated with prevention activities for those who are HIV negative. To do so for everyone who needs the services, there must be a scale up to achieve universal access.

The way forward therefore requires the following:

- Scaling up services to increase coverage in a manner that is equitable
- Finding innovative solutions to address challenges such as human resource constraints and bureaucratic bottlenecks that hamper delivery and scale up of services
- Exploring alternative sustainable sources of funding including coverage of HIV care under the National Health Insurance

Conclusion

Having a responsibility to improve access and equity of access to health care, the government of Ghana and collaborating partners saw HIV/AIDS as one of the greatest challenges to health with the potential of undermining progress made in healthcare delivery. To this end, steps have been taken to plan for and implement an HIV control program, which continues to evolve in response to the demands of the time. Along the way, initiatives were undertaken and procedures instituted. There have been several achievements interspersed with challenges and limitations, some of which prevail as the processes continue. Useful lessons have also come out of these experiences that involved the use of a public health approach within a resource-limited setting. This chapter has sought to capture these issues from a developing country's perspective to contribute to the scope of knowledge on HIV care for sexual and reproductive healthcare students and health professionals.

● ● ● REFERENCES

Addo, N. A., Yawson, A. E., Addo, A. S., Dornoo, B. T., & Seneadza, H. N. A. (2014). A review of national programme data on the HIV epidemic in Ghana 2005-2010. *Postgraduate Medical Journal of Ghana, 3*(2), 73–81.

Academy for Educational Development. (2009). *Strengthening HIV/AIDS response partnerships: Final project report.* Accra, Ghana: Author.

Amofah, G. K. (1992). AIDS in Ghana: Profile, strategies and challenges. *AIDS Analysis Africa, 2*(5), 5.

Asamoah-Adu, C., Khonde, N., Avorkliah, M., Bekoe, V., Alary, M., Mondor, M., . . . Pépin, J. (2001). HIV infection among sex workers in Accra: Need to target new recruits entering the trade. *Journal of Acquired Immune Deficiency Syndromes, 28*(4), 358–366.

AVERT. (2017). *Prevention of mother-to-child transmission (PMTCT) of HIV.* Retrieved from https://www.avert.org/professionals /hiv-programming/prevention/prevention-mother-child

Bjerrum, A. (2016). *Danida's involvement in the Ghanaian health sector 1994-2015.* Retrieved from http://ghana.um.dk/en/news/ newsdisplaypage/?newsID=024751C2-DB08-4C70-8DC1-F55519D9CD59

Centers for Disease Control and Prevention (CDC). (2016). *Global health – Ghana.* Retrieved from https://www.cdc.gov/global health/countries/ghana/default.htm

Côté, A. M., Sobela, F., Dzokoto, A., Nzambi, K., Asamoah-Adu, C., Labbé, A. C., . . . Pépin, J. (2004). Transactional sex is the driving force in the dynamics of HIV in Accra, Ghana. *AIDS, 18*(6), 917–925.

Dapaah, J. M. (2016a). Attitudes and behaviours of health workers and the use of HIV/AIDS health care services. *Nursing Research and Practice,* (2016), ID5172497.

Dapaah, J. M. (2016b). When the clinic becomes a home: Successful VCT and ART services in a stressful environment. *Journal of Social Aspects of HIV/AIDS, 13*(1), 142–151.

Ghana AIDS Commission (GAC). (2001). *Ghana HIV/AIDS strategic framework 2001-2005.* Accra, Ghana: Author.

Ghana AIDS Commission (GAC). (2002). *Ministry of Health 2002-2006 HIV/AIDS strategic plan.* Accra, Ghana: Author.

Ghana AIDS Commission (GAC). (2004). *National HIV/AIDS and STI policy.* Accra, Ghana: Author.

Ghana AIDS Commission (GAC). (2014). *2014 status report for the national HIV and AIDS response.* Accra, Ghana: Author. Retrieved from http://ghanaids.gov.gh/gac1/pubs/2014%20STA-TUS%20REPORT.pdf

Ghana AIDS Commission (GAC). (2016). *National HIV and AIDS Strategic Plan 2016-2020.* Accra, Ghana: Author.

Ghana AIDS Commission (GAC) and Ministry of Health (MOH). (2002). *National Guidelines for the development and implementation of HIV voluntary counseling and testing in Ghana.* Accra, Ghana: Author.

Ghana Social Marketing Foundation (GSMF). (2003). *Stop AIDS, love life.* Accra, Ghana: Author.

Ghana Statistical Service (GSS). (2004). *Ghana demographic and health survey 2003.* Calverton, MD: Author.

Global Fund to Fight AIDS, Tuberculosis, and Malaria (GFATM). (2017), *Ghana - grant portfolio.* Geneva, Switzerland: Author. Retrieved from http://portfolio.theglobalfund.org/en/Grant/List/GHN

Joint United Nations Programme on HIV/AIDS (UNAIDS). (2002). *Report on the global HIV/AIDS Epidemic 2002.* Geneva, Switzerland: Author.

Joint United Nations Programme on HIV/AIDS (UNAIDS). (2009). *UNAIDS calls for a virtual elimination of mother to child transmission of HIV by 2015,* Switzerland: Author. UNAIDS. Retrieved from http://www.unaids.org/en/resources/presscentre/pressrelease andstatementarchive/2009/may/20090521priorityareas

Joint United Nations Programme on HIV/AIDS (UNAIDS). (2011). *Global report: UNAIDS report on the global AIDS epidemic 2010,* Switzerland: Author.

Joint United Nations Programme on HIV/AIDS (UNAIDS). (2016). *Global AIDS update: UNAIDS report.* Retrieved from http://www .who.int/hiv/pub/arv/global-aids-update-2016-pub/en/

Joint United Nations Programme on HIV/AIDS (UNAIDS) & World Health Organization (WHO). (2004). *UNAIDS and WHO policy statement on HIV testing.* Geneva, Switzerland: Author. Retrieved from www.who.int/hiv/pub/vct/statement/en/

Joint United Nations Programme on HIV/AIDS (UNAIDS) & World Health Organization (WHO). (2009). *AIDS epidemic update, November 2009,* Switzerland: Author.

Lamptey, P., Wigley, M., Carr, D., & Collymore, Y. (2002). Facing the HIV/AIDS pandemic. *Population Bulletin 57.* Retrieved from http://www.prb.org/Publications/Reports/2002/FacingtheHIVAIDS PandemicPDF786KB.aspx

Merson, M. H. (2006). The HIV–AIDS pandemic at 25 — the global response. *New England Journal of Medicine, 354,* 2414–2417.

Ministry of Health Ghana (MOH). (1988). *Medium term plan for the prevention and control of AIDS 1989–1993.* Accra, Ghana: Author.

Ministry of Health Ghana (MOH). (2002a). *Guidelines for antiretroviral therapy in Ghana.* Accra: MOH Ghana.

Ministry of Health Ghana (MOH). (2002b). *Guidelines for management of opportunistic infections and other related HIV diseases.* Accra, Ghana: Author.

Ministry of Health Ghana (MOH). (2003). *Prevention of mother-to child transmission of HIV in Ghana: A manual for health workers.* Accra: MOH Ghana.

Ministry of Health Ghana (MOH). (2006). *Towards universal access to antiretroviral therapy: Ghana national ART scale up plan: 2006 -2010.* Accra, Ghana: Author.

Ministry of Health Ghana (MOH). (2010). *Prevention of mother-to-child transmission of HIV in Ghana: Scale-up plan 2011-2015.* Accra, Ghana: Author.

Ministry of Health. (2013). *National Guidelines for the Clinical Use of Blood and Blood Products.* Retrieved from nbsghana.org /wp-content/uploads/2015/07/National-Guidelines-for-the -Clinical -Use-of-Blood-and-Blood-Products-e-version.pdf

Ministry of Health Ghana (MOH). (2014). *National guidelines for prevention of mother-to-child transmission of HIV*. Accra, Ghana: Author. Retrieved from https://aidsfree.usaid.gov/sites /default/files/tx_ghana_pmtct_2014.pdf

National AIDS/STI Control Program Ghana (NACP). (2003a). *AIDS surveillance report: Reported AIDS cases in Ghana*. Accra, Ghana: Author.

National AIDS/STI Control Program Ghana (NACP). (2003b). *NACP bulletin: Quarterly technical bulletin on HIV/AIDS-STIs in Ghana, December 2003*. Accra, Ghana: Author.

National AIDS/STI Control Program Ghana (NACP). (2004a). *HIV/AIDS in Ghana: Current situation, projections, impacts, interventions*. Accra, Ghana: Author.

National AIDS/STI Control Program Ghana (NACP). (2004b). *NACP bulletin: Quarterly technical bulletin on HIV/AIDS-STIs in Ghana, July 2004*. Accra, Ghana: Author.

National AIDS/STI Control Program Ghana (NACP). (2004c). *NACP bulletin: Quarterly technical bulletin on HIV/AIDS-STIs in Ghana, December 2004*. Accra, Ghana: Author.

National AIDS/STI Control Program Ghana (NACP). (2005). *NACP bulletin: Quarterly technical bulletin on HIV/AIDS-STIs in Ghana, June 2005*. Accra, Ghana: Author.

National AIDS/STI Control Program Ghana (NACP). (2006a). *2005 annual report*. Accra, Ghana: Author.

National AIDS/STI Control Program Ghana (NACP). (2006b). *NACP bulletin: Quarterly technical bulletin on HIV/AIDS-STIs in Ghana, March 2006*. Accra, Ghana: Author.

National AIDS/STI Control Program Ghana (NACP). (2007a). *2006 HIV sentinel survey report*. Accra, Ghana: Author.

National AIDS/STI Control Program Ghana (NACP). (2007b). *NACP bulletin: Quarterly technical bulletin on HIV/AIDS-STIs in Ghana, May 2007*. Accra, Ghana: Author.

National AIDS/STI Control Program Ghana (NACP). (2008a). *2007 annual report*. Accra, Ghana: Author.

National AIDS/STI Control Program Ghana (NACP). (2008b). *2007 HIV sentinel survey report*. Accra, Ghana: Author.

National AIDS/STI Control Program Ghana (NACP). (2008c). *Sexually transmitted infections: Guidelines for management*. Accra; NACP Ghana.

National AIDS/STI Control Program Ghana (NACP). (2008d). *NACP bulletin: Quarterly technical bulletin on HIV/AIDS-STIs in Ghana, March 2008*. Accra, Ghana: Author.

National AIDS/STI Control Program Ghana (NACP). (2008e). *National guidelines for the implementation of HIV counseling and testing in Ghana*. Accra, Ghana: Author.

National AIDS/STI Control Program Ghana (NACP). (2009a). *NACP bulletin: Quarterly technical bulletin on HIV/AIDS-STIs in Ghana, November 2009*. Accra, Ghana: Author.

National AIDS/STI Control Program. (2009b). *NACP bulletin: Quarterly technical bulletin on HIV/AIDS-STIs in Ghana, March 2009*. Accra, Ghana: Author.

National AIDS/STI Control Program Ghana (NACP). (2009a). *2008 annual report*. Accra, Ghana: Author.

National AIDS/STI Control Program Ghana (NACP). (2009b). *End of project and grant closure. Round one component of Global Fund to Fight AIDS, TB and Malaria, Ghana 2008*. Accra, Ghana: Author.

National AIDS/STI Control Program Ghana (NACP). (2010a). *2009 Annual report on the national HIV drug resistance prevention and assessment strategy in Ghana*. Accra, Ghana: Author.

National AIDS/STI Control Program Ghana (NACP). (2010b). *NACP bulletin: Quarterly technical bulletin on HIV/AIDS-STIs in Ghana, January 2010*. Accra, Ghana: Author.

National AIDS/STI Control Program Ghana (NACP). (2010c). *NACP bulletin: Quarterly technical bulletin on HIV/AIDS-STIs in Ghana, August 2010*. Accra, Ghana: Author.

National AIDS/STI Control Program Ghana (NACP). (2011a). *2010 annual report*. Accra, Ghana: Author.

National AIDS/STI Control Program Ghana (NACP). (2011b). *2010 HIV Sentinel Survey Report*. Accra, Ghana: Author.

National AIDS/STI Control Program Ghana (NACP). (2011c). *National HIV prevalence & AIDS estimates report 2010-2015*. Accra, Ghana: Author.

National AIDS/STI Control Program Ghana (NACP). (2013). *National HIV and AIDs, STI Policy*. Retrieved from https://www .healthpolicyproject.com/pubs/153_Policyfinal.pdf

National Aids Control Program (NACP). (2017). *Released 2016 HIV Sentinel Report*. Retrieved from https://www.ghanabusinessnews.com/2017/05/11 /national-aids-control-programme-releases-2016-hiv-sentinel-report/

Neequaye, A. R., Neequaye, J. E., & Biggar, R. J. (1991). Factors that could influence the spread of AIDS in Ghana, West Africa: Knowledge of AIDS, sexual behavior, prostitution, and traditional medical practices. *Journal of Acquired Immune Deficiency Syndrome, 4*(9), 914–919.

Neequaye, A. R., Neequaye, J. E., Biggar, R. J., Mingle, J. A., Drummond, J., & Waters, D. (1997). HIV-1 and HIV-2 in Ghana, West Africa: Community surveys compared to surveys of pregnant women. *West African Journal of Medicine, 16*(2), 102–108.

Quinn, T. C. (2001). AIDS in Africa: A retrospective. *Bulletin of the World Health Organization, 79*(12), 1156–1167.

Reece, R., Norman, B., Kwara, A., Flanigan, T., & Rana, A. (2015). Retention to care of HIV-positive postpartum females in Kumasi, Ghana. *Journal of the International Association of Providers of AIDS Care, 15*(5), 406–411.

United Nations. (2001). *Declaration of commitment on HIV/ AIDS. global crisis — global action*. New York, NY: Author. Retrieved from http://www.un.org/ga/aids/coverage/FinalDecla-rationHIVAIDS.html

United Nations. (2006). *Resolution adopted by the General Assembly: 60/262. Political declaration on HIV/AIDS*. New York, NY: Author. Retrieved from http://data.unaids.org/pub /report/2006/20060615_hlm_politicaldeclaration_ares60262_en.pdf

United Nations. (2010). *Population and HIV/AIDS 2010*. New York, NY: Author. Retrieved from http://www.un.org/esa/population /publications/population-hiv2010/population-hiv2010chart.pdf

United Nations Development Program. (2010). *Human develop-ment report 2010*. New York, NY: Author.

United Nations AIDS (UNAIDS). (2016). *Country Factsheets Ghana 2016*. Retrieved from www.unaids.org/en/regionscountries /countries/ghana

U.S. Department of State. (2015). *Ghana country operational plan: COP 2015 strategic direction summary*. Retrieved from https://www.pepfar.gov/documents/organization/250288.pdf

U.S. Department of Health and Human Service [DHHS]. (2017). *Global HIV/AIDS overview: The global HIV/AIDS epidemic.* Retrieved from https://www.hiv.gov/federal-response/pepfar -global-aids/global-hiv-aids-overview

WHO Country Office in Ghana (WCO). (2008). *Experiences of delivering HIV and AIDS services in Ghana: A public-private partnership experience of Odorna Clinic.* Accra, Ghana: Author.

WHO Country Office in Ghana (WCO). (2009a). *Perspectives, experiences, innovations, challenges and lessons learnt: Prevention of mother-to-child transmission of HIV in the treatment acceleration program in Ghana.* Accra, Ghana: Author.

WHO Country Office in Ghana (WCO). (2009b). *Documentation of practices and experiences in home based care in the six TAP sites of national Catholic health service in Ghana.* Accra, Ghana: Author.

World Health Organization | Regional Office for Africa. (2015). *Update Ethiopia: HIV/AIDS Progress in 2014.* Retrieved from www.afro.who.int/sites/default/files/2017-05/ethiopia_update -sheet-on-hiv---aids-programme_2014_final.pdf

World Health Organization (WHO). (2003a). *Global health-sector strategy for HIV/AIDS: 2003-2007: Providing a framework for partnership and action.* Geneva, Switzerland: Author.

World Health Organization (WHO). (2003b). *Treat 3 million by 2005 initiative: Treating 3 million by 2005: Making it happen: The WHO strategy.* Geneva, Switzerland: Author.

World Health Organization (WHO). (2004). *Investing in a Comprehensive Health Sector Response to HIV/AIDS: Scaling up Treatment and Accelerating Prevention: WHO HIV/AIDS plan, January 2004-December 2005.* Geneva, Switzerland: Author.

World Health Organization (WHO). (2007). *Training modules for the syndromic management of sexually transmitted infections* (2nd ed.). Geneva, Switzerland: Author.

World Health Organization (WHO). (2010a). *Accelerating progress towards the health-related Millennium Development Goals.* Geneva, Switzerland: Author. Retrieved from http://www.who.int/topics /millennium_development_goals

World Health Organization (2010b). *Priority interventions HIV/AIDS prevention, treatment and care in the health sector.* Geneva, Switzerland: Author.

World Health Organization (WHO). (2015a). *Guideline on when to start antiretroviral therapy and on pre-exposure prophylaxis for HIV, September 2015.* Geneva: WHO. Box 21-9 Survey Findings and Decision-Making.

World Health Organization (WHO). (2015b). *Number of deaths due to HIV/AIDS: Situation and trends.* Global Health Observatory. Geneva, Switzerland: Author.

World Health Organization (WHO). (2017). *Preventing HIV during pregnancy and breastfeeding in the context of PrEP.* Retrieved from www.who.int/hiv/pub/toolkits/prep-preventing-hiv-during -pregnancy/en/

Glossary of Terms and Acronyms

A

Abstraction of data Process of summarizing and condensing a large amount of findings. Allows for creating a condensed version of the details from the research reports. Use of specific tested, approved pro-forma is recommended.

Accelerated partner therapy Partner notification practices that speed up treatment of sexual partners. Usually follows a sexual health/medical assessment by an authorized sexual health practitioner or pharmacist. Term applied in the United Kingdom.

Accountability Being answerable regarding specific responsibilities.

Active referral See *provider referral.*

Alcolator An online self-assessment tool to ascertain safe alcohol intake. Designed by T. Keogh, Alcohol and Drugs Support Worker at Sandyford.

Allocation concealment Process applied to the allocation of participants to comparison groups by secrecy so that no one knows which group an individual will be placed in. Applied to randomized controlled trials.

Analysis of intention to treat Including participants in an analysis whether or not they did receive the research intervention and despite what happened afterward. Including the total number of participants regardless of whether outcomes were collected.

Anonymity Concealing and protecting an individual's secrecy.

Antimicrobial agents Medications and chemical substances that kill or inhibit the growth of specific microorganisms, such as the organisms that cause the different STIs.

Antimicrobial resistance Change in a microorganism making it nonresponsive to antimicrobial agents or antibiotic drug treatments.

Appraising Reviewing and evaluating or assessing the quality of the material.

Archway Scotland's first sexual assault referral center. A service for anyone over the age of 14 who has been raped or sexually assaulted. Patients are given a full forensic examination and offered counseling and emotional support together with treatment for STIs.

Atresia Degeneration of ovarian follicles.

Attachment theory The work of John Bowlby and Mary Ainsworth in identifying the different forms of attachment established in infancy and how these can continue to impact throughout life.

Attenuation Process by which a strain of pathogenic virus or bacterium becomes less virulent.

Autonomy Self-determination, independence, personal control, and individuality in the making of personal decisions.

B

Bartholin's glands Secretory glands lying near the entrance of the vagina.

Bias Persistent errors in the design of the study that leads to overstatement or understatement of the intervention effect. Biases lead to the risk of poor designs turning out or yielding results that consistently deviate from what is actually true.

Biomedical interventions The implementation of multiple medical and public health principles in a composite or integrated approach to limiting the transmission and spread of STIs and HIV infection.

Blinding Process applied in keeping the participants, researchers, and assessors of outcomes from knowing which individuals are placed in the intervention or control groups.

Bulbourethral glands Accessory structures in the male reproductive tract that produce pre-ejaculatory fluid.

C

Capacitation Change undergone by sperm in the female tract that enables them to fertilize an oocyte.

Cathelicidins Naturally occurring molecules with anti-microbial activity.

cGMP Cyclic guanosine monophosphate.

Choose Life A national strategy and action plan to prevent suicide in Scotland.

Chorionamnionitis Inflammation of the chorionic and amniotic membranes and may be caused by ascending reproductive tract infection during pregnancy. Associated with adverse maternal and fetal morbidity.

Clinical care interventions Medical treatment, clinical care, therapeutic procedures, and other general management procedures.

Clinical effectiveness A means of measuring the effectiveness of treatment interventions, patient/client outcomes, and the related economic upshots. It also allows for measuring and reporting the efficiency or effectiveness of the system of management.

Clinical governance The accountability of the NHS organizations for improving the service provision while also maintaining the standards of high quality care provision in an appropriate environment of professional practice. Essentially a system that recognizes an integrated scheme of management of inputs, structures, and processes.

Clinical outcome routine evaluation A client self-report questionnaire completed before, after, and during therapy to ascertain well-being, risk, functioning, and problems.

Coexistent STI infections The acquisition of more than one sexually transmitted infection occurring because of asymptomatic and untreated infection; missed or inadequately treated primary infection with another newly acquired STI superimposed upon it.

Coiled seminiferous tubule Duct in the testis that is site for sperm production.

Commissioning Authorization and contracting.

Comparator The specific intervention such as the customary or conventional treatment, a placebo, an alternative, or no treatment, with which the research intervention is compared in a controlled trial.

Compliance Adhering to or conforming to a prescribed regime. This may involve self-discipline or personal capability to follow the instructions and keeping to the regime.

Conceptual framework A representation to explain the links or interconnections between specific factors identified to be investigated in a study. These should have direct relation to a research problem/phenomenon. The framework guides the direction of the investigation.

Concordance rates Statistical calculation indicating the probability that an identified clinical condition such as infection acquired by particular individuals would affect those individuals who share with them a specific common factor, for example, couples or twins.

Conditional referral Involves a combination of referral actions. The initial patient referral is backed by provider referral after a consented period of time if partner fails to respond.

Confidence intervals The range of values within which the value of the true measure of an intervention lies. Represent the distribution of the probability of random errors.

Confidentiality Respecting and safeguarding an individual's privacy.

Confounders The unexpected or unexplainable factors that affect the outcomes of interventions. Confounders may influence the outcome being assessed and alter the effect measures causing misinterpretation.

Confounding variables Unknown factors affecting the outcome of an experimental intervention.

Contact tracing Term used in the practice of partner notification to describe locating of sexual partners.

Continuous data Outcomes of measures with countless continuous data with constant/countless number of values within the particular range.

Corpus albicans Regressed form of the corpus luteum.

Corpus luteum Hormone-secreting ovarian structure succeeding the ovarian follicle.

Credibility The extent of detail and thoroughness applied at all stages of the study to achieve trustworthiness of the findings, conclusions, and recommendations.

Cytokines Class of molecules secreted by and active upon immune cells.

D

Data abstraction Process of summarizing and condensing the specific pertinent details about research evidence; a condensed outline of the similarities and differences.

Data extraction Identification and recording of specific information that characterize key elements in the research reports.

De novo mutation Newly occurring DNA alteration.

Descriptive studies Studies that allow for observing, examining, and explaining as well as recording and presenting an account of an existing situation without making changes to alter it.

Dichotomous data Measures with only two possible values that indicate presence or absence.

Dopamine A neurotransmitter.

Ductus epididymis Fine duct within scrotum that matures and stores sperm cells.

E

Effect size An estimate of effect or a statistical summary indicating the measure of an observed association or relationship between an intervention and the outcome.

Empiric treatment Administration or commencement of treatment such as antimicrobial therapy prior to laboratory confirmation of the actual causative organism.

Empirical research Investigative study involving observation and measurement of events and experiences through quantitative and qualitative processes. Extensive data collection is required and methodical processing of the information obtained allows for producing substantiated evidence.

Endogenous infection Multiplication and invasion of opportunistic microorganisms that exist within specific tissue cells as normal bacterial flora.

Epidemiology Study of the determinant factors or causes of disease conditions or infections and the associated effects as it manifests. Also involves studying the course of the disease or infection among the particular population group and the impact of long-term consequences. A comprehensive epidemiologic data may also include studying and reporting the modes of acquisition, transmission, and pattern of spread. Monitoring of STIs allows for examining the pattern and trend of outbreaks of infections and the efficacy of the treatment interventions in relation to an identified microorganism.

Etiologic diagnosis Diagnosis based on identification of the specific microorganism or toxin that causes a specific infection or disease condition.

Evidence-based practice An approach involving identifying, interpreting, and combining convincing research and other substantiated evidence for making sound clinical decisions and judgments to improve care and service provision. It requires that account be taken of clinician-observed evidence, professional expertise, and the expressed needs, preferences, and values of the patient/client. Essentially EBP involves integration of best available research other evidence in in professional practice.

Expedited partner therapy Process aimed at offering an index patient's sexual partner(s) a package of information and prescribed medication, which is delivered to them by the index patient (thus described as *patient-delivered partner therapy*). Term used in the United States.

Experiential learning The process of acquiring knowledge, skills, and values and deriving meaning from exposure to the environment of learning and/or the sources of knowledge and competence acquisition experiences.

Extraction of data The stage-by-stage process of pulling out and recording the key components identified in the research reports. Use is recommended of specific tested and approved pro-forma purposefully developed to provide precise and clearly formulated criteria pertinent to the key components of the research reports. The criteria serve as a guide for distinguishing between the specific factors that determine the directly related studies that should be selected for inclusion in the review and those that should be excluded.

F

Flowback Leakage of semen from the vagina.

Forensic services The use of scientific testing and information gathering to determine the cause and impact of injuries and to assist in the identification of the assailant.

G

Generalizability The extent to which the results of a study remain consistent in other settings and can be applied to other population groups exposed to similar conditions in similar contexts.

H

Health The status of physical, mental, and social well being and not just the absence of disease or illness. Within the context of health promotion, health can be considered in terms of the capability to perform normal physiological and other functions independently, as well as having accessible social and economic resources.

Heterogeneity The variations occurring between studies. Clinical heterogeneity refers to variability between studies attributed to population, patient or participant characteristics, the intervention, or the outcomes. Methodological heterogeneity refers to variations in the design of the studies. Statistical heterogeneity refers to the statistical differences in the effects estimates.

Hierarchical ranking A grading order on a continuum from the highest, strongest, or most significant to the lowest, weakest, or least significant.

Homogeneity The similarities occurring between the research studies selected for systematic review.

Hypothalamus Region of the forebrain that coordinates many homeostatic systems of the body.

Hypothesis Theories or suppositions that can be tested by quantitative research methods using statistical techniques with the aim of proving or disproving the assumption. *Directional hypotheses* indicate a predicted change either positive or negative when one factor has an effect on another factor. *Nondirectional hypotheses* do not predict the type of change or effect that may happen as a result of one factor acting on another.

I

Incidence The number of people who are newly affected by a particular disease or infection during a given period of time, for example, during a particular month or year.

Independent reviews Reviews conducted in a way that avoids alignment and conferring between one reviewer and another.

Index patient The individual (patient/client) who attends the sexual health clinic with sexually transmitted infection to seek treatment and advice.

Informed consent Agreement, permission, or authorization given by an individual or by a legal guardian without coercion after receiving and understanding the information about a specific drug treatment or care procedure.

In-house training activities Enhancing performance by development of required training or other specific needs of the specific group within an identified practice setting.

Integrity Refers to exactness in terms of how accurate and truthful are the results and the researcher's claims or inferences.

Internal validity Accuracy of the results and findings from a study in direct relation to the factors measured.

Interpretive process The researcher's attempt to gain insight and understanding of the lived experiences of people and the particular meanings or subjective connotations that they attach to their life experiences. The process allows for theory building. It depicts the real world of the particular population and their particular life experiences and involves construction of distinguishing or characteristic features.

Intervention In an experimental study, refers to the specific treatment or condition to which the experimental sample group is exposed in order to measure predicted effect or outcome.

Intramural Study activities implemented within the particular organization and/or the specific practice setting.

In vitro studies Research studies involving scientific experimentation on tissue cells taken from parts of the body.

L

Leukocyte A circulating cell of the immune system.

Longitudinal cohort studies Investigations in which an identified population group is assessed for the effect(s) of a specific factor over a given period of time.

M

Macrophage A large phagocytic cell type found at the site of infection.

Manipulation Creating special conditions for an experimental study.

Meta-analysis A statistical technique of combining and contrasting the findings from numerous research studies that applied similar designs and methods in investigating similar questions. It allows all the information collected to be used to produce a convincing summary of the treatment effect for strengthening the predictions of specific treatments and outcomes.

Meta-regression A statistical technique that is employed for exploring how variations in study characteristics impact on study results in terms of the size of effects observed. Essentially, the impact of heterogeneity.

Meta-synthesis A qualitative data processing that pools together the findings from numerous qualitative research studies to develop a new interpretation. The new theory or interpretation can then be tested. In this way a new theory can be built, tested, and clearly explained.

Methodological rigor The degree of thoroughness of the investigative procedure.

Methodology The general principles and approach employed in conducting a research investigation.

Mindfulness The practice of being able to focus awareness on the present moment while also being aware of emotions, thoughts, and bodily sensations.

Moderator variables Variables or factors that can alter the main effects being examined in the review.

Monitoring of STIs Allows for examining the pattern and trend of outbreaks of infections and the efficacy of the treatment interventions in relation to an identified microorganism.

Multidisciplinary team Comprises members of staff from varied backgrounds of healthcare professional disciplines working together.

Myometrium The smooth muscle tissue of the uterus.

N

Nerve plexus A network of intersecting nerves.

Nonsystematic review Reviews that do not necessarily apply the methodical processes from problem identification to reporting, nor do they adhere to any review protocol. This type of review generally presents a discussion of the findings from the research reports and may represent the reviewer's interpretation of the findings with some degree of subjectivity in the conclusions.

O

Obligate The situation where organisms survive only inside living cells.

Odds ratio The ratio of the odds of occurrence in the research study groups. Essentially the number of participants who show the outcome compared to the number of participants who do not show the outcome.

Oocyte Ovarian cell that undergoes division to form the ovum (egg).

Operational definition Explanation of the specific variables, for example, what exactly is meant by the independent variable and what is meant by the dependent or outcome variable. Furthermore, it indicates what precise measurements would be taken in the study to ensure that all the researchers measure the specific factors in the same way on each of the groups of study participants. In essence it allows for defining a variable or term in relation to a specific process and/or outcome.

Outcome The specific change or aspect of health/clinical state of the participants that is caused by the intervention.

Outcome measures The calculated values used to assess the effects or outcomes of the research intervention. They provide information about predicted effects and a means of assessing the success of interventions. It requires the baseline state to be established.

Outliers Observations in the data values that are distinctly separate and lie distant from the range of calculated or projected values.

Ovarian follicle Fluid-filled ovarian structure containing the oocyte.

P

Paradigm Predetermined or set principles forming the ethos, framework, or philosophy that underpins the way a research study is conducted. The concept encompasses the belief, theory, and reasoning that forms the basis and construct or model by which expert researchers and subject specialists endorse the conduct of specific investigative studies.

Partner notification Process of locating and informing sexual partners of patients/clients diagnosed with STIs and/or HIV of their exposure to the infection. Entails providing advice, care, and support to the sexual partners and involves alternative referral systems.

Partner referral/Patient referral A referral option in partner notification in which the index patient accepts the responsibility of informing the sexual partner regarding the possibility of having been exposed to sexually transmitted infection. The index patient is responsible for referring the partner to the relevant services.

Patient-delivered partner therapy Process in which the index patient is given the prescribed medication and additional written information for the sexual partner.

Perusal The process of critically reading and examining articles and documents. In the team context the articles may be placed in files and catalogued to enable easy access, returning, and replenishment with new articles.

Pituitary Major endocrine gland of the body controlling several physiological processes.

Polygenic Trait caused by more than one gene.

Positivist paradigm A quantitative approach to research that assumes that reality is concrete or definite and can be tested or measured by factual processes and objectivity without bias. This involves use of statistical techniques.

Post-traumatic stress disorder A psychological response to trauma, which is often experienced in disturbing bodily sensations including flashbacks.

Postal home sampling Process involving the use of postal testing kit to collect the necessary sample to be sent for laboratory testing. The sample collection occurs within the individual's preferred environment of privacy.

Prevalence The proportion or absolute number of people in a given community or the general population estimated or calculated as having contracted a particular condition, infection, or disease or as being at high risk. Usually described in relation to the trend or pattern of distribution and spread among the population groups over a given period of time. Provides an indication of the predominance or how widespread is the particular condition or infection among the specific community.

Prevalence assessment Use of surveys to determine what percentage of the population is affected by a particular condition disease or infection. The process allows for examining the trends of the condition among population sub-groups, outbreaks, course, and duration of the infection. The information collected allows for planning and developing effective programs of intervention.

Prevention Precautionary and protective measures used for safeguarding individuals or groups from the risk of contracting an infection, becoming reinfected, or acquiring a disease.

Priapism Unwelcome, persistent, and painful erection of the penis.

Primary research study The original research study in which the data collection took place.

Prostaglandins Fatty acid molecules that promote uterine contractions.

Protocols Outline of set plans showing key aspects or components of, for example, a research study. Thus the title, aims, and rationale are stated and the methods of participant recruitment, process of the investigation with data collection, and technique for analyzing the data are outlined. A review protocol provides a practical useful guide to the review process and indicates the intended use to which the findings may be put. The protocol may enclose a participant information sheet and consent form.

Provider referral A referral process in which the sexual health professional or other designated healthcare professional is responsible for contacting sexual partners of an index patient to inform them of their possible exposure to sexually transmitted infection.

Psychosex The application of psychological approaches to understand and overcome sexual difficulties.

Psychotherapy Techniques of managing mental distress; emotional, personality, and behavioural problems; and psychiatric disorders through verbal nonverbal communication interventions. Essentially psychotherapy involves interactive interventions through a range of talking therapies rather than drug treatment.

P-value A way of describing statistical significance. The *P*-value relates to the null hypothesis (the assumption that there is no effect of the intervention being tested). The *P*-value argues the probability that the observed effect or very small extreme *P*-values might have occurred by chance. Thus it is explained as the probability of an observed difference having occurred by chance. In a review of effectiveness the *P*-value may be an indication of a finding being more unusual than that calculated. Commonly a *P*-value < 0.05 is considered as a value of statistical significance. However, this may depend on what is being measured and the sample size. In translating the significance of effects, *P*-values are explained together with confidence intervals.

Q

Qualitative research Investigative study that entails interpretation and theory building from the accounts and responses relating to specific life experiences. For that reason, qualitative research is considered as lacking credibility due to the limitation or shortcoming of the personal or subjective preconceptions in the researchers' interpretations.

Quantitative research Investigative study that entails use of statistical techniques for numerical measures of the specific factors being examined. Such studies are considered to represent more exactness, rigor, and objectivity.

R

Randomized controlled trial A study design that involves testing and evaluating the effectiveness of a specific drug treatment, care intervention, procedure, or policy on an identified patient/client group with a specific clinical condition. Factors indicating the outcomes of the treatment are carefully measured on the sample groups of study participants. The findings from the treatment/ interventional group are compared to a similar sample group from the same population of patients/clients who were not exposed to the specific intervention.

Relative risk ratio A ratio of <1 suggests that the intervention is successful in reducing the risk of an unfavorable outcome.

Replication In terms of organisms, refers to copying and reproducing increasing amount of the virus-carrying cells such as HIV-carrying cells in the genital tract of females through inflammatory processes involving the genital epithelial cells.

Replication risk ratio The ratio of risk of an occurrence in the intervention group to the risk of an occurrence in the control group.

Research replication Repetition of the entire processes of a previous research investigation.

Researcher reflexivity This concept refers to the researcher's deep thoughts and consideration of the conduct of the study and how personal assumptions, decisions, and actions could be impacting on the investigation. Reflexivity may help to gain important new insight that may influence the progress of the study. Researcher reflexivity may occur at the beginning and end of the study.

S

Sampling A process of selecting a representative group of a relatively small proportion from an identified population in a way that allows for making justifiable conclusions to be drawn. *Probability sampling* involves meticulous processes of random selection with statistical calculations used to ensure accurate size and representation of identified characteristics in the population. *Nonprobability sampling* may be purposive involving deliberate selection process using a particular plan to target and choose certain subjects from the general population in order to obtain specific data.

Screening A program of testing applied to a target population in order to identify individuals who are at risk of developing a particular disease.

Seroprevalence Refers to the number of people in the population who test positive to an acquired infection based on the serological tests that determine the presence of specific antibodies in the blood.

Serotonin A neurotransmitter.

Sexual health Defined by the World Health Organization as "a state of physical emotional mental and social well-being in relation to sexuality. A positive and respectful approach to sexuality and sexual relationships."

Sexual risk-taking behaviors Relate to improper and unsafe sexual practices that increase the vulnerability of the sexual partners to acquire sexually transmitted infections, including HIV. Examples include multiple and concurrent sexual partners, frequent casual and unprotected sexual intercourse, and inconsistent and incorrect use of condoms and other barrier methods.

Social cognition The attributes for processing, storing, and applying information. These influence individuals' perceptions, attitudes, behaviors, and reactions to other people.

Social marketing Represents a system involving development, integration, and publicizing of ideas together with promotion of certain products in an attempt to entice people to adopt these for particular applications and practices for which they are purported.

Social model of health An approach to health that is not limited to the medical model and seeks to embrace the fullest sense of what it means to be human but in the context of relevant social structures that have an impact on health.

Social network analysis Process of studying patterns of spread of an identified infection during an outbreak. Entails breakdown and categorization of information obtained from infected patients/clients and through the partner notification process. Useful for identifying clusters of population groups, specific communities in certain geographical areas where an identified infection prevails.

Spermatogenesis Production of sperm cells.

Spermatogonium Stem cells that produce early stages of sperm cell.

Stakeholders An organization, party, or group that has special concern or stake in influencing the conditions, arrangements, or actions for their own ends. This may relate to interest in a particular aspect of healthcare and service provision and there may be implications of economic and political privileges and benefits.

Steve Retson Project (SRP) A sexual health and counseling service for gay men, bisexual men, and men who have had sex with other men.

Steve Retson Project Choices (SRP Choices) A counseling service using cognitive behavioral therapy for gay men who seek to balance taking risks with having a healthy sex life.

Stratification Process involving identification of characteristic traits/features among the target population in order to select a representative sample.

Sub-group analysis Analysis of intervention effects in particular subsets of the research participants.

Surveillance of STIs and antimicrobial resistance Allows for examining and tracking changes to specific microorganisms and allows for detecting resistant strains. The information gathered allows for prompt action to be taken in reporting trends and outbreaks and forms the basis for developing policy recommendations and guidelines. Allows for assessing the effect of specific antimicrobial drugs and to examine the impact of the interventions implemented to control the resistance.

Survivor Scotland Network An initiative of the Scottish Government to oversee the National Strategy for survivors of childhood sexual abuse.

Syndromic case management Management based on the characteristic symptoms associated with a particular STI.

Syndromic diagnosis Diagnosis based on the manifestation of clinical symptoms and signs presented by the patient. This is usually substantiated by appropriate laboratory tests.

Synopsizing Process of summarizing and condensing the findings or evidence from several research studies.

Synthesizing Merging together and integrating the findings of the selected and included research evidence.

Systematic appraisal This process involves detailed assessment and evaluation of a research study. A related term is *critique*.

Systematic review Detailed methodical examination of carefully selected research evidence on an identified problem/clinical phenomenon or topic. This is performed to answer specific review question(s) that should be clearly formulated. The process involves application of specific approved set of inclusion and exclusion criteria and specific rules for identifying, selecting, and appraising relevant primary studies, and then extracting, condensing, and reporting the findings.

T

The Place Sexual health and counseling for young people within Sandyford.

Theoretical framework A representation of the broad relation between the key elements in an identified phenomenon explored through research.

Theory An abstract reasoning that may be used for explaining social relations. Theory may provide a basis for research investigation through the deductive process, which starts from broad and progresses to specific ideas and concepts. Research may also provide a basis for theory development through the inductive process that starts from the particular or specific notions and progresses to general or broad conceptions.

Tight junction Region of close contact between adjacent cells that restricts molecular movement.

Thrive Counseling team within Sandyford to support men who have been sexually abused in childhood.

Transgender A term used to describe a person whose gender identity, expression, or behavior is different to that of the gender assigned to them at birth.

Translation into practice Converting theoretical concepts into practical terms for application in care and service provision.

Transparent Clearly explained and understandable details that can be realistically applied to actual processes or situations.

V

Construct validity Refers to outcome measures relating to a particular phenomenon or occurrence that has been speculated or hypothesized and confirmed in previous studies.

External validity Refers to how the findings from the study sample can be applicable to larger population groups with similar characteristics.

Internal validity Refers to the direct application of observable effects and measurements to the study participants.

Validity Degree of accuracy and thoroughness of research results and truthful interpretation of the findings influenced by correct methods of data collection and accurate analysis. Different dimensions of validity are described.

Variables Variables are specific identified factors that are tested and measured in the investigation. A variable may be described as an independent, causal, or input factor that can bring about change in the dependent/outcome variable. The specific change is carefully studied and measured.

Vas deferens Thick-walled sperm-carrying duct.

W

Weighting Process used in meta-analysis for determining the relative contribution of each study to the overall result. Inverse of the variance is a flexible method used for combining the effect estimates of the individual studies to calculate a weighted average or the mean of the estimate of effects. In this way, studies carrying large amounts of statistical information make relatively greater contribution and are more heavily weighted.

Window period The incubation period of an infection, the time taken for the infective organism to show on the relevant test. It is still possible for an infected person to transmit the infection to another person.

Acronyms

3TC – Lamivudine

A

ABC – Abacavir

ACA – Affordable Care Act

AHPs – Allied health professionals

AHRQ – Agency for Healthcare Research and Quality

AIDS – Acquired Immune Deficiency Syndrome

AMR – Antimicrobial resistance

ANI – Asymptomatic neurocognitive impairment

APA – American Psychological Association

APRNs – Advanced practice registered nurses

APV – Amprenavir

ART – Antiretroviral therapy

ARV – Antiretroviral drugs

ATV – Atazanavir

AZT – Zidovudine

B

BACP – British Association for Counselling and Psychotherapy

BASHH – British Association of Sexual Health and HIV

BASW – British Association of Social Workers

BBV – Blood-borne virus

BCA – Bichloroacetic acid

BHIVA – British HIV Association

BIS – British Infection Society

BMD – Bone mineral density

BNF – British National Formulary

BPAS – British Pregnancy Advisory Service

BV – Bacterial vaginosis

C

CAMHTs – Child and Adolescent Mental Health Teams

cART – Combination antiretroviral therapy

CBT – Cognitive behavioral therapy

CCGs – Clinical commissioning groups

CCR5 – C-C chemokine receptor 5

CCT – Controlled clinical trial

CD4 – Cluster of differentiation 4

CDC – Centers for Disease Control and Prevention

CDPH – California Department of Public Health

CE – Clinical effectiveness

CGPED — Committee of General Practice Education Directors

CHC — Combined hormonal contraception

CMHTs – Community mental health teams

CMS – Centers for medicare and medicaid services

CNO – Chief nursing officer

CNS – Central nervous system

COBI – Cobicistat

COC — Combined oral contraception

CORE – Clinical outcome routine evaluation

COSHH – Control of substances hazardous to health

CPD – Continuing professional development

CQC – Care Quality Commission

CRD – Centre for Reviews and Dissemination

CRHP – Council for Regulation of Health Professions

CSA – Childhood sexual abuse

CSF – Cerebrospinal fluid

CSP – Chartered Society of Physiotherapy

Cu IUD — Copper intrauterine device

CVD – Cardiovascular disease

CXCR4 – C-X-C Chemokine Receptor 4

CYP450 – Cytochrome P450

D

d4T – Stavudine

ddI – Didanosine

DEXA – Dual-energy X-ray absorptiometry

DFA – Direct fluorescent antibody

DFA-TP – Direct fluorescent antibody test for *Treponema pallidum*

DGI – Disseminated gonococcal infection

DH – Department of Health, United Kingdom

DHHS – Department of Health & Human Services, United States

DHT – Dihydrotestosterone

DLV – Delavirdine

DMPA– Depot medroxyprogesterone acetate [trade name DepoProvera]

DNA – Deoxyribonucleic acid

dNTPs – Deoxynucleotide triphosphates

DRV – Darunavir

E

EBH – Evidence-based health care

EBM – Evidence-based medicine

EBP – Evidence-based practice

ECDC – European Centre for Disease Control

ED – Erectile dysfunction

EIAs – Enzyme immuneassays

ELISA – Enzyme linked immunosorbent assay

EMDR – Eye movement desensitisation and reprocessing

EPPI – Evidence for Policy and Practice Information

EPT – Expedited partner therapy

EST – Empirically supported treatment

ETV – Etravirine

EVG – elvitegravir

F

FASD – Fetal alcohol spectrum disorder

FCU – First catch urine

FGM – Female genital mutilation

FI – Fusion inhibitors

FPA – Family planning association

FPV – Fosamprenavir

FSH – Follicle-stimulating hormone

FSRH – Faculty of Sexual and Reproductive Health Care

FTA-ABS – Fluorescent treponemal antibody absorbed

FTC – Emtricitabine

G

GMC – General Medical Council

GnRH – Gonadotrophin-releasing hormone

GP – General practitioner

gp – Glycoprotein

GRASP – Gonococcal Resistance to Antimicrobials Surveillance Programme

GSCC – General social care council

GUM – Genitourinary medicine

GUMCAD – Genitourinary medicine clinic activity dataset

H

HAART – Highly active antiretroviral therapy

HAD – HIV-associated dementia

HAND – HIV-associated neurocognitive disorders

HARS – HIV and AIDS Reporting System

HBcAg – Hepatitis B core antigen

HBM – Health belief model

HBsAg – Hepatitis B surface antigen

HBV – Hepatitis B virus

HCPC – Health and Care Professions Council

HCV – Hepatitis C virus

HIPAA – Healthcare Insurance Portability and Accountability Act of 1996

HIV – Human immunodeficiency virus

HIVAN – HIV-associated nephropathy

HNIG – Human normal immunoglobulin

HPA – Health Promotion Agency

HPV – Human papillomavirus

HRA – Health Research Authority

HRT – Hormone replacement therapy

HSC – Health Service Circular

HSDD – Hypoactive sexual desire disorder

HSE – Health and safety executive

HSV – Herpes simplex virus

I

IBBSs – Integrated biological and behavioral surveys

IDUs – Injecting drug users

IMB – Intermenstrual bleeding

INSTI – Integrase strand transfer inhibitors

IPV – Intimate partner violence

IRIS – Immune reconstitution inflammatory syndrome

ITHBC – Integrated theory of behavior change

ITT – Analysis of intention to treat

IUD – Intrauterine contraceptive device

IUS – Intrauterine system

IUSTI – International Union Against Sexually Transmitted Infections

IVF – In vitro fertilization

J

JHWSs – Joint health and well-being strategies

JSNAs – Joint strategic needs assessments

K

KSF – Knowledge, skills framework

L

LAM – Lactational amenorrhea method

LARC – Long-acting, reversible contraception

LE – Listening Ear

LGBT – Lesbian, gay, bisexual, and transgender

LGBTQ – Lesbian, gay, bisexual, transgender, transsexual, and questioning

LH – Luteinizing hormone

LNG-IUS – Levonorgestrel intrauterine system

LPV – Lopinavir

LVG – Lymphogranuloma venereum

M

MAAGs – Medical audit advisory groups

MHRA – Modern Humanities Research Association

MI – Motivational interviewing

MND – Mild neurocognitive disorder

MSM – Men who have sex with men

MVC – Maraviroc

N

NAATs – Nucleic acid amplification tests

NAGCAE – National Advisory Group on Clinical Audit and Enquiries

NCHHSTP – National Center for HIV/AIDS, Viral Hepatitis, STD, and TB Prevention

NCSP – National Chlamydia Screening Programmes

NES – NHS Education for Scotland

NF-κB – Nuclear factor kappa-light-chain-enhancer of activated B cells

NFV – Nelfinavir

NGU – Nongonococcal urethritis

NHS – National Health Service, United Kingdom

NHS CB – National Health Service Commissioning Board

NHSGGC – National Health Service of Greater Glasgow and Clyde

NHSREC – National Health Service Research Ethics Committee

NHSS – National HIV Surveillance System

NIAID – National Institute of Allergy and Infectious Diseases

NICE – National Institute for Health and Care Excellence

NIHR – National Institute for Health Research

NMAHP – Nurse, midwife, and allied health professional

NMC – Nursing and Midwifery Council

NNRTI – Non-nucleoside reverse transcriptase inhibitors

NOFAS — National Organization on Fetal Alcohol Syndrome

NPs — Nurse practitioners

NQB – National Quality Board

NQS — National Quality Strategy

NRES — National Research Ethics Service

NRLS – National Reporting and Learning System

NRTI — Nucleoside/nucleotide reverse transcriptase inhibitors

NSF – National Service Framework

NVP – Nevirapine

P

PCB – Post-coital bleeding

PCMHTs – Primary care mental health teams

PCOS – Polycystic ovarian syndrome

PCP – Primary care physician

PCR – Polymerase chain reaction

PCTs – Primary care trusts

PDPT – Patient-delivered partner therapy

PEP – Post-exposure prophylaxis

PGDs – Patient group directions

PGEA – Postgraduate educational allowance

PHE – Public Health England

PI – Protease inhibitors

PICO – Population, intervention, comparators, and outcome. An additional element relates to the study design and thus PICOS.

PID – Pelvic inflammatory disease

PIPT – Psychodynamic interpersonal psychotherapy

PLD – People with learning disability

PLHIV – People living with HIV

PMS – Premenstrual syndrome

PMTCT – Prevention of mother-to-child transmission

POMs – Prescription only medicines

POP – Progestogen-only pill

PPACA – Patient Protection and Affordable Care Act

PPDP – Personal and professional development plan

PREP – Post-registration education and practice

PrEP – Pre-exposure prophylaxis

PRISMA – Preferred reporting items for systematic reviews and meta-analysis

PTG – Post-traumatic growth

PTSD – Post-traumatic stress disorder

pVL – Plasma viral load

Q

QIS – Quality Improvement Scotland

QOF – Quality and Outcomes Framework

R

RAL – Raltegravir

RCGP – Royal College of General Practitioners

RCT – Randomized controlled trial

RECs – Research ethics committees

RGF – Research governance framework

RITA – Recent infection testing algorithm

RNA – Ribonucleic acid

RPR – Rapid plasma regain

RPS – Royal Pharmaceutical Society

RPV – Rilpivirine

RT-PCR – Real-time polymerase chain reaction

RTI – Reproductive tract infection

RTV – Ritonavir

S

SAMHSA – Substance Abuse and Mental Health Services Administration

SARA – Sexually acquired reactive arthritis

SARC – Sexual Assault Referral Center

SBI – Screening and brief interventions

SCASS – Sandyford Counseling and Support Services

SFT – Solution-focused therapy

SHA – Sexual health adviser

SHASTD – Society of Health Advisers in Sexually Transmitted Diseases

SIGN – Scottish Intercollegiate Guidelines Network

SOPHID – Survey of prevalence HIV infections diagnosed

SQV – Saquinavir

SRE – Sex and relationships education

SRH – Sexual and reproductive health care

SRP – Steve Retson Project

SRY – Y-linked testis determining gene

SSA – Sub-Saharan Africa

SSHA – Society of Sexual Health Advisers

STD – Sexually transmitted disease

STIs – Sexually transmitted infections

SUD – Substance use disorders

T

TCA – Trichloroacetic acid

TDF – Tenofovir

TESSy – The European surveillance system

TPB – Theory of planned behavior

TPHA – *Treponema pallidum* haemagglutination assay

TPPA – *Treponema pallidum* particle agglutination assay

TRA – Theory of reasoned action

TTM – Transtheoretical model

U

UAI – Unprotected anal intercourse

UNAIDS – Joint United Nations Programme on HIV/AIDS

UPSI – Unprotected sexual intercourse

UTI – Urinary tract infection

V

VAERS – Vaccine Adverse Event Reporting System

VCT – Voluntary counseling and treatment

VDRL – Venereal disease research laboratory

vLARC – Very long-acting reversible contraception

VVC – Vulvovaginal candidiasis

W

WHO – World Health Organization

WSW– Women who have sex with women

HIV Trial Acronyms

BENCHMARK – Long-term efficacy and safety of raltegravir combined with optimized background therapy in treatment-experienced patients with drug-resistant HIV infection.

DAD study – Data collection of Adverse events of anti-HIV Drugs.

DUET trials – Etravirine in the management of treatment-experienced HIV-1-infected patients.

HPTN 052 – Randomized trial to evaluate the effectiveness of antiretroviral therapy plus HIV primary care versus HIV primary care alone to prevent the sexual transmission of HIV-1 in serodiscordant couples.

MERIT – Efficacy and safety of maraviroc and efavirenz, both with zidovudine/lamivudine.

MOTIVATE – Maraviroc therapy in antiretroviral treatment-experienced HIV-1-infected patients.

SMART trial – Strategies for Management of Antiretroviral Therapy trial.

START – Strategic Timing of Antiretroviral Treatment.

TORO _1 and _2 – Durable efficacy of enfuvirtide over 48 weeks in heavily treatment-experienced HIV-1-infected patients in the T-20 versus optimized background regimen only 1 and 2 clinical trials.

Index

Note: Page numbers followed by *f*, or *t* indicate material in figures, or tables, respectively.